MINERALS, VITAMINS and FOOD SUPPLEMENTS

Written and Authored By
Dr. Richard Olree

ISBN 978-0-9892992-0-6

PUBLISHED BY
LANCASTER AG PRODUCTS
60 NORTH RONKS RD
RONKS, PA 17572

PRINTED BY
EXECUTIVE PRINTING CO. INC.
656 W. NEWPORT RD.
ELM, PA 17521

Acknowledgments

This book is in fond memory of the late Chuck Walters, founder of ACRESusa, the premier organic information magazine. Chuck and I wrote the book entitled "Minerals for the Genetic Code". Without Chuck my understanding of minerals and genetics would not have ever been published. Without Chuck's help, I would have never been published in any way, shape or form as Chuck was the great man that pushed my creative abilities to the limits.

I would like to thank Betty Jo Bruder. Bj is an author herself, with a book entitled *Grandma's Burr Dress.* Bj is the mother of our two highly intelligent, capable young adults. Her ability to condense and translate from Dr. Duke's book *Medicinal Herbs of the Bible* was most valuable. I would also like to thank our children, Abby and Richard III, for their patience, as this book has taken away some valuable time with the family for quite awhile.

I would like to thank some other folks that have made this book possible. Dr. Allen Hoaglund and Betty Duncan made the writing possible with their proofreading skills. Dr. Allen is a seasoned Doctor of Chiropractic who practices in Mt. Eaton, Ohio. Over the years our friendship has grown. He is also a veteran fishing partner with many tales to be told only at fish camp in Canada. Allen's insight from years of experience in nutrition was most invaluable in the production of this book.

Betty Duncan is a college-educated elementary teacher. Betty's contribution toward this book was her work at bringing my style of writing, which is about grade 18, to a level of everyday readability. Her ability to smooth out all my unreadable writing and keep the thoughts flowing was very important!

It would be improper not to give mention to a dedicated personal friend that has proven to be invaluable in keeping the health food store operating with high integrity and professionalism. Suzy Bruder is the dedicated wife of Ryon Bruder and proud mother of two fine young adults, Zach and Rena. Without Suzy's assistance the health food store would not be the same.

Also, hats off to Dr. James Duke and his wife Peggy! This book would not be possible without a lifetime of dedicated work in his field. It is with my deepest appreciation for all of his trail-blazing efforts in understanding of the herbs of the Bible and of the world.

Most importantly, I would like to take the time to praise the God almighty for all the abilities He has granted me and the direction my life has taken to make this possible only through Him.

DR. RICHARD N OLREE JR. D.C.

Dr. Olree graduated from Logan College of Chiropractic in 1981 with a bachelor's degree in Biology and a Doctorate in Chiropractic and has served Northern Michigan for the past 31 years. He sees an average of 30-50 people every day. He also owns a health food store that not only serves the local clientele but ships anywhere within the US, Canada and any free country.

For ten years Dr. Olree has been making house visits to the Mio/Fairview Michigan Amish and Mennonite communities. For the last ten years he has been also serving the local Ossineke area Amish community as well.

Dr. Olree and Chuck Walters, founder of Acres U.S.A., an organic farming magazine, worked together to write the book "Minerals for the Genetic Code" and Dr Olree has written the book entitled "Amishman's Handy Guide To Minerals, Vitamins and Food Supplements" to be published soon. "Minerals for the Genetic Code" was published in 2006 with over 3,000 copies sold worldwide and is currently on the second edition. Dr. Olree's contribution to the book focuses on a chart of the spine he developed that overlays the Standard Genetic Chart and lectures on the usage of trace minerals.

Richard N. Olree Jr. D.C., B.S.
Doctor of Chiropractic

Private Practice:	**Other Businesses:**	
Olree Chiropractic Centre	Hillman Health Foods	A1 A2 Genetic Testing Service
311 State Street	311 State Street	P.O. Box 550
Hillman, MI. 49746	Hillman, MI. 49746	Hillman, MI. 49746
989/742/4242	989/742/2561	989/742/2561
1981-present (32 continuous years)	www.emineral.info	

National Board Certification:

NBCE National Board of Chiropractic Examiners 1981

Education:

Oakland Community College
1. Associates in Liberal Arts 1974-1977

Logan College of Chiropractic 09/1977 –01/1981
1. Bachelor of Science in Human Biology – Logan College of Chirpractic 9/79
2. Doctor of Chiropractic – Maturation date 1/81

Hospital Affiliation:

Onaway Community Hospital
Radiological and Co-admission privileges
1981-1987

Cheboygan Community Memorial Hospital
Radiological privileges/ CT scan and plain films of the human spine
1987-present

Alpena Regional Medical Center formerly Alpena General Hospital
MRI, CT scan and plain films of the human spine
1989-present

Major Professional Societies:

Past members of the following societies
1. ACA American Chiropractic Association
2. ICA International Chiropractors Association
3. MCC Michigan Chiropractic Council / District 6 President
4. MCA Michigan Chiropractic Association
5. MSCA Michigan State Chiropractic Association / Chairman of the Hospital Relations Committee

Current member of the following society
1. Michigan Association of Chiropractors

Publications:

1. *Minerals for the Genetic Code*
    May 2006 published by Acres US
2. Many artiles published by AcresUSA magazine

Table of Contents

Dr. Richard N Olree Jr. D.C. 2

Forward 23

Disclamer 24

Introduction 25

The Nervous System 26
    What Is The Vertebral Subluxation? 26

Water - H_2O 30
    Water and Human Health 30
    Hard Water 32
    Soft Water 32
    Bottled Water 32
    Ground Water 32

The Human Immune System 33

Probiotics 34
    Probiotic Strains 36
    Probiotic Descriptions 36
        Bacillus Subtilis - (B. Subtilis) 36
        Bifidobacterium Bifidum - (B. Bifidum) 36
        Bifidobacterium Infantis - (B. Infantis) 36
        Bifidobacterium Longum - (B. Longum) 36
        Enterococcus Faecium - (E. Faecium) 37
        Lactobacillus Acidophilus - (L. Acidophilus) 37
        Lactobacillus Brevis - (L. Brevis) 37
        Lactobacillus Bulgaricus - (L. Bulgaricus) 37
        Lactobacillus Casei - (L. Casei) 37
        Lactobacillus Plantarum - (L. Plantarum) 37
        Lactobacillus Rhamnosus - (L. Rhamnosus) 38
        Lactobacillus Salivarius - (L. Salivarius) 38
        Streptococcus Thermophilus - (S. Thermophilus) 38
    Benefits of bacterial combinations 38
        L. Acidophilus, L. Rhamnosus 38
        L. Rhamnosous, L. Acidophilus, B. Lactis, Streptococcus Thermophilus, L. Bulgaricus 38
        L. Casei, L. Rhamnosus, L. Acidophilus, B. Longum 39
        Culturelle Lactobacillus GG: Lactobacillus GG. 39

Vitamins 40
    Vitamin B_1 - Thiamine 42
    Vitamin B_2 - Riboflavin 43
    Vitamin B_3 - Niacin 44

Vitamin B$_6$ - Pyridoxine	46
Vitamin B$_7$ - Biotin	47
Vitamin B$_8$ - Inositol Hexaphosphate	48
Vitamin B$_9$ - Folic Acid / Folate	49
Vitamin B$_{12}$ - Cyanocobalamin	51
Vitamin B$_{13}$ - Orotic acid	52
Vitamin B$_{15}$ - Pangamic Acid	53
Vitamin B$_{17}$ - Laetrile	54
Vitamin B$_p$ - Choline	56
Vitamin C - Ascorbic acid	58
Vitamin D - Cholecalciferol	60
Vitamin E - Tocopherols	62
Vitamin F - Essential fatty acids	63
Vitamin P - Flavonoids	69
Minerals and Human Health	**70**
Minerals Testing thru Hair Biopsy Analysis	72
Aluminum	73
Antimony	75
Arsenic	77
Barium	80
Boron	82
Cadmium	86
Calcium	88
Chlorine	91
Chromium	94
Cobalt – Please see vitamin B$_{12}$	97
Fluorine	101
Germanium	103
Iodine	104
Iron	108
Lead	112
Lithium	114
Magnesium	116
Manganese	120
Mercury	123

Molybdenum	128
Nitrogen	130
Phosphrus	131
Potassium	134
Rubidium	136
Selenium	137
Silicon	140
Sodium	144
Sulfur	148
Vandiuim	150
Zinc	152

Soil Nutrients 155

Genetically Modified Organisms (GMO) 164

True Food Shopper's Guide 166
- Tips for avoiding GM crops 166
- Fruits & Vegetables 167
- Eggs 167
- Fish 167
- Meat & Fowl 168
- Dairy Products & Alternative Dairy Products 168
- Baby Foods & Infant Formula 169
- Cereals & Breakfast Bars 170
- Energy Bars 171
- Grains, Beans & Pasta 171
- Canned Foods 171
- Frozen Foods 172
- Condiments, Oils, Dressings & Spreads 173
- Snack Foods 173
- Sweeteners 174
- Candy & Chocolate Products 174
- Sodas, Juices & Other Beverages 175

Protein = Amino Acids 176
- Alanine 176
- Arginine 177
- Aspartic Acid, also known as Asparagine 178
- Cysteine - Cystine 179
- Glutamic Acid 180
- Glutamine 181
- Glycine 182
- Histidine 183
- Isoleucine 184

Leucine	185
Lysine	185
Methionine	186
Phenylalanine	187
Proline	188
Selnocysteine	189
Serine	190
Threonine	191
Tryptophan	192
Tyrosine	193
HEALTHFOOD STORE SUPPLEMENTS	**196**
ALA – (Alpha-Linolenic Acid)	196
AMP – (Adenosine Monophosphate)	197
Amylase Inhibitors	198
Apple Cider Vinegar	198
Bach Essence Flowers	204
Agrimony - (Agrimonia Eupatoria)	206
Aspen - (Populus Tremula)	206
Beech - (Fagus Sylvatica)	207
Centaury - (Centaurium Umbellatum)	207
Cerato - (Ceratostigma Willmottiana)	208
Cherry Plum - (Prunus Cerasifera)	208
Chestnut Bud - (Aesculus Hippocastanum)	209
Chicory - (Cichorium Intybus)	209
Clematis - (Clematis Vitalba)	210
Crab Apple - (Malus Pumila)	210
Elm - (Ulmus Procera)	211
Gentian - (Gentiana Amarella)	211
Gorse - (Ulex Europaeus)	212
Heather - (Calluna Vulgaris)	212
Holly - (Ilex Aquifolium)	213
Honeysuckle - (Lonicera Caprifolium)	213
Hornbeam - (Carpinus Betulus)	214
Impatiens - (Impatiens Glandulifera)	214
Larch - (Larix Decidua)	215
Mimulus - (Mimulus Guttatus)	215
Mustard - (Sinapis Arvensis)	216
Oak - (Quercus Robur)	216
Olive - (Olea Europaea)	217
Pine - (Pinus Sylvestris)	217
Red Chestnut - (Aesculus Carnea)	218
Rock Rose - (Helianthemum Nummularium)	218
Rock Water - (Aqua Petra)	219
Scleranthus - (Scleranthus Annuus)	219
Star of Bethlehem - (Ornithogalum Umbellatum)	220

Sweet Chestnut - *(Castanea Sativa)*	220
Vervain - *(Verbena Officinalis)*	221
Vine - *(Vitis Vinifera)*	221
Walnut - *(Juglans Regia)*	222
Water Violet - *(Hottonia Palustris)*	222
White Chestnut - *(Aesculus Hippocastanum)*	223
Wild Oat - *(Bromus Ramosus)*	223
Wild Rose - *(Rosa Canina)*	224
Willow - *(Salix Vitellina)*	224
Rescue Remedy	225
Rescue Remedy Sleep	225
Bee Pollen	226
Beta-Carotene	226
Beta-Glucan	227
Betaine	228
Beta-Sitosterol	228
Biochemical Cell Salts	229
Calcium Fluoride	232
Calcium Phosphate	232
Calcium Sulphate	232
Iron Phosphate	232
Magnesium Phosphate	232
Potassium Chloride	232
Potassium Phosphate	232
Potassium Sulphate	232
Silica	232
Sodium Chloride	233
Sodium Phosphate	233
Sodium Sulphate	233
Borage Oil	233
Bovine Cartilage	234
Bovine Colostrum	234
Brewer's Yeast	235
Bromelain	236
Capsaicin	236
Chitosan	237
Chlorophyll	238
Chondroitin	238
CLA – *(Conjugated Linoleic Acid)*	239
CoEnzyme Q_{10} – *(CoQ_{10})*	240
DHA – *(Docosahexaenoic Acid)*	240
DHEA – *(Dehydroepiandrosterone)*	241
DMAE – *(Dimethylaminoethanol)*	242
EGCG – *(Epigallocatechin Gallate)*	243
Essential Oils	244

Aniseed - *(Pimpinella Anisum)*	244
Anise Star - *(Illicium Verum)*	245
Bacopa – *(Bacopa monnieri)*	245
Basil Sweet - *(Ocimum Basilicum)*	247
Bay - *(Laurus Nobilis)*	247
Benzoin - *(Styrax Benzoin)*	248
Bergamot - *(Citrus Bergamia)*	248
Birch Sweet - *(Betula Lenta)*	249
Blood Orange - *(Citrus Sinensis)*	249
Cajeput - *(Melaleuca Cajeputi)*	250
Camphor - *(Cinnamomum Camphora)*	250
Caraway - *(Carum Carvi)*	251
Cassia - *(Cinnamomum Cassia)*	252
Cedarwood - *(Cedrus Atlantica)*	253
Cedarwood - *(Cedrus Deodora)*	253
Cedarwood - *(Cupressus Funebris)*	254
Cedarwood - *(Juniperus Virginiana)*	255
Chamomile - *(Matricaria Chamomilla)*	255
Cinnamon Bark - *(Cinnamomum Cassia)*	256
Cinnamon Bark - *(Cinnamomum Zeylanicum)*	256
Cinnamon Leaf - *(Cinnamomum Verum)*	257
Citral - *(Litsea Cubeba)*	257
Citronella - *(Cymbopogon Nardus)*	258
Clary Sage - *(Salvia Sclarea)*	258
Clove Bud - *(Syzygium Aromaticumum)*	259
Clove Leaf - *(Syzgium Aromaticum)*	259
Coffee - *(Coffea Arabica)*	260
Coriander - *(Coriandrum Sativum)*	260
Cypress - *(Cupressus Sempervirens)*	261
Eucalyptus – *(Eucalyptus Globules)* , *(Eucalyptus Polybractea)*, *(Eucalyptus Radiata)*	261
Eucalyptus Lemon - *(Eucalyptus Polybractea)*	262
Fir Needle - *(Abies Siberica)*	262
Frankincense - *(Boswellia Serrata)*	263
Ginger Root - *(Zingiber Officinalis)*	264
Helichrysum – *(Helichrysum Italicum)*	265
Jasmine - *(Jasminum Grandiflorum)* , *(Jasminum Sambac)*	265
Juniper Berry – *(Juniperus Communis)*	266
Lavandin Abrialis – *(Lavandula Intermedia var Abrialis)*	266
Lavandin Grosso – *(Lavandula Intermedia var Grosso)*	267
Lavender – *(Lavandula Officinalis)*	267
Lavender Bulgarian – *(Lavandula Angustifolia)*	268
Lavender French – *(Lavandula Dentate)*	268
Lavender Population – *(Lavandula Angustifolia)*	269
Lavender South African – *(Lavandula Angustifolia)*	270
Lavender Spanish – *(Lavandula Stoechas)*	270
Lemon - *(Citrus Limonum)*	271
Lemongrass - *(Cymbopogon Flexuosus)*	271
Lime - *(Citrus Aurantifolia)*	272
Marjoram - *(Origanum Marjorana)*	273
Melissa Leaf - *(Melissa Officinalis)*	274
Menthol - *(Mentha Arvensis)*	274
Myrrh – *(Commiphora Myrrha)*	275

Nutmeg - *(Myristica Fragrans)* 276
Orange – *(Citrus Sinensis)* 276
Origanum - *(Origanum Vulgare)* 277
Patchouli – *(Pogostemon Cablin)* 278
Pepper Black - *(Piper Nigrum)* 278
Peppermint - *(Mentha Arvensis)* 279
Peppermint - *(Mentha Piperita)* 279
Peru Balsam - *(Myroxylon Pereira)* 280
Petitgrain - *(Petitgrain Bigarde)* 280
Pine Scotch - *(Pinus Sylvestris)* 281
Rose - *(Rosa Damascene)* 281
Rosemary - *(Rosmarinus Officinalis)* 282
Rosewood - *(Aniba Rosaeodora)* 282
Sandalwood - *(Santalum Album)* 283
Spearmint - *(Mentha Spicata)* 283
Spikenard - *(Nardastachus Jatamansi)* 284
Tangerine - *(Citrus Reticulata var Tangerina)* 284
Tea Tree - *(Melaleuca Alternifolia)* 285
Thyme - *(Thymus Vulgaris)* 285
Vanilla - *(Vanilla Planifolia)* 286
Vetiver - *(Vetiveria Zizanoides)* 286
Wintergreen - *(Gaultheria Procumbens)* 287
Ylang Ylang - *(Cananga Odorata)* 288

Evening Primrose Oil 289

Fish Oil 289

Fumaric Acid 290

GLA – (Gamma-Linolenic Acid) 291

Glucomannan 291

Grape Seed Extract 292

Grapefruit Seed Extract 293

HMB – (Hydroxyl-Beta-Methylbultyrate) 295

Hydroxycitric Acid 295

Indole – (Indole-3-Carbinol) 296

Insoluble Fiber 297

Ipriflavone 297

Lactase 298

Lecithin 299

Lipase 300

Lutein 300

Lycopene 301

Malic Acid 302

Mannose 302

Medicinal Herbs of the Bible 304

African Myrrh – (*Commiphora Africana*)	307
Aleppo Pine – (*Pinus Halepensis*)	308
Almond – (*Prunus Dulcis*)	309
Aloe – (*Socotrine Aloe*)	311
Apricot – (*Prunus Armeniaca*)	312
Balsam – (*Commiphora Opobalsamum*)	314
Barley – (*Hordeum Vulgare*)	315
Bitter Apple – (*Citrullus Colocynthis*)	316
Black Cumin – (*Nigella Sativa*)	317
Black Mulberry – (*Morus Nigra*)	319
Black Mustard – (*Brassica Nigra*)	320
Blackberry – (*Rubus Sanctus*)	322
Blue Mallow – (*Malva Sylvestris*)	323
Box – (*Buxus Longifolia*)	324
Broadbean – (*Vicia Faba*)	325
Brutian Pine – (*Pinus Brutia*)	327
Butcher's Broom – (*Ruscus Aculeatus*)	328
Camel Thorn – (*Alhagi Camelorum*)	329
Caper – (*Capparis Spinosa*)	330
Carob – (*Ceratonia Siliqua*)	331
Castor Bean – (*Ricinus Communis*)	332
Cattail – (*Typha Australis*)	334
Cedar of Lebanon – (*Cedrus Libani*)	335
Ceylon Cinnamon – (*Cinnamomum Verum*)	336
Chicory – (*Cichorium Intybus*)	338
Cocklebur – (*Xanthium Spinosum*)	340
Common Reed – (*Phragmites Australis*)	341
Coriander – (*Coriandrum Sativum*)	342
Corn Cockle – (*Agrostemma Githago*)	344
Costus Oil – (*Saussurea Lappa*)	345
Cotton – (*Gossypium Herbaceum*)	346
Crown of Thorns – (*Paliurus Spina*)	347
Cucumber – (*Cucumis Sativus*)	348
Cumin – (*Cuminum Cyminum*)	349
Cyprus Turpentine – (*Pistacia Terebinthus*)	350
Dandelion – (*Taraxacum Officinale*)	351
Darnel – (*Lolium Temulentum*)	353
Date Palm – (*Phoenix Dactylifera*)	354
Date-Plum – (*Diospyros Ebenum*)	356
Desert Date – (*Balanites Aegyptiaca*)	357
Dill – (*Anethum Graveolens*)	358
Dyer's Oak – (*Quercus Aegilops*)	360
Eaglewood – (*Aquillaria Agallocha*)	361
Ebony Persimmon – (*Diospyros Melanoxylum*)	362
Egyptian Marjoram – (*Origanum Maru*)	363
Endive – (*Cichorium Endivia*)	364
English Walnut – (*Juglans Regia*)	365
Euphrates Aspen – (*Populus Euphratica*)	367
European Box Thorn – (*Lycium Europaeum*)	368
European Rock Rose – (*Cistus Creticus*)	369
Fenugreek – (*Trigonella Foenum*)	370
Field Mustard – (*Sinapis Arvensis*)	372

Fig Tree – (*Ficus Carica*)	373
Flax – (*Linum Usitatissimum*)	375
Frankincense – (*Boswellia Carteri*)	377
Galbanum – (*Ferula Galbaniflua*)	378
Garden Rue – (*Ruta Graveolens*)	379
Garlic – (*Allium Sativum*)	380
Giant Reed – (*Arundo Donax*)	382
Glasswort – (*Salicornia Europaea*)	383
Glasswort – (*Salsola Kali*)	384
Gopher Wood – (*Cupressus Sempervirens*)	385
Grecian Juniper – (*Juniperus Excelsa*)	386
Hemlock – (*Conium Maculatum*)	387
Henna – (*Lawsonia Inermis*)	388
Holly Oak – (*Quercus Ilex*)	390
Horsemint – (*Mentha Longifolia*)	391
Hyacinth – (*Hyacinthus Orientalis*)	392
Ivy – (*Hedera Helix*)	393
Jericho Rose – (*Anastatica Hierochuntica*)	394
Judas Tree – (Cercis Siliquastrum)	395
Judean Sage – (*Salvia Judaica*)	396
Juniper – (*Cynomorium Coccineum*)	397
Kashmir Willow – (*Salix Fragilis*)	398
Kermes Oak – (Quercus Coccifera)	399
Lentil – (*Lens Culinaris*)	400
Lettuce – (*Lactuca Sativa*)	401
Loveapple – (*Mandragora Officinarum*)	402
Madonna Lily – (*Lilium Candidum*)	403
Manna Ash – (*Fraxinus Ornus*)	404
Mastic – (*Pistacia Lentiscus*)	405
Milk Thistle – (*Silybum Marianum*)	406
Millet – (*Panicum Miliaceum*)	407
Mulberry Fig – (*Ficus Sycomorus*)	408
Muskmelon – (*Cucumis Melo*)	409
Myrrh – (*Commiphora Myrrha*)	410
Myrtle – (*Myrtus Communis*)	411
Narcissus – (*Narcissus Tazetta*)	413
Nettles – (*Acanthus Syriacuss*)	414
Olive – (*Olea Europea*)	415
Onion – (*Allium Cepa*)	417
Onycha – (*Styrax Benzoin*)	419
Palestine Buckthorn – (*Rhamnus Palaestina*)	420
Papyrus – (*Cyperus Papyrus*)	421
Phoenician Rose – (*Rosa Phoenicia*)	422
Pistachio Nut – (*Pisticia Vera*)	423
Plane Tree – (*Platanus Orientalis*)	424
Pomegranate – (*Punica Granatum*)	425
Poppy Seed – (*Papaver Somniferum*)	427
Poplar – (*Populus Alba*)	429
Red Saunders – (*Pterocarpus Santalinus*)	430
Roman Nettle – (*Urtica Pilulifera*)	431
Rose – (*Nerium Oleander*)	432
Russian Olive – (*Elaeagnus Angustifolia*)	433

Saffron – (*Crocus Sativus*) 434
Saigon Cinnamon – (*Cinnamonum Cassia*) 435
Sandarac – (*Tetraclinis Articulata*) 436
Sea Purslane – (*Atriplex Halimus*) 437
Sea-Wrack – (*Zostera Marina*) 438
Sheep Sorrel – (*Rumex Acetosella*) 439
Shittim Wood – (*Acacia Tortilis*) 440
Sodom Apple – (*Solanum Incanum*) 441
Soft Rush – (*Juncus Effusus*) 442
Sorghum – (*Sorghum Bicolor*) 443
Spelt – (*Triticum Spelta*) 444
Spikenard – (*Nardostachys Jatamansi*) 445
Stacte – (*Styrax Officinalis*) 447
Star of Bethlehem – (*Ornithogalum Umbellatum*) 448
Star Thistle – (*Centaurea Calcitrapa*) 449
Stinging Nettle – (*Urtica Dioica*) 450
Sugarcane – (*Saccharum Officinarum*) 451
Sweet Bay – (*Laurus Nobilis*) 452
Syrian Christ Thorn – *(Ziziphus Spina)* 453
Tamarisk – (*Tamarix Aphylla*) 454
Thorn Bush – (*Acacia Nilotica*) 455
Tragacanth – (*Astragalus Gummifer*) 456
Vetiver – (*Vetiveria Zizanioides*) 457
Vine Grape – (*Vitis Vinifera*) 458
Vine of Sodom – (*Solanum Sodomeum*) 460
Water Lily – (*Nymphaea Alba*) 461
Watercress – (*Nasturtium Officinale*) 462
Watermelon – (*Citrullus Lanatus*) 464
Weeping Willow – (*Salix Babylonica*) 466
Wheat Corn – (*Triticum Aestivum*) 467
White Broom – (*Retama Raetam*) 468
White Whistling Wood – (*Acacia Seyal*) 469
Wild Grape – (*Vitis Orientalis*) 470
Willow – (*Salix Alba*) 471
Windflower – (*Anemone Coronaria*) 472
Wormwood – (*Artemisia Herba*) 473
Yellow Flag – (*Iris Pseudoacorus*) 474

Common Herbs 475
Aikal Skullcaps - (*Scutellaria Lateriflora*) 475
Albizia – (*Albizia Lebbeck*) 475
Andrographis – (*Andrographis Paniculata*) 476
Anise - (*Pimpinella Anisum*) 477
Arnica - (*Arnica Montana*) 478
Ashwagandha, Withania – (*Withania Somnifera*) 478
Astragalus - (*Astragalus Membranaceus*) 479
Avocado - (*Persea Americana*) 479
Basil - (*Ocimum Basilicum*) 480
Bay - (*Laurus Nobilis*) 480
Bearberry - (*Arctostaphylos Uva-Ursi*) 481
Beggar's Lice - (*Desmodium Styracifolium*) 481
Bilberry - (*Vaccinium Myrtillus*) 482

Bishop's Weed - (*Aegopodium Podagraria*)	482
Bitter Gourd - (*Momordica Charantia*)	483
Black Cohosh - (*Actaea Racemosa L. var. Racemosa aka Black Bugbane*)	483
Black Haw - (*Viburnum Prunifolium*)	484
Black Horehound - (*Ballota Nigra*)	485
Black Nightshade - (*Solanum Nigrum*)	485
Black Walnut - (*Juglans Nigra*)	486
Blackberry - (*Rubus Fructicosus*)	486
Bloodroot - (*Sanguinaria Candensis*)	487
Blue Cohosh - (*Caulophyllum Thalictroides*)	487
Blueberry - (*Vaccinium Corymbosum*)	488
Borage - (*Borago Officinalis*)	488
Broom Weed - (*Amphiachyris Dracunculoides*)	489
Buchu – (*Barosma Betulina*)	489
Bugleweed (aka- Gypsywort)- (*Lycopus Europaeus*)	491
Bupleurum – (*Bupleurum Falcatum*)	492
Burdock - (*Arctium Lappa*)	492
Burnet Saxifrage - (*Pimpinella Saxifraga*)	493
Butcher's Broom - (*Ruscus Aculeatus*)	494
Calendula aka Marigold - (*Calendula Officinalis*)	494
Californian Poppy – (*Eschscholtzia Californica*)	495
Camu-Camu - (*Myrciaria Dubia*)	495
Cankerroot - (*Coptis Trifolia*)	496
Capers - (*Capparis Spinosa*)	496
Cardamom - (*Elletaria Cardamom*)	497
Carob - (*Caroba Jacaranda Procera*)	498
Cascara – (*Rhamnus Purshiana*)	498
Cat's Claw - (*Uncaria Tomentosa*)	499
Catnip - (*Nepeta Cataria*)	499
Cayenne – (*Capsicum Annuum*)	500
Celandine - (*Chelidonium Majus*)	501
Celery Seed - (*Apium Graveolens*)	501
Chamomile - (*Matricaria Chamomilla*)	502
Chamomile - (*Matricaria Recutita*)	502
Chaparral - (*Larrea Divaricata*)	503
Chaste Berry - (*Vitex Agnus-Castus*)	504
Chickweed - (*Stellaria Media*)	504
Chicory - (*Cichorium Intybus*)	505
Chinese Angelica - (*Angelica Sinensis*)	506
Chinese Skullcap, Baical Skullcap – (*Scutellaria Baicalensis*)	506
Chiso aka beefsteak plant - (*Perilla Frutescens*)	507
Cinchona - (*Cinchona Officinalis*)	508
Cinnamon - (*Cinnamomum Zeylanicum*)	509
Citronella - (*Cymbopogon Nardus*)	509
Citrus Fruits	510
Chinese Angelica aka Dong Quai–(*Angelica Sinensis*)	512
Cleavers – (*Galium Aparine*)	512
Clove - (*Syzygium Aromaticum*)	513
Cocoa – (*Theobroma Cacao*)	513
Codonopsis – (*Codonopsis Pilosula*)	514
Coleus – (*Coleus Forskohlii*)	514
Comfrey - (*Symphytum Officinale*)	515

Table of Contents

- Coriander - (*Coriandrum Sativum*) 515
- Corydalis – (*Corydalis Ambigua*) 516
- Couchgrass - (*Agropyron Repens*) 516
- Country Mallow - (*Sida Cordifolia*) 517
- Cramp Bark – (*Viburnum Opulus*) 517
- Cranberry - (*Vaccinium Macrocarpon*) 518
- Crataeva – (*Crataeva Nurvala*) 519
- Cubeb - (*Piper Cubeba*) 519
- Damiana – (*Turnera Diffusa*) 520
- Dragon's Blood - (*Daemonorops Draco*) 521
- Echinacea - (*Echinacea Angustifolia*) 521
- Echinacea - (*Purpurea Purpurea*) 522
- Eggplant - (*Solanum Melongena*) 523
- Elderberry - (*Sambucus Nigra*) 524
- Elecampane - (*Inula Helenium*) 524
- Eleuthero – (*Eleutherococcus Senticosus*) 525
- English Walnut - (*Juglans Regia*) 526
- Ephedra - (*Ephedra Sinica*) 526
- Eucalyptus - (*Eucalyptus Globulus*) 527
- Euphorbia – (*Euphorbia Hirta*) 528
- Evening Primrose - (*Oenothera Biennis*) 528
- Eyebright – (*Euphrasia Officinalis*) 529
- False Unicorn – (*Chamaelirium Luteum*) 530
- Fava Bean - (*Vicia Faba*) 530
- Fennel - (*Foeniculum Vulgare*) 531
- Fenugreek - (*Trigonella Foenum-Graecum*) 532
- Feverfew - (*Tanacetum Parthenium*) 532
- Forsythia - (*Forsythia Suspensa*) 533
- Fringe Tree – (*Chionanthus Virginica*) 533
- Gentian - (*Gentiana Lutea*) 534
- Ginger - (*Zingiber Officinale*) 534
- Ginkgo - (*Ginkgo Biloba*) 535
- Ginseng - (*Panax Ginseng*) 535
- Globe Artichoke – (*Cynara Scolymus*) 536
- Goldenrod - (*Oligoneuron Small*) 537
- Goldenrod – (*Solidago Virgaurea*) 538
- Goldenseal – (*Hydrastis Canadensis*) 538
- Gotu Kola - (*Centella Asiatica*) 539
- Green Tea – (*Camellia Sinensis*) 540
- Grindelia – (*Grindelia Camporum*) 541
- Guava - (*Psidium Guava*) 542
- Gymnema - (*Gymnema Sylvestre*) 543
- Hawthorn - (*Crataegus Monogyna*) 543
- Hemidesmus – (*Hemidesmus Indicus*) 544
- Holy Basil – (*Ocimum Tenuiflorum*) 545
- Honeysuckle - (*Lonicera Caprifolium*) 545
- Hops - (*Humulus Lupulus*) 546
- Horehound - (*Marrubium Vulgare*) 546
- Horse Chestnut - (*Aesculus Hippocastanum*) 547
- Horsebalm aka Stone Root - (*Collinsonia Canadensis*) 547
- Horseradish - (*Armoracia Rusticana*) 548
- Horsetail aka Indian Almond - (*Equisetum Arvense*) 549

Ipecac - (*Cephaelis Acuminata*)	550
Jaborandi - (*Pilocarpus Microphyllus*)	551
Jewelweed - (*Impatiens Capensis*)	551
Kaffir Potato - (*Plectranthus Esculentus*)	552
Kelp - (*Fucus Vesiculosus*)	553
Khella - (*Ammi Visnaga*)	554
Kudzu - (*Pueraria Lobata*)	555
Lemon Balm - (*Melissa Officinalis*)	556
Lemongrass - (*Cymbopogon Citratus*)	556
Lesser Periwinkle - (*Vinca Minor*)	557
Licorice - (*Glycyrrhiza Glabra*)	557
Malabar Nut Tree, Adhatoda – (*Adhatoda Vasica*)	559
Marshmallow aka Mallow - (*Althaea Officinalis*)	560
Meadowsweet - (*Filipendula Ulmaria*)	561
Milk Thistle - (*Silybum Marianum*)	562
Mints - Peppermint, Spearmint, Apple Mint, and Pineapple Mint	562
Mistletoe – (*Viscum Album*)	563
Motherwort – (*Leonurus Cardiaca*)	564
Mullein - (*Verbascum Thapsus*)	564
Myrrh – (*Commiphora Molmol*)	565
Mustard aka Indian Mustard - (*Brassica Juncea*)	565
Neem - (*Azadirachta Indica*)	566
Nuts - (*Cyperus Rotundus*)	567
Oats – (*Avena Sativa*)	568
Oregano - (*Origanum Vulgare*)	569
Oregon Grape – (*Berberis Aquifolium*)	570
Pansy - (*Viola Tricolor*)	570
Parsley - (*Petroselinum Crispum*)	571
Partridge Berry - (*Mitchella Repens*)	572
Pasque Flower – (*Pulsatilla Vulgaris*)	572
Passionflower - (*Passiflora Incarnata*)	573
Pau d'Arco- (*Tabebuia Avellanedae*)	574
Pineapple - (*Ananas Comosus*)	574
Plantain - (*Plantago Major*)	575
Pleurisy Root – (*Asclepias Tuberose*)	576
Poke Root – (*Phytolacca Decandra*)	577
Prickly Ash – (*Zanthoxylum Clava-Herculis*)	577
Psyllium - (*Plantago Psyllium*)	578
Pumpkin - (*Cucurbita Pepo*)	579
Purslane - (*Portulaca Oleracea*)	580
Pygeum - (*Prunus Africana*)	580
Quevrancho - (*Aspidosperma Quebracho-Blanco*)	581
Red Clover - (*Trifolium Pratense*)	582
Rehmannia – (*Rehmannia Glutinosa*)	582
Reishi - (*Ganoderma Lyceum*)	583
Rhodiola – (*Rhodiola Rosea*)	584
Rhubarb - (*Rheum Palmatum*)	585
Rosemary - (*Rosmarinus Officinalis*)	586
Rough Pigweed - (*Amaranthus Hybridus*)	586
Safflower - (*Carthamus Tinctorius*)	587
Saffron - (*Crocus Sativus*)	588
Sage - (*Salvia Officinalis*)	588

Herb	Page
Sarsaparilla – (*Smilax Ornata*)	589
Saw Palmetto - (*Serenoa Repens*)	590
Saw Palmetto – (*Serenoa Serrulata*)	591
Schisandra - (*Schisandra Chinensis*)	591
Self Heal - (*Prunella Vulgaris*)	592
Sesame - (*Sesamum Orientale*)	593
Shatavari – (*Asparagus Racemosus*)	593
Shepherd's Purse – (*Capsella Bursa-Pastoris*)	594
Shiitake – (*Lentinula Edodes*)	595
Slippery Elm - (*Ulmus Rubra*)	595
Soapwort - (*Saponaria*)	596
Spiny Jujube, Zizyphus – (*Zizyphus Spinosa*)	596
Stemona – (*Stemona Sessilifolia*)	597
St. John's Wort - (*Hypericum Perforatum*)	598
Sunflower - (*Helianthus Annuus*)	598
Sweet flag - (*Acorus Calamus*)	599
Sweet Violet - (*Viola Odorata*)	600
Tea Tree - (*Leptospermum Scoparium*)	600
Thyme - (*Thymus Vulgaris*)	601
Tienchi Ginseng – (*Panax Notoginseng*)	602
Tribulus – (*Tribulus Terrestris*)	603
Turmeric - (*Curcuma Longa*)	604
Valerian - (*Valeriana Officinalis*)	605
Verbena - (*Sisambiguation*)	605
Wheatgrass	606
White Peony – (*Paeonia Lactiflora*)	607
Wild Angelica - (*Angelica Sylvestris*)	607
Wild Bergamot - (*Monarda Fistulosa*)	608
Wild Yam - (*Dioscorea Villosa*)	609
Willow Bark – (*Salix Purpurea*)	609
Wintergreen - (*Gaultheria Procumbens*)	610
Witch Hazel - (*Hamamelis Virginiana*)	611
Wolfberry - (*Lycium Barbarum*)	612
Wormseed - (*Chenopodium Ambrosioides*)	613
Wormwood – (*Artemisia Absinthium*)	613
Yellow Dock – (*Rumex Crispus*)	614
Yellowroot - (*Xanthorhiza Simplicissima*)	615
Yohimbe - (*Pausinystalia Yohimbe*)	616

Conditions that can be affected by herbs: *617*

Aging (Senescence)	617
Allergy	617
Altitude sickness (Soroche)	617
Alzheimer's disease (A/O Senile dementia)	617
Amenorrhea	617
Angina	617
Ankylosing spondylitis	617
Arthritis	617
Asthma	617
Athlete's foot	617
Backache	618
Bad breath	618

Table of Contents

Baldness (Alopecia)	618
Body odor	618
Breast enlargment (Micromastia)	618
Bronchitis	618
Bruises	618
Bunions	618
Bursitis and tendinitis	619
Cancer prevention	619
Canker sores	619
Cardiac arrhythmia	619
Cataracts	619
Chronic fatigue syndrome	619
Colds and flu	619
Constipation	619
Corns	619
Coughing	619
Cuts, scrapes, abscesses	619
Dandruff	619
Depression	620
Diabetes	620
Diarrhea	620
Diverticulitis	620
Dizzness (Vertigo)	620
Dry mouth	620
Earache (Otalgia)	620
Emphysema	620
Endometriosis	620
Erection problems (Impotence)	620
Fainting (Syncope)	620
Fever	620
Flatulence (Gas)	620
Fungal infections (Mycoses)	621
Gallstones and kidney stones	621
Gential herpes and cold sores	621
Gingivitis	621
Glaucoma	621
Gout (Podagrao)	621
Graves disease	621
Hangover	621
Headache	621
Heartburn	621
Heart disease	621
Hemorrhoids	621
High blood pressure	621
High cholesterol	622
Hives	622
HIV infection	622
Hypothyroidism	622
Indigestion (Dyspepsia)	622
Infertility	622
Inflammatory bowel disease (IBS)	622
Inhibited sexual desire in women (Frigidity)	622

Insect bites and stings (Bugbites)	622
Insomnia	622
Intermittent claudication	622
Intestinal parasites	622
Laryngitis	622
Lice	623
Liver problems (Hepatosis)	623
Lyme's disease	623
Macular degeneration	623
Menopause	623
Menstral cramps (Dysmenorrhea)	623
Morning sickness	623
Motion sickness	623
Multiple sclerosis	623
Nausea	623
Osteoporosis	623
Overweight (Obesity)	623
Pain	623
Pneumonia	624
Poison ivy, poison oak, and poison sumac	624
Pregnancy and delivery	624
Prostate enlargement (BPH) (Prostatitis)	624
Psoriasis	624
Raynaud's disease	624
Scabies	624
Sciatica	624
Shingles	624
Sinusitis	624
Skin problems (Dermatoses)	624
Smoking	624
Sores	625
Sore throat	625
Sties	625
Stroke	625
Sunburn	625
Swelling	625
Tinnitus	625
Tonsillitis	625
Toothache	625
Tooth decay (Caries)	625
Tuberculosis	625
Ulcers	625
Vaginitis	625
Varicose veins	626
Viral infections	626
Warts	626
Worms	626
Wrinkles	626
Yeast infections	626

Melatonin 627

Methoxyisoflavone 628

Milk	628
Cow's Milk	628
Almond Milk	629
Coconut Milk	630
Goat Milk	630
Hemp Milk	631
Soy Milk	631
Rice Milk	632
Naringin	632
Octacosanol	633
Oryzanol	634
Oligosaccharides	634
Olive Leaf Extract	635
Phosphatidylserine	636
Phytic Acid	636
Policosanol	637
Propolis	638
Psyllium – (Psyllium Seed)	638
Quercetin	639
Resveratrol	640
Soluble Fiber	641
Spirulina	642
Sulforaphane	642
Velver Antler (Deer – Elk)	643
Definitions of Human Conditions	644
Sourcing the Elements	**656**
Plants Containing Aluminum	656
Plants Containing Antimony	657
Plants Containing Arsenic	657
Plants Containing Barium	658
Plants Containing Boron	659
Plants Containing Bromine	662
Plants Containing Calcium	664
Plants Containing Cesium	673
Plants Containing Chlorine	674
Plants containing Chromium	675

Plants Containing Cobalt	*678*
Plants Containing Copper	*680*
Plants Containing Fluorine	*687*
Plants Containing Germanium	*688*
Plants Containing Iodine	*688*
Plants Containing Iron	*688*
Plants Containing Lanthanum	*698*
Plants Containing Lithium	*698*
Plants Containing Lutetium	*699*
Plants Containing Magnesium	*699*
Plants Containing Manganese	*708*
Plants Containing Molybdenum	*716*
Plants Containing Nitrogen	*718*
Plants Containing Phosphorus	*720*
Plants Containing Potassium	*727*
Plants Containing Rubidium	*737*
Plants Containing Scandium	*739*
Plants Containing Selenium	*739*
Plants Containing Silicon	*742*
Plants Containing Sodium	*745*
Plants Containing Strontium	*751*
Plants Containing Sulfur	*753*
Plants containing Vanadium	*755*
Plants Containing Yttrium	*756*
Plants Containing Zinc	*757*
Sourcing the Amino Acids	**765**
Plants Containing Alanine	*765*
Plants Containing Arginine	*768*
Plants Containing Asparagine	*771*
Plants Containing Cysteine	*772*
Plants Containing Glutamic Acid	*772*
Plants Containing Glycine	*775*
Plants Containing Histidine	*778*
Plants Containing Isoleucine	*781*
Plants Containing Leucine	*784*
Plants Containing Lysine	*788*

Plants Containing Methionine *791*

Plants Containing Phenylalanine *794*

Plants Containing Proline *797*

Plants Containing Serine *801*

Plants Containing Threonine *804*

Plants Containing Tryptophan *807*

Plants Containing Tyrosine *810*

Plants Containing Valine *813*

INDEX *817*

FORWARD

All of life is a gift of God. Although we can break down foods to the essential building blocks and provide insight and information as well as supply things as vitamins, minerals, herbs, and amino acids, it is truly better to obtain good nutrition through proper wholesome foods. But it gets harder and harder to find food that has not been adulterated by men of greed.

The food chain is full of genetically altered foods. In plain and simple language, man has taken the code of one of God's life forms and combined it into another code of life. Man has sought to act like God and create new genetic codes, and then insert them into the food chain and present these new codes as viable forms of food fit for human consumption. Animals that have had to endure consumption of these new types of food do not fair so well in the short or the long run. The stomach, kidneys, and reproductive organs fail to the point that animals are not able to reproduce more than three or four generations. This is shear madness at best and unspeakable at worst.

By letting food be your medicine it is one sure way to eliminate various forms of sickness. Good food is one of the best ways of prevention. An ounce of prevention is worth a pound of cure. It is always good to read the labels of the foods that you buy. If the wording on the side of any package has unpronounceable words, it would be good not to consume any of these products.

Artificial sweeteners should be avoided like the plague as well as any genetically modified organisms (GMO) such as GMO soy, corn, sugar beets, and alfalfa. These foods not only contain the codes of two different life forms, they contain up to 12 times the chemicals that kill all life that have not been genetically modified to withstand the chemicals.

By man's way of thinking, he can create new life forms to feed the masses of people based solely for profit. This will be man's downfall and many will tumble. With the demise of the small farmer and farm life, most food is being raised on what is called "factory farms." Animals are raised never to see the sun, enjoy fresh air or get exercise which has become the norm, not the exception. Most foods have been broken down and reconstituted. The only logic is, Humpty Dumpty sat on a wall, Humpty Dumpty had a great fall, all the kings' horsemen and all the kings' men couldn't put Humpty Dumpty together again. Many have never learned the lessons from this childhood tale.

The day has come that man cannot save seeds for the next harvest with the Genetically Modified Seeds (GMO). Large corporations lay papers on folks that do indeed collect seeds for the next harvest. Currently a farmer is committing suicide every 60 seconds worldwide over crop failure with GMO seeds. The madness needs to someday end, the sooner the better.

Credits and disclaimer

I would like to acknowledge the following different governmental branches whose information was critical in the gathering of information and the pictures utilized in this book.

1. USDA United States Department of Agriculture – Agricultural Research Service Grand Forks North Dakota Human Nutrition Research Center – Nutriton Research for Rural America

2. Plants Database – USDA United States Department of Agriculture – Natural Resources Conservation Service

3. Centers for Disease Control and Prevention

4. USDA United States Department of Agriculture – Agricultural Research Service Dr. Duke's Phytochemical and Ethnobotanical Databases

5. United States Geological Survey

DISCLAMER

There is nothing more important than health during one's lifetime. This book is written strictly for those who desire Self-Applied Prevention. Thirty years of experience has gone into assembling this book. The information presented in this book is not intended to replace professional health care.

Those who are not educated in vitamins, minerals, amino acids, herbs and health food store supplements in general should seek care of a competent health care provider. Asking a Medical Doctor (MD), Osteopathic Doctor (DO), Nurse Practitioner (NP), or Physician's Assistant (PA) for guidance in this area of nutrition with no formal schooling may not be in the best interest of healthcare prevention. Seeking out an alternative health care provider who has training in nutrition may be better suited for a prevention style of life. Many Doctors of Chiropractic, Naturopathic Doctors, Nutritionist, Herbalists, Homeopathy, and a Midwife, may be better suited for a preventive lifestyle.

Please don't misunderstand the above paragraph. There are many fine MDs, DOs and other allopathic practitioners that have alternative-based practices, but this is not the general rule, only the exception. Many allopathic doctors are shunned by their professional peers for having views contrary to training and utilize alternative thoughts of mind.

The information presented in this book is only "suggestions," as each person has the right of choices in the health and welfare of their family. It is suggested that many books should be read on Self-Applied Prevention so each family can make educated decisions for those who wish to participate in their family's health.

The methods and products have not been tested or approved by the Federal Food and Drug Administration, and in no way is this book meant to replace any professional care. All those who freely desire to read and apply this information can do so. However, the author will assume no responsibility. Please exercise your God-given rights and seek education and opinions of those who have experience. This book may not be reproduced without permission from the author.

Introduction

American families are constantly flooded with misleading information about the importance of vitamins and minerals. For instance, breakfast cereals claim that they are full of vitamins and minerals, and sports drinks brag about their ability to rev up fading energy with a jolt of vitamins or minerals.

It is a known fact that vitamins and minerals are good for the body, but which ones do our bodies really need? In addition, is it possible to get too much of a good thing?

With all of these products making confusing claims to be "good and healthy," Dr. Olree explains some myths and facts about vitamins and minerals.

Vitamins are substances occurring in small amounts in foods and may or may not be created within the body.

Vitamins work together and they need to be supplied to the body from food. Each vitamin carries out a specific job in relation to minerals.

Vitamins are needed for specific regulatory function and maintenance of life and growth.

Vitamins do not actually make energy but create reactions for the body to use energy.

Dr. Olree explains that vitamins fall into two categories: fat-soluble and water-soluble. The body stores fat-soluble vitamins (vitamins A, D, E, and K) for somewhat longer periods. Water-soluble vitamins, C, and the B-complex vitamins are stored in a range of tissues of the body, so they need to be replenished more often. Any vitamin C or B that your body does not use as it passes through your system is lost (mostly when you urinate). For that reason, you need a fresh supply of these vitamins every day.

Minerals are identified as two groups: macro-minerals and trace minerals. Macro-minerals like calcium, phosphorus, potassium, sulfur, sodium, chlorine, and magnesium are required in large amounts daily for normal body development.

Trace minerals, on the other hand, are required in small amounts for normal body development and growth. These minerals include iron, iodine, zinc, manganese, copper, chromium, selenium, cobalt, molybdenum, and fluorine.

People can get vitamins and minerals from their everyday diet and supplements. To get all the vitamins and minerals each day, as well as the right balance of carbohydrates, proteins, fats, and calories, one should eat a variety of foods. Fresh fruits and vegetables, whole grains, low-fat dairy products, lean meats, fish, and poultry. Whole or unprocessed foods are the best choices for providing the nutrients the body needs to stay healthy and grow properly.

Since nutrients work together in the body as a team, it should be remembered that they should be supplied in the recommended amounts.

Vitamins and minerals are as equally important as carbohydrates, protein, and fats because they also all work together as a team. A person cannot live only on vitamin and mineral supplements for survival. People need food and the other nutrients. With proper planning and selection, foods are good sources of vitamins and minerals.

In conclusion, for good nutrition, eat with variety, balance, and moderation in mind.

The Nervous System

The first priority in obtaining good health is a properly maintained nervous system.

Chiropractors are remarkably unique in the health care field as they are the only health care professionals trained to detect and treat a condition referred to as the "Vertebral Subluxation Complex." Chiropractors have found vertebral subluxations to be responsible for and contribute to a number of spinal and extra-spinal disorders.

What Is The Vertebral Subluxation?

The vertebral subluxation is the term applied to a vertebra which has lost its normal position and/or motion in relation to neighboring vertebrae. Vertebrae that do not function properly within the spinal framework generate mechanical stress. This accelerates the wear and tear on the surrounding spinal muscles, ligaments, discs, joint and other spinal tissues. Pain, palpatory tenderness, inflammation, decreased spinal mobility, and muscle spasm will eventually follow.

Additionally, because of the direct mechanical and physiological relationship between the spinal column and the spinal nerve roots, vertebral subluxation as well as other spinal abnormalities have the potential to impair proper nerve functioning. Once nerve functioning is compromised, communication within the body becomes less effective, jeopardizing the overall health and wellness of the individual.

Through extensive research and study, chiropractors have identified five components of the vertebral subluxation. Collectively, these elements are known as the "subluxation complex."

1. Kinesiopathology – The loss of normal vertebral positioning and motion in relation to neighboring vertebrae above and below.

2. Myopathology – Pathological changes occurring in the spinal musculature, which includes hypertonicity, spasms, fibrosis, weakness, and improper or inappropriate functioning.

3. Neuropathology – Irritation or injury to spinal nerve roots through compression, stretch, or more commonly chemical irritation from nearby spinal structures.

4. Histopathology – Pathological changes that occur to the spinal tissues such as abnormal bony growths, of the vertebral bodies and joints, fibrosis and adhesions of spinal muscles and ligaments as well as dehydration and degeneration of spinal discs.

5. Pathophysiology – The biochemical changes taking place in the spinal region which include inflammatory biochemical's from injured tissues and biochemical waste products.

Each component of a subluxation must be eliminated for proper healing to occur and for the rehabilitation process to be successful. While full understanding of all components is not necessary, you should be aware of the complexity involved. Patients should also be aware that pain is but a small element of most diseases and disorders. Pain is a very poor indicator of your need for further treatment as pain generally subsides well before tissue healing and mechanical normalization has completed.

What causes subluxation?
Vertebral subluxation has a great number of different causes, all of which, the average individual is exposed to daily. These causes can be described in terms of physical, chemical, and emotional causes.

Physical causes include acute trauma to the body, repetitive motions affecting the spine, bad postural habits, improper workstation habits and design, and weak or imbalanced spinal musculature.

Chemical causes include poor dietary and nutritional practices, drug and alcohol use and abuse, and the ingestion of chemical toxins in the foods we eat, air we breathe, and water we drink. Chemicals that are harmful to the body decrease the body's ability to function optimally and reduce the ability to successfully adapt to and withstand internal and external stresses–making us more susceptible to spinal subluxations and the consequences of these subluxations.

Emotional causes associated with stress.

Excessive stress or inadequate stress management skills can deplete the body of the ability to sustain normal functions. Medical research has much documentation on the impact of emotional stress upon physical health and its devastating effects on the immune system, making the body susceptible to injury and disease.

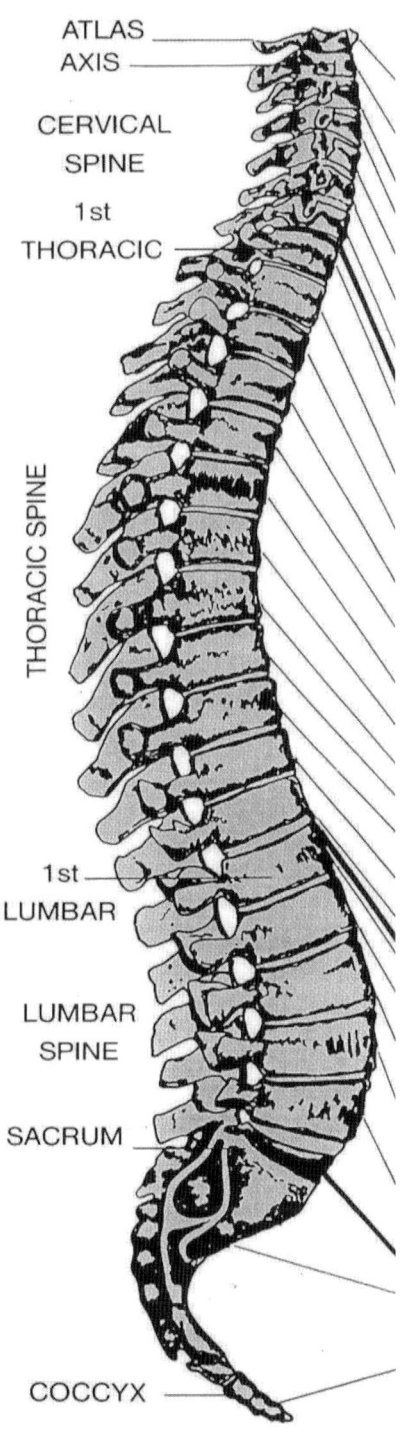

Hillman Health Food Store call 855-Amish-Dr (855-264-7437) www.emineral.info Vitamins and Minerals for Better Living

SYMPTOMS OF SPINAL MISALIGNMENT QUESTIONNAIRE

"The nervous system controls and coordinates all organs and structures of the human body." (*Gray's Anatomy*, 29th Ed., page 4). Misalignments of spinal vertebrae and discs may cause irritation to the nerves which could affect the areas listed. Please help us help you by placing a check mark in the appropriate box under the "Possible Effects" column to indicate your symptoms.

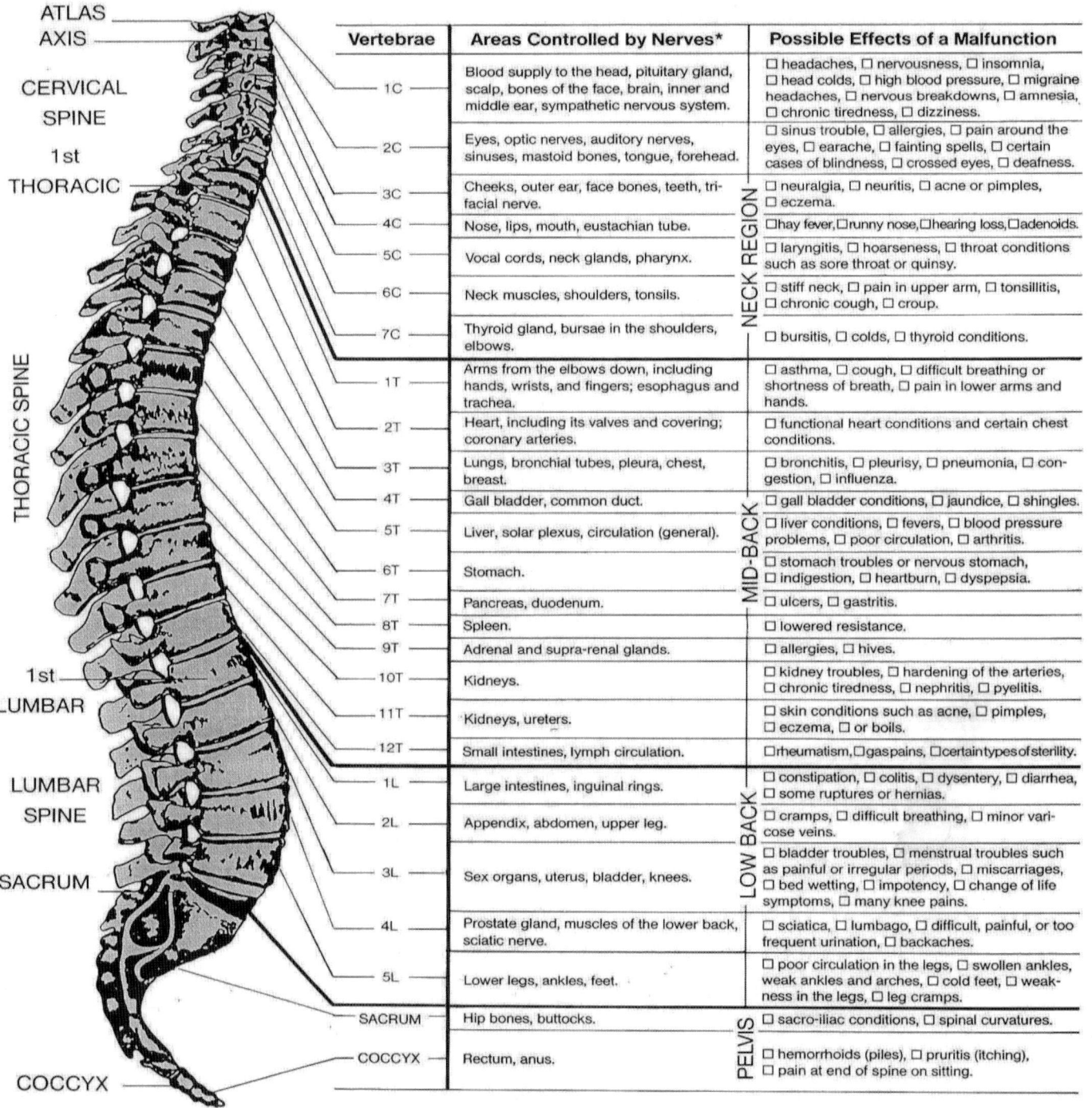

Vertebrae	Areas Controlled by Nerves*	Possible Effects of a Malfunction
1C	Blood supply to the head, pituitary gland, scalp, bones of the face, brain, inner and middle ear, sympathetic nervous system.	☐ headaches, ☐ nervousness, ☐ insomnia, ☐ head colds, ☐ high blood pressure, ☐ migraine headaches, ☐ nervous breakdowns, ☐ amnesia, ☐ chronic tiredness, ☐ dizziness.
2C	Eyes, optic nerves, auditory nerves, sinuses, mastoid bones, tongue, forehead.	☐ sinus trouble, ☐ allergies, ☐ pain around the eyes, ☐ earache, ☐ fainting spells, ☐ certain cases of blindness, ☐ crossed eyes, ☐ deafness.
3C	Cheeks, outer ear, face bones, teeth, tri-facial nerve.	☐ neuralgia, ☐ neuritis, ☐ acne or pimples, ☐ eczema.
4C	Nose, lips, mouth, eustachian tube.	☐ hay fever, ☐ runny nose, ☐ hearing loss, ☐ adenoids.
5C	Vocal cords, neck glands, pharynx.	☐ laryngitis, ☐ hoarseness, ☐ throat conditions such as sore throat or quinsy.
6C	Neck muscles, shoulders, tonsils.	☐ stiff neck, ☐ pain in upper arm, ☐ tonsillitis, ☐ chronic cough, ☐ croup.
7C	Thyroid gland, bursae in the shoulders, elbows.	☐ bursitis, ☐ colds, ☐ thyroid conditions.
1T	Arms from the elbows down, including hands, wrists, and fingers; esophagus and trachea.	☐ asthma, ☐ cough, ☐ difficult breathing or shortness of breath, ☐ pain in lower arms and hands.
2T	Heart, including its valves and covering; coronary arteries.	☐ functional heart conditions and certain chest conditions.
3T	Lungs, bronchial tubes, pleura, chest, breast.	☐ bronchitis, ☐ pleurisy, ☐ pneumonia, ☐ congestion, ☐ influenza.
4T	Gall bladder, common duct.	☐ gall bladder conditions, ☐ jaundice, ☐ shingles.
5T	Liver, solar plexus, circulation (general).	☐ liver conditions, ☐ fevers, ☐ blood pressure problems, ☐ poor circulation, ☐ arthritis.
6T	Stomach.	☐ stomach troubles or nervous stomach, ☐ indigestion, ☐ heartburn, ☐ dyspepsia.
7T	Pancreas, duodenum.	☐ ulcers, ☐ gastritis.
8T	Spleen.	☐ lowered resistance.
9T	Adrenal and supra-renal glands.	☐ allergies, ☐ hives.
10T	Kidneys.	☐ kidney troubles, ☐ hardening of the arteries, ☐ chronic tiredness, ☐ nephritis, ☐ pyelitis.
11T	Kidneys, ureters.	☐ skin conditions such as acne, ☐ pimples, ☐ eczema, ☐ or boils.
12T	Small intestines, lymph circulation.	☐ rheumatism, ☐ gas pains, ☐ certain types of sterility.
1L	Large intestines, inguinal rings.	☐ constipation, ☐ colitis, ☐ dysentery, ☐ diarrhea, ☐ some ruptures or hernias.
2L	Appendix, abdomen, upper leg.	☐ cramps, ☐ difficult breathing, ☐ minor varicose veins.
3L	Sex organs, uterus, bladder, knees.	☐ bladder troubles, ☐ menstrual troubles such as painful or irregular periods, ☐ miscarriages, ☐ bed wetting, ☐ impotency, ☐ change of life symptoms, ☐ many knee pains.
4L	Prostate gland, muscles of the lower back, sciatic nerve.	☐ sciatica, ☐ lumbago, ☐ difficult, painful, or too frequent urination, ☐ backaches.
5L	Lower legs, ankles, feet.	☐ poor circulation in the legs, ☐ swollen ankles, weak ankles and arches, ☐ cold feet, ☐ weakness in the legs, ☐ leg cramps.
SACRUM	Hip bones, buttocks.	☐ sacro-iliac conditions, ☐ spinal curvatures.
COCCYX	Rectum, anus.	☐ hemorrhoids (piles), ☐ pruritis (itching), ☐ pain at end of spine on sitting.

*Directly or indirectly controlled

For further explanation of the conditions shown above, and information about those not shown, ask your Doctor of Chiropractic.

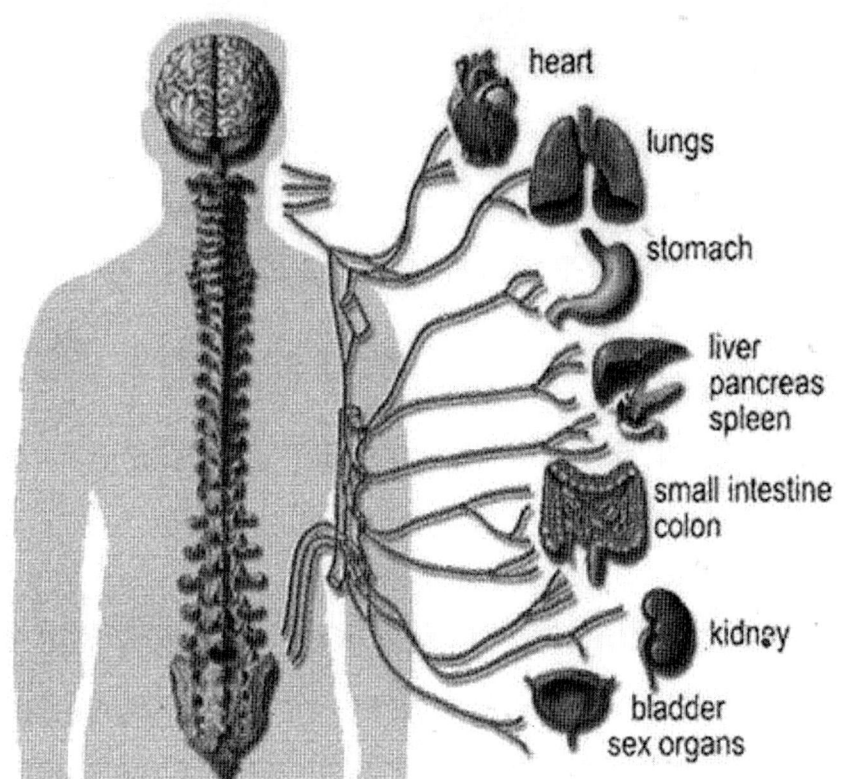

Water - H_2O

Water and Human Health

True health cannot occur without proper hydration of the body. We need to drink half our body weight in ounces of water each day. For instance, if you weigh 200 pounds, you should consume 100 ounces of water. Every organ in the body heavily depends on water to function properly and to its capacity. We are mostly water. The human body is 69% water. The brain is 85% water, bones 35% water, blood 83% water, and the liver 90% water.

A mere 2% drop in our body's water supply can trigger signs of dehydration: fuzzy short-term memory, trouble with basic mental calculations, and difficulty focusing on smaller print, such as this page. Are you having trouble reading this? Drink up! Mild dehydration is also one of the most common causes of daytime tiredness. Just a 5% drop in body fluids will cause a 25% to 30% loss of energy. An 11%+ drop in body fluids will cause death.

What does water have to do with human health? Water is a basic human need. We need water to survive, and we can live for only a few days without it. When we get sick with flu-like symptoms, we usually blame the food we ate as being the cause of our illness. In urban areas of developed countries, many people would never think to consider that they may have become ill from the water that they drank. But many people in developing countries and people living in rural areas of developed countries do not take safe drinking water for granted. They understand the relationship that exists between safe drinking water and good health, because they have experienced waterborne disease firsthand. That is not to say that urban centers have not experienced waterborne illnesses. In Milwaukee, Wisconsin, for instance, in 1993, an outbreak of cryptosporidium killed 110 people and made around 403,000 people ill. Another instance, in Walkerton, Ontario, in 2000, seven people died and around 2,300 people became ill when E. coli contaminated the local water supply. Yet another instance, in North Battleford, Saskatchewan, in 2001, approximately 8,000 people became ill when cryptosporidium contaminated a local water supply.

Drinking refreshing, clean water plays a major role in reducing the risk of certain diseases. Drinking eight glasses of water daily can decrease the risk of colon cancer by 45%, bladder cancer by 50%, and it can potentially even reduce the risk of breast cancer. Adequate water intake will help prevent headaches, constipation, and kidney damage. And those are just a few examples!

Water suppresses the appetite and helps the body metabolize stored fat. Studies have shown that a decrease in water intake causes fat deposits to increase; therefore, increasing water input reduces fat. Why? The answer is because the kidneys need water to function properly. Without sufficient water for the kidneys, the kidneys cannot work adequately and so this affects some of the water going to the liver. One of the primary functions of the liver is to metabolize fat into energy for the body. If the liver needs to do some of the work of the kidneys, the liver cannot work as it should to metabolize fat and so more fat is stored in the body, increasing weight and not using the fat as energy.

If you are not drinking enough water, your body will store as much water as possible as a defense mechanism. Retained water adds to your weight. If you have a water retention problem, drink more water! It may sound crazy, but once the body is trained to expect a regular supply, it will store less, leading to a reduction in your weight.

On a global scale, 1.1 billion people do not have access to safe drinking water and 2.6 billion people do not have access to adequate sanitation. Eighty percent of all illnesses in developing countries are attributed to unsafe drinking water and the spread of waterborne diseases. There are 2.2 million deaths each year that result from unsafe drinking water, 90 percent of whom are children under five years of age.

Water is of major importance to all living things; in some organisms, up to 90% of their body weight comes from water. Up to 60% of the human body is water, the brain is composed of 70% water, and the lungs are nearly 90% water. Lean muscle tissue contains about 75% water by weight, as does the brain; body fat contains 10% water; and bone has 22% water. About 83% of our blood is water, which helps digest our food, transport waste, and control body temperature. Each day humans must replace 2.4 litres of water, some through drinking and the rest taken by the body from the foods eaten.

Fourteen gallons of water! That's how much water we walk around with in body mass. Imagine carrying 120 pounds of water–that's three nearly-full 5-gallon water jugs—around with you all day long, every day of the year. You can do this math for yourself. An average adult's body is 60-70% water; for children it's closer to 75% but it can get as low as 45% if you're overweight. Take your body weight and multiply it by the appropriate percentage of water and you'll see how many pounds of water you're packing. If you want to convert those pounds of water into gallons, just divide by 8.4. Add another 24 pounds of skin and what you've basically got is hundreds of thousands of years of human evolution producing an ambulatory water balloon wrapped in flesh.

During a normal day, we breathe, urinate, and sweat out about three quarts of water, amounting to 5-10% of our body's water. Note that if you're running the 150-mile Marathon Des Sables across the Saharan Desert in Morocco, you're likely leaking more than 12 quarts a day. If you're not continuously replenishing your body's water, you can run into trouble in a hurry.

With a water deficit of as little as one quart you're likely going to start losing some cognitive function, alertness, and ability to concentrate. If you lose a gallon, you'll start feeling pretty lethargic, and you'll likely have a bad headache. If you're down two gallons, you're going to be sick enough to be in the hospital. Three gallons, and you're in the ground.

Yet our water needs are so much greater than simply keeping our bodies hydrated, and therein lies the great water challenge of the 21st century. We use water to grow our food, generate our electricity, and manufacture our clothes. If you visit National Geographic's Water Footprint Calculator, you'll see that it takes about 2,000 gallons of water per person each day to support an American lifestyle. That places a lot of strain on the freshwater systems of our planet.

"THE RIVERS FLOW NOT PAST, BUT THROUGH US"

Water is a chemical substance with the chemical formula H_2O. A water molecule contains one oxygen and two hydrogen atoms. Water is a liquid at ambient conditions, but it often co-exists on earth with its solid state (ice) and gaseous state (water vapor or steam).

Water covers 70.9% of the Earth's surface, and is vital for all known forms of life. On Earth, 96.5% of the planet's water is found in oceans, 1.7% in groundwater, 1.7% in glaciers and the ice caps of Antarctica and Greenland, a small fraction in other large water bodies, and 0.001% in the air as vapor, clouds (formed of solid and liquid water particles suspended in air), and precipitation. Only 2.5% of the Earth's water is freshwater, and 98.8% of that water is in ice and groundwater. Less than 0.3% of all freshwater is in rivers, lakes, and the atmosphere, and an even smaller amount of the Earth's fresh water (0.003%) is contained within biological bodies and manufactured products.

Safe drinking water is essential to humans and all other life forms. Access to safe drinking water has improved over the last decades in almost every part of the world. Approximately 70% of the fresh water used by humans goes to agriculture.

Water is a good solvent and is often referred to as the universal solvent. Water can dissolve many different substances, giving it varying tastes and odors. Humans and other animals have developed senses that enable them to evafluate the potability of water by avoiding water that is too salty or putrid. The taste of spring water and mineral water, often advertised in marketing of consumer products, derives from the minerals dissolved in it. However, pure H₂O is tasteless and odorless. The advertised purity of spring and mineral water refers to absence of toxins, pollutants and microbes, not the absence of naturally occurring minerals.

HARD WATER

Hard water has high mineral content of calcium and magnesium. Hard water is generally not harmful to one's health, but can pose serious problems; hard water is often indicated by a lack of suds formation when soap is agitated in water. Wherever water hardness is a concern, water softening is commonly used to reduce hard water's adverse effects.

SOFT WATER

Soft water softening is the reduction of the concentration of calcium, magnesium, and certain other metal cations in hard water. Water softening methods mainly rely on the removal of Ca^{2+} and Mg^{2+} from a solution or the sequestration of these ions, i.e. binding them to a molecule that removes their ability to form scale or interfere with soaps. Removal is achieved by ion exchange and by precipitation methods. Sequestration entails the addition of chemical compounds called sequestration (or chelating) agents.

BOTTLED WATER

Bottled water drinking water (e.g., city water, well water, distilled water, or spring water) packaged in plastic or glass water bottles.

Pitfalls of plastic bottled water:

Anitmony – a heavy metal released from the plastic (age related)

Bisphenol-A – A female mimicking hormone that causes early development of reproductive organs in young girls

Entrance of whatever is in the city water that the bottled water maker's filters do not remove

A compound found in polycarbonate plastics. Used in manufacture of compact disks, plastic bottles, lining of metal food cans, and dental sealants

Bisphenol-A has estrogenic influences-binds to ER+ breast cancer cells

Bisphenol-A causes a decreased sperm count, increases prostate size

GROUND WATER

Not all ground water is created equal. There are many wells that are naturally toxic due to mineral deposits that are in the water aquifer. The worst case scenario is in the Ganges Delta of Bangladesh, India, where the World Health Organization provided 3 million people with the necessary equipment to pump their own water from the ground. The problem was, no one tested the water and the entire county's population was provided with arsenic. Chronic exposure to arsenic has been linked to serious medical conditions, including hypertension, cardiovascular disease, and a variety of cancers thoughout this entire part of the country.

Where you live will determine what minerals will be present in your ground water. One person with a tissue mineral analysis (hair) was found to have high levels of uranium in the sample tested. His wife was then tested and she also had high levels of uranium. They had inherited the farm from grandparents who both died from leukemia.

A new and present danger to the ground water is from widespread usage of glyphosate (Roundup®). In a paper dated June of 2011 entitled *"Roundup® and birth defects Is the public being kept in the dark?"* by Michael Antoniou, Mohamed Ezz El-Din Mostafa Habib, C. Vyvyan Howard, Richard C. Jennings, Carlo

Leifert, Rubens Onofre Nodari, Claire Robinson, and John Fagan. Men and women with impeccable standings in the scientific communities have taken to task to bring some of the problems with with the usage of glyphosate as it appears to have a half-life of over twenty-two years. If one pound is applied to the ground today, twenty-two years from now there will be one-half pound in the soil, if the glyphosate does not leach into the drinking water.

One needs to have their drinking water analyzed to be sure of what they are consuming. If the water needs to be filtered, it needs to be filtered! There are many water filtration systems on the market and the ones that remove the worst stuff from your water are the reverse osmosis systems. The City of Tampa, Florida, has one of the biggest reverse osmosis systems in the world. They take ocean water and process it though reverse osmosis to obtain pure water without any of the minerals from the ocean present in the water.

The Human Immune System

Changes in the normal mixture of micro flora–bacteria and fungi in the gastrointestinal tract–can intensify the immune system's reaction to common allergens, like pollen or animal dander. Research indicates that micro flora lining the walls of the gastrointestinal tract are a major underlying factor responsible for the immune system's ability to function.

Eighty percent (80%) of the human immune system is the one hundred trillion (100,000,000,000) bacteria that occupy your intestines. There is another ten trillion (10,000,000,000) bacteria that live on your skin. This equates to ten bacteria for every one human cell. What you feed your bacteria will determine what your immunity will be. Changes in gut micro flora caused by widespread use of antibiotics and a modern high-fat, high-sugar, low-fiber diet is responsible for a major increase in all diseases.

Autism was diagnosed in 1996 to be one in ten thousand (1 in 10,000), and today the numbers are a staggering one in 85. Celiac disease was diagnosed in 1996 to be one in ten thousand (1 in 10,000), and today the numbers are a staggering one in 135 persons. The recent increase in allergies and asthma has been attributed to what's called the "hygiene hypothesis," the idea that children in western countries are not exposed to enough infections early in life to prevent the immune system from reacting to harmless stimulus.

In 1996, genetically modified foods (GMO) were released for human consumption. Man has taken God's code instilled in every living plant and creature and started mixing them up, creating new living plants which works the GMO up the food chain including humans. Herbicides have been developed to kill the soil bacteria so plants cannot absorb minerals thus starving the plants to death. Crop plants have been genetically modified to live without trace minerals creating an "empty harvest."

Changes in the human intestine that alter the bacteria have profound effects on human health. Changes in soil will eventually have an impact on human health.

Dr. Mark Holbreich, an allergist in Indianapolis, has been treating Amish communities in Indiana for two decades, but he noticed that very few Amish actually had any allergies. As studies on the farm effect in Europe began to emerge several years ago, Holbreich wondered if the same phenomenon might be found in the United States.

He teamed up with European colleagues to compare Swiss farming children and non-farming children to Amish children in Indiana. Amish families, who can trace their roots to Switzerland, typically use farming methods from the 1800s, and they do not own cars or televisions. The researchers surveyed 157 Amish families, about 3,000 Swiss farming families, and close to 11,000 Swiss families who did not live on a farm–all with children between the ages of six and 12.

They found that just five percent of Amish children had been diagnosed with asthma, compared to 6.8 percent of Swiss farm kids and 11.2 percent of the other Swiss children. Similarly, among 138 Amish children given a skin-prick test to determine whether they were predisposed to having allergies, only 10 children–or seven percent–had a positive response.

In comparison, 25 percent of the farm-raised Swiss children and 44 percent of the other Swiss children had a positive test. The researchers reported these findings in the *Journal of Allergy and Clinical Immunology*. The study did not determine why the children who grew up on farms were less likely to develop asthma and allergies, but other research has pointed to exposure to microbes and contact with cows, in particular, to partially explain the farm effect.

Drinking raw cow's milk also seems to be involved, Holbreich said. The going theory is this early exposure to the diverse potential allergens and pathogens on a farm trains the immune system to recognize them, but not overreact to the harmless ones. As for why the Amish children have even lower allergy and asthma rates than the other farming children, "that piece of the puzzle we really haven't explained," Holbreich explains. He speculated that it could be at least partly a result of the Amish having larger families or spending even more time outside or in barns than people on more modern working farms.

Feeding your gut bacteria is the utmost reason for eating food. What you eat will have a direct effect on your health. You are what you eat. Let food be your medicine.

PROBIOTICS

What are probiotics?

Also known as "good" bacteria or intestinal flora, probiotics refers to a group of bacteria found in the intestines that play an important role in digestion and 80% of human immunity.

What to look for in a probiotic:

- Probiotic Strains
- Probiotic Descriptions
- Combinations

One hundred trillion microorganisms (bacteria) live inside and on us; most are good, some are harmful. Beneficial ones are known as "probiotic microorganisms." They improve the environment of the intestinal tract. The use of good probiotics is important in healing many chronic gastrointestinal (GI) problems that are so often associated in those with Autism Spectrum Disorders (ASD). Some experts feel that ASD children need several times the amount of probiotics than those without GI problems, due to the frequency of dysbiosis (overgrowth of yeast, bacteria, etc.) and "Leaky Gut" (intestinal permeability problems).

Scientific studies over the last 50 years show that probiotic organisms can improve the nutritional quality of foods, produce antibiotics, anticarcinogens, and substances that break down and recycle toxins for their human host.

The major benefits of adding probiotic organisms to the diet: boosts immune system, inhibits disease-causing organisms, improved digestion, vitamin synthesis, detoxification and protection from toxins, prevents diarrhea from various causes, reduces risk of irritable bowel syndromes, cancer-protective effects, increases nutrient absorption, improves resistance to allergies, reduces yeast and other infections.

Lactobacillus acidophilus bacteria reside mostly in the small intestine, and bifidobacterium bifidum in the large intestine (colon). Whether taking a mixed-species product or a single species is better has not been determined. There are mixed opinions on the subject. Some people choose a single strain of friendly flora because of the proven effectiveness of that particular probiotic strain. Taking this strain for its specific properties can be very helpful. However, over extended time, you may want to include a variety of strains.

Capsules are the preferred way to take probiotics because there is more protection from contamination, oxygen, and moisture, and capsules maintain organism integrity. Dairy products that contain added organisms like lactobacillus provide a mild dose of probiotics, if you can consume dairy.

Generally, higher more therapeutic doses of probiotics are needed when first addressing GI symptoms. Probiotic strength is measured in CFUs (colony forming units) per capsule. You may want to take one or several daily. For therapeutic benefits, references vary widely from 250 million to 20 billion viable organisms per day. It is best to check with your doctor, or you can start slowly and build-up to a level you feel is most beneficial.

Talk to others about quality issues, and what works best. Choose a probiotic that has been extensively researched with a great deal of scientific support behind it. Do not buy any product unless it has the manufacture date right on the bottle. Probiotic products, especially lactobacillus and bifidobacterium, lose a lot of potency after 4-10 months. Products last longer when they are refrigerated, although some products do not require refrigeration.

When to take probiotics varies by brand. Always check the label and follow the recommendation of the manufacturer. Some say to take on an empty stomach; some say with food so the food can buffer the organisms; some say in the morning because of stomach acid content; some can be taken anytime. The acid and salts in the gut will harm certain probiotics. Manufacturers consider this when designing a formulation and preparing the capsules. Some capsules are specially coated so the microorganisms will safely reach their destination. Others need to be taken at certain times for optimum performance for that product. Probiotics are not adversely affected by the use of enzymes. They can both be taken during at mealtime.

Fructooligosaccharides and Inulin (FOS) are non-digestible oligosaccharides that help promote the growth and activity of friendly bacteria in the intestinal tract. These oligosaccharides are non-caloric compounds that cannot be broken down by our digestive enzymes and therefore do not adversely affect blood sugar levels. Research has shown that both FOS and inulin enhance the growth of lactic bacteria, especially bifidobacteria, and inhibit the growth of a variety of undesirable organisms. Some people have allergic reactions to FOS in the form of a loose stool. Using probiotics simultaneously with antibiotics may be ineffective as the antibiotic will kill off much of the probiotic. If taking probiotics with antibiotics, it is recommended that the two be taken as far apart as possible to lessen the killing effect the antibiotic has on the probiotic.

PROBIOTIC STRAINS

This is a list of most common strains of probiotics used.

Lactobacillus Acidophilus	Bifidobacterium Bifidum
Lactobacillus Brevis	Bifidobacterium Breve
Lactobacillus Bulgaricus	Bifidobacterium Infantis
Lactobacillus Casei subspecies Casei	Bifidobacterium Licheniformis
Lactobacillus Casei, subspecies Paracasei	Bifidobacterium Longum
Lactobacillus Casei, subspecies Rhamnosus	Bacillus Subtilis
Lactobacillus Fermentum	Bifidobacterium Subtilus
Lactobacillus Rhamnosus	Enterococcus Faecium
Lactobacillus Caucasicus	Fructooligosaccharides
Lactobacillus Helveticus	Streptococcus Cremoris
Lactobacillus Lactis	Streptococcus Faecium
Lactobacillus Plantarum	Streptococcus Infantis
Lactobacillus Reuteri	Streptococcus Thermophilus

PROBIOTIC DESCRIPTIONS

BACILLUS SUBTILIS - (B. SUBTILIS)
B. subtilis is needed for the synthesis of vitamin B_2.

BIFIDOBACTERIUM BIFIDUM - (B. BIFIDUM)
B. bifidum is a prominent probiotic microorganism that takes up residence primarily in the mucous membrane lining of the large intestines and the vaginal tract. B. bifidum prevents the colonization of invading pathogenic bacteria by attaching to the intestinal wall, crowding out, and taking nutrients from these unfriendly bacteria and yeast. B. bifidum produces lactic and acetic acids, which lower the intestinal pH and further inhibit the undesirable bacteria from growing. Research on bifidobacteria has established that these organisms enhance the assimilation of minerals such as iron, calcium, magnesium, and zinc.

BIFIDOBACTERIUM INFANTIS - (B. INFANTIS)
Bifidobacterium infantis is an important organism shown to stimulate production of immunomodulating agents such as cytokines. Bacteriocidal activity is also observed against such pathogens as clostridia, salmonella, and shigella.

BIFIDOBACTERIUM LONGUM - (B. LONGUM)
Bifidobacterium longum is a very abundant organism found in the large intestine. It plays a role in preventing the colonization of invading pathogenic bacteria by attaching to the intestinal wall and crowding out unfriendly bacteria and yeast. Along with other microorganisms, it produces lactic and acetic

acids that lower the intestinal pH and further inhibit the undesirable bacteria. B. longum has, in clinical studies, been found to reduce the frequency of gastrointestinal disorders (diarrhea, nausea, etc.) during antibiotic use.

ENTEROCOCCUS FAECIUM - (E. FAECIUM)
E. faecium has been shown to be important in the nutritional support of diarrheal diseases, especially in cases where pathogenic microbes, such as rotavirus, invade the bowel. This particular organism only transiently colonizes the GI tract. A recent study indicated that an E. faecium-containing yogurt was able to significantly lower LDL cholesterol. E. faecium is safe and has been researched extensively by the World Health Organization.

E. Faecium

This probiotic has become so popular with health professionals over the years because of the proven therapeutic value of E. faecium. This species shows strong activity against a variety of pathogenic organisms. In several studies, it has proven resistant to a wide variety of antibiotics and, in one study, proved more effective than L. acidophilus in shortening the duration of diarrheal episodes. E. faecium is a natural resident of the human intestinal tract.

LACTOBACILLUS ACIDOPHILUS - (L. ACIDOPHILUS)
L. acidophilus is one of the most important microorganisms found in the small intestines. It is known to implant itself on the intestinal wall, and in the lining of the wall of the vagina, cervix, and urethra. It performs many critical functions including inhibiting pathogenic organisms and preventing them from multiplying and colonizing. It is well documented that L. acidophilus produces natural antibiotics like lactocidin, acidophilin, etc., which enhances resistance or immunity. L. acidophilus has known antimicrobial activity against staphylococcus aureus, salmonella, E.coli, and candida albicans.

LACTOBACILLUS BREVIS - (L. BREVIS)
Lactobacillus brevis is a lactic acid producing organism important in the synthesis of vitamins D and K.

LACTOBACILLUS BULGARICUS - (L. BULGARICUS)
Lactobacillus bulgaricus is considered a transient microorganism that does not implant in the intestinal tract, but still provides an important protective role. This organism is used extensively in the commercial fermentation of yogurt. Production of lactic acid by the bacterium provides a favorable environment for the growth of other lactobacilli and bifidobacteria residing in the intestine. Studies indicate that certain strains of L. bulgaricus stimulate production of interferon and tumor necrosis factor, thus establishing a potential role in modulating the immune system.

LACTOBACILLUS CASEI - (L. CASEI)
Lactobacillus casei is closely related to the L. rhamnosus and L. acidophilus strains with some of the same immuno-modulating effects as other Lactobacilli. L. casei has several health-promoting effects provided through the production of bacteriocins, compounds that inhibit the growth of pathogenic bacteria in the small intestine.

LACTOBACILLUS PLANTARUM - (L. PLANTARUM)
Lactobacillus plantarum secretes the naturally occurring antibiotic lactolin, and is known to have the ability to synthesize the amino acid Lysine, which has beneficial anti-viral activities. L. plantarum also produces glycolytic enzymes shown to degrade cyanogenic glycosides and is effective in eliminating nitrate while producing nitric oxide. This probiotic can preserve key nutrients, vitamins, and antioxidants, eliminate toxic components from food, and eradicate pathogens such as S. Aureus from fermented food. L.

plantarum-fermented oat given to healthy volunteers significantly reduced a number of potential pathogens in the gut intestines.

Lactobacillus Rhamnosus - (L. Rhamnosus)

Lactobacillus rhamnosus is primarily found in the small bowel and vaginal tract and is beneficial in inhibiting those bacteria involved in vaginal and urinary tract infections. L. rhamnosus is very prolific in growth, has a high tolerance (resistance) to bile salts, adheres to the intestinal mucosa, and protects the intestinal tract against the invasion of harmful microorganisms. Additionally, this organism favorably affects lactose intolerance. A recent double-blinded, placebo-controlled study suggests that these probiotic bacteria may down-regulate hypersensitivity reactions and intestinal inflammation in patients with atopic eczema and food allergies. L. rhamnosus has been found to have significant benefits in the nutrition and well-being of infants and in the elderly. According to research with this strain, administration of L. rhamnosus is most helpful in inhibiting early intestinal infections in infants. This species of Lactobacillus does not only colonize, acidify and protect the small intestine, but it can quickly establish itself in the large intestine, inhibit the growth of streptococci and clostridia, create anaerobic conditions which favor the implantation of bifidobacteria, and produce biologically desirable lactic acid.

Lactobacillus Salivarius - (L. Salivarius)

Lactobacillus salivarius is important in normalizing the gut flora of those dealing with chronic bowel conditions and shows potential as an effective inhibitor of H. pylori, an organism associated with the occurrence of ulcers.

Streptococcus Thermophilus - (S. Thermophilus)

S. thermophilus, in combination with L. bulgaricus, is used commercially to produce yogurt. This organism is known to be efficient in breaking down lactose by producing the enzyme lactase. Those who are lactose-intolerant may be greatly helped by supplementation with this particular strain. Cytokine production is stimulated in tissue-cultured cells by this bacterium.

Benefits of Bacterial Combinations

L. Acidophilus, L. Rhamnosus

Many researchers now believe the myriad health benefits of L. acidophilus are also attributable to L. rhamnosus. These two species are perhaps the most important lactobacilli in the small intestine.

L. Rhamnosous, L. Acidophilus, B. Lactis, Streptococcus Thermophilus, L. Bulgaricus

These are five extensively researched strains of friendly bacteria. These strains maintain viability in acidic environments such as the one that may be found in the stomach, and are tolerant to compounds found in the intestine such as bile. Clinical research has documented the usefulness of these probiotic strains as an adjunct to the management of gastrointestinal disorders, including:

- Antibiotic-associated decrease in friendly bacteria
- Prevention of Clostridial colonization
- Traveler's diarrhea
- Diarrhea associated with rotaviral gastroenteritis
- Acute non-specific diarrhea
- Constipation
- Enhancement of immune response to rotaviral infection and Adjuvant to rotavirus vaccine
- Alleviation of intestinal inflammation and permeability
- Amelioration of food allergies, especially lactose intolerance
- Enhancement of the intestine's immunological barrier function
- Intestinal production of short-chain fatty acids

L. CASEI, L. RHAMNOSUS, L. ACIDOPHILUS, B. LONGUM

Important studies have demonstrated the immune-enhancing properties of lactic acid bacteria. L. casei has been named in a significant number of these studies. L. rhamnosus, until recently, was included under the heading of L. casei and likely possesses similar immune-potentiating characteristics as L. casei. A strain of L. rhamnosus was also recently shown to mitigate the effects of food allergy on infants with atopic dermatitis–a reduction in intestinal inflammation was considered a key factor in bringing about the improvements observed. Numerous studies have shown probiotic organisms to be effective in:

Reducing lactose intolerance
Relieving constipation
Preventing gastrointestinal infections

Enhancing immune activity
Reducing cholesterol

CULTURELLE LACTOBACILLUS GG: LACTOBACILLUS GG.

Culturelle is the only probiotic supplement containing lactobacillus GG. In 1985, Drs. Sherwood Gorbach and Barry Golden isolated a new strain of lactobacillus that appears to be ideal for use in humans. The strain, named lactobacillus GG (after the surnames of its inventors), is resistant to stomach acid and bile, allowing it to survive its passage through the digestive tract and reach the large intestine intact. Once there it shows an exceptional ability to adhere to the intestinal mucosa and proliferate.

VITAMINS

In 1913 thiamin was discovered as the first vitamin, the "vital amine" necessary to prevent the deficiency disease beriberi. Listed below are all of the currently known vitamins to date. "Amine" means nitrogen, as most all vitamins contains nitrogen. Nitrogen is 76% of the air we breathe and is needed for plants to grow.

Vitamin A - Retinol, Retinal, Retinoic acid

Vitamin A is a chemical that is needed for the bodies to develop and to maintain human life. It was discovered in 1913 by Elmer V. McCollum and was the first fat-soluble vitamin to be recognized. This came about because of its ability to prevent night blindness and the drying and hardening of the arteries. There are three forms of vitamin A:

Retinal   Retinoic acid   Retinol (stored in liver)

Why do we need vitamin A?

Vitamin A is a family of fat-soluble compounds that play an important role in vision, bone growth, reproduction, cell division, and cell differentiation (in which a cell becomes part of the brain, muscle, lungs, etc.). Vitamin A helps regulate the immune system, which helps prevent or fight off infections by making white blood cells that destroy harmful bacteria and viruses. Vitamin A also may help lymphocytes, a type of white blood cell, fight infections more effectively.

Vitamin A promotes healthy surface linings of the eyes and the respiratory, urinary, and intestinal tracts. When those linings break down, it becomes easier for bacteria to enter the body and cause infection. Vitamin A also helps maintain the integrity of skin and mucous membranes, which also function as a barrier to bacteria and viruses.

Retinol is one of the most active, or usable, forms of vitamin A and is found in animal foods such as liver and whole milk and in some fortified food products. Retinol is also called preformed vitamin A. It can be converted to retinal and retinoic acid, other active forms of the vitamin A family.

Provitamin A carotenoids are darkly-colored pigments found in plant foods that can be converted to vitamin A. In the United States, approximately 26% and 34% of vitamin A consumed by men and women, respectively, is provided by provitamin A carotenoids. Common carotenoids found in foods are beta-carotene, alpha-carotene, lutein, zeaxanthin, lycopene, and cryptoxanthin. Of the 563 identified carotenoids, fewer than 10% are precursors for vitamin A. Among these, beta-carotene is most efficiently converted to retinol. Alpha-carotene and beta-cryptoxanthin are also converted to vitamin A, but only half as efficiently as beta-carotene. Lycopene, lutein, and zeaxanthin are carotenoids that do not have vitamin A activity but have other health-promoting properties. The Institute of Medicine encourages consumption of carotenoid-rich fruits and vegetables for their health-promoting benefits.

Some carotenoids, in addition to serving as sources of vitamin A, have been shown to function as antioxidants in laboratory tests. However, this role has not been consistently demonstrated in humans. Antioxidants protect cells from free radicals, which are potentially-damaging by-products of oxygen metabolism that may contribute to the development of some chronic diseases.

What are good food sources of vitamin A?

Apricot	Cream	Peas
Asparagus	Eggs	Pumpkin
Broccoli	Kale	Spinach
Broccoli leaves	Leafy vegetables	Sweet potatoes
Butter (not margarine)	Liver	Winter squash
Cantaloupe	Mango	Yellow squash
Carrots	Melon	
Collard greens	Papaya	

What can happen if we do not get enough vitamin A? People experience night blindness, dry hair and skin, frequent colds, respiratory infections, and skin disorders (such as acne). Cancer and weight loss have also been attributed to vitamin A shortages. Children are most at risk of having a vitamin A shortage because they have not yet developed the ability to store vitamin A.

Vitamin B_1 - Thiamine

Vitamin B_1 is also known as Thiamine.

Vitamin B_1, the first B vitamin, was discovered in 1926 and was named thiamine. In 1936, its complete chemical formula was understood. It was recognized to cure Beriberi, the classic Thiamine Deficiency Syndrome. This syndrome occurs worldwide including the U.S. and most often affects severely underfed infants and weak elderly people. Constant dieting to attempt weight loss, alcoholism, and diets primarily based on processed, refined carbohydrate foods are causes of vitamin B_1 deficiency. One U.S. Department of Agriculture study showed that 45% of the U.S. population does not get enough B_1. Vitamin B_1 is a water-soluble vitamin and it is not stored in body fat. Since it is not stored in the body fat, after the body uses what it needs, any excess vitamin B_1 leaves the body in urine.

Why do we need it? Like most of the B vitamins, vitamin B_1 plays many roles in the human body. It is most important task is to help cells change sugar into the fuel the body runs on. Its also involved in metabolic activities relating to the heart, brain, and muscles, and it helps ensure correct nerve cell function.

How much vitamin B_1 should I take?

According to the National Academy of Science, the recommended daily allowance for vitamin B_1 is as follows:

Adult men: 1.5 milligrams/day
Adult women: 1.1 milligrams/day
Children aged 7-10: 1 milligram/day

Infants: 0.4 milligrams/day
Pregnant/lactating women: 1.6 milligrams/day

What are some good sources of vitamin B_1?

Vitamin B_1 is found in almost all foods, but the best sources are pork and other lean meats. Other good sources include:

- Beans
- Cauliflower
- Cereals
- Corn
- Nuts
- Oatmeal
- Sunflower seeds

What can happen if we do not get enough vitamin B_1? Deficiency can result in edema and abnormal heart rhythm. Having a severe B_1 shortage is rare in the U.S., but can occur in very underfed people, alcoholics, or people on long-term dialysis. Symptoms may include paralysis, loss of balance, loss of feeling in the legs and feet, visual problems, and congestive heart failure.

What can happen if I take too much vitamin B_1? To date, no toxic effects have been reported for vitamin B_1. Because it is water-soluble and is not stored in the body, the chances of excess B_1 building up to toxic levels are highly unlikely. Most people taking multivitamins with high levels of B_1 or eating foods rich in amounts of B_1 do not need to worry about toxicity.

Vitamin B₂ - Riboflavin

Vitamin B_2 is also known as riboflavin.

In 1923, Paul Gyorgi of Heidelberg was investigating egg white injury in rats. Mr. Gyorgi decided to test the effect of vitamin B_2 deficiency in a rat and then enlisted the service of Wagner-Jauregg. In 1933, Kuhn, Gyorgi, and Wagner called it vitamin B_2.

Vitamin B_2 is a water-soluble vitamin. Since it is not stored in body fat, after the body uses what it needs, any excess vitamin B_2 leaves the body in urine or sweat.

Why do we need it? Vitamin B_2 works with the other B vitamins in maintaining body growth and the making of red blood cells. Like vitamin B_1, it helps turn carbohydrates into energy. Some studies have shown that vitamin B_2 may protect against cataracts, migraine headaches, and sickle cell anemia.

How much vitamin B_2 should I take?

According to the National Academy of Sciences, the recommended daily allowance for vitamin B_2 is as follows:

Adult men: 1.7 milligrams/day
Adult women: 1.3 milligrams/day
Children aged 7-10: 1.2 milligrams/day

Infants: 0.5 milligrams/day
Pregnant/lactating women: 1.8 milligrams/day

What are some good sources of vitamin B_2?

Broccoli	Eggs	Lean meats	Spinach
Cheese	Fortified cereals	Milk	Yogurt

Because vitamin B_2 can be destroyed by exposure to light, foods that contain vitamin B_2 should not be stored in glass containers that are exposed to light.

What can happen if we do not get enough vitamin B_2? Deficiencies are quite uncommon with vitamin B_2 found in so many foods of the average diet. However, people who do not get enough vitamin B_2 can suffer from dry or cracked skin, especially around the lips or corners of the mouth. Other symptoms include skin rashes and eye irritation. Severe deficiencies may lead to depression or hysteria.

What can happen if I take too much? Excess consumption of vitamin B_2 may cause a person's urine to become bright yellow, but to date no toxic side effects have been reported. Because it is water-soluble and is not stored in the body, the chances of enough vitamin B_2 building up to toxic levels are highly unlikely. Most people taking multivitamins with high levels of vitamin B_2 or eating foods rich in vitamin B_2 do not need to worry about toxicity.

Vitamin B$_3$ - Niacin

Vitamin B$_3$ is also known as niacin.

An American scientist, Conrad Elvehjem, discovered niacin in 1937. It is a water-soluble vitamin absorbed in the intestines and carried throughout the body in the bloodstream. After the body uses what it needs, any excess vitamin B$_3$ leaves the body in urine.

Why do we need it? Vitamin B$_3$ helps break down blood sugar for energy. It also acts as a vasodilator. This means it widens blood vessels, which helps increase blood flow. Some health experts have prescribed vitamin B$_3$ supplements for helping people lower high cholesterol or triglyceride levels as it plays a major role in protecting against cardiovascular disease.

How much vitamin B$_3$ should I take?

According to the National Academy of Sciences, the recommended daily allowance for vitamin B$_3$ is as follows:

Adult men: 19 milligrams/day
Adult women: 15 milligrams/day
Children aged 7-10: 13 milligrams/day

Infants: 6 milligrams/day
Pregnant/lactating women: 19 milligrams/day

Some good food sources of vitamin B$_3$ include:

Avocados
Chicken
Eggs
Fish

Mackerel
Milk
Nuts
Salmon

Salmon
Swordfish
Veal

What can happen if we do not get enough vitamin B$_3$? Vitamin B$_3$ deficiency causes pellagra, a disease characterized by skin eruptions, digestive and nervous disturbances, and mental decline. The condition can usually be reversed by taking vitamin B$_3$.

What can happen if I take too much vitamin B$_3$? Vitamin B$_3$ toxicity can lead to a range of conditions. Even mildly high doses can cause a dilation of the blood vessels and lead to a potentially painful tingling about the face and shoulders called the "niacin flush," as well as headaches, itchiness and stomach problems. Larger doses may cause diarrhea, nausea, ulcers, gout, diabetes and in rare cases, liver damage. Most of these conditions (with the exception of liver damage) can usually be reversed when taking high doses is stopped.

Vitamin B_5 - Pantothenic Acid

Vitamin B_5 is also known as pantothenic acid. Dr. Roger Williams discovered vitamin B_5 in 1933. He named it after the Greek word pantothen, which means "everywhere." He found this name fits because it is present in all cells. Besides being present in a number of food sources, it is also made in the human body by bacteria in the intestines. Since B_5 is not stored in body fat, after the body uses what it needs, any excess vitamin B_5 leaves the body in urine or sweat.

Why do we need it? Vitamin B_5 provides an important role in cellular metabolism and participates in the release of energy from carbohydrates, fats, and proteins. It is also important for the synthesis of cholesterol, steroids, fatty acids, and assists in the function of other vitamins, especially vitamin B_2. Studies have shown vitamin B_5 to reduce blood cholesterol levels in diabetic patients. Other studies have shown it to stimulate adrenal glands and increase the production of cortisone and other adrenal hormones important for healthy skin and nerves. Vitamin B_5 may also play a protective role against hair loss and rheumatoid arthritis.

How much vitamin B_5 should I take?

According to the National Academy of Sciences, the recommended daily allowance for vitamin B_5 is as follows:

Adult men: between 4-7 milligrams/day
Adult women: between 4-7 milligrams/day
Children aged 7-10: between 4-5 milligrams/day

Infants: 3 milligrams/day
Pregnant/breast-feeding women: between 4-7 milligrams/day

Some good food sources of vitamin B_5 include:

Beans	Eggs	White potatoes
Broccoli	Milk	Whole grains
Cabbage	Sweet potatoes	

What can happen if we do not get enough vitamin B_5? Because the body produces vitamin B_5 naturally, shortages are rare. A person lacking vitamin B_5 may experience upset stomach, increased risk of upper respiratory infections, tiredness, irritability, burning sensations in the feet and sleep disorders.

What can happen if I take too much? Being water-soluble, the body usually excretes any excess vitamin B_5 through sweat or urine. However, very high dosages (over 6 grams per day) may cause diarrhea in humans and have been shown to cause liver damage in rats.

Vitamin B_6 - Pyridoxine

Vitamin B_6 is also known as pyridoxine.

In 1934 Paul Gregory discovered vitamin B_6 a water-soluble vitamin absorbed by the intestines and carried throughout the body in the bloodstream. Since it is not stored in body fat, after the body uses what it needs, any excess vitamin B_6 leaves the body in urine or sweat.

Why do we need vitamin B_6? Vitamin B_6 is considered the "master vitamin" in the processing of amino acids. Vitamin B_6 helps build up and break down amino acids and is needed to make hormones: serotonin, melatonin, and dopamine. It also helps in the production of red and white blood cells. Also converts a substance called tryptophan into vitamin B_3, and plays a role in the metabolism of proteins and fats. Large doses of B_6 may reduce the symptoms of premenstrual syndrome, carpal tunnel syndrome, and depression.

How much vitamin B_6 should I take? According to the National Academy of Sciences, the recommended daily allowance for vitamin B_6 is as follows:

Adult men: 2 milligrams/day
Adult women: 1.6 milligrams/day
Children aged 7-10: 1.4 milligrams/day
Infants: 0.6 milligrams/day
Pregnant/lactating women: 2.2 milligrams/day

Some good food sources of vitamin B_6 include:

- Avocados
- Bananas
- Brewers's yeast
- Carrots
- Leafy green vegetables
- Legumes
- Meats
- Oily fish (especially tuna)
- Potatoes (with skins)
- Poultry
- Watermelon

What can happen if we do not get enough vitamin B_6? Vitamin B_6 deficiency is rare. However, alcohol and tobacco have been shown to impair absorption of B_6. Deficiency can cause skin problems, and nervous system disorders including impaired memory and concentration. A lack of vitamin B_6 has also been linked with increased levels of the chemical homocysteine, which in turn has been connected to heart disease, birth defects, Alzheimer's disease, and possibly dementia. A person may be able to reduce their homocysteine levels by increasing the number of fruits and vegetables eaten.

What can happen if I take too much vitamin B_6? Taking very high doses (over 2,000 mg per day) of vitamin B_6 for months or years can cause numbness in the feet and hands, which may be permanent in some cases. Supplementation should be stopped at once if any of these symptoms begin to develop. Vitamin B_6 also reduces the effects of L-dopa, a drug used to treat Parkinson's disease.

Vitamin B$_7$ - Biotin

Vitamin B$_7$ is also known as biotin.

In 1927, biochemist M.A. Boas was the first scientist to discover vitamin B$_7$. Vitamin B$_7$ is obtained from certain foods and formed by bacteria in the intestines. Since vitamin B$_7$ is not stored in body fat, after the body uses what it needs, any excess leaves the body in urine.

Why do we need vitamin B$_7$? Vitamin B$_7$ plays a number of roles in the human body. Like other B vitamins, it is necessary for metabolism of proteins and carbohydrates into energy. This vitamin is also involved in the production of amino acid proteins and fatty acids. It helps in the combining of hormones and cholesterol, and in the growth of healthy skin and hair follicles.

How much vitamin B$_7$ should I take?

Although no recommended daily allowances have been established for vitamin B$_7$, most health experts generally agree on the following amounts:

Adult men: between 30-100 milligrams/day
Adult women: between 30-100 milligrams/day
Children aged 7-10: 30 milligrams/day

Infants: 15 milligrams/day
Pregnant/breast-feeding women: between 30-100 milligrams/day

Some good food sources of vitamin B$_7$ include:

Bananas
Brewer's yeast
Broccoli
Eggs

Lean beef
Milk
Mushrooms
Nuts

Sweet potatoes
Tomatoes
White potatoes
Whole-grain cereals

What can happen if we do not get enough vitamin B$_7$? Vitamin B$_7$ deficiency is almost unheard of; however, shortages can be caused by surgical removal of the stomach, or by being on a bizarre diet. Raw egg whites, for instance, bind vitamin B$_7$ and make it unavailable for absorption. Alcohol and tobacco also decrease vitamin B$_7$ absorption. Vitamin B$_7$ shortage may lead to dermatitis, brittle nails, and hair loss. Having a severe shortage can lead to high blood cholesterol levels and heart problems.

What can happen if I take too much vitamin B$_7$? There is no evidence of toxicity with vitamin B$_7$. Because it is water-soluble and is not stored in the body, the chances of excess buildup to toxic levels are highly unlikely. Most people taking a good B-Complex vitamin with high levels of vitamin B$_7$ or eating foods rich in amounts of vitamin B$_7$ do not need to worry about toxicity.

Vitamin B_8 - Inositol Hexaphosphate

Vitamin B_8 is also known as inositol hexaphosphate.

Vitamin B_8 is one of the basic substances that make up our cells. Vitamin B_8 is an important molecule that plays a role in energy production and metabolism. It is also a precursor to uric acid. Uric acid is a naturally occurring substance that is believed to neutralize some free radicals and may prevent the development of multiple sclerosis. Vitamin B_8 is believed to play a helpful role in many bodily functions, including the release of insulin, protein synthesis, and oxygen metabolism. Studies conducted in Europe suggest that vitamin B_8 may enhance oxygen delivery to the muscles that can result in increased endurance and may be of benefit to athletes. Vitamin B_8 may also work together with other chemicals to remove a buildup of lactic acid in the blood that could possibly improve energy production and exercise performance.

How much vitamin B_8 should I take?

The amount of vitamin B_8 to be taken depends on the condition being treated. Generally, some practitioners will recommend 500-2,000 milligrams of vitamin B_8 in supplement form, taken 30 minutes before exercising. Some studies have used doses ranging up to 6 grams per day, taken for several weeks.

What forms of vitamin B_8 are available?

Brewer's yeast   Various animal organ meats

What can happen if I take too much vitamin B_8? Are there any interactions that I should be aware of taking vitamin B_8? What precautions should I take? Vitamin B_8 appears to be well tolerated in individuals taking relatively large doses (5-6 grams per day) for extended periods (over 26 weeks). While no side effects have been reported with the use of vitamin B_8, unused vitamin B_8 can be changed by the body into uric acid, which may cause problems for people at risk of developing gout. High amounts of uric acid may lead to conditions such as arthritic joints and toes. As of this writing, there are no well-known drug interactions linked with vitamin B_8. As always, make sure to speak with a licensed health care provider before taking vitamin B_8 or any other herbal remedy or dietary supplement.

Vitamin B$_9$ - Folic Acid / Folate

Vitamin B$_9$ is also known as folic acid / folate.

Vitamin B$_9$ was first noticed by Lucy Willis in 1930 and isolated by Henry K. Mitchell in 1941. Vitamin B$_9$ is considered a "brain food." It is especially important in pregnancy because it helps to control embryonic and fetal nerve cell formation, which is important to normal development. Vitamin B$_9$ is also needed for energy production and the formation of red blood cells, and it strengthens immunity by helping in proper formation and functioning of white blood cells.

Some good food sources of vitamin B$_9$ include:

Asparagus	Cheese	Kidney beans
Baked beans	Chicken	Lentils
Barley	Chickpeas	Pasta
Brewer's yeast	Citrus fruits and juices	Rice
Brown rice	Cornmeal	Seafood (salmon, tuna)
Brussel sprouts	Dates	Spinach
Spinach	Flour	Whole grains

What can happen if I do not get enough vitamin B$_9$? A common sign of vitamin B$_9$ shortage is a sore, red tongue. Anemia, tiredness, graying hair, growth impairment, and weakness are also common signs. Many studies have also shown that women who get plenty of vitamin B$_9$ (during their childbearing years, not just while pregnant) can help lessen the risk of birth defects, including spina bifida and anencephaly.

Vitamin B_{10} - Para-aminobenzoic acid

Vitamin B_{10} is also known as para-aminobenzoic acid (PABA).

E. T. Krebs discovered B_{10} vitamin in 1943. It is actually a water-soluble vitamin similar to other B vitamins. Vitamin B_{10} has a protective effect on many parts of the body. It is used as an ingredient in various sunscreens to protect the skin against sunburn, aging, and some types of skin cancer that can be caused by too much exposure to sunlight. Vitamin B_{10} also helps in the production of red blood cells and vitamin B_{10} is used in the metabolism of certain proteins. It is also believed to play a role in the fertility levels of males, although research on this subject has yet to be conducted thoroughly. There is also unreliable evidence that oral supplementation with Vitamin B_{10} can help restore gray hair to a darker color.

How much vitamin B_{10} should I take? Most studies that have examined vitamin B_{10} have used dosages ranging between 300 milligrams to 12 grams per day. Any person taking amounts of vitamin B_{10} larger than 400 milligrams per day should speak to a licensed health care provider.

What foods contain vitamin B_{10}?

Bran	Liver	Wheat germ
Grains	Molasses	Yeast

What can happen if I take too much vitamin B_{10}? Are there any interactions I should be aware of? What precautions should I take?

While no serious side-effects have been noted in patients taking between 300 and 400 milligrams of vitamin B_{10}, larger amounts may cause low blood sugar, skin irritations, and in some instances, liver damage. Vitamin B_{10} may also cause allergic reactions on the skin. Extremely large doses (more than 20 grams per day) may be fatal in small children.

Vitamin B_{10} seems to interfere with the activities of certain antibiotics known as "sulfa drugs." Therefore, it should not be taken when these medications are being used. As always, make sure to speak with a licensed health care provider before taking vitamin B_{10} or any other herbal remedy or dietary supplement.

Vitamin B_{12} - Cyanocobalamin

Vitamin B_{12} is also known as cyanocobalamin.

In 1956 English physicist Dorothy Hodgkin completed the mapping of the B_{12} chemical structure. Robert Burns Woodward produced vitamin B_{12} after a ten-year effort. Vitamin B_{12} is a water-soluble vitamin absorbed in the intestines and carried throughout the body in the bloodstream. Since it is not stored in body fat, after the body uses what it needs, any excess B_{12} leaves the body in urine or sweat.

Why do we need vitamin B_{12}?

Vitamin B_{12} is essential for the production of red blood cells. It plays a role in the digestion of proteins, fats, and the blending of myelin, a fatty substance that encases nerve fibers like insulation. Vitamin B_{12} also shows some antioxidant properties working with vitamin B_9 to change the amino acid homocysteine into methionine, a substance that helps prevent cells from becoming malignant. Vitamin B_{12} injections have also been rumored to increase energy, although at present, there has been no scientific evidence to prove this claim.

B_{12} is responsible to bring a host of trace minerals into the body, which includes the following:

- Chromium
- Copper
- Germanium
- Iron
- Manganese
- Molybdium
- Nickel
- Vanadium
- Zinc

How much vitamin B_{12} should I take?

According to the National Academy of Sciences, the recommended daily allowance for vitamin B_{12} is as follows:

Adult men: 2-2.4 micrograms/day
Adult women: 2-2.4 micrograms/day
Children aged 7-10: 1.4 micrograms/day
Infants: 0.5 micrograms/day
Pregnant/breast feeding women: 2.6 micrograms/day

What are some good food sources of vitamin B_{12}?

- Cheese
- Clams
- Cod
- Eggs
- Fish
- Meats
- Milk
- Oily fish
- Sardines
- Tuna
- Yogurt

What can happen if I do not get enough vitamin B_{12}? Vitamin B_{12} shortages are rare in young people. The elderly may have trouble absorbing vitamin B_{12} and may require supplements. Symptoms of vitamin B_{12} deficiency can include memory loss, instability, disorientation, nerve damage, decreased reflexes, and possible hearing loss. Deficiency of B_{12} has also been linked with increased levels of homocysteine, associated with heart disease, birth defects, and Alzheimer's disease.

A genetic defect of having no protein called the gastric intrinsic factor may also result in vitamin B_{12} deficiency. In such cases, a condition known as pernicious anemia can develop. The condition must be treated with vitamin B_{12} injections, or damage to nerves can occur.

What can happen if I take too much vitamin B_{12}? To date, no reports of toxicity have been linked with high intake levels of vitamin B_{12}. Because it is water-soluble and is not stored in the body, the chances of enough vitamin B_{12} building up to toxic levels are very unlikely.

Vitamin B_{13} - Orotic acid

Vitamin B_{13} is also known as orotic acid.

Biscaro and Belloni discovered B_{13} in milk in 1905. Intestinal bacteria make vitamin B_{13}, mostly used in connection with vitamin B_9 and vitamin B_{12}. It helps the absorption of essential nutrients especially calcium, magnesium and helps the production of genetic material. It may be beneficial after a heart attack and has been used in conditions such as multiple sclerosis and chronic hepatitis, reported to prevent liver-related complications and premature aging.

Some good sources of vitamin B_{13} are:

Beef	Potatoes	Whey
Carrots	Root vegetables	
Fresh cow's milk	Turnips	

Vitamin B_{13} has been attached to such minerals as:

Calcium	Potassium	Magnesium

This is easily absorbed and utilized by the body. It also helps in treating the symptoms of multiple sclerosis and chronic hepatitis. Deficiency of vitamin B_{13} may cause:

Liver disorders	Cell degeneration	Premature aging

It is an important indicator of ammonia disorder metabolism, which can lead to sickness or death in individuals.

Vitamin B_{15} - Pangamic Acid

Vitamin B_{15} is also known as pangamic acid.

Russia has been the most progressive country using B_{15}, believing it to be a very important nutrient treating a multitude of symptoms and diseases. Russian research has shown a reduction of lactic acid buildup in athletes, thereby decreasing muscle fatigue and increasing endurance.

Used regularly in Russia for many health issues, including:

- Aging and senility
- Alcoholism
- Autism
- Chemical poisonings
- Drug addiction
- Heart disease
- High blood pressure and diabetes
- Liver disease
- Schizophrenia
- Skin diseases

Vitamin B_{15} is found in:

- Apricot kernels
- Beef blood
- Brewer's yeast
- Pumpkin and sunflower seeds
- Whole grains such as brown rice

B_{15} helps in the formation of specific amino acids such as methionine. It plays a role in the oxidation of glucose in cell respiration. Like vitamin E, it acts as an antioxidant helping to lengthen cell life through its protection from oxidation. B_{15} mildly stimulates the endocrine and nervous systems, and by enhancing liver function, it helps in the detoxification process.

B_{15} has been shown to lower blood cholesterol, improve circulation and general oxygenation of cells and tissues, and is helpful for arteriosclerosis and hypertension. In Europe, vitamin B_{15} has been used to treat premature aging because of both its circulatory stimulus and its antioxidant effects. It helps protect the body from pollutants, especially carbon monoxide.

The most common form of B_{15} is calcium pangamate. B_{15} is often taken with vitamin E and vitamin A. A common amount of DMG is 50-100 mg. taken twice daily, usually with breakfast and dinner. This level of intake may improve general energy levels, support the immune system, and reduce alcohol cravings, making it very helpful in moderating chronic alcohol problems.

Vitamin B_{17} - Laetrile

Apricot kernels are the richest source of B_{17}. Ernst Krebs is the world's leading authority on the relationship between cancer and nitrilosides, and the discovery of laetrile.

Apricot kernels are known to prevent and cure cancer, even though the medical establishment has worked night and day and even lied to suppress it. Vitamin B_{17} is found in most all fruit seeds such as the apple, peach, cherry, orange, nectarine, and apricot. It is found in some beans and many grasses such as wheat grass. The hard wooden pit in the middle of the peach is not supposed to be thrown away. In fact, the wooden shell is strong armor protecting one of the most important foods known to man, the seed.

It is one of the main courses of food in cultures such as the Navajo Indians, the Hunzas, the Abkhasians, and many more. Did you know that within these tribes there has never been a reported case of cancer?

We don't need to make the seed a main course but we do need the equivalent of about seven apricots seeds per day to improve our odds for a cancer-free life. The kernel or seed contains the highest amounts of vitamin B_{17}.

One of the most common nitrilosides is amygdalin. This nitriloside occurs in the kernels of seeds of practically all fruits. The seeds of apples, apricots, cherries, peaches, plums, nectarines, and the like carry this factor, often in the extraordinary concentration of 2 to 3 percent. The rule of thumb when eating seeds is to eat the fruit along with the seeds. For example, you do not want to extract the seeds from 50 apples and eat only those seeds; however, eating a few apples every day along with their seeds is perfectly safe.

Since the seeds of fruits are possibly edible, it may be proper to designate the non-toxic water soluble accessory food factor or nitriloside that they contain as vitamin B_{17}. The presence of nitriloside in the diet produces specific physiologic effects and leaves as metabolites specific chemical compounds of a physiologically active nature. The production by a non-toxic, water-soluble accessory food factor of specific physiological effects as well as identifiable metabolites suggests the vitamin nature of the compound.

Vitamin B_{17} is a relatively simple compound found in much of our food supply. It is most abundant in the seeds of non-citrus fruits. Most commercially prepared amygdalin is extracted from the seeds of the apricot. Amygdalin is composed of two molecules of glucose (a sugar), one molecule of benzaldehyde (an analgesic) and one molecule of hydrocyanic acid (an anti-neoplastic compound). Thiocyanate is excreted in the urine.

Foods that contain vitamin B_{17} are listed below:

Alfalfa sprouts	Buckwheat	Garbanzo sprouts
Apple seeds	Buckwheat sprouts	Gooseberries
Apricot kernels	Cane syrup	Huckleberries
Bamboo shoots	Cashews	Lentil sprouts
Barley	Cherry kernels	Lentils
Beet tops	Cranberries	Lima beans
Bitter almond	Currants	Linseed meat
Blackberries	Eucalyptus leaves	Loganberries
Boysenberries	Fava beans	Macadamia nuts
Brewer's yeast	Flax seeds	Millet
Brown rice	Garbanzo beans	Millet seed

Mung bean sprouts	Raspberries	Watercress
Peach kernels	Sorghum	Wheatgrass
Pecans	Spinach	Yams
Plum kernels	Strawberries	
Quince	Walnuts	

Vitamins

Vitamin B_p - Choline

Vitamin B_p is also known as choline, was discovered by Adolph Strecker in 1864, and was chemically synthesized in 1866. In 1998 B_p was classified as an essential nutrient by the Food and Nutrition Board of the Institute of Medicine. Choline's importance as a nutrient was first appreciated in the early research on insulin functions when B_p was found to be the necessary nutrient in preventing fatty liver. In 1975 scientists discovered that the administration of B_p increased the synthesis and release of acetylcholine by neurons. These discoveries lead to the increased interest in dietary B_p and brain function.

Today, we know B_p to be a dietary nutrient important for all cells to function normally. B_p is required for synthesis of essential components of membranes and is an important source of labile methyl groups.

A study in Nov 2010 by Leslie M. Fischer, Kerry Ann da Costa, Lester Kwock, Joseph Galanko, and Steven Zeisel was to test postmenopausal women with low estrogen levels and see if they were more susceptible to the risk of organ dysfunction if not given a sufficient B_p filled diet. When deprived of B_p in their diet almost 80% of the men and postmenopausal women developed liver or muscle damage. The study also found that young women can supply more B_p because pregnancy is a time when the body's demand for choline is highest. B_p is particularly used to support the fetus's developing nervous system.

B_p and its metabolites are needed for three main physiological purposes:

- Structural integrity
- Signaling roles for cell membranes
- Cholinergic neurotransmission
- Major source for methyl groups via its metabolite Trimethylglycine (betaine) which participates in the S-adenosylmethionine (SAMe) synthesis pathways

B_p deficiency signs

Most common signs of B_p deficiencies are fatty liver and hemorrhagic kidney necrosis. Dietary intake of a B_p full diet can reduce the severity of the deficiency. A study of this on animals has created some controversy due to the inconsistency in dietary modifying factors.

B_p deficiency in animals compromises renal function. B_p low diets can also cause:

- Atherosclerosis
- Bone abnormalities
- Elevated level of the liver enzymes
- Growth impairment
- Hypertension
- Infertility
- Liver disease
- Neurological disorders

B_p deficiency is considered to both initiate and promote cancer activities. Required B_p levels in diet were determined by feeding healthy humans a B_p deficient diet until they developed biochemical changes consistent with B_p deficiency.

Fish odor syndrome: trimethylaminuria

B_p is a precursor to trimethylamine, which some persons are not able to break down due to a genetic disorder called trimethylaminuria. Persons suffering from this disorder may suffer from a strong fishy or otherwise unpleasant body odor, due to the body's release of odorous trimethylamine. A body odor will occur even on a normal diet–i.e., one that is not particularly high in B_p. Persons with trimethylaminuria is advised to restrict the intake of foods high in B_p; this may help to reduce the sufferer's body odor.

Groups at risk for B_p deficiency: Vegetarians, vegans, endurance athletes, and people who drink a lot of alcohol may be at risk for B_p deficiency and may benefit from B_p supplements.

In general, people who do not eat many whole eggs may have to pay close attention and get enough B_p in their diets. Studies on a number of different populations have found that the average intake of B_p was below the adequate intake.

The adequate intake of B_p is 425 mg (milligrams) per day for adult women; higher for pregnant and breast-feeding women. A human infant consumes a great amount of B_p from breast milk. It is particularly important for pregnant women to get enough B_p, since low B_p intake may raise the rate of neural tube defects in infants, and may affect their child's memory. One study found that higher dietary intake of B_p shortly before and after conception was associated with a lower risk of neural tube defects. The amount allowed for adult men is 550 mg/day.

Sources of B_p in animal and plant foods:

Almonds	Grapefruit	Soybeans, dry
Beef liver	Kidney beans	Spinach
Brown rice	Large hardboiled egg	Wheat germ
Cauliflower	Lecithin	
Chicken	Milk, 1% fat	
Cod fish	Peanuts	

VITAMIN C - ASCORBIC ACID

Vitamin C is also known as ascorbic acid. Vitamin C is one of several antioxidants shown to play a key role in the prevention of many types of cancers. Vitamin C maintains collagen, a protein needed for the formation of skin, ligaments, and bones. Also enhancing the immune system, it helps heal wounds, mend fractures, and aids in resisting some types of bacterial and viral infections.

Dr. Linus Pauling, often known as the "Father of Vitamin C," twice awarded the Nobel Prize, declared that large intakes of up to 10 grams of ascorbic acid each day aids anti-cancer activity within the body and also assists in repairing damaged arteries and removing arterial plaque (atherosclerosis) for heart disease sufferers. Pauling lived to be 94. Today, much higher doses of vitamin C are used by many practitioners for cancer/heart/stroke patients in nutritional therapy who believe Pauling was right and that the popular nutrient is indispensable to the body in its fight to regain health from cancer.

Vitamin C, is an important component of a healthy diet. The history of vitamin C revolves around the human disease scurvy, probably the first human illness to be recognized as a deficiency disease. Its deficiency symptoms include exhaustion, massive hemorrhaging of flesh and gums, general weakness and diarrhea. Resultant death was common. Scurvy is a disease unique to guinea pigs, various primates, and humans.

As early as 1536, Jacques Cartier, a French explorer, reported the amazing curative effects of infusions of pine bark and needles used by Native Americans. These items are now known to be good sources of ascorbic acid. However, some 400 years were to pass before vitamin C was isolated, characterized, and synthesized. In the late 1700s, the British Navy ordered the use of limes on ships to prevent scurvy. This practice was, for many years, considered quackery by the merchant marines, and the Navy sailors became known as "Limeys." At that time, scurvy aboard sailing vessels was a serious problem with often up to 50% of the crew dying from scurvy on long voyages.

Heat destroys vitamin C. This means that for every meal you cook, 100% of the vitamin C content has been destroyed. Many go through an entire winter cooking their food because they like something warm. Humans cannot make vitamin C in their bodies, unlike most mammals, so our only source of this valuable complex is dietary.

If you are sick, put 20-30 g of vitamin C powder in water and then drink throughout the day. Replenish when necessary. This ensures high potency dosage is delivered on a regular basis simultaneously with water intake. Vitamin C is very safe for kids and highly effective when they get fevers or childhood ailments. For adults, mega-dose vitamin C is effective for all forms of infection, flu, muscle weakness, muscle pain, chronic lower back pain, general pain management, and periodontitis.

Vitamin C recommendations are to take daily preventive doses of 10,000 to 15,000 milligrams/day. Parents are advised to give their children their age in vitamin C grams (1 gram = 1,000 milligrams). That would be 2,000 milligrams/day for a two-year-old, 9,000 milligrams/day for a nine-year-old, and for older children; level off at about 10,000 milligrams/day.

There are many good reasons to give large quantities of vitamin C to a cancer patient. Ascorbic acid strengthens the collagen "glue" that holds healthy cells together and retards the spread of an existing tumor. The vitamin also strengthens the immune system and provides a surprising level of pain relief. Vitamin C has been shown to be preferentially toxic to cancer cells.

Plant sources of vitamin C:

Acerola	Cucumber	Parsley
Apple	Eggplant	Passion fruit
Apricot	Elderberry	Pawpaw
Asparagus	Fig	Peach
Avocado	Garlic	Pear
Banana	Grape	Persimmon
Beetroot	Grapefruit	Persimmon (native, raw)
Bilberry	Guava (common, raw)	Pineapple
Blackberry	Horned melon	Plum
Blackcurrant	Kakadu plum	Potato
Blueberry	Kale	Raisin
Broccoli	Kiwifruit	Raspberry
Brussels sprouts	Lemon	Red pepper
Cabbage (raw green)	Lettuce	Redcurrant
Camu Camu	Lime	Rose hip
Carrot	Loganberry	Seabuckthorn
Cauliflower	Mandarin orange	Spinach
Cherry	Mango	Strawberry
Chili pepper (green)	Melon, cantaloupe	Tangerine
Chili pepper (red)	Melon, honeydew	Tomato
Choke cherry	Mica Muro	Tomato, red
Cloudberry	Onion	Watermelon
Crabapple	Orange	Wolfberry (Goji)
Cranberry	Papaya	

What can happen if I do not get enough vitamin C? A person with vitamin C deficiency can develop scurvy as well as hemorrhages, loose teeth, gingivitis, bad breath, bone disease, bleeding gums, increased chance for infection and colds or respiratory infections. Taking too much vitamin C may cause diarrhea.

VITAMIN D - CHOLECALCIFEROL

Vitamin D is also known as cholecalciferol. Vitamin D is called "The Sunshine Vitamin" because our bodies can not make this vitamin without sunlight. Vitamin D is actually a term for a group of hormones that are stored mainly in the liver, as well as fat and muscle tissue. It is one of three vitamins naturally manufactured by the body, and it is produced by a chemical reaction to the ultraviolet radiation contained in sunlight.

Why do we need it? Vitamin D increases the body's absorption and metabolism of calcium and phosphorus. This makes it very important in maintaining strong, healthy bones and teeth. If all people knew their vitamin D levels, hundreds of thousands or millions or billions of dollars would not be spent on needless sickness and it could all be prevented by a simple vitamin D test. In my opinion, low vitamin D levels are connected with every sickness.

How much vitamin D should I take?

According to the National Academy of Sciences, the recommended daily allowance for vitamin D is as follows:

Adult men: 200 international units (5 micrograms)/day
Adult women: 200 international units (5 micrograms)/day
Adults age 51-70: 400 international units (10 micrograms)/day
Adults 71 and over: 600 international units (15 micrograms)/day

Children aged 7-10: 200 international units (5 micrograms)/day
Infants: 200 international units (5 micrograms)/day
Pregnant/lactating women: 200 international units (5 micrograms)/day

In the opinion of many health care doctors, the above numbers are extremely low. My recommendation is 2000 international units every day for everybody and even more if there is sickness.

What are some good sources of vitamin D? Exposure to sunlight is the easiest way to build up stores of vitamin D. By exposing the face, hands and forearms for between 15-20 minutes two or three times per week, most people can manufacture all the vitamin D they need. Vitamin D is also found in a number of food products, most notably vitamin D-fortified milk.

Other sources include:

Cheese
Egg yolks

Fish
Fortified cereals

Liver

What can happen if I do not get enough vitamin D? Having a vitamin D shortage can result in bone related disorders such as rickets in children and osteomalacia in adults. A Vitamin D shortage also increases the risk of hip fractures in postmenopausal women and has been linked to higher numbers of prostate cancer and breast cancer.

What can happen if I take too much vitamin D? High doses of vitamin D can be very toxic. In children, large doses can cause mental retardation, stunted growth, and kidney failure. In older children and adults, too much vitamin D can result in:

Anorexia	Diarrhea	Weakness
Changes in a person's mental state	Nausea	

With the exception of kidney failure, low-calcium intake and avoidance of vitamin D from a person's diet can usually reverse these side effects. It is important to know your own blood levels!

Vitamin E - Tocopherols

Vitamin E is also known as tocopherol.

Two scientists, Bishop and Evans, discovered vitamin E in 1932. They isolated the pure substance from wheat germ in 1936 and described its structure in 1938. They gave it the name Tocopherol that comes from the Greek word: tokos, meaning offspring and phero, meaning to bring forth. It was determined that this substance was required for reproduction in rats and was referred to as the anti-sterility vitamin. Vitamin E is a fat-soluble vitamin stored in the liver. It is one of three vitamins, which also act as antioxidants.

There are eight different E vitamins:

- Alpha-tocopherol
- Beta-tocopherol
- Delta-tocopherol
- Eta-tocopherol
- Gamma-tocopherol
- Theta-tocopherol
- Zada-tocopherol

Why do we need it? In its role as an antioxidant, vitamin E helps lessen the effect of unstable particles called "free radicals" which damage cell membranes. It slows the oxidation of "bad" cholesterol, which may reduce the risk of plaque buildup in our arteries. It may reduce the risk of stroke and heart attacks. Vitamin E plays an important role building red blood cells and using vitamin K. Some studies show vitamin E may raise resistance to infectious diseases and protect against cataracts. Vitamin E requires selenium to function.

How much vitamin E should I take? Never take a stand-alone vitamin E unless you know how many other E vitamins are present. It must say, "Mixed Tocophero,l" on the supplement bottle.

According to the National Academy of Sciences (NAS), the recommended daily allowance for vitamin E is as follows:

- Adult men: 10 milligrams/day
- Adult women: 8 milligrams/day
- Children aged 7-10: 7 milligrams/day
- Infants: 4 milligrams/day
- Pregnant/lactating women: 12 milligrams/day

In addition to the NAS guidelines, some groups recommend much higher doses (between 70-130 milligrams/day).

Some good food sources of vitamin E:

- Avocados
- Egg yolks
- Green leafy vegetables
- Nuts
- Peas
- Sunflower seeds
- Sweet potatoes
- Sunflower seeds
- Wheat germ oil

What can happen if I do not get enough vitamin E? Deficiencies of vitamin E have been linked to heart disease. People with very low blood levels of vitamin E may also be at higher risk for cancer.

What can happen if I take too much? Some people taking huge amounts of vitamin E have reported experiencing fatigue, nausea, and diarrhea. Too much vitamin E may also cause bleeding problems, mostly in people taking anti-clotting medications.

VITAMIN F - ESSENTIAL FATTY ACIDS

Essential fatty acids (EFAs) are fats that humans must ingest because the body requires them for good health but cannot be made by the body. Fatty acids are essential for our cells to function normally and stay alive. The cell membranes allow the passage of necessary minerals and molecules in and out of our cells. Healthy cell membranes discourage dangerous chemicals and organisms like bacteria, viruses, moulds and parasites from entering the cell. These membranes also maintain chemical receptor sites for hormones, the body's crucial messengers. Fatty acids are involved in countless chemical processes in our bodies and are used as building blocks for certain hormones.

When the two essential fatty acids were first discovered in 1923, they were designated Vitamin F. In 1930 work by Burr, Burr and Miller showed that the two essential fatty acids are better classified with the fats than with the vitamins. Fatty acids are the building blocks of fats, and the different types are distinguished based on their chemical structure.

Only two essential fatty acids are known for humans:

1. Alpha-linolenic acid (an omega-3 fatty acid) which include EPA (eicosapentaenoic acid) and DHA (docosahexaenoic acid)
2. Linoleic acid (an omega-6 fatty acid) which includes gamma-linolenic acid, dihomo-gamma-linolenic acid and arachidonic acid

Types of fats in food:

1. Saturated fats - Avoid this type of fat. Saturated fat is the main dietary cause of high blood cholesterol. The American Heart Association recommends that you limit your saturated fat intake. If you have coronary heart disease or your LDL cholesterol level is 100 mg/dL or greater, your doctor should recommend the lifestyle change in relationship to diet.

2. Unsaturated fats - Unsaturated fats contain fewer hydrogen atoms, and one or more pairs of carbon atoms are linked by double chemical bonds. A fatty acid with one double bond is called monounsaturated.

3. Monounsaturated fat - Monounsaturated fat is found in olive, peanut and canola oils, avocados and most nuts. This fat lowers LDL cholesterol.

4. Polyunsaturated fat - Polyunsaturated fat. This is found in vegetable oils such as safflower, sunflower, corn, soy and cottonseed oil. This fat also helps lower LDL cholesterol. But polyunsaturated fat is more susceptible to chemical changes that may influence the risk of some diseases.

5. Trans fat - Stay away from this type of oil. Trans fat, which is also called hydrogenated or partially hydrogenated vegetable oil. Trans fat is found in margarine and shortening and foods such as cookies, crackers and other commercially baked goods made with these ingredients. Trans fat raises LDL cholesterol and lowers high-density lipoprotein (HDL), the "good" cholesterol. Since trans- fats don't occur in nature, our bodies don't know how to deal with them effectively and they act as poisons to crucial cellular reactions.

6. Cis fat - Stay away from this type of oil. Naturally occurring fatty acids contain double bonds of a particular configuration, referred to as "cis-" by biochemists. The cis- causes the molecules to be bent so that the two hydrogen atoms are on the same side of the double bond. This means the bonds between the molecules are weaker due to their irregular shape, resulting in a lower melting point, in supermarket shopper lingo, they are "solid at room temperature."

Other fatty acids that are only "conditionally essential" include:

1. Lauric acid (a saturated fatty acid)
2. Palmitoleic acid (a monounsaturated fatty acid)

The biological effects of the omega-3 and omega-6 fatty acids are mediated by their mutual interactions. In the body, essential fatty acids serve multiple functions. In each of these, the balance between dietary omega-3 and omega-6 strongly affects function. They are modified to make the classic eicosanoids which affects inflammation and many other cellular functions and the endocannabinoids which affects mood, behavior and inflammation.

Omega-9 fatty acids are not essential in humans, because humans generally possess all the enzymes required for their synthesis.

Store-bought margarine is oil with hydrogen processed into the oil. This is called hydrogenation. A side-effect of hydrogenation is that a residue of toxic metals, usually nickel and aluminium, is left behind in the finished product. These metals are used as catalysts in the reaction, but they accumulate in our cells and nervous system where they poison enzyme systems and alter cellular functions, endangering health and causing a wide variety of problems. These toxic metals are difficult to eliminate without special detoxification techniques, and our 'toxic load' increases steadily with small exposures over time. Since they are increasingly found in our air, food and water, the cumulative doses can add up to dangerous levels over time.

Food sources:

Almost all the polyunsaturated fat in the human diet is from essential fatty acid. Some of the food sources of omega-3 and omega -6 fatty acids are:

Canola (rapeseed) oil (non GMO)	Hemp oil	Soya oil (non GMO)
Chia seeds	Leafy vegetables	Sunflower seeds
Fish	Pumpkin seeds	Walnuts
Flaxseed (linseed)	Shellfish	

Essential fatty acids play a part in many metabolic processes, and there is evidence to suggest that low levels of essential fatty acids, or the wrong balance of types among the essential fatty acids, may be a factor in a number of illnesses, including osteoporosis.

Plant sources of omega-3 contain neither eicosapentaenoic acid (EPA) nor docosahexaenoic acid. The human body can (and in case of a purely vegetarian diet often must, unless certain algae or supplements derived from them are consumed) convert α-linolenic acid to eicosapentaenoic acid and subsequently docosahexaenoic acid. This however requires more metabolic work, which is thought to be the reason that the absorption of essential fatty acids is much greater from animal rather than plant sources.

Human health conditions that can be affected with essential fatty acid:

1. Diet and heart disease - Almost all the polyunsaturated fats in the human diet are EFAs. Essential fatty acids play an important role in the life and death of cardiac cells.

2. Essential fatty acid deficiency results in dermatitis similar to that seen in zinc or biotin deficiency.

3. Treatment for depression - Research suggests that high intakes of fish and omega-3 fatty acids are linked to decreased rates of major depression. Omega-3 fatty acids, such as docosahexaenoic acid and eicosapentaenoic acid are important for enzymatic pathways required to metabolize long-chain polyunsaturated fatty acids. Low plasma concentrations of docosahexaenoic acid predict low concentrations of cerebrospinal fluid 5-hydroxyindoleacetic acid. It is found that low concentrations of 5-HIAA in the brain is associated with depression and suicide.

4. There are high concentrations of docosahexaenoic acid in synaptic membranes of the brain. This is critical for synaptic transmission and membrane fluidity. The omega-6 fatty acid to omega-3 fatty acid ratio is important to avoid imbalance of membrane fluidity. Membrane fluidity affects function of enzymes such as adenylate cyclase and ion channels such as calcium, potassium, and sodium, which in turn affects receptor numbers, and functioning, as well as

serotonin neurotransmitter levels. It is evident that western diets are deficient in omega-3 and excessive in omega-6, and balancing of this ratio would confer numerous health benefits.

5. function of the Vision - Docosahexaenoic acid is found at very high concentrations in the cell membranes of the retina; the retina conserves and recycles docosahexaenoic acid even when omega-3 fatty acid intake is low. Animal studies indicate that DHA is required for the normal development and retina. Moreover, these studies suggest that there is a critical period during retinal development when inadequate docosahexaenoic acid will result in permanent abnormalities in retinal function. Recent research indicates that docosahexaenoic acid plays an important role in the regeneration of the visual pigment rhodopsin, which plays a critical role in the visual transduction system that converts light hitting the retina to visual images in the brain.

6. Nervous System - The phospholipids of the brain's gray matter contain high proportions of docosahexaenoic acid and alpha-linolenic acid, suggesting they are important to central nervous system function. Brain docosahexaenoic acid content may be particularly important, since animal studies have shown that depletion of docosahexaenoic acid in the brain can result in learning deficits. It is not clear how docosahexaenoic acid affects brain function, but changes in docosahexaenoic acidcontent of neuronal cell membranes could alter the function of ion channels or membrane-associated receptors, as well as the availability of neurotransmitters

7. Clinical signs of essential fatty acid deficiency include a dry scaly rash, decreased growth in infants and children, increased susceptibility to infection, and poor wound healing.

Eating a balanced diet should ensure a person a daily amount of essential fatty acids. Consult your family physican for advice as to which supplements would be right your family.

Vitamin H - Biotin

Vitamin H is also known as biotin.

All B vitamins help the body to convert food (carbohydrates) into fuel (glucose), which is used to produce energy. These B vitamins, often referred to as B complex vitamins, also help the body metabolize fats and protein. B complex vitamins are needed for healthy skin, hair, eyes, and liver. They also help the nervous system function properly.

Your body needs biotin to metabolize carbohydrates, fats, and amino acids, the building blocks of protein. Biotin is often recommended for strengthening hair and nails and it's found in many cosmetic products for hair and skin.

Like all B vitamins, it is a water-soluble vitamin, meaning the body does not store it. However, bacteria in the intestine can make biotin. It is also available in small amounts in a number of foods. Biotin is also important for normal embryonic growth, making it a critical nutrient during pregnancy.

It is rare to be deficient in biotin. Symptoms include:

Cracking in the corners of the mouth	Fatigue	Swollen and painful tongue that is magenta in color
Depression	Hair loss	
Dry eyes	Insomnia	
Dry scaly skin	Loss of appetite	

People who have been on parenteral nutrition (nutrition given through an IV) for a long period of time, those taking antiseizure medication or antibiotics long-term, and people with conditions like Crohn's disease that make it hard to absorb nutrients are more likely to be deficient in biotin.

Hair and nail problems: Evidence suggests that biotin supplements may improve thin, splitting, or brittle toe and fingernails, as well as hair. Biotin, combined with zinc and topical clobetasol propionate, has also been used to combat alopecia areata in both children and adults.

Cradle cap (seborrheic dermatitis): Infants who don't have enough biotin often develop this scaly scalp condition. However, no studies have shown that biotin supplements, given in formula or breast milk, effectively treat cradle cap. Always ask your doctor before taking any vitamin, herb, or supplement if you are breastfeeding.

Diabetes: Preliminary research indicates that a combination of biotin and chromium might improve blood sugar control in some people with type 2 diabetes, but biotin alone doesn't seem to have the same effect. More research is needed to know for sure whether biotin has any benefit.

Peripheral Neuropathy: There have been reports that biotin supplements improve the symptoms of peripheral neuropathy for some people who developed this condition from either diabetes or ongoing dialysis for kidney failure. Peripheral neuropathy is nerve damage in the feet, hands, legs, or arms. Numbness, tingling, burning or strange sensations, pain, muscle weakness, and trouble walking are some symptoms. However, there aren't any studies that evaluate whether biotin really helps treat peripheral neuropathy.

Dietary sources:

- Almonds
- Bananas
- Beans
- Blackeye peas
- Brewer's yeast
- Cauliflower
- Cooked eggs, especially egg yolk
- Legumes
- Mushrooms
- Peanuts
- Pecans
- Sardines
- Soybeans
- Walnuts
- Whole grains

Raw egg whites contain a protein called avidin that interferes with the body's absorption of biotin. Food-processing techniques can destroy biotin. Less-processed versions of the foods listed above contain more biotin.

Available Forms: Biotin is available in multivitamins and B-vitamin complexes, and as individual supplements. Standard preparations are available in 10 micrograms, 50 micrograms, and 100 micrograms tablets and contain either simple biotin or a complex with brewer's yeast.

How to take it: Adequate daily intakes for biotin from food, according to the National Academy of Sciences, are listed below:

Pediatric
Infants
Birth - 6 months: 5 micrograms
7 - 12 months: 6 micrograms

Children
1 - 3 years: 8 micrograms
4 - 8 years: 12 micrograms
9 - 13 years: 20 micrograms

Adolescents
14 - 18 years: 25 micrograms

Adult
19 years and older: 30 micrograms

Pregnant
Women: 30 micrograms
Breast-feeding women: 35 micrograms

Precautions: With that said, biotin has not been associated with side effects, even in high doses, and is considered to be non-toxic.

Possible interactions: Although there is no evidence that biotin interacts with any medication, there are some medications that may lower biotin levels. If you are being treated with any of the following medications, you should not use biotin without first talking to your health care provider.

Antibiotics: Long-term antibiotic use may lower biotin levels by destroying the bacteria in the gut that produces biotin.

Antiseizure medications: Taking antiseizure or anticonvulsants medications for a long time can lower biotin levels in the body. Valproic acid can cause biotinidase deficiency, which may be helped by biotin supplements. Ask your doctor before taking any supplements, however.

Anticonvulsant medications include:

Carbamazepine (Carbatrol)
Phenobarbital
Phenytoin (Dilantin)

Vitamin K - Primidone

Vitamin K is also known as Primidone. Vitamin K represents a family of fat soluble molecules, which are widely known as vitamin K_1 (phylloquinone), K_2 (primidone), and K_3 (menadione). Vitamin K is a fat-soluble vitamin. The "K" is derived from the German word "koagulation." Coagulation refers to the process of blood clot formation. While vitamin K_3 does not have a significant biological role, both K_1 and K_2 are biologically active. Vitamin K_2 consists of a small group of molecules called menaquinones. Vitamin K is stored in the liver and the body's fat reserves. Vitamin K is created by the probiotics that line the gastrointestinal tract.

Why do we need it? Vitamin K's most important role is in making many of the proteins responsible for blood clotting. It also helps make a protein called osteocalcin, which plays a key role in keeping healthy bones, healing bone fractures and preventing osteoporosis. Some studies show that it helps in maintaining strong bones in the elderly.

How much vitamin K should I take?

According to the National Academy of Sciences, the recommended daily allowance for vitamin K is as follows:

Adult men: 80 micrograms/day
Adult women: 65 micrograms/day
Children aged 7-10: 30 micrograms/day

Infants: 10 micrograms/day

Pregnant/lactating women: 65 micrograms/day

Some good food sources of vitamin K:

Beef liver	Citrus fruits	Non-GMO soybean oil
Bran	Eggs	Spinach
Broccoli	Green leafy vegetables	Turnip greens
Cabbage	Milk	

What can happen if I do not get enough vitamin K? Because vitamin K is a naturally occurring substance (it is made by bacteria in the intestines and stored in the liver), having a shortage is very uncommon. However, shortages may occur in people who have trouble absorbing fats, are on long-term antibiotic therapy, or take other medications such as warfarin and phenobarbital. Symptoms found in people who have a vitamin K shortage include easy bruising and ruptured capillaries. A low intake of vitamin K may also increase the risk of hip fractures in women.

What can happen if I take too much? Allergic-type reactions, including skin rashes and itching, have been reported in those people taking high doses of vitamin K. People taking an anticoagulant called coumadin (also known as warfarin) should not take vitamin K supplements without first speaking with a health care profesional.

VITAMIN P - FLAVONOIDS

Vitamin P, otherwise known as flavonoids, enhances the use of vitamin C by improving absorption and protecting from oxidation. Flavonoids are referred to as "Super Antioxidants." There are no daily recommended daily allowances for this vitamin. No overdose symptoms are expected.

Flavonoids are shown to have effects such as:

Antiallergic
Anti-inflammatory
Antithrombogenic

Anticarcinogenic
Antiviral

Flavonoids scavenge for free radicals associated with oxygen and iron; or by inhibiting oxidative enzymes. Over 4000 flavanoids have been found, and fall in four different groups:

Anthocyanins
Catechins

Flavones
Flavanones

How this vitamin works in your body:

Anti-inflammatory properties acting against histamines
Capillary fragility
Help protects against infection and blood vessel disease
Improves capillary strength
Inhibits tumor growth
Lowers blood pressure by relaxing smooth muscle of cardiovascular system
Lowers cholesterol levels

Prevents accumulation of atherosclerotic plaque
Prevents hemorrhoids
Prevents miscarriages
Prevents nosebleed
Promotes blood vessel health
Promotes estrogen-like activity
Retinal bleeding in people with diabetes and hypertension

Foods where vitamin P is found:

Apricots
Bilberry
Black currants
Broccoli
Buckwheat
Cherries

Citrus fruits
Ginkgo
Grapes
Green pepper
Green tea
Hawthorn

Milk thistle
Onions
Red wine
Rose hips
Tomatoes
Yarrow

MINERALS AND HUMAN HEALTH

There are 92 elements found in nature. In the table listed below are the quantities of elements found in the earth's crust, oceans, and atmosphere. These are the elements our body must draw upon to survive. It becomes increasingly evident when studying the relationship of minerals to human health that keeping the level of minerals in balance in every tissue, fluid, cell, and organ, in the human body may be the key to maintaining human health.

Elements found in the earth's crust, oceans and atmosphere:

Earth's Crust (by mass)	Oceans (by mass)	Atmosphere (volume of dry air)
Oxygen 46.5%	Oxygen 85.79%	Nitrogen 78.08%
Silicon 28.0%	Hydrogen 10.67%	Oxygen 20.95%
Aluminum 8.1%	Chlorine 2.07%	Argon 0.93%
Iron 5.1%	Sodium 1.14%	Carbon Dioxide 0.03%
Calcium 3.5%	Magnesium 0.14%	Neon 0.0018%
Sodium 3.0%	All others 0.19%	Helium 0.0005%
Potassium 2.5%		Krypton 0.0001%
Magnesium 2.2%		Xenon 0.000008%

Through geophysical forces, mixing of the earth's crust with water can provide virtually every mineral our body requires to maintain health. This explains why the noted nutritionists, Ruth L. Pike and Myrtle L. Brown stated in *Nutrition: An Integrated Approach* (John Wiley &Sons, 1984, p.197) that: "Water is compatible with more substances than any known solvent, and therefore it is an ideal medium for transporting nutrients in the cells and for the chemical reactions of cellular metabolism to take place." Table 2 lists 66 elements that have been identified to date to be in sea water. A few surviving inland seas such as the Great Salt Lake of Utah have concentrated many of the same minerals found in the sea through geothermal and evaporative processes. These natural sources of the elements can provide a rich source of minerals compatible to human physiological needs.

Table 2 - Decreasing average concentration of 66 elements in sea water (mg/l)

Oxygen	Molybdenum	Thorium
Hydrogen	Zinc	Gallium
Chlorine	Nickel	Mercury
Sodium	Arsenic	Lead
Magnesium	Copper	Zirconium
Sulfur	Tin	Bismuth
Calcium	Uranium	Lanthanum
Potassium	Krypton	Gold
Bromine	Manganese	Niobium
Carbon	Vanadium	Thallium
Strontium	Titanium	Hafnium
Boron	Cesium	Helium
Silicon	Cerium	Selenium
Fluorine	Antimony	Tantalum
Argon	Silver	Beryllium
Nitrogen	Yttrium	Protactinium
Lithium	Cobalt	Radium
Rubidium	Neon	Radon
Phosphorus	Cadmium	
Lodine	Tungsten	
Barium	Selenium	
Aluminum	Germanium	
Iron	Zeon	
Indium	Chromium	

These are average concentrations. Variations will exist depending on the collection site of the sample. Ref. Handbook of Chemistry and Physics, 65th Ed. 1984-1985, CRC Press, Boca Raton, Fl., p. F-149

Yttrium   Zinc   Zirconium

These are average concentrations. Variations will exist depending on the collection site of the sample. Ref. *Handbook of Chemistry and Physics*, 65th Ed. 1984-1985, CRC Press, Boca Raton, Fl., p. F-149

Hillman Health Food Store call 855-Amish-Dr (855-264-7437) www.emineral.info Vitamins and Minerals for Better Living

MINERALS TESTING THRU HAIR BIOPSY ANALYSIS

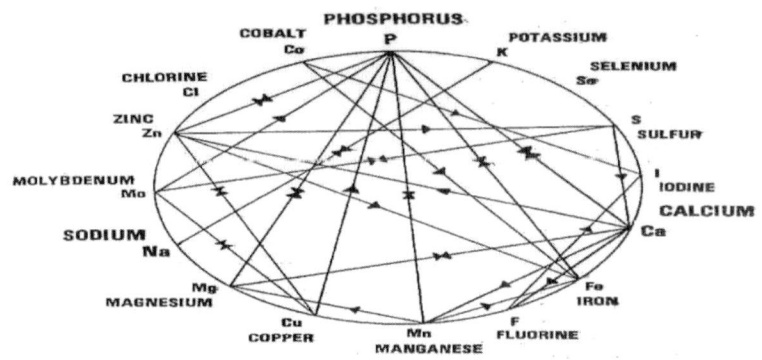

Hair tissue mineral analysis is a soft tissue mineral biopsy that uses hair as the sampling tissue. A biopsy is an analysis of a body tissue. Hair is considered a soft tissue, and hence hair analysis is a soft tissue biopsy. The test measures the levels minerals in the hair with an accuracy of plus or minus about 3%. This is about the same level of accuracy as most blood tests, or a little better.

Why use hair for measuring minerals?

Hair makes an excellent biopsy material for many reasons:

1) Sampling is simple and non-invasive.

2) Hair is a stable biopsy material that remains viable for years, if needed, and requires no special handling.

3) Mineral levels in the hair are about ten times that of blood, making them easy to detect and measure accurately in the hair.

4) Hair is a fairly rapidly growing tissue. The body often throws off toxic substances in the hair, since the hair will be cut off and lost to the body.

Hair mineral values often vary by a factor of ten or much more, making measurement easier and providing a tremendous amount of accurate knowledge about the cells and the soft tissue of our bodies.

5) Toxic metals are easier to detect in the hair than in the blood. They are not found in high concentrations in the blood except right after an acute exposure. However, most tend to accumulate in the soft tissues such as the hair, as the body tries to move them to locations where they will do less damage.

The following minerals are currently being tested -

1) Essential elements

Boron (B)	Iron (Fe)	Rubidium (Rb)
Calcium (Ca)	Lithium (Li)	Selenium (Se)
Chromium (Cr)	Magnesium (Mg)	Sodium (Na)
Cobalt (Co)	Manganese (Mn)	Strontium (Sr)
Copper (Cu)	Molybdenum (Mo)	Sulfur (S)
Germanium (Ge)	Phosphorus (P)	Vanadium (V)
Iodine (I)	Potassium (K)	Zinc (Zn)

2) Toxic Minerals

Aluminum (Al)	Cadmium (Cd)	Thallium (Tl)
Antimony (Sb)	Lead (Pb)	Thorium (Th)
Arsenic (As)	Mercury (Hg)	Tin (Sn)
Barium (Ba)	Nickel (Ni)	Titanium (Ti)
Beryllium (Be)	Platinum (Pt)	Uranium (U)
Bismuth (Bi)	Silver (Ag)	Zirconium (Zr)

Please contact a qualified health coach to obtain a hair test.

Aluminum

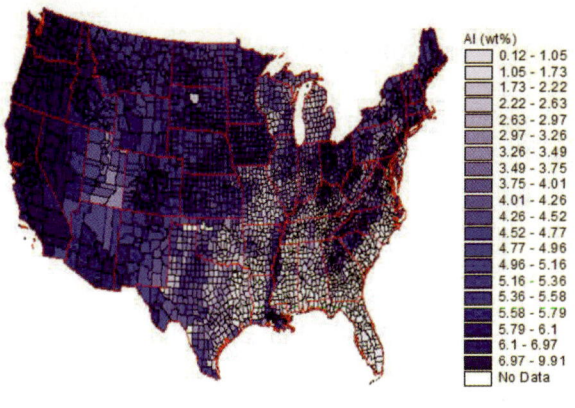

Aluminum is the most abundant metal in the earth's crust and widely distributed. It is used to make beverage cans, pots, pans, airplanes, siding, roofing, and foil. Powdered aluminum metal is used in explosives and fireworks. Aluminum compounds are used in many diverse and important industrial applications such as alums (aluminum sulfate) in water-treatment and alumina in abrasives and furnace linings.

Aluminum can be found in consumer products including:

Antacids
Antiperspirants

Astringents
Buffered aspirin

Cosmetics
Food additives

How can I be exposed to aluminum?

Food is the primary source of exposure. Unprocessed foods like fresh fruits, vegetables, and meat contain very little aluminum.

Aluminum compounds may be added during processing of foods, such as:

Anticaking agents
Baking powder
Coloring agents

Flour
Table salt

City water is sometimes treated with aluminum salts while it is processed to become drinking water for its "sparkling effects." People are exposed to aluminum in some cosmetics, antiperspirants, and pharmaceuticals such as antacids and buffered aspirin. Antacids have 300–600 milligrams aluminum hydroxide (approximately 104–208 milligrams of aluminum) per tablet, capsule, or 5-milliliter (mL) liquid dose. Buffered aspirin may contain 10–50 milligrams of aluminum per tablet. Vaccines may contain small amounts of aluminum compounds. An amount may enter through your skin when you are exposed to aluminum. Hopefully, most aluminum in food, water, and medicines leaves your body quickly in the feces.

How can aluminum affect my health?

Some workers who breathe aluminum-containing dusts or aluminum fumes have decreased performance in some tests that measure functions of the nervous system. Studies show that people exposed to high levels of aluminum may develop Alzheimer's disease. Some people who have kidney disease store a lot of aluminum in their bodies. The kidney disease causes less aluminum to be removed from the body in the urine. Sometimes, these people developed bone or brain diseases that doctors think were caused by the excess aluminum. Although aluminum containing over the counter oral products are considered safe in healthy individuals at recommended doses, some adverse effects have been observed following long-term use in some individuals. Studies in animals show that the nervous system is a sensitive target of aluminum toxicity. The animals did not perform as well in tests that measured the strength of their grip or how much they moved around.

How can aluminum affect children?

This section discusses potential health effects in humans from exposures during the period from conception to maturity at 18 years of age. Brain and bone disease caused by high levels of aluminum in the body have been seen in children with kidney disease. Bone disease has also been seen in children taking some medicines containing aluminum. In these children, the bone damage is caused by aluminum in the stomach preventing the absorption of phosphate, a chemical compound required for healthy bones.

Aluminum is found in breast milk. Small amounts of aluminum will enter the infant's body through breastfeeding. Typical aluminum concentrations in human breast milk are also found in soy-based infant formula and milk-based infant formula. Very young animals appeared weaker and less active in their cages and some movements appeared less coordinated when their mothers were exposed to large amounts of aluminum during pregnancy and while nursing. In addition, aluminum also affected the animal's memory. These effects are similar to those that have been seen in adults.

How can families reduce the risk of exposure to aluminum? It is hard to avoid exposure to aluminum because it is so common and widespread in the environment. Exposure to aluminum is naturally present in food, water, pots, and pans and in soil. Eating large amounts of processed food containing aluminum additives or frequently cooking acidic foods in aluminum pots may expose a person to higher levels than a person who generally consumes unprocessed foods and uses pots made of other materials (e.g., stainless steel or glass).

Limiting your intake of any quantities of aluminum-containing antacids and buffered aspirin and using these medications only as directed is the best way to limit exposure to aluminum from these sources. As a precaution, such products should have childproof caps or should be kept out of reach of children so that children will not accidentally ingest them. Aluminum is necessary for the human body but in the utmost small quanties found only through natural foods.

Food sources for aluminum:

Asparagus
Black bean
Black cherry
Butter bean
Carrot
Chickweed
Common-thyme
Cucumber
Devil's claw
Dwarf bean
Echinacea
Field bean
Flageolet bean
French bean
Garden bean
Garden-thyme
Gotu kola
Grape
Green bean
Haricot bean
Haricot vert
Honey buchu
Kidney bean
Lima bean
Mullein
Navy bean
Pea bean
Peach
Pennyroyal
Pop bean
Popping bean
Sassafras
Smooth sumac
Snap bean
String bean
Tomato
Wax bean
Wild cherry

ANTIMONY

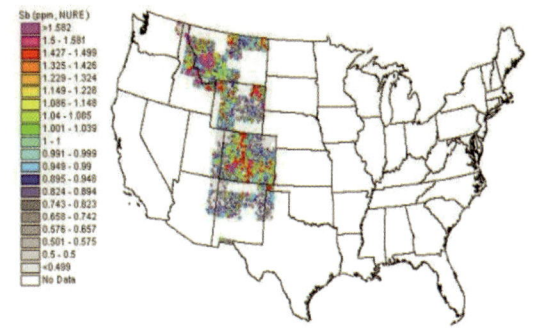

Antimony is a toxic metal and is released from plastic containers including bottled water.

Antimony is a silvery white metal of medium hardness that breaks easily. Small amounts of antimony are found in the earth's crust. Antimony oxide is a white powder that does not evaporate, but a small amount of it will dissolve in water and be absorbed in the body. Most antimony oxide produced is added to textiles and plastics to prevent their catching on fire.

Little or no antimony is mined in the United States. Antimony ore and impure metals are brought into this country from other countries for processing. Small amounts of antimony are also released into the environment by incinerators and coal-burning power plants.

How might I be exposed to antimony? You may be exposed to antimony by breathing air, drinking water, and eating foods that contain it. You also may be exposed by skin contact with soil, water, and other substances that contain antimony. Plastic water bottles are a constant source of antimony as they leach into the drinking water bottle. Food usually contains small amounts of antimony. You eat and drink about 5 micrograms (five millionths of a gram) of antimony every day. The average concentration of antimony in meats, vegetables, and seafood is 0.2–1.1 parts per billion.

How can antimony enter and leave my body? Antimony can enter your body when you drink water or eat food, soil, or other substances that contain antimony. Antimony can also enter your body if you breathe air or dust containing antimony. We do not know if antimony can enter your body when it is placed on your skin. A small amount of the antimony you eat or drink enters the blood after a few hours. The amount and the form of antimony in the food or water will affect how much antimony enters your blood. After you eat or drink very large doses of antimony, you may vomit. This will prevent most of the antimony from entering through the stomach and intestines into your blood. Antimony in your lungs will enter your blood after several days or weeks. After antimony enters your blood, it goes to many parts of your body. Most of the antimony goes to the liver, lungs, intestines, and spleen. The amount of antimony that will enter your blood from your lungs is not known; however, it will leave your body in feces and urine over several weeks.

How can antimony affect my health?

Exposure to antimony for a long time can irritate your eyes, skin, and lungs. Breathing antimony for a long time can cause problems with the lungs, heart problems, stomach pain, diarrhea, vomiting, and stomach ulcers. We do not know if antimony can cause cancer, birth defects or affect reproduction in humans. Antimony can have beneficial effects when used for medical reasons. It has been used as a medicine to treat people infected with parasites. Persons who have had too much of this medicine or are sensitive to it when it was injected into their blood or muscle have experienced adverse health effects like diarrhea, joint and/or muscle pain, vomiting, problems with anemia and heart problems showing up on electrocardiograms.

Foods that contain trace amounts of antimony:

Almond	Butternut	Pea bean
Asparagus bean	Cashew	Pecan
Black walnut	Coconut	Pistachio
Brazil nut	English filbert	Yardlong bean

Minerals & Human Health

ARSENIC

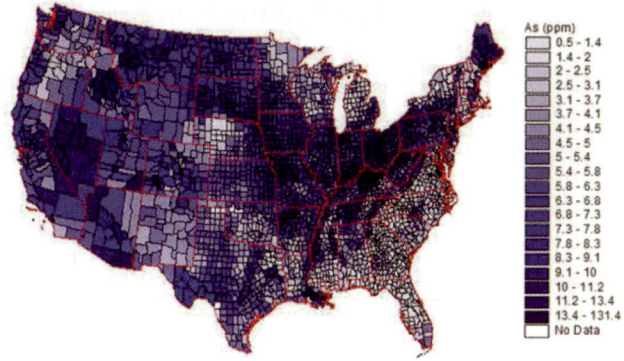

Arsenic is necessary. If measurable in the human body, you have too much. A naturally occurring element is widely distributed in the Earth's crust. Usually found in the environment combined with other elements such as oxygen, chlorine, and sulfur. Arsenic combined with these elements is called inorganic arsenic. When combined with carbon and hydrogen, it is referred to as organic arsenic. You usually cannot tell if arsenic is present in your food, water, or air.

In the past, inorganic arsenic compounds were predominantly used as pesticides, primarily on cotton fields and orchards. Inorganic arsenic compounds can no longer be used in agriculture; however, organic arsenic compounds, namely cacodylic acid, disodium methyl arsenate (DSMA), and monosodium methyl arsenate (MSMA), are still used as pesticides, primarily on cotton. Some organic arsenic compounds are used as additives in animal feed. Small quantities of elemental arsenic are added to other metals to form metal mixtures or alloys with improved properties. The greatest use of arsenic in alloys is in lead-acid batteries for automobiles. Another important use of arsenic compounds is in semiconductors and light-emitting diodes.

How might I be exposed to arsenic?

Since arsenic is found naturally in the environment, you will be exposed to some arsenic by eating food, drinking water, or breathing air. You normally take in small amounts of arsenic in the air you breathe, water you drink, and food you eat. Of these, food is usually the largest source of arsenic. The predominant dietary source of arsenic is seafood, followed by rice/rice cereal, mushrooms, and poultry. While seafood contains the greatest amounts of arsenic, fish, and shellfish, is mostly in an organic form of called arsenobetaine that is much less harmful. Some seaweeds may contain arsenic in inorganic forms that may be more harmful. Children are likely to eat small amounts of dust or soil each day, exposing them to arsenic.

How can arsenic enter and leave my body?

If you swallow arsenic in water, soil, or food, most of the arsenic may quickly enter your body. The amount that enters will depend on how much you swallow and the kind of arsenic you swallow. This is the most likely way for you to be exposed near a waste disposal site. If you breathe air that contains arsenic dust, many of the particles settle onto the lining of the lungs. Most of these particles are taken up from the lungs into the body. You might be exposed in this way near waste disposal sites where arsenic-contaminated soils are allowed to blow into the air, or if you work with arsenic-containing soil or products. If you get arsenic-contaminated soil or water on your skin, only a small amount will go through your skin into your body.

Both inorganic and organic forms leave your body in the urine. Most inorganic arsenic will be gone within several days, although some will remain in your body for several months or even longer. If exposed to organic arsenic, most of it will leave your body within several days.

How can arsenic affect my health?

Scientists use many tests to protect the public from harmful effects of toxic chemicals and to find ways for treating persons who have been harmed. Inorganic arsenic has been recognized as a human poison since ancient times, and large oral doses (above 60,000 parts per billion in water, which is 10,000 times higher than 80% of U.S. drinking water arsenic levels) can result in death. If you swallow lower levels of inorganic arsenic, you may experience irritation of your stomach and intestines, with symptoms such as stomach ache, nausea, vomiting, and diarrhea. Other effects you might experience from swallowing inorganic arsenic include decreased production of red and white blood cells, which may cause fatigue, abnormal heart rhythm, blood-vessel damage resulting in bruising, and impaired nerve function causing a "pins and needles" sensation in your hands and feet.

Perhaps the single-most characteristic effect of long-term oral exposure to inorganic arsenic is a pattern of skin changes. These include patches of darkened skin and the appearance of small "corns" or "warts" on the palms, soles, and torso, and are often associated with changes in the blood vessels of the skin. Skin cancer may also develop. Swallowing arsenic has also been reported to increase the risk of cancer in the liver, bladder, and lungs. The Department of Health and Human Services (DHHS) has determined that inorganic arsenic is known to be a human carcinogen (a chemical that causes cancer). The International Agency for Research on Cancer (IARC) and EPA has determined that inorganic arsenic is carcinogenic to humans.

How can arsenic affect children?

This section discusses potential health effects in humans from exposures during the period from conception to maturity at 18 years of age. Children are exposed to arsenic in many of the same ways that adults are. Since arsenic is found in the soil, water, food, and air, children may take in arsenic in the air they breathe, the water they drink, and the food they eat. Since children tend to eat or drink less of a variety of foods and beverages than do adults, ingestion of contaminated food or juice or infant formula made with arsenic-contaminated water may represent a significant source of exposure. In addition, since children often play in the soil, put their hands in their mouths, and sometimes intentionally eat soil, ingestion of contaminated soil may be a more important source of arsenic exposure for children than for adults. In areas of the United States where natural levels of arsenic in the soil and water are high, or in areas in and around contaminated waste sites, exposure of children to arsenic through ingestion of soil and water may be significant. In addition, contact with adults who are wearing clothes contaminated with arsenic (e.g., with dust from copper- or lead-smelting factories, from wood-treating or pesticide application, or from arsenic-treated wood) could be a source of exposure. Because of the tendency of children to taste things that they find, accidental poisoning from ingestion of pesticides is also a possibility. Although most of the exposure pathways for children are the same as those for adults, children may be at a higher risk of exposure because of normal hand-to-mouth activity.

Children who are exposed to inorganic arsenic may have many of the same effects as adults, including irritation of the stomach and intestines, blood vessel damage, skin changes, and reduced nerve function. Thus, all health effects observed in adults are of potential concern in children. There is also some evidence that suggests that long-term exposure to inorganic arsenic in children may result in lower IQ scores. We do not know if absorption of inorganic arsenic from the gut in children differs from adults. There is some evidence that exposure to arsenic in early life (including gestation and early childhood) may increase mortality in young adults.

There is some evidence that inhaled or ingested inorganic arsenic can injure pregnant women or their unborn babies, although the studies are not definitive. Studies in animals show large doses of inorganic arsenic-causing illness in pregnant females can also cause low birth weight, fetal malformations, and even fetal death. Arsenic can cross the placenta between mother and child and has been found in fetal tissues. Arsenic is found at low levels in breast milk.

Animals exposed to organic arsenic compounds can also cause low birth weight, fetal malformations, and fetal deaths. The dose levels that cause these effects also result in effects in the mothers.

Cancer: Arsenic has been associated with certain types of skin cancer. Some studies also show a possible link with lung, bladder, liver, colon, and kidney cancers.

Plants that contain trace amounts of arsenic are listed from the most to least amounts:

Antler herb	Ginseng	Orange
Apple	Grape	Parsley
Banana	Grapefruit	Plum
Bladderwrack	Hawthorn	Potato
Broadbean	Horsetail	Red currant
Carrot	Irish moss	Rice
Clubmoss	Kelp	Safflower
Corn	Knotweed	Skullcap
Cucumber	Kudzu	Spinach
Dogwood	Lettuce	Tangerine
Dulse	Licorice	Water lotus
Faba bean	Magnolia vine	White currant
Ginger	Mulberry	Wolfberry

BARIUM

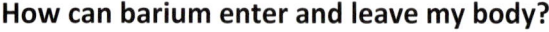

Barium should not be detectable in the body.

Barium is a silvery-white metal that takes on a silver-yellow color when exposed to air, occurring in nature as many different forms called compounds.

How might I be exposed to barium?

Background levels of barium in the environment are very low. The air that most people breathe contains about 0.0015 parts of barium per billion parts of air. The highest amount measured from water wells has been 10 parts per million. The amount of barium found in soil ranges from about 15 to 3,500 parts per million. Some foods, such as Brazil nuts, seaweed, fish, and certain plants, may contain high amounts of barium. The amount in food and water usually is not high enough to be a health concern. However, information is still being collected to determine if long-term exposure to low levels of barium causes any health problems.

How can barium enter and leave my body?

Barium enters your body when you breathe air, eat food, or drink water containing barium. It may also enter your body to a small extent when you have direct skin contact with barium compounds. The amount of barium that enters the bloodstream after you breathe, eat, or drink depends on the barium compound and is removed mainly in feces and urine. Most barium that enters your body is removed within 1–2 weeks, while the small amount of that stays in your body is mainly found in the bones and teeth.

How can barium affect my health?

The health effects associated with exposure to different barium compounds depend on how well the specific barium compound dissolves in water or in the stomach. For example, barium sulfate does not easily dissolve in water and causes few harmful health effects. Doctors sometimes give barium sulfate orally or by placing it directly in the rectum of patients for purposes of making x-rays of the stomach or intestines. The use of this particular barium compound in this type of medical test is not harmful to people.

Eating or drinking very large amounts of barium compounds that dissolve in water or in the stomach can cause changes in heart rhythm or paralysis in humans. Some people who did not seek medical treatment soon after eating or drinking a very large amount of barium have died. After eating or drinking somewhat smaller amounts of barium for a short period of time, you may experience vomiting, abdominal cramps, diarrhea, difficulties in breathing, increased or decreased blood pressure, numbness around the face, and muscle weakness. One study showed that people who drank water containing as much as 10 ppm of barium for 4 weeks did not have increased blood pressure or abnormal heart rhythms.

The health effects of barium have been studied more often in experimental animals than in humans. Rats that ate or drank barium over short periods had swelling and irritation of the intestines, changes in organ weights, decreased body weight, and increased numbers of deaths. Rats and mice that drank barium over long periods had damage to the kidneys, decreases in body weight, and decreased survival. We have no information about the ability of barium to affect reproduction in humans; a study in experimental animals did not find reproductive effects.

Some studies of humans and experimental animals exposed to barium in the air report damage to the lungs, other studies have not found these effects. We have no reliable information about the health effects in humans or experimental animals that are exposed to barium by direct skin contact.

Barium has not been shown to cause cancer in humans or in experimental animals drinking it in water. The Department of Health and Human Services (DHHS) and the International Agency for Research on Cancer (IARC) have not classified barium as to its carcinogenicity. The EPA has determined that barium is not likely to be carcinogenic to humans following ingestion and there is insufficient information to determine whether it will be carcinogenic to humans following inhalation exposure.

Listed below are 50 foods that contain trace amounts of barium:

Allspice	Cone pepper	Mugwort
Almond	Corn	Muskmelon
American persimmon	Cucumber	Navy bean
Apple	Dandelion	Orange
Asparagus	Dwarf bean	Paprika
Asparagus bean	Dwarf sumac	Pea bean
Beet	Eggplant	Pear
Beetroot	Endive	Pecan
Bell pepper	Field bean	Pistachio
Black bean	Filbert	Plum
Black cherry	Flageolet bean	Potato
Black walnut	French bean	Red cabbage
Brazil nut	Garden bean	Sassafras
Butterbur	Garden beet	Sassafras
Butternut	Grape	Smooth sumac
Cabbage	Grapefruit	Soybean
Cantaloupe	Green bean	Sugar beet
Carrot	Green pepper	Sweet pepper
Cashew	Haricot	Sweetgum
Cherry pepper	Haricot bean	Tomato
Chinese cabbage	Haricot vert	White cabbage
Cinnamon	Japanese cinnamon	Wild cherry
Clover	Kidney bean	Willow oak
Coca	Lettuce	Winged sumac
Coconut	Melon	Yardlong bean

BORON

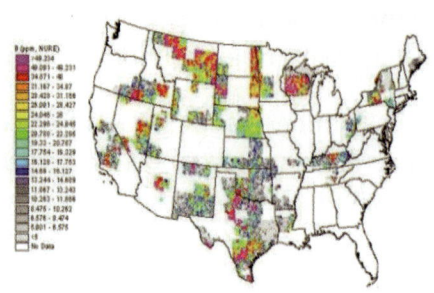

Gay-Lussac, Thenard, and Davy discovered boron in 1808. It is element number 8 on the atomic periodic table. Boron, a trace mineral, was recognized as an essential micronutrient for human consumption in the 1980s, known to be essential for plants since the early 1900s. Recent research is showing that it plays a critical role in metabolism and bone health.

Boron exerts an influence on cellular response to hormones. It seems to modulate cell signaling by assisting in transmembrane ion movement. Boron is found in the front part of the brain.

Boron plays an important role in the metabolism of calcium and magnesium, also a regulator effect of estrogens and testosterone production within the body. The synthesis of estrogens and testosterone require hydroxylation, a biochemical process adding hydroxide (OH) groups to precursor substances.

There seems to be many ways that boron has an influence on bone health, by reducing urinary calcium loss. One study showed a 44% reduction in urinary excretion of calcium when boron supplementation was given to boron-deficient women. Boron may also have an effect on the synthesis of vitamin D. Another study showed an increased incidence of osteoarthritis in areas with low boron levels in the soil.

Other Facts:

Meat and fish are poor sources of boron. Fruits and vegetables need to be grown in soil with adequate amounts of boron. Water core of an apple is a boron deficiency.

Boron promotes:

Cellular response to hormones
Metabolism of calcium
Metabolism of magnesium

Bone health
Healthy teeth

Boron protects against:

Abnormal estrogen metabolism
Abnormal testosterone metabolism

Urinary calcium loss
Urinary magnesium loss

No drugs have been identified to deplete boron. Boron is a mineral, cannot be destroyed, is not depleted by cooking, and is found in most fruits, vegetables, and nuts. No foods are known to be fortified with Boron.

Recommended dietary allowance:

There is no set recommended daily allowance for boron. Usual dose to correct deficiency is 1 to 9 milligrams a day.

Infants
Ages 0.0-0.5: breast milk only

Ages .5 thru 1.0: 3milligrams is the upper limit

Children
Ages 1-3: 3milligrams is the upper limit

Ages 4 thru 8: 6 milligrams is the upper limit

Males and females
Ages 9 thru 13: 11milligrams is the upper limit

Ages 19 thru 90: 20 milligrams is the upper limit

Ages 14 thru 18: 17 milligrams is the upper limit

Pregnant - There is no recommended daily allowance for boron.

Breast feeding – Lactating - There is no recommended daily allowance for boron.

Toxic doses: The average South Korean resident ingests 45 milligrams a day. No adverse side effects have been reported with dietary intake up to 41 milligrams a day. Larger amounts have caused nausea, vomiting, diarrhea, skin rashes, and fatigue.

Food sources for boron:

American persimmon	Dandelion	Red cabbage
Apple	Dill	Red currant
Apricot	Fig	Red mangrove
Asparagus	Ginseng	Rutabaga
Asparagus bean	Grape	Sour cherry
Beet	Lamb's lettuce	Strawberry
Beetroot	Lettuce	Sugar beet
Black cherry	Marjoram	Sweet marjoram
Black currant	Parsley	Sweetgum
Brussels sprouts	Pea bean	Tomato
Cauliflower	Peach	White cabbage
Celery	Pear	White currant
Coca	Plum	Wild Cherry
Corn salad	Poppyseed	Yardlong bean
Cumin	Radish	

Bromine

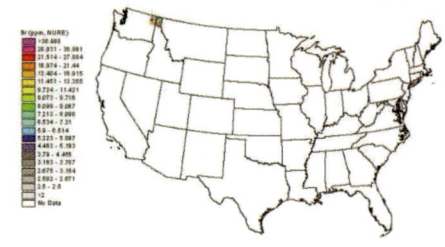

Bromine is a naturally occurring element that is a liquid at room temperature. It has a brownish-red color with a bleach-like odor, and it dissolves in water. Bromine is found naturally in the earth's crust and seawater in various forms. Bromine can also be found as an alternative to chlorine in swimming pools. Products containing bromine are used in agriculture, sanitation, and fire retardants (chemicals that help prevent things from catching fire). Some bromine-containing compounds were historically used as sedatives (drugs that can make people calm or sleepy). However, these drugs for the most part are no longer for sale in the United States.

Following the release of bromine into water, you could be exposed by drinking or eating contaminated water or food. Following release of bromine gas into the air, you could be exposed by breathing the fumes. Skin exposure to bromine could occur through direct contact with bromine liquid or gas. Bromine gas is heavier than air, so it would settle in low-lying areas.

Exposure to bromine is by directly irritating the skin, mucous membranes, and tissues. The seriousness of poisoning caused by bromine depends on the amount, route, and length of time of exposure, as well as the age and preexisting medical condition of the person exposed.

Immediate signs and symptoms of exposure to bromine are having a cough, having trouble breathing, headache, having irritation of your mucous membranes (inside your mouth, nose, etc.), dizzy, or watery eyes. Getting bromine liquid or gas on your skin could cause skin irritation and burns. Liquid bromine that touches your skin may first cause a cooling sensation that is closely followed by a burning feeling.

Swallowing bromine-containing compounds (combinations of bromine with other chemicals) would cause different effects depending on the compound. Swallowing a large amount of bromine in a short period would likely cause nausea and vomiting (gastrointestinal symptoms).

Survivors of serious poisoning caused by breathing in bromine may have long-term lung problems. People who survive serious bromine poisoning may also have long-term effects from damage done by what is called systemic poisoning, for example, kidney or brain damage from low blood pressure.

Protective and preventive exposure steps to take:

Protect yourself from exposure by avoiding bread, soda pop, bedding, and household furniture that contains bromine. If the bromine release was indoors, get out of the building. If you are near a release of bromine, emergency coordinators may tell you to either leave the area or to "shelter in place" (stay where you are) inside a building to avoid being exposed to the chemical. If you think you may have been exposed to bromine, you should remove your clothing, rapidly wash your entire body with soap and water, and get medical care as quickly as possible.

As you take off clothing that may have bromine on it, any clothing that has to be pulled over your head should be cut off your body instead of being pulled over your head. If you are helping other people remove their clothing, try to avoid touching any contaminated areas, and remove the clothing as quickly as possible. As fast as possible, wash any bromine from your skin with large amounts of soap and water. Washing with soap and water will help avoid further chemicals from harming your body. If your eyes are burning or your vision is blurred, rinse your eyes with plain water for 10 to 15 minutes. If you wear contacts, remove them and put them with the contaminated clothing. Do not put the contacts back in your eyes (even if they are not disposable contacts). If you wear eyeglasses, wash them with soap and water. You can put your eyeglasses back on after you wash them.

After you have washed yourself, place your clothing inside a plastic bag. Avoid touching contaminated areas of the clothing. If you cannot avoid touching contaminated areas, or you are not sure where the contaminated areas are, wear rubber gloves or put the clothing in the bag using tongs, tool handles, sticks, or similar objects. Anything that touches the contaminated clothing should also be placed in the bag. If you wear contacts, put them in the plastic bag, too. Seal the bag, and then seal that bag inside another plastic bag. Disposing of your clothing in this way will help protect you and other people from any chemicals that might be on your clothes. When the local or state health department or emergency personnel arrive, tell them what you did with your clothes. The health department or emergency personnel will arrange for further disposal.

Foods that contain bromine:

Almond	Field bean	Pea
Banana	Flageolet bean	Pistachio
Beet	French bean	Pop bean
Beetroot	Garden bean	Popping bean
Bell pepper	Garden beet	Potato
Black bean	Giant knotweed	Red cabbage
Bladderwrack	Green pepper	Rhubarb
Brazil nut	Haricot vert	Snap bean
Butterbur	Haricot bean	Stinging nettle
Cabbage	Horseradish	String bean
Carrot	Kelp	Sugar beet
Cherry pepper	Kidney bean	Sweet pepper
Cinnamon	Mugwort	
Cone pepper	Navy bean	White cabbage
Dandelion	Onion	
Dill	Paprika	Wax bean
Dwarf bean	Parsley	

CADMIUM

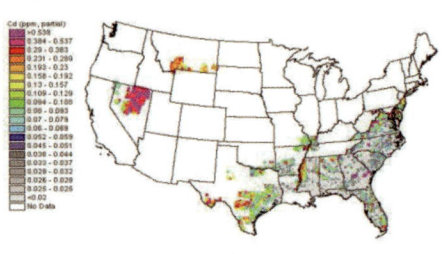

Description - Metal found in the earth's crust, associated with zinc, lead, and copper ores.

Cadmium is used for the following:

1) Batteries (83%)
2) Pigments (8%)
3) Coatings and platings (7%)
4) Stabilizers for plastics (1.2%)
5) Nonferrous alloys, photovoltaic devices, and other uses (0.8%)

What happens to cadmium when it enters the environment?

Cadmium is emitted to soil, water, and air by non-ferrous metal mining and refining, manufacture and application of phosphate fertilizers, fossil fuel combustion, and waste incineration and disposal. Cadmium can accumulate in aquatic organisms and agricultural crops. Cadmium and its compounds may travel through soil, but its mobility depends on several factors such as pH and amount of organic matter, which will vary depending on the local environment. Generally, cadmium binds strongly to organic matter where it will be immobile in soil and be taken up by plant life, eventually, entering the food supply.

How might I be exposed to cadmium? Food and smoking-primary source of exposure. In the United States, for nonsmokers the primary source of cadmium exposure is from the food supply. In general, leafy vegetables such as lettuce and spinach, potatoes and grains, peanuts, soybeans, and sunflower seeds contain high levels of cadmium, approximately 0.05- 0.12 mg cadmium/kg. Tobacco leaves accumulate high levels of cadmium from the soil.

Elevated cadmium levels in water sources in the vicinity of cadmium emitting industries (historical and current) have been reported. Aquatic organisms will accumulate cadmium, possibly entering the food supply. People who fish in local waters as a means of food should be cautious and abide by any advisories.

How can cadmium enter and leave my body?

1) Inhalation, about 5-50% of the cadmium you breathe will enter your body through your lungs.

2) Ingestion, A small amount of the cadmium in food and water (about 1-10%) will enter your body through the digestive tract. If you do not have enough iron or other nutrients in your diet, you are likely to take up more cadmium from your food than usual.

3) Skin contact, virtually no cadmium enters your body through your skin.

Leave your body, most of the cadmium that enters your body goes to your kidney and liver and can remain there for many years. A small portion of the cadmium that enters your body leaves slowly in urine and feces. Your body can change most cadmium to a form that is not harmful, but too much cadmium can overload the ability of your liver and kidney to change the cadmium to a harmless form.

How can cadmium affect my health?

Breathing air with very high levels of cadmium can severely damage the lungs and may cause death. Breathing air with lower levels of cadmium over long periods of time (for years) results in a build-up of cadmium in the kidney, and if sufficiently high, may result in kidney disease.

Eating food or drinking water with very high cadmium levels severely irritates the stomach, leading to vomiting and diarrhea, and sometimes death. Eating lower levels of cadmium over a long period of time can lead to a build-up of cadmium in the kidneys. If the build-up of cadmium is high enough, it will damage the kidneys. Exposure to lower levels of cadmium for a long time can also cause bones to become fragile and break easily. Kidney and bone effects have also been observed in laboratory animals ingesting cadmium. Anemia, liver disease, and nerve or brain damage have been observed in animals eating or drinking cadmium. We have no good information on people to indicate what cadmium levels people would need to eat or drink to result in these diseases, or if they would occur at all.

Lung cancer has been found in some studies of workers exposed to cadmium in the air and studies of rats that breathed in cadmium. The U.S. Department of Health and Human Services (DHHS) has determined that cadmium and cadmium compounds are known human carcinogens. The International Agency for Research on Cancer (IARC) has determined that cadmium is carcinogenic to humans. The EPA has determined that cadmium is a probable human carcinogen.

How can cadmium affect children? The health effects seen in children from exposure to toxic levels of cadmium are expected to be similar to the effects seen in adults (kidney and lung damage). Harmful effects on child development or behavior have not generally been seen in populations exposed to cadmium, but more research is needed. A few studies in animals indicate that younger animals absorb more cadmium than adults. Animal studies also indicate that the young are more susceptible than adults to a loss of bone and decreased bone strength from exposure to cadmium. Cadmium is found in breast milk and a small amount will enter the infant's body through breastfeeding. The amount of cadmium that can pass to the infant depends on how much exposure the mother may have had.

In birth defects, studies in animals exposed to high enough levels of cadmium during pregnancy have resulted in harmful effects in the young. The nervous system appears to be the most sensitive target. Young animals exposed to cadmium before birth have shown effects on behavior and learning. There is also some information from animal studies that high enough exposures to cadmium before birth can reduce body weights and affect the skeleton in the developing young.

How can families reduce the risk of exposure to cadmium? Do not smoke tobacco products, cadmium accumulates in tobacco leaves. The national geometric mean blood cadmium level for adults is 0.376 µg/L. Mean blood cadmium levels for heavy smokers have been reported as high as 1.58 µg/L. Children can be exposed to cadmium through parents who work in cadmium-emitting industries. Therefore, good hygiene practices such as bathing and changing clothes before returning home may help reduce the cadmium transported from the job to the home.

Avoid cadmium contaminated areas and food.

Detecting exposure

Cadmium can be measured in blood, urine, hair, or nails. Urinary cadmium has been shown to accurately reflect the amount of cadmium in the body. The amount of cadmium in your blood shows your recent exposure to cadmium. The amount of cadmium in your urine shows both your recent and your past exposure. Cadmium levels in hair or nails are not as useful as an indication of when or how much cadmium you may have taken in, partly because cadmium from outside of your body may attach to the hair or nails.

CALCIUM

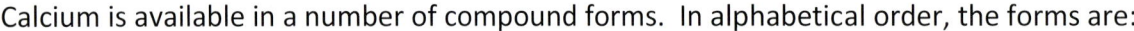

Humphrey Davy discovered the element calcium in 1808 when he separated it from a salt. It is element number 20 on the atomic periodic table.

An essential macronutrient, it is the most abundant mineral in the body and 99% of it is in the bones and teeth. The rest is in the cells and body fluids. It is estimated the average adult has between 2 and 3 pounds calcium in their body. It is the fifth most common substance found in humans. This crystalline compound gives bones and teeth rigidity and strength.

Calcium is available in a number of compound forms. In alphabetical order, the forms are:

Calcium ascorbate
Calcium aspartate
Calcium carbonate
Calcium citrate
Calcium glycinate
Calcium lactate
Calcium maleate
Calcium phosphate

Calcium promotes:

Colon health
Healthy blood
Normal blood clotting
Normal muscle contractions
Normal nerve transmissions
Strong bones
Strong teeth
Vitamin D metabolism

Calcium protects against:

Blood vessel stiffness
Bowel inflammation
Brittle nails
Colon dysfunction
Cramps
Diarrhea
Indigestion
Insomnia
Irregular heartbeat
Muscle injury
Osteoporosis
Periodontal disease
PMS symptoms
Weak bones

Deficiency symptoms: The soft bones and teeth of Ricketts is the most often seen calcium deficiency disease in children and are closely associated with vitamin D deficiency. Osteoporosis and osteomalacia are the maladies caused by calcium deficiency in adults. Calcium depletion should be considered in persons with complaints of muscle twitching and cramps and symptomatic blood pressure elevations such as headache and dizziness.

Symptoms of calcium deficiency include:

Back and leg pain
Insomnia
Headaches (tension type)
Heart palpitations
High blood pressure
Muscle cramps
Tooth decay

A lack of exercise can decrease calcium absorption. Inflammatory bowel disease can interfere with the assimilation of calcium into the body.

Drugs that deplete: Caffeine is the most widely used drug that can reduce calcium. High doses of magnesium, phosphorous and zinc can prompt excessive urinary excretion and thus depletion. Alcohol, rightly so a drug, depletes calcium. It will leach calcium from the bones. Some antibiotics, anti-seizure medications, diuretics, and steroids can cause depletion. Mineral oil can interfere with calcium absorption and should be dosed if prescribed at a time 1/2 hour before or 2 hours after calcium supplementation or a meal.

Function in the body: The time of greatest need for consistent, adequate amounts of calcium in the diet is during times of rapid growth as in childhood, pregnancy, and lactation to ensure healthy development and maintenance of bones and teeth. Calcium metabolism is dependent on many other substances. The presence of vitamin D in the form of calciferol is vital for calcium to be absorbed from the intestines. One study looking at calcium supplementation and increases in bone density found when given with vitamins and other minerals, absorption increased almost three times over just calcium supplementation alone. This needs to be a consideration in the treatment of osteoporosis.

Three regulatory mechanisms control serum calcium, the blood calcium level. This is very tightly controlled in a very narrow range controlled by the kidneys.

Low levels of calcium can cause hypertension by decreasing the vasodilatory response of blood vessels. This is the type of hypertension effectively treated by calcium supplements and checking a serum calcium level on newly diagnosed hypertension is an important part of the initial workup. Calcium supplementation may help but is not a recommended treatment for other forms of hypertension.

Calcium plays a vital role in the muscle contraction-relaxation cycle. The most important muscle in the body, the heart, is dependent on calcium for healthy functioning. Calcium regulates cell wall permeability and the passage of fluids through cell membranes.

Calcium activates enzymes involved in fat digestion and protein metabolism. A recent study showed a decrease in rates of obesity in persons taking calcium supplements on a regular basis.

Other facts: Phosphorous displaces calcium. It increases urinary calcium excretion. As serum, calcium levels go down because of this, calcium is leached from bones and teeth eventually weakening them. The number one source of phosphorous in the American diet is carbonated soft drinks also known as phosphinated sodas. Animal protein is a lesser source of phosphorous.

Cow's milk is the number one dietary source for calcium in the U.S. Many people suffer a food allergy to bovine milk proteins due to the 7-beta-casomorphin that is in about 50% of American dairy cows. This is frequently unrecognized. If digestive difficulties are thought to be dairy related, it is also a lactose intolerance problem. In those where allergy to the protein is identified, other sources of dietary calcium need to be sought perhaps along with supplementation as well. This is also true for those with lactose intolerance who find the altered "lactose reduced" products unacceptable. Another consideration in the appropriateness of cow's milk as a source of calcium is that of an enzyme, bovine xanthine oxidase, which can cause damage to arterial membranes. Antibodies to this enzyme have been found in the blood of people with atherosclerosis. Pasteurized milk measures the absence of the enzyme alkaline phosphatase to consider milk successfully pasteurized. This very enzyme is need for calcium absorption, therefore raw milk is recommended over store bought, pasteurized milk. Whatever the reason for avoidance of dairy products in the diet, appropriate calcium supplementation needs to be taken.

Calcium is a macro mineral, as is magnesium, and the amount needed by the body per day is much higher than the micro minerals, such as copper and zinc. As such, the macro minerals can interfere with the absorption of the micro minerals. The bulk of the macro minerals are probably best taken at a time separate from any micro mineral supplementation that has been recommended.

Recommended daily allowance: For more than fifty years, nutrition experts have produced a set of nutrient and energy standards known as the Recommended Daily Allowances (RDA). A major revision is currently underway to replace the RDA. The revised recommendations are called Dietary Reference Intakes (DRI) and reflect the collaborative efforts of the U.S. and Canada. Until 1997, the RDA was the only standards available and they continue to serve health care professionals until the DRI can be established for all nutrients.

1997 Dietary Reference Intakes (DRI): IOM Committee on Dietary Reference Intakes:

Age (YRS) Amount in milligrams

Infants
Ages 0.0 thru 0.5: 210 milligrams/day
Ages 0.5 thru 1: 270 milligrams/day

Children
Ages 1 thru 3: 500 milligrams/day
Ages 4 thru 8: 800 milligrams/day

Females and males
Ages 9 thru 13: 1300 milligrams/day
Ages 31 thru 50: 1000 milligrams/day
Ages 14 thru 18: 1300 milligrams/day
Ages 51 thru 70: 1200 milligrams/day
Ages 19 thru 30: 1000 milligrams/day
Ages over 71: 1200 milligrams/day

Toxic doses: Doses of calcium larger than 1500-2000mg a day are not readily absorbed and usually excreted by the kidneys. In some cases, this excretion may cause excess accumulation in the soft tissues and interfere with the absorption of copper, iron, magnesium, and zinc.

Food cannot grow without calcium so all the foods in the world could be listed!

Foods that contain calcium:

- Barberry
- Basil
- Black bean
- Black cherry
- Bladderwrack
- Butterbur
- Cauliflower
- Celery
- Chicory
- Collard
- Crampbark
- Dandelion
- Dill
- Dwarf bean
- Field bean
- Flageolet bean
- French bean
- Garden bean
- Green bean
- Haricot
- Haricot vert
- Haricot bean
- Horsetail
- Irish moss
- Kelp
- Kidney bean
- Lettuce
- Licorice
- Mango
- Mulberry
- Navy bean
- Neem
- Oregano
- Papaya
- Pau D'Arco
- Pop bean
- Popping bean
- Radish
- Rhubarb
- Snap bean
- Stinging nettle
- String bean
- Sweet marjoram
- Thyme
- Tomato
- Vanilla
- Watercress
- Wax bean
- Wild cherry
- Wolfberry

CHLORINE

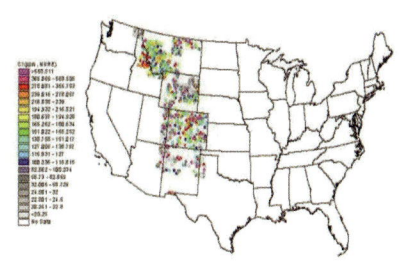

Karl Scheele discovered chlorine in 1774, but believed it to be an oxide of another yet to be discovered element. Humphrey Davy recognized the elemental quality of this halogen in 1810.

Chloride composes about 3% of the total body mineral content. It is one of the main ions balancing osmotic pressure in body fluids. Chloride, potassium, and sodium are the body's three major electrolytes. These particles are called electrolytes as they have an electronic charge. They are found in the body's fluids both intracellularly (within cells) and extracellularly (outside of cells) as fully dissociated ions. The solubility and enhancement of bioavailability of proteins and other substances is influenced by their ionic strength.

Chloride, like the other electrolytes, is absorbed easily when present throughout the intestinal tract. It is then controlled in its activity by hormonal communication primarily from the adrenal cortex and the anterior pituitary. The kidneys excrete chloride.

Deficiency symptoms: Chloride deficiency in America is rare due to the ease of availability and widespread use of salt (NaCl) in the diet of most people. Deficiency can cause nausea, vomiting, and diarrhea. These gastrointestinal disturbances can also cause chloride depletion if protracted and left unchecked.

Excessive sweating and exposure to high altitudes can cause chloride depletion. Replacing electrolytes promptly and frequently in those situations is very important to avoid serious disturbances in fluid homeostasis.

Other causes of chloride deficiency include adrenal insufficiency, systemic acidosis (low pH) which can occur for a variety of reasons, and long-term use of diuretics with neither unchecked nor replaced excessive electrolyte loss. Acid/base pH imbalances can occur, the effect of these maladies.

Chloride promotes:
Energy production
Excretion of metabolic waste
Fluid balance
Normal digestion
Normal nerve transmission
Normal water distribution
PH balance

Chloride protects against:
Fatigue
Muscle weakness
Palpitations
Stomach problems
Swelling

There is no recommended daily allowance for chloride, but 1 gram a day is adequate.

Drugs that deplete: Diuretics (water pills) can deplete chloride in persons that are sensitive to these losses, or excessive use and abuse with serum electrolyte evaluations and replacement.

Food preparation to retain chlorine: Heat does not destroy or alter the molecular structure of chloride found predominantly in sodium chloride (table salt). Processed foods contain large amounts of chloride. Excessively salting one's food does the same.

Function in the body: Chloride ions are dispersed through the fluids of the body. Between 80-90% are maintained in the extracellular (outside cells) fluids where the primary anion function occurs. This function, along with sodium and potassium, maintains normal osmotic equilibrium. This result in water being properly distributed and this balance maintained in the body. The extracellular fluids include blood, lymph, and fluids between cells. The rest of the chloride is in the intracellular (inside the cells) fluids.

Chloride ions play a significant role in the excretion of carbon dioxide (CO_2) waste from metabolic energy production in each cell. A chloride-bicarbonate interaction allows plasma to transport CO_2 as bicarbonate to the lungs to be expired.

Normal nerve transmission and muscle contractility and relaxation are dependent on chloride along with the other electrolytes as well as calcium and magnesium.

Acid/base pH balance in the body is maintained primarily by chloride along with phosphate and sulfate. This is tightly regulated as a slight shift to acidic or the opposite alkaline state can greatly impede system functions.

Chloride is necessary to maintain normal digestion. Adequate amounts of gastric hydrochloric acid keep the proper acidity in the stomach that is needed to break down the food ingested to the smallest macronutrient molecules for healthy nutrition. Most people diagnosed as having acid reflux actually are low in hydrochloric acid. This occurs because the already low stomach acid does not break down food fast enough, leading to fermentation in the stomach and a different acid created which gives the reflux of acid feeling. Suppressing acid reflux with antacids further increases the need for normal stomach acid. There will be symptom relief taking antacids, but the problem will be like riding a roller coaster up and down with symptoms. Using more hydrochloric acid in supplement form can properly fix the problem. In addition, minerals need strong stomach acid to be properly absorbed. Long-term antacid use will lead to mineral deficiencies because of inabilities to absorb without proper stomach acid.

Other facts: Hypochlorhydria is a state of low gastric hydrochloric acid levels from inadequate secretion of gastric acid by the parietal cells in the stomach wall. It is an undervalued, under recognized clinical component of many digestion related health disorders. These disorders may not necessarily manifest with symptoms in the gastrointestinal tract but will still be at the root of some neuron, immunological and metabolic syndromes. Hypochlorhydria is much more common today than thirty years ago.

Recommended daily allowance: There is no RDA any DRI (dietary reference intake) for chloride but it is estimated that the average healthy adult can safely consume from 1.5 to 5 grams per day on a regular basis.

Toxic doses: Chloride is so efficiently excreted by the kidneys that accumulations to toxic levels are unknown.

Food sources: Table salt (sodium chloride, NaCl) is the primary source of chloride in the American diet and mostly throughout the world.

Foods that contain chlorine:

Almond	Butternut	Date palm
Asparagus	Cashew	Eggplant
Bean	Chaparral	English filbert
Banana	Chickweed	Faba bean
Black pepper	Cinnamon	Flax
Brazil nut	Coconut	Habas
Broadbean	Corn	Lentil
Buckwheat	Dandelion	Lettuce
Butterbur		

Linseed	Pineapple	Tomato
Mango	Pistachio	Walnut
Mugwort	Potato	Wheat
Mungbean	Red currant	White currant
Oats	Soybean	White pepper
Orange	Spinach	Yardlong bean
Pea	Stinging nettle	
Pea bean	Sweet potato	
Pecan	Tangerine	

CHROMIUM

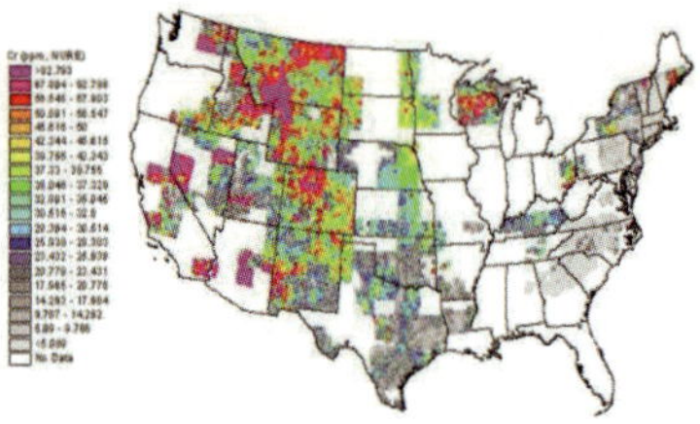

Chromium is a metal that was discovered by Vanquelin in 1790. It is number 24 on the atomic periodic table.

Chromium, an essential trace mineral, plays an important role in the effectiveness of insulin (blood sugar levels). The average healthy adult has only 4-6 milligrams in their body. It is estimated that it is very frequently deficient in the American diet. Chromium is notorious for its poor absorption into the body. It is estimated that 90% of the U.S. population consumes less than adequate amounts of chromium. In addition, high sugar consumption can lead to chromium deficiency because sugar raises serum chromium levels, pulling it from other tissues in the body. This prompts the kidneys to excrete the excess and if this is repeated and sustained, deficiency results, particularly when intake does not keep up with output.

Chromium is only active in the body in a trivalent state with which it can combine with other organic compounds. Trivalent chromium combines with vitamin B_3, glycine, glutamic acid and cysteine to form glucose tolerance factor (GTF) identified as chromium III dinicotinic acid-glutathione complex.

Chromium is available in a number of compounds listed below:

Chromium chloride
Chromium enriched nutritional yeast
Chromium picolinate
Chromium polynicotin

Chromium promotes:

Balanced lean tissue to fat ratio
Decreased cortisol levels
Increased immunoglobulins
Normal blood sugar
Normal cholesterol
Normal glucose tolerance
Normal triglycerides

Chromium protects against:

Abnormal lipid levels
Central obesity
Depressed mood
Insulin resistance

Deficiency symptoms: The effects of chromium deficiency can produce the symptoms of insulin resistance including glucose intolerance, elevated blood sugar levels, and numbness and tingling in the extremities, and/or disturbances of protein and lipid metabolism. Sustained low levels of chromium have been associated with cardiovascular disease.

Food preparation to retain chromium: Refined and processed foods are low in chromium. Cooking acidic food in stainless steel cookware increases chromium content.

Food sources of chromium:

Barberry	Catnip	Dulse
Barley	Chickweed	Echinacea
Bayberry	Cilantro	Feverfew
Bearberry	Cinnamon	Garlic
Black cohosh	Coriander	Ginger
Blessed thistle	Dandelion	Ginseng
Blue cohosh	Devil's claw	Gotu kola
	Grapple plant	

Great burdock	Mullein	Smooth sumac
Horsetail	Nutmeg	Sorrel
Irish moss	Oats	Stevia
Juniper	Peach	Thyme
Lemongrass	Poppyseed poppy	Valerian
Lettuce	Pumpkin	Wheatgrass
Licorice	Raspberry	White mustard
Marshmallow	Red clover	Wild yam
Milk thistle	Safflower	Yarrow
Mugwort	Sarsaparilla	

Recommended daily allowance (RDA): There is no established RDA for chromium. The Estimated Safe and Adequate Daily Dietary Intake (ESADDI) established by the National Research Council in 1989 is 50 to 200 micrograms per day for adults. The scientific literature repeatedly reports pharmacological doses of 200 to 400 micrograms/day being used.

Table of Adequate Intake (Food and Nutrition Board of the National Academy of Science):

Age (YRS) amount in micrograms

Infants
Ages 0.0 thru 0.5:   0.2 micrograms/day   Ages 0.5 thru 1:   5.5 micrograms/day

Children
Ages 1 thru3:   11 micrograms/day   Ages 4 thru 8:   15 micrograms/day

Females
Ages 9 thru 13: 21 micrograms/day   Ages 31 thru 50: 25 micrograms/day
Ages 14 thru 18: 24 micrograms/day   Ages 51 thru 70: 20 micrograms/day
Ages 19 thru 30: 25 micrograms/day   Ages over 71:   20 micrograms/day

Males
Ages 9 thru 13:   25 micrograms/day   Ages 31 thru 50: 35 micrograms/day
Ages 14 thru 18:   35 micrograms/day   Ages 51 thru 70: 30 micrograms/day
Ages 19 thru 30:   35 micrograms/day   Ages over 71:   30 micrograms/day

Pregnant and breast-feeding
Ages under 18 months old: 19 micrograms/day
Ages over 18 months old: 29 micrograms/day

Toxic doses:

There are no reports found that describe the occurrence of toxicity from properly manufactured chromium supplements taken within the safe range. One potential effect of excess ingestion is mild gastrointestinal upset. Recent anecdotal reports for products labeled chromium picolinate describe anemia, memory loss, and DNA damage. The manufacturing practices of the suppliers were not reported.

Some research has shown supplemental chromium in the picolinate form broke down DNA, which is thought to generate mutations and possibly cancer. A Dartmouth University study demonstrated that chromium picolinate was absorbed into the cells in its intact form within a test tube and caused chromosomal DNA breaks in hamster ovarian cells. Other chromium salts did not do this. Examples of the other forms are nicotinate (chromium polynicotinate) or the chloride version, which has a low gastrointestinal absorption rate.

COBALT – PLEASE SEE VITAMIN B_{12}

COBALT IS THE MAIN MINERAL THAT IS CONTAINED IN VITAMIN B_{12}.

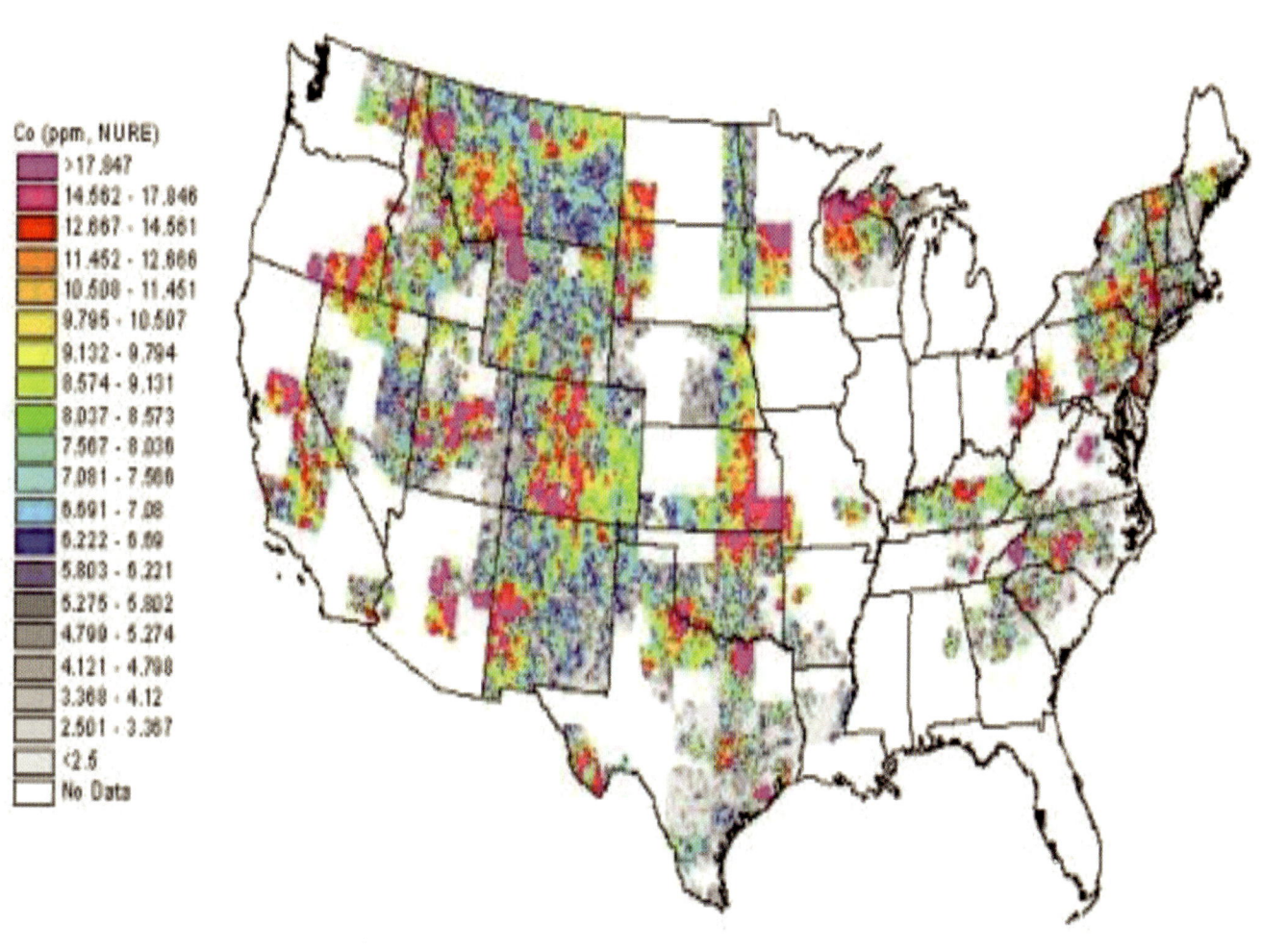

Copper

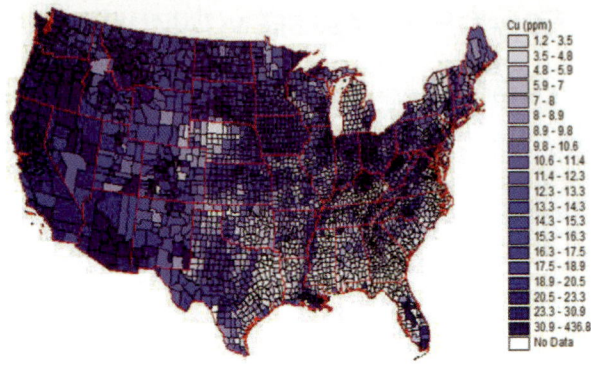

Copper is an elemental metal that is found in its pure form in nature that was known to prehistoric and ancient people. It is number 29 on the atomic period table.

Copper, an essential trace mineral, is a cofactor of many enzymes throughout the body including 11 oxidase systems.

Copper is absorbed in the small intestines and transported to the liver by transcuprein and albumin. It is there that it is incorporated into certain enzymes, secreted into the blood on ceruloplasmin, a protein that is an important antioxidant in the blood.

Some surveys suggest that the typical American diet provides about half of the RDA for copper.

The available copper compounds for supplementation and treatments include:

Copper amino acid chelate
Copper citrate
Copper gluconate
Copper glycinate

Copper lysinate
Copper sebacate
Copper sulfate

Deficiency symptoms:

Mild deficiency is common but severe deficiency is rare. Menkes' Disease is a genetic defect inhibiting copper absorption and resulting in steely hair, small stature, cardiovascular abnormalities, progressive mental decline, and premature death.

Deficiency symptoms include:

Anemia
Breakdown of connective tissue
Brittle, wiry hair
Decreased cardiac output
Fatigue

Impaired neuron function
Loss of hair color
Low body temperature
Pale skin

Copper promotes:

Anti-inflammatory activity
Antioxidant help
Hair color
Healthy blood vessels
Healthy bones
Healthy lungs

Healthy skin
Healthy tendons
Hemoglobin function

Iron absorption

Copper protects against:

Anemia
Arthritis flares
Dull hair Free radicals damage
Free radicals damage

Poor collagen formation
Poor elastin formation

Drugs that deplete: Antiretroviral medications and some antibiotics can deplete copper.

Food preparation to retain copper: Processing strips copper from many foods.

Foods that contain copper:

Artichoke	Fennel	Pistachio
Asparagus	Field bean	Plum
Asparagus pea	Filbert	Pop bean
Bell pepper	Flageolet bean	Popping bean
Black bean	French bean	Poppyseed
Black cherry	Garden bean	Pumpkin
Burdock	Green bean	Red cabbage
Cabbage	Haricot	Sassafras
Cacao	Haricot bean	Scotch kale
Cashew	Haricot vert	Sesame
Cauliflower	Kale	Snap bean
Cherry pepper	Kidney bean	Spinach
Coconut	Kitchen kale	String bean
Collards	Lettuce	Tomato
Cucumber	Navy bean	Wax bean
Curly kale	Oats	White cabbage
Dwarf bean	Peach	Wild cherry

Fortified foods available: No copper fortified foods known.

Function in the body:

1. Antioxidant Activity: Copper-zinc superoxide dismutase (SOD) is one of the body's most important antioxidant enzymes. Copper is also a component in dopamine beta-hydroxylase, which oxidizes vitamin C. This enzyme is a key in norepinephrine synthesis as well.
2. Anti-Inflammatory Activity: Some copper chelates have this effect and help to relieve some forms of arthritis.
3. Cardiovascular Disease: Studies have shown that an imbalance, either high or low, in copper levels can increase the incidence of cardiovascular abnormalities.
4. Collagen formation is dependent on copper. Proper collagen synthesis insures the integrity of bone, cartilage, fascia, skin, and tendons.
5. Elastin formation requires adequate amounts of copper. Elastin is a protein that provides the elasticity of lung, blood vessel, and skin tissue.
6. Oxygen transporting in the body depends on copper, as it is necessary for the synthesis and function of the helix hemoglobin. Copper stimulates the absorption of iron.
7. Melanin, the protein that produces the color in hair and skin, requires copper for its production.

Other facts: Excessive calcium inhibits the absorption of copper.

A family history of Wilson's disease or hemochromatosis, copper pipes in the home, excessive intake of foods high in copper or high supplementation can lead to the severe brain, triple negative breat cancer, kidney, and/or liver damage of sustained copper toxicity.

Recommended dietary allowance (RDA): The RDA for copper is 2 milligrams per day. The scientific literature reports use of pharmacologic dosing of 2 to 4 milligrams a day.

RDA/AI (Adequate Intake): Age (YRS) Amount in micrograms/day

Infants
Ages 0.0 thru 0.5:   200 micrograms/day   Ages 0.5 thru 1: 220 micrograms/day

Children
Ages 1 thru 3:   340 micrograms/day   Ages 4 thru 8:   440 micrograms/day

Females
Ages 9 thru 13: 700 micrograms/day   Ages 31 thru 50: 900 micrograms/day
Ages 14 thru 18: 890 micrograms/day   Ages 51 thru 70: 900 micrograms/day
Ages 19 thru 30: 900 micrograms/day   Ages over 71:   900 micrograms/day

Males
Ages 9 thru 13:   700 micrograms/day   Ages 31 thru 50:   900 micrograms/day
Ages 14 thru 18:   890 micrograms/day   Ages 51 thru 70:   900 micrograms/day
Ages 19 thru 30:   900 micrograms/day   Ages over 71:   900 micrograms/day

Pregnant and breast-feeding
Ages under 18 months old: 1000 micrograms/day   Ages over 18 months old: 1300 micrograms/day

Toxic doses: Copper toxicity with measurable tissue elevations occur when about 500% of the normal ingestion occurs. In these cases of elevated copper levels, most of the difficulties arise because of the interference with the absorption of other metal ion minerals.

Symptoms of toxicity include:

Dizziness   Headache   Salivation
Gastrointestinal upset   Metallic taste   Weakness

FLUORINE

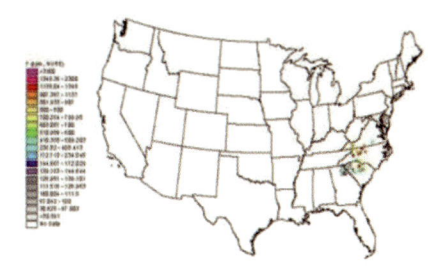

Fluoride is found in foods, however man has hyper-accumulated this mineral. This mineral displaces the most important mineral of the human body namely iodine. To be healthy, fluorine should be avoided like the plague. One only has to read your toothpaste label if it contains fluoride: Contact an emergency room if the toothpaste is swallowed.

The Fluoride Conspiracy

"Fluoridation is the greatest case of scientific fraud of this century." - Robert Carlton, Ph.D, former EPA scientist, 1992

The history of forcing fluoride on humans through the fluoridation of drinking water is wrought with lies, greed, and deception. Governments that add fluoride to drinking water supplies insist that it is safe, beneficial, and necessary; however, scientific evidence shows that fluoride is not safe to ingest and areas that fluoridate their drinking water supplies have higher rates of cavities, cancer, dental fluorosis, osteoporosis, and other health problems. Because of the push from the aluminum industry, pharmaceutical companies and weapons manufacturers, fluoride continues to be added to water supplies all over North America and due to recent legal actions against water companies that fluoridate drinking water supplies, precedent has been set that will make it impossible for suits to be filed against water suppliers that fluoridate. There is a growing resistance against adding toxic fluoride to our water supplies.

The "dental carries prevention myth" associated with fluoride originated in the United States in 1939, with a scientist named Gerald J. Cox. Mr. Cox was employed by ALCOA, the largest producer of toxic fluoride waste and at the time being threatened by fluoride damage claims, fluoridated some lab rats, concluded that fluoride reduced cavities and claimed that it should be added to the nation's water supplies. In 1947, Oscar R. Ewing, a long time ALCOA lawyer, was appointed head of the Federal Security Agency, a position that placed him in charge of the Public Health Service. Over the next three years, eighty-seven new American cities began fluoridating their water, including the control city in a water fluoridation study in Michigan, thus eliminating the most scientifically objective test of safety and benefit before it was ever completed.

American "education and research" was funded by the Aluminum Manufacturing, Fertilizer and Weapons Industry looking for an outlet for the increasingly mounting fluoride industrial waste while attaining positive profit increase. The "discovery" that fluoride benefited teeth was paid for by industry that needed to be able to defend "lawsuits from workers and communities poisoned by industrial fluoride emissions" (Bryson 1995) and turn a liability into an asset. Fluoride, a waste constituent in the manufacturing processes of explosives, fertilizers and other "necessities," was expensive to dispose of properly and until a "use" was found for it in America's water supplies, the substance was only considered a toxic, hazardous waste. Through sly public re-education, fluoride once a waste product, became the active ingredient in fluorinated pesticides, fungicides, rodenticides, anesthetics, tranquilizers, fluorinated pharmaceuticals, and a number of industrial and domestic products, fluorinated dental gels, rinses and toothpastes. Fluoride is so much a part of a multibillion-dollar industrial and pharmaceutical income, that any withdrawal of support from pro-fluoridationists is financially impossible, legally unthinkable, and potentially devastating for their career and reputation.

Despite growing evidence that it is harmful to public health, U.S. federal and state public health agencies and large dental and medical organizations such as the American Dental Association, continue to promote fluoride. Water fluoridation continues, despite the Environmental Protection Agency's own scientists, whose union, Chapter 280 of the National Treasury Employees Union, has taken a strong stand against it. Dr. William Hirzy, vice president of Chapter 280, stated that "fluoride (that is added to municipal water) is a hazardous waste product for which there is substantial evidence of adverse health effects and, contrary to public perception, virtually no evidence of significant benefits"(Mullenix 1998). Although fluoride is up to 50 times more toxic than sulfur dioxide, the American Clean Air Act does not regulate it as an air pollutant. Thousands of tons of industrial fluoride waste are added into drinking water supplies all over North America. Supposedly to encourage gleaming smiles in our children, big industry in the U.S. has the benefit of emitting as much fluoride waste into the environment as they like with absolutely no requirement to measure emissions and no way of being held accountable for poisoning people, animals and vegetation.

In a society where products containing asbestos, lead, beryllium, and many other carcinogens have been recalled from the marketplace, it is surprising that fluoride is embraced so thoroughly and blindly. It seems absurd that we would consider paying the chemical industry to dispose of their toxic waste by adding it to our water supply. Hiding the hazards of fluoride pollution from the public is a capitalist-style con job of epic proportions that has occurred because a powerful lobby wishes to manipulate public opinion in order to protect its own financial interests. Flourine is needed by the human body only in trace amounts and from food.

Foods that contain fluorine:

- Allspice
- Almond
- Apple
- Bell pepper
- Black currant
- Black walnut
- Brazil nut
- Butternut
- Cabbage
- Carrot
- Cashew
- Cauliflower
- Cherry pepper
- Clover
- Coconut
- Cone pepper
- Dill
- Dwarf bean
- Field bean
- Flageolet bean
- French bean
- Garden bean
- Garden dill
- Ginger
- Green bean
- Green pepper
- Haricot
- Haricot vert
- Haricot bean
- Horseradish
- Black bean
- Kidney bean
- Lettuce
- Navy bean
- Paprika
- Parsley
- Pecan
- Pistachio
- Pop bean
- Popping bean
- Red cabbage
- Red currant
- Rhubarb
- Snap bean
- Spinach
- Stinging nettle
- String bean
- Tomato
- Wax bean
- White cabbage
- White currant

GERMANIUM

Other common names for germanium:

Germanium sesquioxide
Germanium 132
GE OXY 132

Organic germanium
Oxy-G2
Pro-oxyge

Vitamin O

Small amounts of organic germanium are found in some plant-based foods. Inorganic germanium is mined and widely used as a semiconductor in the electronics industry. Both organic and inorganic germanium has been sold as dietary supplements, though the organic forms are more commonly used today. Ge-132 is a compound that contains germanium, carbon, hydrogen, and oxygen. It is often called organic germanium, because chemists refer to carbon-containing compounds as organic.

Available scientific evidence does not support claims that germanium supplements are effective for preventing or treating cancer in humans, and numerous reports show that it may be harmful. A study conducted by the U.S. Food and Drug Administration (FDA) reported that supplements containing germanium are potentially a hazard to humans. As a result, the FDA issued an "Import Alert," which allows germanium imports to be seized if they are to be used as a food supplement. However, the amount and type of germanium naturally found in foods does not appear to be toxic.

Germanium supplements are available in health food stores and over the Internet in powdered form and capsules ranging from 35 to 500 milligrams. There is no standardized dose.

The late Dr. Kazuhiko Asai of Japan began investigating the biological properties of germanium after reading reports from Russia that said the mineral had tremendous therapeutic value. In 1969, Dr. Asai founded the Asai Germanium Research Institute. He reported that he had developed a way to produce germanium that was chemically identical to the germanium extracted from plants. Dr. Asai also found germanium in many common herbal remedies including ginseng, garlic, comfrey, and aloe.

Dr. Otto Warburg, a Nobel Prize winning biochemist, stated that germanium helped to increase the delivery of oxygen to cells. He believed that boosting the oxygen supply to healthy cells slowed the growth of tumors.

Germanium may interfere with certain medicines and make seizures worse. Drugs for which side effects include kidney problems may cause harm if taken with germanium. Very little testing during pregnancy has been reported, but at least one form of germanium caused ill effects on fetuses in animal tests. Women who are pregnant or breast-feeding should not take germanium. At this time, germanium is not recommended as a dietary supplement for anyone due to the potential for serious health hazards.

Iodine

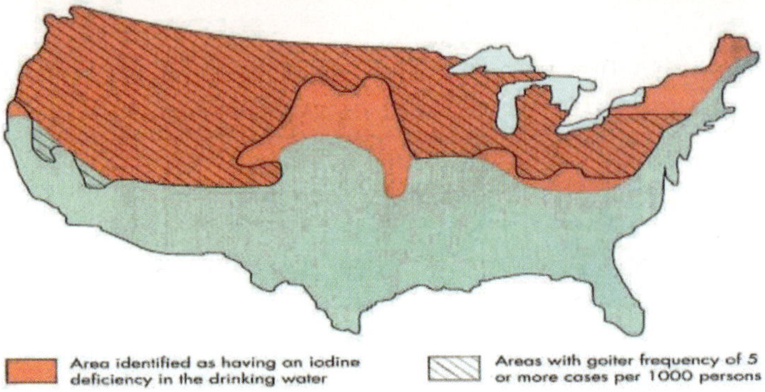

The above picture is called a goiter belt (enlarged thyroid), highlighted in red showing low iodine levels in the soil or air. This is one of the most important minerals for the body.

Iodine is a solid halogen discovered by Bernard Courtois in 1811. It was extracted from seaweed. Number 53 on the atomic periodic table, Iodine is considered an essential trace mineral. Only known to be utilized as a component of thyroid hormones, these hormones are diiodotyrosine, triiodothyronine (T3), and thyroxine (T4) which are found in every cell of the body. Iodine is converted to iodide in the gastrointestinal tract where it is then absorbed and transported to the thyroid gland. It is then stored in the thyroid on tyrosine protein which is part of a protein complex called tyroglobulin until it is needed for production of hormones.

Iodized salt has potassium iodide added and provides the equivalent of about 400 micrograms per teaspoon.

Deficiency symptoms: Depletion or insufficient ingestion and/or absorption of iodine decreases thyroid hormone synthesis. Hypothyroid activity can cause these symptoms:

Basal metabolism slowing	Dry skin	Thickening of the skin
Brittle hair or hair loss	Fatigue	Weight gain
Constipation	Fluid retention	
Depressed mood	Sleep disturbance	

Disease states:

1. Cretinism: Persistent low levels of thyroid hormone during pregnancy can cause cretinism, resulting in both mental and physical retardation.

2. Goiter: Enlargement of the thyroid gland from a lack of iodine. Called simple goiter and becoming very large and prominent in the front of the neck, it can be prevented and cured by ingestion of iodine. There are naturally occurring substances in some foods that promote goiter. These are contained in brussel sprouts, raw cabbage, cauliflower, peanuts, soybeans, and turnips. Cooking destroys these substances, but if iodine-deficient persons ingest excessive amounts of the raw forms, goiter is promoted.

3. Myxedema: Iodine deficiency is just one cause of this severe hypothyroid state. This condition is life threatening, needs medical intervention, and thyroid replacement therapy. It is marked by a very slow metabolic rate with psychomotor slowing, anemia, liver enlargement and abnormal function, fluid retention, thickening of the skin, and/or enlarged tongue with slowing of the speech.

Function in the body:

The effects of iodine are those of the thyroid gland hormones. These effects are far reaching, regulating basal metabolism, cellular oxygen consumption, and overall energy production in the body. As a result, body temperature, synthesis of proteins, physical growth, and reproduction are dependent upon these hormones.

Thyroid gland suppression or damage will cause it to have alterations in its production ability, most commonly to under produce or unable to produce the hormones. There are a number of scenarios where this will happen.

Taking oral thyroid replacement hormone at higher than needed doses will suppress whatever thyroid function remains. There is a complex "feedback" communication system in place to regulate a balance in the hormone levels of the body. Damage from infection, chemicals, radiation, tumors or the body's own immune system (in the case of autoimmune destruction) can adversely alter the amount of hormone produced by any of the glands involved in this "feedback" system. This in turn could cause an underproduction or in some cases an overproduction of thyroid hormones and the utilization of iodine in the body.

In a hypothyroid state, the basal metabolism can go down as much as 50%. In a hyperthyroid state, it can more than double causing palpitation, tremor, diarrhea, sweating, and anxiety.

Other facts: There is a sensitive, complicated communication system between hormones in general and specific hormones in particular that controls and regulates hormone production in the body. This communication system is referred to as negative feedback hormone control.

A decline in serum thyroid hormone levels, occurring for any number of reasons, triggers the hypothalamus gland to release thyroid-releasing hormone. The thyroid-releasing hormone signals the pituitary gland to release thyroid-stimulating hormone. A rise in thyroid-stimulating hormone stimulates the thyroid gland to take up more iodine, produce more enzymes to cleave thyroglobulin, produce more thyroid hormones, and to release these hormones into the circulation to be transported to the cells throughout the body. Bioavailability of iodine is an integral part of this whole process.

Three clinical trials involving 1,551 pregnant women taking iodine supplements were reviewed and shown a marked reduction of early infancy death and incidence of cretinism by age four in areas where there were high levels of cretinism. There also were much better scores on psychomotor and neurological function testing between early infancy and two years of age.

Poor iodine status should be suspected if recurrent bacterial infections occur in the presence of other symptoms of iodine deficiency.

Iodine promotes:

Healthy reproduction	Stable body temperature
Healthy weight	Stable normal metabolism
Physical growth	Thyroid hormones

Iodine protects against:

Cold intolerance	Waxy skin
Fatigue	Weight gain
Low thyroid hormones	

Recommended dietary allowances for adults range from 150 to 200 micrograms a day.

Foods that contain iodine (soil must contain iodine to be in the plants):

Almond	Date palm	Pecan
Apple	English filbert	Pineapple
Apricot	Fava bean	Pistachio
Black pepper	Fennel	Potato
Black walnut	Garlic	Rye
Bladderwrack	Ginseng	Sesame
Brazil nut	Horseradish	Sorrel
Broad bean	Hyssop	Spinach
Buckwheat	Jerusalem artichoke	Strawberry
Butterbur	Kelp	Sunflower
Butternut	Lentil	Swamp cabbage
Cashew	Mango	Sweet potato
Cinnamon	Mangrove	Tomato
Coca	Mugwort	Water spinach
Coconut	Non-GMO soybean	White pepper
Corn	Oats	
Dandelion	Pea	

Drugs that deplete iodine:

1. Fluoride-based drugs, fluoride toothpaste, dental floss with fluoride, teflon frying pans, bromine, and bromine-related products can and will decrease iodine. Fluoride containing insecticide sprayed on our vegetables and fruits take iodine out of the body.

2. Please READ your bread labels and make sure there is no bromine which will be listed a bromated or bromated vegetable oil. The label may have the words bromated or bromated vegetable oil present as this give bread a constant pattern of flour.

Food preparation to retain iodine: Most processing of food is done with salt that usually adds iodine.

Food sources: The most common source of iodine in the U.S. diet is iodized salt, but watch out for the addition of aluminum and this will appear as silicoaluminate. The best organic source of iodine is Sea Kelp that is available in health food stores.

1989 Recommended Dietary Allowances (RDA) -

National Academy of Sciences:

Age (YRS) Amount in micrograms

Infants
Ages 0.0 thru 0.5:   40 micrograms/day   Ages 0.5 thru 1:   50 micrograms/day

Children
Ages 1 thru 3:   70 micrograms/day   Ages 7 thru 10:   100 micrograms/day
Ages 4 thru 8:   50 micrograms/day

Females
Ages 9 thru 13:   150 micrograms/day   Ages 31 thru 50:   150 micrograms/day
Ages 14 thru 18: 150 micrograms/day   Ages 51 thru 70:   150 micrograms/day
Ages 19 thru 30: 150 micrograms/day   Ages over 71:   150 micrograms/day

Males
Ages 9 thru 13:   150 micrograms/day   Ages 19 thru 30:   150 micrograms/day
Ages 14 thru 18: 150 micrograms/day   Ages 31 thru 50:   150 micrograms/day

Ages 51 thru 70: 150 micrograms/day		Ages over 71: 150 micrograms/day

Pregnant
All ages under 18 months old: 17 micrograms/day
Ages over 18 months old: 13 micrograms/day
Lactating women: 200 micrograms/day

Toxic doses: There has been no recorded harm done at supplementation doses as high as 20 times the normal amount needed daily. Mega doses of iodine are discouraged as excessive intake can cause enlargement of the thyroid-resembling goiter and is actually called iodine goiter.

Please consult your healthcare provider for proper dosing of iodine.

Iron

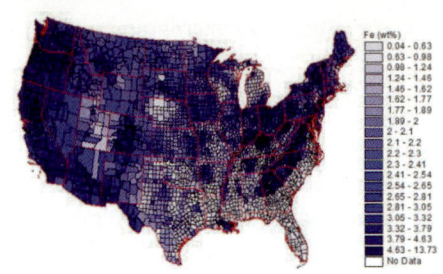

Iron use and the Iron Age were underway by 1000 BC. Since then, the history of civilization has been the history of iron. It is a transition metal and is number 26 on the periodic table.

Iron, an essential trace mineral, plays a role in many critical biochemical reactions within the body. It is primarily a component of the oxygen transport system in hemoglobin. About 80% of total iron is in the blood of a healthy individual.

Also involved in metabolism of serum glucose to energy within the cell, iron is part of many enzymes that cascade in the process of making new cells and amino acids, the building blocks of protein. These enzymes are also involved in the production of hormones and neurotransmitters.

Compounds of iron that are available include:

- Ferrous ammonium citrate
- Ferrous fumarate
- Ferrous gluconate
- Ferrous glycinate
- Ferrous sulfate

Deficiency symptoms: Loss of blood is the leading cause of iron depletion because more than 3/4 of the total amount of iron is in the blood. Trauma victims, menstruating women, and those with bleeding disorders like gastrointestinal ulcers or tumors in certain parts of the body lose iron at varying rates. Iron deficiency anemia can occur. This is an anemia where red blood cells contain less hemoglobin and have a diminished oxygen carrying capacity.

Symptoms of iron deficiency anemia are:

- Breathlessness (particularly with exertion)
- Brittle nails (can flatten out and begin to appear spoon like)
- Fatigue
- Hair loss
- Headache
- Pallor

Other conditions can lead to iron deficiency. Hypochlorhydria is a decrease in the production of and lack of hydrochloric acid in the stomach. This occurs from genetic abnormalities, some medications, and with age. Gastric hydrochloric acid is necessary for iron absorption.

Diarrhea and other gastrointestinal conditions that result in greater motility can decrease absorption.

Iron promotes:

- Energy
- Hemoglobin formation
- Metabolism of fatty acids
- Oxygen transport

Iron protects against:

- Anemia
- Breathlessness
- Fatigue
- Pallor

Iron supplements are only indicated if there is iron depletion. A simple blood test can measure iron levels and iron's ability to be bound in the body for utilization. Iron is a free radical and can cause harm if supplementation is taken in the presence of normal iron levels.

Function in the body: Oxygen transport throughout the body in hemoglobin is the major biological function of iron. Each hemoglobin molecule contains four iron atoms. These are contained in the heme segment. Heme picks up oxygen in the lungs as the blood passes by the alveoli in the lungs. Myoglobin in the muscles is an iron protein that accepts the oxygen from the hemoglobin and stores it until the muscles are ready to use it.

Oxygen is either stored or released by signals from electron transportation and the ability of iron to transport electrons is the key in the biological exchange. Iron is able to convert back and forth easily between its reduced state, the ferrous state (Fe++ or FE^{+2}) and its oxidized state, its ferric state (Fe+++ or FE^{+3}). This electron transport feature of iron is the prime biological activity of many enzymes. Iron is part of the synthesis process of carnitine, which is a hydrophilic amino acid derivative and is part of the production of carnitine acyltrasferase, essential in the metabolism of fatty acids.

Other facts: Vitamin E inhibits the absorption of iron and as such iron deficiency is a potential but not probable. Still, it would be advisable not to take supplemental vitamin E with doses of iron if iron replacement therapy supplements have been prescribed to correct anemia.

Hypochlorhydria (low levels of the hydrochloric acid digestive juices) and diminished digestive enzymes may inhibit absorption of iron. These gastrointestinal states occur primarily with the elderly, but the incidence is on the rise with the increased use of "antacids" in our society.

Hemochromatosis is a disorder that results in too much iron being absorbed from the gastrointestinal tract in the body.

There are two forms of hemochromatosis: primary and secondary.

Primary hemochromatosis is usually caused by a specific genetic problem that causes too much iron to be absorbed. When people with this condition have too much iron in their diet, the extra iron is absorbed in the gastrointestinal tract and builds up in the body tissues, particularly the liver. The result is liver swelling. Primary hemochromatosis is the most common genetic disorder in the United States, affecting an estimated 1 of every 200 to 300 Americans.

Secondary or acquired hemochromatosis can be caused by diseases such as thalassemia or sideroblastic anemia, especially if the person has received a large number of blood transfusions. Occasionally, it may be seen with hemolytic anemia, chronic alcoholism, and other conditions.

Hemochromatosis affects more men than women. It is particularly common in Caucasians of western European descent. Symptoms are often seen in men between the ages of 30 and 50 and in women over 50, although some people may develop problems by age 20. You have a higher risk of hemochromatosis if someone else in your family has or had the condition.

Symptoms include:

- Abdominal pain
- Fatigue
- Generalized darkening of skin color (often referred to as bronzing)
- Joint pain
- Lack of energy
- Loss of body hair
- Loss of sexual desire
- Weight loss
- Weakness

Signs and tests: A physical examination shows liver and spleen swelling, and skin color changes. Blood tests may help make the diagnosis.

Treatment of hemochromatosis: The goal of treatment is to remove excess iron from the body and treat any organ damage. A procedure called phlebotomy is the best method for removing excess iron from the body. One-half liter of blood is removed from the body each week until the body iron level is normal. This may require many months or even years to accomplish. After that, less frequent phlebotomy is needed to maintain normal iron levels. How often you need this procedure depends on your symptoms and your levels of hemoglobin and serum ferritin, and how much iron you take in your diet.

If you are diagnosed with hemochromatosis, you should follow a special diet to reduce how much iron is absorbed from your diet. The diet prohibits alcohol, especially for patients who have liver damage. You will also be told to avoid iron pills or vitamins containing iron, vitamin supplements, iron cookware, raw seafood (cooked is fine), or fortified processed foods such as 100% iron breakfast cereals.

Drugs that deplete iron: Non-steroidal anti inflammatory medication like aspirin, ibuprophen, etc, and the steroids can cause gastro intestinal ulceration and subsequent bleeding. Antacids, Histamine 2 blockers (H2) and proton pump inhibitors (PPI's) can interfere with iron bioavailability.

Food preparation to retain iron: Processing grains removes some iron.

Foods that contain iron:

American persimmon	Field bean	Milk thistle
Barberry	Flageolet bean	Mullein
Black bean	French bean	Navy bean
Black cherry	Garden bean	Oats
Blue cohosh	Garden thyme	Pennyroyal
Butter bean	Ginger	Pop bean
Butterbur	Great burdock	Popping bean
Catnip	Green bean	Raspberry
Chickweed	Haricot	Red clover
Common thyme	Haricot vert	Safflower
Coneflower	Haricot bean	Sassafras
Corn salad	Horsetail	Snap bean
Dandelion	Kidney bean	String bean
Devil's claw	Lamb's lettuce	Thyme
Dwarf bean	Lima bean	Wax bean
Echinacea	Marjoram	Wild cherry
Eggplant	Marshmallow	

1989 Recommended Dietary Allowances (RDA)—National Academy of Sciences:

Infants
Ages 0.0 thru 0.5: 6 milligrams/day   Ages 0.5 thru 1: 10 milligrams/day

Children
Ages 1 thru 3: 10 milligrams/day   Ages 7 thru 10: 10 milligrams/day
Ages 4 thru 8: 10 milligrams/day

Females

Ages 9 thru 13: 15 milligrams/day
Ages 14 thru 18: 15 milligrams/day
Ages 19 thru 30: 15 milligrams/day

Males
Ages 9 thru 13:   12 milligrams/day
Ages 14 thru 18: 12 milligrams/day
Ages 19 thru 30: 10 milligrams/day

Pregnant
All ages: 30 milligrams/day

Ages 31 thru 50: 15 milligrams/day
Ages 51 and over: 15 milligrams/day

Ages 31 thru 50: 10 milligrams/day
Ages 51 and over: 10 milligrams/day
Ages over 71: 150 milligrams/day

Lactating women: 15 milligrams/day

Lead

Human Health and Lead

Lead is a naturally-occurring element that can be harmful to humans when ingested or inhaled, particularly to children under the age of six. Lead poisoning can cause a number of adverse human health effects, but is particularly detrimental to the neurological development of children. To learn more about the effects of lead poisoning and EPA's role in reducing the presence of lead in the environment, visit EPA Lead.

For hundreds of years, lead has been mined, smelted, refined, and used in products (e.g., as an additive in paint, gasoline, leaded pipes, solder, crystal, and ceramics). Natural levels of lead in soil range between 50 parts per million (ppm) and 400 ppm. Mining, smelting, and refining activities have resulted in substantial increases in lead levels in the environment, especially near mining and smelting sites. For example, near some types of industrial and municipal facilities, and adjacent to highways (Chaney et al., 1984; Shacklette et al., 1984) soil lead concentrations have been reported to be more than 11,000 ppm (National Research Council, 1980).

Lead particles in the environment can attach to dust and be carried long distances in the air. Such lead-containing dust can be removed from the air by rain and deposited on surface soil, where it may remain for many years. In addition, heavy rains may cause lead in surface soil to migrate into ground water and eventually into water systems.

Possible ways to be exposed to lead: Everyone is exposed to "background levels" of lead, given its widespread distribution. Possible routes of lead exposure include:

1) Ingestion of lead-contaminated water, soil, paint chips, or dust;

2) Inhalation of lead-containing particles of soil or dust in air; and

3) Ingestion of foods that contain lead from soil or water.

Symptoms of Lead Exposure - Lead poisoning can be a serious public health threat with no unique signs or symptoms. Early symptoms of lead exposure may include:

1) Persistent fatigue
2) Irritability
3) Loss of appetite
4) Stomach discomfort and/or constipation
5) Reduced attention span
6) Insomnia

Failure to treat lead poisoning in the early stages can cause long-term or permanent health damage, but because of the general nature of symptoms at early stages, lead poisoning is often not suspected.

In adults, lead poisoning can cause:

1) Hearing and vision impairment
2) Increased blood pressure
3) Nerve damage to the sense organs and nerves controlling the body
4) Poor muscle coordination
5) Reproductive problems (e.g., decreased sperm count)
6) Retarded fetal development even at relatively low exposure levels

In children, lead poisoning can cause:

1) Anemia
2) Behavioral problems
3) Damage to the brain and nervous system
4) Hearing loss
5) Hyperactivity
6) Liver and kidney damage

Although the effects of lead exposure are a potential concern for all humans, young children (less than seven years old) are most at risk. This increased vulnerability results from a combination of the following factors:

1) Children typically have higher intake rates (per unit body weight) for environmental media (such as soil, dust, food, water, air, and paint) than adults, since they are more likely to play in dirt and put their hands and other objects in their mouths.
2) Children tend to absorb a higher fraction of ingested lead from the gastrointestinal tract than adults.
3) Children tend to be more susceptible than adults to the adverse neurological and developmental effects of lead.
4) Nutritional deficiencies of iron or calcium, which are common in children, may facilitate lead absorption and exacerbate the toxic effects of lead.

Medical Tests for Lead Exposure

If you have concerns about possible lead exposure, contact your personal physician or county/state health department. Your doctor can conduct blood tests to determine lead concentrations in your blood. Blood tests are inexpensive and sometimes free; however, please consult your insurance provider to determine coverage of such tests. Lead in bone and teeth can be measured using x-ray techniques, but this test is not used very often. In communities where houses are old and deteriorating, residents are encouraged to take advantage of available screening programs offered by local health departments and to have children living in the residence checked regularly for lead poisoning. Because the early symptoms of lead poisoning are similar to those of other illnesses, it is difficult to diagnose lead poisoning without medical testing.

Lithium

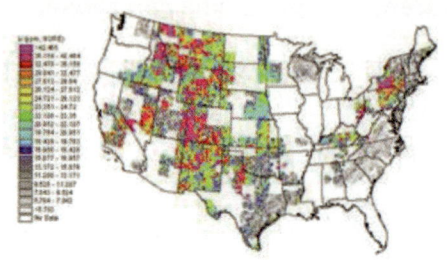

Lithium is a naturally-occurring mineral similar to sodium and potassium. Small amounts are present in most foods. Large amounts are used in the treatment of manic depression-also called bipolar disorder. The Wayne State team was studying lithium's effects on manic depression when they discovered that this remarkable mineral could protect brain cells from premature death. Lithium may even cause brain cells to regenerate after a loss from disease. After four weeks of lithium treatment researchers were surprised to find that the patients' brain gray matter increased by an average of 3 percent. Data show that lithium plays a vital role in maintaining neural health.

Benefits of lithium

Lithium offers both short-and long-term benefits for the health of the nervous system. Prof. Bjorksten demonstrated that lithium was an effective aluminum chelator and lithium continues to be the most effective electrolyte for aluminum detachment.

Lithium in the diet

There is growing evidence that lithium may be an essential mineral in the human diet. Animals on low-lithium diets have shown reproductive problems, shorter life spans, poor lipid metabolism, and behavioral abnormalities. In epidemiological studies of humans, low levels of lithium in drinking water have been correlated with a higher incidence of mental hospital admissions, violent crime, suicide, drug addiction, and heart disease. Levels in the scalp hair of violent criminals and heart disease patients have been found to be lower than those in healthy volunteers. Lithium is not that minuscule. In terms of atoms, lithium is more abundant in the body than six of the minerals that are commonly taken in food supplements.

Lithium salts

Lithium, like sodium, occurs naturally in a number of different salts. Lithium carbonate and lithium citrate are approved as prescription forms of lithium. The citrate and carbonate salts are only slightly soluble in water, and are poorly absorbed by the cells. Another form of lithium—lithium orotate—is a highly bioavailable form of lithium that is available as an over-the-counter dietary supplement. Because of its superior bioavailability, lower doses of lithium orotate than lithium carbonate (or lithium citrate) may be used to achieve therapeutic brain lithium concentrations and relatively stable serum concentrations.

Lithium orotate, is a salt of vitamin B_{13} and lithium. It requires 8 times less lithium orotate than lithium carbonate, thereby lessening concerns of potential impaired kidney function. Lithium orotate has been promoted as an alternative to lithium carbonate, which because it must be used in high doses, is potentially toxic. Lithium orotate is heavily touted by Dr. John Gray, among others, as a low toxicity alternative. It is marketed as a dietary supplement used in small doses to treat certain medical conditions - stress, bipolar disorder, alcoholism, ADHD, ADD, aggression, PTSD, Alzheimer's and to improve memory. Lithium orotate is sold under a wide variety of brand names and is available at some drugstores and health food stores. Although a few psychiatrists prescribe lithium orotate to their patients, it is most often naturopaths and other alternative health practitioners who recommend this lithium compound to their patients.

Lithium orotate has also been demonstrated to be of benefit in the treatment of alcoholics, and proved useful in alleviating alcohol-related symptoms of liver dysfunction, seizure disorders, headaches, hyperthyroidism, Meniere's syndrome, liver and lung cancers.

Conclusion

Lithium orotate is a safe nutritional supplement that may help to prevent Alzheimer's disease, alcoholism (and related conditions) and other neurodegenerative conditions. Because of its superior bioavailability, lower (and safer) doses of lithium orotate are as effective as the much higher doses found in prescription lithium.

Foods that contain lithium:

- Asparagus
- Beet
- Beetroot
- Bell pepper
- Black bean
- Buck bush
- Cantaloupe
- Carrot
- Cherry pepper
- Chinese cabbage
- Common thyme
- Cone pepper
- Cucumber
- Dwarf bean
- Endive
- Field bean
- Flageolet bean
- French bean
- Garden bean
- Garden beet
- Garden thyme
- Grapefruit
- Green bean
- Green pepper
- Haricot
- Haricot bean
- Haricot vert
- Kidney bean
- Lettuce
- Melon
- Muskmelon
- Navy bean
- Onion
- Orange
- Paprika
- Parsley
- Peach
- Plum
- Pop bean
- Red cabbage
- Snap bean
- String bean
- Sugar beet
- Sweet pepper
- Thyme
- Tomato
- Wax bean
- White cabbage

MAGNESIUM

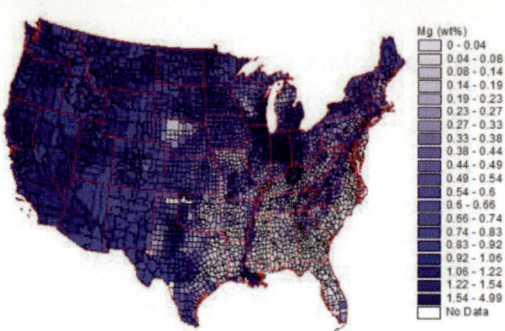

Magnesium is a flammable, lightweight earth alkali. Joseph Black discovered the element in 1755 in Scotland, and Humphrey Davy produced the pure metal with his electrolytic apparatus in 1808. It is number 12 on the atomic periodic table.

Magnesium, an essential trace mineral, plays a critical role in the synthesis of DNA and RNA, energy production, nerve impulse transmission, muscular contraction and relaxation, temperature regulation, bone and teeth formation, and cardiovascular functioning. It is a cofactor in more than 300 enzymes and proper functioning of all tissues is dependent on it.

Approximately 50% of the total amount of magnesium in the body is in bone. Most of the remaining magnesium is in cells of soft tissues, muscles, and organs predominantly. Only about 1% is found in the blood and there are mechanisms in place to keep very tight control on the serum magnesium level. If the serum magnesium level is low, the intercellular level is quite depleted in most cases. After ingestion, magnesium is absorbed into the body in the small intestines. The kidneys excrete it.

The amount of elemental magnesium in each compound varies. The amount of elemental magnesium in each molecule of a compound is not as important as its bioavailablity, which has far greater influence on the effectiveness of the magnesium supplement.

Magnesium compounds are available in:

1) Magnesium oxide (60%)
2) Magnesium carbonate (45%)
3) Magnesium hydroxide (42%)
4) Magnesium citrate (16%)

5) Magnesium lactate (12%)
6) Magnesium chloride (12%)
7) Magnesium sulfate (10%)

Deficiency symptoms: Severe magnesium deficiency is rare in the U.S. and is associated with hypocalcaemia (low calcium levels) and hypokalemia (low potassium levels). The combination of these can cause serious cardiac dysfunction and death.

Early signs of magnesium deficiency include:

Anorexia
Anxiety/panic
Depression
Fatigue

Gastrointestinal distress (nausea/vomiting)
Muscle cramping
Numbness/tingling (extremities/face)

Deficiency will cause worsening of these symptoms plus arrhythmias (abnormal heart rhythms), coronary artery spasms (a potential for heart attack), and seizures.

Kidney stones and osteoporosis can develop with persistent magnesium deficiency. Research has shown a correlation between low magnesium levels and development or advancing diabetes. Vasodilatation can be impaired by diminishing magnesium and blood pressure elevations can be the result.

Function in the body: Magnesium is a cofactor in oxidative phosphorylation during production of adenosine triphosphate (ATP) in the Kreb's Cycle (energy production). It is required for the metabolism of the macronutrients, carbohydrates, fats, and proteins. It participates in at least 300 intermediary enzyme reactions.

Magnesium increases oxygenation to muscle fibers and improves contractility. Muscle fibers of the heart damaged by infarction or lethal arrhythmia are reduced by the administration of intravenous magnesium soon after the injury has occurred. If given within the early stages of the heart attack, death rates have been reduced by 70%.

It can also lower blood pressure by its action of blood vessel relaxation however; it is not effective as a primary treatment for essential hypertension. Magnesium is involved in calcium metabolism, vitamin D synthesis, crystallization of bone minerals and part of the process that binds calcium to tooth enamel.

Other facts: Several clinical studies have looked at the effect of supplemental magnesium on overall metabolic control of type 2 diabetes. One study administered oral supplements equivalent to 300 milligrams elemental magnesium per day and after four months, blood sugar, and blood pressure significantly improved over the placebo control group. Another study used magnesium oxide in two strengths equal to 600 milligrams and 300 milligrams elemental magnesium. The blood sugar control did not improve significantly in either group despite the fact that the magnesium levels did go up in the 600 milligram group. More research is needed using bioavailable compounds and supplements that are manufactured to ensure purity and quality.

Be aware that most in-home water purification systems such as reverse osmosis or distillation, remove valuable nutrients such as magnesium as well as other healthful minerals. Most "purified" bottled waters have no or low levels of natural minerals. Bottled water in the U.S. has average magnesium content of 2.7milligrams per liter, about one-seventh as much as the historic levels in U.S. drinking water sources.

Magnesium is a macro mineral, as is calcium, and the amount needed by the body per day is much higher than the micro minerals, such as zinc, copper and selenium. As such, the macro minerals can interfere with the absorption of the micro minerals. The bulk of the macro minerals are probably best taken at a time separate from any micro mineral supplementation recommended.

Magnesium promotes:

Blood vessel flexibility
Bone health
Bowel motility
Calcium metabolism
Calm mood
Heart tissue function

Metabolism of carbohydrates, fats, and proteins
Muscle function
Normal blood pressure
Strength
Tooth enamel strength

Magnesium protests against:

Achy muscles
Anxiety
Bone loss
Constipation
Death during a heart attack

Demineralized bones
Dental cavities
Fatigue
Muscle weakness
Thin tooth enamel

Drugs that deplete magnesium:

Diuretics and cancer chemotherapeutic agents are the most frequently cited drugs that cause excessive loss of magnesium. Antibiotics, steroids, and hormones, including birth control pills, can cause depletion as well.

Food preparation to retain magnesium: Food processing is the major cause of magnesium depletion. Refined white flour has 85% less magnesium than whole wheat; white rice has 65% less magnesium than brown rice.

Foods that contain magnesium vary due to soil conditions:

Asparagus	Garden bean	Oats
Black bean	Green bean	Pop bean
Black cherry	Haricot	Poppyseed
Bladderwrack	Haricot bean	Red clover
Borage	Haricot vert	Sassafras
Butter bean	Irish moss	Skullcap
Chives	Kelp	Snap bean
Cilantro	Kidney bean	Spinach
Cucumber	Lettuce	Spinach
Dill	Licorice	Stinging nettle
Dwarf bean	Lima bean	String bean
Field bean	Linseed	Wax bean
Flageolet bean	Mangrove	Wheat
Flax	Navy bean	Wheatgrass
French bean	Neem	Wild cherry

Recommended dietary allowance: For more than fifty years, nutrition experts have produced a set of nutrient and energy standards known as the recommended dietary allowances. A major revision is currently underway to replace the RDA. The revised recommendations are called Dietary Reference Intakes (DRI) and reflect the collaborative efforts of the U.S. and Canada. Until 1997, the RDA was the only standards available and they continue to serve health care professionals until the DRI can be established for all nutrients.

1997 Dietary Reference Intakes (DRI):

IOM Committee on Dietary Reference Intakes
Age amount in milligrams:

Infants
Ages 0.0 thru 0.5: 30 milligrams/day   Ages 0.5 thru 1: 75 milligrams/day

Children
Ages 1 thru3: 80 milligrams/day   Ages 7 thru 10: 140 milligrams/day
Ages 4 thru 8: 130 milligrams/day

Females
Ages 9 thru 13:   240 milligrams/day   Ages 31 thru 50:   320 milligrams/day
Ages 14 thru 18: 360 milligrams/day   Ages 51 and older: 320 milligrams/day
Ages 19 thru 30: 310 milligrams/day

Males
Ages 9 thru 13:   240 milligrams/day
Ages 14 thru 18: 210 milligrams/day
Ages 19 thru 30: 400 milligrams/day

Ages 31 thru 50:   420 milligrams/day
Ages 51 and over: 420 milligrams/day

Lactating women: add 15 milligrams/day   Pregnant: add 40 to age specific amount.

Toxic doses: Toxicity is rare. Renal impairment that decreases the effectiveness of the kidneys in excreting excess magnesium can lead to harmful elevations. One of the most common side effects of elevating levels of magnesium is diarrhea. This is not an indicator of toxicity, but if persistent could indicate impending magnesium toxicity.

A magnesium toxic state results in many of the same symptoms as magnesium depletion/deficiency.

These symptoms may include:

Heart failure
Hypotension
Loss of reflexes

Mental status change
Muscle weakness and flaccidity

MANGANESE

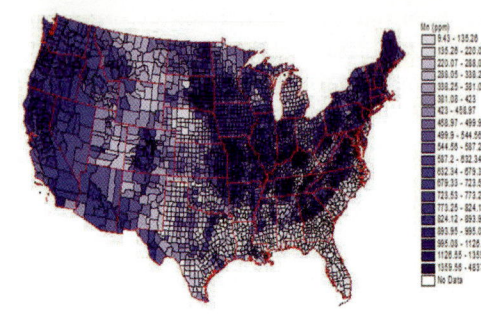

Manganese is a transition metal. In 1770, it was discovered by Ignatius Kaim, then investigated by Bergman and Scheele and finally isolated by a Swedish mineralist named Johann Gottlieb Gahn. It is number 25 on the atomic periodic table.

Manganese, an essential trace micro mineral, is a cofactor in the activation of a wide variety of enzymes that influence many biological activities. It is needed for bone growth and fatty acid and protein metabolism. Food grown with glyphosate in the soil has reduced manganese levels.

The average human body contains only 18 to 20 mg of manganese total, most of which is contained within the bone matrix. Small amounts are distributed in the pituitary gland. The liver, pancreas, ligaments, and intestinal tissues have miniscule amounts.

It is absorbed in the small intestines. Supplements should be prescribed and closely monitored by a licensed health care professional.

Deficiency symptoms: Symptoms of manganese deficiency are extremely rare as magnesium can substitute for manganese. Symptoms of manganese deficiency are:

Abnormal skeletal structures   Weak ligaments
Loss of muscle coordination

Hypocholesterolemia (low cholesterol) may be associated with low manganese levels, as it is needed for biosynthesis of the various cholesterols. There have been low levels found in some epileptics, schizophrenics, and women with osteoporosis.

Manganese promotes:

Dopamine production	Healthy mitochondria	Thyroid function
Healthy cartilage	Inner ear development	Vibrant hair color
Healthy connective tissues	Normal blood clotting	

Manganese protects against:

Abnormal bleeding	Dull hair	Rough skin
Arthritis	Low energy production	Stiff joints
Cravings	Low thyroid hormone levels	

Manganese can be neurotoxic producing a syndrome similar in symptoms to Parkinson's disease.

Function in the body:

1. Manganese is necessary for the synthesis of glycoproteins, lipoproteins, and mucopolysaccharides. These are building blocks for cartilage and connective tissue. It also has an influence on the activity of osteoblasts and osteoclasts and the mineralization of bone. Manganese containing enzymes play a role in the synthesis of prothrombin and so has a role in blood clotting regulation.

2. The manganese-containing enzyme, mitochondria super oxide dismutase, is one of the prime antioxidant defense systems against the toxic effects of oxygen during energy production within each cell.

3. Manganese is needed for thyroxin (T4), the main hormone of the thyroid gland, dopamine, a major neurotransmitter, and melanin, a protein giving color and flexibility to hair and skin.

4. The embryonic developments of the otoliths of the inner ear necessary for equilibrium depend on manganese. During pregnancy, food sources should be part of the diet.

Other facts: Miners of manganese as well as welders who work without adequate safety or protective gear; risk inhalation and toxicity that could lead to manganism. The dust from the mining activity and aerosolized manganese from the welding rod is inhaled when not properly masked. In 1993, the National Institute of Health issued a statement concerning manganese and manganism: "Occupational exposure to manganese for six months to two years can result in manganism, a disease of the central nervous system characterized by psychogenic and neurological disorders with symptoms resembling Parkinson's disease."

A diet low in iron and high in manganese, particularly in a person with depleted iron stores, will deplete iron further as manganese competes with iron for absorption. Vegetarians should be careful with manganese supplementation for this reason.

Increased levels of manganese have been found in the brains of some persons with amyotrophic lateral sclerosis (ALS, Lou Gerig's Disease).

Drugs that deplete: None known

Food preparation to retain manganese: None known

Foods that contain manganese:

Artichoke	Garden bean	Oats
Bilberry	Garden dill	Parsley
Black bean	Ginger	Pineapple
Blue cohosh	Ginseng	Pop bean
Buchu	Grape	Raspberry
Catnip	Green bean	Red clover
Cinnamon	Haricot	Saffron
Clove	Haricot bean	Sage
Cranberry	Haricot vert	Sassafras
Dill	Kidney bean	Sorrel
Dwarf bean	Ladyslipper	Spinach
Dwarf sumac	Lettuce	Stinging nettle
Fennel	Mangrove	Sumac
Field bean	Mugwort	Sweetflag
Flageolet bean	Navy bean	
French bean	Oats	

Fortified Foods Available: None

Recommended dietary allowance (RDA): There is no RDA for manganese. Suggested dietary intake has been 2 to 5 milligrams a day. Guildelines are as follows:

Infants
Ages 0.0 thru 0.5:   0.003 milligrams/day   Ages 0.5 thru 1: 0.06 milligrams/day

Children
Ages 1 thru3: 1.2 milligrams/day   Ages 7 thru 10:   1.6 milligrams/day
Ages 4 thru 8: 1.5 milligrams/day

Females
Ages 9 thru 13: 1.6 milligrams/day
Ages 14 thru 18: 1.6 milligrams/day
Ages 19 thru 30: 1.8 milligrams/day

Ages 31 thru 50: 1.8 milligrams/day
Ages 51 and older: 1.8 milligrams/day

Males
Ages 9 thru 13:   1.9 milligrams/day
Ages 14 thru 18: 2.2 milligrams/day
Ages 19 thru 30: 2.2-2.3 milligrams/day

Ages 31 thru 50: 2.2-2.3 milligrams/day
Ages 51 and over: 2.38 milligrams/day

Pregnant
All ages: 2.0 milligrams/day

Lactating women: 2.6 milligrams/day

Toxic doses: Manganese can be neurotoxic. Excessive intake, either inhaled or ingested, can produce manganism, with permanent neuro damage and symptoms similar to those of Parkinson's disease. High levels of manganese can interfere with iron absorption.

Toxicity symptoms include:

Dementia	Mask like face	Psychosis
Gait alterations	Neuromuscular dysfunction	Tremor

Minerals & Human Health

MERCURY

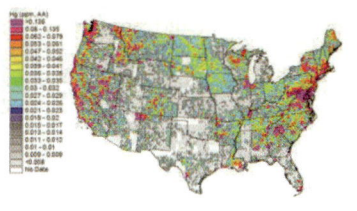

Methylmercury poisoning has made it clear that adults, children, and developing fetuses are at risk from dietary exposure to methylmercury. During these poisoning outbreaks some mothers with no symptoms of nervous system damage gave birth to infants with severe disabilities and it became clear that the developing nervous system of the fetus may be more vulnerable to methylmercury than is the adult nervous system. Mothers who are exposed to methylmercury and breast-feed their babies may also expose their infant children through their milk. This advice was for women who might become pregnant; women who are pregnant; nursing mothers; and young children. The advisory provides three recommendations for selecting and eating fish or shellfish to ensure that women and young children will receive the benefits of eating fish and shellfish and be confident that they have reduced their exposure to the harmful effects of methylmercury.

Consumption of fish with higher methylmercury levels can lead to elevated levels of mercury in the bloodstream of unborn babies and young children and may harm their developing nervous system. These disabilities have been documented in ability to use language, to process information, and in visual/motor integration. Nearly all methylmercury exposures in the U.S. occur through eating fish and shellfish. Microscopic organisms convert inorganic mercury into methylmercury, which accumulates up the food chain in fish, fish-eating animals, and people.

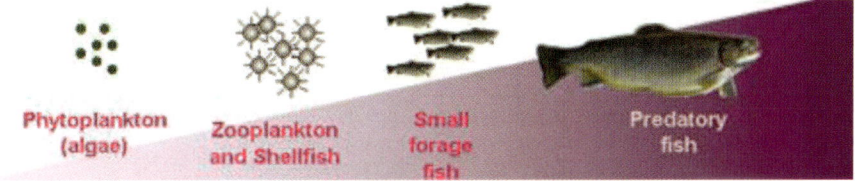

Elemental mercury exposure - When elemental mercury is spilled or a device containing mercury breaks, the exposed elemental mercury can evaporate and become an invisible, odorless toxic vapor. This is especially true in warm or poorly-ventilated rooms or spaces.

Elemental or metallic mercury is the liquid metal used in thermometers, barometers, and thermostats and other electrical switches. Metallic mercury is often found in school laboratories as well as in thermometers, barometers, switches, thermostats, and other devices found in school science labs. There are some necklaces imported from Mexico that contain a glass pendant that contains mercury. The mercury-containing pendants can come in various shapes such as hearts, bottles, balls, saber teeth, and chili peppers. If broken, they release metallic mercury to the environment.

Dental amalgam - Mercury is used in dentistry in dental amalgam. Dental amalgam is a direct filling material used in restoring teeth. It is made up of approximately 40-50% mercury, 25% silver and 25-35% a mixture of copper, zinc and tin. Amalgam use is declining because the incidence of dental decay is decreasing and because improved substitute materials are now available for certain applications.

Mercury in Drug and Biologic Products

Thimerosal content for biological products can be found at 'Thimerosal in Vaccines and Mercury in Plasma-Derived Products'.

Manufacturer	Name of Product	Manufacturer	Name of Product
Akorn Inc.	AK Spore Ophthalmic Solution	American International Chemical	Thimerosal (bulk chemical)
Akorn Inc.	AK Spore HC Ophthalmic Combo Drops	American International Chemical	Thimerosal USP 97% (bulk chemical)
Akorn Inc.	Fluoracaine Ophthalmic Solution	American Pharmaceutical	12 Hour Nasal Solution
Akorn Inc.	AK Spore HC Otic Suspension	Appletree Markets	Long Lasting Nasal Spray
Alcon Laboratories	Profenal 1% Ophthalmic Solution	Bausch & Lomb	Flurbiprofen Sodium Ophthalmic Solution
Alcon Laboratories	Adsorbonac 2% Ophthalmic Solution	Bausch & Lomb	Neomycin & Polymyxin B Sulfates & Gramicidin Ophthalmic Solution
Alcon Laboratories	Adsorbonac 5% Ophthalmic Solution	Bausch & Lomb	Neomycin & Polymyxin B Sulfates & Hydrocortisone Otic Suspension
Allergan America	Ocufen Ophthalmic Solution	Bausch & Lomb	Sulfacetamide Sodium & Prednisolone Sodium Phosphate Ophthalmic Solution 10%/.23%
Allergan America	Poly Pred Ophthalmic Suspension	Bristol-Myers Squibb	Fungizone Lotion
Allergan Inc.	Blephamide SOP Ophthalmic Ointment	Bristol-Myers Squibb	Fungizone Cream
Allergan Inc.	Bleph-10 Ophthalmic Ointment 10%	C.O. Truxton Inc.	Bio-Cot Otic Suspension
Allergan Inc.	FML SOP Ophthalmic Ointment 0.1%	C.O. Truxton Inc.	Decongest Nasal Spray
Allergan Inc.	Poly Pred Ophthalmic Suspension	Cheshire Pharmaceutical	Otocort Otic Suspension
Altaire Pharmaceuticals	Nasal Relief 12 Hour Spray	American International Chemical	Thimerosal (bulk chemical)
American Assn. Retired Persons	Oxymetazoline Nasal Spray	Cheshire Pharmaceutical	Ocutricin Ophthalmic Solution
Cheshire Pharmaceutical	Sulfapred Ophthalmic Solution	Foxmeyer Drug Co.	Nasal Spray Pump
CVS	Nasal Spray Pump	Global Source	Nasin Long Acting Nasal Spray
CVS Revco DS Inc.	12 Hour Decongestant Pump Nasal Spray	Harco Drug	Mercurochrome Aqueous Solution
Dolder Ltd.	Thimerosal (bulk chemical)	Harris-Teeter	Oxymetazoline Nasal Spray
Dorex International Corp.	Long Acting Nasal Spray	Hi Tech Pharmacal Co.	Long Acting Nasal Spray
Drug Guild Distributors	Long Acting Nasal Spray Kolex LA	Hudson Corp.	Nasal Spray Extended Relief
DRX Pharmaceutical	Blephamide Ophthalmic Ointment	Hurst Pharmaceutical	Duomycin-HC Otic Suspension
DRX Pharmaceutical	Cortisporin Ophthalmic Suspension	K and B Distributors	Mercurochrome Aqueous Solution

DRX Pharmaceutical	Neomycin Polymyxin B Sulfates Hydrocortisone Ophthalmic Suspension	King Pharmaceuticals	Cortisporin Ophthalmic Suspension
DRX Pharmaceutical	Neomycin Polymyxin B Hydrocortisone Otic Suspension	King Pharmaceuticals	Neosporin Ophthalmic Suspension
DRX Pharmaceutical	Neomycin Polymyxin B Gramicidin Ophthalmic Solution	King Pharmaceuticals	Viroptic Ophthalmic Solution
DRX Pharmaceutical	Vasocidin Ophthalmic Solution	King Pharmaceuticals	Neomycin Polymyxin B Sulfates Hydrocortisone Otic Suspension
DRX Pharmaceutical	Colymycin S Otic Suspension	King Pharmaceuticals	Pediotic Suspension
DRX Pharmaceutical	Pediotic Otic Suspension	King Pharmaceuticals	Cortisporin Otic Suspension
Dysers Sal	Thimerosal (bulk chemical)	Kinray	Oxymetazoline Nasal Spray
Family Independent Pharmacy	12 Hour Nasal Decongestant Spray	Laboratori Derivati	Adrenal Cortex Injection
Family Independent Pharmacy	Long Acting Nasal Spray	Leader	12 Hour Nasal Spray
Farm Fresh Inc.	Hemorrhoid Relief Ointment	Leader	Nasal Pump Spray
Fays Drug Services	12 Hour Nasal Spray Pump	LS Raw Materials Ltd.	Mercurochrome NF 12 100% (bulk chemical)
Federated Foods	Long Acting Nasal Spray	Major Pharmaceuticals	Cortomycin Ophthalmic Suspension
Fleming Companies	12 Hour Nasal Spray		
Major Pharmaceuticals	Sulfacetamide Sodium & Prednisolone Sodium Phosphate Ophthalmic Solution	Physicians Total Care Inc.	Viroptic Ophthalmic Solution
Major Pharmaceuticals	Cortomycin Otic Suspension	Physicians Total Care Inc.	Cortisporin Ophthalmic Suspension
Major Pharmaceuticals	Neocidin Ophthalmic Solution	Physicians Total Care Inc.	Ocufen Ophthalmic Solution
Martin Surgical Supply	Testosterone Injection Suspension 50 mg	Physicians Total Care Inc.	Vasocidin Ophthalmic Solution
Martin Surgical Supply	Testosterone Injection Suspension 100 mg	Ping On Ointment Co. Ltd.	Ping On Topical Ointment
Mays Drug Stores	Hemorrhoid Relief Ointment	Prime Natural Health	12 Hour Nasal Spray
Medalist Laboratories	Long Lasting Nasal Spray Pump	Primedics Laboratories	Testerone Injection Suspension 50 mg
Meyers Supply Inc.	Long Acting Nasal Spray	Publix Inc.	Long Acting Nasal Spray
Navresso	Long Acting Nasal Spray	Publix Supermarkets	Long Acting Decongestant Nasal Spray
Omicron Quimica SA	Thimerosal USP 97% (bulk chemical)	Qualitest Pharmaceuticals	Nasal Spray Solution
Parade (Grocer's Supply)	Oxymetazoline Nasal Spray	Qualitest Pharmaceuticals	Antibiotic HC Otic Suspension
Parkedale Pharmaceuticals	Coly-Mycin S Otic Suspension	RDS Acquisition Corp.	12 Hour Nasal Spray
Pay N Save Corp.	Decongestant Nasal Spray	Republic Drug Co.	12 Hour Nasal Spray

Pharmedix	Bleph 10 Ophthalmic Solution 10%	Schering-Plough Animal Health	Gentocin Durafilm Ophthalmic Solution (for dogs only)
Pharmedix	Viroptic Ophthalmic Solution 1%	Scrivner, Inc.	Hemorrhoid Relief Ointment
Pharmedix	Blephamide Ophthalmic Ointment	Sight Pharmaceuticals	Neomycin Polymyxin B Sulfates Hydrocortisone Otic Suspension
Pharmedix	Triple Antibiotic Ophthalmic Solution	Sight Pharmaceuticals	Sulfacetamide Sodium & Prednisolone Sodium Phosphate Ophthalmic Solution
Pharmedix	Colymycin S Otic Solution	Spectrum Quality Products	Merbromin (bulk chemical)
Pharmedix	Neo Poly with HC Otic Suspension	Spectrum Quality Products	Mercuric Oxide Yellow (bulk chemical)
Physicians Total Care Inc.	Neomycin Polymyxin B Sulfates Hydrocortisone Ophthalmic Suspension	Spectrum Quality Products	Thimerosal (bulk chemical)
Spectrum Quality Products	Thimerosal (bulk chemical)	US Ophthalmics	Sulf-10 Ophthalmic Solution
Super Laboratories	Long Acting Nasal Spray	US Ophthalmics	Vasocidin Ophthalmic Solution
Taro Pharmaceuticals	Taro Nasal Decongestant Spray	US Ophthalmics	Phenylephrine HC1 Ophthalmic Solution 10%
Teral Laboratories	Oticin HC Otic Suspension	USCO Logistics	Procofen Ophthalmic Solution
Thames Pharmacal Co.	12 Hour Nasal Spray	USCO Logistics	Profenal Ophthalmic Solution
Thrifty Payless Inc.	Nasal Spray Pump Formula	VEDCO Inc.	Tribiotic Ophthalmic Solution
Thrifty Payless Inc.	Decongestant Nasal Spray Pump	Waldbaum Inc.	Hemorrhoidal Ointment
United Research Labs	Antibiotic Ear Suspension	Weeks and Leo Co. Inc.	Long Acting Nasal Spray Solution
United Research Labs	Neomycin Polymyxin B Sulfates Gramicidin Ophthalmic Solution	Whitehall-Robins	Dristan 12-Hour Nasal Spray
US Ophthalmics	Fluorescein Sodium Ophthalmic Solution		

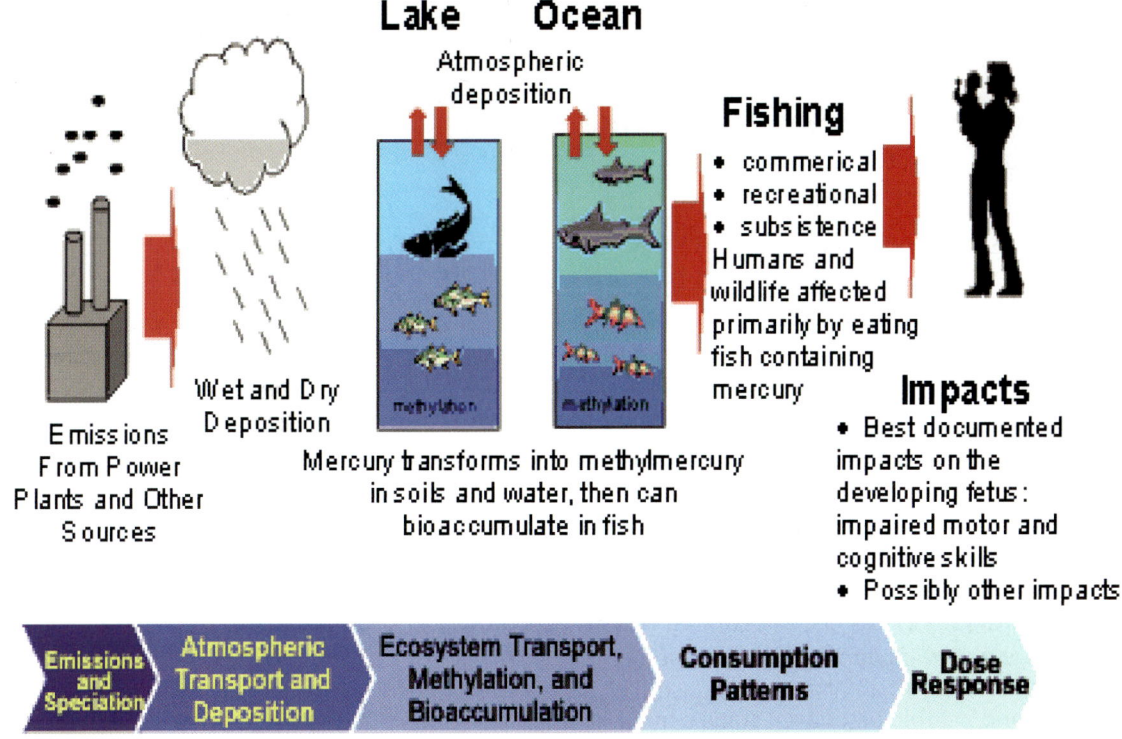

MOLYBDENUM

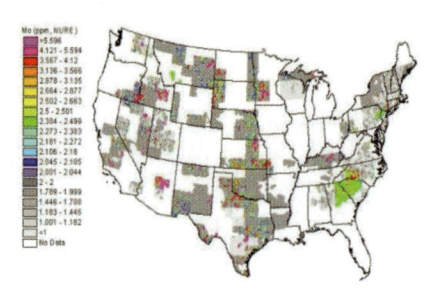

Molybdenum is an essential trace element for virtually all life forms. It functions as a cofactor for a number of enzymes that catalyze important chemical transformations in the global carbon, nitrogen, and sulfur cycles. Thus, molybdenum-dependent enzymes are not only required for human health, but also for the health of our ecosystem.

Function: The biological form of molybdenum, present in almost all molybdenum-containing enzymes (molybdoenzymes), is an organic molecule known as the molybdenum cofactor. In humans, molybdenum is known to function as a cofactor for three enzymes:

1) Sulfite oxidase catalyzes the transformation of sulfite to sulfate, a reaction that is necessary for the metabolism of sulfur-containing amino acids (methionine and cysteine).

2) Xanthine oxidase catalyzes the breakdown of nucleotides (precursors to DNA and RNA) to form uric acid, which contributes to the plasma antioxidant capacity of the blood.

3) Aldehyde oxidase and xanthine oxidase catalyze hydroxylation reactions that involve a number of different molecules with similar chemical structures. Xanthine oxidase and aldehyde oxidase also play a role in the metabolism of drugs and toxins.

Of these three enzymes, only sulfite oxidase is known to be crucial for human health.

Nutrient interactions include copper. Excess dietary molybdenum has been found to result in copper deficiency in grazing animals (ruminants). In ruminants, the formation of compounds containing sulfur and molybdenum, appear to prevent the absorption of copper.

Deficiency: Dietary molybdenum deficiency has never been observed in healthy people.

The Recommended Dietary Allowance (RDA): The recommended dietary allowance for molybdenum was most recently revised in January 2001. The RDA values for molybdenum are listed in the table below in micrograms/day by age and gender. Adequate intake levels were set for infants based on mean molybdenum intake from human milk, exclusively.

Recommended dietary allowance for molybdenum:

Infants
Ages 0.0 thru 0.5: 2 micrograms/day   Ages 0.5 thru 1: 3 micrograms/day

Children
Ages 1 thru 3: 17 micrograms/day   Ages 7 thru 10: 34 micrograms/day
Ages 4 thru 8: 22 micrograms/day

Females and males
Ages 9 thru 13:   34 micrograms/day   Ages 19 and older: 50 micrograms/day
Ages 14 thru 18: 43 micrograms/day

Pregnant
All ages: 50 milligrams/day   Lactating women: 50 milligrams/day

Foods that contain molybdenum:

Asparagus	Endive	Parsley
Asparagus bean	Field bean	Pea
Bell pepper	Flageolet bean	Pea bean
Black bean	French bean	Plum
Black cherry	Garden bean	Pop bean
Buckwheat	Ginseng	Potato
Butter bean	Green bean	Red cabbage
Cabbage	Green pepper	Snap bean
Cauliflower	Haricot bean	String bean
Cauliflower	Haricot vert	Sweet pepper
Cherry pepper	Kidney bean	Tomato
Cone pepper	Lettuce	Wax bean
Corn	Lima bean	White cabbage
Corn salad	Navy bean	Wild cherry
Cucumber	Non-GMO soybean	Yardlong bean
Dwarf bean	Onion	
	Paprika	

NITROGEN

The chemical element nitrogen is a colorless, odorless gas that was discovered in 1772 by Daniel Rutherford, uncle of Sir Walter Scott, of Scotland, and independently by Joseph Priestley and Henry Cavendish of England and Carl W. Scheele of Sweden. The French chemist Antoine L. Lavoisier proved that it was an element. The name nitrogen is derived from the Greek words nitron and genes, which mean, "saltpeter producing," because one of the most important nitrogen compounds then known was saltpeter (potassium nitrate).

Occurrence: Nitrogen is the most abundant uncombined element. Air is 78.06% nitrogen gas by volume. Nitrogen is found in gases from volcanoes, springs, and mines. The many important and useful organic nitrogen compounds include proteins, urea, and vitamins such as vitamin(s) B_1, B_2, B_3, B_4, B_5, B_6, B_7, B_9, B_{10}, B_{11}, B_{12}, B_{15}, and B_{17}.

Foods that contain nitrogen:

Achiote	Garden bean	Pop bean
Beet	Garden beet	Popping bean
Beetroot	Garden dill	Radish
Bell pepper	Ginger	Red cabbage
Black bean	Green bean	Rutabaga
Cabbage	Green pepper	Saffron
Cauliflower	Haricot	Snap bean
Cauliflower	Haricot bean	Sorrel
Cherry pepper	Haricot vert	Spinach
Common indigo	Horseradish	Stinging nettle
Cone pepper	Kidney bean	String bean
Cucumber	Lettuce	Sugar beet
Dill	Navy bean	Tomato
Dwarf bean	Paprika	Wax bean
Field bean	Parsley	White cabbage
Flageolet bean	Pea	
French bean	Pineapple	

PHOSPHRUS

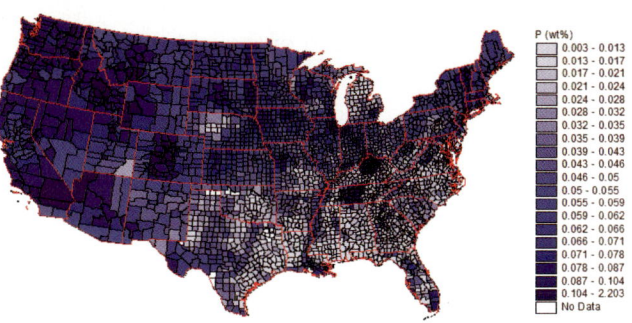

Phosphorus is a flammable, solid, nonmetallic, nitrogen group element with color variations of white, red, or black. Hennig Brand of Germany discovered it in 1669 when he precipitated it from urine. It is number 15 on the atomic periodic table.

Phosphorous, an essential trace, nonmetallic element, is the second most abundant mineral in the body following calcium. It is found primarily in bones, muscles, nerves, and teeth. About 80% of it is in the skeleton and the rest is very metabolically active in every cell of the body, primarily as phosphatidylcholine, also known as lecithin, a phospholipid. Phosphatidylcholine is a component of cell membranes, most importantly the brain, and other soft tissues. Phospholipids are important transporters of other substances such as neurotransmitters, across cell membranes.

Phosphorous is necessary for the assimilation of carbohydrates and fats as well as activation of many enzymes. Phosphorous is a component of adenosine triphosphate, the primary energy source for the body's cells. Phosphorous participates in more biological processes than any other mineral and is involved in every metabolic process in the body, acting as a buffer in the blood and body tissues.

Phosphorous in supplements is usually in combination with other minerals. Examples of these forms are: dipotassium phosphate, also known as phosphoric acid and dicalcium phosphate sometimes referred to as calcium hydrogen phosphate, or tricalcium phosphate.

Deficiency symptoms: Phosphorous depletion is rarely seen in humans. Those at risk include alcoholics, dialysis patients, people with celiac or Crohn's disease (malabsorption syndromes), and those on extreme diets lacking phosphorous rich foods.

Function in the body:

1. Phosphorous is regulated through renal absorption, interaction with calcium, parathyroid hormone, and vitamin D.

2. Phosphorous plays a role in the function of bones and teeth which is needed to form calcium phosphate, the crystallized substance that provides strength and rigidity.

3. Buffering System: buffers and maintains pH balance in blood and other fluids, indispensable portion of the acid alkaline balance of the body.

4. Cellular Energy: There is phosphate groups in adenosine triphosphate, the "packets" of energy produced in the mitochondria of cells throughout the body.

5. Cellular reproduction as part of DNA and RNA synthesis.

6. Enzymes that activate or is one of many activating substances in co-enzymes and enzymatic reactions.

7. Lipids which are part of phospholipids and lipid metabolism.

8. Protein Synthesis: as part of the enzymes involved in amino acid availability as building blocks for the body.

Other facts: Lecithin is phosphotidylcholine and is a phospholipid. Brain cell membrane levels of phosphotidylcholine decline with age. It has been proposed that supplementing with lecithin improves cognition and memory. Studies of elderly with cognitive defects and dementia have not demonstrated this in a consistent way and are inconclusive. The same kind of results emerged from studies of Parkinson's disease, stroke, and specific impaired memory syndromes. A recent literature review of published, peer-reviewed research concluded that lecithin supplementation "appears useful for improving the structural integrity and functionality of the neuronal membrane that may assist membrane repair." More investigation is underway in attempts to determine if supplementation improves cognitive ability, memory, and/or mobility in certain subsets of populations with impairments in these areas.

Symptoms could include:

Bone abnormalities
Cognitive deficits

Fatigue
Memory impairment

Wasting

Phosphorus promotes:

Accurate genetic code replication
Availability of building blocks for the body
Calcium metabolism
Energy
Healthy bones

Normal lipid metabolism
PH balance of blood, body fluids
Strong teeth
Thyroid function
Vitamin D production

Phosphorus protects against:

Abnormal amino acid synthesis
Abnormal cell replication
Bone abnormalities

Diminished phospholipids
Fatigue
Fluid imbalances

Soft teeth
Wasting

Foods that contain phosphorus:

Almond
Asparagus
Barley
Barley grass
Beetroot
Bitter melon
Black bean
Butter bean
Cauliflower
Coca
Cucumber
Dwarf bean
Field bean
Flageolet bean
Flax

French bean
Garden bean
Garden beet
Garden cress
Green bean
Haricot bean
Haricot vert
Horsetail
Kidney bean
Lambs quarter
Lettuce
Lima bean
Linseed
Navy bean
Oats

Pop bean
Poppyseed
Pumpkin
Radish
Sesame
Snap bean
String bean
Sugar beet
Swamp cabbage
Water spinach
Watercress
Watermelon
Wax bean

Drugs that deplete: Phosphorous is depleted by aluminum containing antacids, diuretics, and some cardiac and antihypertensive drugs. Iron can inhibit the absorption of phosphorous. Mineral oil and excessive magnesium can interfere with the absorption of phosphorous if administered at the same time.

Food preparation to retain phosphorus: Food processing removes phosphorous from grains and may remove it from soy.

An unhealthy source of phosphorous in the American diet and unfortunately increasingly around the world is phosphinated soda, the many carbonated soft drinks.

Fortified foods available:

| Dairy | Flour | Grain products |

Recommended dietary allowance:

Infants
Ages 0.0 thru 0.5:   100 milligrams/day   Ages 0.5 thru 1: 275 milligrams/day
Children
Ages 1 thru 3: 460 milligrams/day   Ages 7 thru 10: 800 milligrams/day
Ages 4 thru 8: 500 milligrams/day

Females and males
Ages 9 thru 13: 1250 milligrams/day   Ages 31 thru 50: 700 milligrams/day
Ages 14 thru 18: 1250 milligrams/day   Ages 51 and older: 700 milligrams/day
Ages 19 and older: 700 milligrams/day

Pregnant: the same as for non-pregnant women of comparable age

Lactating: the same as for non lactating women of comparable age

Toxic Doses: Too much phosphorous interferes with calcium absorption and can produce bone abnormalities such as osteoporosis occurring in people who drink phosphinated sodas in large quantities on a daily basis.

Excess phosphorous can worsen hyperthyroidism.

POTASSIUM

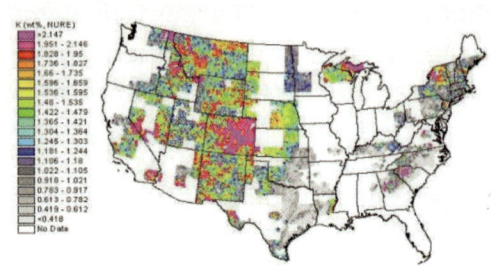

Potassium, also known as kalium, is a soft alkali metal and one of the most active metals known. Humphrey Davy electrolyzed "fused potash" to form pure potassium in 1807.

Potassium, an essential trace macro mineral is one of the body's major electrolytes. Electrolytes carry an electronic charge that provides strong influence over the solubility of substances. The electrolytes regulate osmotic pressures in the body fluids and potassium is the one that is predominate in electrolyte activity within all the cells. In fact, cells contain more potassium than any other mineral. Approximately 98% of total potassium in the body is within the cells.

Hormones of adrenal and pituitary glands maintain tight control over the potassium level in the serum of blood. These hormones regulate a proper balance between all the electrolytes. The kidneys excrete excess potassium. Potassium works most closely with sodium to achieve homeostasis with normal water distribution. The third major electrolyte with which potassium and sodium closely relate is chloride.

Supplemental forms of potassium are dominated by potassium chloride, a salt used as a sodium chloride (regular table salt) substitute for many people on sodium restricted diet.

Other compounds include:

Potassium acetate	Potassium citrate	Potassium proteinate
Potassium bicarbonate	Potassium gluconate	

Deficiency symptoms: Protracted vomiting, and/or diarrhea, diabetic ketoacidosis, extreme weight loss dieting, kidney disease, malnutrition, and starvation can cause potassium deficiency. Potassium depletion can occur with the ingestion of alcohol, caffeine, large amounts of sodium chloride (table salt) or sugar, and water intoxication. Chronic stress has been shown to cause electrolyte disturbance probably secondary to excessive, sustained adrenal stimulation, and has produced hypokalemia, the term for low potassium levels.

Symptoms of low potassium (hypokalemia) include:

Arrhythmias	Disorientation	Muscle spasms
Blood pressure disturbance	Dizziness	Muscle weakness
Constipation	Edema (swelling)	Neuron misfiring
Polydipsia (excessive thirst)		

Potassium promotes:

Fluid balance throughout the body	Muscle function
Heart tissue function	Nerve function

Potassium protects against:

Abnormal nerve function	Muscle cramping
Fatigue	Muscle weakness
Irregular heart rate	Swelling

Function in the body: Potassium works in concert with sodium to balance osmotic pressures and intracellular and extracellular water distribution throughout the body. Potassium has important roles in critical neuromuscular impulse transmissions. The function of the heart, other muscles, and nerves are dependent on normal levels of this electrolyte.

Other facts: Maintaining normal levels of potassium by eating a potassium rich diet of fresh fruits and vegetables each day has been shown to decrease the incidence of stroke.

There is no recommended dietary allowance for potassium. Adults need about 2 to 5 grams a day.

Drugs that deplete potassium: Diuretics and cancer chemotherapeutic agents deplete potassium most frequently. Depletion of this electrolyte occurs with use of some antibiotics, antihypertensive medications, laxatives, and steroids.

Foods that contain potassium:

Asparagus	Dwarf bean	Lettuce
Beet	Endive	Navy bean
Beetroot	Field bean	Parsley
Bitter melon	Flageolet bean	Pop bean
Black bean	French bean	Radish
Bok	Garden bean	Rhubarb
Borage	Garden beet	Snap bean
Carrot	Garden cress	Spinach
Cauliflower	Garden dill	String bean
Celery	Green bean	Sugar beet
Chinese Cabbage	Haricot	Tomato
Cilantro	Haricot bean	Watercress
Cucumber	Haricot vert	Wax bean
Dandelion	Kidney bean	
Dill	Lambs quarter	

Fortified foods available: None

Toxic doses: Renal failure (diminished kidney function) causes serum potassium levels to raise, a condition known as hyperkalemia that is essentially potassium toxicity and constitutes a medical emergency in the acute stage and with escalating levels. Patients with chronic renal failure many times will have chronic mild hyperkalemia for which their body compensates. Over time, these compensations produce untold effects such as calcification of the soft tissues. Some long time dialysis patients will have more calcium in their aorta than in their bones as the mineral shifts in their bodies are so profound.

Symptoms of acute hyperkalemia can include:

Arrhythmias	Dyspnea (shortness of breath)
Cardiac arrest	Muscular rigidity or flaccidity
Decreased heart output	Parasthesias (decreased sensation)
Disorientation	

RUBIDIUM

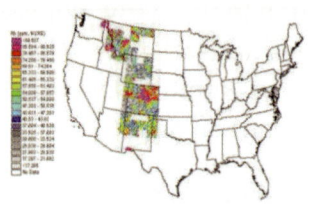

A German scientist, Gustav Kirchhoff, with Robert Bunsen discovered rubidium in 1861. A soft, silvery-white metallic element that seemed to ask more questions than the two could answer, and science is still awaiting more answers. The Mendeleyev Chart assigns it the number 37.

Research tells us the average human being has about 350 milligrams of rubidium in the body. Rubidium competes with potassium ions for entry into the body. Rubidium chloride accelerates cyclic energy synthesis in the cortex of a rat brain and changes circadian rhythms of sleep in short.

Imbalance: Very high rubidium partnered with low potassium can put muscles into a state of semi-paralysis. Rubidium will take the place of potassium in the sodium-potassium pump.

Depression: The mere mention of depression suggests a near epidemic in America. Its link to rubidium and mainstream medicine's preference to rely on pharmaceuticals rather than nutrition for treatment may one day be seen as a medical tragedy on par with the ignorance of vitamin C that condemned generations of seamen to die of scurvy.

Test animal results reveal that absence of rubidium in diets results in higher urea nitrogen in plasma, potassium in blood, kidneys and tibia bone, magnesium in muscles and tibia, iron in muscles and excess copper in kidneys, while lower rubidium concentration in tissues, sodium in muscles, potassium in testicles, phosphorous and calcium in spleen, zinc in plasma and testicles, copper in heart, liver and spleen.

Pharmaceutical medicine expects depression to be answered with a plethora of fluoride laced antidepressant drugs. Rubidium has a long half-life, for which reason providers of this supplement rely on medical physicians and natural health providers to counsel patients, package directions being absolute. Extensive research approves administration of oral rubidium. As with many if not all trace minerals, it can become toxic, only if concentration in muscles reaches 30 percent of the potassium levels.

In the case of rubidium, it is better to reach for some Brazil nuts. Well-disciplined research tells us that the Finnish diet usually contains 4.5 micrograms of rubidium per day. The English seem to consume 1.4 milligrams a day, and Americans have a 2.51 milligram intake of this vital element. The best source of rubidium is unprocessed Brazil nuts.

Foods that contain rubidium:

Almond	Coconut	Plum
Apple	Cone pepper	Potato
Asparagus bean	Cucumber	Radish
Banana	Dandelion	Red cabbage
Beet	English filbert	Red currant
Beetroot	Garden beet	Rhubarb
Bell pepper	Garden dill	Rutabaga
Bilberry	Grapefruit	Spinach
Black currant	Green pepper	Stinging nettle
Butterbur	Mugwort	Sugar beet
Carrot	Paprika	Sweet pepper
Cashew	Parsley	Tomato
Cauliflower	Parsnip	White cabbage
Cherry pepper	Pea bean	White currant
Cinnamon	Pear	Yardlong bean
Cloudberry	Pecan	

SELENIUM

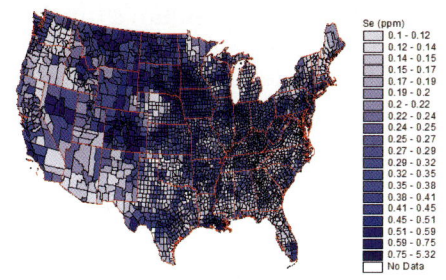

J. J. Berzelius discovered selenium in Sweden in 1817 and named after Selene, the Greek Goddess of the Moon. It is number 34 on the atomic periodic table. Selenium, an essential trace micro mineral, was thought to be very toxic. Over the past half century, it has been found to be a key in antioxidant enzymes. These enzymes are made up of selenium proteins that are important in detoxification of free radicals and thus play a role in prevention of chronic diseases. They provide some of the defense mechanisms of the immune system and also helps regulate thyroid function.

The forms that are available for supplementation include organic and inorganic compounds. The organic compound and the one thought to be best absorbed and utilized in the body is selenomethionine, an analogue of the amino acid methionine. Another seleno amino acid is selenocysteine. There are some specialty yeasts that have as much as 2000 micrograms of selenium per gram, which is mostly the organic compound. Most supplements of selenium are made of, in total or part, the inorganic sodium selenite and sodium selenate. These are bioavailable, but to a lesser degree and may be involved in the development of type 2 diabetes.

Deficiency symptoms: Selenium deficiency is rare in the U.S. as most of the North American continent has selenium in the growing soil although farming practices can deplete this. China has had high rates of selenium deficiency primarily because of the low levels of selenium occurring naturally in the soil.

The Keshan district of China had high rates of childhood cardiomyopathies (enlarged, poor functioning hearts) until selenium supplementation was started. This type of cardiomyopathy is called Keshan Disease and research indicates a certain viral infection in the presence of low selenium levels may cause this.

Another condition of selenium deficiency is Kashin-Beck Disease. This is a degenerative joint disease called an osteoarthropathy and progresses with crippling effects.

Another syndrome from selenium deficiency is myxedematous endemic cretinism. This results in mental retardation.

Severely injured persons or those suffering major intestinal inflammation may have interference with selenium absorption and resultant deficiency. Those on total parenteral nutrition (intravenous feeding) need selenium and other micronutrients added in forms that are compatible with blood components.

Selenium promotes:

Anti-inflammatory activity
Detoxification
Immune function
Thyroid function
Vitamin E utilization
White blood cell production

Selenium protects against:

Cardiac inflammatory disorders
Cataracts
Heavy metal toxicity
Lowered thyroid hormone
Other Inflammatory disorders
Premature aging

Function in the body: Selenium's function in the body has:

1. Anti-inflammatory effect that is provided by glutathione peroxidase, an important selenoprotein enzyme.

2. Antioxidant effect of glutathione peroxidase is powerful, one of the most effective antioxidant enzymes of the immune system.

3. Anticarcinogenic activity by preventing free radical damage to DNA and RNA within the nucleus of cells.

4. Antiviral effect by boosting certain white blood cells - the T lymphocytes and natural killer cells.

5. Detoxifying properties that reduce the effects of damaging ions from heavy metal and some cancer chemotherapeutic agents.

6. Thyroid hormone conversion activity changing thyroxin (T4) to triiodothyronine (T3). A selenoprotein enzyme called deiodinase mediates this conversion. Deiodinase is a peroxidase enzyme that is involved in the activation or deactivation of thyroid hormones.

7. Vitamin E potentiation, boosting its antioxidant activity.

Other facts: A diet for infants of strictly cow's milk with no supplementation will result in low selenium levels and resultant deficiency syndromes. Cow's milk has 60% less selenium than human milk.

White rice has approximately 1500% less selenium than brown rice.

A diet rich in selenium or selenium supplementation may help to decrease the risk of cancer because of its role in DNA repair. It may also help prevent heart disease and help to control asthma symptoms.

Drugs that deplete selenium: Steroids deplete selenium.

Food preparation to retain selenium: Processing removes significant amounts of selenium from grain based foods.

Food Sources: All plant foods grown in selenium rich soil. Selenium in food varies depending on the region from which it was grown and harvested. Whole grains are the best source. Dairy products and eggs as well as seafood and liver are good animal sources. Brazil nuts can be extremely high in selenium content.

Fortified foods available: None known.

1989 recommended dietary allowances (RDA):

Infants
Ages 0.0 thru 0.5:   10 micrograms/day   Ages 0.5 thru 1: 15 micrograms/day

Children
Ages 1 thru 3:   20 micrograms/day   Ages 7 thru 10:   30 micrograms/day
Ages 4 thru 8:   20 micrograms/day

Females and males
Ages 9 thru 13:   40-50 micrograms/day   Ages 19 and older: 55 micrograms/day
Ages 14 thru 18: 55 micrograms/day

Pregnant
All ages: 65 micrograms/day   Lactating women: 75 micrograms/day

Toxic doses: Blood levels of selenium that exceed 100 microgram per deciliter cause risk of a condition called seleninosis. The symptoms are:

Brittle blotchy nails	Hair loss
Could lead to neurological damage	Halitosis
Diarrhea	Irritability
Fatigue	Nausea/vomiting

One incident of manufacturing error led to excess amounts of selenium in a supplement that was many times greater than the label intended. Industrial accidents have caused excessive amounts of selenium and toxicity.

Foods that contain selenium if selenium is found in the soil:

Aloe	Echinacea	Lemongrass
Barberry	Fennel	Marshmallow
Barley	Feverfew	Milfoil
Barley grass	Garden thyme	Oats
Black cohosh	Garlic	Pennyroyal
Black walnut	Gentian	Peppermint
Bladderwrack	Ginseng	Psyllium
Blessed thistle	Grape	Pumpkin
Blue cohosh	Hawthorn	Raspberry
Brazil nut	Honey buchu	Safflower
Burdock	Hops	Sarsaparilla
Catnip	Horsetail	Slippery elm
Chaparral	Indian sorrel	Stinging nettle
Common thyme	Irish moss	Thyme
Coneflower	Kelp	Valerian
Crampbark	Lady's thistle	White mallow
Curly dock	Hawthorn	
Dulse	Ladyslipper	

SILICON

Silicon is also known as silica. There is no life without silica! In 1939, the Nobel Prize winner for chemistry, Professor Adolf Butenant, proved that life could not exist without silica. According to his research conducted at Columbia University in 1972, silica is an essential nutrient and must be supplied continuously from food sources. Silica plays an important role in many body functions and has a direct relationship to mineral absorption. The average human body holds approximately seven grams of silica, a quantity far exceeding the figures for other important minerals such as iron.

Many studies that prove the favorable influence of vegetable silica on the development of animals have been under-taken. Silica is essential to the development and mineralization of the skeleton. The absence of silica results in skeletal deformities. Hormonal disturbances in the human organism are often due to a calcium-magnesium imbalance, several studies have shown that silica can restore this delicate balance. Silica also benefits the assimilation of phosphorous. Thus, it may be considered a catalyst in the use of other elements.

Osteoporosis is a symptom of the aging process. As calcium in our body system leaches, our bones become brittle and weak. Taking only a calcium supplement cannot correct or stop this threatening and crippling disease because the body cannot assimilate and make use of the calcium without the presence of silica. Evidence suggests, instead of building bone, supplemental calcium by itself, accelerates the leaching of bone calcium. This hastening worsens osteoporosis and similar diseases, affecting supportive and connective tissues in the body.

For osteoporosis, silica can stop the pain and even restore the body's self-repair process. Osteoporosis symptoms attack women primarily after menopause but the degenerative process starts much earlier in their younger days. More women are dying of fractures caused by osteoporosis than of cancer of the breast, cervix, and uterus combined. In osteoporosis, thinning of the bones occur due to insufficient production of the surrounding protein medium in which calcium salts first deposit. A lack of calcium in the bone matrix leads to enlargement of canals and spaces in the bones, giving the bones a porous, thinned appearance. The weakened bone becomes fragile and may be broken by a minor injury. The bones may even fracture from normal pressure or stress. For purposes of remineralizing damaged bones, it is recommended that a sufficient silica supplement be taken daily. Bones are mainly made of phosphorus, magnesium, and calcium but also contain silica. Silica is responsible for deposition of minerals in the bones, especially calcium. It speeds up healing of fractures and reduces scarring at the site of a fracture.

Tissue degeneration accelerates due to aging when connective tissue develops an increasing inability to retain moisture when left unassisted. Silica can help slow the degenerative process of connective tissue. With silica, vitality and life are often lost as the years accumulate, but can be naturally maintained or restored to your skin. Connective tissue consists of collagen, elastin, mucopolysaccharides, and mucous carbohydrates that help moisture retention. Their ability to retain moisture keeps the connective tissue bouncy and has obvious importance in the prevention of premature aging. All these important molecules house large quantities of silica. Collagen, largely made up of silica, is the "glue" that holds us together. If our body has enough silica glucosaminoglycans, the collagen will make us look younger.

If you regularly follow a silica regimen, your skin will keep its young look. However, do not expect instant results. It is a good idea to start organic vegetable silica supplementation years before the collagen in your body has deteriorated to the point where it shows wrinkles on your face and body. A good silica supplementation program works far better than other products for maintaining healthier and longer lasting collagen.

Hair is nature's greatest beauty enhancer. It makes us sexually attractive and serves to protect us. Hair deserves to be pampered. Hair at 90 micrograms per gram of silica is almost as rich as healthy bones, containing 100 micrograms per gram. Silica is a major component of hair. Using a good silica supplement should be part of your ongoing hair care program for revitalizing hair. Silica helps to prevent baldness, stimulates healthier hair growth, and assures beautiful shine, luster, and strength.

By hardening the enamel, silica prevents cavities and preserves teeth. Silica also prevents bleeding gums, gum atrophy, and recession causing loosening of teeth, which could ultimately lead to tooth loss. Vegetable silica effectively fights caries (ulceration and the decay of a bone or of a tooth) and inflammation.

Your nail plates are complex protein structures that grow four to five millimeters per month on average. In case of deficiency, the rate of growth slows. Therefore, your fingernails can be the first indicators of silica deficiency. Demineralization of nails precedes by far any decalcification of bones. It is possible to start silica supplementation in time to prevent bone loss. With silica supplementation, fragile nails become normal within a short period of time. Silica will beautify the appearance of your nails and improve hardness, making them shinier and less prone to breaking.

The restorative effects of silica will be most noticeable on hair, skin, nails, and teeth. Skin and hair require silica essentially for the same purpose, as do other tissues. As we know, the supporting collagen underneath the skin enhances elasticity and beauty. Collagen owes that quality to silica, which provides a beautiful complexion that is more than skin deep.

Silica can be helpful to us in the following ways:

1. Silica has inhibitory effects on coronary diseases.

2. Organic vegetable silica supplementation helps repair, maintain vital lung tissues, and protects them from pollution. By maintaining or restoring the elasticity of lung tissues, silica reduces inflammation in bronchitis.

3. It acts as a cough decreasing agent. Silica tones the upper respiratory tract (nose, pharynx, and larynx), reducing swelling because of its positive action on the lymphatic system.

4. Silica supplementation helps prevent many unwanted side effects of menopause keeping women free of stress and reducing development of osteoporosis.

5. Silica works with other antioxidants to prevent premature aging and to preserve youthfulness.

6. New researches have found that antioxidants, like organic vegetable silica, protect against harmful radiation.

7. Silica can help prevent kidney stones and heal infections of the urinary tract. It is a natural diuretic that can increase excretion of urine by 30 percent, thus flushing the water-excreting system and restore normal function to these vital organs.

8. The presence of sufficient silica in the intestines reduces inflammation and can cause disinfection in the case of stomach and intestinal catarrh and ulcers. Silica can prevent or clear up diarrhea and its opposite, constipation.

9. Vegetable silica will help normalize hemorrhoidal tissues.

10. In regulating and normalizing the bowels, silica has a pleasant side effect; it can alleviate lower back pain, which often troubles the elderly.

11. Silica proves effective with female discharge, abscesses, and ulcers in the genital area and cervix, as well as mastitis (especially for breast-feeding mothers).

12. The intake of silica acts as a supportive treatment for inflammation of the middle ear.

13. Because of the beneficial effectiveness on the lymphatic system, silica can be used for swelling of lymph nodes in the throat.

14. Silica can stimulate the immune system.

15. Silica can normalize circulation and regulate high blood pressure (hypertension).

16. Silica can decrease vertigo, headache, tinnitus (buzzing of the ears), and insomnia.

17. Silica can help diabetes by promoting synthesis of elastase inhibitor by the pancreas.

18. Silica can help arterial disease by strengthening the blood vessels.

19. Silica can help prevent tuberculosis.

20. By improving the elasticity of the joints, silica helps rheumatism.

21. Silica can help avoid or alleviate Alzheimer's disease by preventing the body from absorbing aluminum and may flush aluminum out from the tissues.

22. Silica can stimulate cell metabolism and division.

23. Silica delays the aging process of the tissues. In younger people, tissues typically contain more silica than that of older people.

24. Silica increases mobility and reduces pain in osteoarthritis and sclerotic conditions.

25. Silica beautifies hair with shine, elasticity, and strength.

26. Silica prevents wrinkles.

Dosage: According to Professor Loeper, daily silica needs of humans are 20-30milligrams. Supplemental use of organic vegetable silica extracted from spring time horsetail ensures that an adequate amount of silica is continuously available to the body.

With adequate intake, enough assimilation of the vital nutrient can be assured even when the body's ability to assimilate is impaired. Any excess silica not needed by the body is automatically eliminated through the blood stream, kidneys, and intestines.

All of us need silica, regardless of our age. It is as important to give the body dietary sources of silica early in life as it is during the aging process when levels in tissue usually drop off steeply. Silica has a direct influence on absorption of all minerals that the body requires to maintain health, adding to the quality of life, and improving stamina and appearance.

For remineralization, purposes, such as bone mending, four to eight times that amount (20-30mg) should be ingested until silica therapy has proven successful. This is best done under the supervision of your physician.

Scientists believe that silica exists in three forms within the body:

1. A soluble form, accounting for ten percent of the body's silica.

2. A form combined with lipids and accounting for thirty percent.

3. A form combined with proteins accounting for the remaining sixty percent. This explains why our daily requirement of silica is quite high. In order for us to now lay down the foundations for shaping and building our body five, ten or even thirty years down the road; we should turn to foods and supplements that furnish us with our daily requirement of 20-30 milligrams of silica.

Finding the right silica may be confusing at times. Make sure that the vegetable silica you use is 100 percent pure aqueous extract. Also, be sure that it is from spring horsetail (*Equisetum Hymale.*)

Foods that contain silica:

Almond	Eyebright	Parsley
Banana	Field bean	Pineapple
Black bean	Flageolet bean	Pistachio
Black walnut	French bean	Pop bean
Brazil nut	Garden bean	Popping bean
Burdock	Garden dill	Radish
Butternut	Ginger	Red currant
Cashew	Goldenseal	Snap bean
Coconut	Grape	Spinach
Coneflower	Green bean	Stinging nettle
Corn	Haricot	Strawberry
Cucumber	Haricot bean	String bean
Date palm	Haricot vert	Wax bean
Dulse	Horsetail	Wheatgrass
Dwarf bean	Kidney bean	White currant
Echinacea	Lettuce	
English filbert	Navy bean	

Sodium

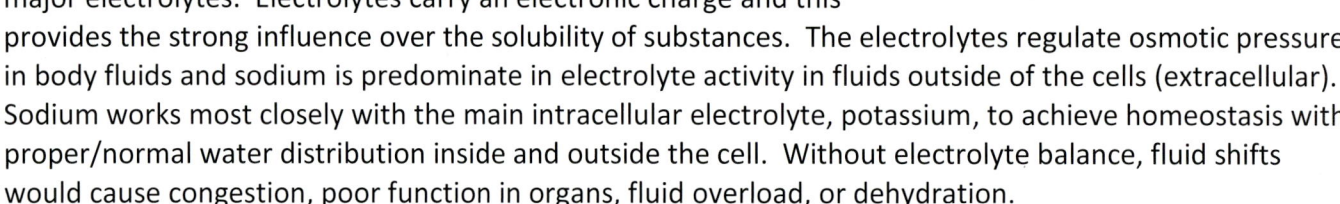

Humphrey Davy discovered sodium in 1807. It is an alkali metal and the 11th element on the atomic periodic table.

Sodium, an essential trace macro mineral, is one of the body's major electrolytes. Electrolytes carry an electronic charge and this provides the strong influence over the solubility of substances. The electrolytes regulate osmotic pressure in body fluids and sodium is predominate in electrolyte activity in fluids outside of the cells (extracellular). Sodium works most closely with the main intracellular electrolyte, potassium, to achieve homeostasis with proper/normal water distribution inside and outside the cell. Without electrolyte balance, fluid shifts would cause congestion, poor function in organs, fluid overload, or dehydration.

The kidneys, master chemists of the body, excrete excess sodium if present in the body. The American diet contains far more sodium than needed or healthy. Up to 3000% more sodium in the form of sodium chloride (table salt) is consumed daily, mostly used in food processing, preservation and packaging in convenience, snack, or "junk" food. One teaspoon of salt is the equivalent of 2400 milligrams of sodium. Indiscriminant addition of salt to prepared food at the table can substantially add to the amount consumed.

Besides sodium chloride, there are other far less occurring sodium compounds available. One example is sodium fluoride that is highly toxic and found in most American toothpaste.

Function in the body: Fluid homeostasis (balance) is the primary physiologic role of sodium. The blood volume within blood vessels known as the intravascular volume is most dependent on sodium. Without adequate levels in the blood, fluids leak out of blood vessels into the spaces in, around, and between organs and tissues, causing swelling. With too much sodium, the intravascular volume increases causing blood pressure elevations and other types of fluid shifts that can jeopardize health.

Other facts: An eight-ounce can of "soda pop" type soft drink contains approximately between 35 and 55 milligrams of sodium; a glass of milk, with all its superior nutritional power, contains over 100 milligrams.

Deficiency symptoms: Some conditions can cause sodium depletion and deficiency. Dehydration caused by excessive sweating, severe vomiting, and diarrhea, and/or decreased intake of water for sustained periods. Some cancers, such as lung cancer, can cause sodium deficiency.

Sodium deficiency symptoms can include:

Appetite loss
Dehydration
Dyspnea (shortness of breath)
Edema (swelling)

Fatigue
Memory and concentration impairment
Muscle fatigue (ease of exhaustion)

Sodium promotes:

Blood pressure stability
Blood vessel stability

Cardiac function
Fluid balance in whole body

Sodium protects against:

Fatigue
Irregular heart rate
Low blood pressure
Swelling

The average American has far too much sodium in their diet. There is no RDA for sodium; however, it is suggested not to exceed 3 grams a day.

Drugs that deplete sodium: Diuretics cancer chemotherapeutic agents and steroids deplete sodium most readily. Other drugs that can cause depletion are some antihypertensive drugs, antibiotics, and gout medications. Aspirin can deplete sodium. More than not, sodium is added to the food preparatory and packaging process.

Food sources: Table salt (sodium chloride) is the number one source for sodium in the U.S. diet and increasing in diets throughout the world. It is used not only at the table but in massive quantities in food processing-in canning and bottling, in preparing foods for freezing, in convenience and "fast" foods, in sauces, dressings and condiments, in snack and "treat" foods, in dried and specialty meats, and in packaged foods in general.

Sodium occurs naturally in much smaller quantities in "raw" food. Meat and dairy foods contain more sodium than raw or unsalted cooked vegetables and whole grains. Fresh fruit is very low in sodium.

Fortified foods available: Sodium is added to many foods, not to avoid depletion syndromes, but for preservation purposes. Naturally occurring salts such as the pink tinged, Redmond Real Salt (mined in Redmond Utah) or Pink Himalayan Salt have several dozen other minerals in their makeup, not just sodium and chloride. These other mineral rich salts are healthier than regular table salt and have been shown to normalize high blood pressures compared to regular, white table salt.

Recommended dietary allowance (RDA): No RDA exists for sodium but intake is said to not exceed three grams a day under dietary guidelines.

Toxic doses: Renal failure, failure of the function of the kidneys, can lead to dangerously high serum sodium levels that can cause serious fluid shifts in the body and cause fluid accumulation in areas such as the lungs and heart. These could become life threatening.

Foods that contain sodium:

Artichoke	Endive	Red cabbage
Beet	Garden beet	Sage
Beetroot	Ginseng	Scotch kale
Black mustard	Irish moss	Soybean
Bladderwrack	Kale	Spinach
Bok	Kelp	Spinach
Borage	Kitchen kale	Stinging nettle
Carrot	Lettuce	Sugar beet
Celery	Licorice	Tomato
Cilantro	Mangrove	Turmeric
Collards	Oats	Watercress
Comfrey	Olive	White cabbage
Curly kale	Parsley	Wild indigo
Dandelion	Pennyroyal	Wolfberry
Dulse	Radish	

Strontium

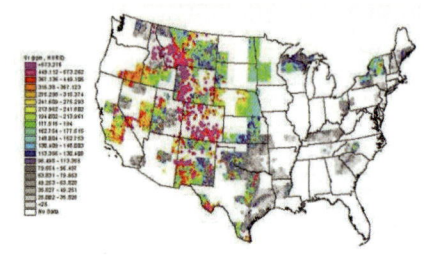

Strontium is named after the Scottish village of Strontian, having been discovered in the ores taken from the lead mines. In 1790, Adair Crawford, a physician engaged in the preparation of barium, recognized that the Strontian ores exhibited different properties to those normally seen.

Research on strontium goes back almost 50 years, when in 1959 a groundbreaking clinical trial was conducted at the world-renowned Mayo Clinic. Physicians treated a group of patients suffering from severe, painful bone loss with strontium—and found that every single person experienced improvement.

Why is strontium able to make your bones so much stronger and more resistant to fracture? This is because unlike any other mineral, strontium stimulates the rapid formation of bone tissue. Strontium has been safely used as a medicinal substance for more than a hundred years. It was first listed in *Squire's Companion to the British Pharmacopoeia* in 1884. Subsequently, strontium was used therapeutically in the United States and Europe. As late as 1955, strontium compounds were still listed in the Dispensatory of the United States of America.

The processes of bone resorption and formation are tightly governed by a variety of systemic and local regulatory agents. In addition, minerals and trace elements affect bone formation and resorption through direct or indirect effects on bone cells or bone mineral. Some trace elements closely related to calcium chemically, such as strontium have pharmacological effects on bone when present at levels higher than those required for normal cell physiology. The human body contains approximately 320 to 400 mg of strontium in bone, and connective tissue. If we look at clinical studies, indeed, strontium was found to exert several effects on bone cells. In addition to its antiresorptive activity, strontium was found to have anabolic activity in bone, and thus may have significant beneficial effects on bone balance in normal and osteopenic animals. Accordingly, strontium has been thought to have potential in the treatment of osteoporosis.

In a three-year, randomized, double-blind, placebo controlled study using 680 milligrams of strontium daily, women suffering from osteoporosis experienced a 41 percent reduction in risk of a vertebral fracture, compared with placebo. Overall, vertebral density in the strontium group increased by 11.4 percent but there was a 1.3 percent decrease in the placebo group.

In a second study, 353 women who had suffered at least one vertebral fracture due to osteoporosis took varying levels of a prescription medication of strontium referred to as strontium ranelate or a placebo. The women who took 680 milligrams of strontium daily had an increase in lumbar bone mineral density of approximately 3 percent per year, significantly greater than placebo. By the second year of the study, there was a significant decrease in additional fractures in the strontium group as compared with the placebo group.

These studies, the benefits of strontium ranelate (reducing risk fracture by as much as 50%) and the history of strontium in medical practice were discussed as an editorial in the *New England Journal of Medicine,* January 29, 2004.

Further, scientists are looking into the benefits of strontium for osteoarthritis because researchers hypothesized that strontium might also improve cartilage metabolism. In addition, benefits for dental caries since 10% of subjects had no dental caries in a 10-year study sponsored by the U.S. Navy, resided in a small town that had unusually high levels of strontium in the municipal water supply. In clinical research strontium gluconate was absorbed better than strontium carbonate.

The form of strontium ranelate has been demonstrated to increase bone mass through its stimulatory effect of osteoblasts (which increases bone formation), and its inhibitory effect of osteoclasts (which cause bone loss through bone resorption). At the recommended daily dosage of 2 grams in granules form, strontium ranelate has shown a significant reduction of vertebral fractures and hip fractures in clinical trials, with decreased back pain and decreased body height loss compared to the placebo group. At this time, it is primarily recommended for post-menopausal women, but not pregnant, or breast-feeding females.

Strontium is available as:

Strontium carbonate	Strontium citrate	Strontium ranelate
Strontium chloride	Strontium gluconate	Strontium sulfate

Foods that contain strontium:

American persimmon	Field bean	Orange
Asparagus	Flageolet bean	Parsley
Black bean	French bean	Pop bean
Black cherry	Garden bean	Red cabbage
Buck bush	Grapefruit	Sassafras
Butter bean	Green bean	Smooth Sumac
Butterbur	Haricot	Snap bean
Carrot	Haricot bean	String bean
Chinese cabbage	Haricot vert	Sweetgum
Coca	Kidney bean	Tomato
Cucumber	Knotweed	Wax bean
Dandelion	Lettuce	White cabbage
Dwarf bean	Lima bean	Wild cherry
Dwarf sumac	Navy bean	Willow oak
Endive	Onion	Winged sumac

SULFUR

Sulfur is a yellow, non-metal and known through the ages; it is in the chalcogen group and number 16 on the atomic table.

An essential minor mineral, the body must have sulfur predominantly to determine the structure and shape as well as function of proteins. Sulfur-containing amino acids strengthen and stabilize proteins by creating links between them formed by disulfide bonds. The four sulfur-containing amino acids in the body are cysteine, cystine, methionine, and taurine. Keratine, a protein of hair, skin, and insulin are the most sulfur prevalent proteins although all proteins in the body contain some sulfur.

Collagen is a mucopolysaccharide whose structure is dependent on sulfur. Chondrointin sulfate, another mucopolysaccharide compound is found at high levels in joint tissues.

The liver synthesizes anticoagulant proteins containing sulfur to prevent hypercoagulability of the blood and unwanted clot formation, heparin is one of these.

Function in the body:

1. Two disulfide bonds forming insulin join two polypeptide chains of specific sequencing of amino acids.
2. An important component of Coenzyme A, Sulfur is essential for metabolism and generation of body energy.
3. It is part of the biochemical activity of vitamin B_1, B_5 as well as lipoic acid. Lipoic acid is an important antioxidant protecting cell membranes as it interacts with vitamin C and essential in mitochondrial dehydrogenase reactions in production of energy.

Other facts: Elemental sulfur is not taken as a supplement, but is a component of many dietary compounds. Some of the B complex vitamins contain sulfur as well as some amino acids. Certain foods such as garlic and onions attribute their strong smell to large amounts of sulfur.

Burning flesh, hair, nails, and feathers smell of sulfur released from their proteins.

Deficiency symptoms: In the advanced stages of starvation with profound muscle destruction, sulfur deficiency can occur. Proteins in general would not be available for tissue, enzyme, and hormone generation and organ failure would be eminent without sulfur.

Sulfur promotes:

Antioxidant activity	Normal insulin
Cell membrane health	Vitamin B synthesis
Energy production	

Sulfur protects against:

Fatigue	Low vitamin B_1 and vitamin B_7 levels
Insulin resistance	

The predominant source for this mineral is protein rich foods.

Drugs that deplete sulfur: No drugs have been identified as depleting the nutrient.

Food preparation to retain sulfur: Not destroyed by cooking or processing, it is released in burning protein material.

Foods that contain sulfur:

Almond	English filbert	Pea
Beet	Garden beet	Pistachio
Beetroot	Garden cress	Radish
Bell pepper	Garden dill	Red cabbage
Black pepper	Grapefruit	Rutabaga
Black walnut	Green pepper	Sorrel
Butterbur	Horseradish	Spinach
Butternut	Lettuce	Stinging nettle
Cabbage	Mango	Sugar beet
Cashew	Mugwort	Sunflower
Cauliflower	Non - GMO soybean	Sweet pepper
Cherry pepper	Oats	Tomato
Chickweed	Onion	Wheat
Cone pepper	Paprika	White cabbage
Cucumber	Parsley	White pepper
Dandelion	Parsnip	

Fortified foods available: None

Recommended dietary allowance: There is no set recommended dietary allowance for sulfur.

Toxic doses: No toxicity is found with sulfur. The excesses are cleared by the kidneys and excreted in the urine.

VANDIUIM

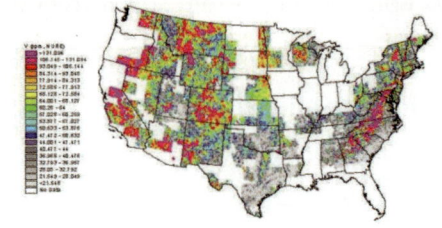

Named after the Norse goddess Vanadis, of beauty and fertility, vanadium was first discovered by Andres Manuel del Rio in 1801 as he was preparing salts from material contained in "brown lead." Del Rio suspected he discovered a new element and intended to call it "Panchromium" (Greek for many colored), an appropriate name, given the various oxides of vanadium are differently colored.

Whether the element vanadium plays any nutritional, biochemical, or biologic role in the human is a question that has been extremely difficult to answer. At the turn of the century, French physicians used vanadium as a cure-all, but only for a short time because some thought it was quite toxic. The question of its role in humans, if any, has been up in the air ever since.

Vanadium may act as a co-factor for enzymes in blood sugar metabolism, lipid/cholesterol metabolism, bone/tooth development, fertility, thyroid function, hormone production, and neurotransmitter metabolism.

Vanadium deficiency has not been described in man. Deficiency in animals causes:

Infertility	Poor bone, tooth, and cartilage formation
Iron metabolism defects	Reduction in red blood cell production leading to anemia

Vanadium is an essential element in the diets of chickens; deficiency affects bones, feathers, and blood. It is possible that deficiency in humans may lead to high cholesterol and triglyceride levels along with increased susceptibility to heart disease and cancer.

Vanadium can easily be toxic if taken in synthetic form. It may cause:

Blood vessel damage	Liver damage	Stunted growth
Diarrhea	Loss of appetite	
Kidney failure	Nerve damage	

Excess vanadium in humans has been suggested as a factor in bipolar disorder. Animal experiments have shown that vanadium can mimic the effects of insulin, reducing blood sugar levels from high to normal. These benefits are seen with low doses and there have been limited clinical trials with vanadium salts in Type II diabetes patients, indicating vanadium may have therapeutic potential treatment for diabetes.

Since 1980 when research first showed this trace mineral could lower blood sugars, tantalizing results have been found in studies of rodents and a limited number of human studies. Unfortunately, no one has been "cured;" while very serious concerns have been raised about the potential damage this mineral might create.

Vanadium can improve sensitivity to insulin in both Type I and Type II diabetes. It has been shown in human studies to have some ability to lower cholesterol levels and blood pressure. Areas of the world where vanadium (and selenium) levels are high in the soil have lower rates of heart disease. After oral intake, effects of the mineral are seen weeks to months later due to its accumulation in tissues of kidneys and bone.

Vanadium has been shown to lower growth of human prostate cancer cells in tissue cultures, and reduce bone and liver cancer in animals. These widespread effects on cancer and diabetes, along with the protective effect seen with another trace mineral, selenium, on certain cancers, suggest that trace minerals are likely to come under more scrutiny for potential health benefits and toxicity.

Unfortunately, vanadium's effects are not all positive. Vanadium works by blocking dozens of enzymes, including ribonucleases, mutases, kinases, and synthases. This indiscriminate blocking action has the potential to be both positive and negative.

There is no RDA for vanadium. A daily intake of 10 to 100 micrograms is likely safe and adequate.

Foods that contain vanadium:

Allspice	English filbert	Pea bean
Almond	European filbert	Pear
Asparagus	Field bean	Pecan
Asparagus bean	Flageolet bean	Pistachio
Black bean	Flax	Pop bean
Black cherry	French bean	Popping bean
Black walnut	Garden bean	Red cabbage
Brazil nut	Ginseng	Sassafras
Butter bean	Green bean	Sassafras
Butternut	Haricot	Snap bean
Cabbage	Haricot bean	String bean
Cashew	Haricot vert	Tomato
Clover	Kidney bean	Wax bean
Coconut	Lettuce	White cabbage
Corn	Lima bean	Wild cherry
Dwarf bean	Navy bean	Yardlong bean

ZINC

Most frequently found to be a gray color, this transition metal was known for its metallurgical properties in ancient Asia and early Europe. Zinc is number 30 on the atomic periodic table, an essential mineral and plays a vital role in numerous biochemical processes.

Zinc is found in cells throughout the body with highest amounts in the tissue of the kidneys, liver, pancreas as well as the musculoskeletal system. Zinc is also found in the eye, skin, hair, nails, prostate gland, and sperm.

Deficiency symptoms: Many symptoms could be the signal of zinc deficiency. The level of depletion determines not only the severity of symptoms but also which systems in the body will suffer adverse effects. This is the result of the extensive range of biological activities dependent on zinc.

Zinc deficiency may be associated with:

Acne
Anomalies of the skin nails and hair (dandruff, hair loss)
Anorexia
Depression
Frequent infections

Joint pain
Menstrual disturbance secondary to ovulatory delays
Night blindness
Nystagmus (involuntary eye movements)
Sensory deficits in smell and taste

Lifelong depletion and deficiency can cause dwarfism, hypogonadism, and sexual immaturity.

Zinc deficiency in pregnancy, a time of greater need, can cause birth defects and low weights in neonates and maternal stretch marks may be more enhanced with deficiency.

Many patients with chronic diseases of rheumatoid arthritis and diabetes mellitus Type 2 have been found zinc deficient. HIV depletes zinc as does smoking.

It is a commonly held view that many Americans are somewhat zinc deficient is because the standard American diet is low in zinc as food processing removes it.

Function in the body:

1. Zinc's most profound function in the body is its role in genetic expression and cellular division. It is necessary for protein and DNA/RNA synthesis, therefore necessary for normal growth and development.

2. It is important as a functioning component of many enzymes with a wide array of activities, assisting in numerous hormone activities and critical to immune function.

3. Zinc a factor in insulin production does not influence on the activity of insulin. The prompting sequence that starts the conversion of thyroxine (T4) to triiodothyronine (T3) is dependent on zinc. Growth hormones rely on zinc.

Other actions: Zinc regulates vitamin A release from liver stores to maintain adequate levels. It also regulates the activity of T lymphocytes, natural killer cells, interleukin 2, and all critical components of the immune system. Necessary for some sensory perceptions such as salt-taste and dark adaptation in night vision, zinc has anti-inflammatory effects and should be supplemented if deficient in patients with inflammatory states or diseases. Zinc facilitates wound healing, particularly burns. It is important for prostate health and preventing benign prostatic hypertrophy (BPH), an enlargement of the prostate that causes urinary flow difficulties. Critical to fertility, zinc not only has a role on sperm production but also in ovulation.

Other facts: Zinc supplementation may prolong the lives of those suffering with cataracts and age related macular degeneration. An ongoing study called the Age-Related Eye Disease Study, reported in a 2004 issue of the *Archives Of Ophthalmology*, enrolled 4,757 persons with a median age of 69, and randomized them into groups. One group was given zinc with antioxidants, zinc oxide 80 milligrams, cupric oxide 2 milligrams, vitamin C 500 milligrams, vitamin E 400 IU, B-carotene 15 milligrams. The other groups were given zinc with cupric oxide 2 milligrams, the antioxidants alone, or placebo. Of the total, 4,753 had follow up data for mortality. The zinc with antioxidants and then the zinc group alone had slowed the progression of these eye diseases and a reduction on mortality over a 6.25 year period.

Zinc can leach into water supplies when lying in galvanized pipes of older plumbing systems thus becoming a source of zinc. Modern plumbing has eliminated this source.

Galvanized cookware could be a possible source for zinc when acidic foods are cooked.

Zinc promotes:

Accurate replication of genetic code
Anti-inflammatory effect
Energy production
Immune health
Normal cellular division
Normal growth and development
Normal hormone function

Normal insulin production
Prostate health
Reproductive health
Skin and hair health
Thyroid function
Vitamin A utilization
Wound healing

Zinc protects against:

Brittle hair and nails
Diminished antioxidant enzymes
Fatigue
Impotence
Infection

Joint ache
Sore throats
Weak immune barrier in intestines
White spots in nails

Drugs that deplete: Some antihypertensive medications, diuretics, hormones, steroids, and gastric acid drugs (H2 blockers), also some of the HIV antiretroviral therapeutics can deplete zinc.

Food preparation to retain zinc: Heat does not destroy zinc. Food processing or "refining" does remove zinc.

Foods that contain zinc:

Aloe	Cucumber	Haricot
Asparagus	Dill	Haricot bean
Black bean	Dwarf bean	Haricot vert
Black cherry	Endive	Hyacinth bean
Bonavist bean	Field bean	Kidney bean
Brussel	Flageolet bean	Lablab bean
Butter bean	French bean	Lettuce
Cauliflower	Garden bean	Lima bean
Cauliflower	Garden dill	Mugwort
Celery	Ginseng	Navy bean
Collards	Green bean	Parsley

Plum	Sesame	Swamp cabbage
Pop bean	Snap bean	Tomato
Popping bean	Soybean	Water spinach
Poppyseed	Spinach	Wax bean
Pumpkin	Stinging nettle	Wild cherry
Sassafras	String bean	

Fortified foods available: None known.

1989 Recommended Dietary Allowances (RDA)–National Academy of Sciences

Infants
Ages 0.0 thru 0.5:   5 milligrams/day   Ages 0.5 thru 1: 5 milligrams/day

Children
Ages 1 thru 3:   10 milligrams/day   Ages 7 thru 10:   10 milligrams/day
Ages 4 thru 8:   10 milligrams/day

Females
Ages 9 thru 13:   12 milligrams/day   Ages 19 and older: 12 milligrams/day
Ages 14 thru 18:   12 milligrams/day

Males
Ages 9 thru 13:   15 milligrams/day   Ages 19 thru 71:   15 milligrams/day
Ages 14 thru 18:   15 milligrams/day

Pregnant
All ages: 15 milligrams/day
Lactating women: 1st 6 month   19 milligrams/day   2nd 6 months 16 milligrams/day

Toxic doses: Zinc toxicity is rare. Ingesting large quantities (>80milligrams a day) can induce copper deficiency if sustained more than a few weeks.

Symptoms would include:

Diarrhea	Lethargy	Muscle fatigue
Dizziness	Nausea	Vomiting

Zinc levels in the body that are too high can depress immune function, interestingly so can levels that are too low.

SOIL NUTRIENTS

By Reuben Stoltzfus

Reuben is a researcher, speaker, leader in sustainable agriculture, and CEO of Lancaster Agriculture Products in Ronks PA. Reuben is very passionate about the positive impact that healthy soil and plants have on animals and humans.

What is the relationship between herbs and soil?

Pungent and potent, we as home gardeners and market growers of herbs pay close attention to these two words. In order to produce tasty herbs that contribute to overall human health, we must also pay close attention to the soil in which we grow our herb plants. Preparing the soil so that microorganisms, nutrients, good bacteria, and soil life are alive and well and part of the mix is of utmost importance. They do the work in the soil that allows the plants to take the needed minerals and nutrients up through their roots.

It is known that herbs grow best when soils have adequate organic matter. By focusing on trace minerals, bacteria in the soil, cover crops, manure management, re-mineralizing the soil and working with natural resources such as colloidal minerals and rock powders, we as gardeners and growers will have the organic matter to make our herbs vibrant and give them health-producing qualities.

What is the definition of good soil?

> The soil is a dynamic body,
> teeming with microorganisms
> whose activities vary from day to day
> and from season to season
> with changes in temperature,
> moisture, and food supply.

Soil is the material on the earth's surface that can support the roots of plants and provide nutrients for plant life. Plants are dependent on water, the sun, and the soil's nutrients to give them energy for vegetative growth and reproduction. The health, vitality, and yield of the plants are directly related to the nutrient content of the soil in which they are grown.

Healthy Soil

The condition of our soils is important because all life on earth is dependent on soil. A close look at healthy soil reveals that it is teeming with life and activity. It is rich in organic matter, insects, earthworms, air, water, and nutrients. Healthy soil retains nutrients and has a texture that allows water and air to permeate it. The four major components of soil are mineral matter, organic matter, water, and air. The mineral matter such as stones and rock powders usually originates from the bedrock that lies beneath the soil. Organic matter (humus) is the decayed remains and waste products of plants and animals.

Fertile Soil

Healthy soil must be fertile and for soil to be fertile, it must have nutrients readily available and a pH value at a recommended level for the plants that will be grown in it. The pH level of the soil refers to its acidity or alkalinity and each plant has it own preferred value range. Soil pH is one of the most important soil properties that affect the availability of nutrients. In the desired pH range of 6.5 to 6.8, nutrients are more readily available to plants and microbial populations in the soil increase.

Minerals in the Soil

It is important to note that the mineral composition of the soil is what makes the difference between rich fertile soil and poor infertile soil. Plants need minerals to be in an available and balanced form. Minerals are what create sweetness, flavor, and nutrition in fruits, grains, and vegetables. Without balanced minerals, it is possible to achieve high production, but not the highest quality nutritional food.

The same holds true for herbs and their medicinal values. When adequate soil nutrients are supplied in forms of minerals and rock powders, herb plants can produce to the maximum potential that God has designed for them.

Nutrition brings the highest genetic potential.

What is the history of soil and nutrition in our country?

In the western movement of farmers to the American frontier, the search was always for good fertile land. Virgin soils were the most continuous attraction drawing people to the wilderness in the west. Those pioneers who were the most successful in finding the best soil actually felt, smelled, and tasted it before putting down stakes.

Year by year the farmers lived on the soil and eventually discovered that their non-rotated crops diminished their returns. They had not replenished the soil nutrients their crops had used up. With the offer of virgin soil farther west at nominal prices, many farmers moved on after a few years. Unfortunately the economics favored using up the nutrients in the soil without replacing them. They had not learned the lesson that soils are dynamic. They were not committed to maintaining soil fertility by encouraging soil life and replacing the nutrients and minerals their crops had used.

Today in America sustainable farmers and growers are very aware of the importance of building healthy, balanced, nutrient-dense soil for their present use and also for succeeding growers. They know that the health of their soil correlates directly with the mineral density of the crops and produce they harvest. They also know there is a strong connection between soil, food, dinner plate, and human health. Healthy soil results in healthy food and healthy food results in healthy humans.

There is a link between soil quality and nutritional decline. Unfortunately, from 1940 to 1991, the produce quality in the United States has dropped. The USDA confirms this loss of nutrients. On the average, fruit lost 60% of its mineral density and vegetables lost nearly 80%.

We need to work hard at reversing this trend of declining nutrition in our foods and make sure that we grow nutritious, wholesome foods. The number one goal for growers must be the production of top quality herbs, fruits, and vegetables that are full of nutrients and vitality and taste delicious.

The largest sphere of influence with which to raise the quality of our current produce is the soil. In the end, we must garden and farm from the bottom up. The beginning of great gardens and produce acres that produce healthy, nutrient-dense produce is the soil.

How do we manage soil well?

The road back to healthy soil includes managing residue and seeding cover crops, both done in the fall after harvest.

Residue management is an excellent way to incorporate nutrients back into the soil. This involves chopping or shredding the stalks of the previous season's plants immediately after harvesting them. These stalks have pulled many minerals out of the soil to nourish the plants. Minerals, nitrogen, sugars, protein, and saps are left in the stalks and it is beneficial to return them to the soil.

Digestion in the soil is as important as digestion in the human body. Just as human bodies need enzymes to break down food, so the soil needs microbes to break down the corn stalks, vines, and other plants that were growing in gardens. The residue needs to be turned back into the soil because it contains nutrients for next year's crop.

Use a good microbial package for fall application and distribute across residue and entire garden to aid digestion in the soil. A bacteria product, that contains enzymes, will break down the residue. Shallow incorporate the plant residue into the soil by tilling no more than 6-inches deep. There are several tillage methods that work well.

Seeding a cover crop before putting a garden to bed for the winter adds many benefits to the soil. After incorporating the residue, seed a cover crop such as Jerry Forage Oats. The cover crop's roots will hold the nutrients that were just applied. It is a way to feed soil by providing readily available nutrients when residue goes into the soil, thus adding nitrogen and organic matter. Plus, a cover crop also prevents wind, water, and soil erosion during the winter months.

In the spring, inoculate cover crops with compose. Then turn under the cover crops well ahead of planting time. The nutrition in cover crops is now available in the soil for spring plants.

What do trace minerals do in the soil?

> Minerals in the soil need to be
> plentiful, available, balanced, and diverse

Minerals are as essential to soils and plants as air is to young infants when they begin to breathe. No one would think of closing off an infant's airway, but that is in essence what we are doing by not applying minerals to our soils.

Minerals are important for beneficial bacteria to flourish in the soil, fungi to form, algae to develop, plant root exudates to grow, and roots to elongate. All of these are needed for increased plant and herb resistance to stresses from disease, insects and weeds, and an increased ability of the plants to efficiently use soil water.

Plants have a marvelous immune system, similar to a human's immune system. When that immune system is supplied with resources such as minerals, it will combat diseases and ward off insects. Thus, it is possible to control diseases and insects with nutrition instead of relying on fungicides and insecticides.

A focus on disease and insect prevention through nutrition requires a balance of trace minerals. It is important to plan for ways to get trace minerals back into the soil because plants that have trace minerals applied along with their general fertilizer program will have better health and more sustainability. A major benefit will be higher quality herbs with more potency and pungency.

The lack of trace minerals in soils will definitely have an adverse effect on plants. They will be starving for these nutrients if trace minerals are not put in the soils every year to feed the soil biology. Soil nutrient deficiencies need to be addressed so that this trend can be reversed. Feeding soil life with full nutrition and a broad spectrum of trace minerals is the place to start.

Trace minerals determine the quality of the plants grown and that has an ongoing domino effect on humans who consume the plants. These minerals are very vital for humans to survive, function, and enjoy good health. Thus, to improve human health, our soils need to be improved with trace minerals.

What are the most important soil nutrients and minerals?

Here is a listing of soil nutrients and minerals that will improve our soils and preserve this rich natural resource for future generations. The following entries that describe soil nutrients will help us on our sustainable journey to a greener tomorrow.

Soil Nutrients

The three essential nutrients in soil for proper herb plant growth are nitrogen (leaf growth), phosphorus (root growth), and potassium (overall health). Plants use large amounts of these primary nutrients for their growth and survival and they must be replaced in order to maintain the proper soil conditions for ongoing herb production.

Also important in soil are these nutrients; calcium, magnesium, and sulfur. Large amounts of calcium and magnesium are added when limestone and rock powders are applied to acidic soils. Sulfur is produced by the microbial life in the soil in a form that plants can use. The slow decomposition of soil organic matter helps to keep the proper amount of sulfur in the soil.

Calcium: an essential part of plant cell wall structure, provides for normal transport and retention of other elements, gives strength to the plant, counteracts the effect of alkali salts and organic acids in the plant

Magnesium: essential for photosynthesis, activates many plant enzymes needed for growth

Sulfur: produces protein, improves root growth and seed production, aids in chlorophyll formation, promotes development and activity of enzymes and vitamins, helps with vigorous plant growth and resistance to cold

Trace Minerals

In all there are 40 minerals that plants need for proper, healthy growth. Many of these are needed in only very small quantities. We call these trace minerals. Many are abundantly available in the soil, but they need the action of microbes to make them usable by the plants. The following are five of the most essential trace minerals in the soil.

Boron: essential for seed and fruit development, helps in the use of nutrients such as in calcium uptake in the tissues, regulates other nutrients, aids in the production of sugar and carbohydrates, required so that calcium can perform its metabolic chore.

Copper: important for reproductive growth, key to elasticity in the plant, controls mold, interacts with iron and manganese

Iron: draws energy to the plant leaf by absorbing heat from the sun; essential for the formation, maintenance, and synthesis of chlorophyll and RNA metabolism in the chloroplasts

Manganese: breaks down carbohydrates; aids in nitrogen metabolism; is synergistic with iron; brings the electrical charge into the seed, creating the magnetic force to draw the other elements into the seed

Zinc: regulates plant growth and consumption of sugars, essential for the transformation of carbohydrates, contributes to test weight, helps to make acetic acid in the root to prevent rotting

We are awed by the complexity of the many elements needed in the soil for good healthy life to exist at that level. It is interesting to note that all of these elements are supplied through the natural system in amounts that are adequate and balanced. When we neglect the natural system, deplete the soil, or add detrimental ingredients, we upset the balance of nature and create a domino effect of problems that begins in our soils and consequently extends to our herb plants and eventually to our own human health.

Additional Details about Important Nutrients

Carbon

Carbon is a non-metal element that occurs in all organic life and is the basis of organic chemistry. It is a basic element of our life-sustaining universe. Carbon is contained in all proteins, sugars, starches, and other carbohydrates. Without carbon, there would be no fats, oils, vitamins, amino acids, enzymes, or hormones. Carbon is so linked to all of life's processes that life cannot exist without it. It has the interesting chemical property of being able to bond to itself as well as to a wide variety of other elements, forming almost 10 million known compounds. Some compounds give flavor to many fruits.

Calcium

Calcium is the king of nutrients. Since it has the responsibility of moving the soil's nutrients up into the plant, calcium must be present in the soil in sufficient quantities so that plants receive the proper quantities of calcium, phosphorus, and all other nutrients. Proper amounts of calcium are present if calcium levels are at 70-75% of the soil exchange capacity. This will improve the root system, the stem, and the leaves of the plants.

Proper levels of calcium improve soil texture (flocculation) by causing the soil particles to be loosely bonded to each other, rather than sticking closely to one another. Soil that is properly flocculated allows more air and water to enter the soil structure. When air and water enter the soil structure, they provide oxygen and nitrogen as well as other nutrients to the soil. A proper level of calcium ensures an environment that is conducive to the life of soil microorganisms.

Effects of low calcium - In most plants, calcium deficiency is first observed in the roots of the plant. The root growth is reduced and root rotting occurs before there are symptoms in the vegetative part of the plant. When calcium deficiencies are severe, growing points are distorted, look spotted, fail to grow, and even die.

Magnesium

Magnesium should occupy 10-20% of the soil's exchange capacity. It is a key element in photosynthesis, because it resides at the heart of the pigment that contains molecular chlorophyll. If photosynthesis declines, crop quality and yield will also decline. Magnesium is a constituent of chlorophyll, aids in phosphate metabolism, and activates several enzyme systems. Along with calcium, magnesium is the key to proper air and water in the soil, plus it helps to hold the soil together and tightens it up.

Effect of low magnesium – Result is poor crop growth. An effective solution is to apply magnesium sulfate.

Effects of high magnesium – Results are low levels of nitrogen, weeds, and heavy and tight soil. This can be corrected by applying gypsum.

Phosphorus

Phosphorus is the catalyst of life. A catalyst is something that must be present for the consumption of other things; however, the catalyst itself does not become completely used up in the process. All nutrients, with the exception of nitrogen and sometimes potassium, must be compounded with phosphorus to be provided to the plant. It is the job of phosphorus to compound all these nutrients, combining them with it so that calcium can carry everything into the plant. Organic phosphates are the compounds that provide the energy for most of the chemical reactions that occur in living cells. Therefore, enriching soils with phosphorus enhances plant growth and contributes to root, flower, and fruit development.

Phosphorus is contained in all tissues, is the workhorse of plant nutrition, and is responsible for cell division, cell growth, and photosynthesis. Phosphorus is used in a 1:1 ratio with potassium. Soil must have good phosphorus uptake to build good sugar levels in plants.

Effect of low phosphorus - Retards soil life and contributes to low sugar levels in plants. It also results in poor quality produce because phosphorus is needed to move other nutrients in the plant. Solution is to apply soft rock phosphate. Colloidal sources of phosphorus will not leach out of the soil.

Potassium

Potassium is a catalyst in chlorophyll production; a governor for taking free nutrients from the air such as carbon, hydrogen, and oxygen; and is needed so that plants can make starches, sugars, proteins, vitamins, enzymes, and cellulose. In addition, potassium is essential for protein synthesis and formation. Potassium improves the flavor and color of fruits and vegetables and promotes drought tolerance, winter hardiness, and disease and insect resistance. It contributes to stem and root growth and is necessary for the translocation of sugars, the proper color of fruit, and the bulk (size) of a crop.

Effects of low potassium - Results in low energy for crops, lack of drought tolerance, smaller stalks, and lower yields. Complacency about potassium levels in the soil is dangerous.

Effects of high potassium - Too much potassium from excessive manure application results in grassy weeds, reduced calcium uptake in plants, lower plant health and quality, and poor livestock health. This can be corrected with high calcium limestone and/or gysum.

Sulfur

Sulfur is a constituent of proteins and resembles oxygen, but is less active and more acidic. It is essential for formation of sulfur-containing proteins and its release in the soil is governed by the size of the organic matter held in reserve.

Sulfur remains a key element in crop proteins: it is necessary for the formation of high-quality protein. It is a requirement for nitrogen fixation in legumes and is vital to vitamin synthesis in all plants. These two actions are important determinants of crop quality. Sulfur gives onions, garlic and mustard their distinctive flavors.

Effects of low sulfur - Plant proteins will be incomplete, humus will not form properly, and soils will have low energy. To remedy, add gypsum or sulfate of potash-magnesia.

How does food serve as medicine?

Nutrition brings healing.
Nutrition brings genetic expression.
Nutrition brings us to healthy living.

A comprehensive approach including both medicine and nutrition needs to be taken when human health issues occur. There is more in food that will help our bodies than previously thought, even superseding the benefits of pharmaceutical drugs. Amazingly enough, health conditions and illnesses improve when specific wholesome foods are carefully chosen and properly prepared to match the needs of the human body. In this way, food becomes our medicine.

Organic food that is chemical free is not enough. We need to go well beyond that concept to food that is also abundantly full of life and packed with nutrients. In other words, we need mineral-dense and nutrient-dense organic food.

It is possible to grow herbs, fruits, and vegetables that add quality to life and minimize pain and sickness. Paying attention to minerals, vitamins, and nutrients in food is a great first step to avoiding serious illnesses and expensive medical treatments. Even many physicians and university professors are discovering that there is more to prevention than there is to treatment and are calling for good nutrition.

Unfortunately, the commercially purchased food in the USA no longer has the adequate nutritional value to sustain life at the cellular level. The decline of agriculture has come slowly and our dependence on medicine has increased gradually. If America wants to restore human life at the human health cellular level, we must have good food and complete nutrition.

There is a strong and direct connection between
the soil, food, dinner plate,
and human health.

Growers and gardeners know that when they grow their own herbs, fruits, and vegetables in their back yards, they have full control over the nutrients in the soil, what is applied to the plants, and how they are grown. The healthier the plant, the healthier the human. A number one reason to put effort into gardening is to edify human health.

Diversity is important when it comes to nutrition and the mineral profile that plants bring to humans. For example, one should not depend on meat and potatoes alone as a daily diet. The basics of meat and potatoes need to be accompanied by herbs, leafy greens, garden salads, peas, broccoli, cauliflower, zucchini, squash, root vegetables such as carrots, a wide assortment of fruits, and the list goes on.

The goal lies in this phrase, "Eating your color." Eat as many wide and diverse colors (reds, greens, whites, oranges, etc.) as possible, this helps to ensure a healthy, wholesome, and nutritious food appearance on America's dinner plates.

Now is the time to turn to food as medicine.

- Food to prevent illnesses and diseases
- Food for a better quality of life
- Food for joy and pleasure
- Food for being all that God intended us to be

My primary focus is on nutrition as we develop the multiple steps in our growing programs. Through many years of research we have found that these various steps are what will stabilize the peaks and valleys in plant production. My focus is growing programs use trace minerals, solid protein, biology, and vitamins. Our goal is to constantly feed plants a diverse flow of minerals, which support the immune system of the plant and help the plant avoid disease and insect pressures.

The Importance of Soil Analysis

The purpose of soil testing is to determine the nutrient density of the soil and the relation of the different nutrients to each other. A soil test is used as a road map for treatment of your soils. By reading this road map, you can understand where you presently are and gain a vision for what you need to do in the future. With regular soil testing and recordkeeping, you can see the changes and the nutrients that you used to bring about the changes. Under normal conditions we recommend that soil samples be taken every two or three years.

Have your soil samples sent out for evaluation, for the major and minor minerals. Based on the results of these soil samples, we are able to give specific recommendations for which fall dry blends to use and its application rate. If needed, we can make custom mixes tailored to specific soil samples.

The Start of a Healthy Plant is in the Soil

We have developed the highest quality dry and liquid blends that add an array of nutrients and trace minerals to the soil. Based on the results of soil samples, we can recommend just the right blends for specific soil situations. The rate of application is determined by the balance and level of fertility in the soil. These Blends work hard to properly align the calcium, magnesium, phosphorus, potassium, trace minerals, and pH in the soil. They stimulate the ability of herb plants to take up more nutrients and supplement the needs of growing plants.

Fall Season

This season of the year is very important for improving soil in gardens and produce rows. The months from August to December are the prime times to put nutrients back into the soil and prepare it for next year's plants and herbs before the ground freezes. Adding nutrients in the fall allows the soil to make improvements over the winter and begins the process of making the nutrients available for the following spring and summer.

Fall Dry Blends

Fall dry blends will put nutrients back into the soil and prepare it for next year's crops. These Blends are specially designed to improve the nutrient balance and content in the soil and are formulated with ingredients that are friendly to soil's microorganisms.

By offering these fall dry blends, we help growers attain the goal of balanced soil that is biologically alive. When there is a high, balanced nutrient reserve in the soil, the result will be potent and tasty herb plants that are disease and insect resistant and fruits and vegetables that are high quality, nutrient-dense food. By giving plants the resources they need, they will grow into what God, the Creator, designed them for.

Soil Management

As a foundational practice for all soils, I highly recommend the following:

- In the fall apply one of our Dry Blends that we specifically recommend for you
- Plant a cover crop
- Next spring inoculate your soil for proper breakdown of residue and the cover crop
- Incorporate your cover crop
- Start spring fertilization before planting. It is important that plants have immediate nutrients as soon as they are placed in the ground!

The Basics of Herb Gardening

- Cultivating: work the ground during optimal soil conditions (not too wet) so that it is porous and air and water can move through it.
- Weeding: persevere throughout the growing season, using the method of your choice.
- Side-dressing: apply organic liquid biological near the base of your herbs during growth spurts.
- Foliar feeding: apply liquid fertilizer directly to the leaves of your herbs to stimulate plant growth
- Irrigation: consistently regulate water irrigation since water is the most important nutrient you can apply to herbs

GENETICALLY MODIFIED ORGANISMS (GMO)

A Genetically modified organism (GMO) is an organism that has been forcibly changed at a genetic level. GMO's are also known as genetically engineered food/animals. GMO's were made to help growers use less pesticide, increase crop yield, and reduce world hunger. The question is, are GMO's safe for consumption?

A GMO is created by inserting a foreign gene into the DNA of a plant. This process is nothing like natural or cross breeding methods. The process starts by cutting out a section of E. coli bacteria DNA, leaving a gap that is filled with the foreign DNA pieces, when mixed together. Once the modified cell is created it cannot just be put into the host cell. The cells of the original plant will reject the foreign gene that is being introduced. Because of the rejection, there are three ways to implant the foreign gene into the cell of the host plant called invasion technology.

1. A soil bacterium is used that causes tumors in plants to carry the normally rejected cell into the nucleus of the plant. Changing the DNA structure to the desired result.
2. Electricity is used to create tiny holes in the plants cell structure for the foreign cell in enter the host cell.
3. A gene gun is used to blast small particles of gold coated with the foreign DNA in to the host cell.

A common illustration would be a farmer grows tomatoes in a cold region. He loses part of his crop to the cold temperature. A gene is isolated and removed from the Atlantic flounder fish that makes the able to withstand the cold temperatures. That gene is spliced together with the DNA of E. coli bacteria then injected, by one of the three methods, in to the tomato host cell. Then a cold weather resistance tomato grows and the farmer yields a full crop. There are unexpected results from this kind of gene modification. Like persons who are have a fish allergy would now be allergic to this modified tomato, unknowingly.

Over all it sounds like a good idea to make improvements on an already good, natural system. Unfortunately little testing has been done and no one really knows the full effects these modified crops will have on humans, animals, and the earth. Dr. Charles M. Benbrook, former Director, Board of Agriculture National Academy of Science, tells us that people have concerns about using bacteria and viruses to modify gene structures. Some studies have indicated that a result is smaller crop yields, not larger ones like expected. Studies with GM soy, showed animals when given the choice, gravitate to non-GMO feed. Also there is a direct link between deceased fertility and low birth weight in GM-fed mice, according to a 2008 study published at www.responsibletechnology.org. Laboratory mice fed GM soy show liver cell damage, altered gene expression, and higher metabolic activity, article from Cell structure and Function, 2002. As well as their testicular cell structure was altered. A Russian study shows rats fed GM soy based feed had infant mortality rate of over 55 percent and some were not able to conceive at all. Lancett, 1999 says, that rats fed GM potatoes developed potentially pre-cancerous cell growth in the digestive tract, smaller brains, liver, testicles, and immune system damage. Ninety-days into a Monsanto study showed rats which ate BT corn indicated toxicity in the liver and kidneys, had blood pressure problems, allergies, infections and disease, higher blood sugar, and anemia. According to animal science in 2006, Rabbits fed roundup ready soy (for 40 days) had increased cell metabolism and changed enzymes levels in the kidneys, heart and liver.Soon after GM soy was introduce in the United Kingdom soy allergies skyrockets by 50 percent.

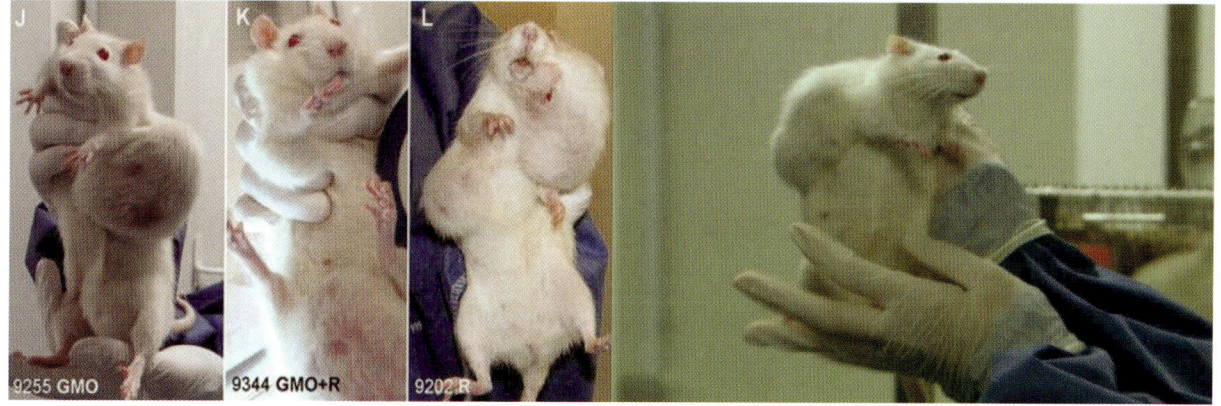

A insect resistant bacteria natural found in soil was genetically introduced into a corn crop in the Philippians. The corn grew its own pesticide with in the cells of the corn and killed invading bugs. The pesticide that grew from the corn became airborne. After blood testing 39 people who lived close to the corn field showed their immune system was affected. These people had skin, intestinal, and respiratory problems directly related to the pesticide growing corn. If that is the results from breathing the air around the fields, what will happen when we eat the pesticide growing corn over a long period of time?

There is a danger to organic farmers as well. Over 70 percent of soy, canola, corn, and sugar beets are genetically modified. These altered crops are now cross contaminating natural and organic crops through bees or wind transporting the pollen. This ruins the value and purity of organic crops. Trucks, grain elevators, and store houses are not set up to receive natural and GM crops, and often are mixed. Some countries have refused to purchase GM crops, resulting in further loss to the farming economy. There is no stopping cross contamination, it will only continue. Most foods that are processed contain GMO's at their sources, from pasta to cereal and much more. Since there is no labeling required we do not really know how many foods are really affected.

How will eating GMO's food affect our future generations? Cancer, organ failure, sterility are all very real possibilities from eating these modified foods. There are plans to add more nutrients and even vaccines in to our food supply through GMO's technology. It is already being added to animal feeds, again without proper testing. Such animals as cows, pigs, and salmon have become a GM through cloning or invasion technology.

There needs to be more testing and research done on GM food and animals. Awareness in the U.S. about GMO food is surprisingly low. Since there is little to no regulation or labeling on GMO's, be sure to ask questions at your grocery store, farm market, and seed supplier. Buy organic and look for products labeled non-GMO. Know what you are buying, eating, and growing. Avoid at risk ingredients.

Hillman Health Food Store call 855-Amish-Dr (855-264-7437) www.emineral.info Vitamins and Minerals for Better Living

TRUE FOOD SHOPPER'S GUIDE
How to Avoid Foods Made with Genetically Modified Organisms [GMOs]

GMO Free?

The True Food Network is CFS's grassroots action network where concerned citizens can voice their opinions about critical food safety issues, and advocate for a socially just, democratic and sustainable food system. To join the network and receive free action alerts visit www.truefoodnow. org and stand up for True Food!

To learn more about GMOs, consult the book *Your Right to Know: Genetic Engineering and the Secret Changes in Your Food* by Andrew Kimbrell. Information on GMOs is also available at www.centerforfoodsafety.org

SPECIAL NOTE: This guide was compiled based on companystatements, not genetic testing. Any product labeled as Non-GMO indicates that its manufacturing process is designed to avoid GMOs, but consumers should be aware that GM contamination is possible due to natural pollen movement, weather events, seed contamination, or human error. Hence there is no guarantee such products are 100% free of GMOs.

The Center for Food Safety works to protect human health and the environment by curbing the proliferation of harmful food production technologies and by promoting organic and other forms of sustainable agriculture. CFS has offices in Washington, DC and San Francisco, CA.
Contact: info@truefoodnow.org
660 Pennsylvania Avenue, SE, Suite 302, Washington, DC 20003
www.centerforfoodsafety.org

How to avoid brands made with genetically modified organisms (GMOs)

Genetic Engineering (GE) or Genetic Modification (GM) of food involves the laboratory process of artificially inserting genes into the DNA of food crops or animals. The result is called a genetically modified organism or GMO. GMOs can be engineered with genes from bacteria, viruses, insects, animals, or even humans. Most Americans say they would not eat GMOs if labeled, but unlike most other industrialized countries, the U.S. does not require labeling. This Non-GMO Shopping Guide is designed to help reclaim your right to know about the foods you are buying, and help you find and avoid GMO foods and ingredients.

TIPS FOR AVOIDING GM CROPS

TIP #1: BUY ORGANIC
Certified organic products are not allowed to contain any GMOs. Therefore, when you purchase products labeled "100% organic," "organic," or "made with organic ingredients," all ingredients in these products are not allowed to be produced from GMOs. For example, products labeled as "made with organic ingredients" only require 70% of the ingredients to be organic, but 100% must be non-GMO.

Lancaster Agriculture Products 717-687-9222 www.lancasterag.com Naturally Interested in Your Future

TIP #2: LOOK FOR "NON-GMO" LABELS

Companies may voluntarily label products as "non-GMO." Some labels state "non-GMO" while others spell out "Made Without Genetically Modified Ingredients." Some products limit their claim to only one particular "At-Risk" ingredient such as soy lecithin, listing it as "non-GMO."

TIP #3: AVOID AT-RISK INGREDIENTS

Avoid products made with any of the crops that are GM. Most GM ingredients are products made from the "Big Four:" corn, soybeans, canola, and cottonseed, used in processed foods. Some of the most common genetically engineered Big Four ingredients in processed foods are:

Corn
- Corn flour, meal, oil, starch, gluten, and syrup
- Sweeteners such as fructose, dextrose, and glucose
- Modified food starch*

Soy
- Soy flour, lecithin, protein, isolate, and isoflavone
- Vegetable oil* and vegetable protein*

Canola Canola oil (also called rapeseed oil)
Cotton Cottonseed oil

*May be derived from other sources

Additionally, GM sugar beet sugar recently entered the food supply. Look for organic and non-GMO sweeteners, candy and chocolate products made with 100% cane sugar, evaporated cane juice, agave, or organic sugar, to avoid GM beet sugar.

TIP #4: BUY PRODUCTS LISTED IN THIS SHOPPING GUIDE

Keep this Guide with you whenever you shop. Store it inside your reusable shopping bag, put it into your coupon holder or check book, or leave it in your car.

FRUITS & VEGETABLES

Very few fresh fruits and vegetables for sale in the U.S. are genetically modified. Novel products such as seedless watermelons are NOT genetically modified. Small amounts of zucchini, yellow crookneck squash, and sweet corn may be GM. The only commercialized GM fruit is papaya from Hawaii-about half of Hawaii's papayas are GM.

EGGS

Eggs: Non-GMO

Egg Innovations Organic
Eggland's Best Organic
Land O'Lakes Organic
Nest Fresh Organic

Organic Valley
Pete and Jerry's Organic Eggs
Wilcox Farms Organic

FISH

FDA is currently considering approval of the first GE animal intended for human consumption, a genetically engineered Atlantic salmon. This approval is pending despite overwhelming consumer opposition and unacceptable risks to human health, the marine environment, wild salmon populations and fishing economies. There are several other GE fish in the pipeline as well. To make matters worse, FDA argues that these GE fish don't even need to be labeled! Check out our new campaign website at www.ge-fish.org to learn more and find out what you can do to help stop GE fish.

MEAT & FOWL

No genetically modified fowl or livestock is yet approved for human consumption. However, plenty of non-organic foods are produced from animals raised on GM feed such as grains. Look for 100% grass-fed animals.

ALTERNATIVE MEAT PRODUCTS

Many alternative meat products are processed and include ingredients that can be genetically engineered, so give the ingredient lists close attention to avoid the Big Four at-risk ingredients, especially soy.

Non-GMO	May contain GMO ingredients
365 Brand (Whole Foods)	Boca, unless labeled organic (Kraft)
Amy's	Gardenburger
Bountiful Bean	Morningstar Farms, Natural Touch, Worthington, Loma Linda unless labeled organic (Kellogg)
Small Planet Tofu	
Sunshine Burger	
The Simple Soyman	
Vitasoy	
Wildwood	
White Wave	
Woodstock Farms	

DAIRY PRODUCTS & ALTERNATIVE DAIRY PRODUCTS

Some U.S. dairy farms inject the genetically engineered hormone rBGH, also called rBST, into their cows to boost milk production—so be sure to purchase products with a label that indicates cows free of rBGH or rBST. Many alternative dairy products are made from soybeans and may contain GM materials.

Dairy Products: Non-GMO
Certified Organic
Alta Dena Organics
Butterworks Farm
Harmony Hills Dairy
Horizon Organic
Kirkland Organic
Lactaid Organic (Organic only)
Morningland Dairy
Nancy's Organic Dairy
Natural by Nature
Noris Organic
Oregon Ice Cream Company (Alden's, Julie's)
Organic Valley Dairy
Pacific Village
Radiance Dairy
Rogue Creamery
Safeway Organic Brand
Seven Stars Farm
Straus Family Creamery
Stremick's Heritage organic
Stonyfield Farm
Trader Joe's (organic line)
Wallaby
Whole Foods organic line

Wisconsin Organics
Woodstock Farms

Produced Without rBGH National
Albertson's
Alta Dena
Ben & Jerry's Ice Cream
Brown Cow Farm
Crowley Cheese of Vermont
Dannon
Darigold
Double Rainbow ice cream
Franklin County Cheese
Grafton Village Cheese
Great Hill Dairy
Lactaid milk (milk only)
Lifetime Dairy
Lochmead
Market Pantry (Target)
Nancy's Natural Dairy
Safeway (Dairy Glen and Lucerne)
Trader Joe's store brand
Walmart Great Value store brand
Whole Foods and 365 brands
Yoplait

Lancaster Agriculture Products 717-687-9222 www.lancasterag.com Naturally Interested in Your Future

West Coast
Alpenrose Dairy
Beecher's butter
Berkeley Farms
Bravo Farms cheese
Clover Stornetta Farms
Cowgirl creamery
Eberhard
Fred Meyer
Mountain Dairy
Joseph Farms Cheese
Mallories
Market of Choice
Oregon Gourmet cheese
Rogue Creamery
Rose Valley butter
Sunshine Dairy Foods
Tillamook Cheese
Trader Joe's store brand
Umpqua
Western Family
Wilcox Family Farms
Willamette Valley cheese
Yami

Midwest and Gulf States
Chippewa Valley Cheese
Chippewa Valley Cheese
Erivan Dairy Yogurt
Promised Land Dairy
Westby Cooperative Creamery

East Coast
Blythedale Farm Cheese
Crescent Creamery
Derle Farms (milk with "no rBST" label only)
Erivan Dairy Yogurt
Farmland Dairies
Oakhurst Dairy
Trader Joe's store brand
Wilcox Dairy (rBST-free dairy line only)

May contain GMO ingredients
Colombo (General Mills)
Dannon
Kemps (aside from "Select" brand)
Kraft
Land O' Lakes
Lucerne
Parmalat
Sorrento
Yoplait (General Mills)

Alternative Dairy Products Non-GMO
Belsoy
EdenSoy
Imagine Foods/Soy Dream
Nancy's Cultured Soy
Organic Valley Soy
Pacific Soy
Silk
Soy Delicious
Sun Soy
Stonyfield Farm O'Soy
Tofutti
Trader Joe's brand
VitaSoy/Nasoya
WestSoy
WholeSoy
WholeSoy
Yves The Good Slice
Zen Don

May contain GMO ingredients
8th Continent

BABY FOODS & INFANT FORMULA

Milk or soy protein is the basis of most infant formulas. The secret ingredients in these products are often soy or milk from cows injected with rBGH. Many brands also add GMO-derived corn syrup, corn syrup solids, or soy lecithin.

Non-GMO
Baby's Only
(certified organic products)
Earth's Best
Gerber products
HAPPYBABY
 Mom Made Meals
Organic Baby
Plum Organics
Tastybaby

May contain GMO ingredients
Enfamil (Mead Johnson)
Good Start (Gerber/Nestle)
Nestle brands (Gerber/Nestle)
Similac/Isomil – except Similac
Organic (Abbott Labs/Abbott Nutrition)

BAKED GOODS
While baking ingredients such as wheat flour, rice, kamut, and oats are not genetically modified, many packaged breads and bakery items contain other GMO ingredients such as corn syrup.

Non-GMO
Alvarado Street Bakery
Arrowhead Mills (organic line)
Bakery on Main
Berlin Natural Bakery
Bob's Red Mill (organic line)
Dr. McDougall's Right Foods
Dr Oetker Organics
Eden
French Meadow
Natural Ovens Bakery
(organic line)
Nature's Path
Rudi's Organic Bakery
Rumford Baking Powder
Safeway O brand (organic)
Trader Joe's brand

May Contain GMO Ingredients
Aunt Jemima
(Quaker Oats/Pepsico)
Betty Crocker (General Mills)
Bisquick (General Mills)
Calumet Baking Powder (Kraft)
Duncan Hines (Pinnacle Foods)
Hungry Jack (Smucker's)
Pillsbury (Smucker's)

CEREALS & BREAKFAST BARS
Cereals and breakfast bars are very likely to include GMO ingredients, because they are often made with corn and soy products.

Non-GMO:
Ambrosial Granola
Barbara's (organic line)
Cascadian Farms
Eden
EnviroKidz
Golden Temple
Grandy Oats
Health Valley (organic line)
Lundberg® Purely Organic
Rice Cereal
Nature's Path
Nonuttin'
Omega Smart Bars
Peace Cereal Organic
Ruth's
Safeway O brand (organic)
Simple Sweets
Sunridge Farms
Trader Joe's brand
Whole Foods 365

May Contain GMO Ingredients
General Mills
Kellogg
Post (Kraft)
Quaker

ENERGY BARS

Non-GMO
Clif Bar
Divine Foods
Genisoy Bars
GoodOnYa Bar
Lara Bar
Luna Bar
Macrobars
MacroLife Naturals
Mojo (Clif Bar)
Nature's Path
Nutiva
Odwalla
Organic Food Bar
Ruth's
Optimum Energy Bar
Organic Food Bar
Weil by Nature's Path Organic
Z Bars (Clif Bar)

May Contain GMO Ingredients
Balance Bar
Nature Valley snack bars and granola bars (General Mills)
Nabisco Bars (Kraft)
PowerBar (Nestle)
Quaker Granola Bars

GRAINS, BEANS & PASTA

Other than corn, no GM grains are sold on the market. Look for 100-percent wheat pasta, couscous, rice, quinoa, oats, barley, sorghum, and dried beans (except soybeans).

Non-GMO
Amy's
Annie's
Bob's Red Mill, organic line
Casbah (Hain-Celestial)
Dr. McDougall's Right Foods
Eden certified organic grains
Fantastic Foods
Field Day
Ian's Natural Foods
Kamut
Lotus Foods
Lundberg Family Farms
Organic Planet
Rising Moon
Seeds of Change (organic meals)
Sensations
Sunridge Farms
Trader Joe's store brand
Vita-Spelt pasta
Whole Foods 365

May Contain GMO Ingredients
Betty Crocker meals (General Mills)
Knorr (Unilever)
Kraft Macaroni & Cheese meals
Near East (Quaker Oats Company / Pepsico)
Pasta Roni and Rice-A-Roni meals (Quaker Oats Company/Pepsico)

CANNED FOODS

Look for less processed canned foods and foods packed only in water or olive oil (not corn, soybean, canola or cottonseed), and avoid canned foods containing corn syrup, sugar not labeled as "cane sugar" and soy ingredients which could be derived from GM crops.

Non-GMO
Amy's
Annie's
Eden
ShariAnn's certified organic beans
Trader Joe's store brands
Westbrae certified organic beans
Whole Foods 365
Woodstock Farms
Yves Veggie Cuisine (Hain Celestial)

May Contain GMO Ingredients
Chef Boyardee
Dinty Moore, Stagg, Hormel
Franco-American (Campbell's)

Hillman Health Food Store call 855-Amish-Dr (855-264-7437) www.emineral.info Vitamins and Minerals for Better Living

SOUPS & SAUCES

Many soups and sauces are highly processed, so give the ingredient lists close attention to avoid the Big Four at-risk ingredients. Canned foods can be simply vegetables or fruits packed in water, but many canned foods also contain corn syrup or sugar which could be derived from GM crops. Look for less processed canned foods and foods packed only in water or olive oil (not corn, soybean, canola or cottonseed), and avoid canned foods containing corn syrup, sugar not labeled as "cane sugar" and soy ingredients.

Non-GMO	May Contain GMO Ingredients
Amy's	Bertolli (Unilever)
Annie's	Campbell products (including Healthy Request, Chunky,
Eden	Simply Home, and Pepperidge Farm)
Emerald Valley Kitchen	Chef Boyardee (Con Agra)
Fantastic Foods	Chi-Chi's (Hormel)
Field Day	Classico (Heinz)
Green Mountain Gringo	Del Monte
Hain	Healthy Choice (ConAgra)
Health Valley/Westbrae	Hormel products
Imagine Natural	Hunt's (ConAgra)
Muir Glen Organic	Old El Paso (General Mills)
Rising Moon	Pace (Campbell 's)
ShariAnn's Organics	Prego (Campbell's)
Seeds of Change	Progresso products
Trader Joe's store brands	(General Mills)
(Trader Joe's, Trader Jose's,	Ragu (Unilever)
Trader Giotto's)	
Walnut Acres	
Whole Foods 365	

FROZEN FOODS

Many frozen foods are highly processed. Keep an eye out for the Big Four at-risk ingredients and stay away from frozen foods that contain them, unless they are marked organic or non-GM.

Frozen Food Non-GMO	May Contain GMO Ingredients
A.C. LaRocco	Banquet (ConAgra)
Amy's Kitchen	Bertolli (Unilever)
Cascadian Farms Organic frozen	Boca, unless labeled organic (Kraft)
meals and vegetables	Celeste (Pinnacle Foods)
Cedarlane	Eggo Waffles (Kellogg)
Helen's Kitchen	Gardenburger
Ian's Natural Foods	Green Giant frozen meals (General Mills)
Linda McCartney frozen meals	Healthy Choice (ConAgra)
Mom Made Meals	Kid's Cuisine (ConAgra)
Morningstar Farms	Lean Cuisine (Nestle)
(Organic line ONLY)	Marie Callender's (ConAgra)
Rising Moon	Morningstar Farms, Morningstar
The Simple Soyman	Farms Natural Touch, unless
Trader Joe's store brands	labeled organic (Kellogg)
Woodstock Farms	Rosetto Frozen Pasta (Nestle)
	Stouffer's (Nestle)
	Swanson (Campbell's)
	Tombstone (Kraft)
	Totino's (Smucker's)
	Voila! (Birds Eye/Unilever)

CONDIMENTS, OILS, DRESSINGS & SPREADS

Unless labeled explicitly, corn, soybean, cottonseed, and canola oils probably contain genetically modified products. Choose pure olive, coconut, sesame, sunflower, safflower, almond, grapeseed, and peanut oils. Also choose preserves, jams, and jellies with cane sugar, not corn syrup.

Non-GMO
- Annie's
- Bountiful Bean
- Bragg's liquid amino
- Carrington Farms Flax Seed
- Crofter's Organic
- Drew's salad dressing
- Eden
- Emerald Cove
- Emperor's Kitchen
- Emerald Valley Kitchen
- Field Day
- Follow Your Heart
- Harvest Moon Mushrooms
- I.M. Health SoyNut Butters
- Ian's Natural Foods
- Krazy Ketchup
- Maranatha Nut Butters
- Miso Master
- Muir Glen organic tomato ketchup
- Nasoya
- Newmans Own Organic
- Ruth's
- The Simple Soyman
- Spectrum oils and dressings
- SushiSonic Asian Condiments
- Trader Joe's store brands
- Tropical Traditions
- Vegan by Nature Buttery Spreads
- Vigoa Cuisine
- Whole Foods 365
- Wholemato
- Woodstock Farms

May Contain GMO Ingredients
- Crisco (Smucker's)
- Del Monte
- Heinz
- Hellman's (Unilever)
- Kraft condiments and dressings
- Mazola
- Pam (ConAgra)
- Peter Pan (ConAgra)
- Skippy (Unilever)
- Smucker's (except their "Simply 100% Fruit" line of preserves)
- Wesson (ConAgra)
- Wish-Bone (Unilever)

SNACK FOODS

Look for snacks made from wheat, rice, or oats, and ones that use sunflower or safflower oils. There is no GM popcorn on the market, nor is there blue or white GM corn.

Non-GMO
- Barbara's (organic line)
- Bearitos/Little Bear Organics (Hain Celestial)
- Earthly Treats
- Eco-Planet
- Eden
- Field Day
- FritoLay Lay's Naturals potato chips ("Naturals" potato chips ONLY)
- Garden of Eatin'
- Grandy Oats
- Hain Pure Snax/Hain Pure Foods
- Health Valley
- Ian's Natural Foods
- Kettle Foods
- Kopali Organics
- Late July Organic Snacks
- Mary's Gone Crackers
- Namaste Foods
- Nature's Path Organic
- Newman's Own Organics & Newman's Own (except salad dressing)
- Peeled Snacks
- Plum Organics Tots
- Revolution Foods
- Revolution Foods
- Ruth's
- Simple Sweets
- Sunridge Farms
- Safeway O organic brand
- Trader Joe's store brand
- Woodstock Farms, organic

May Contain GMO Ingredients
FritoLay (Lay's, Ruffles, Doritos, Cheetos, Tostitos)
Hostess Products (Interstate Brands)
Keebler (Kellogg's)
Kraft (Nabisco, Nilla Wafers, Oreos, Ritz, Nutter Butter, Honey Maid, SnackWells, Teddy Grahams, Wheat Thins, Triscuit)
Pepperidge Farm (Campbell's)
Pringles
Quaker Oats Company

SWEETENERS

Many sweeteners, and products like candy and chocolate that contain them, can come from GMO sources. Look for organic and non-GMO sweeteners, candy and chocolate products made with 100% cane sugar, evaporated cane juice or organic sugar to avoid GM beet sugar, and watch out for soy lecithin in chocolates and corn syrup in candies.

The sweetener aspartame is derived from GM microorganisms. It is also referred to as NutraSweet® and Equal® and is found in over 6,000 products, including soft drinks, gum, candy, desserts, yogurt, tabletop sweeteners, and some pharmaceuticals such as vitamins and sugar-free cough drops.

Sweetners Non-GMO
Sweeteners, Non-GMO:
C&H Pure Cane Sugar
Brer Rabbit molasses
Eden
Florida Crystals (organic, natural and demerara)
Grandma's Best Molasses
Sweet Cloud
Tropical Traditions
Trader Joe's brand (Pure cane sugar, raw sugar, brown sugar, organic sugars)
Wholesome Sweetners (organic sugars, molasses, blue agave syrups, Organic Zero)
Woodstock Farms (organic)

May Contain GMO Ingredients
Crystal Sugar (American Crystal)
Big Chief sugar (Michigan Sugar Company)
Equal
GW sugar (Western Sugar)
Nutrasweet
Pioneer sugar (Michigan Sugar Company)
White Satin sugar (Snake River/Amalgamated Sugar)

CANDY & CHOCOLATE PRODUCTS

Chocolate Non-GMO
Chocolove
Endangered Species Chocolate
Ghirardelli Chocolate
Green & Black's Organic Chocolate
Kopali Organics
Lindt Chocolate
Newman's Own
Nonuttin'
Woodstock Farms (organic)

May Contain GMO Ingredients
Hershey's
Mars, Inc.
Nestlé (Crunch, Kit Kat, Smarties)
Toblerone (Kraft)

Candy Non-GMO
Jelly Belly
Pure Fun Confections
Reed's Crystallized Ginger candy (certified organic)
St. Claire Organic
Sunridge Farms

May Contain GMO Ingredients
Hershey's
Lifesaver (Kraft)
Mars (Wrigley's, Skittles, Starburst)
Nestlé

SODAS, JUICES & OTHER BEVERAGES

Most juices are made from GMO-free fruit (avoid papaya though, as it could be GMO), but the prevalence of corn-based sweeteners—e.g. high-fructose corn syrup—in fruit juices is cause for concern. Many sodas are primarily comprised of water and corn syrup. Look for 100-percent juice blends.

Non-GMO	May Contain GMO Ingredients
After the Fall organic juices	Coca-Cola (Fruitopia, Minute Maid, Hi-C, NESTEA)
Big Island Organics	Dr. Pepper Snapple Group (Dr. Pepper, 7Up, A&W, Snapple,
Blue Sky	Hawaiian Punch, Sunkist, Crush, Canada Dry, Mott's juice, Squirt, Sun Drop,
Cascadian Farm	Schweppes ginger ale, Vernors, Country Time, Clamato, IBC root beer,
Crofters Organic	Nantucket Nectors, Stewart's, Orangina, Diet Rite, Hires root beer)
Eden	Hansen Beverage Company
Odwalla	Hawaiian Punch (Procter and Gamble)
Quinoa Gold	Kraft (Country Time, Kool-Aid, Crystal Light, Capri Sun, Tang)
R.W. Knudsen organic juices	Libby's (Nestlé)
and spritzers (Smucker's)	Ocean Spray
Santa Cruz Organic (Smucker's)	Pepsi (Tropicana, Frappuccino, Gatorade, SoBe, Dole)
Sea20 Organic Energy Drink	Sunny Delight (Procter and Gamble)
Teeccino Herbal Caffe	Swiss Miss (Con Agra)
Walnut Acres Organic Juices	

The Center for Food Safety's Shoppers' Guide is now available for iPhone and Android operating systems on your mobile phone! You can now download our free application to your phone and always have your Shoppers' Guide on hand. The app also has shopping tips, a "what's new" section to keep you up to date on our most recent activities, an "action" section to take urgent actions on the go, and it even allows you to call or email companies still using GE ingredients right from the app! You can also share CFS's actions and articles on Facebook or Twitter right from the app. In addition, CFS has just launched our mobile activists list. You can join from the app—and soon from our website—to receive action alerts via text message. Visit our website, iTunes, or Android Marketplace to download your free True Food Shoppers Guide app today! The iPhone app works on iPhone, iPod Touch and iPad, and the Android app works on all Android-based phones.

Hillman Health Food Store call 855-Amish-Dr (855-264-7437) www.emineral.info Vitamins and Minerals for Better Living

Protein = Amino Acids

All protein is made up of amino acids. Proteins regulate nearly every biochemical reaction in the body. Amino acids account for 75% of dry body weight (total weight minus water weight). 100% of neurotransmitters, such as norepinephrine, serotonin, Gamma amino butyric acid, acetylcholine, aspartate, glutamate, are made of amino acids. 100% of hormones are made up of amino acids. Sex hormones are made up of amino acids plus fat or lipids. 100% of neuropeptides, the substances the brain releases with every thought, are amino acids. 100% of peptides are made up of amino acids. 95% of muscle is made up of amino acids. 95% of the heart is made up of amino acids. There are approximately 1,000 different kinds of "information molecules" made up of amino acids. RNA and DNA require amino acids. In other words, amino acids are necessary for our genes to function properly. While vitamins and minerals are important, they only make up 1.5% of dry body weight. You need the right vitamins and minerals, but if your amino acids are out of balance, you will not be healthy. Glucose and oxygen are the primary fuels for the amino acid miracle that we are. Given these numbers, do you think that amino acids might have something to do with health, illness and recovery?

Amino acids are the necessary building blocks of all protein. Required by every cell in the body in the correct balance, our diet of processed and chemically enriched foods still falls far short of the required amounts of these nutrients. The information in this section can help you determine which of these essentials you may be missing in your diet. The amino acids regarded as essential for humans are phenylalanine, valine, threonine, tryptophan, isoleucine, methionine, leucine, lysine, and histidine. Additionally, cysteine (or sulphur-containing amino acids), tyrosine (or aromatic amino acids), and arginine are required by infants and growing children. Essential amino acids are "essential" not because they are more important to life than the others, but because the body does not synthesize them, making it essential to include them in one's diet in order to obtain them. In addition, the amino acids arginine, cysteine, glycine, glutamine, histidine, proline, serine, selenocysteine, and tyrosine are considered conditionally essential, meaning they are not normally required in the diet, but must be supplied exogenously to specific populations that do not synthesize it in adequate amounts.

The following amino acids will be discussed:

1. Alanine
2. Arginine
3. Aspartic Acid
4. Cysteine
5. Glutamic Acid
6. Glutamine
7. Glycine
8. Histidine
9. Isoleucine
10. Leucine
11. Lysine
12. Methionine
13. Phenylalanine
14. Proline
15. Selnocysteine
16. Serine
17. Threonine
18. Tryptophan
19. Tyrosine
20. Valine

ALANINE

Alanine is an important source of energy for muscle and a major part of connective tissue. Alanine is primary amino acid in sugar metabolism. It boosts the immune system by producing antibodies.

Alanine deficiencies are seen in:

Elevated insulin and glucagon levels
Fatigue
Hypoglycemia
Muscle breakdown
Viral infections

Alanine excess is seen in:

Diabetes mellitus   Low insulin and glucagon levels   Starvation

Food sources: Food that contains alanine:

Asparagus	Garden bean	Pop bean
Black bean	Garden thyme	Poppyseed
Bonavist bean	Green bean	Pumpkin
Broad bean	Haricot bean	Purslane
Butter bean	Haricot vert	Sesame swamp
Butternut	Hyacinth bean	Snap bean
Cabbage water	Kidney bean	Spinach
Carob locust	Lamb's lettuce	Spinach white
Cauliflower	Lambs quarter	String bean
Chives	Lentil	Sunflower
Corn	Lentil	Sweet acacia
Dwarf bean	Lima bean	Watercress
Faba bean	Lupine chaya	Watermelon
Field bean	Navy bean	Wax bean
Flageolet bean	Pea bean	White mustard
French bean	Pigweed	Yardlong bean

ARGININE

Arginine is a nonessential amino acid, which means that it is manufactured from other amino acids in the liver. Arginine is required for proper elimination of urea from the body.

Main functions:

Essential for normal immune system activity

Necessary for wound healing

Assists with regeneration of damaged liver

Necessary for production and release of growth hormone

Most potent amino acid

Increasing release of insulin and glucagon

Precursor to gamma-aminobutyric butyric acid, an important inhibitory neurotransmitter

Decreases size of tumors

Necessary for sperm formation

Indispensable for optimum growth

Important to muscle metabolism

Acts as a vehicle for transport

Storage and excretion of nitrogen

Increases muscle mass while decreasing the amount of body fat

Plays an important role in post-injury problems of weight changes and tissue healing

Increases collagen, the main supportive fibrous protein in bones, cartilage and other connective tissues

Combats physical and mental fatigue

Promotes the detoxification of ammonia that is poisonous to living cells

Arginine deficiencies seen in:

Candidiasis (yeast infection) Immune deficiency syndromes
Gulf War Syndrome

Caution: Because of arginine's powerful boost to the immune system, people suffering from a great variety of illnesses may be tempted to experiment with it. Before doing so, make sure you do not have any acute or chronic viruses, such as Epstein-Barr, C_y cytomegalovirus, H_u human herpes virus VI, or H_E herpes simplex I or II. Arginine will speed up the rate of viral growth, which can prove to be dangerous. The amino acid, lysine has the opposite effect on viruses, slowing down their growth.

Excellent food sources of arginine include dairy products, meat, poultry, fish, nuts, and chocolate.

The following are foods that contain arginine:

Almond	Faba bean	Pea
Aloe	Fennel	Pistachio
Asparagus pea	Field bean	Pop bean
Black bean	Flageolet bean	Popping bean
Black caraway	French bean	Poppy seed
Black mustard	Garbanzo	Pumpkin
Brazil nut	Garden bean	Sesame
Broad bean	Great scarlet	Snap bean
Buffalo gourd	Green bean	String bean
Butternut	Haricot bean	Sunflower
Carob	Haricot vert	Swamp cabbage
Chaya	Kidney bean	Sweet acacia
Chickpea	Lentil	Watercress
Chinese foxglove	Lentil	Watermelon
Chives	Locust bean	Wax bean
Cowage	Mung bean	White lupine
Dwarf bean	Navy bean	

Those people with kidney or liver disease should speak with a health care provider before taking arginine supplements. Patients with herpes should not take arginine because it may cause the virus to multiply.

Large amounts of arginine may both promote and/or interfere with the growth of cancer. While beginning research has shown that arginine stimulates the immune system, a high intake has also been linked with increased cancer cell growth in humans. As of this writing, it remains unclear whether arginine is helpful or harmful for people with cancer. Arginine research has also shown benefits for reducing arterial plaguing associated with coronary heart disease by helping the lining of blood vessels remain more non-stick like a Teflon coating.

ASPARTIC ACID, ALSO KNOWN AS ASPARAGINE

Aspartic acid, readily available in protein foods, is very active in many body processes, including the formation of ammonia and urea and their disposal from the body. It is found in high levels throughout the human body, especially in the brain, where it performs an excitatory function.

Main functions:

Aspartic acid is interconvertible with asparagine; therefore, the two amino acids have many functions in common.

Builds up the immune system

Endurance

Increases resistance to fatigue

Involved in the formation of RNA and DNA, the chemical bases of heredity and carriers of genetic information

Protects the liver and promotes normal cell function

Aspartic acid deficiency is seen in: Deficiencies are seen with calcium and magnesium deficiencies or imbalances. Because of this connection, low aspartic acid levels should lead the doctor to test for calcium and/or magnesium deficiencies.

Aspartic acid excess is seen in:

Amyotrophic Lateral Sclerosis (ALS or Lou Gehrig's disease)

Epilepsy, especially right after a seizure

Stroke (brain attack)

Food sources: The following are foods that contain asparagines:

Apple
Asparagus
Bell pepper
Black caraway
Black cumin
Black currant
Burning bush
Cayenne
Celery
Cherry pepper
Chili
Chinese boxthorn
Chinese matrimony vine
Chinese wolfberry
Clubmoss
Coffee
Comfrey

Cone pepper
Cut leaf
Date palm
Elephant garlic
Fennel
Giant taro
Ginger
Ginkgo
Grapefruit
Green pepper
Hops
Horseradish
Hot pepper
Licorice
Lily
Lucid asparagus
Marshmallow
Milfoil

Onion
Orange
Paprika
Pineapple
Red chili
Spur pepper
Strawberry
Sugar beet
Sweet pepper
Tabasco
Tangerine
Tarragon
Tea
Tomato
Water lotus
Yarrow

CYSTEINE - CYSTINE

Cystine is a stable form of the amino acid cysteine. The body is capable of converting one to the other as required and in metabolic terms they can be thought of as the same. Both cystine and cysteine are rich in sulphur and can be readily synthesized by the body. Cystine is found abundantly in hair keratin, insulin and certain digestive enzymes. As a detoxification agent Cystine has been shown to protect the body against damage induced by alcohol and cigarette smoking.

Main functions:

Antioxidant protective against radiation, pollution, ultra-violet light and other causes of increased free radical production

Essential in growth, maintenance, and repair of skin

Key ingredient in hair and one of the 3 main sulfur-containing amino acids, along with taurine and methionine

Major constituent of glutathione, an important tripeptide made up of cystine, glutamic acid, and glycine

Natural detoxifier

Precursor to chondroitin sulfate, the main component of cartilage

Precursor to the amino acid taurine

Two molecules of cysteine make cystine.

Cysteine/Cystine deficiency is seen in:

Chemical Sensitivity

Food Allergy

The following are foods that contain cysteine:

Ashwagandha	Ginseng	Sickle pod
Buffalo gourd	Indian fig	Soybean
Carrot	Lime	Sunflower
Coffee	Linseed	Tea
Date Palm	Onion, shallot	Watermelon
Flax	Prickly pear	Wheat
Ginkgo	Rice	

GLUTAMIC ACID

Glutamic acid (glutamate) is simply converted to glutamine and is synthesized from arginine, ornithine, and proline. Glutamic acid, which is important to brain function, is the only amino acid metabolized in the brain. The conversion of glutamic acid to glutamine helps clear potentially toxic ammonia. Glutamic acid, with the help of vitamin B_6 and manganese, is also a precursor of gaba (gamma-aminobutyric acid), an important neurotransmitter in the central nervous system.

Main functions:

Accelerates wound and ulcer healing

Detoxifies ammonia in the brain and plays major role of building DNA in the brain

Glutamic acid is a precursor to two nerve transmitters: glycine and gamma amino butric acid

Helps stop alcohol and sugar cravings

Increases blood sugar level

Increases energy

Metabolizes sugars and fats

Transports potassium across the blood-brain barrier

Used in the treating hypoglycemia

Toxicity: Monosodium glutamate also known as MSG is a food additive that should be avoided at all times.

Food sources: Large amounts of glutamic acid can be found in meat, poultry, fish, eggs, and most dairy products.

The following are foods that contain glutamic acid:

Almond	French bean	Popping bean
Asparagus	Garden bean	Poppyseed
Asparagus bean	Goa bean	Pumpkin
Asparagus pea	Green bean	Sesame
Black bean	Habas pea	Snap bean
Bok	Haricot bean	Soybean
Bonavist bean	Hyacinth bean	String bean
Broadbean	Kidney bean	Sweet acacia
Butternut	Lablab bean	Tomato
Carob	Lentil	Watermelon
Chaya	Locust bean	Wax bean
Chinese foxglove	Mungbean	Wheat
Chives	Navy bean	White mustard
Dwarf bean	Pea bean	Winged bean
Faba bean	Pigeon pea	Yardlong bean
Field bean	Pistachio	
Flageolet bean	Pop bean	

GLUTAMINE

Glutamine is the most abundant amino acid in the body, but deficiencies can occur during metabolic stress. Glutamine is the preferred fuel for the sensitive, fast growing cells that make up your gastrointestinal (GI) tract as well as your immune system.

Main functions:

An important glycogenic amino acid, that is essential for helping maintain normal and steady blood sugar levels

Essential to gastrointestinal function; provides energy to the small intestines

Gamma amino butric acid is an inhibitory neurotransmitter that produces serenity and relaxation

Glutamine has the highest blood concentration of all the amino acids

Glutamine is a precursor to the neurotransmitter gamma amino butric acid

Glutamine is involved with muscle strength and endurance

Involved in DNA synthesis

Precursor to the neurotransmitter amino acid glutamate (glutamic Acid)

The intestines are the only organ in the body that uses glutamine as its primary source of energy

Used treating alcoholism and protects against alcohol poisoning, used in the treatment of schizophrenia and senility

Glutamine deficiency seen in:

Alcoholism   Anxiety and panic disorders   Chronic fatigue syndrome

Glutamine excess is seen with the use of some anti-convulsing medications.

The following are foods that contain glutamine:

Aloe vera	Date palm	Sickle pod
Apple	Orange	
Black currant	Pineapple	

GLYCINE

Glycine is required by the body for the mainainence of the central nervous system, and in men glycine plays an essential role in maintaining healthy prostate functions. Glycine also plays an important function in the immune system were it is used in the synthesis of other non-essential amino acids.

Main functions:

Builds up the immune system

Effective for hyperacidity (used in many gastric antacid agents)

Enzymes involved in energy production

Inhibits sugar cravings

Involved in glucagon production, assisting in glycogen metabolism

Is a main inhibitory neurotransmitter in the brain and spinal cord. The other is gamma amino butric acid.

One of the 3 critical glycogenic amino acids, along with serine and alanine

Part of the structure of hemoglobin

Glycine deficiency is seen in:

Anemia	Chronic fatigue syndrome	Viral Infections
Candidiasis (yeast infection)	Hypoglycemia	

Glycine excess is seen in starvation.

The following are foods that contain glycine:

Almond	Fennel	Navy bean
Asparagus	Field bean	Pigweed
Asparagus pea	Flageolet bean	Pistachio
Black bean	French bean	Pop bean
Black caraway	Garden bean	Popping bean
Black cumin	Goa bean	Poppyseed
Bonavist bean	Green bean	Pumpkin
Broadbean	Haricot bean	Sesame
Buffalo gourd	Horseradish	Snap bean
Butternut	Hyacinth bean	Soybean
Carob	Jew's mallow	Spinach
Chives	Kidney bean	String bean
Dwarf bean	Lablab bean	Sunflower
Faba bean	Lambs quarter	Swamp cabbage

Sweet acacia
Water spinach
Watercress

Wax bean
White lupine
White mustard

Winged bean

HISTIDINE

In the brain, histamine regulates a wide variety of physiological processes, including water and food intake, sleep-wake cycles, endocrine homeostasis, locomotion, and memory and learning.

Main functions:

Assists in maintaining proper blood pH

Associated with allergic response and used to treat allergies

Has been used to treat rheumatoid arthritis

High concentrations in hemoglobin

Precursor to histamine

Useful in treating anemia due to relationship to hemoglobin

Histidine deficiency is seen in:

Anemia

Dysbiosis (Imbalance of intestinal bacterial flora)

Rheumatoid arthritis

Histidine excess is in:

High histidine levels are associated with low zinc levels and low histidine levels are associated with high zinc levels. Thus, abnormal histidine levels are an indicator that zinc levels should be tested.

Pregnancy

The following are foods that contain histidine:

Asparagus bean
Asparagus pea
Black bean
Bonavist bean
Broadbean
Buffalo gourd
Butter bean
Butternut
Carob
Dwarf bean
Faba bean
Field bean
Flageolet bean
French bean
Garden bean
Green bean

Green gram
Haricot bean
Hyacinth bean
Jew's mallow
Kidney bean
Lablab bean
lambs quarter
Lentil
Lentil
Lima bean
Locust bean
Mungbean
Mungbean
Navy bean
Pea bean
Pop bean

Popping bean
Pumpkin
Sesame
Snap bean
Spinach
String bean
Sunflower
Sweet acacia
Velvet bean
Watercress
Watermelon
Wax bean
White mustard
Winged bean
Yardlong bean

ISOLEUCINE

In the human body Isoleucine is concentrated in the muscle tissues. Isoleucine is necessary for hemoglobin formation and in stabilizing and regulating blood sugar and energy levels.

Main functions:

One of the 3 major Branched-Chain Amino Acids, the other 2 being leucine and valine, all of which are involved with muscle strength, endurance, and muscle stamina

Branched-Chain Amino Acids levels are significantly decreased by insulin. Translation: High dietary sugar or glucose intake causes release of insulin, which, in turn, causes a drop in Branched-Chain Amino Acids levels.

Therefore, right before exercise, it is not wise to ingest foods high in glucose or other sugars, as the Branched-Chain Amino Acids, including isoleucine will not be readily available to muscles

Muscle tissue uses Isoleucine as an energy source

Required in the formation of hemoglobin

Isoleucine deficiency is seen in:

Acute hunger
Chronic fatigue syndrome
Hyperinulinemia

Kwashiorkor (starvation)
Obesity
Panic disorder

Isoleucine excess is seen in:

Diabetes mellitus with kenotic hypoglycemia

Essential to the formation of hemoglobin

Primarily metabolized in muscle tissue

Should always be in well-balanced proportion with leucine and valine

The following are foods that contain isoleucine:

Asparagus	Garden bean	Pigweed
Asparagus pea	Goa bean	Pop bean
Black bean	Green bean	Popping bean
Black mustard	Green gram	Pumpkin
Bok	Haricot bean	Sesame
Bonavist bean	Hyacinth bean	Snap bean
Broadbean	Jew's mallow	Spinach
Buffalo gourd	Kidney bean	String bean
Butter bean	Lablab bean	Sunflower
Carob	Lamb's lettuce	Swamp cabbage
Chives	Lambs quarter	Sweet acacia
Corn salad	Lentil	Velvet bean
Dwarf bean	Lettuce	Water spinach
Faba bean	Lima bean	Wax bean
Field bean	Mungbean	Wheat
Flageolet bean	Navy bean	Winged bean
French bean	Pea	

LEUCINE

Leucine is an essential amino acid which cannot be synthesized by the body but must always be acquired from dietary sources and is essential for growth. Leucine also promotes the healing of bones, skin and muscle tissue.

Main functions:

As one of the 3 branched-chain amino acids (the other 2 being Isoleucine and Valine), leucine has all of the properties discussed with Isoleucine, as it pertains specifically to the branched-chain amino acid functions.

Potent stimulator of insulin

Helps with bone healing

Helps promote skin healing

Leucine deficiency seen in:

Acute hunger
Chronic fatigue
Depression
Hyperinsulinemia
Ketosis
Leucine excess seen in:
Lowers elevated blood sugar levels

Metabolized in muscle tissue
Promotes healing of skin and broken bones
Should always be in well-balanced proportion with valine and isoleucine
Starvation
Vitamin B_{12} deficiency in pernicious anemia

The following are foods that contain isoleucine:

Asparagus bean	Flageolet bean	Popping bean
Asparagus pea	French bean	Pumpkin
Black bean	Garden bean	Sesame
Black caraway	Green bean	Snap bean
Black cumin	Green gram	Spinach
Bonavist bean	Haricot bean	String bean
Broadbean	Hyacinth bean	Sunflower
Buffalo gourd	Kidney bean	Sweet acacia
Butter bean	Lablab bean	Velvet bean
Butternut	Lambs quarter	Watercress
Carob	Lentil	Watermelon
Chives	Lima bean	Wax bean
Cowage	Navy bean	Wheat
Dwarf bean	Pea	Winged bean
Faba bean	Pea bean	Yardlong bean
Fennel	Pigweed	
Field bean	Pop bean	

LYSINE

L-Lysine was heralded in early 80's as a treatment for mouth blisters and cold sores due to its effects on viral growth and reproduction. L-Lysine aids in the production of antibodies, hormones and enzymes, maintains the body's nitrogen balance, aids calcium absorption and is instrumental in the formation of collagen.

Amino Acids

Main functions:

Inhibits viral growth and as a result is used in the treatment of herpes simplex, viruses associated with chronic fatigue syndrome, such as: Epstein-Barr virus, cytomegalo virus, and HHV6

Carnitine is formed from lysine and vit-C

Helps form collagen, the connective tissue in bones, ligaments, tendons, and joints

Assists in the absorption of calcium

Essential for children, critical for bone formation

Involved in hormone production

Lowers serum triglyceride levels

Anti-fatigue effect

Promotes bone growth by helping form collagen, the fibrous protein which makes up bone

Lysine deficiency is seen in:

AIDS
Anemia
Chronic fatigue syndrome

Epstein-Barr virus
Hair loss
Herpes

Irritability
Weight loss

Lysine excess is seen in:

Excess of ammonia in the blood

The following are foods that contain of lysine:

Asparagus
Asparagus bean
Asparagus pea
Black bean
Black caraway
Black cumin
Bok
Bonavist bean
Broadbean
Butter bean
Carob
Cowage
Dwarf bean
Faba bean
Fennel
Field bean
Flageolet bean

French bean
Garden bean
Green bean
Green gram
Green gram
Habas
Haricot bean
Hyacinth bean
Kidney bean
Lablab bean
Lambs quarter
Lentil
Lentil
Lima bean
Mungbean
Mungbean
Navy bean

Parsley
Pea
Pea bean
Pop bean
Popping bean
Pumpkin
Snap bean
Spinach
String bean
Sweet acacia
Velvet bean
Watercress
Wax bean
Wheat
Winged bean
Yardlong bean

METHIONINE

Methionine is an essential amino acid that is not synthesized by the body and must be obtained from food. It is one of the sulphur containing amino acids and is important in many body functions.

Main functions:

Assists in breakdown of fats

Precursor of the amino acids cysteine, cystine, and taurine

Helps reduce blood cholesterol levels

Assists in the removal of toxic wastes from the liver

One of the sulfur-containing amino acids (the others being cysteine and the minor amino acid, taurine)

The sulfur-containing amino acids act as anti-oxidants that neutralize free radicals

Helps prevent disorder of hair, skin, and nails due to sulfur and anti-oxidant activity

Precursor to carnitine, melatonin (the natural sleep aid) and choline (part of the neurotransmitter, acetylcholine)

Involved in the breakdown of epinephrine, histamine, and nicotinic Acid

Required for synthesis of RNA and DNA

Natural chelating agent for heavy metals - lead and mercury

Methionine deficiency is seen in:

Chemical exposure
Multiple chemical sensitivity
Vegan and or vegetarians

Methionine excess is seen in individuals who eat an abundant amount of red meat.

The following are foods that contain methionine:

Asparagus	Flageolet bean	Pumpkin
Asparagus bean	French bean	Sesame
Asparagus pea	Garden bean	Snap bean
Barley	Goa bean	Spinach
Barley grass	Great scarlet poppy	String bean
Black bean	Green bean	Sunflower
Black caraway	Haricot bean	Swamp cabbage
Black cumin	Kidney bean	Sweet acacia
Brazil nut	Locust bean	Water spinach
Buffalo gourd	Navy bean	Watercress
Butternut	Oats	Watermelon
Carob	Pea bean	Wax bean
Chaya	Pigweed	Wheat
Chives	Pistachio	White mustard
Dwarf bean	Pop bean	Winged bean
Fennel	Popping bean	Yardlong bean
Field bean	Poppy	

PHENYLALANINE

Phenylalanine is one of the amino acids which the body cannot manufacture itself, but must acquire from food. Phenylalanine is a precursor of tyrosine, and together they lead to the formation of thyroxine or thyroid hormone, and of epinephrine and norepinephrine which is converted into a neurotransmitter, a brain chemical which transmits nerve impulses. This neurotransmitter is used by the brain to manufacture norepinephrine which promotes mental alertness, memory, elevates mood, and suppresses the appetite very effectively.

Main functions:

DL-Phenylalanine is useful in reducing arthritic pain

Enhances mood, clarity of thought, concentration, and memory

Major part of collagen formation

Powerful anti-depressant

Precursor to the hormone Thyroxine

Precursor to Tyrosine, which is the precursor to neurotransmitters: Dopamine and excitatory neurotransmitters Norepinephrine and Epinephrine

Suppresses appetite

Suppresses appetite

Used in the treatment of Parkinson's disease

While the L-form of all of the other amino acids is the one that is beneficial to people, the D and DL forms of Phenylalanine have been useful in treating pain

Phenylalanine deficiency is seen in:

AIDS	Depression	Parkinson's disease
Cancer	Obesity	

Caution: Phenylalanine should be avoided in:

High blood pressure	Pigmented melanoma	Pregnancy
Panic disorder/anxiety attacks	PKU (phenylketonuria)	

The following are foods that contain phenylalanine:

Asparagus bean	French bean	Pop bean
Asparagus pea	Garden bean	Popping bean
Black bean	Goa bean	Pumpkin
Black caraway	Green bean	Snap bean
Black cumin	Haricot bean	Spinach
Bonavist bean	Hyacinth bean	String bean
Buffalo gourd	Kidney bean	Sunflower
Butter bean	Lablab bean	Swamp cabbage
Butternut	Lamb's lettuce	Sweet acacia
Carob	Lentil	Water spinach
Corn salad	Lima bean	Watercress
Dwarf bean	Mungbean	Watermelon
Fennel	Navy bean	Wax bean
Field bean	Pea bean	Winged bean
Flageolet bean	Pistachio	Yardlong bean

PROLINE

Proline is synthesized by the body from the amino acids glutamine. It is one of the main components of collagen, the connective tissue structure that binds and supports all other tissues. It is most effective in this regard when combined with vitamin C supplementation.

Main functions:

Critical component of cartilage, and health of joints, tendons, and ligaments

Involved in keeping heart muscle strong

Proline excess is seen in:

A major constituent of collagen, the main fibrous protein found in bone, cartilage, and connective tissue

Acute alcohol intake

The main precursor to proline is glutamate. The secondary precursor to proline is ornithine (minor amino acid)

Works with vitamin C in keeping skin and joints healthy

Chronic liver disease sepsis (infection of the blood)

Glycogenic (energy storage of glucose in the liver and muscles)

The following are foods that contain proline:

Almond	Flageolet bean	Pumpkin
Asparagus	French bean	Purslane
Asparagus bean	Garbanzo	Red cabbage
Asparagus pea	Garden bean	Sesame
Black bean	Goa bean	Snap bean
Black caraway	Green bean	Spinach
Black cumin	Haricot bean	String bean
Broadbean	Kidney bean	Sweet acacia
Carob	Lambs quarter	Velvet bean
Chickpea	Lentil	Watercress
Chives	Navy bean	Wax bean
Cowage	Okra	Wheat
Dwarf bean	Pea bean	White cabbage
Faba bean	Pigweed	White mustard
Fennel	Pop bean	Winged bean
Field bean	Popping bean	Yardlong bean

SELNOCYSTEINE

Selenocysteine exists in the cell. Selenocysteine is found in every domain of life on Earth. Selenocysteine amino acid has the same structure as that of cysteine. But here sulphur atom is replaced by selenium. Proteins having more than one selenocysteine residues are called selenoprotein. There is no single free pool of selenocysteine amino acid that exists within cells to be used. So it means it is an essential amino acid which is needed to be provided through food via gut probiotics.

Sources of selenocysteine

Selenocysteine is found in proteins and in variety of foods of either animal origin or plant origin.

Selenocysteine animal sources are:

Cheese	Fish	Seafood
Chicken	Meat	Turkey
Egg	Poultry	

Functions of selenocystein:

The important functions of selenocysteine in proteins are its anti-oxidant activity.

It is also used in the preparation of variety of vitamins and lots of other supplements.

It is also fortified with livestock feeds.

Our body utilizes selenocysteine to form selenium, which is believe to play important role in preventing mercury toxicity as well as enhance liver functions.

People deficient with selenium have lean body mass, prone to premature aging or to heart diseases.

SERINE

Serine is synthesized by the body from the amino acids glycine or threonine. Its production requires adequate amounts of vitamin B_7, B_6, and B_9. It is needed for the metabolism of fats and fatty acids, muscle growth and a healthy immune system.

Main functions:

One of the 3 most important glycogenic amino acids, the others being alanine and glycine

Critical in maintaining blood sugar levels

Boosts immune system by assisting in production of antibodies and immunoglobulins

Myelin sheath (the fatty acid complex that surrounds the axons of nerves is derived from serine) acts like an insulator

One variation of serine namely phosphotidyl serine, a minor amino acid serves several important functions within the central nervous system, including development of the myelin sheath

Multiple sclerosis is one of the so-called "de-myelinating diseases."

Required for growth and maintenance of muscle

The amino acid glycine is a precursor to serine and the two are interconvertible

Serine deficiency is seen in:

Candidiasis
Total body gamma and neutron irradiation Hypoglycemia

Serine excess is seen in:

Serine excess is seen in vitamin B_6 deficiency.

The following are foods that contain serine:

Asparagus	Chives	Green gram
Asparagus bean	Cowage	Haricot bean
Asparagus pea	Dwarf bean	Hyacinth bean
Black bean	Faba bean	Kidney bean
Bonavist bean	Field bean	Lablab bean
Broad bean	Flageolet bean	Lambs quarter
Butter bean	French bean	Lentil
Butternut	Garden bean	Lima bean
Carob	Goa bean	Mungbean
Cauliflower	Green bean	Navy bean

Pea	Sesame	Velvet bean
Pea Bean	Snap bean	Water spinach
Pigweed	Soybean	Watermelon
Pistachio	Spinach	Wax bean
Pop bean	String bean	White lupine
Popping bean	Swamp cabbage	Winged bean
Pumpkin	Sweet acacia	

THREONINE

Threonine, an essential amino acid, is not manufactured by the body and must be acquired from food. It is an important constituent in many body proteins and is necessary for the formation of tooth enamel protein, collagen and elastin.

Main functions:

Required for formation of collagen

Helps prevent fatty deposits in the liver

Aids in production of antibodies

Can be converted to glycine (a neurotransmitter) in the central nervous system

Acts as detoxifier

Needed by the gastrointestinal tract for normal functioning

Provides symptomatic relief in amyotrophic lateral sclerosis, Lou Gehrig's disease

In laboratory animal experiments, increases thymus weight

Threonine is often low in depressed patient and helpful in treating depression

Threonine deficiency is seen in:

AIDS	Depression	Muscle spasticity
Amyotrophic lateral sclerosis	Epilepsy	Vegetarianism

Threonine excess is seen in:

Alcohol ingestion
Liver cirrhosis
Pregnancy

Those treated with sedative anti-convulsing medication (animal studies)
Vitamin B_6 deficiency

The following are foods that contain threonine:

Aba bean	Chinese foxglove	Green bean
Asparagus	Chives	Haricot bean
Asparagus pea	Corn salad	Hyacinth bean
Asparagus pea	Cowage	Kidney bean
Black bean	Dwarf bean	Lablab bean
Bok	Field bean	Lamb's lettuce
Bonavist bean	Flageolet bean	Lambs quarter
Buffalo gourd	French bean	Lentil
Butter bean	Garden bean	Lentil
Carob	Goa bean	Navy bean

Amino Acids

Oats	Spinach	Watermelon
Pigweed	String bean	Wax bean
Pop bean	Swamp cabbage	White lupine
Popping bean	Sweet acacia	White mustard
Road bean	Velvet bean	Winged bean
Sesame	Water spinach	Winged bean
Snap bean	Watercress	

TRYPTOPHAN

Tryptophan an essential amino acid, is one of the amino acids which the body cannot manufacture itself, but most acquire from food. It is the least abundant in proteins and also easily destroyed by the liver. Tryptophan is necessary for the production of the vitamin B_3, which is essential for your brain to manufacture the key neurotransmitter serotonin.

Main functions:

Precursor to the key neurotransmitter, serotonin, which exerts a calming effect

Effective sleep aid, due to conversion to serotonin

Reduces anxiety

Effective in some forms of depression

Treatment for migraine headaches

Stimulates growth hormone

Effective in lowering cholesterol levels along with lysine, carnitine, and taurine

Can be converted into vitamin B_3

Lowers risk of arterial spasms

The only plasma amino acid that is bound to protein

Tryptophan deficiency is seen in:

ALS
Chronic fatigue syndrome
Depression

Food and drug administration ban of Tryptophan
Insomnia

Tryptophan excess is seen in:

Increased blood levels of free fatty acids
Increased intake of salicylates (aspirin)

Sleep deprivation
Vitamin B_3 intake

Caution: Simultaneous treatment with Tryptophan and Prozac (and other SSRI anti-depressants, such as Paxil and Zoloft) can produce a permanent brain disorder called serotonin syndrome. Serotonin syndrome, or serotonin toxicity, is a rare condition but can be potentially life threatening. This treatment combination is to be avoided.

The following are foods that contain tryptophan:

Almond	Field bean	Navy bean
Asparagus	Flageolet bean	Pigweed
Asparagus pea	French bean	Pop bean
Black bean	Garbanzo	Popping bean
Black mustard	Garden bean	Pumpkin
Bonavist bean	Goa bean	Sesame
Butternut	Green bean	Snap bean
Cauliflower	Green gram	Spinach
Chickpea	Haricot bean	String bean
Chicory	Horseradish	Sunflower
Chives	Hyacinth bean	Watercress
Collards	Kidney bean	Wax bean
Corn salad	Lablab bean	White mustard
Dwarf bean	Lamb's lettuce	Winged bean
Evening Primrose	Mungbean	

TYROSINE

Tyrosine is an amino acid which is synthesized from phenylalanine in the body. It is a precursor of the important brain neurotransmitters epinephrine, norepinephrine and dopamine, which transmit nerve impulses and are essential to prevent depression. Dopamine is vital to mental function and seems to play a role in sex drive. Tyrosine is also used by the thyroid gland to produce one of the major hormones, Thyroxin.

Main functions:

Precursor to neurotransmitters dopamine, norepinephrine, epinephrine (adrenaline), and melanin

Effective anti-depressant for norepinephrine-deficient depressions

Tyrosine is preferred over phenylalanine, which is also a precursor to all of the above neurotransmitters

Phenylalanine is one-step removed from the metabolic process, and can aggravate high blood pressure

Precursor to thyroxine and growth hormone

Increases energy, improves mental clarity and concentration requires pyridoxal-5-phosphate (P5P) a form of vitamin B_6 to be converted into norepinephrine P5P deficiency will lower norepinephrine levels, even if tyrosine levels are normal

Tyrosine deficiency is seen in:

Chronic fatigue
Depression
Drug addiction and dependency

Hypothyroidism
Parkinson's disease
Syndrome Gulf War Syndrome

Tyrosine excess is seen in:

Hyperthyroidism

Chronic liver disease and or cirrhosis

The following are foods that contain tyrosine:

Asparagus bean	Flageolet bean	Sesame
Asparagus pea	French bean	Snap bean
Black bean	Garden bean	Spinach
Black caraway	Green bean	String bean
Black cumin	Habas	Swamp cabbage
Black mustard	Haricot bean	Sweet acacia
Bonavist bean	Hyacinth bean	Velvet bean
Broadbean	Kidney bean	Water lotus
Butternut	Lablab bean	Water spinach
Carob	Lambs quarter	Watercress
Chaya	Navy bean	Watermelon
Chives	Oats	Wax bean
Cowage	Pea	Wheat
Dwarf bean	Pea bean	White lupine
Faba bean	Pop bean	Winged bean
Fennel	Popping bean	Yardlong bean
Field bean	Pumpkin	

Valine

Valine is one of the amino acids which the body cannot for manufacture itself but must acquire from food sources. Valine has a stimulant effect. Healthy growth depends on it. A deficiency results in a negative hydrogen balance in the body.

Main functions:

Valine is one of the 3-major branched-chain amino acids . . . the other 2 being leucine and isoleucine . . . all of which are involved with muscle strength, endurance, and muscle stamina

Branched-chain amino acid levels are considerably decreased by insulin. High dietary sugar or glucose intake causes release of insulin, which, in turn causes a drop in branched-chain amino acid levels and competes with tyrosine and tryptophan in crossing the blood-brain barrier. The higher the valine level, the lower the brain levels of tyrosine and tryptophan. One of the implications of this competition is that tyrosine and tryptophan nutritional supplements need to be taken at least an hour before or after meals or with supplements that are high in branched chain amino acids.

Actively absorbed and used directly by muscle as an energy source

Is not processed by the liver before entering the blood stream

Any acute physical stress (including surgery, sepsis, fever, trauma, starvation) requires higher amounts of valine, leucine, and isoleucine

During a period of valine deficiency, all of the other amino acids (and protein) are less well absorbed by the GI tract

Valine deficiency is seen in:

Elevated insulin levels	Kwashiorkor	Obesity
Hunger	Neurological deficit	

Valine excess is seen in:

Glycogenic (energy storage source of glucose in the liver and muscles), metabolized in muscle

Ketotic hypoglycemia

Used in the treatment of severe amino acid deficiencies caused by addictions

Valine always be in well-balanced proportion with leucine and isoleucine

Visual and tactile hallucinations

The following are foods that contain valine:

Asparagus	Flageolet bean	Popping bean
Asparagus pea	French bean	Poppyseed
Asparagus pea	Garden bean	Pumpkin
Black bean	Goa bean	Sesame
Black mustard	Goa bean	Snap bean
Bok	Green bean	Spinach
Broadbean	Haricot bean	String bean
Buffalo gourd	Horseradish	Sunflower
Butter bean	Kidney bean	Swamp cabbage
Butternut	Lamb's lettuce	Velvet bean
Carob	Lambs quarter	Water spinach
Chives	Lentil	Watercress
Corn salad	Lima bean	Wax bean
Cowage	Navy bean	White mustard
Dwarf bean	Pea	Winged bean
Faba bean	Pistachio	Winged bean
Field bean	Pop bean	

HEALTHFOOD STORE SUPPLEMENTS

(ALPHBETICAL LISTING)

ALA – (Alpha-Linolenic Acid)

Alpha-linolenic acid (ALA) is an essential fatty acid that comes from plants. Considered an essential nutrient, it is used as a source of energy by the body. ALA is considered a "parent" fatty acid; it is converted by the body into omega-3 fatty acids, which are found in fish oils. Omega-3 fatty acids perform a number of regulatory functions in the body including heart rate, blood pressure, immune response, and breakdown of fats. Essential fatty acids such as ALA are also used to make brain and nervous tissue. Small studies have shown that ALA may prevent coronary heart disease and stop artherosclerosis. Other researchers have begun studying ALA's anti-inflammatory and immunologic effects for conditions such as migraine headaches and depression. Currently, ALA is used to reduce cholesterol levels, treat allergic and inflammatory conditions, and fight autoimmune diseases such as multiple sclerosis and lupus.

How much ALA should I take? There is no recommended daily allowance of ALA. However, a healthy diet should include less saturated fats and more essential fatty acids. Before taking ALA supplements, discuss your situation with your health care provider.

What are some good sources of ALA?

Flaxseed	Mackerel	Walnut
Flaxseed oil	Pumpkin	
Linseed oil	Salmon	

What can happen if I do not get enough ALA? As previously stated, there is no recommended daily allowance of ALA. If you have questions or concerns, talk with your health care provider about ALA and ALA supplements.

What can happen if I take too much? Are there any side effects I should be aware of? ALA supplements are usually high in calories; therefore, excess amounts may lead to unwanted weight gain. Flaxseed oil (a source of ALA) may increase the body's need for vitamin E. Make sure to talk with your health care provider for more information.

Alpha-Lipoic Acid

Alpha-lipoic acid (ALA) is an antioxidant manufactured in the body. It is sometimes referred to as the universal antioxidant because, unlike most antioxidants, it is soluble in both fat and water. In addition to being created by the body, it can be found in some foods and supplements (see below). ALA has several benefits, particularly for people with diabetes. It enhances glucose uptake in people with type-2 diabetes, delays the process of glybosylation (in which sugar molecules attach themselves to proteins), and can reduce nerve damage and pain caused by diabetes. Early evidence suggests that ALA can improve visual function in people with glaucoma. Test-tube studies show that ALA can stop the HIV virus from replicating, but whether ALA supplements can help people infected with HIV remains unclear at this point.

How much alpha-lipoic acid should I take? As of this writing, there is no clear evidence that any particular dose of ALA provides a benefit for any particular condition. In the glaucoma study that was previously mentioned, researchers provided subjects with 150 mg of ALA per day. Other studies typically use between 750 and 800 milligrams per day. Some practitioners recommend 20-50 mg of alpha-lipoic acid daily to provide general antioxidant protection.

What are some good sources of alpha-lipoic acid? What forms are available? The body produces small amounts of alpha-lipoic acid naturally. Some red meats, particularly liver, are believed to be good sources of ALA; supplements are also available.

What can happen if I do not get enough alpha-lipoic acid? What can happen if I take too much? Are there any side effects I should be aware of? Because alpha-lipoic acid is produced naturally in the body, shortages are not known to occur in humans. However, for people who take large doses of ALA supplements, some side effects may occur, including skin rash, and diabetics run the risk of suffering hypoglycemia. Long-term use of alpha-lipoic acid in animals has been shown to interfere with the actions of the vitamin B_7, but research on humans has yet to be carried out. As always, make sure to speak with a licensed health care provider before you begin taking alpha-lipoic acid or any other herbal remedy or dietary supplement.

AMP – (ADENOSINE MONOPHOSPHATE)

AMP is short for adenosine monophosphate. It's a substance formed by the body during certain metabolic processes and is found within the bodies of cells. It is related to adenosine, a molecule that affects a person's heartbeat.

Although the exact purpose of AMP remains unclear, some studies suggest that it may relieve pain associated with shingles, research suggests that people with shingles may have low levels of AMP in the blood. A study that was carried out in the mid 1980s found that AMP injections relieved the pain connected with shingles more quickly than a placebo, and helps future skin lesions from appearing. Another study showed that AMP could treat a skin condition that causes certain people to become extremely sensitive to light.

How much AMP should I take? Because the body creates AMP normally, the exact amount to be taken on a daily basis remains unknown. The photosensitivity study mentioned above used between 160 and 200 milligrams of AMP per day, while research regarding AMP and shingles has used a specially formulated gel. People with herpes simplex or herpes zoster may have low levels of AMP, but the exact cause and impact has yet to be decided.

What forms of AMP are available? AMP is created by the body during certain metabolic processes. It is also available as a supplement, but can be rather difficult to obtain.

What can happen if I take too much AMP? Are there any interactions I should be aware of? What precautions should I take? Although studies of AMP have not reported any side effects, some scientists believe that supplementing with large doses of AMP may result in increased levels of adenosine, which may interfere with the body's immune system. In addition, there is evidence that intravenous injections of AMP could alter the heart's rhythm. As such, only a licensed physician should perform injections of AMP. As of this writing, there are no well-known drug interactions associated with AMP. As always, make sure to speak with a licensed health care provider before taking AMP or any other herbal remedy or dietary supplement.

Amylase Inhibitors

Amylase inhibitors are substances that prevent certain starches from being absorbed by the body. Developed decades ago, amylase inhibitors are extracted from plants that belong to the legume family, such as kidney beans, then altered and sold as dietary supplements. The main use for amylase inhibitors is weight loss. Recent studies have shown that highly concentrated versions of amylase inhibitors may block the absorption of certain starches, which could lead to lower carbohydrate consumption and in theory, cause a person to lose weight. Other studies have shown that purified amylase inhibitor extracts, taken with a starchy meal, can lower blood sugar levels in both healthy people and people diagnosed with diabetes. This has led some researchers to believe that amylase inhibitors may be helpful in controlling blood sugar levels.

How much amylase inhibitor should I take? The amount of amylase inhibitor to be consumed depends on the potency of the substance. Recommended doses are between 1,500 milligrams and 6,000 milligrams, depending on the substance's purity and potency.

What forms of amylase inhibitors are available? Amylase inhibitors are made from certain members of the legume family, such as white kidney beans. Amylase inhibitors can also be extracted from wheat

What can happen if I take too many amylase inhibitors? Are there any interactions I should be aware of? What precautions should I take?

High amounts of amylase inhibitors may cause diarrhea in some people. In addition, because amylase inhibitors can have an effect on blood sugar levels, they should not be taken by diabetics who are currently taking medications to lower their blood sugar without first speaking with a licensed health care provider. As always, make sure to speak with a licensed health care provider before taking amylase inhibitors or any other herbal remedies or dietary supplements.

Apple Cider Vinegar

Apple cider vinegar has been used for centuries as a folk remedy for a selection of ills. The ancient Egyptians, as far back as 3000 B.C., and even the father of modern medicine, Hippocrates, 400 B.C sang the praises of this unique, yet humble, product. Apple cider vinegar has been highly regarded throughout history. The saying, "An apple a day keeps the doctor away," comes from the medieval English saying. This saying actually says: "To eat an apple before going to bed will make the doctor beg for his bread."

Fermenting apple juice to alcoholic apple cider, and then letting the oxygen interact with it, turns the alcohol into acetic acid—one of the "magic" ingredients in the finished product. To help this process along from the alcoholic base, "mother" is added—that being the spider web look-alike bacteria foam that forms during the fermentation process. Some people complain that it might be too acidic to drink, but that is really a fallacy since the acidity is lower than that of commercial cola!

Benefits that may be achieved by using apple cider vinegar for:

Arthritis	Cramps	Heart
Asthma	Diabetes	Indigestion
Blood pressure	Diarrhea	Kidney Stones
Bones	Depression	Metabolism
Cancer	Eyes	Muscles
Candida	Fatigue	Nasal congestion
Cholesterol	Food poisoning	Sore throat
Colds	Gallstones	Stiff joints
Constipation	Headaches	Ulcers

Substances in apple cider vinegar are:

Minerals   Vitamins

NO REFRIGERATION REQUIRED.

Internal benefits and external benefits are:

Helps control weight	Helps remove body sludge toxins	Rich in enzymes and potassium
Helps maintain healthy skin	Helps soothe dry throats	Soothes irritated skin
Helps promote youthful, healthy bodies	Promotes digestion and ph Balance	Support a healthy immune system
	Relieves muscle pain from exercise	Weight loss

I had always heard about apple cider vinegar... everyone in the world should be drinking this on a daily basis! This would be hard to believe in our modern day world, where our health is kept together and disease is kept at bay by a battery of doctors, ranging from:

Cardiologists	Internists	Pathologists
Dermatologists	Neurologists	Radiologists
Gynecologists	Oncologists	

Minerals in apple cider vinegar:

Boron	Fluorine	Potassium
Calcium	Iron	Silicon
Chlorine	Magnesium	Sodium
Copper	Phosphorous	Sulfur

Vitamins in apple cider vinegar:

Provitamin beta-carotene	Vitamin B_2	Vitamin E
Vitamin A	Vitamin B_6	Vitamin P
Vitamin B_1	Vitamin C	

Hillman Health Food Store call 855-Amish-Dr (855-264-7437) www.emineral.info Vitamins and Minerals for Better Living

These minerals and vitamins are useful in:

Well-functioning metabolism

Reducing cholesterol (the dangerous LDL cholesterol type)

Regulating the water content in the cells and body

Reducing water retention in the body

Reducing excess sodium from the body

Helps with regulating blood pressure

Assists in preventing circulatory problems

Helps with diminishing premature calcification of the arteries

Helps increase concentration and memory

Assists in blood circulation, body temperature as well as vitality and energy

Help from chronic health conditions such as: Arthritis This is the condition of inflammation of the joints and is a major chronic disease in the West. It is believed to be partly caused by a build-up of toxic wastes in the tissues, causing irritation. It is thought that these metabolic toxic wastes can be contained by eliminating food allergies as well as unhealthy lifestyles such as smoking, not exercising and being obese. Arthritis suffers have reported a positive influence that apple cider vinegar has on the pain experienced as well as slowing down the progression of this disease. Most people using it as a therapy for this problem ingest it four times a day.

Asthma - Although orthodox medicine might not agree with this remedy, some people have found relief from asthma by ingesting apple cider vinegar, as well as applying pads soaked in apple cider vinegar under pressure to the inside of the wrists.

Blood pressure - The potassium in apple cider vinegar is said to be beneficial to both the heart and blood pressure, and in some quarters this remedy is said to assist in making the blood thinner, and thereby assisting with blood pressure and in the prevention of a stroke.

Bones - The manganese, magnesium, silicon (and calcium) found in apple cider vinegar has been linked in sustaining bone mass, which is important in the fight against osteoporosis. A supplement of apple cider vinegar could for this reason be valuable to consider should you suffer from a calcium shortage, have a problem with osteoporosis, or if you are entering your postmenopausal stage where a risk of bone loss could cause a problem.

Cancer - Although apple cider vinegar cannot cure cancer, it is a valuable ally to have around to help fight free radicals in the body which have been shown to be indicative in the formation of various cancers. Beta-carotene, found in apple cider vinegar, is a powerful antioxidant, which helps in neutralizing the free radicals formed in our bodies through oxidation. To prevent these free radicals and to keep them in check, we need antioxidants in our system to rid our bodies of these potentially dangerous compounds. If free radicals are left alone to have the run of our bodies, they cause major damage by severely damaging cells, which leads to aging and degeneration. The pectin in apple cider vinegar adds fiber to the diet, and even the American Cancer Society promotes a high fiber diet to help with preventing cancer, especially colon cancer. The reason for this is that fiber binds with certain cancer-causing (carcinogenic) compounds in the colon, and speeds up their elimination from the body.

Candida - Although there are different factors influencing the formation of candida (which is a yeast infection), a disturbance of your diet as well as an intake of antibiotics must be looked at when you experience such an episode of candida flare-up. These factors must be considered because they can throw the yeast balance in your body out of sync. A selection of topical creams and lotions are available, but a cheap alternative can be found by douching twice a day with a solution of apple cider vinegar until the symptoms disappear. The solution is made from 2 tablespoons of apple cider vinegar to a quart of lukewarm water–this solution will assist in restoring the acid balance.

Cholesterol - A good warning system for heart disease is the presence of high blood cholesterol in the system. To help prevent this, follow a lifestyle which includes eating a diet high in fruits and vegetables, maintaining your ideal weight, and getting enough exercise while avoiding processed foods, junk foods and hydrogenated oils. Another way is to add fiber to your diet, especially water-soluble fiber–such as the pectin found in apple cider vinegar. Water-soluble fiber soaks up water, which adds bulk, and interacts with your body, and also keeps on working longer than non water-soluble fiber. Fiber also soaks up fats and cholesterol in the body and then is excreted instead of being reabsorbed. Non water-soluble fiber soaks up moisture in the body, but cannot interact with the body. The amino acids contained in apple cider vinegar have also shown promise in neutralizing some of the harmful oxidized LDL cholesterol.

Colds - It has been found that the pH factor (the acidity factor) of the body becomes a bit more alkaline prior to a cold or flu striking you down. When you take apple cider vinegar it helps to rebalance the acid level of your body. Another remedy for colds and flu and said to be specifically beneficial for chest complaints during the winter is to soak a piece of brown paper with apple cider vinegar and place pepper on one side of the paper. Then, tie the paper (pepper side down) onto your chest and leave on for 25 - 30 minutes.

Constipation - Not having proper bowel movements is blamed for many illnesses and diseases which befall us. The logic behind it stating that should the waste products from our bodily functions be retained in the body for longer than what nature intends, it will cause toxins to be absorbed back into the system. As we age our bodies produce less and start to lag behind in the manufacture of digestive acids (hydrochloric acid), pepsin and digestive enzymes–which can cause constipation. When we add fiber to our diet, such as the pectin in apple cider vinegar, we assist our body by having regular bowel movements and proper elimination.

Cramps - If you have never woken up in the middle of the night with cramps tearing through your calves, feet or legs, you would not understand the agony. A useful remedy to assist with this is to take apple cider vinegar. *See Muscles below.

Diabetes - This disease is becoming more and more common. Now, there may be various reasons for this phenomenon, but it must be remembered that it is not only extremely serious but needs proper medical supervision. One should also practice strict adherence to dietary rules and medication as prescribed by your medical practitioner. It is, however, interesting to note that added dietary fiber, such as contained in apple cider vinegar, is beneficial in controlling blood glucose levels.

Diarrhea - There are various causes for diarrhea. Although it should not be left untreated, it sometimes is a way for the body to rid itself of harmful compounds and ingested materials. The pectin in apple cider vinegar is great to take when suffering from this problem, since this water-soluble fiber swells up and forms bulk. It is also an effective ingredient to use against certain bacteria which causes diarrhea and the intestinal flora also transforms pectin into a protective coating which soothes the irritated lining of the colon. Next time you have a problem, consider this most humble treatment.

Depression - Although prescribing apple cider vinegar for depression would be classified as extremely alternative, some Eastern medicines believe that depression is the symptom of a "stagnant" or tired liver. If you believe in this philosophy, then apple cider vinegar would help to fight depression because it is a great medium to help detoxify and clean the liver.

Eyes - Cataract development in the eye is associated to oxidation of the lens of the eye due to alterations caused by free radicals changing the structure of the lens. With this in mind apple cider vinegar can be of use with this problem because the antioxidant properties of beta-carotene contained in apple cider vinegar are great in combating free radicals.

Fatigue - Lactic acid is released in the body during exercise as well as periods of stress, and this can lead to fatigue, which in turn can be combated by the amino acids contained in apple cider vinegar. The enzymes, as well as the potassium contained in apple cider vinegar can also be of great help in the quest for more energy and vitality.

Food poisoning - Because of the great disinfectant qualities inherent in apple cider vinegar, some people use it when suffering from mild cases of food poisoning and find it beneficial. If you suffer from violent symptoms and suspect serious food poisoning, please contact your medical practitioner immediately.

Gallstones and kidney stones - A theory exists that the acids found in apple cider vinegar are beneficial in breaking up kidney stones and gallstones by softening or dissolving them. Since there are so many other influencing factors, we cannot guarantee any results, but should you be suffering from gallstones or kidney stones it might be worth your while to supplement your diet with apple cider vinegar.

Headaches - The cause of headaches can be stress, allergies, tiredness, and problems with your gallbladder, liver, kidneys, or a variety of other factors. Although apple cider vinegar cannot be touted as a headache treatment, it has been found that people have slightly more alkaline urine when suffering from a headache, and, therefore, apple cider vinegar could be effective since it will assist in bringing your body's acid level back into sync. The inhalation of apple cider vinegar could also assist with a headache. Inhalation can be achieved by adding some apple cider vinegar to boiling water in a big pan, removing it from the stove and carefully inhaling the vapor.

Heart - Since apple cider vinegar is used to promote the health of veins and capillaries, it is by implication also useful in assisting in the health of the heart and blood pressure. The potassium found in the apple cider vinegar is also beneficial to the heart.

Indigestion - When people start talking about indigestion, they immediately start referring to the "excess" stomach acid that they have! In most cases it is NOT a case of an excess of stomach acid, but a shortage of it. Hydrochloric acid and pepsin, an enzyme working in an acid environment, are needed to break down the food effectively. A shortage of these two ingredients will lead to a sluggish digestion of food and resultant indigestion. Taking apple cider vinegar may assist in effecting a remedy.

Metabolism - The quest for achieving the ideal weight always will include effective and efficient metabolism. Without it, your dietary intake will not be metabolized correctly, and the nutrients will not be available to the body and will result in excess weight being added to the body frame. Apple cider vinegar has been used for centuries in aiding the liver to detoxify the body and to help with digesting rich, fatty and greasy foods, and for proper metabolizing of proteins, fats and minerals. If the food cannot be broken down into the absorbable form, the body cannot assimilate the required nutrients needed from the diet. An added extra to help with this is the malic acid and tartaric acid found in apple cider vinegar because they help to bring the acid content into balance, while killing off unwanted and unfriendly bacteria in the digestive tract.

Muscles - Lactic acid in muscles is the cause of the muscles feeling sore and stiff. By adding some apple cider vinegar to your diet, it could assist the body to get rid of it at a faster pace. This is because it will help to break down the acid crystals and make it much easier to be flushed out the body.

Nasal congestion - A constant draining of mucus from the sinus cavities can both be sore and uncomfortable. It is best to cut out or eat as little as possible of mucus forming food—which traditionally and in most cases would be dairy products. Many sufferers of nasal congestion have experienced relief by adding apple cider vinegar to their diet.

Sore throat - A gargle made from apple cider vinegar and water could prove to be a great relief for a sore throat—be it that of a bacterial or virus infection. The solution is a 50/50 mixture, and it is best to spit out the solution after gargling, which should be repeated every hour. After gargling rinse the mouth with clean water to prevent the acid from eroding the enamel on your teeth.

Stiff joints - A shortage of potassium in the body may cause stiff joints. Since apple cider vinegar is a good source of potassium, it could help in relieving this problem. Another remedy is to relax in a warm tub with some apple cider vinegar added to the water.

Ulcers - Apple cider vinegar is showing great promise in helping to heal alcohol-induced ulcers. The reason behind this is that it activates the body to start its own defensive mechanism. This, together with other indicators, suggests that apple cider vinegar may in the near future be drawn into the fold of alternative ulcer preventing remedies.

Weight loss - Apple cider vinegar has been used as a weight loss remedy for centuries, and although the mechanics are not always clear on how it works, it really does work. It has been suggested that the apple cider vinegar works because it makes the body burn calories better and reduces the appetite or simply that it gets the entire metabolism working at top efficiency. Whatever the reason, the fact remains that it has stood the test of time as a fat-busting supplement, and has helped countless people to achieve their ideal weight.

"An apple a day keeps the doctor away!"

Bach Essence Flowers

Dr. Edward Bach was an English physician and homeopathic doctor and worked in a homeopathic hospital and was also a successful conventional doctor. He continually searched for the purest methods of healing and became unsatisfied with the limitations of orthodox medicine and their focus on curing symptoms insted of gettin to the bottom of the problem. While walking in the garden, he discovered that each dewdrop on a flower acquires the vibration of that plant, essentially giving water a memory.

In 1930 Dr. Bach went to Wales where he developed 12 healers and 7 helpers. In 1934 he moved to Mount Vernon Oxford and found a remaining 19 remedies. In 1936 he died at the age of 50.

Dr. Bach felt that there are blockages between the subconscious and the soul direction. The following quotes are from his book entitled *Free Thysel*. "Health and happiness result from being in harmony with our own nature, and doing the work for which we are individually suited." "Disease is entirely the result of a conflict between our spiritual and mortal selves." "Disease is the re-action to interferences. This is temporary failure and unhappiness and this occurs when we allow others to interfere with our purpose in life and implant in our minds doubt, or fear, or indifference."

His remedies are completely safe and can be used on babies and infants as well as horses, dogs, and cats. In fact, vets are now using his remedies. (Placebo effect impossible) You can even use them with plants themselves.

There are 38 Bach Essences. They are divided into these groups:

Abnormal fears
Decision mMaking
Discouraging events

Inability to stay focused in the present
Relationship with others
Relationship with self

Relationship with self:

Larch – Lack of self esteem
Pine – Self blame, guilt
Willow – Resentment
Agrimony – Can't face own feelings
Rock water – Rigid personal regime

Elm – Overwhelmed by responsibility
Crab apple – Feeling unclean
Hornbeam – Monday morning feeling
Oak – Pursuit of duty

Relationship with others:

Beech – Judgmental
Centaury – Submissive
Chicory – Possessive
Heather – Needy
Holly – Envy or hatred

Impatiens – Impatient
Vervain – Over enthusiastic
Vine – Dictatorial
Water violet – Aloofness
Vervain – Over enthusiastic

Decision making:

Cerato – Keep asking others
Chestnut bud – Repeating mistakes
Wild oat – Too many choices

Scleranthus – Torn between 2 choices
Walnut – Others smother change

Discouraging events:

Gentian – Doubt by any setback
Gorse – Hopelessness

Mustard – Gloom for unknown reason
Sweet chestnut – Anguish

Abnormal fears:

Aspen – Unknown fear
Cherry Plum – Losing control
Mimulus – Known fear

Red Chestnut – Fear for loved ones
Rock Rose – Terror
Star of Bethlehem – Shock

Inability to stay focused in the present:

Clematis – Ungrounded
Honeysuckle – Living in past
Wild Rose – Resignation

Olive – Mental and physical exhaustion
White Chestnut – Obsessive thoughts

THE 38 BACH FLOWER REMEDIES

INDICATIONS	BACH FLOWER	POSITIVE QUALITIES
	AGRIMONY - (AGRIMONIA EUPATORIA)	
Mental torment and worry hidden behind a cheerful appearance. Avoiding emotional pain. Can't face own feelings.	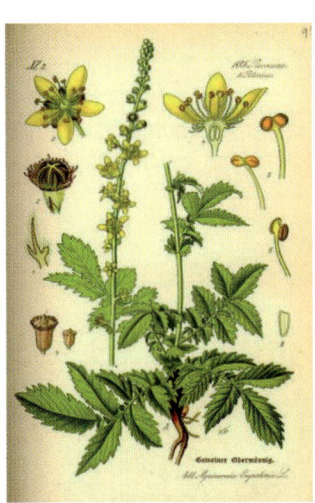	Emotional honesty and inner peace.
	ASPEN - (POPULUS TREMULA)	
Vague fears and apprehension of unknown origin. Unconscious anxieties.	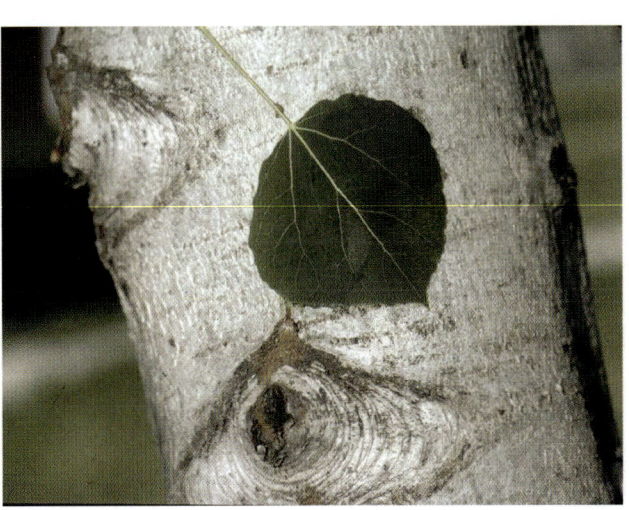	Fearlessness and trust.

INDICATIONS	BACH FLOWER	POSITIVE QUALITIES

BEECH - *(FAGUS SYLVATICA)*

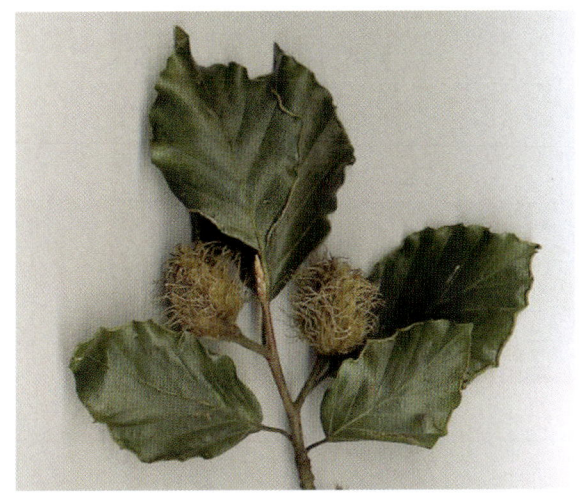

Intolerance, criticism, passing judgements. Perfectionism.

Sympathy and tolerance. Acceptance of others.

CENTAURY - *(CENTAURIUM UMBELLATUM)*

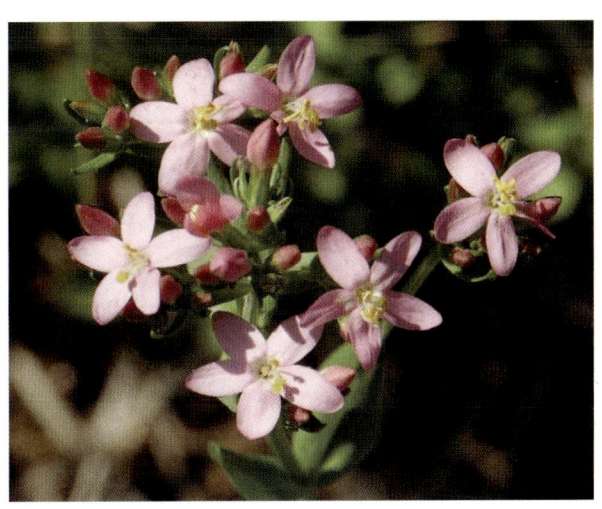

Weak-willed, easily influenced, self-neglect. Doormats.

Self-determination and self-recognition. Inner strength.

Bach Essence Flowers

INDICATIONS	BACH FLOWER	POSITIVE QUALITIES

Cerato - (Ceratostigma Willmottiana)

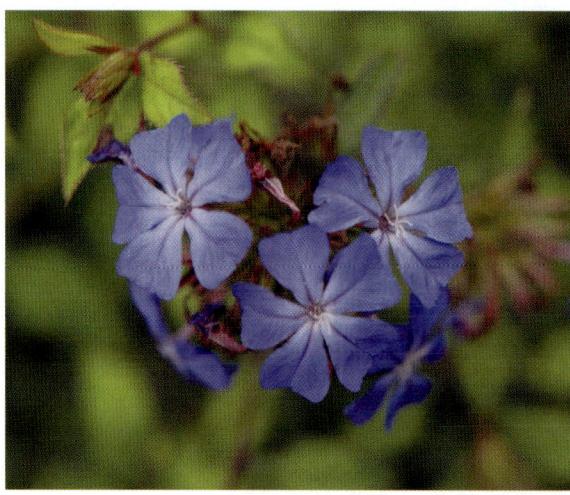

Self-distrust, self-doubt and uncertainty. Seeking advice from others.

Inner knowing (intuition) and self-trust. Self-confidence.

Cherry Plum - (Prunus Cerasifera)

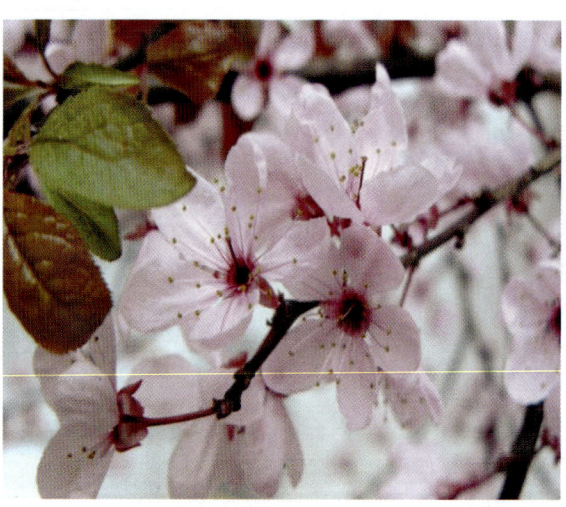

Fear of mental/emotional breakdown and loss of control. Desperation and destructive impulses.

Spiritual surrender and composure. Trust in God or the Divine.

| INDICATIONS | BACH FLOWER | POSITIVE QUALITIES |

CHESTNUT BUD - *(AESCULUS HIPPOCASTANUM)*

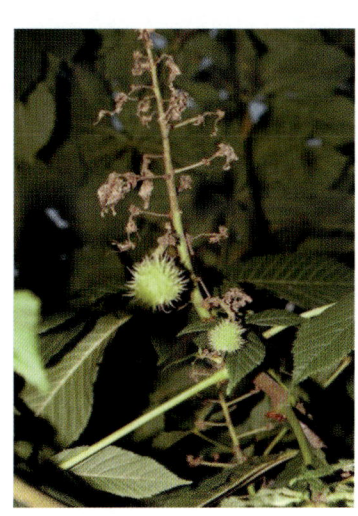

Repeating mistakes and failure to learn from experience. Habitual behavior.

Breaking old patterns. Understanding life's lessons. Wisdom.

CHICORY - *(CICHORIUM INTYBUS)*

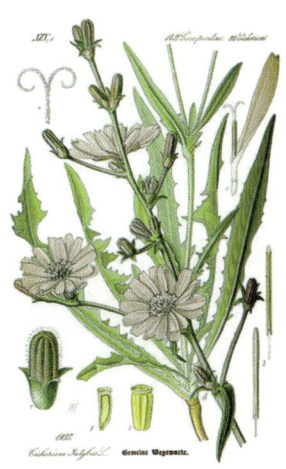

Self-centeredness and self-pity. Possessive and demanding. Emotional neediness.

Selfless love given freely. Respecting the freedom of others.

Bach Essence Flowers

| INDICATIONS | BACH FLOWER | POSITIVE QUALITIES |

CLEMATIS - *(CLEMATIS VITALBA)*

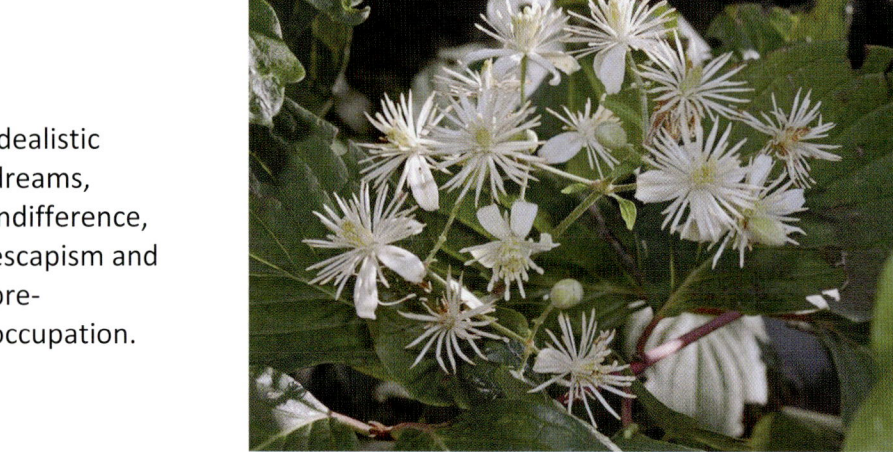

Idealistic dreams, indifference, escapism and pre-occupation.

Expressing inspiration in practical life. Creative idealism.

CRAB APPLE - *(MALUS PUMILA)*

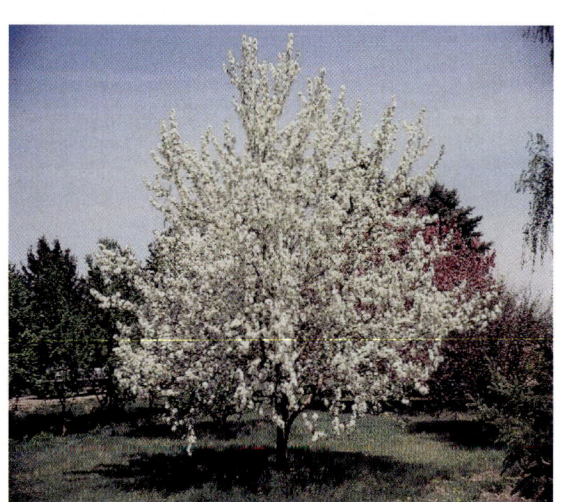

Self-dislike and self-disgust. Obsessed with impurity and imperfection.

The Cleansing Remedy. Self-acceptance and perspective.

| INDICATIONS | BACH FLOWER | POSITIVE QUALITIES |

ELM - (ULMUS PROCERA)

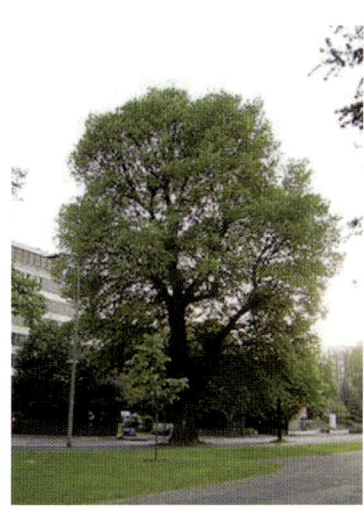

Overwhelmed by responsibility. Temporary inadequacy and despondency.

Self-assurance and confidence to complete one's tasks.

GENTIAN - (GENTIANA AMARELLA)

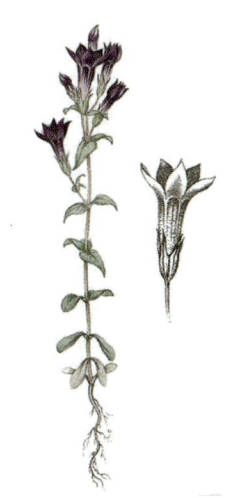

Discouragement after a setback. Reactive depression and doubt.

Faith and perseverance despite difficulties.

INDICATIONS	BACH FLOWER	POSITIVE QUALITIES

GORSE - (ULEX EUROPAEUS)

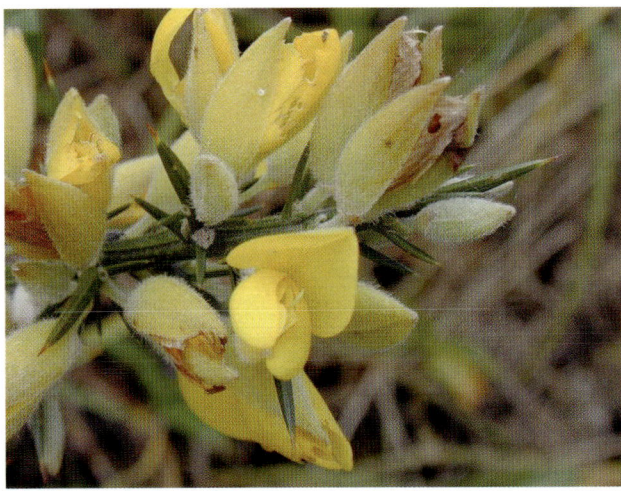

Overwhelming despair, hopelessness and resignation. Chronic illness.

New hope, faith and optimism. Recovery.

HEATHER - (CALLUNA VULGARIS)

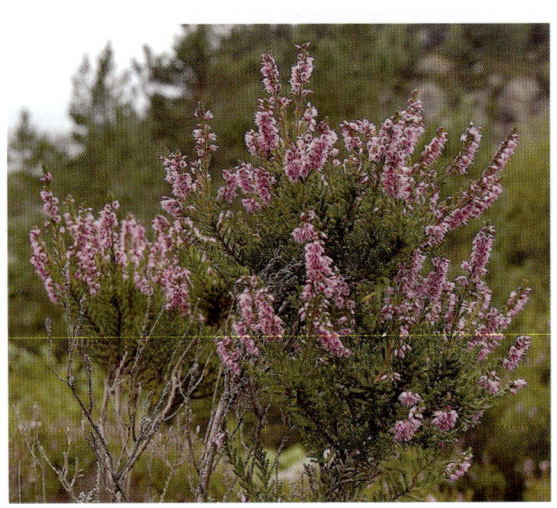

Self-centeredness, self-concern, incessant talkers. The Needy Child.

Emotional self-sufficiency and compassion for others.

INDICATIONS	BACH FLOWER	POSITIVE QUALITIES

HOLLY - (ILEX AQUIFOLIUM)

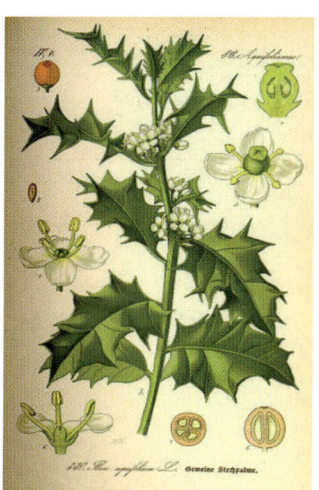

Hatred, jealousy, envy, suspicion, anger, and separativeness.

Love, the greatest healing elixir. Compassion and an open heart.

HONEYSUCKLE - (LONICERA CAPRIFOLIUM)

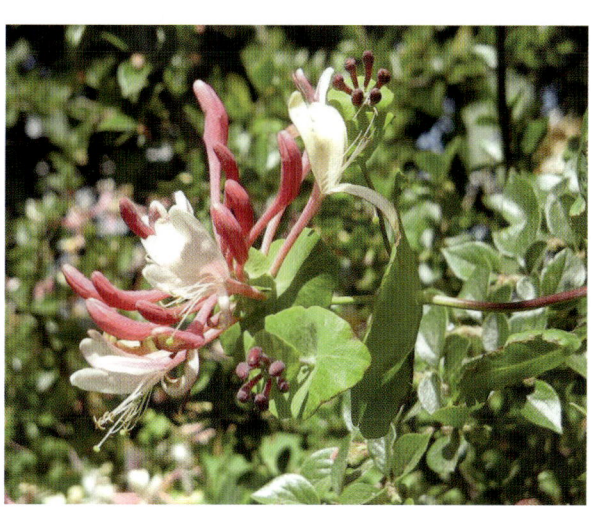

Living in the past, regrets from the past, nostalgia, and homesickness.

Letting go and moving on. Emotional freedom.

Bach Essence Flowers

INDICATIONS	BACH FLOWER	POSITIVE QUALITIES

HORNBEAM - (CARPINUS BETULUS)

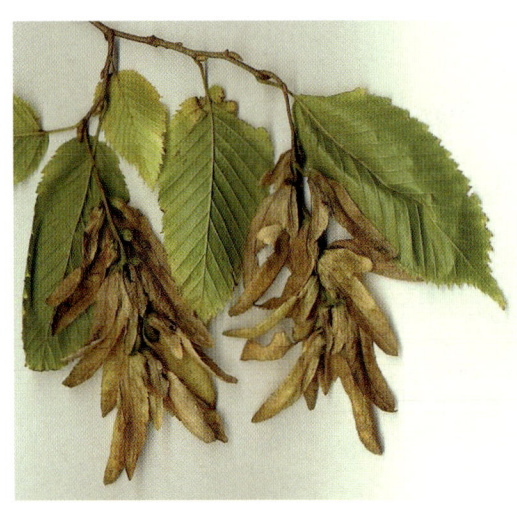

Mental and physical exhaustion. Tiredness. Boredom with daily routine.

Revitalization, enthusiasm, and energy.

IMPATIENS - (IMPATIENS GLANDULIFERA)

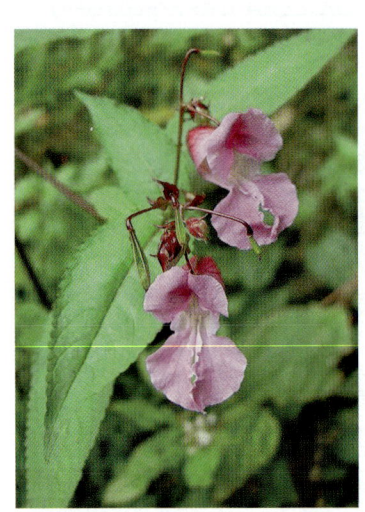

Impatience, irritability, frustration, and extreme mental tension.

Patience, acceptance, and gentleness.

| INDICATIONS | BACH FLOWER | POSITIVE QUALITIES |

LARCH - (LARIX DECIDUA)

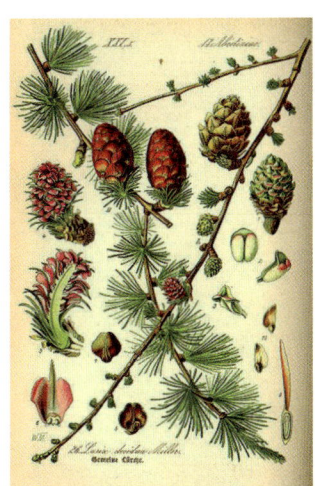

Lack of confidence. Anticipation of failure. Feelings of inferiority.

Self-confidence, spontaneity, and creative expression.

MIMULUS - (MIMULUS GUTTATUS)

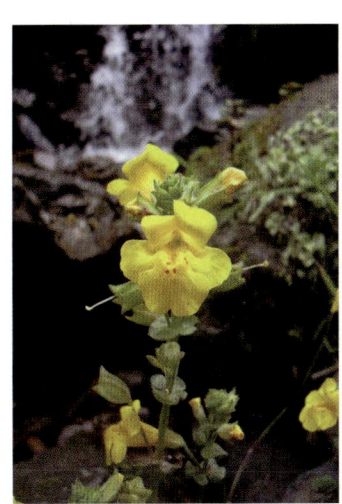

Fear and anxiety of known origin. Shyness and timidity. Introversion.

Courage and confidence.

| INDICATIONS | BACH FLOWER | POSITIVE QUALITIES |

Mustard - (Sinapis Arvensis)

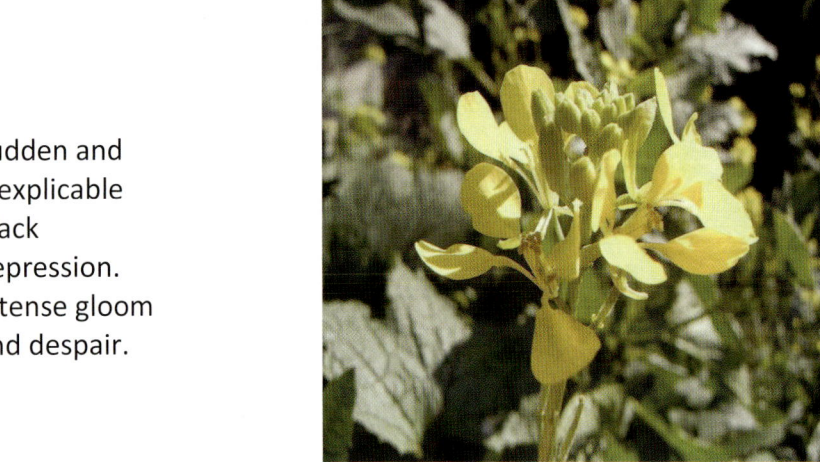

Sudden and inexplicable black depression. Intense gloom and despair.

Joy and inner serenity. Peace and equanimity.

Oak - (Quercus Robur)

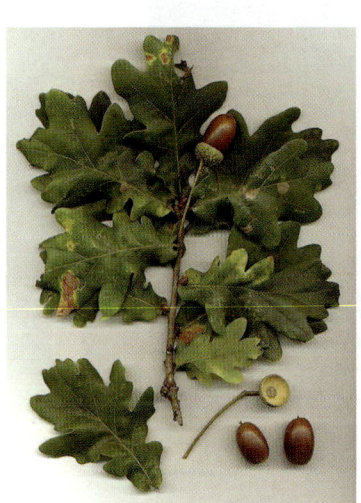

Depression due to overwork. Inflexible struggle against mental/physical odds.

Renewed strength and stability. Accepting limits. Knowing when to surrender.

| INDICATIONS | BACH FLOWER | POSITIVE QUALITIES |

OLIVE - (OLEA EUROPAEA)

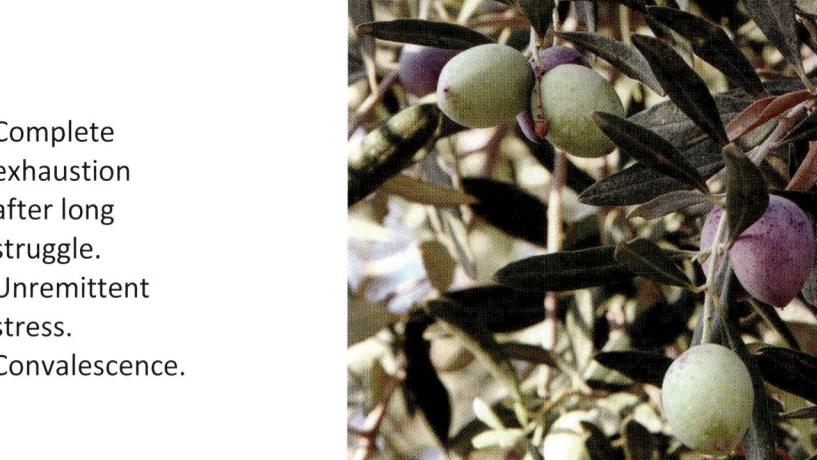

Complete exhaustion after long struggle. Unremitting stress. Convalescence.

Rejuvenation and regeneration. Energy and nourishment.

PINE - (PINUS SYLVESTRIS)

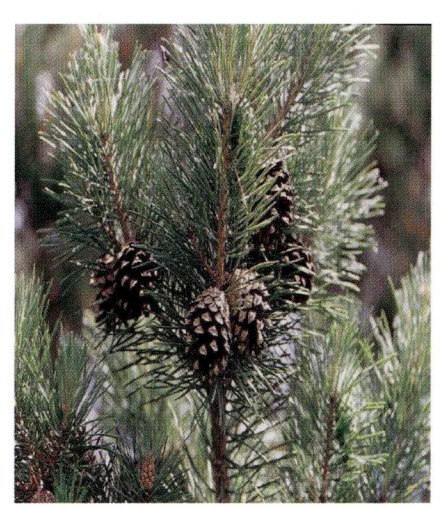

Guilt, self-blame, and self-criticism. Regret and remorse.

Self-forgiveness and self-acceptance.

| INDICATIONS | BACH FLOWER | POSITIVE QUALITIES |

RED CHESTNUT - (AESCULUS CARNEA)

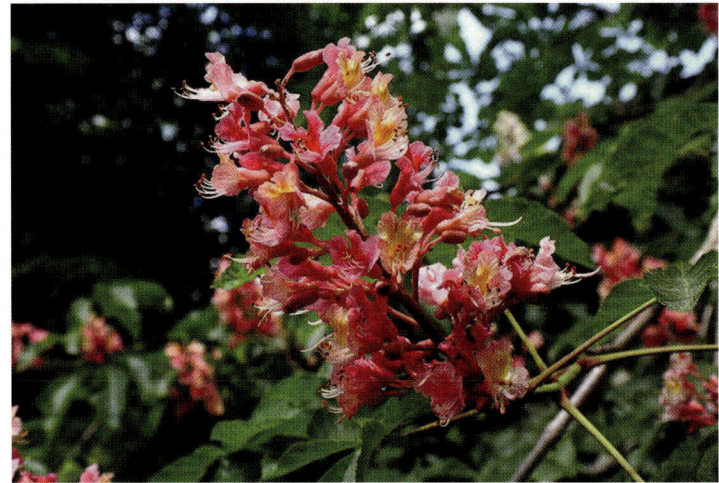

Excessive fear, worry, and anxiety for others, especially loved ones.

Objective caring and concern. Inner peace. Trust in the unfolding of life.

ROCK ROSE - (HELIANTHEMUM NUMMULARIUM)

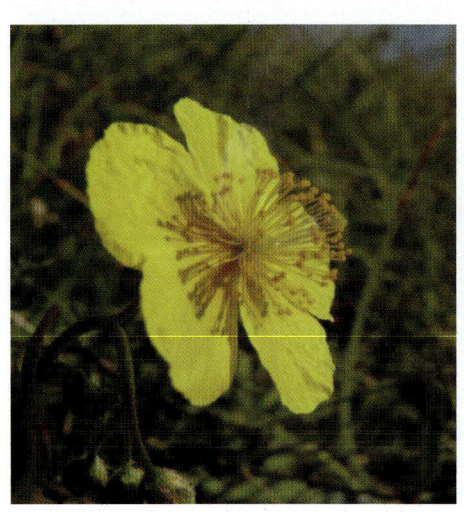

Shock, terror, panic, and extreme fright. Nightmares. Acute crisis.

Self-forgetting, self-transcendence, and courage. Steadfastness in the face of challenge.

Bach Essence Flowers

| INDICATIONS | BACH FLOWER | POSITIVE QUALITIES |

Rock Water - (Aqua Petra)

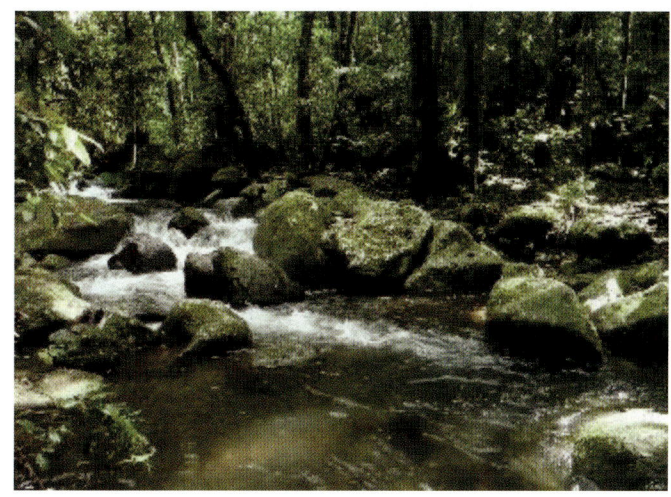

Self-martyrdom, self-repression, and self-denial. Rigidity.

Flexibility and inner freedom. Opening to feelings.

Scleranthus - (Scleranthus Annuus)

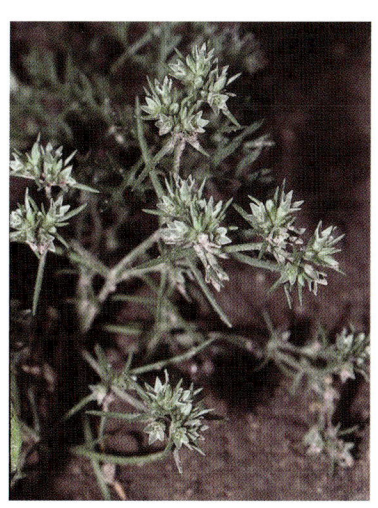

Uncertainty, indecision, and vacillation. Lack of balance.

Balance and poise. Decisiveness and inner resolve.

Bach Essence Flowers

| INDICATIONS | BACH FLOWER | POSITIVE QUALITIES |

Star of Bethlehem - *(Ornithogalum Umbellatum)*

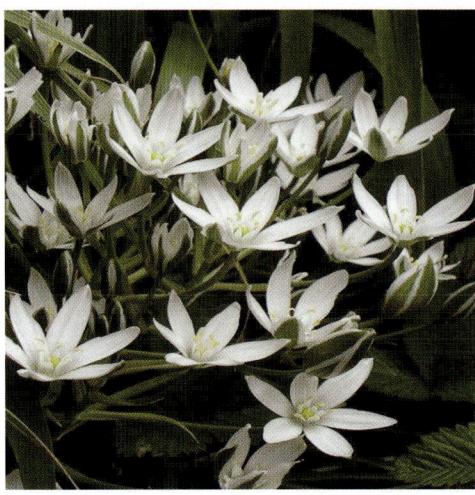

Mental/physical shock. Recent or past trauma.

Soothing and calming. Comforting and healing. Awakening and reorientation.

Sweet Chestnut - *(Castanea Sativa)*

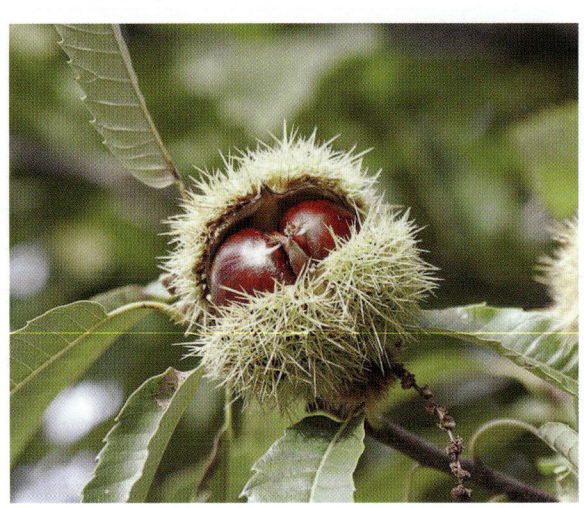

Extreme mental anguish and despair. "Dark Night of the Soul."

Courage and strength. Faith in self.

| INDICATIONS | BACH FLOWER | POSITIVE QUALITIES |

VERVAIN - (VERBENA OFFICINALIS)

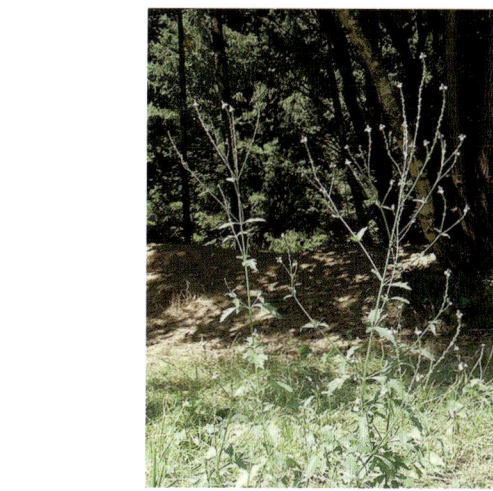

Strain, stress, tension, over-enthusiasm. Extremism and fanaticism.

Moderation and tolerance. Self-discipline and restraint.

VINE - (VITIS VINIFERA)

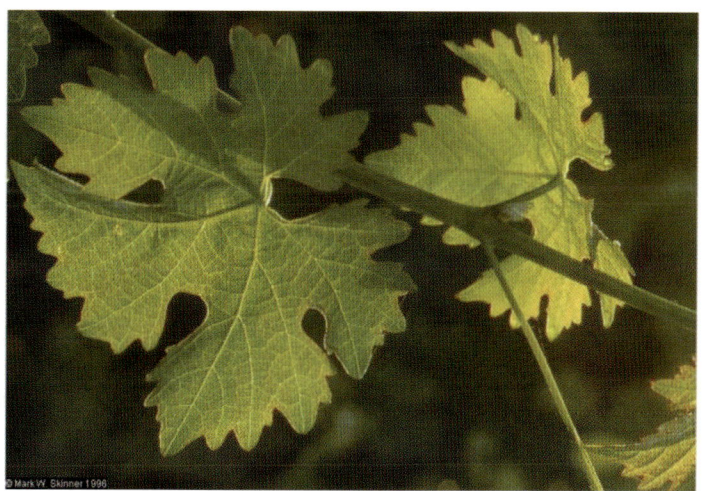

Dominating, ruthless, and inflexible. Ambitious and tyrannical. Aggressiveness.

Positive leadership qualities. Tolerance and selfless service. Humility.

INDICATIONS	BACH FLOWER	POSITIVE QUALITIES

WALNUT - (Juglans Regia)

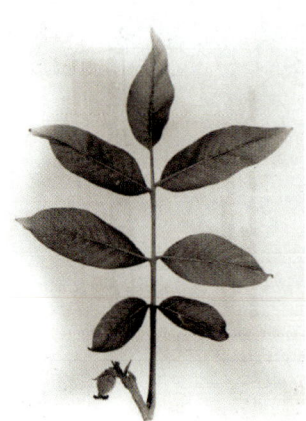

Life changes. Over-sensitivity to ideas and influences. "The Link-Breaker."		Protection. Freedom and courage to follow own path. Letting go of the past.

WATER VIOLET - (Hottonia Palustris)

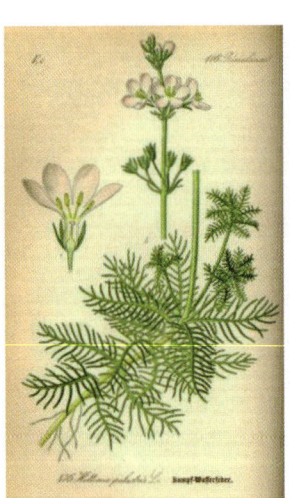

Proud, disdainful, aloof and tense. Physical stiffness.		Ability to share one's gifts with others. Gentleness and sympathy.

Bach Essence Flowers

| INDICATIONS | BACH FLOWER | POSITIVE QUALITIES |

WHITE CHESTNUT - (AESCULUS HIPPOCASTANUM)

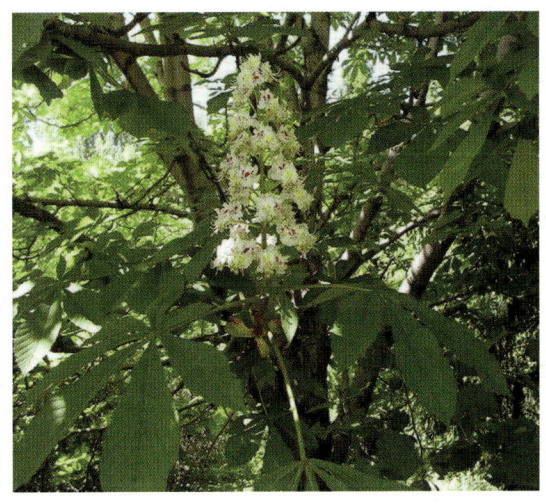

Worry and mental arguments. Persistent unwanted thoughts. Mind stuck in a rut.

Mental tranquillity and calmness. Clarity and inner peace.

WILD OAT - (BROMUS RAMOSUS)

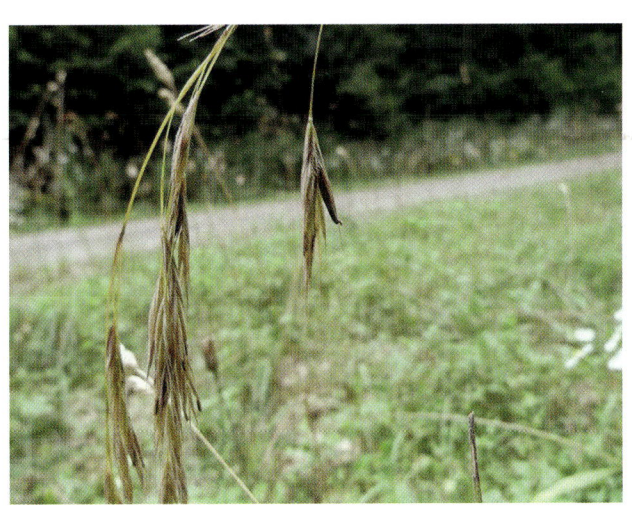

Uncertainty about life direction. Dissatisfied and unfulfilled.

Sense of vocation and purposefulness. Self-actualization. Work as expression of inner calling.

Bach Essence Flowers

| INDICATIONS | BACH FLOWER | POSITIVE QUALITIES |

WILD ROSE - (ROSA CANINA)

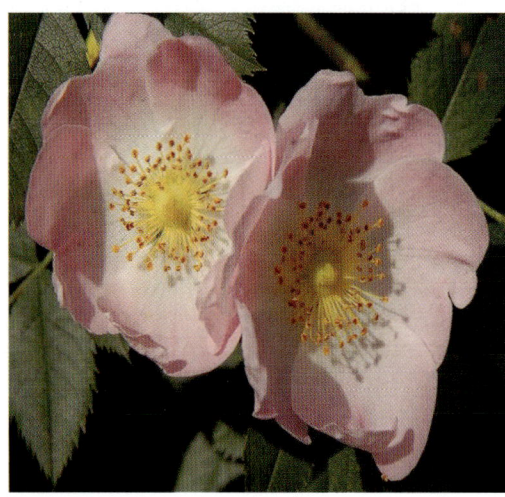

Apathy and resignation. Negative conditions. Giving up on life.

Vitality, interest, and joy in life. Inner motivation.

WILLOW - (SALIX VITELLINA)

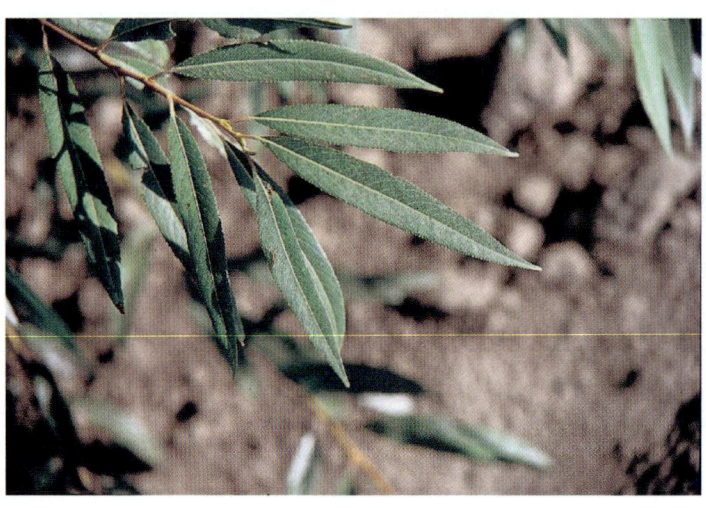

Resentment and bitterness. Blaming others. Negative and destructive thoughts.

Forgiveness. Acceptance of personal responsibility. Positive thoughts, optimism and faith.

INDICATIONS	BACH FLOWER	POSITIVE QUALITIES

RESCUE REMEDY

INDICATIONS	BACH FLOWER	POSITIVE QUALITIES
Combination remedy for emergencies, accidents, shock, trauma (short-term or deep-seated), panic and unconsciousnes. All conditions of extreme stress.	Cherry plum Clematis Impatiens Rock rose Star of Bethlehem	Calm and stability in any emergency or time of high stress.

RESCUE REMEDY SLEEP

INDICATIONS	BACH FLOWER	POSITIVE QUALITIES
Combination remedy for emergencies, accidents, shock, trauma (short-term or deep-seated), panic and unconsciousnes. All conditions of extreme stress.	Cherry plum Clematis Impatiens Rock rose Star of Bethlehem	Calm and stability in any emergency or time of high stress.

Bach Essence Flowers

Bee Pollen

Bee pollen is a fine, powder-like substance produced by flowering plants. It serves as the male element in the fertilization of plants and is often carried and collected by bees returning to their hives. This is when the pollen is harvested for commercial use. It contains carbohydrates, fats, proteins, and some vitamins and minerals. Beginning research from the Ukraine shows that pollen may help people with rheumatoid arthritis and can treat disorders of the liver, gallbladder, stomach, and intestines. Pollen extracts are sometimes used to help people desensitize plants to which they are allergic. In addition, melbrosia, a mixture of fermented bee pollen, flower pollen, and royal jelly, may treat menopausal symptoms in women, including headaches and urinary incontinence.

How much bee pollen should I take? The optimal dose of bee pollen is unknown. However, a generally recommended dose is 500 milligrams, taken two to three times per day.

What are some good sources of bee pollen? What forms are available? Most flowering plants that grow naturally produce pollen. While it is not clear which plants produce the best pollen, some of the most common pollens used commercially come from timothy crass, corn, rye, and pine. Bee pollen is usually harvested directly from beehives.

What can happen if I do not get enough bee pollen? What can happen if I take too much? Are there any side effects I should be aware of? Because bee pollen is not an essential nutrient, pollen shortages do not occur in humans. Many people have allergies to natural pollens that are inhaled; reactions to ingested pollen have also been reported, sometimes with serious outcomes. Aside from the allergic reactions, no other major side effects have been reported. As of this writing, there are no known drug interactions with bee pollen. As always, however, make sure to speak with a licensed health care provider before taking bee pollen or any other dietary supplement or herbal remedy.

Beta-Carotene

Beta-carotene is an antioxidant, a substance that minimizes the damage to the body caused by free radicals. It is present in plants (giving them their coloring) and is changed by the body into vitamin A. In addition to its naturally occurring form, some manufacturers also make synthetic beta-carotene that does not appear to have antioxidant properties. The synthetic form should be avoided until research can prove its effectiveness. Studies have shown that beta-carotene can protect the body from developing a variety of harmful conditions. It helps prevent symptoms of asthma in some people while performing exercise. It may help improve vision in some people with poor sight and help people who suffer from night blindness. It also boosts the immune system, helping fight off infections. Specifically, beta-carotene can guard against heart disease, prevent certain forms of cancer and many precancerous conditions.

How much beta-carotene should I take? The typical beta-carotene supplement contains approximately 25,000 international units, or 15 milligrams.

What forms of beta-carotene are available?

Broccoli
Cantaloupe
Carrots

Dark green and orange-yellow vegetables
The darker the color, the higher the level of beta-carotene present

What can happen if I take too much beta-carotene? Are there any interactions I should be aware of? What precautions should I take? Because the body excretes any beta-carotene that it does not use, it is virtually impossible to overdose on it. However, patients who take extremely high amounts of beta-carotene for extended periods of time may experience a yellowing or orange tint to the skin, particularly on the soles of the feet and the palms of the hands. The color will eventually fade with decreased beta-carotene intake; if this occurs, consult a health care provider. Research has shown that beta-carotene supplements may actually increase the risk of lung cancer in smokers. Whether natural or synthetic, beta-carotene should not be consumed by smokers; synthetic forms of the substance should be avoided altogether. Animal research suggests that beta-carotene combined with heavy alcohol use may cause liver damage; therefore, alcoholics or people who take alcohol on a daily basis should not take beta-carotene supplements. As always, make sure to speak with a licensed health care provider before taking beta-carotene or any other dietary supplement or herbal remedy.

BETA-GLUCAN

Beta-glucan is a fiber-like polysaccharide (a complex sugar) that comes from the walls of baker's yeast, oats, barley and some mushrooms, while different varieties of beta-glucan come from different food sources. Beta-glucan is used most often to strengthen the immune system and lower blood cholesterol levels. Research conducted as far back as the 1960s has shown that beta-glucan can stir up the activity of white blood cells, particularly macrophages and neutrophils, which provide a first line of defense against foreign bacteria. However, since most studies of beta-glucan have been performed on animals, its success in humans remains undecided. As for blood cholesterol, studies show that beta-glucan derived from oats or yeast is effective in reducing levels of LDL, or "bad" cholesterol, while increasing levels of HDL ("good") cholesterol.

How much beta-glucan should I take? The amount of beta-glucan being taken depends on the condition being treated. To lower cholesterol levels, trials have used doses ranging from 2,900 milligrams to 15,000 milligrams per day. Effective amounts have yet to be determined to increase one's immune system. However, many makers (and some practitioners) usually recommend between 50 milligrams and 1,000 milligrams daily, taken on an empty stomach.

What forms of beta-glucan are available? Beta-glucan can be derived from a variety of cereals and cereal fibers, including oats, wheat, and barley. Supplements of beta-glucan are also available, usually in liquid, capsule and tablet form.

What can happen if I take too much beta-glucan? Are there any interactions I should be aware of? What precautions should I take? Because beta-glucan is not considered an essential nutrient, deficiency and toxicity levels have not been decided. As of this writing, there are no well-known drug interactions with beta-glucan. As always, make sure to speak with a licensed health care provider before taking beta-glucan or any other dietary supplement or herbal remedy.

Betaine

Also known as trimethylglycine or TMG, betaine is a chemical compound similar to choline, vitamin B_9, and SAMe. Together, these compounds work as "methyl donors" that carry methyl molecules throughout the body and so they help in the completion of several vital chemical processes. As a nutritional supplement, betaine's main role is to support and improve how the liver works. Mostly, it does a good job of helping the liver process fats or lipids; animal studies have shown that betaine helps protect the liver from chemical damage and can improve or even reverse a condition called fatty liver disease caused by high intake of alcohol. Betaine has also been shown to be useful in controlling homocysteine levels in the blood and so it may help to reduce the rate at which atherosclerosis and osteoporosis occurs. There is sketchy evidence that betaine can help improve a condition called dry mouth.

How much betaine should I take? To help treat fatty liver disease caused by alcohol intake, many practitioners recommend between 1,000 and 2,000 milligrams of betaine supplements taken three times daily. Lower amounts are often taken as a general supplement and to improve the overall function of the liver.

What forms of betaine are available? Betaine can be obtained through the foods a person eats, including fish, beets, and beans. Betaine is also available as a dietary supplement, usually as betaine hydrochloride, in capsule or tablet form.

What can happen if I take too much betaine? Are there any interactions I should be aware of? What precautions should I take? As of this writing, there are no known side effects or drug interactions linked to betaine. As always, make sure to speak with a licensed health care provider before taking betaine or any other herbal remedy or dietary supplement.

Beta-Sitosterol

What is beta-sitosterol? Why do we need it? Beta-sitosterol is one of a group of organic compounds found in plants and animals called sterols. Not considered an essential nutrient, studies have shown that beta-sitosterol is effective in reducing the symptoms of benign prostatic hyperplasia, a precursor to prostate disease. Some athletes also take beta-sitosterol and other sterols to enhance athletic performance and reduce the risk of infection.

How much beta-sitosterol should I take? The amount of beta-sitosterol to be taken depends on the condition being treated. Most clinical trials of the supplement in treating blood cholesterol have used daily levels ranging from 500 milligrams to 10 grams. Some studies have shown that daily doses of 60 to 130 milligrams can reportedly reduce the symptoms of benign prostatic hyperplasia.

What forms of beta-sitosterol are available?

Rice bran
Wheat germ

Corn oils
Wheat germ Peanut

What can happen if I take too much beta-sitosterol? Are there any interactions I should be aware of? What precautions should I take? As of this writing, there are no known side effects from taking large amounts of beta-sitosterol; there also are not any well-known drug interactions. As always, make sure to speak with a licensed health care provider before taking beta-sitosterol or any other dietary supplement or herbal remedy.

BIOCHEMICAL CELL SALTS

Schüessler cell salts, also called tissue salts, were developed by Dr. Wilhelm Heinrich Schüessler, who was born in Zwischenahn, Germany, in 1821. Dr. Schüessler was born and raised at a time when the conflict of material science (study of physical science; of things made by man and of non-living systems, i.e., computers, chemistry, earth science) and natural science (study of living things, i.e., biology, medicine) was at its peak–materialism vs. vitalism.

Influences on Schuessler

Justus von Liebig - developed the understanding of the law of minimum, also called Liebig's law, which states that growth is controlled not by the total of resources available, but by the scarcest resource (limiting factor).

Rudolf Virchow - the founder of cellular pathology, who taught that all illnesses are based upon a change in function or condition of cells in the body.

Jacob Moleschott (1822 -1893) - taught physiological chemistry. His prime focus was the totality of all biochemical processes that run in the body or cell, with all their intermediate steps within the metabolism. Moleschott was a materialist in his approach.

As Schüessler was exposed to homeopathic teachings as well as material science and the biomedical workings of the organism, he was in the unique position to take all aspects into consideration.

In 1874, Schüessler's "Abridged Therapeutics, founded upon histology and cellular pathology," was printed and released. This text details his understanding of the role of the cell. Also, at the time, Dr. Schüessler undertook studies to see which mineral elements would remain after a person or animal had died. He burned cadavers and examined the contents, establishing that 12 minerals would remain, and depending on the state of health of the cadaver before its death, certain minerals would be lacking.

The remedies have been used by millions of people for over 120 years worldwide. They have proven to be helpful in balancing many conditions in the body. These remedies have the most important place in alternative practice worldwide. The strong point of using the cell salts is building up the constitutional health of a person over long period of time. They are used to rebuild the organs and tissues. The cell salts are equilibrium remedies. This means they are used to balance excess and deficiency. Furthermore, cell salts work well with herbs and with vitamin supplements.

The cell salts are great for people of any age. The two groups of people who benefit the most from using the cell salts are children between the ages of 0 – 3 years because this is a period when there is rapid growth. In children you can really build them up especially during growth. During growth periods you can use them for extended periods of time giving them daily for 1 to 2 years at a time. The elderly benefit because while the cell salts nourish and balance deficiency they are gentle.

Dosing: Remedies are generally taken as 4 tablets, 4 times a day but they can be used acutely much more frequently. For example: Mag Phos is one of the best remedies for hiccups and can be taken every 5 minutes as needed. You can be very flexible with the doses depending on the circumstances.

The cell salts are broken into 6 groups.

1) Calcium group

A) Calc Flor (calcium fluoride)   B) Calc Phos (calcium phosphors)   C) Calc Sulph (calcium sulphur)

2) Sodium group

A) Nat Mur (sodium chloride)   B) Nat Phos (sodium phosphate)   C) Nat Sulph (sodium sulphate)

3) Potassium group

A) Kali Mur (potassium chloride)   B) Kali Phos (sodium phosphate)   C) Kali Sulph (potassium sulphate)

4) Magnesium group

A) Mag Phos (magnesium phosphate

5) Iron Group

A) Ferrum Phos (iron phosphate)

6) Sand group

A) Silica

Of the original biochemical cell salts, sodium, potassium, and calcium are in 9 of the 12 remedies. Sulphur is in 3 remedies.

Dr. Schüessler's practitioners developed fifteen additional cell salts. They were discovered as part of the body after Dr. Schüessler's lifetime. These salts are called additional or supplement cell salts. Three of these supplement salts came even later than the salts from 13 to 24 and, hence, are not recognized by all practitioners. The additional cell salts can't be found everywhere. In some countries (i.e. USA) there are only a few vendors who offer them.

Now, there have been another 15 cell salts added which are as follows:

1) Arsenic iodide — (arsenic - iodine)
2) Aurum chloratum natronatum — (gold - sodium - chloride)
3) Calcium carbonate — (calcium - carbon - oxygen)
4) Calcium sulphide — (calcium - sulfur)
5) Copper arsenite — (copper - arsenic)
6) Lithium chloride — (lithium - chlorine)
7) Manganese sulphate — (manganese - sulfur)
8) Potassium aluminium sulfuricum — (potassium - aluminum - sulfur)
9) Potassium arsenite — (potassium - arsenic)

10) Potassium bromide   (potassium - bromine)
11) Potassium dichromate   (potassium - chromium)
12) Potassium iodide   (potassium - iodine)
13) Selenium   (selenomethionine)
14) Sodium bicarbonate   (sodium - hydrogen - carbon - oxygen)
15) Zinc chloride   (zinc - chloride)

The list of all cell salts that are related to various body tissues are as follows:

Cell Salt	Related Body Tissues
Arsenic iodide	Skin, allergies
Aurum chloratum natronatum	Day and night rhythm, female reproductive organs
Calcium carbonate	Vitality, anti aging
Calcium fluoride	Connective tissue, skin, joints
Calcium fluoride	Connective tissue, skin, joints
Calcium phosphate	Bones and teeth
Calcium phosphate	Bones and teeth
Calcium sulphate	Joints, pus
Calcium sulphide	Vitality, body weight
Copper arsenite	Digestive system, kidneys
Iron phosphate	Immune system
Lithium chloride	Rheumatism, nerves
Magnesium phosphate	Muscles
Manganese sulphate	Iron system
Potassium aluminium sulfuricum	Digestive system, nervous system
Potassium arsenite	Skin, vitality
Potassium bromide	Nervous system, skin
Potassium chloride	Mucous membranes
Potassium dichromate	Blood, sugar metabolism
Potassium iodide	Sign gland
Potassium phosphate	Nervous system
Potassium sulphate	Metabolism
Selenium	Liver, blood vessels, day and night rhythms
Silica	Connective tissue, skin, hair
Sodium bicarbonate	Purification, body acid balance
Sodium chloride	Water regulation
Sodium phosphate	Metabolism
Sodium sulphate	Purification
Zinc chloride	Metabolism, womb, nerves

One possibility to determine the right cell salt to use is to look for certain signs in the face. This approach is called "face analysis" or "facial diagnosis". The facial diagnosis is based on the idea that the absence of certain minerals develops certain signs on the face. The signs to take note of are the coloring of the face or the state and the vigor of the skin.

The face analysis was discovered by Dr. Schüessler and was developed by one of his followers: Kurt Hickethier. Kurt Hickethier led a sanitarium in Ellrich in the Harz (Germany). He wrote a book about the face analysis which is the standard work to the face analysis even today. Hickethier thought the facial diagnosis to be the best method to recognize an illness and the needed cell salts. This contradicted even then the prevailing doctrine and also does not fit into today's image of a diagnosis, because "diagnosis" is used in the modern usage to recognize a certain illness and to name. To avoid conflicts with the usual usage of the word "diagnosis," nowadays one often speaks of "face analysis." Nevertheless, the analysis of the face plays the most important role for the identification of the suitable mineral salts.

In the following list you can find the most important signs in the face to the respective mineral salts.

1) Calcium Fluoride

- Square folds around the eyes
- Diversified folds below the eyes
- Brown black coloring around the eyes
- Burst veins
- Scales in the face
- Cracked lips, corners of mouth, hands, fingers
- Periodontosis
- Shining skin

2) Calcium Phosphate

- Waxy skin
- Skin color like cheese
- White coating of the tongue
- Halitosis
- White noses and auricles
- Sweaty hair
- Rough voice

3) Calcium Sulphate

- Whiteness, alabaster-like skin coloring
- Only few signs in the face
- Brown spots/ liver spots

4) Iron Phosphate

- Reddened forehead, cheeks
- Red, hot ears/chin
- Red tongue
- Blue black shade in the nasal root and under the eyes
- Grey black coloring around the nose
- Pale gums

5) Magnesium Phosphate

- Red, round spots on the cheeks (always or temporarily)
- Red spots in the neck
- Otherwise pale skin
- Convulsions of the corners of mouth
- Twitch of the eyelids

6) Potassium Chloride

- Milky skin/blue white skin color
- Skin like cheese
- Swollen lymphatic knots
- White coating of the tongue
- Mealy skin dandruff
- Stuck together eyes

7) Potassium Phosphate

- Ash-grey skin, mainly in the chin area
- Grey ocular part
- Sunken temples
- Absent expression
- Brown coating of the tongue
- Dry tongue
- Periodontosis
- Gum bleeding
- Halitosis

8) Potassium Sulphate

- Brown-yellow skin
- Dark eyelids
- Yellowish around the mouth
- Freckles
- Dandruff on viscous base
- Sticking head dandruff
- Yellow and slimy coating of the tongue

9) Silica

- Shining skin, as varnished (polished shine)
- Waxy yellow or pale skin Color
- Deep-recumbent eyes
- Slip eyelids
- Laughter lines/crow's-feet
- Convulsions of the eyelids
- Small skin pores
- Vertical wrinkles in front of the ears
- Brittle hair
- Dry nose

10) Sodium Chloride

Humid shine on the upper eyelid, like snail mucus (gelatin shine)
Bright eyelids
Big skin pores

Bloated face/spongy cheeks
Head dandruff
White seclusions of the eyes
Clear coating of the tongue

Salivary vesicles on the edge of the tongue
Skin rash in the upper forehead
Itch/Dry Skin

11) Sodium Phosphate

Greasy, dull shine on the forehead
Greasy nose
Big skin pores

Blackheads/pimples
Pale mucous membranes
Hanging cheeks

Double chin
Tongue is yellowish in the back

12) Sodium Sulphate

Green-yellow complexion, especially forehead and temples
Bluish redness in the nose

Bluish redness in front of the ears
Redness in the external corner of the eye

Tongue looks dirty and greenish

Borage Oil

Borage oil comes from the seeds of the borage plant with large, blue, star-shaped flowers, grown naturally throughout Europe and North Africa, also farmed commercially in the United States. The seeds are removed from the plant, then pressed or processed to obtain their oil. Borage oil's main ingredient is gamma linolenic acid (GLA), a fatty acid that the body changes into prostaglandin E1 or PGE1. PGE1 reduces inflammation, helps to widen blood vessels, and may act as a blood thinner. In scientific studies, long-term use of borage oil has been shown to reduce symptoms of rheumatoid arthritis. Borage oil may also be effective in treating a variety of skin conditions such as atopic dermatitis–scaly skin, dryness, and skin rashes. Studies carried out on infants show that borage oil applied to the skin can reduce skin lesions and seborrheic dermatitis without producing any unpleasant side effects.

How much borage oil should I take? The amount of borage oil to be taken depends on the condition being treated. Internally, most studies have used doses ranging from between 360 milligrams to 2.8 grams daily. Larger amounts may be used if borage oil is being applied topically. Many people in Western societies may have a shortage of GLA due to a variety of factors including aging, glucose intolerance, and dietary fat intake. Certain medical conditions may also prevent the body from making GLA including premenstrual syndrome, diabetes and some skin conditions.

What forms of borage oil are available? Borage oil is mainly found in supplement form. Its main ingredient, gamma linolenic acid, is also available in black currant seed oil and evening primrose oil.

What can happen if I take too much borage oil? Are there any interactions I should be aware of? What precautions should I take? Borage seeds contain small amounts of substances called pyrrolizidine alkaloids, which may cause liver damage. However, scientific studies have not shown that pyrrolizidine alkaloids are present in borage oil. Some minor side effects may be linked with high borage oil intake such as nausea, indigestion, and headache. As of this writing, there are no well-known drug interactions linked with borage oil. As always, make sure to speak with a licensed health care provider before taking borage oil or any other herbal remedy or dietary supplement.

BOVINE CARTILAGE

Bovine cartilage comes from cows, and usually from the cartilage helping form a cow's trachea. Bovine cartilage is also present in cow ears, nose, knees, and other joints. The cartilage is cleaned, dried, and powdered before being used as a supplement. It should not be confused with shark cartilage, which may have different properties and elements. Bovine cartilage has been used medicinally since the 1950s, when early studies suggested that bovine tracheal cartilage could help promote wound healing. In vitro studies have shown that bovine cartilage may shrink the size of certain tumors and help improve the performance of the immune system. It is also believed to be helpful in the treatment of skin diseases like psoriasis and certain forms of arthritis. Very few studies have been conducted on bovine cartilage, and its effectiveness in the treatment of these conditions remains uncertain.

How much bovine cartilage should I take? When using bovine cartilage as a dietary supplement, some practitioners recommend that patients take between 3 and 4 capsules per day in the dosage of 750 milligrams per capsule. The dosage may be increased to treat other conditions, but patients should speak with a licensed health care provider before taking large amounts of bovine cartilage.

What forms of bovine cartilage are available? Bovine cartilage can be found at some health food stores and may be available by mail order as a nutritional supplement. It is usually available as a powder, capsule, tablet or extract and can be taken orally, or through intravenous or intramuscular injections.

What can happen if I take too much bovine cartilage? Are there any interactions I should be aware of? What precautions should I take? Large amounts of bovine cartilage may cause nausea and vomiting along with tiredness, dizziness, and indigestion. Parenteral administration of bovine cartilage can cause inflammation and irritation at the site of the injection. As of this writing, there are no known drug interactions with bovine cartilage. As always, make sure to speak with a licensed health care provider before taking bovine cartilage or any other dietary supplement or herbal remedy.

BOVINE COLOSTRUM

Bovine colostrum is a milky-like fluid produced by cows. It is produced during the first 24 to 48 hours after a cow gives birth and is meant to help young calves in the first few hours after being born. Colostrum contains a variety of antibodies, growth hormones, proteins, enzymes and is considered a potentially important nutritional supplement.

Because of colostrum's high antibody content, it is believed by some to help stimulate the immune system and may help prevent some types of infectious diseases. Research has shown that colostrum may significantly reduce the symptoms of diarrhea in children caused by the rotavirus. There is also evidence that colostrums may be effective in treating diarrhea caused by other bacteria, including H. pylori and clostridium difficile. Bovine colostrum may also be helpful in preventing peptic ulcers, although more research needs to be carried out to confirm these ideas.

How much bovine colostrum should I take? Because bovine colostrum is not an essential element, recommended daily allowances have not been decided yet. However, many product manufacturers recommend between 1,000 milligrams and 4,000 milligrams of bovine colostrum per day to improve immune function and treat infections.

What forms of bovine colostrum are available? Bovine colostrum is available in a variety of forms, including capsules, tablets, liquid extracts and infusions, powders, nutrition bars, and some skin care products. It can be found (in one form or another) at most health food stores and many supermarkets.

What can happen if I take too much bovine colostrum? Are there any interactions I should be aware of? What precautions should I take? As of this writing, there are no known side effects linked with taking large amounts of bovine colostrums. There are also no well-known drug interactions. As always, make sure to speak with a licensed health care provider before taking bovine colostrum or any other herbal remedy or dietary supplement.

BREWER'S YEAST

Brewer's yeast (often-called nutritional yeast) first resulted by what was produced from the brewing of beer. It differs from live baker's yeast in that its live yeast cells have been destroyed, leaving the nutrients behind. Although it is still used to brew certain beverages, brewer's yeast is now grown as a separate product and is prized for its nutritional value. Brewer's yeast is looked upon favorably because it contains high levels of many important nutrients, including most of the B vitamins, 16 amino acids, and 14 different minerals. Brewer's yeast also has a high protein content (one tablespoon provides 4.6 grams of protein), making it a valuable source of protein for vegetarians, has high quantities of phosphorous and chromium, which can lower blood glucose levels and low-density lipoprotein (LDL) levels.

How much brewer's yeast should I take? Brewer's yeast can be taken in juice or water; four tablespoons per day are recommended. Most health care providers suggest that people taking brewer's yeast start with a small amount (one teaspoon), then progress to four tablespoons.

What are some good sources of brewer's yeast? Brewer's yeast can be found at many supermarkets and health food stores. It is available in flake, powder, tablet, and liquid form.

What can happen if I do not get enough brewer's yeast? There are no known studies documenting the lack of brewer's yeast in a normal diet and its impact on the human body.

What can happen if I take too much? Are there any side effects I should be aware of? Large doses (more than four tablespoons per day) may cause gas in some subjects. If you have frequent yeast infections, you should avoid brewer's yeast. People with osteoporosis should avoid brewer's yeast because of its high phosphorous content. If you take a yeast supplement, you should also take extra calcium.

Bromelain

Bromelain is a digestive enzyme found in the stem and fruit of pineapples. It is composed of two proteolytic enzymes (bromelain A and B) and a handful of other substances, including perioxidase, acid phosphatase, protease inhibitors, and calcium. Bromelain has shown usefulness in treating a wide range of conditions, as an anti-inflammatory, it can reduce pain and swelling and speed up the healing process. As a natural protease inhibitor, it may prove useful in AIDS patients by slowing the production of HIV. It can relieve the symptoms of angina pectoris, stop blood clots from forming, improve digestion, and increase the effectiveness of antibiotics and some forms of chemotherapy.

How much bromelain should I take? As a digestive aid, most health professionals recommend 500 milligrams of bromelain taken with meals. Other dosages can be taken depending on the condition:

*Traumatic injuries: 500 milligrams four times a day on an empty stomach

*Cardiovascular disease: 500-750 milligrams three times a day on an empty stomach

*Joint inflammation: 500-2,000 milligrams a day, taken in two doses

As always, make sure to speak with your health care provider before taking bromelain supplements.

What are some good sources of bromelain? Pineapples and other tropical fruits

What can happen if I do not get enough bromelain? No definitive studies have been conducted regarding a lack of bromelain in one's diet.

What can happen if I take too much? Are there any side effects I should be aware of? People who are allergic to pineapples may suffer allergic reactions and asthma if they take bromelain supplements. Large amounts may cause nausea, vomiting, diarrhea, but no serious side effects have been reported in humans. Bromelain can increase your risk of bleeding if taken at the same time as anticoagulants and also enhance the effects of antibiotics such as tetracycline. If you have high blood pressure, you may experience an increased heart rate after taking bromelain.

Capsaicin

Capsaicin is a chemical compound derived from peppers, specifically cayenne peppers. It is extremely hot, somewhat irritating, and bitter. It can be absorbed through the skin and mucus membranes and is usually applied topically. Among its active ingredients are several capsaicinoids, volatile oils, proteins, and carotenoids. External applications of capsaicin in the form of creams and ointments are often used to relieve pain and improve circulation in patients with arthritis, and to treat skin conditions such as psoriasis and pruritis. Applying capsaicin to the nasal cavity may be effective in reducing cluster headaches and allergic rhinitis. Gloves should be used when capsaicin is applied.

How much capsaicin should I take? Capsaicin should not be administered orally. When applied to the skin, most practitioners use a capsaicin cream or ointment in a 0.025% or 0.075% percent solution.

What forms of capsaicin are available? Capsaicin is usually available in the form of a cream or ointment, which can be applied topically. Capsaicin injections are also available, but only a licensed health care provider should administer these.

What can happen if I take too much capsaicin? Are there any interactions I should be aware of? What precautions should I take? Capsaicin can be extremely irritating to the mucus membranes and the eyes; therefore, it should not be applied to the eyes or used on broken skin. Gloves should also be used when capsaicin is administered topically. Side effects from capsaicin may include skin redness and burning after application; in these cases, the use of capsaicin should be discontinued. Capsaicin may interfere with some types of drugs. It can increase the frequency of cough associated with ACE inhibitors, increase the sedating effects of some sedative medications, and interact with some types of antihypertensive medications. As always, make sure to speak with a licensed health care provider before taking capsaicin or any other dietary supplement or herbal remedy.

The following minerals are found in cayenne:

Aluminum	Lithium	Selenium
Boron	Magnesium	Silica
Calcium	Manganese	Sodium
Chromium	Nickel	Titanium
Cobalt	Nitrogen	Zinc
Iron	Potassium	

CHITOSAN

Chitosan is a fiber-like substance at comes from chitin, a polysaccharide found in the exoskeletons of crabs, shrimp and other shellfish. It possesses a positive ionic charge, which gives it the ability to chemically bond with negatively charged fats, lipids and bile.

Unlike dietary fiber, chitosan cannot be digested. However, it appears to have quite a few gastrointestinal benefits. Repeated animal studies (and some beginning human studies) have shown that chitosan supplements can lower LDL ("bad") cholesterol while raising HDL ("good") cholesterol. Other studies suggest that large amounts of chitosan taken with vitamin C may reduce dietary fat absorption.

How much chitosan should I take? At this time, suggested levels have not yet been determined for chitosan. However, most human research has used between 3-6 grams of chitosan per day with meals.

What are some good sources of chitosan? What forms are available? Chitosan is found in the shells and exoskeletons of crustaceans such as shrimp and crab. It is available as a tablet, capsule, or powder.

What can happen if I do not get enough chitosan? What can happen if I take too much? Are there any side effects I should be aware of? Because chitosan is not classified as an essential nutrient, deficiency and toxicity levels have not been decided. In addition, because chitosan absorbs dietary fat, it may also impair the absorption of fat-soluble vitamins, such as vitamins A, D, E, and K. People who are allergic to shellfish, or who have problems absorbing certain vitamins and minerals, should not use chitosan. It should also not be used by children or pregnant women. At present, there is no evidence of any adverse drug reactions with chitosan.

CHLOROPHYLL

Chlorophyll is the substance responsible for giving green plants their color. It uses the sun's energy during photosynthesis and is responsible for a variety of metabolic functions, including perspiration and growth.

Interestingly, the chlorophyll molecule is chemically similar to human blood, except that its central atom is magnesium, while in human blood, the central molecule is iron. It acts as an anti-inflammatory and antioxidant.

Historically, chlorophyll was used to treat gastrointestinal problems and to help the formation of red blood cells and hemoglobin. It has also been used to fight bad breath and reduce the strength of odors related to urine, feces, and infected wounds. There is some beginning evidence that chlorophyll may detoxify substances that could cause cancer.

How much chlorophyll should I take? Because chlorophyll is not considered an essential nutrient, there are no guidelines regarding recommended daily allowance. However, some practitioners recommend 100milligrams of a chlorophyll capsule or tablet taken 2-3 times a day to fight odors.

What are some good sources of chlorophyll? What forms of chlorophyll are available? Chlorophyll is available in a wide variety of forms, from fresh cut herb to tablets, extracts (both fluid and dry), tinctures, and infusions. Most chlorophyll is sold in a water-soluable form. Fat-soluble chlorophyll is more expensive to make, but is a superior source to use and will provide better results.

What can happen if I do not get enough chlorophyll? What can happen if I take too much chlorophyll? Are there any side effects I should be aware of? Since chlorophyll is not an essential nutrient, dietary allowances have yet to be established. However, it is known that individuals who do not get enough green foods in their diet may lack a necessary amount of chlorophyll. As of this writing, there are no known side effects or drug interactions with chlorophyll.

CHONDROITIN

Chondroitin is one of the major building blocks of cartilage. It consists of a series of repeating chains of molecules called glycosaminoglycans, and helps create cartilage's structure. It also holds water and nutrients, and allows other molecules to move through cartilage. It is often taken at the same time as a similar supplement, glucosamine.

Chondroitin sulfate has been proven an effective treatment for osteoarthritis. In osteoarthritis, a person's cartilage wears down, resulting in a loss of chondroitin sulfate. Supplementation with chondroitin has been shown to slow the progression of—and in some cases, reverse—osteoarthritis, while also strengthening and healing bones.

In addition to cartilage, chondroitin is also present in the lining of blood vessels and the urinary bladder. Chondroitin helps to prevent unusual movement of blood or urine between barriers, and to prevent excess blood clotting. Beginning research also suggests that chondroitin sulfate may lower blood cholesterol levels and can prevent atherosclerosis in both humans and animals.

How much chondroitin should I take? The amount of chondroitin to be taken depends on the condition being treated. For atherosclerosis, some researchers have used very high amounts (up to 5 grams, taken twice per day with meals), then reducing the amount over time to 500 milligrams three times per day. For osteoarthritis, many practitioners recommend 400 milligrams of chondroitin sulfate taken three times per day. Oral chondroitin sulfate is absorbed better when it is dissolved in water prior to consumption.

What forms of chondroitin are available? Chondroitin is produced naturally in the body. The most widely used form of chondroitin supplement is chondroitin sulfate. It is available as a tablet, capsule, or powder, and should be dissolved in water before use.

What can happen if I take too much chondroitin? Are there any interactions I should be aware of? What precautions should I take? Some studies have reported that large doses (more than 10 grams per day) may cause some people to feel queasy. No other unpleasant effects have been reported. Unreliable research suggests that men with prostate cancer should not take chondroitin supplements, but this suggestion has not been proven definitively.

As of this writing, there are no known drug interactions with chondroitin. As always, make sure to speak with a licensed health care provider before taking chondroitin or any other dietary supplement or herbal remedy.

CLA – (CONJUGATED LINOLEIC ACID)

CLA stands for conjugated linoleic acid. It is a slightly different version of an essential fatty acid (linoleic acid) and is found in dairy products. In humans, it is produced from linoleic acid by bacteria that live in the intestinal tract.

At present, scientists are unsure exactly what type of protective effects CLA has. Animal studies have shown that CLA supplements can reduce the risks of certain types of cancers, including cancer of the breast, prostate, lung and stomach; these studies have yet to be carried out in humans, however. Other research suggests that CLA can reduce body fat in people who exercise regularly, but not body weight.

How much CLA should I take? At present, the appropriate amount of CLA to be taken on a daily basis has not been decided. Most animal studies have used large amounts, equal to several grams per day for humans; the body fat study mentioned earlier used a dose of 4.2 grams of CLA per day for four weeks.

What forms of CLA are available? CLA is produced in the body by intestinal bacteria, which convert linoleic acid to CLA when needed. CLA can also be found in many dairy products (especially grass-fed dairy), such as eggs, milk, and cheese, along with beef, chicken, and corn oil (non GMO).

What can happen if I take too much CLA? Are there any interactions I should be aware of? What precautions should I take? Because CLA is not an essential nutrient, average daily dosage levels and maximum recommended intake levels have not been decided. Also, as if this writing, the side effects of CLA in humans have not been determined in any published studies. There are also no known interactions with drugs. However, an unpublished study from 1997 noted an increased incidence of gastrointestinal problems in people taking large amounts of CLA. As always, make sure to speak with a licensed health care provider before taking CLA or any other dietary supplement or herbal remedy.

Coenzyme Q_{10} – (CoQ_{10})

Coenzyme Q_{10} is a substance found in the mitochondria of every cell in the body. It plays a role in the process that creates ATP, making it important for energy production. Although CoQ_{10} is classified as an antioxidant, there has been some discussion as to whether it should be reclassified as a vitamin.

There is growing research that suggests CoQ_{10} can play a very important role in the treatment of several conditions, particularly those related to the cardiovascular system. CoQ_{10} can reverse or prevent heart lesions linked with angina, hypertension, and congestive heart failure. Supplementation with CoQ_{10} can reduce high blood pressure in patients with a coenzyme deficiency. It may be beneficial in controlling abnormal heart rhythms and may protect the heart during surgery or a heart attack.

Additional studies have shown that CoQ_{10} supplementation may have a positive effect in the treatment of breast cancer, diabetes, immune deficiency, muscular dystrophy, and periodontal disease. When used along with an exercise routine, CoQ_{10} can improve heart rate and maximal oxygen consumption.

How much coenzyme Q_{10} should I take?

The generally recommended dose for coenzyme Q_{10} is 25 milligrams twice daily. Some researchers have experimented with larger doses for the following conditions:

*Heart disease: 100milligrams a day

*Enhancing athletic performance: 60 milligrams a day for four to eight weeks

*Potential prevention of cancers: 400 milligrams per day

What are some good sources of coenzyme Q_{10}? What forms are available? Coenzyme Q_{10} is found in every plant and animal cell. The best dietary sources include oily fish, organ meats (such as liver) and whole grains. Besides food sources, coenzyme Q_{10} supplements are available in several forms, including gel capsules, hard capsules, tablets, and sprays. Because Q_{10} is oil-soluble, it should be taken with a meal that contains oil.

What can happen if I do not get enough coenzyme Q_{10}? What can happen if I take too much? Are there any side effects I should be aware of? Most people get enough Q_{10} in their diet. However, levels of Q_{10} can decline in elderly people or patients with certain health conditions, so supplementation may be necessary for these subjects. A lack of Q_{10} can, in time, lead to heart failure.

Much documented evidence shows the most widely used drugs, statins, prescribed by allopathic physicians to lower cholesterol levels also depletes CoQ_{10} levels. Reccomended use of CoQ_{10} while using statin drugs is highly recommended. In addition, no definitive studies have been carried out on Q_{10} supplementation during pregnancy or while breast-feeding. Women who are pregnant or lactating should speak with a health care provider before taking Q_{10} supplements.

DHA – *(Docosahexaenoic Acid)*

DHA is short for docosahexaenoic acid. It is a type of fatty acid that belongs to a class of substances called essential fatty acids. It is produced naturally by the body and is present in a wide range of foods.

DHA has been shown to reduce levels of triglycerides in the bloodstream. Studies have shown that DHA can be just as effective as fish oils in lowering triglyceride levels in people at risk for heart disease. It also plays an important role in the prevention of a group of nervous disorders such as Zellwegger's syndrome, which damage the myelin sheaths surrounding nerve cells and is possibly fatal to infants. Double-blind studies have also shown that DHA may improve brain functioning in babies and may help to manage some autoimmune disorders, such as lupus and rheumatoid arthritis. There is also evidence that children with attention deficit disorder and other childhood diseases may have low DHA levels and may benefit from DHA supplementation.

How much DHA should I take? Because DHA is a naturally occurring substance, most healthy people do not take DHA supplements. However, most studies of DHA supplements have used doses ranging from 1 to 3 grams per day–usually coming from fish oil.

What forms of DHA are available? DHA is found mainly in cold-water fish such as mackerel, salmon, sardines, herring, anchovies, and albacore tuna. Cod liver oil contains large amounts of DHA and a similar fatty acid, EPA. Vegetarians can obtain DHA from certain microalgae. DHA is also available as a supplement, usually in capsule or extract form.

What can happen if I take too much DHA? Are there any interactions I should be aware of? What precautions should I take? Premature infants who are not breast-fed usually suffer a shortage of DHA and so DHA supplementation is recommended in these people. Patients with a history of heart disease should talk with their health care provider after taking fish oil supplements for several months, as this may lead to increased blood sugar levels. In addition, while DHA appears to treat some autoimmune disorders, it does so by decreasing the activity of certain immune cells. As a result, patients with autoimmune disorders who are taking large doses of DHA may be at increased risk of infections.

As of this writing, there are no well-known drug interactions with DHA. As always, make sure to speak with a licensed health care provider before taking DHA or any other herbal remedy or dietary supplement.

DHEA – (DEHYDROEPIANDROSTERONE)

DHEA is short for dehydroepiandrosterone, a hormone that is secreted by the adrenal glands and converted into other hormones as needed. It is the most abundant androgen in the body; on average, the adrenals produce between 15 and 30 milligrams of DHEA per day.

Only a small percentage of the body's supply of DHEA is in the active form; the rest moves around in the bloodstream as DHEA sulfate (DHEA-S) and is set aside. Later it can be converted to the active form of DHEA when needed.

DHEA has been linked with positive effects in a number of conditions, ranging from heart disease and obesity to osteoporosis. Other studies have shown that DHEA can improve some of the symptoms of systemic lupus erythematosus, an autoimmune disease, and may play some role in protecting against depression. DHEA is also thought to help build muscle mass and reduce fat. It may also speed up recovery time following injury, which has made it more and more popular with athletes.

How much DHEA should I take? Dosages of DHEA for men and women differ: men seem to be able to handle higher doses. Men have been shown to be able to take doses up to 50 milligrams per day, while in women, the maximum recommended dose is 25 milligrams per day. However, because the long-term effects of DHEA have not been studied thoroughly, its safety and effectiveness has yet to be decided.

What forms of DHEA are available? DHEA is available in either natural or synthetic forms, and is available in capsules, drops, or a type of chewing gum. Most DHEA comes from sterols taken from wild yams and is often marketed as "natural" DHEA. However, it is recommended that only pharmaceutical-grade supplements be used.

What can happen if I take too much DHEA? Are there any interactions I should be aware of? What precautions should I take? DHEA is a precursor of hormones such as estrogen and testosterone, so patients with hormone-sensitive cancers (such as those of the breast, prostate, ovaries, and testes) should avoid DHEA supplements. In addition, it should not be taken by people under 40 unless a person's DHEA levels are low. Because DHEA has a steroid-like effect on the human body, the International Olympic Committee, the National Football League, and other athletic organizations have banned its use.

As of this writing, there are no known drug interactions with DHEA, but it may interact negatively with alcohol. As always, make sure to speak with a licensed health care provider before taking DHEA or any other dietary supplement or herbal remedy.

DMAE – (Dimethylaminoethanol)

DMAE stands for dimethylaminoethanol, a chemical produced naturally in the body, but which is also available from some dietary sources. It plays an important part in many of the brain's chemical processes and may serve as a precursor to the brain chemical acetylcholine. DMAE is believed to play a wide role in many conditions that affect the brain.

Initially, DMAE was marketed as a treatment for attention deficit disorder. Currently, the two main uses of DMAE as a supplement are for the treatment of Alzheimer's disease and tardive dyskinesia, a movement disorder that results from long-term use of antipsychotic medications. Clinical research has yet to show positive proof that DMAE is useful in treating either of these conditions, however.

How much DMAE should I take? Previous studies have used DMAE ranging in doses up to 1,600 milligrams per day. However, because of possible adverse side affects (see below), DMAE supplementation is not recommended as of this writing.

What forms of DMAE are available? In addition to being produced naturally in the body, DMAE is available in supplement form (including tablet, liquid, and capsule), but it is not widely available.

What can happen if I take too much DMAE? Are there any interactions I should be aware of? What precautions should I take? Although DMAE is considered somewhat non-toxic, studies have shown that patients with Alzheimer's disease may experience drowsiness and confusion following DMAE supplementation. In addition, episodes of mania and depression have also been reported as possible side effects, and a study published in the early 1980s suggested that DMAE might actually cause, not prevent, symptoms of tardive dyskinesia. Patients diagnosed with epilepsy or bipolar disorder, or those suffering from kidney or liver disease should not take DMAE.

As of this writing, there are no well-known drug interactions associated with DMAE. As always, make sure to speak with a licensed health care provider before taking DMAE or any other herbal remedy or dietary supplement.

EGCG – (Epigallocatechin Gallate)

EGCG stands for epigallocatechin gallate. It's a chemical substance found in green tea and is thought to be responsible for most of the healthy benefits connected with green tea. In particular, EGCG is a polyphenol, which helps with the production of certain proteins and alkaloids.

EGCG and the other polyphenols in green tea have been shown to have a wide range of positive health benefits. These substances can lower total cholesterol levels, increase antioxidant activity in the blood, and may reduce the number of cavities and rate at which gum disease develops. Several studies have shown that ECGC and other ingredients can fight several forms of cancer. In addition, EGCG and green tea polyphenols may reduce the risk of high blood pressure and alter the makeup of intestinal bacteria, and promote a healthy immune system.

How much EGCG should I take? Most of the research into EGCG and polyphenols has revolved around the consumption of green tea. In many of these studies, a minimum of three cups per day has shown to create some of the health benefits linked to green tea. However, some researchers believe that patients may need to consumer much larger amounts–up to 10 cups per day–to receive the full benefits of EGCG and other ingredients.

What forms of EGCG are available? EGCG and polyphenols can be found in almost any type of green tea. In addition, tablets and capsules containing extracts of EGCG and other polyphenols are available. Some capsules provide concentrations equivalent to drinking four cups of tea; many of these products are decaffeinated.

What can happen if I take too much EGCG? Are there any interactions I should be aware of? What precautions should I take? While there are no particular side effects linked with EGCG, drinking excess amounts of green tea can result in insomnia and anxiety; these conditions are usually caused by the tea's caffeine content. Another study found that green tea extracts could inhibit the absorption of iron in women; therefore, theoretically, large amounts of green tea could lead to iron deficiency in some people.

Certain medications may react negatively to consumption of green tea and/or green tea extracts, including (but not limited to) atropine, cardec, codeine, ephedrine, pseudoephedrine, lomotil, theophylline, and warfarin. Patients taking these medications should talk with a licensed health care provider before consuming green tea or green tea extracts. As always, make sure to speak with a licensed health care provider before taking EGCG or any other dietary supplement or herbal remedy.

ESSENTIAL OILS

What are essential oils?

Essential oils are the subtle, volatile liquids that are distilled from plants. Shrubs, flowers, trees, roots, seeds and petals (roses for example) are used in the distilling process. They are the regenerating, oxygenating, and immune defense properties inherent in all chlorophyll rich plants. They contain the highest known oxygenating molecules transporting the nutrients to the cells of the body. Without oxygen molecules, nutrients cannot be effectively assimilated and utilized by the cells. Not only do therapeutic quality essential oils deliver oxygen and nutrients to the cells, they also aid in the tissue's disposal of toxic waste products.

There is a great deal of evidence pointing to the extra strain infertility can place on individuals and subsequently on the marital relationship itself. Aromatherapy can help alleviate these stresses.

In aromatherapy, the aromas of some essential oils are used in order to stimulate relaxation in the muscles and to relieve tension.

Essential oils are highly concentrated plant substances, distilled from roots, seeds, barks and leaves.

Because essential oils are so concentrated, they should not be applied directly to the skin. Instead, try the following methods:

1. Massage: dilute the essential oil in a base such as grapeseed oil, wheatgerm or almond oil

2. Oil Burner: add 3 to 4 drops of essential oils to a container holding water that is heated by a small candle, allowing the aromas to gently fill the air to smell

3. Baths: add 5 to 10 drops of essential oil to a warm bath

ANISEED - (PIMPINELLA ANISUM)

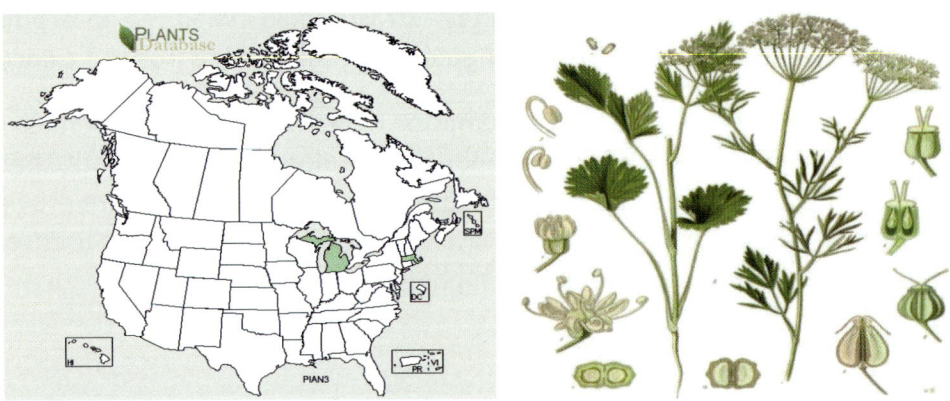

Aniseed is considered to have antiseptic, anti-spasmodic, carminative, diuretic, expectorant, galactagogue, stimulant and stomachic properties. Additionally, it is reputed to control the lice and itch mite.

The oil is very potent and not to be used on sensitive skin. Avoid use during pregnancy.

ANISE STAR - (ILLICIUM VERUM)

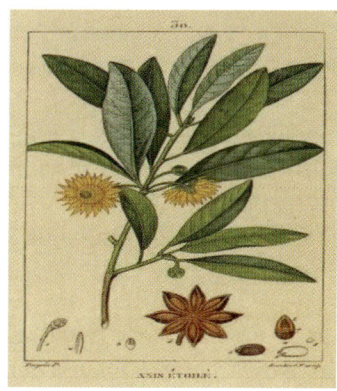

Anise star oil has carminative, stomachic, stimulant and diuretic properties. In the East it is used to combat colic and rheumatism.

Anise star is generally non-toxic and non-irritating.

BACOPA – (BACOPA MONNIERI)

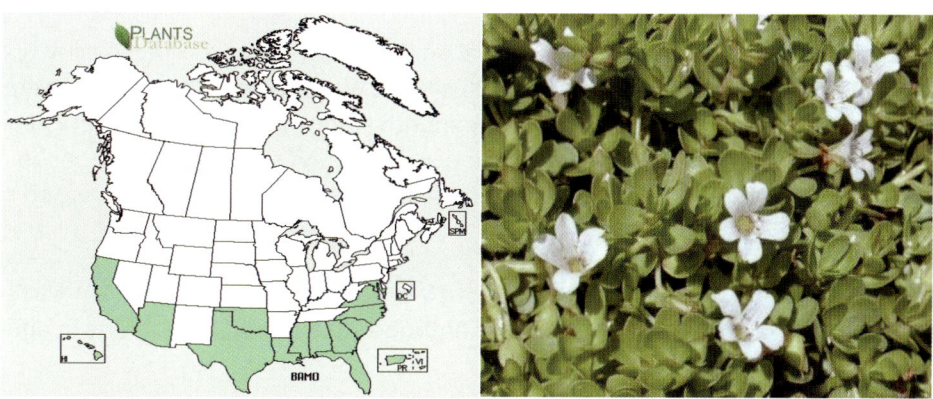

Bacopa was prominently mentioned in Indian texts as early as the 6th Century. Bacopa leaf extract is called brahmi in Ayurvedic medicine and is widely used in India, especially for:

Analgesia (pain relief)	Enhancing memory	Improve mental performance
Asthma	Epilepsy	Mental disorders
Cardiotonic (heart tonic)	Epilepsy	Nerve tonic
Diuretic (increases urine flow)	Hoarseness	

The Effects of Bacopa Monnieri Approved By Clinical Research Trials:

1) Bacopa effects on brain functions: In a double blind randomized placebo-controlled research study in Australia, at the University of Wollongong, bacopa was found to be effective in tests for retention of new information. In another similar study mentioned in Neuropsychopharmacology, its effects were documented for several weeks and various memory functions were tested with levels of anxiety. The study revealed the same bacopa decreases the rate of forgetting of newly acquired information, verbal learning rate and memory consolidation. In yet another study, the chronic administration (3 to 12 weeks) bacopa showed significant improvement in speed of visual information processing by IT task, learning rate and memory consolidation as compared to placebo.

2) Bacopa in mild to moderate mental deficiency: Bacopa was tested on men with mild to moderate mental deficiency. 172 persons received 500 milligrams of bacopa extract three times a day while 114 persons received a placebo for one year. At the end of study, there was improvement in concentration ability, memory span, and overall mental performance in individuals taking the extract as compared with the placebo group. There was improvement in the performance of school children with poor educational performance.

3) Alzheimer's disease and bacopa: Loss of cholinergic activity in hippocampus was the primary cause of Alzheimer's disease. Bacopa showed important antioxidant activity in many brain parts like hippocampus, striatum and the frontal cortex. Further studies showed its protective effect against DNA damage in astrocytes and fibroblast cells. All this suggests its important role in Alzheimer's and at the least it could be useful in checking the progression of this disease to some extent.

4) Bacopa in epilepsy: Despite its mention as an anti-epilepsy role it was found to exert this effect only on very high doses over long periods. The dose near LD50 showed effect against seizures. Research in India found bacopa to exert some anticonvulsant effect.

5) Bacopa improving learning skills: In the above mentioned research trial, the animals were trained in a T maze. One group wasn't given any medicine, a second group was given Diazepam and the third, fourth and fifth group received bacopa. After 10 days there was comparable memory and learning enhancement in the group treated with bacopa. Biochemical studies found the serotonin content of bacopa groups to be more compared to a control group and the other group.

6) Bacopa in stress: In this study on rats, bacopa showed the potential to be effective in stress. The response had been better in the group that was pretreated for one week with 20 to 40 milligrams per kilogram/daily of it even before being exposed to stress.

7) Bacopa for anxiety: Research on rats as models of clinical anxiety showed the anxiolytic activity of its extracts with 25 percent bacosides as comparable to Lorazepam. Plus there were no side effects of Lorazepam, like amnesia. Rather there was a memory enhancing effect. Another one month study on diagnosed anxiety neurosis patients, with syrup of bacopa herb equivalent to 12 grams of crude powder, found significant reduction in anxiety symptoms, level of disability and fatigue. There was an additional increase in immediate memory, decreased respiratory rate and decreased systolic blood pressure.

8) Bacopa for depression: The bacopa extract in the dose of 20 to 40 milligrams per kilogram was given once daily for five days and it was found comparable to the standard anti-depressant drug Imipramine in anti-depressant activity in rodent animals.

9) Bacopa and ADD hyperactive children: Another double blind study at BRD Medical College, at Gorakhpur, India, on children with ADHD (Attention Deficit Hyperactive Disorder) showed benefits after 12 weeks of bacopa use in sentence repetition, logical memory and paired associated learning tasks. The children were given the test four weeks after the bacopa had been withdrawn and it affirms its lasting effect.

Basil Sweet - *(Ocimum Basilicum)*

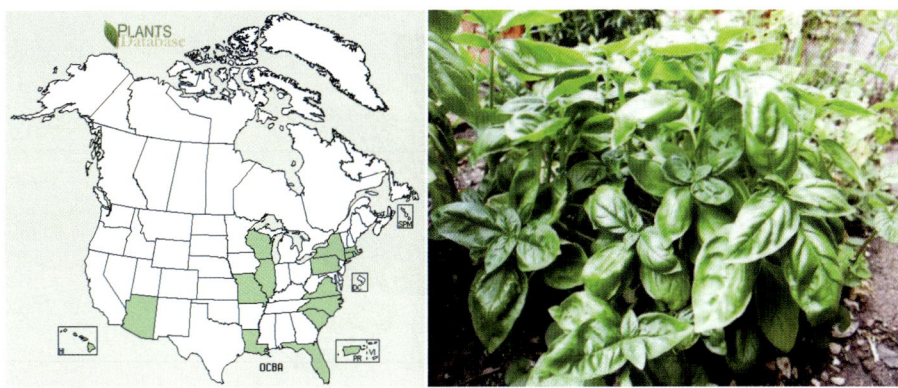

Basil essential oil can be used to clear the sinuses, promote digestion and stimulate circulation, especially in the respiratory system. It is prized in Ayurvedic medicine for its ability to strengthen compassion, faith, and bring clarity. This variety has a sweet vaguely anise-like, mint, smoky odor.

It may irritate sensitive skin. Do not use during pregnancy.

Bay - *(Laurus Nobilis)*

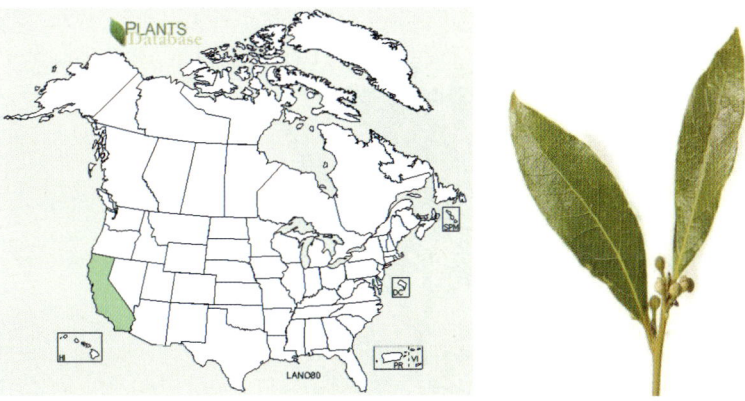

Bay oil is said to have antiseptic, anti-biotic, analgesic, anti-neuralgic, aperitif, astringent, emmenagogue, febrifuge, insecticide and sedative properties. Bay can be used in the treatment of rheumatism, muscular pain, circulation problems, colds, flu, dental infections and skin infections. Bay has a high eugenol content and may irritate the skin and mucus membranes, so use with caution. Avoid during pregnancy.

BENZOIN - *(STYRAX BENZOIN)*

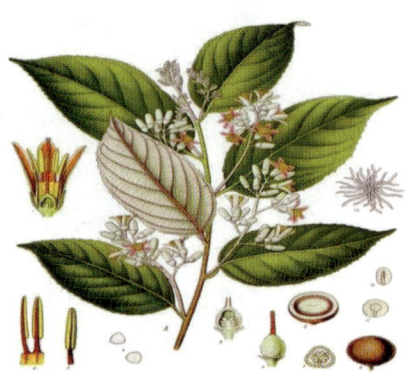

Benzoin oil is reputed to have antiseptic, anti-depressant, anti-inflammatory, carminative, deodorant, diuretic and expectorant properties. Benzoin is widely used as a fixative in perfumes. It can also be used for assisting with respiratory ailments, and skin conditions such as acne, eczema and psoriasis. We would recommend placing the bottle in a very hot water bath, changing the water frequently and once it is back to the liquid state be sure to shake before use.

Benzoin is a non-toxic and non-irritant, but a mild sensitizer and should be avoided if you have sensitive or allergy-prone skin.

BERGAMOT - *(CITRUS BERGAMIA)*

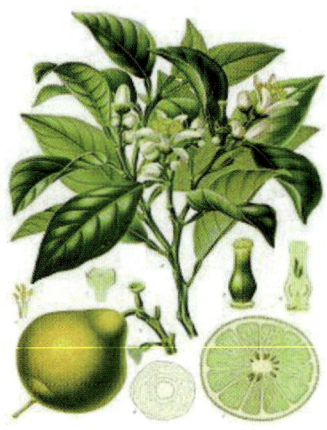

To be used in skin and hair care formulations without worrying about sun exposure after use. Bergamot can be used to treat skin ailments such as psoriasis and eczema and it is considered to relieve stress and anxiety. The aroma is basically citrus, yet fruity and sweet with a warm spicy floral quality.

It may cause sensitivity in some individuals. Avoid use during pregnancy.

Birch Sweet - (Betula Lenta)

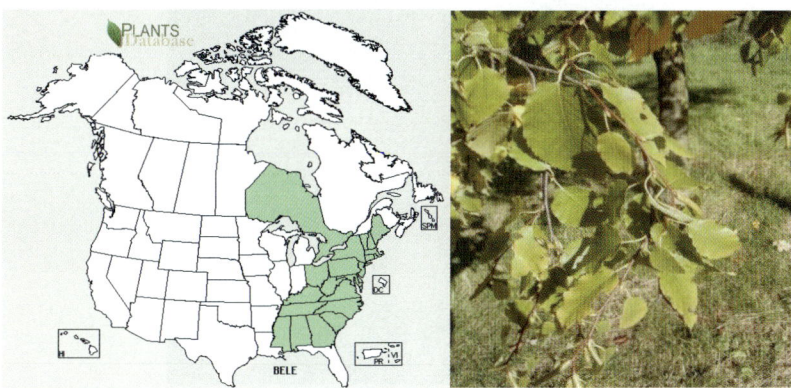

Birch sweet oil is credited with being an analgesic, anti-inflammatory, anti-pryetic, anti-rheumatic, antiseptic, astringent, depurative, diuretic, and tonic. It is an effective addition to massage oil blends for sore muscles, sprains and painful joints because of its anti-inflammatory and antispasmodic properties.

Birch sweet oil is potentially toxic and may cause skin irritation. Use in dilution and avoid during pregnancy.

Blood Orange - (Citrus Sinensis)

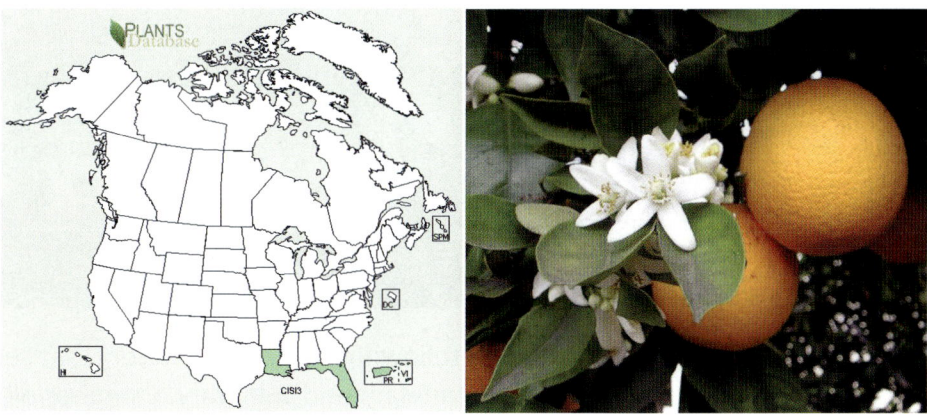

Blood orange oil is considered to have anti-depressant, antiseptic, antispasmodic and aphrodisiac properties. Avoid exposure to sunlight after skin application due to possible photo-toxicity.

CAJEPUT - *(MELALEUCA CAJEPUTI)*

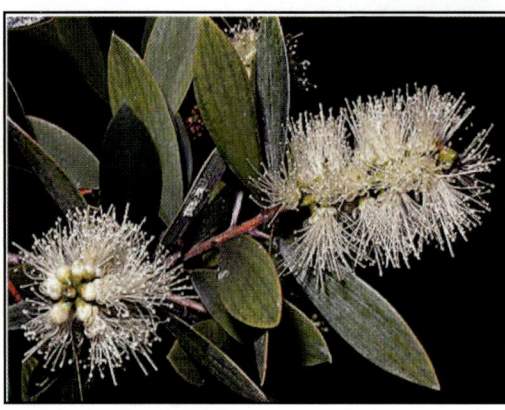

Cajeput oil has antiseptic and anti-microbial properties and is used chiefly as a local application for skin ailments and as a stimulating expectorant. Other properties include being mildly analgesic, anti-neuralgic, antispasmodic, anthelminthic, diaphoretic, carminative, expectorant, febrifuge, insecticide, sudorific and tonic.

There is no known toxicity but avoid during pregnancy.

CAMPHOR - *(CINNAMOMUM CAMPHORA)*

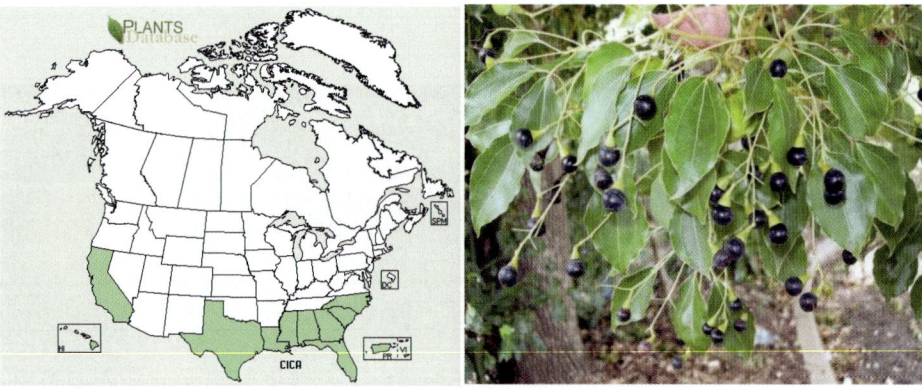

The therapeutic properties of camphor oil include the following: anti-inflammatory, antiseptic, cardiac, carminative, diuretic, febrifuge, insecticide, laxative, stimulant and vulnerary. Camphor oil can be used in the treatment of nervous depression, acne, inflammation, arthritis, muscular aches and pains, sprains, rheumatism, bronchitis, coughs, colds, fever, flu and infectious diseases. It is a well-known preventive of moths and other insects, such as worms in wood.

Camphor oil is powerful oil and should be used with care. Overdosing can cause convulsions and vomiting. Pregnant women or persons suffering from epilepsy and asthma should not use it.

Caraway - *(Carum Carvi)*

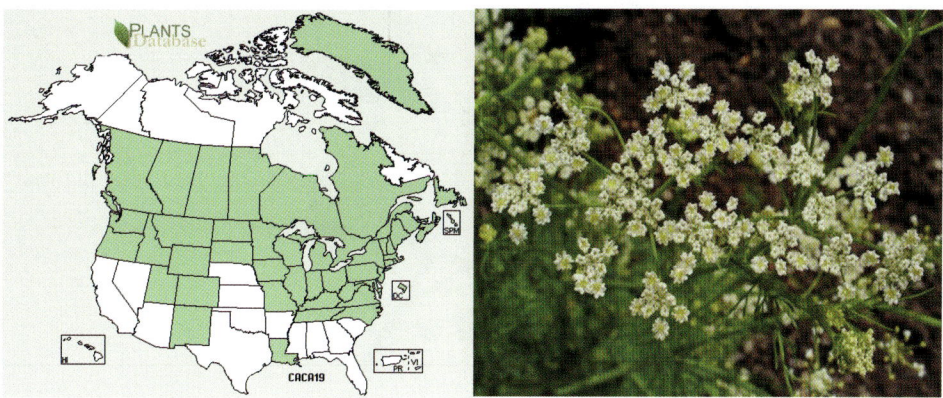

The therapeutic properties of caraway oil include: anti-histaminic, antiseptic, astringent, carminative, digestive, disinfectant, emmenagogue, expectorant, stimulant, stomachic, tonic and vermifuge. As an expectorant it helps to clear bronchitis, bronchial asthma and coughs. It is also helpful in cases of sore throats and laryngitis.

It is non-toxic and non-sensitizing. It may cause skin irritation if used in high concentration. Avoid use during pregnancy.

Carrot Seed - *(Daucus Carota)*

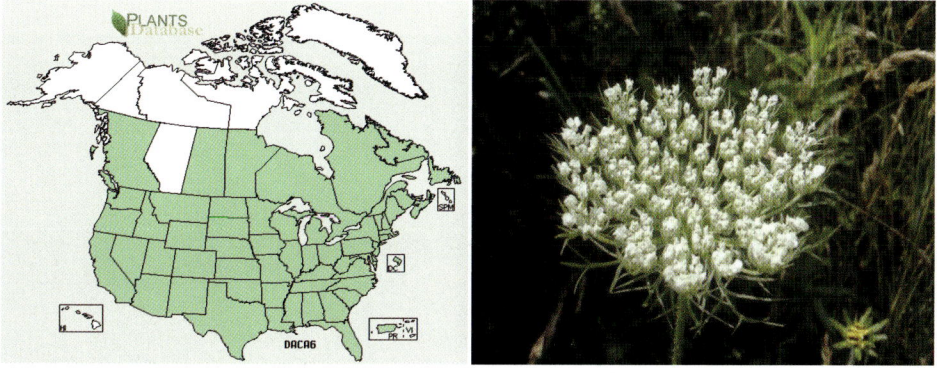

Carrot seed oil is considered one of the best oils for mature skin. It is believed to stimulate cell growth while removing toxins giving the skin a more toned, smooth and youthful appearance. It is reputed to be useful in treating scars, wounds and burns and there are those who believe it can be useful to reduce and even prevent wrinkles. Carrot seed oil is helpful for arthritis, gout, edema, rheumatism and the accumulation of toxins in muscles and joints. It strengthens the mucus membranes in the nose, throat and lungs, thus has a beneficial effect on problems such as bronchitis and influenza.

It is non-toxic, non-irritant, and non-sensitizing. Avoid use during pregnancy.

Cassia - *(Cinnamomum Cassia)*

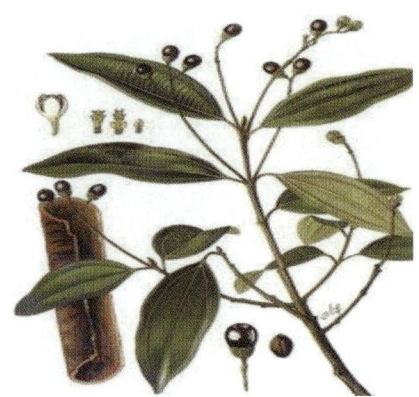

Cassia oil can be used as a tonic, carminative and stimulant. It is used to treat nausea, flatulence and diarrhea. Chinese and Japanese scientists have found that cassia has sedative effects and lowers high blood pressure and fever in experimental animals. The oil has antiseptic properties, killing various types of bacteria and fungi. Cassia oil is used mainly as a carminative (for relieving colic and griping) or as a stomach tonic. It can also be used for colds, influenza, fevers, arthritis and rheumatism.

Cassia oil is a dermal irritant, dermal sensitizer and a mucus membrane irritant and should be avoided in pregnancy.

Catnip - *(Nepeta Cataria)*

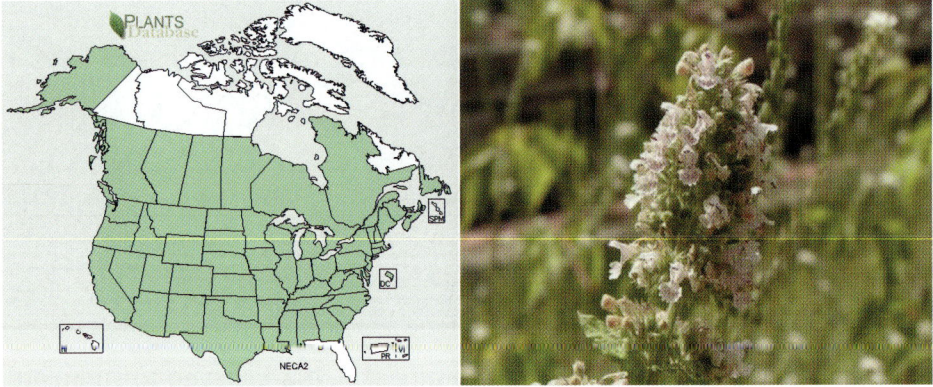

Catnip oil is reputed to have antispasmodic, carminative, diaphoretic, emenagogue, nervine, stomachic, stimulant, astringent and sedative properties. Rubbing catnip oil on the forehead is sometimes employed as a means of easing the pain of a headache. Poultices including catnip oil and leaves are also sometimes used to help with chest congestion. A cloth soaked with catnip oil is said to help slow and even reverse fever when wrapped around the forehead and cheeks.

There is no known toxicity. Avoid use during pregnancy.

CEDARWOOD - *(CEDRUS ATLANTICA)*

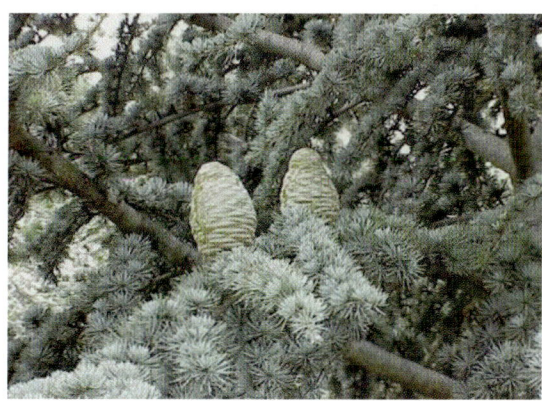

Cedarwood atlas oil can be used to assist with acne, arthritis, bronchitis, coughing, cystitis, dandruff, dermatitis, stress. It has warming, uplifting, and toning properties. Cedarwood oil is considered to be comforting, reviving and an aphrodisiac.

It is non-toxic and non-irritant. Avoid during pregnancy.

CEDARWOOD - *(CEDRUS DEODORA)*

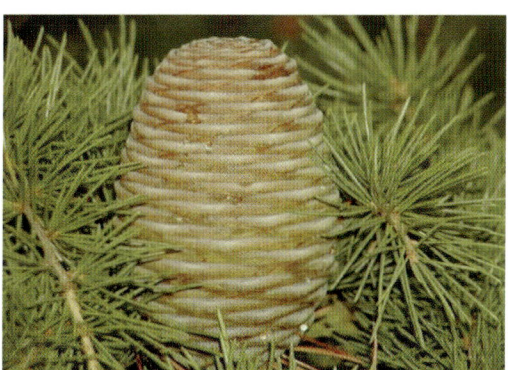

Himalayan cedarwood oil is believed to have the following properties: antiseptic, anti-putrescent, anti-seborrheic, aphrodisiac, astringent, diuretic, expectorant, fungicidal, mucolytic, sedative (nervous), stimulant (circulatory), tonic.

It is non-toxic, non-irritant, and non-sensitizing. Avoid during pregnancy.

CEDARWOOD - (CUPRESSUS FUNEBRIS)

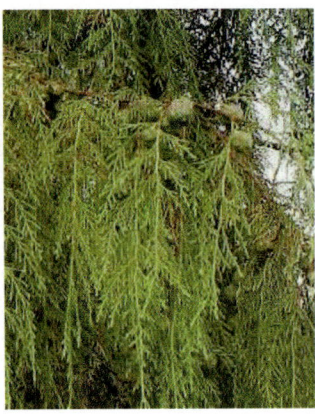

Cedarwood oil has been used for fungal growths, muscular aches and pains, removing warts, rheumatism, skin afflictions, as well as cosmetics, perfumes, and scenting soaps. It is reputed to have antiseptic, anti-putrescent, anti-seborrheic, aphrodisiac, astringent, diuretic, expectorant, fungicidal, mucilytic, sedative (nervous), stimulant (circulatory) and tonic properties.

It is non-toxic, non-irritant, and non-sensitizing. Avoid during pregnancy.

Cedarwood - (Juniperus Ashei)

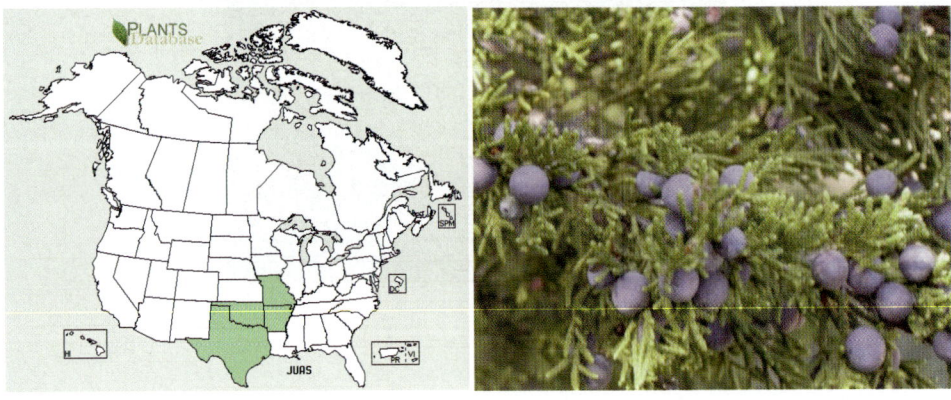

Cedarwood Texas oil is believed to assist with the following ailments: acne, arthritis, bronchitis, catarrh, circulation problems, congestion, coughs, cystitis, dandruff, eczema, greasy hair, leucorrhea, oily skin, psoriasis, sinusitis and water retention. It is also said to possess insect repellent and anti-fungal properties.

It is non-toxic, non-irritant, and non-sensitizing. Avoid during pregnancy.

CEDARWOOD - *(JUNIPERUS VIRGINIANA)*

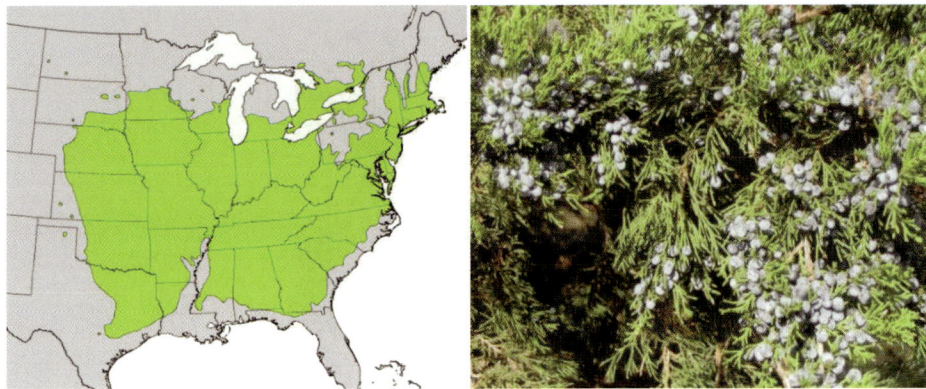

Cedarwood Virginian oil is reputed to calm nervous tension and states of anxiety. It is an expectorant and useful in treating hemorrhoids, deterring moths and other insects, and will act as a mild astringent. It is a very powerful antiseptic, fungicidal and anti-seborrhea (helps with dandruff, hair loss and oily hair). Consumers will also see it in men's toiletries, in products used to combat acne, and in products designed to relieve muscle and joint pain.

It is non-toxic, non-irritan, and non-sensitizing. Avoid during pregnancy.

CHAMOMILE - *(MATRICARIA CHAMOMILLA)*

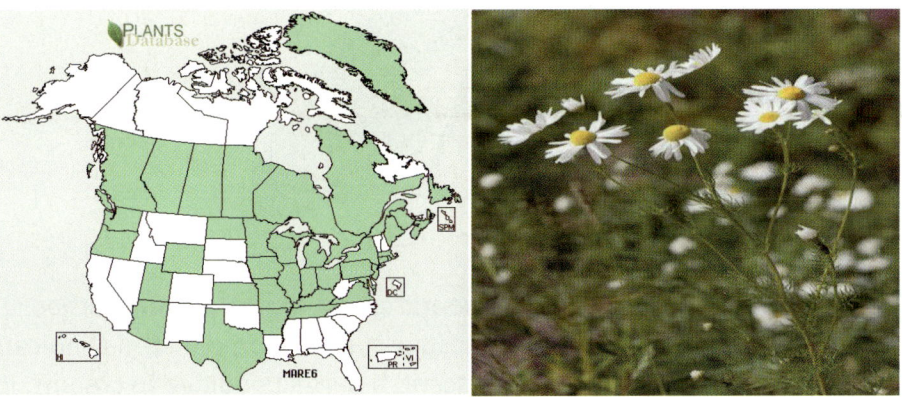

Chamomile oil is effective as an analgesic, anti-allergenic, anti-inflammatory, antispasmodic, antibacterial, carminative, febrifuge, fungicidal, hepatic, nerve sedative, stimulant of leucocyte production, stomachic, sudorific, vermifuge, and as vulnerary agent. This oil is an excellent skincare remedy, providing soothing calming and cleansing benefits useful for burns, blisters, inflamed wounds, dermatitis, eczema, rashes and wounds.

It is non-toxic and non-irritant but causes dermatitis in some individuals. Do not use the essential oil during pregnancy because it is a uterine stimulant.

Cinnamon Bark - (Cinnamomum Cassia)

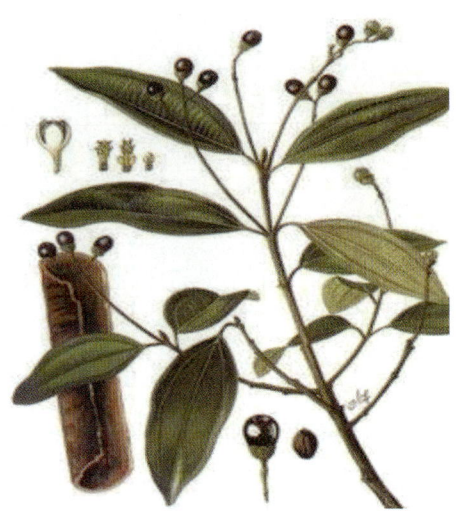

Cinnamon Bark - (Cinnamomum Zeylanicum)

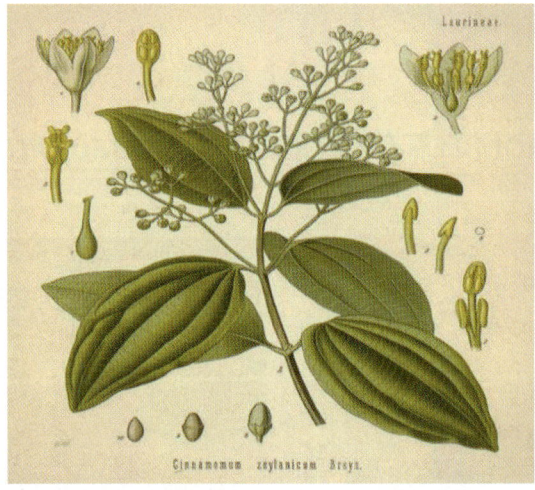

Cinnamon bark oil is highly respected as having antiseptic and antimicrobial properties. It has also been used to treat diarrhea and other problems of the digestive system. Some material indicates that it is perfect in topical applications, and with its pleasant scent, a perfect additive to creams, lotions, and soaps.

Cinnamon bark oil can be irritating to the skin and mucous membranes—particularly in large doses. It should always be used in dilution. Avoid use during pregnancy.

CINNAMON LEAF - *(CINNAMOMUM VERUM)*

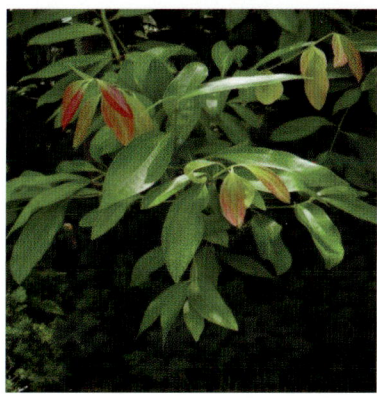

Cinnamon leaf oil is believed to have the following properties: stimulant, antiseptic, antibiotic, astringent, carminative, emmenagogue, and anti-spasmodic. It is also considered to have natural insect repellent properties.

Though non-toxic, it is capable of causing sensitivity–particularly with mucous membranes. It should also be used in proper dilution and avoided during pregnancy.

CITRAL - *(LITSEA CUBEBA)*

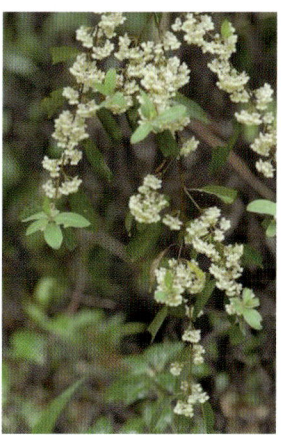

Citral oil is known for its invigorating and antiseptic properties. An excellent anti-depressant, citral tones and fortifies the nervous system and can be used in bath for soothing muscular nerves and pain. It has also been used in treatments of acne, athlete's foot, excessive perspiration, flatulence, insect repellent, muscle aches, oily skin, scabies, and stress.

Avoid in glaucoma and with children. Use caution in prostatic hyperplasia and with skin hypersensitivity or damaged skin. Avoid use during pregnancy.

CITRONELLA - (CYMBOPOGON NARDUS)

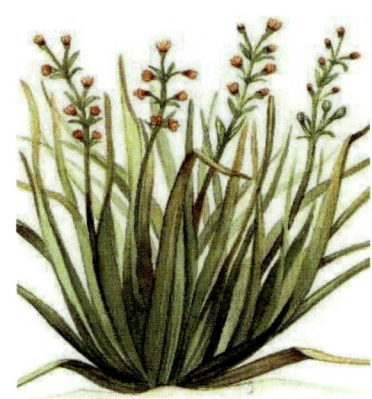

Citronella oil is credited with having therapeutic properties as an antiseptic, deodorant, insecticide, parasitic, tonic and as a stimulant. Nonetheless, most people will associate it with its insecticide properties. It will also be seen in soaps and candles, and it has common applications in massage. This oil can also help with minor infection, but is more commonly known for its ability to assist in combating colds and flu. Citronella can also be used for excessive perspiration and for conditioning oily skin and hair.

Citronella may irritate sensitive skin. Avoid use during pregnancy.

CLARY SAGE - (SALVIA SCLAREA)

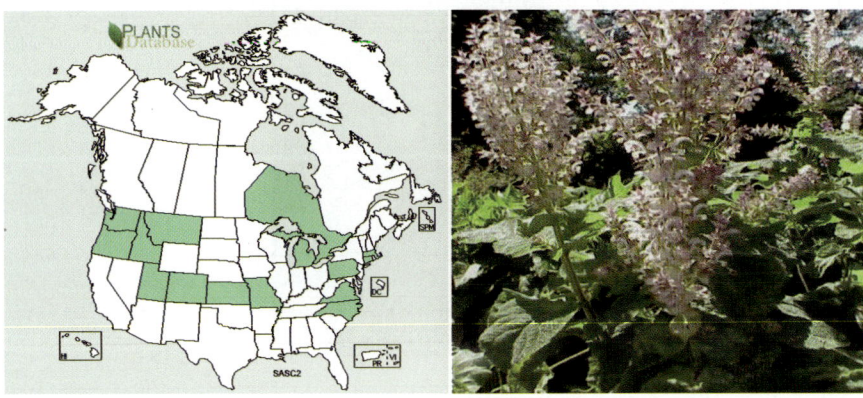

Clary sage oil is viewed by aromatherapists as an antidepressant, antispasmodic, deodorant, emmenagogue, hypotensive, nervine, sedative, tonic and uterine. It is well known for providing a euphoric action, for balancing uterine issues, and as an agent to clean greasy hair. There is also some documentation of its effectiveness in helping to relax the spasms of asthma.

Clary sage oil is non-toxic and non-sensitizing. It is not to be used during pregnancy.

Clove Bud - (*Syzygium Aromaticumum*)

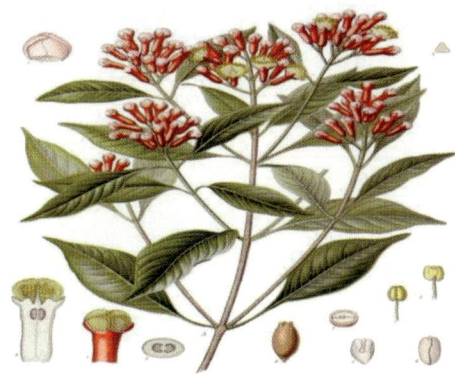

Clove bud oil is an effective agent for minor pains and aches (particular dental pain) and is helpful when battling flu and colds.

Clove bud oil can cause sensitization in some individuals and should be used in dilution. It should also be avoided during pregnancy.

Clove Leaf - *(Syzgium Aromaticum)*

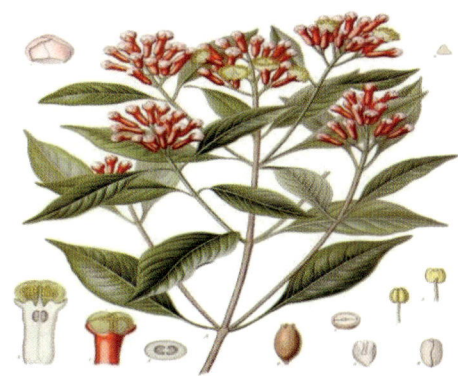

The leaf of this evergreen, indigenous to Southeast Asia, has a long history as being beneficial for skin irritations and digestion, and to counter bad breath. It is often substituted for clove bud in soap and candle manufacturing.

Clove leaf oil can cause sensitization in some individuals and should be used in dilution. It should also be avoided during pregnancy.

COFFEE - *(COFFEA ARABICA)*

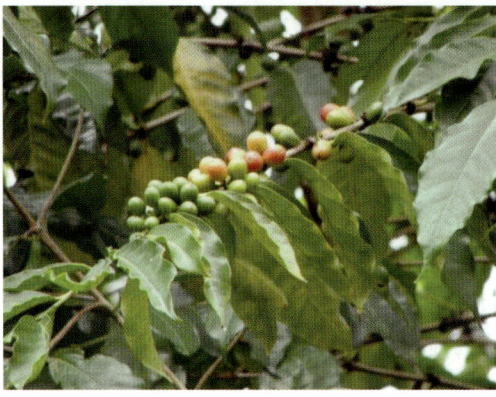

Coffee oil has a multitude of possible uses. It can be burned as a room deodorizer and is considered to be an excellent anti-oxidant. It has also been used to combat depression, respiratory issues, stings, fevers, and general nausea.

Coffee oil should be avoided during pregnancy. It may also cause heart palpitations in some individuals.

CORIANDER - *(CORIANDRUM SATIVUM)*

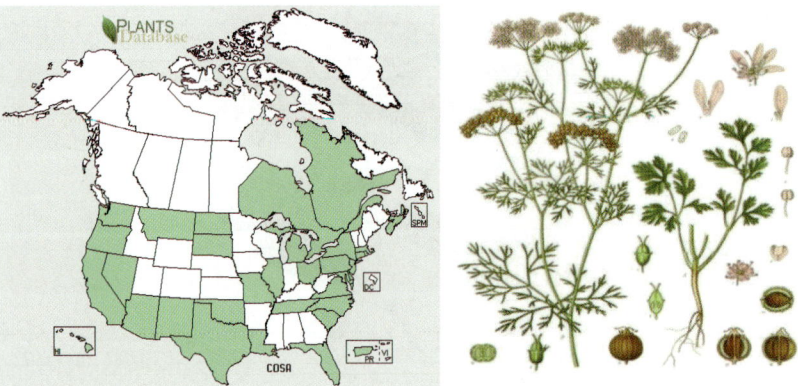

The therapeutic properties of coriander oil include being analgesic, aphrodisiac, antispasmodic, carminative, depurative, deodorant, digestive, carminative, fungicidal, revitalizing, stimulant and stomachic. Coriander oil can be useful to refresh and awake the mind. It can be used for mental fatigue, migraine pain, tension and nervous weakness. This oil's warming effect is also helpful for alleviating pain such as rheumatism, arthritis and muscle spasms. There are some indications that it can also be useful in combating colds and flu.

Avoid use during pregnancy.

CYPRESS - *(CUPRESSUS SEMPERVIRENS)*

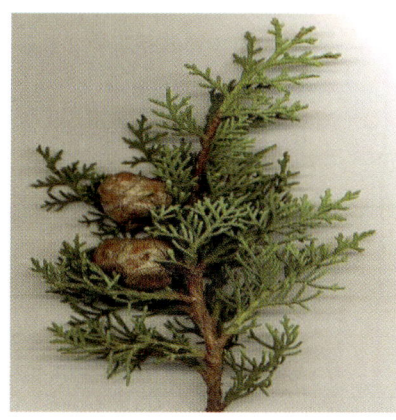

Cypress oil has been used to combat excessive perspiration (particularly feet), hemorrhoids, menorrhagia, oily skin, rheumatism, and varicose veins. Aromatherapists also commonly credit cypress with being a relaxing, nerve soothing essential oil. It has the properties of an astringent and has been used in skin care applications.

This oil is regarded as being very gentle and suitable for all skin types.

EUCALYPTUS – *(EUCALYPTUS GLOBULES)* , *(EUCALYPTUS POLYBRACTEA)*, *(EUCALYPTUS RADIATA)*

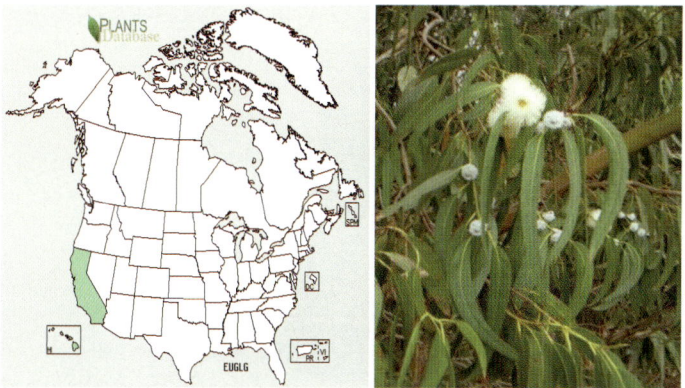

Eucalyptus oil is fantastic on skin ailments. This is used on burns, blisters, wounds, insect bites, lice and skin infections, as well as to combat the effects of colds and the flu. There is also a history of eucalyptus oil being applied to sore muscles and joints.

Eucalyptus oil should be used in dilution, and be avoided during pregnancy. It is considered toxic if taken internally, non-irritant, and non-sensitive. Avoid if you have high blood pressure or epilepsy.

Eucalyptus Lemon - *(Eucalyptus Polybractea)*

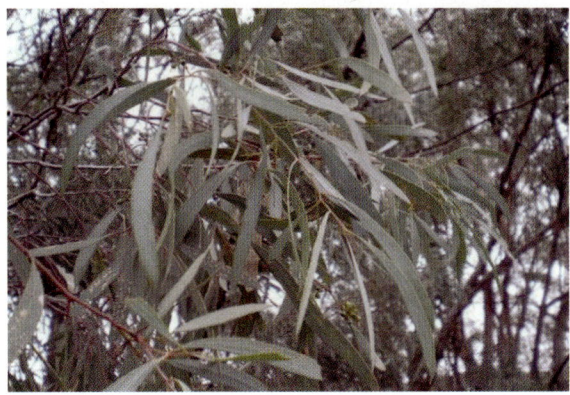

Eucalyptus lemon oil is reputed to assist with ailments such as arthritis, bronchitis, catarrh, cold sores, colds, coughing, fever, flu, poor circulation, and sinusitis.

Eucalyptus lemon oil should be used in dilution, and be avoided during pregnancy. It is considered toxic if taken internally, non-irritant, and non-sensitive. Avoid if you have high blood pressure or epilepsy.

Fir Needle - *(Abies Siberica)*

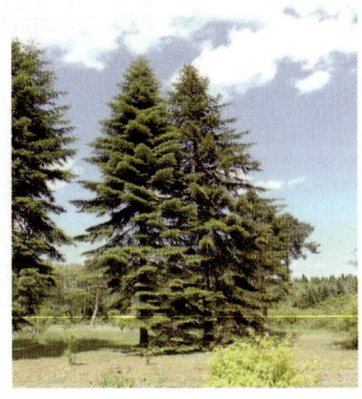

Fir needle oil is reported to help with arthritis, bronchitis, colds, coughs, flu, muscle aches, rheumatism and sinusitis. It is a popular oil used to bring out masculine, outdoorsy attributes in men's fragrances, bath preparations, air fresheners, herbal oils, soaps, and shaving creams.

Fir needle oil is non-toxic, non-irritant, and non-sensitizing. Liquid may cause irritation to the eyes so use well diluted. Avoid use during pregnancy.

FRANKINCENSE - (BOSWELLIA SERRATA)

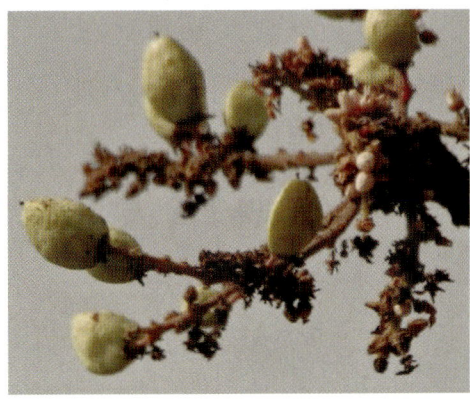

The therapeutic properties of frankincense oil include use as an antiseptic, astringent, carminative, digestive, diuretic, sedative, tonic, and expectorant. Frankincense is said to help rejuvenate the aging skin, and is effective with bacterial and fungal infections. The anti-inflammatory property of this oil is reputed to be an effective treatment for joint pain and arthritis. Frankincense can also be used as an insect repellent and is also widely used in cosmetics and soap manufacturing.

Frankincense oil is non-toxic, non-irritant, and non-sensitizing. Avoid use during pregnancy.

Geranium - (Pelargonium Graveolens)

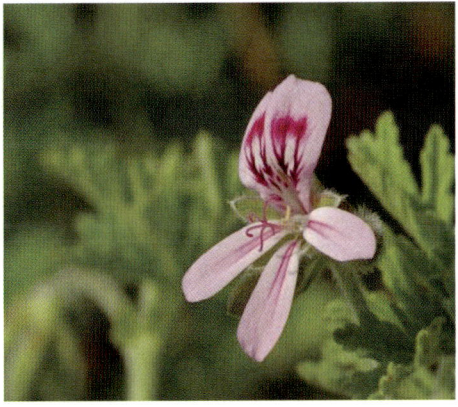

The therapeutic properties of geranium oil include the being used as an astringent, haemostatic, diuretic, antiseptic, anti-depressant, tonic, antibiotic, anti-spasmodic and as an anti-infectious agent. This uplifting oil has a great all-over balancing effect and this extends to the skin, where it helps to create balance between oily and dry skin. Geranium can also be used to relieve feelings of stress and anxiety, promoting a sense of inner peace. The strong smell of this oil is particularly good to ward off mosquitoes and head lice.

Geranium oil is non-toxic and non-irritant and generally non-sensitizing. It can cause sensitivity in some people and due to the fact that it balances the hormonal system, it should be avoided during pregnancy.

GINGER ROOT - *(ZINGIBER OFFICINALIS)*

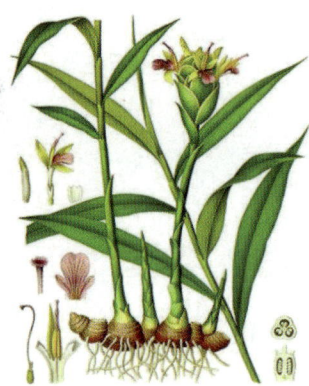

Ginger oil is believed by aromatherapists to be applicable for colds and flu, nausea (motion sickness, morning sickness), rheumatism, coughs, and circulation issues. It also has warming properties that help to relieve muscular cramps, spasms, aches and ease stiffness in joints. Ginger is also viewed as an aphrodisiac and is believed to ease anxiety, renew vitality, and revitalize self-confidence.

Ginger oil can irritate sensitive skin. Avoid use during pregnancy.

Grapefruit (Pink) – *(Citrus Racemosa)*

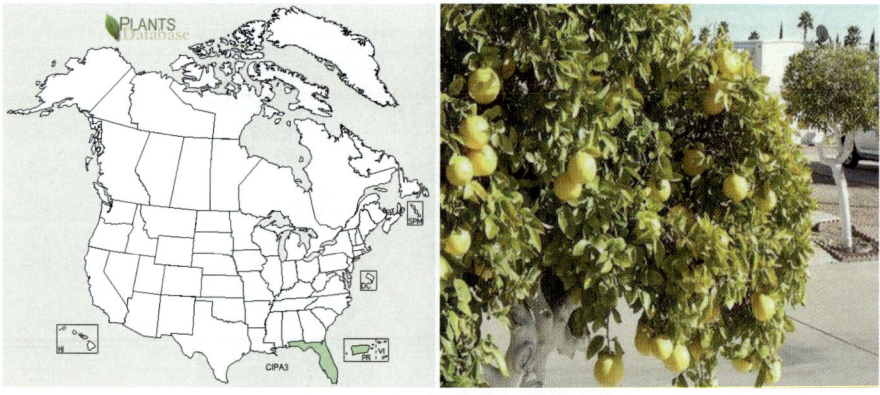

Grapefruit pink oil is believed by aromatherapists to be a spiritual up-lifter, and to ease muscle fatigue and stiffness. It is also a purifier of congested, oily and acne prone skin and is sometimes added to creams and lotions as a natural toner and cellulite treatment. Grapefruit essential oil is reputed to ease nervous exhaustion and relieve depression.

Grapefruit pink oil can cause photosensitivity. Avoid use during pregnancy.

HELICHRYSUM – *(HELICHRYSUM ITALICUM)*

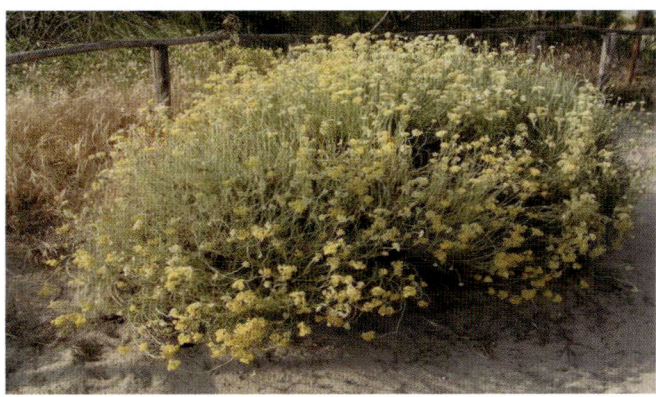

Helichrysum oil is credited by aromatherapists as being effective for acne, bruises, boils, burns, cuts, dermatitis, eczema, irritated skin and wounds. It is said to support the body through post-viral fatigue and convalescence, and can also be used to repair skin damaged by psoriasis, eczema or ulceration. Helichrysum essential oil is believed to soothe away deep emotional stress and diffuse anger and destructive feelings.

Helichrysum oil is non-toxic, non-irritating, and non-sensitizing. Avoid use during pregnancy.

JASMINE - *(JASMINUM GRANDIFLORUM)* , *(JASMINUM SAMBAC)*

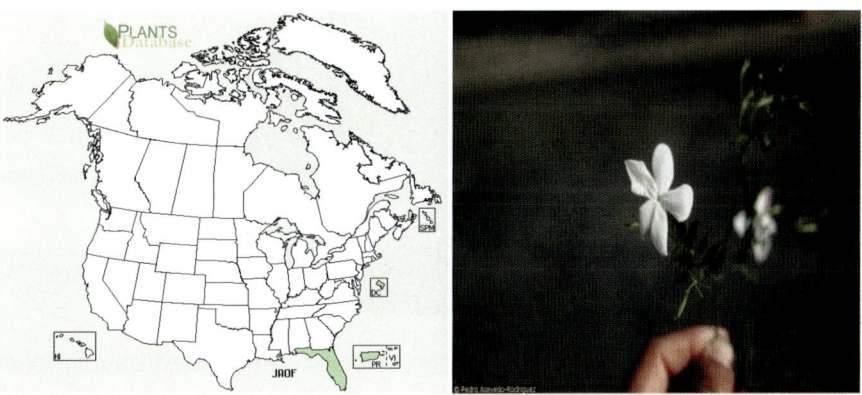

Jasmine oil is well respected for its aphrodisiac properties. It is a sensual, soothing, calming oil that promotes love and peace. It is important to note that all absolutes are extremely concentrated by nature. They should not be evaluated in this state unless you are accustomed to the undiluted fragrance. For those trying jasmine oil for the first time, we strongly recommend they be evaluated in dilution. Otherwise, the complexity of the fragrance–particularly the rare and exotic notes–becomes lost.

JUNIPER BERRY – (JUNIPERUS COMMUNIS)

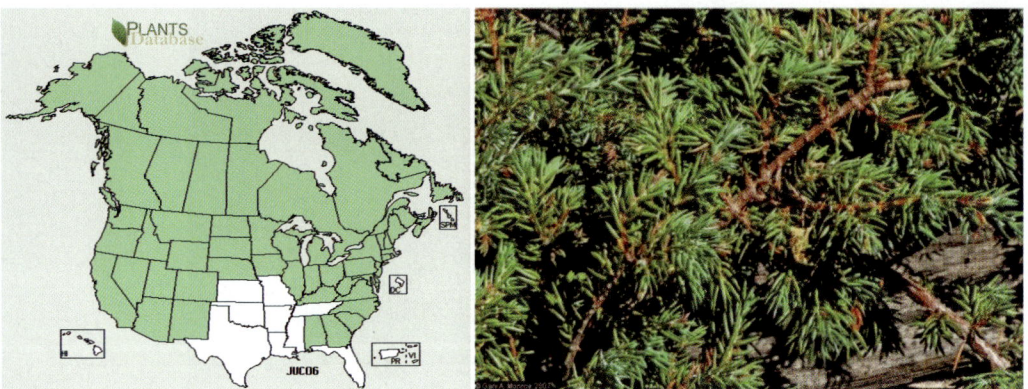

Juniper berry oil is credited as being a supportive, restoring, and a tonic aid. It is excellent for meditation and is a popular oil in weight loss and detoxification blends, because of its diuretic properties. It is also considered purifying and clearing for the mind.

Juniper berry oil is non-irritating and non-sensitizing. Avoid use during pregnancy.

LAVANDIN ABRIALIS – (LAVANDULA INTERMEDIA VAR ABRIALIS)

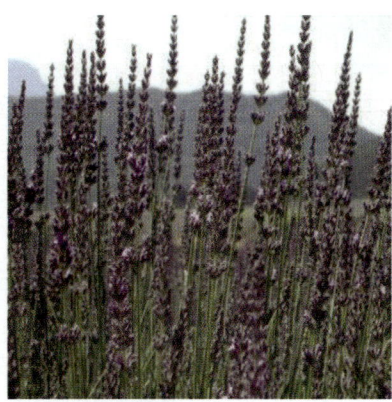

Lavandin abrialis oil is used almost exclusively for scent. It is also reputed to have applications with colds and head congestion.

Due to the high camphor content, lavandin abrialis oil should be avoided during pregnancy and by those with epilepsy.

LAVANDIN GROSSO – (LAVANDULA INTERMEDIA VAR GROSSO)

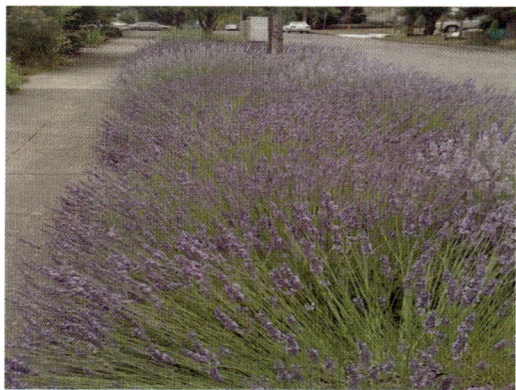

Lavandin grosso oil is used almost exclusively for scent. Due to the high camphor content, lavandin grosso oil should be avoided during pregnancy and by those with epilepsy.

LAVENDER – (LAVANDULA OFFICINALIS)

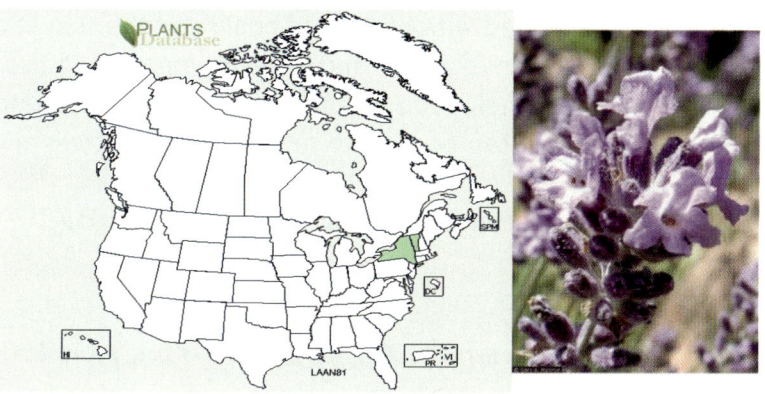

It is recognized as having some strong properties which include:

Analgesic	Choleretic	Parasitical
Anticonvulsant	Cicatrizant	Rubefacient
Anti-depressant	Cordial	Sedative
Anti-microbial	Cytophylactic	Stimulant
Anti-rheumatic	Diuretic	Sudorific
Antiseptic	Emmenagogue	Tonic
Anti-spasmodic	Deodorant	Vermifuge
Anti-toxic	Hypotensive	Vulnerary
Carminative	Insecticide	
Cholagogue	Nervine	

Avoid high doses during pregnancy because it is a uterine stimulant.

LAVENDER BULGARIAN – *(LAVANDULA ANGUSTIFOLIA)*

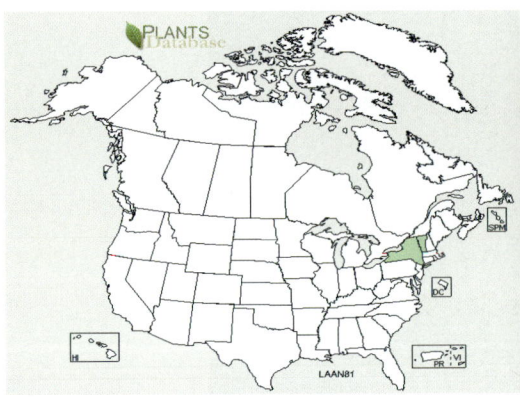 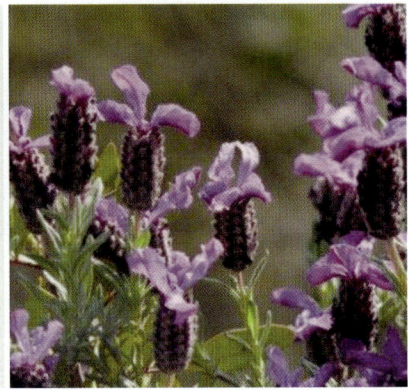

Properties of lavender bulgarian oil include:

Analgesic	Antispasmodic	Cordial
Anti-convulsive	Antiviral	Cytophylactic
Anti-depressant	Bactericide	Decongestant
Anti-phlogistic	Carminative	Deodorant
Antirheumatic	Cholagogue	Diuretic
Antseptic	Cicatrisant	

Herbalists regard lavender as the most useful and versatile essential oil for therapeutic purposes. Lavender is the essential oil most commonly associated with burns and healing of the skin. It also has antiseptic and analgesic properties which will ease the pain of a burn and prevent infection. It also has cytophylactic properties that promote rapid healing and help reduce scarring. The scent of Lavender essential oil is said to have a calming effect on the body and it can be used to reduce anxiety, stress and promote sleep.

Lavender Bulgarian Essential Oil is non-toxic, non-irritating, and non-sensitizing.

LAVENDER FRENCH – *(LAVANDULA DENTATE)*

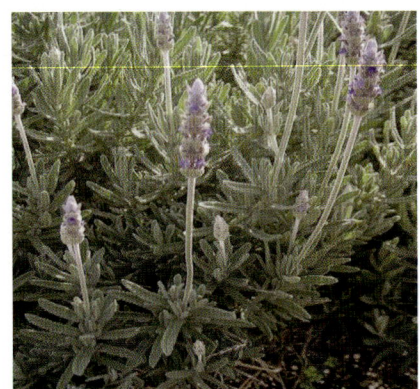

Properties of lavender French oil include:

Analgesic	Antispasmodic	Cordial
Anti-convulsive	Antiviral	Cytophylactic
Anti-depressant	Bactericide	Decongestant
Anti-phlogistic	Carminative	Deodorant
Antirheumatic	Cholagogue	Diuretic
Antseptic	Cicatrisant	

Herbalists regard lavender as the most useful and versatile essential oil for therapeutic purposes. Lavender is the essential oil most commonly associated with burns and healing of the skin. It also has antiseptic and analgesic properties which will ease the pain of a burn and prevent infection. It also has cytophylactic properties that promote rapid healing and help reduce scarring. The scent of lavender is said to have a calming effect on the body and it can be used to reduce anxiety, stress and promote sleep. Lavender French essential oil is a popular choice amongst both aromatherapists and massage therapists for its combination of therapeutic quality and pleasant floral scent

Lavender French oil is non-toxic, non-irritating, and non-sensitizing.

LAVENDER POPULATION – (LAVANDULA ANGUSTIFOLIA)

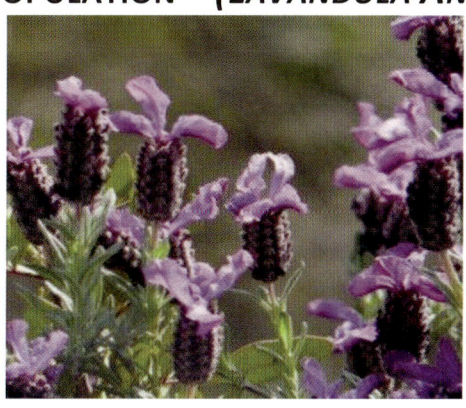

Properties of lavender population oil include:

Analgesic	Antispasmodic	Cordial
Anti-convulsive	Antiviral	Cytophylactic
Anti-depressant	Bactericide	Decongestant
Anti-phlogistic	Carminative	Deodorant
Antirheumatic	Cholagogue	Diuretic
Antseptic	Cicatrisant	

This lavender is grown at a high pristine elevation over 3,500 feet, creating a highly exotic and complex lavender oil. Mellowed by the long daylight hours in high latitude, moderate rainfall and sandy soil, this lavender rivals the best of the world's great lavenders. Herbalists regard lavender as the most useful and versatile essential oil for therapeutic purposes. Lavender is the essential oil most commonly associated with burns and healing of the skin. It also has antiseptic and analgesic properties that will ease the pain of a burn and prevent infection. It also has cytophylactic properties that promote rapid healing and help reduce scarring. The scent of lavender is said to have a calming effect on the body and it can be used to reduce anxiety, stress and promote sleep.

Lavender population oil is non-toxic, non-irritating, and non-sensitizing.

Lavender South African – (Lavandula Angustifolia)

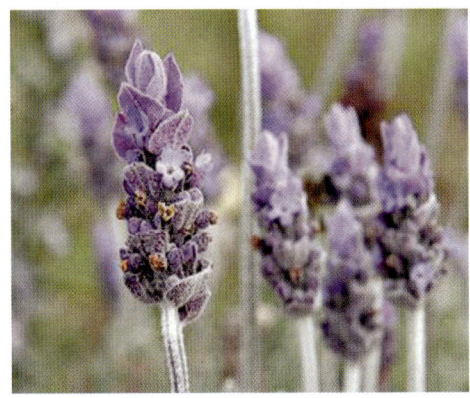

Lavender South African is credited with being an:

Analgesic	Antispasmodic	Cordial
Anti-convulsive	Antiviral	Cytophylactic
Anti-depressant	Bactericide	Decongestant
Anti-phlogistic	Carminative	Deodorant
Antirheumatic	Cholagogue	Diuretic
Antseptic	Cicatrisant	

Lavender is widely used in aromatherapy and in the perfumery industry. The scent has a calming effect which aids in relaxation and the reduction of stress and anxiety. It also has antiseptic and analgesic properties which will ease the pain of a burn, prevent infection and promotes rapid healing. It can be used with massages oils to effectively relieve joint and muscle pain.

Lavender South African oil is non-toxic, non-irritating, and non-sensitizing.

Lavender Spanish – (Lavandula Stoechas)

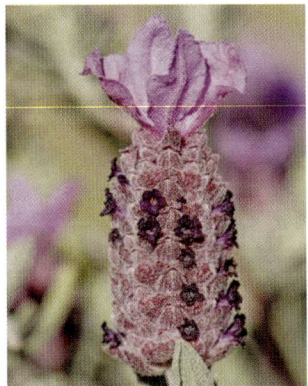

Lavender Spanish oil has similar medicinal properties to common lavender (L. angustifolia). It yields more essential oil than that species but therapeutically not considered as good. The flowers, and the essential oil derived from them, are anti-asthmatic, antiseptic, antispasmodic, digestive and expectorant. Externally, the essential oil is used as an antiseptic wash for wounds, ulcers, sores etc and as a relaxing oil for massage.

Lavender Spanish oil is non-toxic, non-irritating, and non-sensitizing.

LEMON - (CITRUS LIMONUM)

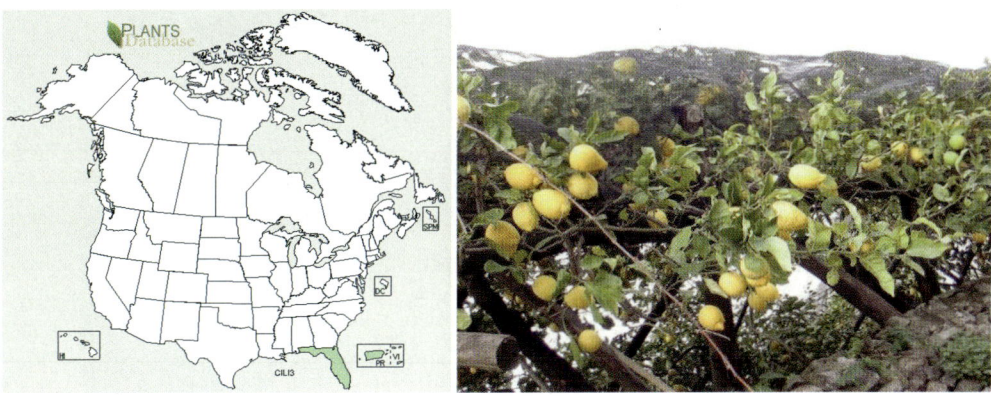

Lemon oil has been historically recognized as a cleanser. It is reputed as being antiseptic, and as having refreshing and cooling properties. On skin and hair it can be used for its cleansing effect, as well as for treating cuts and boils. Research has also shown lemon oil to enhance the ability to concentrate.

Lemon oil is non-toxic, but may cause skin irritation in some. Lemon is also phototoxic and should be avoided prior to exposure to direct sunlight. Avoid during pregnancy.

LEMONGRASS - (CYMBOPOGON FLEXUOSUS)

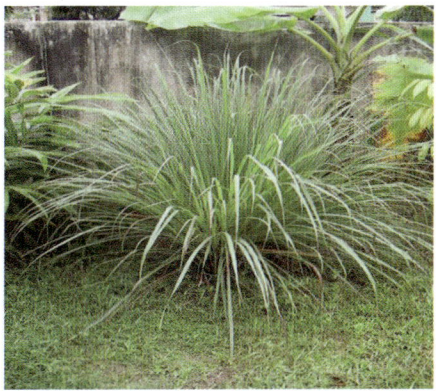

Lemongrass oil is known for its invigorating and antiseptic properties. It can be used in facial toners as its astringent properties help fight acne and greasy skin. An excellent anti-depressant, lemongrass oil tones and fortifies the nervous system and can be used in bath for soothing muscular nerves and pain. Lemongrass shares similar properties with citronella and has a great reputation for keeping insects away.

Lime - *(Citrus Aurantifolia)*

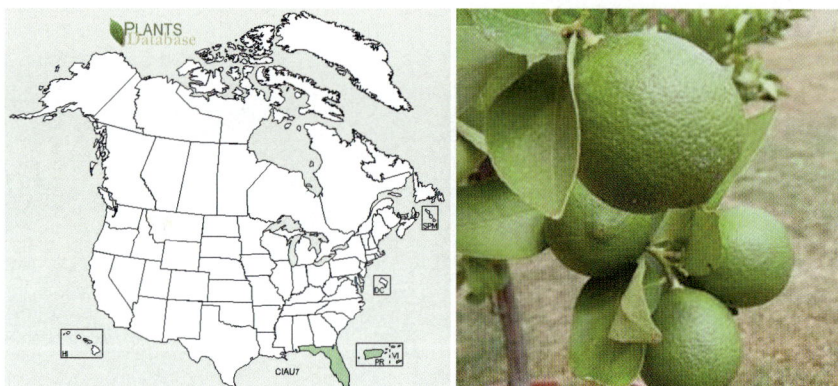

Lime oil has a crisp, refreshing citrus scent that has been used by aromatherapists for its uplifting and revitalizing properties. It can also act as an astringent on skin where it is reputed to help clear oily skin.

Lime oil is considered phototoxic. Users should avoid direct sunlight after application. Avoid use during pregnancy.

Mandarin - *(Citrus Reticulata)*

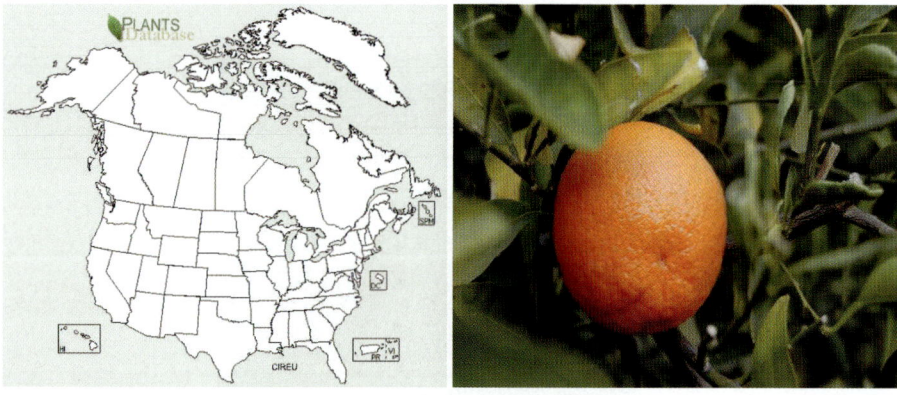

Mandarin oil is often used as a digestive aid, for use against hiccups, anxiety, and to assist the liver functions of the elderly. Mandarin oil is also commonly used in soaps, cosmetics, perfumes and men colognes. It also has many applications in the flavoring industry.

There is some evidence that mandarin essential oil is phototoxic. Direct sunlight should be avoided after use. Avoid use during pregnancy.

Marjoram - (Origanum Marjorana)

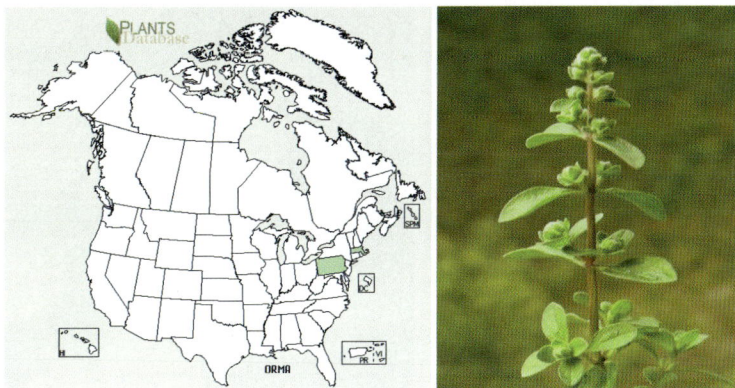

Warming and comforting, marjoram sweet oil can be massaged into the abdomen during menstruation, or added to a warm compress. It is also useful for treating tired aching muscles, and is perfect for use in a sports massage. A few drops on a vaporizer will also encourage sleep, and a few drops can be added to a warm/hot bath at the first signs of a cold. It can also be used in masculine, oriental, and herbal-spicy perfumes and colognes.

Marjoram sweet oil is generally non-toxic, non-irritating, and non-sensitizing. Avoid use during pregnancy.

May Chang - (Litsea Cubeba)

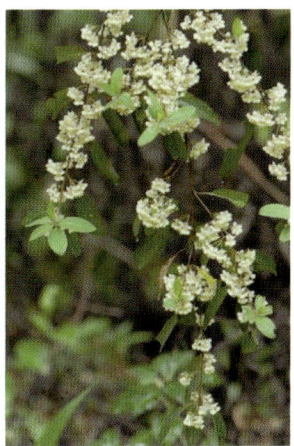

Also known as may chang, litsea cubeba oil is most valued for its calming and anti-inflammatory properties. Other therapeutic properties include being astringent, antiseptic, insecticide, hypotensive, stimulant, and tonic.

Litsea cubeba oil is possible skin irritant. Avoid use during pregnancy.

MELISSA LEAF - *(MELISSA OFFICINALIS)*

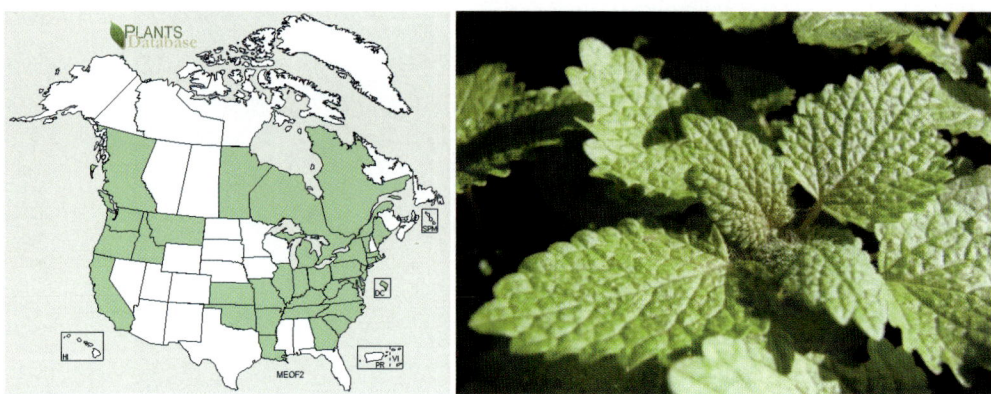

Melissa leaf oil is well known for its anti-depressant and uplifting properties. It is also reported to have uses as an antispamodic, bactericidal, carminative, cordial, diaphoretic, nervine, sedative, stomachic, sudorific, and tonic.

Melissa leaf oil has possible sensitizing and dermal irritating characteristics. Nonetheless, it is viewed by experts as non-toxic. Avoid use during pregnancy.

MENTHOL - *(MENTHA ARVENSIS)*

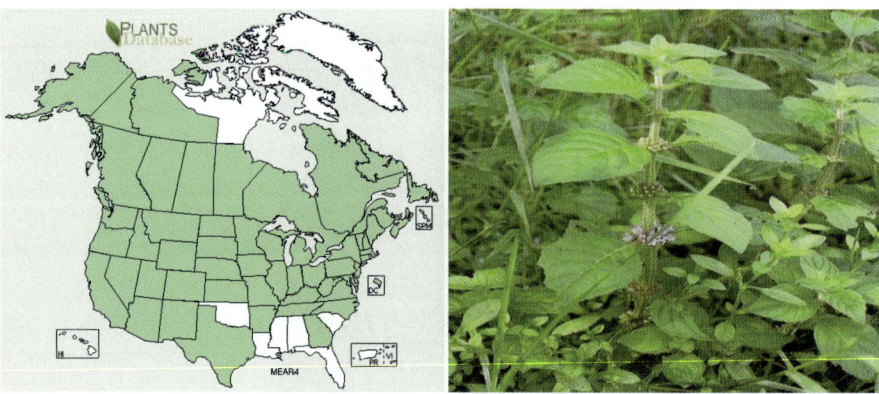

Menthol liquid oil has been used as a flavoring for centuries, but also has applications in aromatherapy when applied to sore muscles or in combination with other products such as in a pain relief balm. It is often referred to as having a cooling effect.

Menthol liquid oil can be sensitizing, particularly in concentrations. Aromatherapists recommend that this product be used in moderation. Avoid use during pregnancy.

Myrrh – (Commiphora Myrrha)

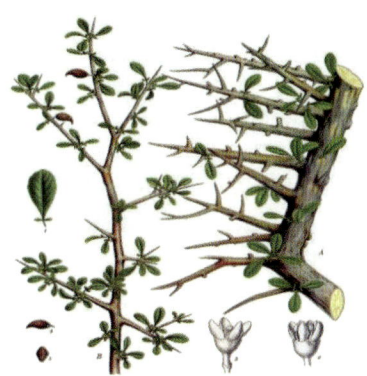

Myrrh oil is thought to enhance spirituality. Aromatherapists use it as an aid in meditation or before healing. Its actions are characterized as the following: antimicrobial, antifungal, astringent and healing, tonic and stimulant, carminative, stomachic, anti-catarrhal, expectorant, diaphoretic, vulnerary, locally antiseptic, immune stimulant, bitter, circulatory stimulant, anti-inflammatory, and antispasmodic.

Myrrh oil can be possibly toxic in high concentrations and should not be used during pregnancy.

Neroli - (Citrus Aurantium Amara)

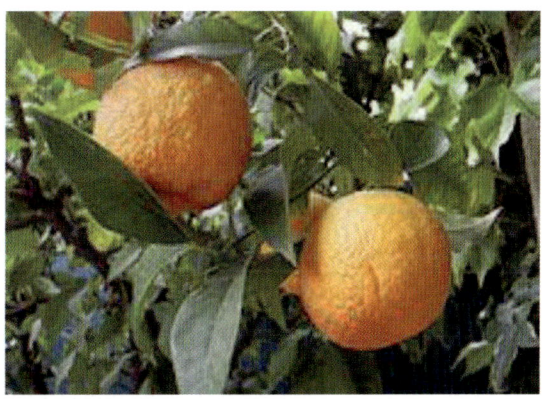

Neroli oil increases circulation and stimulates new cell growth. It can prevent scarring and stretch marks, and has been found useful in treating skin conditions linked to emotional stress. Any type of skin can benefit from this oil, although it is particularly good for dry, irritated or sensitive skin. It regulates oiliness and minimizes enlarged pores. Neroli oil helps to clear acne and blemished skin, especially if the skin lacks moisture. With regular treatment, it can reduce the appearance of fragile or broken capillaries and varicose veins. Other properties include being antidepressant, antiseptic, antispasmodic, aphrodisiac, carminative, cordial, deodorant, digestive, stimulant (nervous) and tonic (cardiac, circulatory).

This oil is non-toxic and non-sensitizing. Avoid use during pregnancy.

NUTMEG - *(MYRISTICA FRAGRANS)*

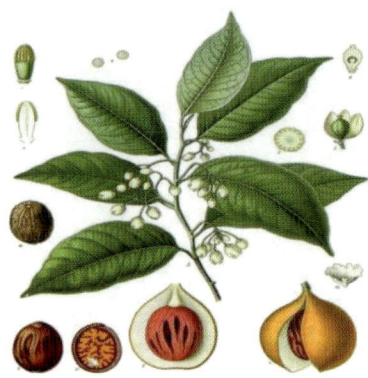

Nutmeg oil can be used as a treatment for the following: arthritis, constipation, fatigue, muscle aches, nausea, neuralgia, poor circulation, rheumatism and slow digestion. It is a valuable addition to many aromatherapy blends, adding warmth, spice and inspiration, when used in very small amounts. Nutmeg oil can be used in soaps, candle making, dental products and hair lotions.

If used in large amounts, nutmeg oil can cause toxic symptoms such as nausea and tachycardia. Avoid use during pregnancy

ORANGE – *(CITRUS SINENSIS)*

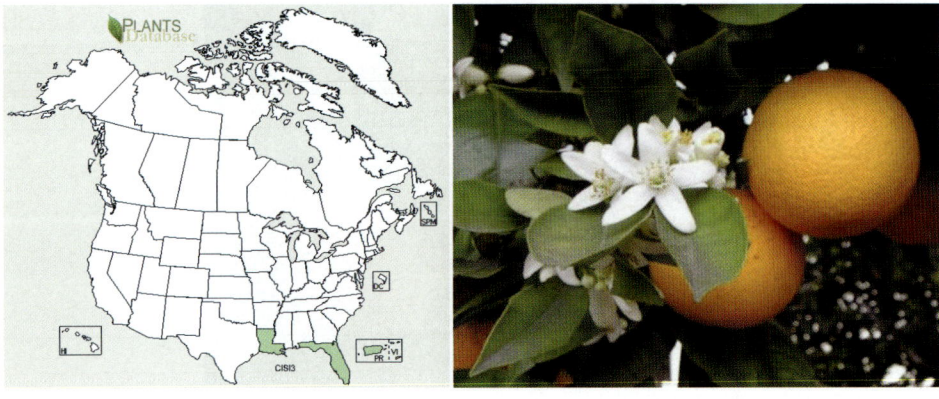

Properties for orange oil are as follows: antidepressant, antiseptic, antispasmodic, aphrodisiac, carminative, cordial, deodorant, digestive, stimulant (nervous) and tonic (cardiac, circulatory). It has also been applied to combat colds, constipation, dull skin, flatulence, the flu, gums, slow digestion, and stress. The increased concentration of the essential oil fragrance makes the oil perfect for soap and candle making.

Some aromatherapists have reported that a small percentage of few people have experienced dermatitis from the limonene content of sweet orange. Orange oil is considered photo-toxic and exposure to sunlight should be avoided. Do not use if pregnant.

Origanum - *(Origanum Vulgare)*

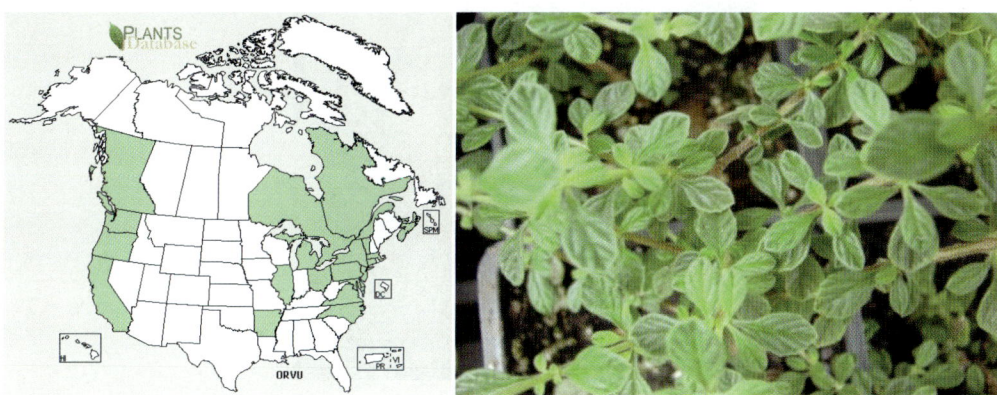

Origanum oil is said to have the following properties: analgesic, anti rheumatic, antiseptic, antispasmodic, antitoxic, antiviral, bactericidal, carminative, choleretic, cytophylactic, diaphoretic, diuretic, emmenagogue, expectorant, febrifuge, fungicidal, parasiticide, rubefacient, stimulant and tonic. Due to high carvacol content, origanum oil is considered to be "nature's cure all" as it is reputed to have one of the best antiseptic and anti-bacterial properties. It can also be used as a fragrance component in soaps, colognes and perfumes, especially men's fragrances.

Origanum oil is both a dermal irritant and a mucous membrane irritant. Avoid use if pregnant.

Palmarosa - *(Cymbopogon Martinii var Motia)*

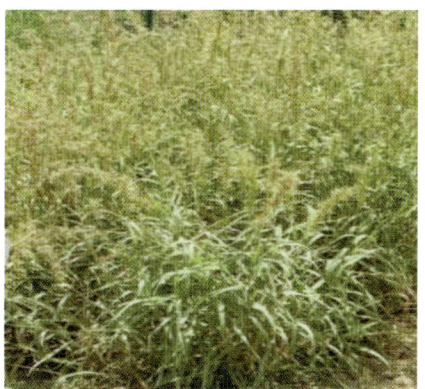

Palmarosa oil properties include use as an antiseptic, bactericidal, cicatrizant, digestive, febrifuge, hydrating, stimulant (digestive, circulatory), and tonic. It is used extensively as a fragrance component in cosmetics, perfumes and especially soaps due to its excellent tenacity. Aromatherapists recommend it as an oil to diffuse during flu epidemics. Its action against viral illnesses and bacteria–coupled with the attractive smell–make it a great oil to use to disinfect a room.

Palmarosa oil is a dermal irritant. Avoid use if pregnant.

Patchouli – (Pogostemon Cablin)

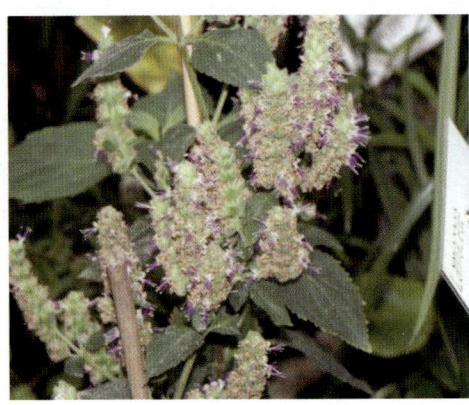

Patchouli oil is recognized by aromatherapists as being effective for combating nervous disorders, helping with dandruff, sores, skin irritations and acne. The specific properties include use as an antidepressant, anti-inflammatory, anti-emetic, antimicrobal, antiphlogistic, antiseptic, antitoxic, antiviral, aphrodisiac, astringent, bactericidal, carminative, deodorant, digestive, diuretic, febrifuge, fungicidal, nerving, prophylactic, stimulating and tonic agent. In the perfumery industry, it is interesting to note that patchouli improves with age, and that the aged product is what is preferred over freshly harvested. In aromatherapy, patchouli is an excellent fixative that can help extend other, more expensive oils.

Cautions: None known

Pepper Black - (Piper Nigrum)

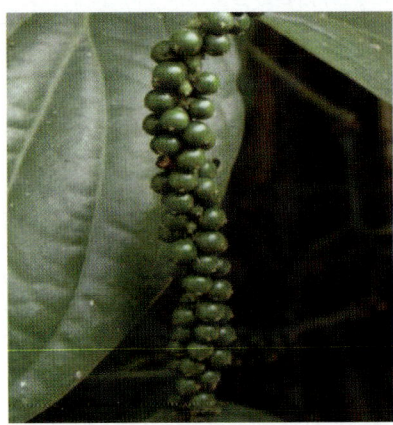

Black pepper oil can be used in the treatment for pain relief, rheumatism, chills, flu, colds, increase circulation, exhaustion, muscular aches, physical and emotional coldness, nerve tonic, and fevers. The therapeutic properties include the following: analgesic, antiseptic, anti-spasmodic, anti-toxic, aphrodisiac, digestive, diuretic, febrifuge, laxative, rubefacient, tonic (especially of the spleen).

Black pepper oil may cause irritation to sensitive skins and using too much could over-stimulate the kidneys and should be avoided in pregnancy due to its possible skin sensitizing effect.

PEPPERMINT - (MENTHA ARVENSIS)

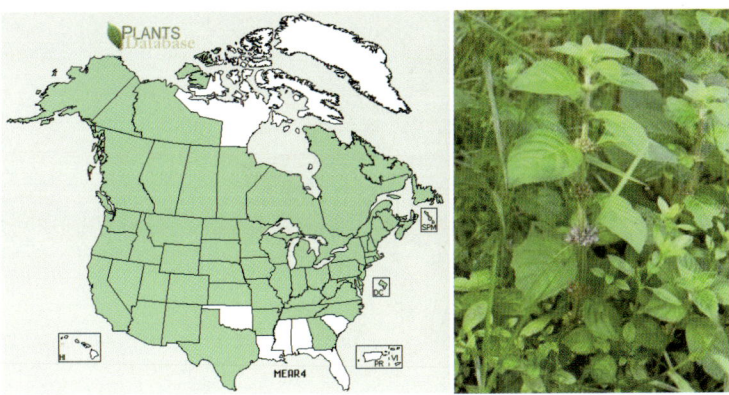

Peppermint oil has long been credited as being useful in combating stomach ailments. It is also viewed as an antispasmodic and antimicrobial agent. Of course, most people will associate it with being a flavoring or scenting agent in foods, beverages, skin and hair care products (where it has a cooling effect by constricting capillaries and helping with bruises and sore joints), as well as soaps and candles.

Peppermint oil can be sensitizing due to the menthol content. Avoid use during pregnancy.

PEPPERMINT - (MENTHA PIPERITA)

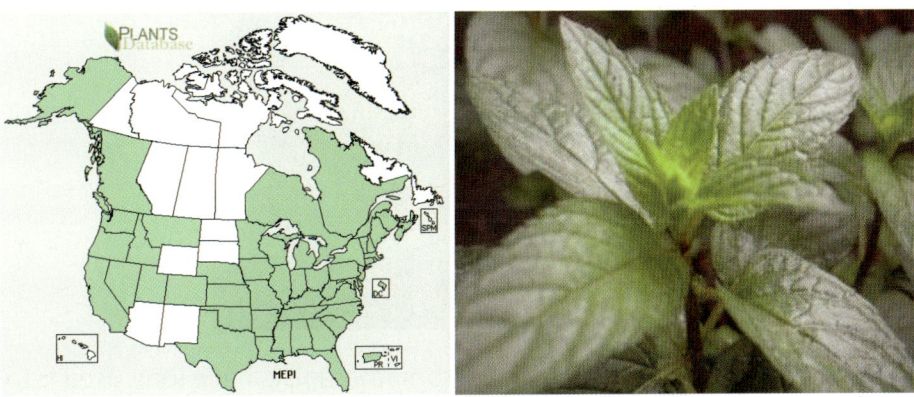

Peppermint oil is widely credited with being a digestive aid. Peppermint leaves contain menthol, which is a proven aid to digestion. The familiar aroma of mentha piperita is known for both its warming and cooling properties. Friendly to the sinuses, peppermint is also useful to the muscular system, especially for women during monthly cycles or menopause. Properties include being refreshing, a mental stimulant and energizing. It relieves bad breath and is a good nerve tonic that helps with mental fatigue and nervous stress.

Peppermint oil should be used well diluted since high concentration can cause a burning sensation and sensitization. Avoid use during pregnancy.

PERU BALSAM - *(MYROXYLON PEREIRA)*

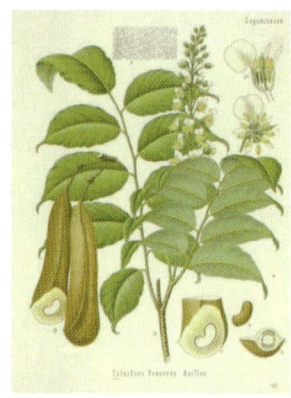

Peru balsam oil has been used by aromatherapists for bronchitis, chapped skin, colds, coughing, eczema, the flu, poor circulation, rashes, sensitive skin, and nervous and stress disorders. It is also believed to promote growth of epithelial cells.

Peru oil may cause skin sensitization in some. Avoid use during pregnancy.

PETITGRAIN - *(PETITGRAIN BIGARDE)*

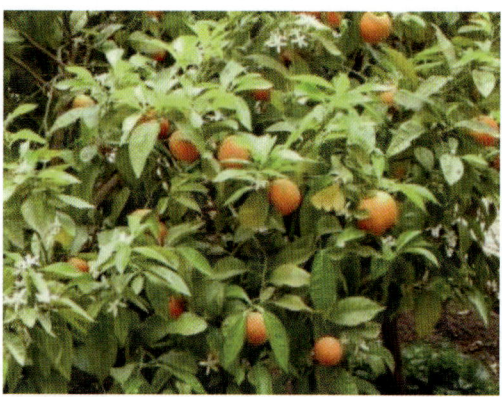

Petitgrain oil is believed to have uplifting properties. Aromatherapists have long used it to calm anger and stress, while it has been used in the skin care industry for acne, oily skin, and as a deodorizing agent.

Petitgrain oil is generally non-toxic, non-irritant, and non-sensitizing. Avoid use during pregnancy.

PINE SCOTCH - *(PINUS SYLVESTRIS)*

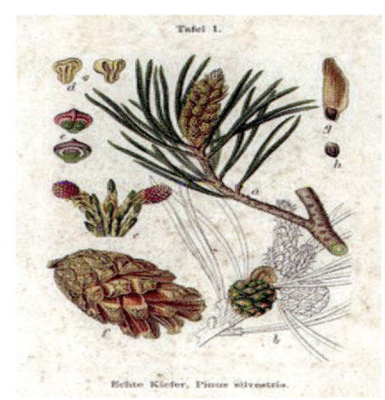

Pine scotch oil is viewed as an analgesic, antibacterial, antibiotic, anti fungal, antiseptic, and as an antiviral. Aromatherapists credit its use for arthritis, asthma, bladder infections, bronchitis, catarrh, cholagogue, as a circulatory agent, for colds, convalescence, coughs, cuts, cystitis, as a decongestant and deodorant. It has also been applied to eczema, those with laryngitis, lice, muscular aches, neuralgia, psoriasis, rheumatism, ringworm, scrapes, and sinusitis. Its versatility is well documented.

Although pine scotch oil is considered safe since it is non-toxic and non-irritant, it should still be used with care on the skin since it can cause irritation in high dosage and may sensitize the skin as well.

ROSE - *(ROSA DAMASCENE)*

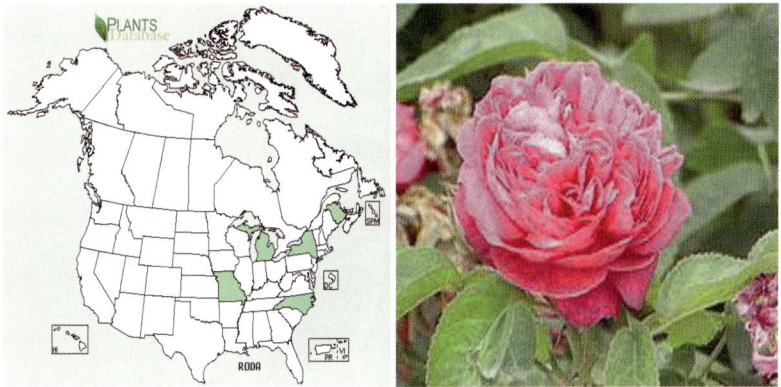

Rose oil is very common oil in the perfume and aromatic industry. Aromatherapists also credit it with being an exotic aphrodisiac, an emollient in skin care products, and a balancer of the spirit.

It is important to note that all absolutes are extremely concentrated by nature. They should not be evaluated in this state unless you are accustomed to the undiluted fragrance. For those trying Absolutes for the first time, we strongly recommend they be evaluated in dilution. Otherwise, the complexity of the fragrance–particularly the rare and exotic notes–becomes lost.

ROSEMARY - (ROSMARINUS OFFICINALIS)

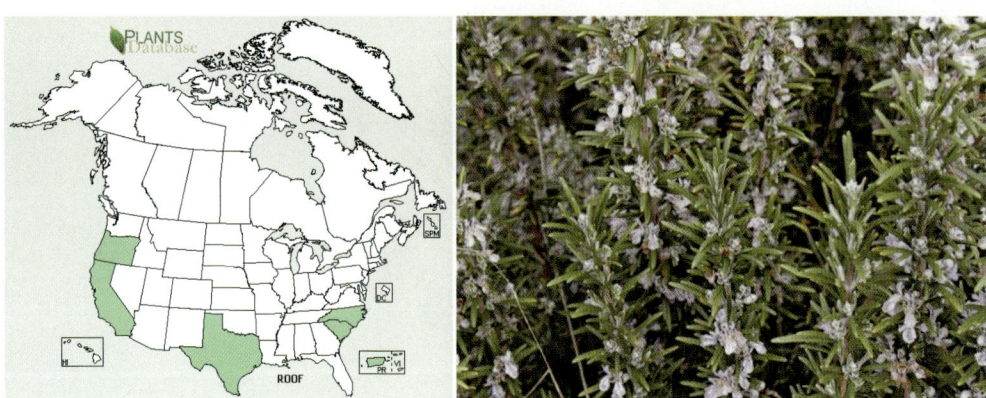

Rosemary oil stimulates cell renewal and improves dry or mature skin, easing lines and wrinkles. It can also clear acne, blemishes or dull dry skin by fighting bacteria and regulating oil secretions. It improves circulation and can reduce the appearance of broken capillaries and varicose veins. Rosemary oil helps to overcome mental fatigue and sluggishness by stimulating and strengthening the entire nervous system. It enhances mental clarity while aiding alertness and concentration. Rosemary oil can help you cope with stressful conditions and see things from a clearer perspective.

Rosemary oil is generally non-toxic and non-sensitizing. It is not suitable for people with epilepsy or high blood pressure. Avoid in pregnancy since it is an emmenagogue.

ROSEWOOD - (ANIBA ROSAEODORA)

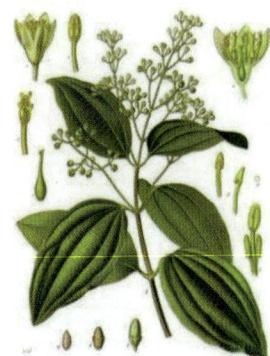

Rosewood oil is credited with being a bactericidal, anti-fungal, antiviral, anti-parasitic cellular stimulant, immune system stimulant, tissue regenerator, tonic, antidepressant, antimicrobial, and as an aphrodisiac. It is also regarded as a general balancer to the emotions. Rosewood oil is rich in linalool, a chemical which can be transformed into a number of derivatives of value to the flavor and fragrance industries. Avoid use in pregnancy. It is a possible irritant to sensitive skin.

SANDALWOOD - *(SANTALUM ALBUM)*

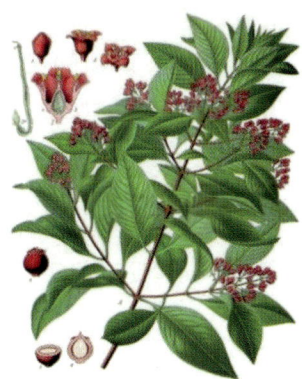

Sandalwood oil is used by aromatherapists to combat bronchitis, chapped and dry skin, depression, laryngitis, leucorrhea, oily skin, scars, sensitive skin, stress, and stretch marks. It also has historical applications as an aid in meditation for religious ceremonies. Sandalwood oil is believed to create an exotic, sensual mood with a reputation as an aphrodisiac. It also has extensive uses in the perfume industry as a fixative, and use in body care products for the fragrance it provides.

Sandalwood oil is considered a non-toxic, non-irritant, and non-sensitizing oil.

SPEARMINT - *(MENTHA SPICATA)*

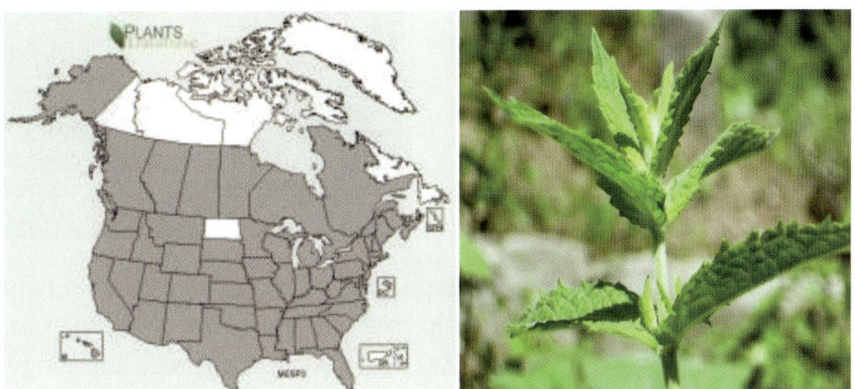

Aromatherapists claim the therapeutic properties of spearmint oil are: as a local/topical anesthetic, antispasmodic, astringent, carminative, decongestant, digestive, diuretic, expectorant, stimulant, and restorative. It is also believed to be an uplifting oil, great for alleviating fatigue and depression.

Spearmint oil may irritate mucous membranes. Avoid use during pregnancy.

Spikenard - *(Nardastachus Jatamansi)*

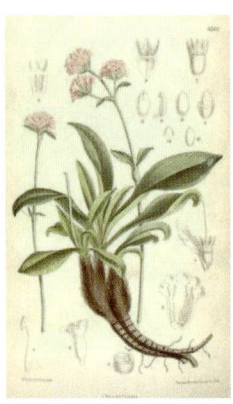

Spikenard oil is used by aromatherapists for rashes, wrinkles, cuts, insomnia, migraines, and wounds.

Spikenard oil should be avoided during pregnancy.

Tangerine - *(Citrus Reticulata var Tangerina)*

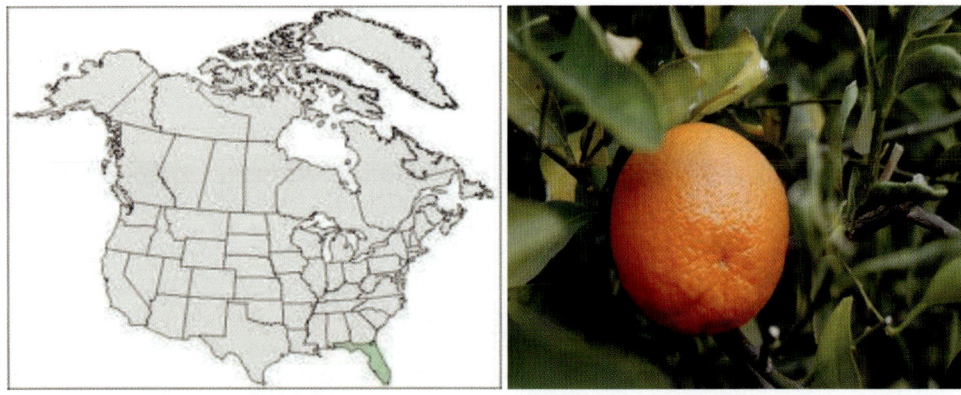

Tangerine oil, like most of the citrus family, can be depended upon for its refreshing and rejuvenating characteristics. Its aroma clears the mind and can help to eliminate emotional confusion. Aromatherapists also consider it to be very comforting, soothing and warming. Users may also see tangerine oil used in perfumes, soaps, and as an antispasmodic, carminative, digestive, diuretic, sedative, stimulant (digestive and lymphatic), and tonic.

Tangerine oil is similar to other essential oils in the citrus family in that it can be photo-toxic. Care should be taken not to expose the skin to sunlight after a treatment. Similarly, the oil should be diluted well before use on the skin. Avoid use during pregnancy.

TEA TREE - *(MELALEUCA ALTERNIFOLIA)*

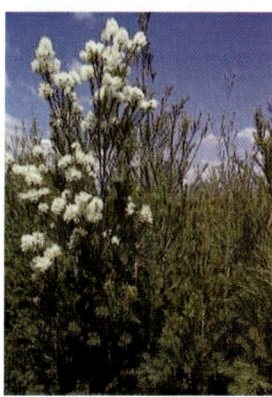

Tea tree oil is best known as a very powerful immune stimulant. It can help to fight all three categories of infectious organisms (bacteria, fungi, and viruses), and there is evidence that tea tree oil massages prior to an operation may help to fortify the body and reduce post-operative shock. Used in vapor therapy, tea tree oil can help with colds, measles, sinusitis, and viral infections. For skin and hair, tea tree has been used to combat acne, oily skin, head lice, and dandruff. As essential oils have become more accepted by the public, the use of tea tree has increased significantly. This can be readily evidenced by the commercial products now using tea tree oil.

Tea tree oil may cause dermal sensitization in some people. Do not take internally.

THYME - *(THYMUS VULGARIS)*

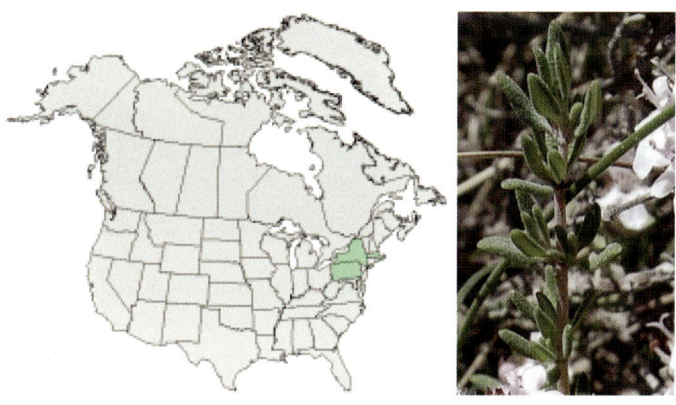

Red thyme oil has been used effectively as a bactericide, antiseptic, antimicrobial, astringent, antispasmodic, antitoxic, diuretic, antifungal, insecticide, tonic, and as an immune stimulant. Thyme oil can assist with nervous complaints, respiratory problems, poor circulation and problems of the digestive system. Red thyme oil should be avoided during pregnancy, or if a history of high blood pressure exists. Thyme contains a high amount of toxic phenols (carvacrol and thymol) that can irritate mucus membranes, cause skin irritation and skin sensitization.

VANILLA - (VANILLA PLANIFOLIA)

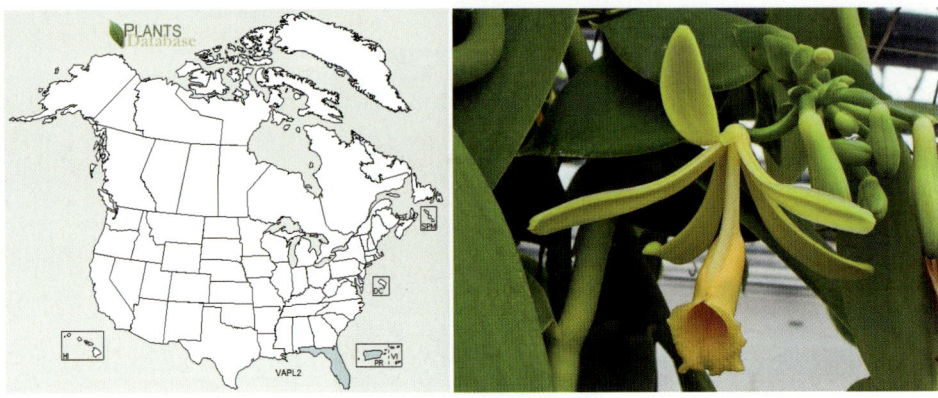

Vanilla oil is considered a premiere sensual aphrodisiac and one of the most popular flavors/aromas. It is comforting and relaxing and is also an ingredient in oriental type perfumes.

There is no known toxicity. Avoid high concentration in pregnancy. This product contains vanillin that will change the color in soaps and body care products. Avoid very high concentrations in skin care. It is not suitable for candle use. It is recommended that this oil be stored in dark amber, blue, or green glass bottles since it has been found to dissolve aluminum bottles.

VETIVER - (VETIVERIA ZIZANOIDES)

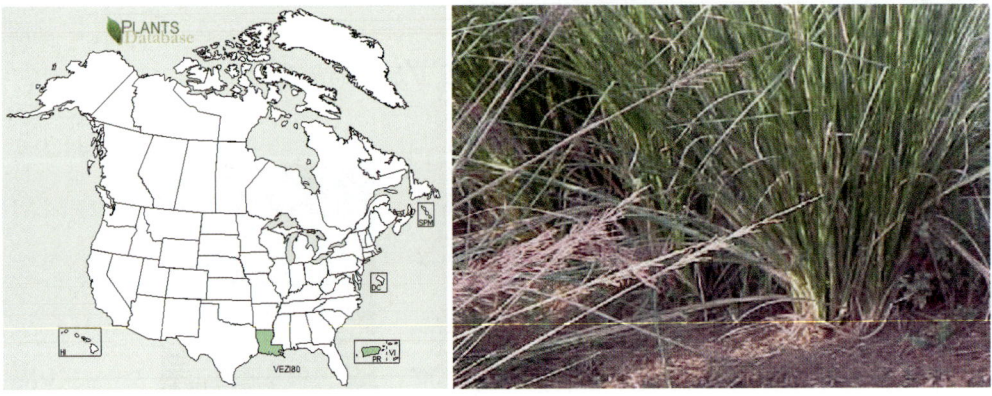

Vetiver oil is said to be deeply relaxing and comforting. It is used as a base note in perfumery and aromatherapy applications.

There is no known toxicity. Avoid high concentration in pregnancy.

WINTERGREEN - (GAULTHERIA PROCUMBENS)

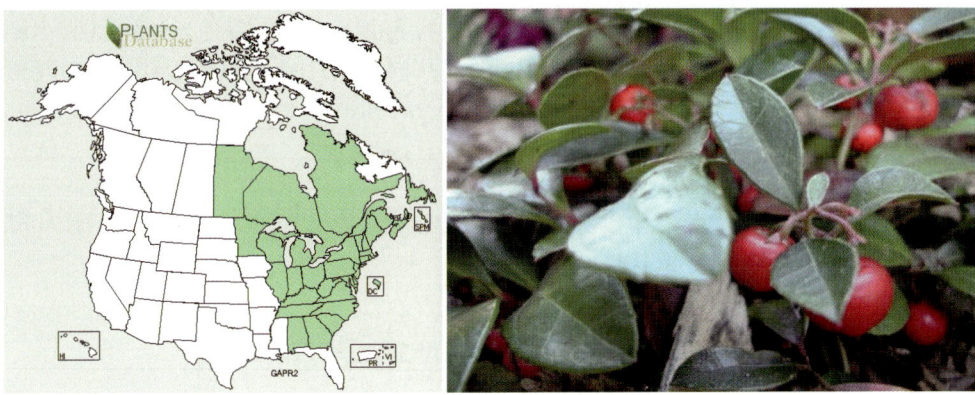

Wintergreen oil has a history of use as a pain reliever. It is also believed to increase the speed of healing for skin disorders, and when added to lotions, acts as a natural moisturizer.

Avoid use if pregnant. Safety in young children, nursing women, or those with severe liver or kidney disease is not known.

Yarrow – (Achillea Millefolium)

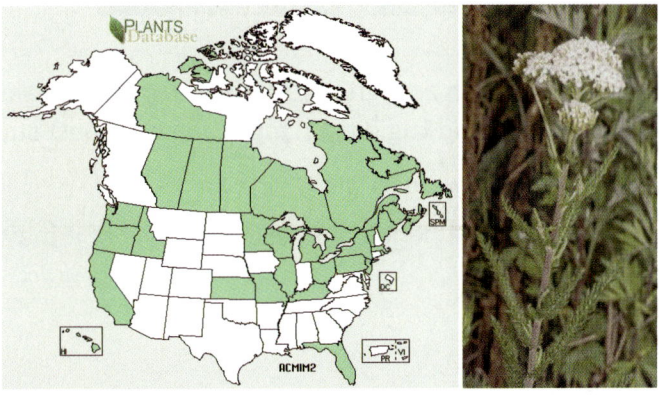

The Latin name achillea refers to the Greek hero Achilles. With this plant, Achilles cured the wounds of his warriors after he had been attended to the blood stopping properties of yarrow. The name millefolium refers to the leaves, mille means thousand and folium means leaves. Yarrow also has fever decreasing properties and was used before instead of quinine. According to the herbalist Vogel, described in a document from 1794, Indian tribes used yarrow to treat incised wound. The Micmacs used it to stimulate transpiration by fever and cold.

Yarrow is a very useful medicinal herb. The juice or dried powder can be applied to bleeding wounds. A strong tea may be taken for internal bleeding. Its anti-inflammatory action will reduce swelling and heal inflamed cuts or wounds. Internally, yarrow acts as a soothing relaxant on the voluntary nervous system. It counteracts cramps and spasm of the stomach, abdomen and uterine system. At the same time, its bitter principles support the digestive system by acting on the gallbladder and liver. Yarrow also supports the urinary system and is an effective anti-inflammatory and diuretic in cases of urinary infections, such as cystitis. It is an excellent women's herb that can bring on delayed menstruation, soothe painful periods and menstrual cramps and reduce excessive bleeding. The fresh juice is recommended as a tonic. Yarrow improves peripheral circulation by dilating the blood vessels. It is indicated for high blood pressure and angina pectoris. It is also one of the best herbs to induce a cooling sweat to reduce fevers. It can also be used for inner cleansing, e.g. prior to a sauna or sweat lodge. Yarrow's overall cleansing and toning properties, combined with its anti-inflammatory action may explain its use in the treatment of rheumatism. Yarrow can be described as a tonic and alterative that over time will improve the overall function of all the main bodily systems, as well as being of excellent service in the treatment of acute problems.

Caution: Some individuals are sensitive to yarrow and may develop allergic reactions with exposure.

YLANG YLANG - (CANANGA ODORATA)

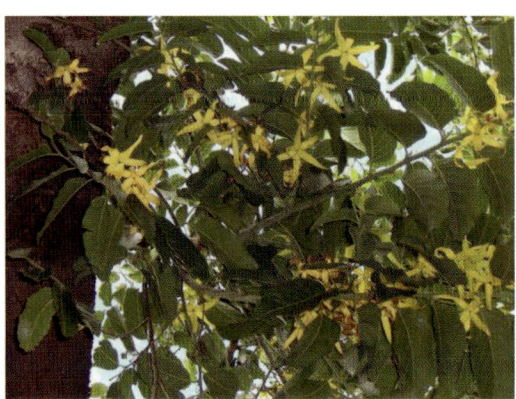

Ylang-ylang oil can assist with problems such as high blood pressure, rapid breathing and heartbeat, nervous conditions, as well as impotence and frigidity. Ylang-ylang oil is best suited for use in the perfumery and skincare industries.

Ylang-ylang oil can cause sensitivity on some people and excessive use of it may lead to headaches and nausea.

EVENING PRIMROSE OIL

Evening primrose oil comes from the seeds of the evening primrose plant. Similar to borage oil, which is discussed elsewhere in this book, evening primrose oil's main ingredient is gamma linolenic acid, a type of fatty acid that the body changes to prostaglandin E1 (PGE1), a hormone-like substance that is important for several chemical processes.

Evening primrose oil has been used mostly to treat diabetes and skin conditions such as itching, redness, eczema, and dry skin. Evening primrose oil also acts as an anti-inflammatory and may be useful in treating conditions such as rheumatoid arthritis. Some studies have shown that evening primrose oil may help reduce cholesterol levels in the blood and cause some cancerous tumors to shrink, but further research into these claims is warranted.

How much evening primrose oil should I take? Because evening primrose oil is not an essential nutrient, recommended intake levels have not been decided. However, most researchers have used between 3,000 and 6,000 milligrams of evening primrose oil in clinical trials, which translates to approximately 270 milligrams to 540 milligrams of gamma linolenic acid.

What forms of evening primrose oil are available? The primary source of evening primrose oil is as a dietary supplement (usually a capsule or extract), which is derived from the seeds of the evening primrose plant. For the body to convert evening primrose into PGE1, several other nutrients are needed, including magnesium, zinc, vitamin C, and vitamin B_6. As a result, some health care providers recommend that these nutrients be taken in with evening primrose oil for optimal health and well-being.

What can happen if I take too much evening primrose oil? Are there any interactions I should be aware of? What precautions should I take? Some studies have shown that evening primrose oil can bring about the symptoms of temporal lobe epilepsy. Patients taking medications for epileptic seizures should talk with their health care provider before taking evening primrose supplements. In addition, it may interfere with the activity of tamoxifen, a well-known breast cancer drug. As always, make sure to speak with a licensed health care provider before taking evening primrose oil or any other herbal remedy or dietary supplement.

FISH OIL

Fish oil is derived from fatty types of fish such as salmon and mackerel. The two main parts of fish oil are eicosapentaenoic acid (EPA) and docosahexaenoic acid (DHA), a pair of omega-3 fatty acids. Both help lower levels of blood triglycerides and may stop the development of atherosclerosis.

EPA and DHA are connected with several other health benefits as well. They can help treat inflammatory conditions such as Crohn's disease and rheumatoid arthritis; are very important in the creation of prostaglandins (which help dilate blood vessels); and may be useful in the treatment of schizophrenia. EPA and DHA also improve the functioning of the immune system. Animal studies have shown that fish oil can prevent some types of cancer in animals, but these results have not been copied in humans.

How much fish oil should I take? Healthy people who frequently eat fatty fish usually do not need to take fish oil supplements. Most researchers who have studied EPA and DHA have used dosages equal to 10 grams of fish oil per day. Some positive effects have been in studies that used larger amounts (up to 21 grams per day).

What forms of fish oil are available? Fish oil comes from oil fish such as mackerel, salmon, herring, sardines, cod, anchovies, and albacore tuna. The largest amounts of EPA and DHA are found in cod liver oil. The typical fish oil supplement contains 18 percent EPA and 12 percent DHA; more purified supplements contain higher amounts of DHA and EPA. Fish oil is available as a capsule, pill, or extract.

What can happen if I take too much fish oil? Are there any interactions I should be aware of? What precautions should I take? Taking more than 3 grams of fish oil per day for several months may increase blood sugar and cholesterol levels. As a result, patients with heart disease and diabetes should speak with a health care provider before taking fish oil supplements. Some research suggests that the increase in blood sugar levels may be decreased by taking vitamin E.

Fish oil may also interact with certain medications, including cyclosporine, pravastatin, and simvastatin. As always, make sure to speak with a licensed health care practitioner before taking fish oil or any other dietary supplement or herbal remedy.

FUMARIC ACID

Much like vitamin D, fumaric acid is formed by the body, in the skin, during exposure to sunlight. It is related to malic acid, and is involved in the making of energy derived from food.

The exact uses of fumaric acid remain unclear. However, evidence suggests the people with psoriasis may have a biochemical disorder that interferes with the body's ability to create enough fumaric acid. As a result, some health care providers recommend fumaric acid to help treat psoriasis and other skin conditions.

How much fumaric acid should I take? The amount of fumaric acid to be consumed depends on the individual being treated. Generally, patients should speak with a dermatologist before using fumaric acid to determine a correct dosage. Most practitioners recommend that patients take small amounts of a fumaric acid supplement (60-100 milligrams per day, orally or topically), with the dosage increasing slowly over several weeks until an effect is seen. Only esterified forms of fumaric should be used.

What forms of fumaric acid are available? Fumaric acid is produced naturally by the body. In addition, fumaric acid is available as a dietary supplement (to be consumed orally) and as a preparation (to be applied topically). As stated before, only esterified forms of fumaric acid should be used, and only after speaking with a dermatologist.

What can happen if I take too much fumaric acid? Are there any interactions I should be aware of? What precautions should I take? Taking large amounts of fumaric acid over a short period of time may result in kidney disorders. Other side effects connected with fumaric acid intake are gastrointestinal distress, irritation of the eyes and flushing of the skin; some small studies have shown that extended use of fumaric acid may lower a person's white blood count, possibly making them more at risk to infection.

As of this writing, there are no well-known drug interactions connected with fumaric acid. As always, make sure to speak with a licensed health care provider before taking fumaric acid or any other herbal remedy or dietary supplement.

GLA – (Gamma-Linolenic Acid)

Gamma-linolenic acid, or GLA, is a type of fatty acid that comes from two main sources: It can be formed in the body from other fatty acids, or it can be derived from the oils of certain plants such as black currant and evening primrose. In fact, evening primrose oil is often marketed as gamma-linolenic acid.

In the body, GLA is used in the production of hormone-like substances called prostaglandins, which are believed to be involved in several metabolic processes, including regulation of the immune system. Laboratory studies have suggested that GLA can shrink the size of cancerous tumors and cause "subjective" improvement in people with cancer, although a difference of opinion has been raised about the results of these studies. GLA has also been suggested as a remedy for a variety of conditions, including arthritis, skin problems, high blood pressure, and premenstrual syndrome.

How much gamma-linolenic acid should I take? As of this writing, the optimal daily intake of gamma-linolenic acid is unknown. Many trials often use dosages of 3,000 to 6,000 milligrams of evening primrose oil, which roughly translates to 270 milligrams to 540 milligrams of GLA.

What forms of gamma-linolenic acid are available? Evening primrose oil (which contains sizable amounts of gamma-linolenic acid) is available primary in supplement form, as is black currant oil. GLA supplements are available in liquid and capsule form; an injectible form is also being studied in Europe. Several substances, in addition to GLA, are necessary for the body to make prostaglandins. As a result, some researchers suggest that people take supplements of magnesium, zinc, vitamin C, vitamin B_3, and vitamin B_6 along with GLA or evening primrose oil.

What can happen if I take too much gamma-linolenic acid? Are there any interactions I should be aware of? What precautions should I take? While gamma-linolenic acid does not appear to be toxic, there have been reports that it can worsen the symptoms of temporal lobe epilepsy. People who use anticonvulsant medications should not take it. Long-term use of GLA may lead to blood clots or decreased immune function. As always, make sure to speak with a licensed health care provider before taking gamma-linolenic acid or any other dietary supplement or herbal remedy.

Glucomannan

Glucomannan is a water-soluble dietary fiber derived from the konjac root, a Japanese plant. The plant is cleaned, and the fiber is purified before being used as a supplement.

The main uses of glucomannan are to promote larger stools and improve digestion. Studies conducted on individuals suffering from constipation have shown that glucomannan supplementation helps produce a bowel movement within 12 to 24 hours. Glucomannan also delays the emptying of stomach contents, which allows for a more steady absorption of dietary sugar, and can bring down blood sugar levels. As a result, some scientists believe that glucomannan can be used to help treat diabetes and related conditions.

Because glucomannan is a soluble fiber, it can bind to certain acids created in the stomach and remove them from the body. In this way, it can help lower blood cholesterol and blood lipid levels. Controlled studies have shown that glucomannan can reduce levels of total blood cholesterol, LDL ("bad") cholesterol, and triglycerides, and may even raise levels of HDL ("good") cholesterol. Glucomannan may also help promote weight loss.

How much glucomannan should I take? The amount of glucomannan to be consumed depends on the condition being treated.

A basic guide for glucomannan supplementation is as follows:

Laxative: 3-4 grams per day
Lowering blood cholesterol: 4-13 grams per day

Controlling blood sugar: 500-700 milligrams per 100 calories in one's daily diet
Weight loss: 1-3 grams before each meal

It is also recommended that patients drink at least eight ounces of water each time they consume any bulk-forming laxative such as glucomannan.

What forms of glucomannan are available? Glucomannan is available as a bulk powder and as a type of capsule. It is not known if any foods contain large amounts of glucomannan.

What can happen if I take too much glucomannan? Are there any interactions I should be aware of? What precautions should I take? Because glucomannan expands rapidly, patients with any disorder of the esophagus should avoid taking glucomannan or any other fiber supplement in pill form. Supplementing with glucomannan may also result in flatulence and abdominal discomfort, especially in people not used to a high-fiber diet. There is also evidence that some people may have an allergic reaction to glucommanan powder. If an allergic reaction occurs, discontinue use.

As of this writing, there are no well-known drug interactions associated with glucomannan. As always, make sure to speak with a licensed health care provider before taking glucomannan or any other herbal remedy or dietary supplement.

GRAPE SEED EXTRACT

Grape seed extract is a nutrient that belongs to the bioflavonoid family. It is derived from the seeds and skin of grapes, which can be green, red, or purple in color.

The active ingredients contained in grape seed extract are believed to act as antioxidants; studies have shown that grape seed extract supplements can raise the amount of antioxidants in the blood dramatically. These antioxidants can neutralize substances called free radicals, and may reduce (or prevent) much of the damage they cause.

Grape seed extract has proven to be valuable in the treatment of poor blood flow in the capillaries and veins; small studies have produced increased capillary strength using as little as 50 milligrams per day, and increased venous blood flow using 150 milligrams per day. Other studies have shown that it improves the aspects of vision in healthy people, including the prevention of age-related macular degeneration and the effects of glare from bright lights.

How much grape seed extract should I take? There is currently no recommended daily allowance (RDA) for grape seed extract. However, an intake of between 50-100 milligrams of grape seed extract is suggested for the prevention of heart disease and circulatory problems; larger doses may be used to treat specific illnesses.

What forms of grape seed extract are available? Grape seed extract can be found either alone or in combination with other nutrients as part of a multivitamin, multiherbal supplement. It can also be found in herbal extracts, capsules, or tablets.

What can happen if I take too much grape seed extract? Are there any interactions I should be aware of? What precautions should I take? Flavonoids in general, and the flavonoids associated with grape seeds, are considered free of side effects. Since they are water-soluble, any excess levels of grape seed extract that are not absorbed by the body are excreted via sweat or urine. However, women who are pregnant or breastfeeding should avoid grape seed extract supplements. As of this writing, there are no known drug interactions with grape seed extract. As always, make sure to speak with a licensed health care provider before taking grape seed extract or any other dietary supplement or herbal remedy.

GRAPEFRUIT SEED EXTRACT

Grapefruit seed extract (GSE), also known as citrus seed extract, is a liquid derived from the seeds, pulp, and white membranes of grapefruit. Self-made natural GSE processed in the laboratory without solvents or synthetic agents is prepared by grinding the grapefruit seed and juiceless pulp, then mixing with glycerin. Commercially available GSE sold to consumers is made from the seed, pulp, glycerin, and synthetic preservatives all blended together. Grapefruit seed extract is sold as a food supplement and used in cosmetics because it is a claimed natural antimicrobial.

An early proponent was Dr. Jacob Harich (1919–1996). A long time promoter of GSE was Aubrey Hampton, the founder of Aubrey Organics. Some marketers of GSE affirm this extract to be a safe, natural, and an effective preservative. This extract has been stated by some practitioners of alternative medicine to possess antibacterial, antiviral, and antifungal properties. It has been recommended by some nutritionists for the treatment of candidiasis, earache, throat infections, and diarrhea.

Grapefruit seed extract, or sometimes called citrus seed extract in some parts of the world, is a liquid extracted from the pulp and seeds of the grapefruit. GSE is commonly consumed as a supplement and used in cosmetics because of its antimicrobial effect. It is generally considered a safe and natural supplement and has become a staple in the artillery of many alternative medicine doctors. It is claimed that grapefruit seed extract contains a natural antimicrobial agent, benzethonium chloride, commonly included in many sore throat medications. This claim has not been conclusively proven, however, and much more studies must be conducted to determine this. Below you will find a much bigger summary of grapefruit seed extract, where and how it is used, and much much more. This information has been written by people, just like you, who had great success with using grapefruit seed extract, this information is not meant to be a medical advice; you must always consult your doctor before starting to take any supplement.

Nature has bestowed us with everything that will help us lead a life free of diseases and disorders. One such thing is grapefruit seed extract. Grapefruit seed extract has many medicinal properties that have been proven very beneficial in fighting various infections, viruses, and harmful germs. It is highly beneficial to the immune system, as it helps in the preservation of the intestinal bacteria that help fight the disease causing germs.

Medicinal properties are highly useful for general well-being. The immune levels of the body increase and help keep away various diseases and infections, such as, candida, sinusitis, and giardiasis just to state a few. Grapefruit extract creams can be applied on all parts of the body to help and maintain the texture and glow of the skin. The liquid can be used as a facial cleanser. The diluted extract can be massaged gently to cleanse all impurities and acne. It is very effective for minor skin problems. Applying the diluted solution on affected areas twice a day can cure the irritation. You can mix some into your shampoo and massage it into your scalp and you can use it to strengthen your nails. It is a very handy solution in the kitchen as well. It is used to wash vegetables, fruits, meat, and poultry. Clean cutting boards, toothbrushes, and all kinds of utensils with it to disinfect them.

Treatments for the following include:

Candida/Yeast Infection Treatment - One of the most common causes of yeast infections is following antibiotic treatment. What prolonged antibiotic usage does is effectively reduce the population of bacterial organisms, both good and parasitic, causing an imbalance of fungi bacteria ratio. Candida infections result in many health conditions, certain ones being more characteristic than others. Common clinical features demonstrated by candida infections include spontaneous fatigue, loss of mental clarity, vaginal discharge or balanitis (swelling [inflammation] of the foreskin and head of the penis) in men.

In recent years, the efficacy of grapefruit seed extract has been studied, with positive results. To begin, grapefruit seed extract was found to be equi-potent to many synthetic antibiotics available to man. The amazing this, about this however, is the fact that it is virtually absent of the ill effects associated with today's antibiotic usage. Candida infections are however fungal in origin, not bacterial, so you might be wondering how this comes into play. Grapefruit seed extract is also a fungicidal agent.

After reviewing many stool samples that were sent to Dr. Data lab, all the test results that were reviewed as bad had one thing in common, all the pathology found was determined to respond to grapefruit seed extract therapy.

The usual starting dose of grapefruit seed extract is around 10 drops taken twice daily in water or selected fruit juices, between meal times. This is done for the first three days, following which the dose is increased to 15 drops twice daily, for a further 7 days. Following this period, until completion the dose is increased to 15 drops three times daily, with a complete clearance of symptoms within the 28 day period. It is very scarce to see a patient requiring continued treatment, but owing to the safe nature of GSE, it may be used for up to 4 to 6 months to eradicate stubborn infections. Because of the bitter taste of GSE liquid extract, overdosing is a rare occurrence, and is one of the primary reasons persons switch to the capsule form instead. Conversion of liquid to capsules is roughly 10 drops to 1 capsule, so if a simple change of dosage from increases patient compliance, by all means try it.

A Natural Antiseptic - To disinfect, simply add ten drops of the liquid extract to visibly clear water, agitate for a short period, then let stand for a couple more minutes. If consuming river water, as much as 25 drops may be needed, once prior filtration has been done.

Natural Alkalinizing Agent - Grapefruit seed extract contains high levels of vitamin C, E, and bioflavonoids, which are considered strong antioxidants and knockout free radicals that damage cells and cause diseased states.

Treats Gingivitis or Bleeding Gums - The logic behind this one is simple, gingivitis is a diseased state of the gum line resulting in inflammation and soreness. Now, the cause of this is bacterial in origin, so GSE's anti-microbial effect is a viable option to combat this problem. Bleeding gums commonly result from a deficiency of vitamin C, so in addition to preventing the foul odour that bleeding gums exude, it is loaded with the vitamin to help improve this condition.

Treatment of Thrush - Thrush is a fungal infection, commonly affecting newborns and persons with immuno-compromised systems. Grapefruit seed extract, apart from possessing immune system bolstering vitamin C.

HMB – (Hydroxyl-Beta-Methylbultyrate)

HMB is short for hydroxyl-beta-methylbultyrate. It is a derivative of leucine, an essential amino acid, and is present in some foods.

Research suggests that HMB plays a role in the making of proteins, including the protein used to build new muscle tissue. A study published in 1996 showed that weightlifters who took three grams of HMB per day showed greater gains in muscle mass and strength over a seven-week period compared to people who took no supplements. However, other studies have shown that HMB does not contribute to increased athletic performance or changes in body composition.

In addition to muscle tissue, evidence suggests that HMB can help contribute to the loss of body fat and control weight. Further studies need to be performed to verify these results, however.

How much HMB should I take? The amount of HMB to be taken depends on the condition being treated. Most studies that have examined the usefulness of HMB have used doses of three grams per day, usually in combination with exercise. Other studies have used weight-specific doses of HMB, in the amount of 17 milligrams per pound of body weight per day.

What forms of HMB are available? Small amounts of HMB are present in some foods, mainly alfalfa and catfish. HMB is also produced in the body as a derivative of the amino acid leucine. In addition, HMB supplements are available at many health food stores, usually as capsules or tablets.

What can happen if I take too much HMB? Are there any interactions I should be aware of? What precautions should I take? As of this writing, there are no known side effects linked with HMB, nor are there any well-known drug interactions. As always, make sure to speak with a licensed health care provider before taking HMB or any other herbal remedy or dietary supplement.

Hydroxycitric Acid

Hydroxycitric acid (HCA) is a chemical compound found in the garcinia cambogia, a small, pumpkin-shaped fruit native to Southeast Asia. The garcinia (also known as the malabar tamarind) is often used as a condiment in curry dishes.

Animal studies suggest that HCA may aid in weight loss. Laboratory studies have shown that HCA reduces the change of excess carbohydrates into fat by preventing certain enzymatic processes from taking place.

HCA also appears to curb appetite and appears to work better on subjects that have high simple-sugar diets as opposed to high-fiber diets. However, the majority of these studies have been carried out in animals. Similar trials in humans have yet to produce definitive results. As a result, the effectiveness of HCA for weight loss remains unclear as of this writing.

How much hydroxycitric acid should I take? Because HCA is not an essential nutrient, the best possible levels and recommended daily allowances have yet to be decided. While some practitioners recommend taking 500 milligrams three times per day (before each meal) to help promote weight loss, this amount is far below that used in clinical animal studies on a pound-for-pound basis.

What forms of hydroxycitric acid are available? HCA is found only in a few plants, the chief of these being garcinia cambogia. Large amounts of HCA are found in the plant's rind. In addition to garcinia, HCA supplements are available in a variety of forms, including powders, capsules, tablets, energy bars, and chewing gum.

What can happen if I take too much hydroxycitric acid? Are there any interactions I should be aware of? What precautions should I take? HCA use has not been linked to any unpleasant effects. High-fiber diets appear to inhibit the absorption of hydroxycitric acid into the body; as a result, people who are on high-fiber diets and are attempting to lose weight may require larger daily HCA supplements. As of this writing, there are no known drug interactions with HCA. As always, make sure to speak with a licensed health care provider before taking hydroxycitric acid or any other dietary supplement or herbal remedy.

INDOLE – (INDOLE-3-CARBINOL)

Indole (also known as indole-3-carbinol) is a chemical found in leafy green vegetables that belong to the cabbage family. It is a member of a group of chemicals called glucosinates and is created whenever cruciferous vegetables are crushed or cooked.

Indole is a powerful antioxidant. It is believed to be responsible for reducing the risk of cancer in people who eat large amounts of broccoli, cabbage, cauliflower, and kale. In animal studies, indole appears to be especially effective against breast and cervical cancers because of its ability to increase the body's breakdown of estrogen. However, until future studies are completed on humans, some researchers have recommended that indole be taken as a dietary supplement only with extreme caution.

How much indole should I take? The amount of indole to be consumed depends on the condition being treated. Most animal studies examining the role of indole in breast cancer have used dosages ranging from 300 milligrams to 400 milligrams per day. Because indole is not an essential nutrient, recommended daily allowances have yet to be established.

What forms of indole are available? Indole is available in a variety of cruciferous vegetables, such as kale, cauliflower, and cabbage. It is available in its highest concentration in broccoli. In addition, indole is available as a dietary supplement and can be found at many health food stores.

What can happen if I take too much indole? Are there any interactions I should be aware of? What precautions should I take? As of this writing, there are no known side effects associated with taking indole, nor are there any known drug interactions connected with indole. Because few studies have been carried out on humans, some researchers have recommended that indole be taken as a dietary supplement only under the supervision of a health care provider. As always, make sure to speak with a licensed health care provider before taking indole or any other herbal remedy or dietary supplement.

INSOLUBLE FIBER

Fiber is divided into two general categories–water soluble and water insoluble. This section will discuss insoluble fiber. Insoluble fiber is a subclass of dietary fiber and is considered "insoluble" because its main components do not readily dissolve in water and are not metabolized by intestinal bacteria. The main ingredients in insoluble fiber are cellulose, hemicellulose, and lignans, which form the structural parts of plants.

Insoluble fiber plays a very important role in digestion. It absorbs water in the intestines and enlarges and softens a person's stools, helping to ease elimination of waste. There is also evidence that insoluble fiber helps to protect people from heart disease and colon cancer; scientists have put forward ideas that the main components of insoluble fiber bind to carcinogens, which are then carried from the body along with the fiber as waste products. Dietary fiber gained from fruits and vegetables is believed to have the most protective effects.

How much insoluble fiber should I take? The amount of fiber in the average Western diet is about 10 grams per day. However, many scientists suggest that people should eat between 40 and 60 grams of a combination of soluble and insoluble fiber daily.

What forms of insoluble fiber are available? High levels of insoluble fiber are found in whole grains, especially brown rice. Bran and other wheat products also have high levels of insoluble fiber. Beans, many fruits, psyllium, and some vegetables contain large amounts of both soluble and insoluble fiber. Insoluble fiber can also be bought as a supplement, usually in powder form.

What can happen if I take too much insoluble fiber? Are there any interactions I should be aware of? What precautions should I take? Because insoluble fiber absorbs water in the intestines, high fluid intake is also required. Some insoluble fibers, such as bran, may reduce the absorption of calcium into the body. Therefore, patients with low calcium levels should speak with a health care provider before taking large amounts of fiber. People diagnosed with scleroderma should also consult a health care provider before taking fiber supplements or beginning a diet high in fiber. In addition, certain medications, such as Lovastatin, Verapamil, and Propoxyphene, may interact with fiber supplements. As always, make sure to speak with a licensed health care provider before taking soluble fiber or any other herbal remedy or dietary supplement.

IPRIFLAVONE

Ipriflavone is a type of flavonoid (a water-soluble plant pigment) that is derived from daidzein, a compound found in soy. Research has shown that it is a very important element that not only helps the body absorb calcium into the bones, but helps prevent those bones from breaking down.

Long-term use of ipriflavone has shown to be safe and successful in stopping bone loss in women who have gone through menopause or who have had their ovaries removed. A 1998 study of women with low bone density showed that compared to a placebo, women given a combination of calcium and ipriflavone had higher vertebral bone density rates. Double-blind studies carried out primarily in elderly women have also confirmed that ipriflavone is effective in improving bone density and reducing the occurrence of fractures and bone-related pain in people with osteoporosis.

How much ipriflavone should I take? For people with low bone density, most practitioners will suggest 200 milligrams of an ipriflavone supplement taken three times per day. Taking the same overall amount of ipriflavone in different doses (i.e., 300 milligrams twice daily) has been shown to be just as helpful.

What forms of ipriflavone are available? Ipriflavone is present in some foods but only in trace amounts. However, ipriflavone is also available as a dietary supplement and can be found in tablet, capsule, and liquid forms.

What can happen if I take too much ipriflavone? Are there any interactions I should be aware of? What precautions should I take? Two small studies have shown that long-term use of ipriflavone may result in a major reduction in lymphocytes (white blood cells), which could increase the risk of infection in some persons. In both studies, white blood cell levels returned to normal after stopping the use of ipriflavone, but only after an extended period of time. As a result, women who take ipriflavone should have their white blood cell levels checked regularly by their health care provider. Patients with severe kidney disease should take lower levels of ipriflavone than those without kidney disease. Some forms of estrogen therapy may increase the need for ipriflavone. Patients taking medications such as Cenestin, conjugated estrogens, esterified estrogens, Estratab, Menest, or Premarin should speak with their health care provider about the effect these drugs can have with ipriflavone. As always, make sure to speak with a licensed health care provider before taking ipriflavone or any other herbal remedy or dietary supplement.

LACTASE

Lactase is a naturally occurring enzyme located in the small intestines. Its function is to digest lactose, the naturally occurring sugar in milk. People who do not produce enough lactase have an impaired ability to digest milk (especially cow milk) and may be diagnosed as being lactose intolerant. Approximately 20 percent of the adult population in the United States is lactose intolerant.

Lactase supplements are usually taken to treat the symptoms of lactose intolerance, such as diarrhea, indigestion, heartburn, and irritable bowel syndrome.

How much lactase should I take? Because lactase is a naturally occurring substance produced by the body, little research has been conducted into the exact amount a lactase-individual should take. In addition, the degree of lactose intolerance can vary widely between people, so larger amounts may be needed by some people to improve the symptoms of lactose intolerance.

What forms of lactase are available? Lactase drops are available at some nutrition stores and from health care providers. They are often added to milk about 24 hours before drinking to remove levels of lactose in the milk. People directly before a meal that contains dairy products or other items high in lactose can also take lactase capsules and tablets orally. The amount of lactase to be taken depends on the individual's intolerance to lactose and the amount of lactose-containing foods to be eaten.

What can happen if I take too much lactase? Are there any interactions I should be aware of? What precautions should I take? Because the body produces it, lactase is considered extremely safe. As of this writing, no known side effects or drug interactions have been noted with lactase supplementation. As always, make sure to speak with a licensed health care provider before taking lactase or any other dietary supplement or herbal remedy.

LECITHIN

Lecithin belongs to a category of fat-soluble substances called phospholipids, which are important parts of cellular membranes.

Lecithin is produced by the liver and is needed by the body to not only create cell membranes, but to transport nutrients into cells and keep the membranes permeable. Without lecithin, the membranes would harden and in time stop working.

Lecithin is composed mostly of phosphoric acid, choline, linoleic acid, vitamin B_8, and several other B vitamins. The choline in lecithin is used to make acetylcholine, a neurotransmitter that is necessary for the brain to function normally, especially in infants. In addition to its natural uses, lecithin is used commercially for items that require emulsifiers (substances that blend fats with water). It acts as a protective covering for many substances and helps keep items in certain processed foods from separating.

Studies have shown that lecithin may be useful in treating a range of neurological disorders, ranging from multiple sclerosis to memory loss. Animal studies have shown that female rats given lecithin have produced offspring with better memory and learning skills. These studies have not been copied in humans. Other research suggests that lecithin can prevent the buildup of fats in the liver and stop gallstones from forming.

How much lecithin should I take? While there are no recommended daily allowances for lecithin, some researchers have suggested a daily supplement of 550 milligrams for men and 425 milligrams for women. Most people receive enough amount of lecithin through their diet.

What forms of lecithin are available? Many animal and plant-based foods contain good amounts of lecithin, including egg yolks (soft, not hard), soybeans (non GMO), liver, peanuts, and oatmeal. Lecithin is also available as a supplement. To boost its absorption, researchers recommend that it be taken with meals.

What can happen if I take too much lecithin? Are there any interactions I should be aware of? What precautions should I take? High doses of lecithin can produce side effects such as nausea, vomiting, and diarrhea. In addition, because lecithin can increase levels of acetylcholine, it should not be taken by people who suffer from bipolar disorder. High levels of acetylcholine can worsen the condition of people in the depressive phase of bipolar disorder. As of this writing, there are no known drug interactions with lecithin. As always, make sure to speak with a licensed health care provider before taking lecithin or any other herbal remedy or dietary supplement.

LIPASE

Lipase is one of three categories of enzymes made by the pancreas. In addition to pancreatic lipase, there is also gastric lipase (produced by the stomach), pharyngeal lipase (produced by the salivary glands), and hepatic lipase (produced by the liver).

Each lipase has different properties. Gastric and pharyngeal lipases, for instance, have lower molecular weights and greater pH stability than pancreatic lipase. Gastric lipase metabolizes food molecules within the stomach and intestine, while pharyngeal lipase breaks down molecules in the mouth and esophagus.

Lipases are used by the body to help in the digestion of fats by breaking them down into free fatty acids and monoglycerides. They can also be used to treat digestive problems and conditions that may cause a person to have trouble absorbing nutrients. Some practitioners believe pancreatic enzyme supplements can treat autoimmune disorders, inflammations, and some food allergies.

How much lipase should I take? Most people already produce plenty of pancreatic lipase. However, to aid in the digestion of fats, some practitioners suggest taking 1-2 capsules of 6,000 LUs (lipase units) before meals.

What are some good sources of lipase? Lipase is made by the body and does not come from one's diet. However, people can take lipase supplements and other pancreatic enzymes, which are available in capsule and tablet form. Before taking any supplements, however, be sure to consult with a certified health professional.

What can happen if I do not get enough lipase? Some people are unable to make certain types of lipase, which can hold back the absorption of some nutrients. Damage to the pancreas or liver can also reduce the production of certain lipases. In these situations, lipase and other enzyme supplements are recommended.

What can happen if I take too much? No side effects or toxicology has been reported in patients taking lipase supplements and other pancreatic enzyme supplements.

LUTEIN

Lutein is a yellow-colored pigment that belongs to the carotenoids family. In humans, it is found in the eyes, in the central area of the retina called the macula, where a person's visual alertness is most sharp.

Lutein reduces age-related macular degeneration and helps filter out damaging light. One study carried out in 1994 found that adults with the highest dietary intake of lutein had a 57% decreased risk of macular degeneration compared to people with the lowest intake. A similar trial conducted in 1992 found a link between intake of lutein and an increased risk of cataracts.

Lutein also functions as an antioxidant. Unreliable evidence suggests it helps protect skin cells against ultraviolet radiation and may fight several forms of cancer, including those that affect the colon, rectum, breast, lungs, and prostate.

How much lutein should I take? People whose eyes appear to be better protected from macular degeneration have taken a minimum of 6milligrams per day. Many practitioners recommend that lutein supplements be taken with food to improve absorption.

What are some good sources of lutein? What forms are available?

Black currant	Kale	Romaine lettuce
Collard greens	Leeks	Spinach
Egg yolks	Peas	

In addition to food sources, lutein is also available as a dietary supplement in capsule or tablet form.

What can happen if I do not get enough lutein? What can happen if I take too much? Are there any side effects I should be aware of? Deficiency and toxicity levels have yet to be established for lutein; however, studies show that people who eat more lutein-containing foods are at a decreased risk of macular degeneration. No unpleasant effects from lutein have been reported; there is currently no evidence of drug interactions with lutein.

LYCOPENE

Lycopene is a substance belonging to the carotenid family. Carotenes are a brightly colored group of fat-soluble plant pigments that display antioxidant properties, which help fight cellular damage in humans. Lycopene is red, which helps give tomatoes their distinctive color.

Many studies have shown lycopene to be effective in fighting certain forms of cancer. A 1995 study by researchers at Harvard University found that men who consumed greater amounts of lycopene had a much lesser chance of developing prostate cancer than those who consumed lesser amounts. Other beginning studies have found that lycopene may offer protection against cancers of the pancreas, colon, rectum, esophagus, oral cavity, breast, and cervix. In Europe, researchers have found a link between lycopene intake and a reduced risk of cardiovascular disease. Lycopene supplements have also improved immune function in the elderly.

How much lycopene should I take? While the Food and Drug Administration has yet to develop a suggested daily allowance for lycopene, the Harvard study showed that men who had the greatest protection against cancer consumed at least 6.5milligrams per day (or ate at least 10 servings of tomato-based foods per week).

What are some good sources of lycopene? What forms are available? Tomatoes and tomato-based foods (such as tomato paste, tomato soup, and tomato juice and pasta sauce) are the best sources of lycopene. Other foods that contain lycopene are watermelon, pink grapefruit, and guava. Lycopene supplements are also available in capsule and tablet form.

What can happen if I do not get enough lycopene? What can happen if I take too much? Are there any side effects I should be aware of? To date, no studies have been carried out on the subject of lycopene deficiency or overdose. At the time of this writing, no adverse effects have been reported concerning the use of lycopene, and no evidence of any drug interactions with lycopene has been reported.

Malic Acid

Malic acid is a naturally forming type of acid, which is produced both in the human body and in some foods. It plays an important role in the way the body produces adenosine triphosphate, a very important source of energy.

Malic acid is also used as a flavoring and is often blended with other acids, sugars, and seasonings to create new tastes in foods and beverages.

Research has suggested that malic acid helps to improve the body's energy production. Some studies have shown that a combination of malic acid supplements and magnesium may help people with fibromyalgia by reducing pain levels and increasing endurance levels. Researchers also believe that malic acid supplements can treat many hypoxia (oxygen-deficient) related conditions, such as respiratory and circulatory problems, and chronic fatigue syndrome. Few studies have been conducted in these areas, however.

How much malic acid should I take? Because malic acid is created naturally in the body, most people do not need to take malic acid supplements. Most studies of malic acid have used supplements ranging from 1,200 to 2,400 milligrams, usually at the same times as magnesium.

What forms of malic acid are available? Malic acid is found in a wide variety of fruits and vegetables. The highest amounts of malic acid are found in apples. As a result, malic acid is sometimes referred to as "apple acid." Malic acid is also available as a dietary supplement.

What can happen if I take too much malic acid? Are there any interactions I should be aware of? What precautions should I take? As of this writing, there are no known side effects or drug interactions that result from taking malic acid. As always, however, make sure to speak with a licensed health care provider before taking malic acid or any other herbal remedy or dietary supplement.

Mannose

Mannose is a simple sugar that is structurally related to glucose. The body absorbs it much slower than glucose; however, when ingested, it is not converted to glycogen or stored in the liver, but rather continues directly into the bloodstream as a source of energy.

While the body metabolizes small amounts of mannose, the greater part of mannose consumed is excreted by the body through urine. Evidence suggests that the E. coli bacteria can attach to mannose molecules, helping to remove it from the body. As a result, some practitioners may recommend mannose to help treat or prevent urinary tract infections. Mannose is also used in veterinary medicine to treat bacterial infections in animals and to detect the presence of salmonella bacteria in animal feed.

How much mannose should I take? To help treat urinary infections, some practitioners recommend 1 teaspoon of mannose, dissolved in water or juice and taken every 2-3 hours.

What forms of mannose are available? Mannose occurs naturally in a variety of fruits, including apples, blueberries, cranberries, oranges, and peaches. It is also available as a dietary supplement, usually as a liquid extract.

What can happen if I take too much mannose? Are there any interactions I should be aware of? What precautions should I take? Test-tube studies have suggested that consuming large doses of mannose may cause birth defects. Although the risk of birth defects resulting from mannose is considered extremely small, pregnant women should nevertheless consult with a licensed health care provider before taking mannose supplements. As of this writing, there are no well-known drug interactions associated with mannose. As always, make sure to speak with a licensed health care provider before taking mannose or any other herbal remedy or dietary supplement.

MEDICINAL HERBS OF THE BIBLE

The Biblical Medicinal Herbs of the Bible was written by Dr. James Duke and his wife Peggy Duke in 1983. With Dr. Duke's written permission to utilize, the following herbs have originated from that source.

Born in Birmingham, Alabama, in 1929, James A. "Jim" Duke is a Phi Beta Kappa PhD (botany, 1961) graduate of the University of North Carolina. Jim, following military service, undertook postdoctoral activities at Washington University and Missouri Botanical Garden in St. Louis, Missouri. There he began studies of neotropical ethnobotany, his overriding interest to this day. From 1963 to 1965, Duke was ecologist with the USDA (Beltsville, Maryland), joining Battelle Columbus Laboratories (1965-71) for ecological and ethnobotanical studies in Panama and Colombia. During this formative period, Duke lived with various ethnic groups, closely observing their deep dependence on forest products. The first of some twenty books, his *Isthmian Ethnobotanical Dictionary* catalogs hundreds of Isthmian plants and their uses. Rejoining USDA in 1971, Duke had assignments relating to crop diversification, medicinal plants, and energy plant studies in developing countries. A popular lecturer on the subjects of ethnobotany, herbs, medicinal plants, and new crops and their ecology, he has taped dozens of TV and radio shows. There is a good biographic sketch in the Sep./Oct. 1991 issue of *EastWest* magazine. The National Agriculture Library has a video history of Dr. Duke's career and development. Duke grows dozens of interesting plants on his six-acre farmette (Herbal Vineyard) with his wife and illustrator, Peggy. On September 30, 1995, he retired after 30 years with the USDA. Before retiring, Dr. Duke brought his Father Nature's Farmacy database online at USDA. It is now, in Duke's retirement, one of the most frequently-consulted databases with the Plant Genome Project at USDA.

Duke has already doubled the data content in the interactive database he maintains as Director, Duke's Herbal Vineyard, Inc. The database is especially useful for determining biological activities and healing potentials of food ands herbs. Fluent in Spanish, Duke has studied and/or lectured widely, concentrating on tropical ecology, medical botany, and crop diversification. Widely travelled, Duke "cut his tropical eye teeth" in Panama where he was resident from 1966-68. While working on an encyclopedia of economic plants, he has collaborated with the National Cancer Institute on both their AIDS and cancer-screening programs and their Designer Food Program (to prevent cancer). His databases on the ecology, nutritional content, folk medicinal uses, and chemical constituents of economic plants are being widely utilized. Duke's major goal lately is to reverse the disdain for alternative medicines in the U.S., where, as in the Third World, a larger and larger percentage of the people can no longer afford first-world pharmaceuticals. Duke has a contagious interest in natural foods and nutritional approaches to preventive medicine. Between 1990 and 1992, Duke was advising the Designer Food Program of the NIH, then under the guidance of Dr. Herb Pierson.

With an total of more then five years in Latin America, Duke has traversed parts of Argentina, Belize, Bolivia, Brazil, Chile, Colombia, Costa Rica, Dominican Republic, Ecuador, Guadelupe, Guatemala, Honduras, Jamaica, Mexico, Panama, Peru, Puerto Rico, and Venezuela. In Asia, he has had lengthy visits in China, India, Indonesia, Pakistan, and quick looks at Burma, Japan, Laos and Vietnam. In the Middle East, he has worked in Iran, Israel, Kuwait, and Syria, with quick looks at the Mediterranean countries of Egypt, Greece, Italy, Portugal, and Spain. His only tours in tropical Africa include Madagascar, Sao Tome, The Ivory Coast, and Zambia. Recently he has been teaching field ethnobotany regularly in Amazonian Peru, Belize, and Costa Rica (mostly in the winter), and in the Maine northwoods (in summer only).

Jim belongs to the American Botanical Council (Trustee), American Herb Association (Life), American Society of Pharmacognosy, Association for Tropical Biology (Life), Council of Agricultural Science and Technology (Cornerstone Life Member), Herb Research Foundation (Advisor), International Association of

Plant Taxonomists (Life), International Society for Tropical Root Crops (Life), International Weed Science Society (Life), Organization for Tropical Studies (Life), Oriental Healing Arts Society (Honorary), Phi Beta Kappa, Sigma Xi, Smithsonian Institution (Collaborator), Society for Conservation Biology (Life), Society for Economic Botany (Life), Southern Appalachian Botanical Club (Life), and the Washington Academy of Sciences (Life).

Dr. Duke serves as a Senior Scientific Adviser to Nature's Herbs and is on the board of trustees of the American Botanical Council, Director, Botanical Products International (Hakalau Hawaii) and Microbotanica, the Scientific Advisory Team of Shaman Pharmaceuticals (San Francisco), Medical Advisory Board of Herbalife (Los Angeles), and serves as Medicinal Plant Adviser to Reader's Digest and Time-Life. He also serves as an advisor or unpaid consultant to ACEER (Amazon Center for Environmental Education and Research), Alternative Medicine Digest, American Health, the Center for Alternative Medicine in Women's Health (NY), Center for Mind-Body Medicine, Center for Plant Conservation, Herb Research Foundation, International Expeditions, National College of Phytotherapy, Rodale Press, Rheumatology Unit (NIH); Supplements/ Dietary Advisory Board (NIH, Bethesda MD), Rosenthal Center for Alternative/Complementary Medicine, TRAMIL, and the World Health Organization (Traditional Medicine Program). He is CEO of a newly formed consulting firm, Duke's Herbal Vineyard Inc, where he is writing the newsletter, *News from the Herbal Village*, and raising several specimen herbs for analysis and study. Routinely queried by editors and writers for several different popular and scientific health-oriented journals, and by producers of radio and television networks, both conservative and liberal, Duke recently has given accredited continuing education lectures on herbal medicine, pros and cons, to chiropractors, nurses, nurse practitioners, pharmacists, and physicians.

In addition to scores of popular and scientific articles, Duke has published several pertinent books:

1. *Handbook of Legumes of World Economic Importance*, Plenum Press, New York, 345 pp., 1981
2. *Medicinal Plants of the Bible*, Trado-Medic Books, Buffalo, New York, 233 pp., 1981
3. *CRC Handbook of Medicinal Herbs*, CRC Press, Inc., Boca Raton, Florida, 704 pp., 1985
4. *Culinary Herbs: A Potpourri*, Trado-Medic Books, Buffalo, New York, 195 pp., 1985
5. *Medicinal Plants of China* (with E. Ayensu), Reference Publications, Algonac, Michigan, 2 vols., 705 pp., 1985
6. *CRC Handbook of Proximate Analysis Tables of Higher Plants* (with A. Atchley), CRC Press, Inc., Boca Raton, Florida, 389 pp., 1986
7. *Isthmian Ethnobotanical Dictionary*, 3rd edition, Scientific Publishers, Jodhpur, India, 205 pp., 1986
8. *Handbook of Northeastern Indian Medicinal Plants*, Quarterman Press, Lincoln, Massachusetts, 212 pp., 1986
9. *Living Liqueurs*, Quarterman Press, Lincoln, Massachusetts, 110 pp., 1987
10. *CRC Handbook of Agricultural Energy Potential for Developing Countries* (with A. Atchley, K. Ackerson, and P. Duke), CRC Press, Inc., Boca Raton, Florida, 4 vols., 1063 pp., 1987
11. *CRC Handbook of Nuts*, CRC Press, Inc., Boca Raton, Florida, 343 pp., 1989
12. *Field Guide to Medicinal Plants*, Houghton-Miflin, Boston MA, 366 pp, 1990
13. *Ginseng, a Concise Handbook*, Reference Publications, Algonac, Michigan, 273 pp., 1990
14. *CRC Handbook of Edible Weeds*, CRC Press, Inc., Boca Raton, Florida, 1992
15. *CRC Handbook (and Database) of Phytochemical Constituents of GRAS Herbs and Other Economic Plants*, 654 pp., 1992 and the *CRC Handbook (and Database) of Biological Activities of Phytochemicals* (1992)

16. **CRC Handbook of Alternative Cash Crops**, (J. A. Duke and J. L. duCellier), CRC Press, Inc., Boca Raton, Florida, 536 pp., 1993
17. **Amazonian Ethnobotanical Dictionary** in 1994
18. **CRC Handbook of Aromathematics**
19. **Green Pharmacy**, Rodale Press, Green Pharmacy for Rodale Press
20. **Synergy in Phytomedicines**, Synergetic Press
21. **Second edition to the CRC Handbook of Medicinal Herbs**

Currently Dr. Duke is retired from the USDA. Dr. Duke is a regular or occasional contributor or editorial adviser to such periodicals as:

Alternative Medicine Digest	The Environmentarian	Journal of Optimal Nutrition
American Health	HerbalGram	Journal or Aromatherapy
Business of Herbs	Herbs for Health	Mind-Body Connection
Complementary Medicine for the Physician	The International Permaculture Species Yearbook	Natural Health
Diversity	The Journal of Alternative & Complementary Medicine	Organic Gardening
Economic Botany		News from the Herbal Village
		Wild Foods Forum

African Myrrh – (Commiphora Africana)

...out of the ground made the Lord God to grow every tree that is pleasant to the sight, and good for food; ...there is bdellium...

Genesis 2

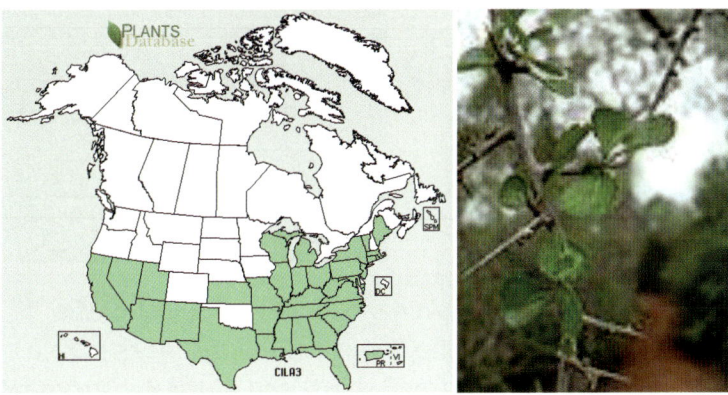

African myrrh is the tree which provides the aromatic gum known as bdellium, and grows in the territory east of Persia. When the bark is incised, the gum that oozes out is "the bigness of a white olive." Gum removed from the bark of the tree would soon harden, become transparent and waxlike, and resemble pearl. In Tabore and Ugugo, Africa, the gum, melted with butter, is applied as a perfume. The women of Egypt carried pouches filled with bdellium, for a delightful perfume. In West Africa the resin is used as an insecticide believed to repel termites. The wood is used for beads, the stems as a chewstick.

Bdellium is a folk cancer remedy for indurations of the liver and sinews, tumors of the spleen, polyps, carcinomata, and scirrhus. In tropical Africa the resinous exudate is sometimes applied as a plaster for fever and spasms. Washed bark mixed with salt is used for snakebite. Pound leaves with millet are taken with milk as a stomachic. Ronga used the remedy for stomach troubles. The plant is regarded as a stomachic and collyrium. West Africans hold their face over the steaming pot for eye inflammations.

ALEPPO PINE – (PINUS HALEPENSIS)
...as for the stork, the fir trees are her house...Psalm 104

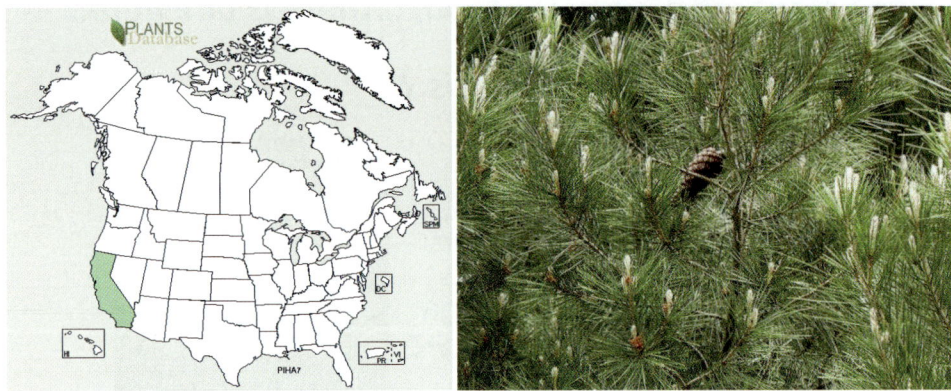

Source of Greek turpentine, the aleppo "pine" is a handsome tree. Most of the "fir tree" references in the Bible are now believed to refer to the aleppo pine, pinus halepensis. As the Bible tells us, the timber was quite useful, for construction (doors, homes, rafters, ships) and musical instruments. The tree is also used for tanning.

The myriad uses of "turpentine" from any species of pine might as well accrue to pinus halepensis turpentine as well. "Turpentine" is loosely defined as the oleoresin obtained from longleaf and slash pines and other pines that yield exclusively terpene oils or the essential oil obtained from the oleoresin. Turpentine from one species or another has been used for catarrh, cough, dysuria, dyschezia, gonorrhea, leucorrhea, and rheumatism. Unquestionably turpentine has antiseptic, counterirritant, and rubefacient properties, and it is apparently also allergenic and tumorigenic, causing albuminuria, coma, cough, erythema, hematuria, headache, insomnia, nausea, and urticaria. Rosin from various pine species has been used for abscesses, boils, and cancers. Pine tar has been used in expectorant cough syrups for bronchitis, catarrh, colds, etc. Rosin has also been used for skin diseases like psoriasis, ringworm, and toothache. In Russia, steroids have been extracted from pine pulps. In Dioscorides day, the seeds were used for cough, the cones for stomach ailments. Algerians use pitch from aleppo pine for hemorrhoids and skin ailments. North Africans apply the powdered bark on wounds as an astringent. Seeds mixed with honey (taken first thing in the morning) spermatogenic."

ALMOND – (PRUNUS DULCIS)

...and carry down the man a present, a little balm, a little honey, spices, and myrrh, nuts, and almonds...Genesis 43

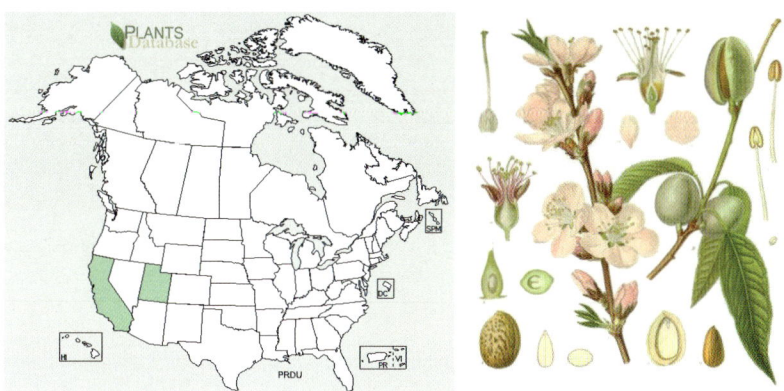

It has been inferred that almond did not grow naturally in Egypt, since Jacob's sons took almonds to Joseph. Nowadays the almond is widespread in the Holy Landand is one of the earliest trees to flower. Almonds are cultivated for the nuts used in candies, baked products, and confectioneries, and for the oils obtained from the kernels. Oil used as a flavoring agent in baked goods, perfumery, and medicines. Much valued in the orient because it furnished very pleasant oil. In Tuscany, almond branches are used as divining rods to locate hidden treasure. To this day modern English Jews carry branches of flowering almonds into the synagogue on spring festival days. There is the legendary story of Charlemagne's troops' spears (almond) sprouting in the ground overnight and shading the tents the next day. Almonds are also valued for their ornamental flowers, one of the first tree flowers in the Palestinian spring. Because of their association with spring, the almond flower is also associated with life after death or immortality.

Considered alterative, astringent, carminative, cyanogenetic, demulcent, discutient, diuretic, emollient, laxative, lithontryptic, nervine, sedative, stimulant and tonic, the almond is a component of folk remedies for asthma, cold, corn, coughs, dyspnea, eruptions, gingivitis, heartburn, internal ulcers, itch, lungs, prurigo, sclerosis (of spleen), skin, sore, spasm, stomatitis, and tumors (especially of the bladder). It is no surprise that the seeds and/or oil (containing amygdalin) are widely aclaimed as folk cancer remedies, for all sorts of cancers and tumors, calluses, condylomata, and corns. Lebanese extract the oil for skin trouble, including white patches on skin; used throughout the Middle East for an emollient; also for itch. Raw oil from the bitter variety is used for acne. Almond and honey was given for cough. Thin almond paste was added to wheat porridge to pass gravel or stone. It is believed by the Lebanese to restore virility. Iranians make an ointment from bitter almonds for furuncles. Ayurvedics consider the fruit, the seed and its oil aphrodisiac, using the oil for biliousness, headache, and the seed as a laxative. Unani use the seed for ascites, bronchitis, colic, cough, delirium, earache, gleet, hepatitis, headache, hydrophobia, inflammation, renitis, skin ailments, sore throat, and weak eyes.

The fruit contains the following minerals:

Aluminum	Iodine	Potassium
Boron	Iron	Silica
Calcium	Magnesium	Sodium
Chlorine	Manganese	Sulfur
Copper	Nitrogen	Zinc

The fruit contains the following amino acids

Alanine	Glutamate	Histidine
Arginine	Glycine	Isoleucine

Leucine	Proline	Tyrosine
Lysine	Serine	Valine
Methionine	Threonine	
Phenylalanine	Tryptophan	

The seed contains the following minerals:

Aluminum	Iron	Potassium
Calcium	Manganese	Sodium
Copper	Nitrogen	Zinc

ALOE – (SOCOTRINE ALOE)
...and brought a mixture of myrrh and aloes...John 19

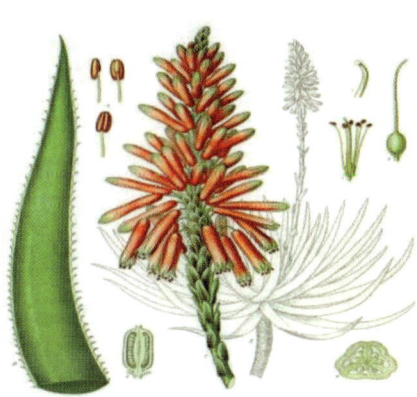

Brought by Nicodemus to embalm Jesus, aloes were also used as a purgative and emmenagogue. Malodorous and bitter, the drug is now used more as a horse medicine. It is still esteemed in the orient for its perfume and its cordial properties and widely used as a medicine for rheumatic complaints. Generally the aloes of the Old Testament are regarded to be aquitaria agallocha or santalum album, while aloes of the New Testament are believed to be aloe pmyi. Plant cultivated for the drug, socotrine, most valued of the commercial types of drug aloe; used as a laxative; milder and less irritating than other drug aloes. Known to the ancient Egyptians who used the inspissate juice as an embalming fluid. Because of its bitter odor, it is now used chiefly by veterinarians, but it could probably be used in all those ways that the more popular Barbados aloes are used. It contains about one-fourth as much aloe emodin as Curacao aloe. The leaves provide a violet dye, not requiring a mordant.

Aloes are popular in folk medicine. The drug is manufactured principally from the pulp of the fleshy leaves, although every part of the plant is purgative. This species is sometimes used in pills for cancer, condyloma, indurations, polyps and tumors (anus, eye, lips, mouth, nose, spleen, tongue). Aloe emodin is reported to have anticancer activity. The peeled gel is applied to inflamed eyes and on skin inflammations, burns, and sores. The pulp is taken internally for intestinal ailments, sore throat, and ulcers. Small doses of the fresh latex serve as a purgative. The emmenagogue socotrine aloe is used for intestinal ailments and as a vermifuge. Recently leaf extracts of aloe species have shown lectin like activity, markedly promoting growth of normal but not tumor cells and also promoting the healing of wounded cells.

APRICOT – (PRUNUS ARMENIACA)
...A word fitly spoken is like apples of gold in pictures of silver...Proverbs 25

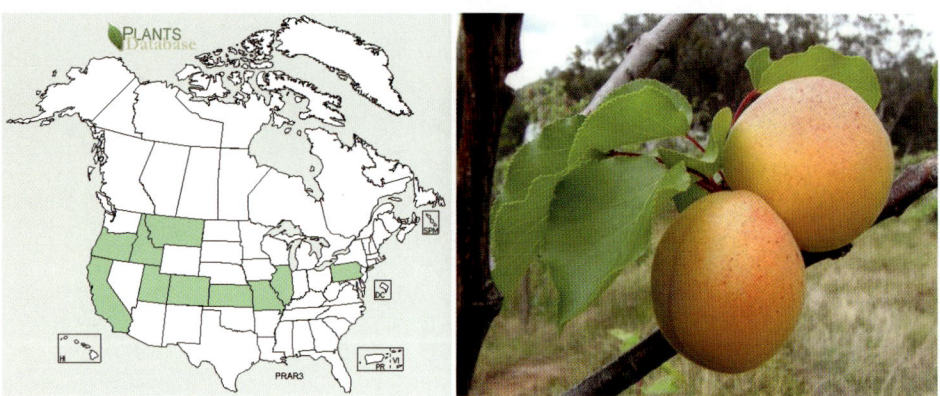

Apricots are cultivated for the fruit, eaten fresh out of hand, or dried, made into conserves or alcoholic beverages. Kernels produce sweet edible oil sometimes used as a substitute for almond oil. Chinese almonds are the seed kernels of several sweet varieties of apricot, used for almond cookies, eaten salted and blanched, or made into gruel or flour. Afghans also use the seeds as almonds. Bitter apricot kernel is highly toxic because of prussic acid present. Expressed oil, known as Persic oil or apricot oil, is used as a pharmaceutical vehicle; it is obtained by the same process as bitter almond oil. Pit shells have been used to prepare activated charcoal, via destructive distillation.

An apple a day keeps the doctor away. In Biblical days, Solomon said, "*Comfort me with apples for I am sick.*" Surely they didn't mean apricot pits in the Garden of Eden. It is the fruit of that forbidden tree whose mortal taste brought death into the world, and all our woe. The pits do contain laetrile like compounds which can cure or kill, depending on dosage.

Considered antidotal, antitussive, aphrodisiac, cyanogenetic, demulcent, emollient, expectorant, preventive, sedative, tonic, vermifuge, vulnerary, apricot is an element in folk medicines for anemia, asthma, bronchitis, catarrh, cold, constipation, cough, eyes, fertility (female), fever, heart, hemorrhage, inflammation, laryngitis, puerperium, rheumatism, spasm, swellings, thirst, and tumors. The fruit is said to be a folk remedy for cancer. Unani use the tonic seed for deafness, earache, hepatitis, pales and worms, the fruit for diarrhea, fever, and thirst. Medicinally, a paste which is obtained by crushing the kernel, is used for inflammation of the eyes, and is considered antispasmodic, demulcent, pectoral, sedative, vulnerary, and anthelmintic. After chewing the fruits, Tibetans apply them in ophthalmia. Ginger and licorice combined with kernels make a confection used as a tussic and expectorant remedy. Another concoction made by fermentation is used as a prophylactic and tonic. Decoction of kernels made into a beverage is used for cough, asthma and catarrhal ailments. Kernel juice is used for hemorrhages. In Chinese medicine, fruit of bitter almond is useful in heart disease. In Korea, the expectorant kernel is used to treat dry throat. POISON: A double kernel is said to be enough to kill a man. If eaten in excess, fruit is believed to harm the bones and muscles, to promote blindness and falling hair, to numb mental facilities, and to injure parturient women.

The fruit contains the following minerals:

Aluminum	Iodine	Potassium
Boron	Iron	Silica
Calcium	Magnesium	Sodium
Chlorine	Manganese	Sulfur
Copper	Nitrogen	Zinc

The seed contains the following minerals:

Aluminum	Iron	Potassium
Calcium	Manganese	Sodium
Copper	Nitrogen	Zinc

The fruit contains the following amino acids:

Alanine	Leucine	Threonine
Arginine	Lysine	Tryptophan
Glutamate	Methionine	Tyrosine
Glycine	Phenylalanine	Valine
Histidine	Proline	
Isoleucine	Serine	

BALSAM – (COMMIPHORA OPOBALSAMUM)
...they traded in thy market wheat of Minnith, and Pannag, and honey, and oil, and balm...Ezekiel 27

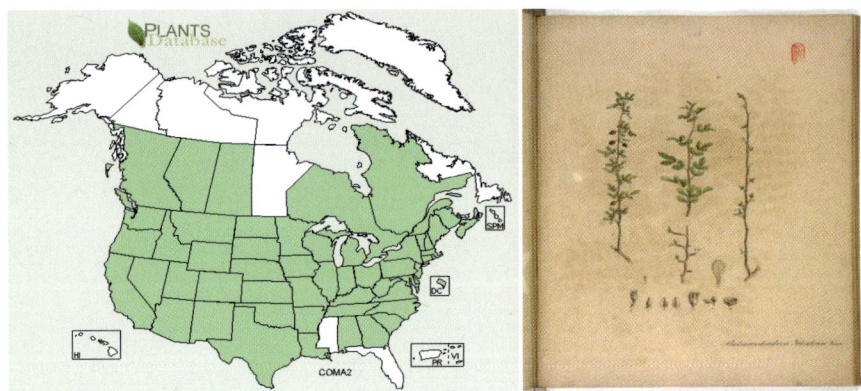

Balm is the gum or thickened juice oozing from the balsam tree that was very prolific in Judea. The balm was an emblem of Palestine, and shrubs in cultivation were protected by guards to keep them safe. The plant is much used in medicine. The tree, native to Yemen, was thought to have been introduced to Palestine by the Queen of Sheba on her famous visit to King Solomon. The species was later cultivated in Palestine, chiefly around Jericho, where it still existed at the time of the Roman conquest. The soldiers carried balm branches back to Rome as symbols of their victory over the Hebrews.

Regarded as astringent, carminative, demulcent, diaphoretic, digestive, diuretic, expectorant, stimulant, stomachic, sudorific, and vulnerary, the balm of Ezekiel is a folk remedy for cacoethes, gonorrhea, sclerosis, and urogenital ailments. Reportedly used for indurations of the liver, spleen and uterus, kidney, bladder, stomach, tumors of the rectum, vagina, carcinomata of the breast, morbid granulations, apostemes in the eye, and cancer of the gums and mouth. In Lebanon the dried fruits are eaten for stomach trouble and flu; the wood is burned to smoke lesions. Christians dissolved bits in wine as a digestive. The gum was poured over open wounds and apparently acted as an antiseptic and protective covering against secondary infections. In Isfahan, a few fruits are swallowed whole for colds and shivering.

BARLEY – (*HORDEUM VULGARE*)
...Let thistles grow instead of wheat, and cockle instead of barley...
Job 31

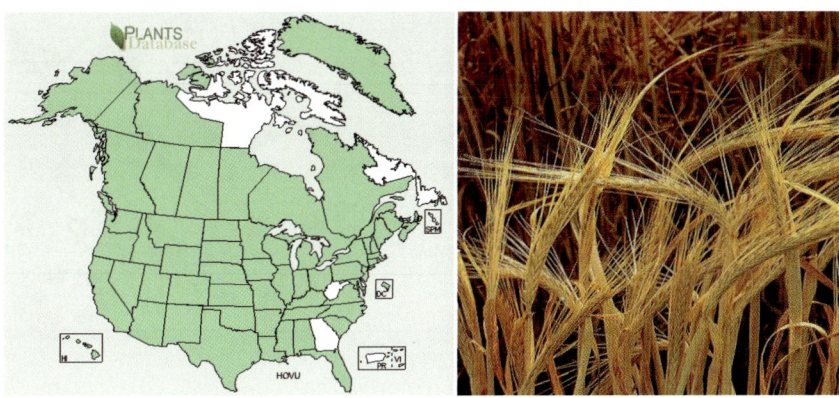

Jewish folklore calls them the "seven species," the barley, wheat, vines, figs, pomegranate, oil (olive), and honey (date) of Deuteronomy. Barley may be less important since the internal combustion engine replaced the horse, but stalks of the wild varieties, the valuable germplasm of the geneticists, still wave on the hills of Galilee and Judea, ancestors of the world's barley. Barley is the fourth most important cereal in the United States, but probably half of the production is used for livestock fodder, a quarter for the brewing industry (80% for beer, 14% distilled alcohol, 6% malt syrup). Winter barley furnishes nutritive pasturage without seriously reducing yields. In Europe, where climate is more temperate, spring forms predominate and are of high malting quality. In India, a cooling drink called sattu is made. Ashes of leaves used in Patna (India) in preparation of cooling sherbets. Ezekiel 4:9 and 12 puts down a recipe I have seen nowhere else. *"Take thou unto thee wheat, and barley, and beans, and lentiles, and millet, and fitches, and put them in one vessel, and make thee bread thereof...And thou shalt eat it as barley cakes..."*

It is considered abortifacient, antilac tagogue, demulcent, digestive, diuretic, emollient, expectorant, febrifuge, preventive (fever, grayhair), and stomachic, barley has been suggested for acrochordons, bladder, bronchitis, burns, cancer, catarrh, chest, chilblains, cholera, cough, debility, diarrhea, dyspepsia, fever, figs, inflammation, measles, phthisis, puerperium, scirrhus, sores, tumors and urogenital ailments, and warts. Barley grain is demulcent and easily assimilable, and used in invalid and convalescent diets. Pearl barley is form commonly used. Powdered parched grains used in form of gruel for painful and atonic dyspepsia. Algerians used barley after trepanning and in poultices for fractures and swollen testicles and abscesses; and applied it to the head in sunstroke. Lebanese regard the cultivated barley for infections and tuberculosis. Barley water with honey prescribed for bronchial coughs, and with gum arabic used for soothing irritations of the bladder and urinary passage. The seed meal is a folk remedy for cancer of the uterus, inflammatory tumors and gatherings, parotid gland tumors, and hard tumors. The seed flour is said to be a cure for anal condylomata, tumors behind the ears, scirrhus of the testicles, and spleen, whitlows and tumors. Seed cataplasms are said to help breast cancers. Lebanese mix barley with olive oil for indolent ulcers.

BITTER APPLE – (CITRULLUS COLOCYNTHIS)
...Behold, I will feed them, even this people, with wormwood, and give them water of gall to drink...Jeremiah 9

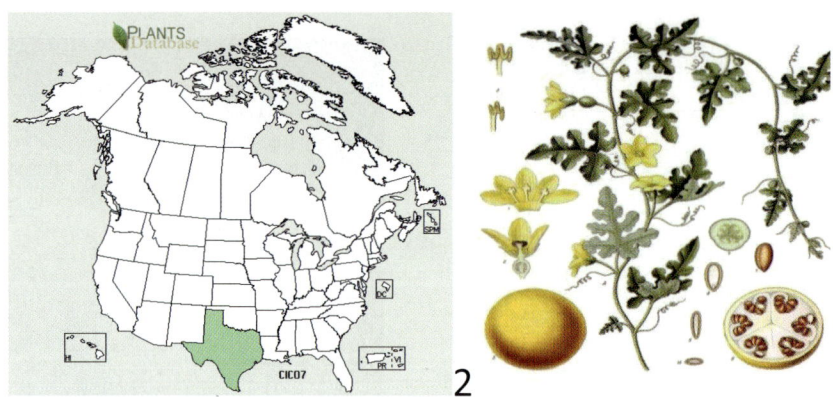

This is the wild gourd of II Kings, gathered in mistake for melons by one of the prophets during the dearth in Gilgal, and shred into a pot of mush making it impotable. When the fruit is ripe its pulp dries to form a powder used as a bitter medicine and drastic purgative. This powder is so inflammable that the Arabs collect it to use as kindling. Arabs smear a bitter black extract of the rind of the fruit onto waterbags to repel camels. The fruit is used to repel moths from wool. Dry fruits are said to kill mites and weevils. In India, the vine is planted as a sand binder. Seed, often removed from the poisonous pulp and eaten in Central Sahara regions, contains a fixed oil, which can be used as an illuminant. It is also used to darken gray hair. In spite of the bitterness, the fruits are eaten by grazing animals and the seecls gathered by desert rodents, even hungry man, after soaking in water. Bedouins are said to be able to survive nearly two weeks on the seed, through probably with diarrhea. Goats and wild game eat the stem and leaves.

Considered cathartic, ecbolic, emmenagogue, febrifuge, hydragogue, purgative, and vermifugal, the colocynth is used for amenorrhea, ascites, bilious disorders, cancer, dropsy, fever, jaundice, leukemia, rheumatism, snakebite, tumors (especially of the abdomen), and urogenital disorders. The purgative action is so drastic as to have caused fatalities. One woman who took 120 grains to induce abortion died in fifty hours. The plant figures into remedies for cancer, carcinoma, endothelioma, leukemia, corns, tumors of the liver and spleen.

The pulp or leaves is a folk remedy for cancerous tumors. A decoction of the whole plant, made in juice of fennel, is said to be a remedy for indurations of the liver. For rheumatism the Bedouins tie a slice of fresh gourd onto the heel before retiring (in the Sinai, I was told that the Bedouins could taste the bitter gourd in the morning as a result). Milk soaked in the empty gourd is said to serve as a vermifuge. A tar like exudate of the seeds is used to treat camels. Arabs use the fruit as an abortifacient. A pinch of powdered colocynth in cider was said to have arrested dropsy in Tripoli. Lebanese used the powdered pulp in resinous gum for piles. In Beirut, the pulp was used for open varicose veins. Lebanese also allude to its use for cancer, gangrene and wounds. In Algeria, colocynth is used as a gargle and mouthwash, a counterirritant in chest cold plasters. The rind with salt is poulticed onto frostbite. Around Rabat, they swallow one seed daily, without chewing, for 21 days for diabetes.

Ayurvedics use the root for arthritic pain, breast inflammation, ophthalmia and uterine pain, the fruit for adenopathy, anemia, ascites, asthma, bronchitis, constipation, dyspepsia, elephantiasis, fetal atrophy, jaundice, leucoderma, splenomegaly, throat diseases, tubercular glands, tumors, ulcers, and urinary discharges. Unani, considering the fruit abortifacient, carminative, and purgative, use it for brain disorders, epilepsy, hemicrania, inflammation, leprosy, and ophthalmia, and weakness of the limbs.

BLACK CUMIN – (NIGELLA SATIVA)
...For the fitches are not threshed with a threshing instrument...but the fitches are beaten out with a staff...Isaiah 28

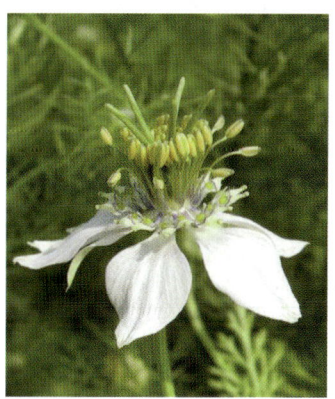

Black cumin is widely cultivated for its aromatic seeds, used whole or ground as a flavoring, especially in oriental cookery. Whole seeds used in Russian rye bread and for flavoring Turkish breads. Seeds may be used as a stabilizing agent for edible fats. Arabs mix the seed with honey as a confectionary. The tiny seeds are very hot to the palate and are sprinkled on food like pepper; in fact, in Europe they are sometimes mixed with real pepper. Ethiopians add them to Capsicum pepper sauces. They are also added to bread and sprinkled on cakes. Seeds can be sprinkled among woolens as a moth repellant.

According to an Arab proverb, "In the black seed is the medicine for every disease except death." Regarded as carminative, digestive, diuretic, emmenagogue, excitant, lactagogue, purgative, resolvent, stimulant, stomachic, sudorific, tonic, and vermifuge, fitches have been suggested as folk remedies for asthma, bilious ailments, bronchitis, calluses, cancer, colic, corns, cough, eruptions, fever, flu, headache, jaundice, myrmecia, orchitis, puerperium, sclerosis, skin, snakebite, stomachache, swellings, tumors of the abdomen and eyes, and warts. Algerians take the roasted seeds with butter for cough, with honey for colic. Nigellone in the oil protects guinea pigs against histamine induced bronchospasms, suggesting the rationale behind its use in asthma, bronchitis, and cough. The lipid portion of the ether extract of the seeds has shown lactagogue activity in rats, verifying its folk usage as a lactagogue. In large quantities the seed are also used to induce abortion. Lebanese took the seed extract for liver ailments. In Indonesia, the seeds are added to astringent medicines for abdominal disorders. In Malaya the seeds are poulticed onto abscesses, headache, nasal ulcers, orchitis, and rheumatism. Ethiopians mix the seed, with melted butter, wrap it in a cloth, and sniff it for headache. Arabian women use the seeds as a galactagogue. With a folk reputation for indurations and/or tumors of the abdomen, eyes and liver, it is not surprising to find that 100 g seed contain 510 mg sterols, of which 63.1% is the antitumor sterol, beta sitosterol. In Ayurvedic medicine, where used as a purgative adjunct, the herb is considered anthelmintic, apertif, aromatic, carminative, and emmenagogue. In Unani, it is further considered abortifacient and diuretic, and used for ascites, coughs, eye sores, hydrophobia, jaundice, paralysis, piles and tertian fever.

The seed contains the following minerals:

Calcium	Potassium
Iron	Sodium

The seed contains the following amino acids:

- Alanine
- Arginine
- Glutamate
- Glycine
- Isoleucine
- Leucine
- Lysine
- Methionine
- Phenylalanine
- Proline
- Serine
- Threonine
- Tyrosine
- Tryptophan
- Valine

BLACK MULBERRY – (MORUS NIGRA)
...And to the end they may provoke the elephants to fight, they shewed them the blood of grapes and mulberry...
I Maccabees 6

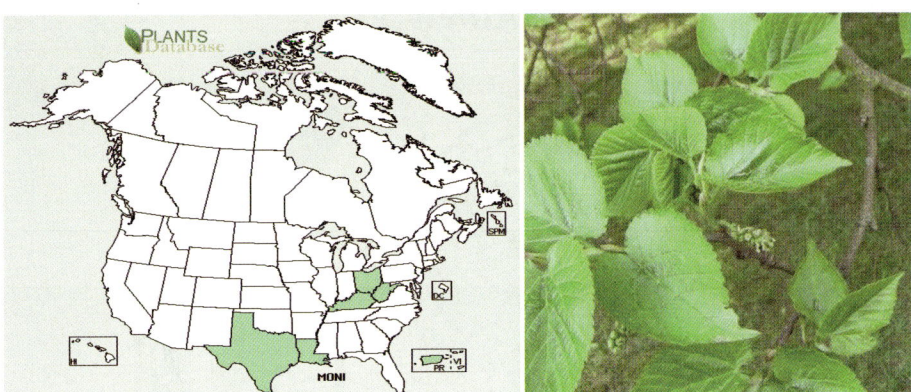

Black mulberry is widely cultivated for its edible fruit, eaten fresh or made into jams, jellies, sherbet, or wine. Fruits may be carefully sun dried and stored as a nutritious winter food. The fruit should be picked very ripe, at which time they are sweet and well flavored. Easily squashed, they stain the skin. To remove stain, juice from unripe fruit is rubbed over the skin. Wild birds, poultry, and hogs are fond of fruits. The red juice was used to incite the elephants of Antioch into battle. Burmans worship the mulberry, while some Europeans believe the devil stains his shoes black therewith. In old Palestine both the black and white mulberries were cultivated to feed silkworms. In parts of China, they make a thick preserve on the 15th day of their first month. Wood is used for joining. Bark contains tannins and is considered purgative and vermifuge. The trees are often planted as ornamentals. The berries are used to fatten sheep after which their meat is believed to be more digestible.

Considered depurative, laxative, purgative, refrigerant, and vermifuge, mulberry has been used in folk remedies for cancers, coughs, dysmenorrhea, fevers, sore throat, swellings, thirst, toothache, and tumors. The juice, boiled in honey for an ointment is said to be a folk remedy for tumors of the fauces. A plaster made from the sap is said to remedy indurations of the viscera. Mulberry is a "remedy" for cold impostumes of the uterus, knots, and tumors of the spleen. Medically, fruits are nutrient, refrigerant, laxative and are used to check thirst and to cool the blood. Philips reports a mixture of cow manure, crushed bilberry leaves and olive oil, wrapped in fresh mulberry leaves, for earache. Bark of the root is used in Iran for dysmenorrhea. Cambodians use the leaves for conjunctivitis.

Hillman Health Food Store call 855-Amish-Dr (855-264-7437) www.emineral.info Vitamins and Minerals for Better Living

Black Mustard – (*Brassica Nigra*)

...The kingdom of heaven is like a grain of mustard seed, which a man took, and sowed in his field: which indeed is the least of all seeds: but when it is grown, it is the greatest among herbs...

Matthew 13

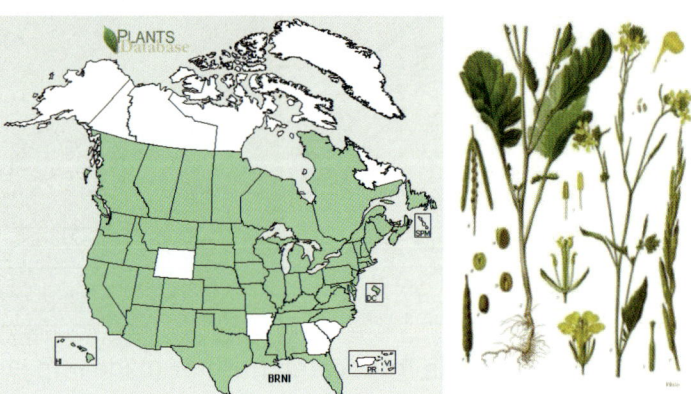

Black mustard is cultivated for its seeds, the source of commercial table mustard, used as a condiment and medicine. Seeds also contain both a fixed and an essential oil, used as a condiment, lubricant, and soap constituent. Black mustard is mixed with white mustard (Sinapis alba) to make mustard flour, used in various condiments as "English mustard" when mixed with water and "continental mustard" with vinegar. The leaves are eaten as a potherb. Mustard flowers are good honey producers. In agriculture mustard is also used as a cover crop. Smoke from burning mustard is said to repel flies and mosquitoes.

Mustard is considered anodyne, apertif, carminative, diuretic, emetic, laxative, rubefacient, stimulant, stomachic, and vesicant. Mustard plaster is used externally for many afflictions, like arthritis and rheumatism. A liquid prepared from the seed, when gargled, is said to be a folk remedy for tumors of the "sinax." In Ethiopia alone, the seed is used for amebiasis, abscesses, bloat, constipation, dysentery, rheumatism, and stomachache as well as for abortion. A decoction or plaster of the seed used in a cataplasm is used for hardness of the liver and spleen. Seeds are also said to help carcinoma and throat tumors. Lately mustards have been shown to contain at least five compounds which inhibit neoplasias induced by polycyclic aromatic hydrocarbons. Mustard relieves congestion by drawing the blood to the surface as in head afflictions, neuralgia, spasms. Hot water poured on bruised seeds makes a stimulant foot bath, good for colds and headaches. Old herbals suggested mustard for alopecia, epilepsy, snakebite, and toothache. Mustard oil is said to stimulate hair growth. Mustard is also recommended as an aperient ingredient of tea, useful in hiccup. Mustard flour is considered antiseptic. The oil is considered useful in pleurisy and pneumonia. Ayurvedics value the leaves for throat complaints and worms, the seeds for cough, external parasites, fever, itch, megalospleny skin ailments, tumors, and worms. Unani also recommend the seeds for boils, ear, eye and nose problems, edema, inflammation, rheumatism and toothache.

Black mustard plant has the minerals:

Calcium	Magnesium	Potassium
Copper	Manganese	Sodium
Iron	Nitrogen	Zinc

Black mustard has the following amino acids:

Arginine	Lysine	Tyrosine
Histidine	Methionine	Tryptophan
Isoleucine	Phenylalanine	Valine
Leucine	Threonine	

BLACKBERRY – (*RUBUS SANCTUS*)
...nor of a bramble bush gather they grapes...Luke 6

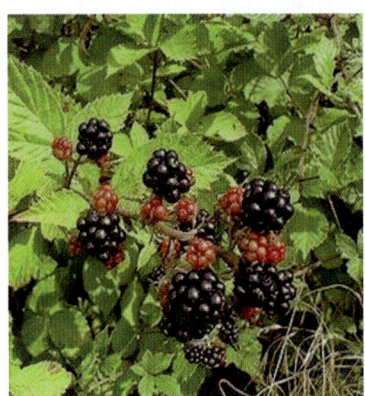

Whether or not this is more or less useful as a hedge, a medicine, an ornamental, or a fruit than other species of blackberry is not clear. The leaves of this bramble are probably as useful an astringent as the leaves of other Rubus species. Lebanese use the berry syrup to calm over-stimulated boys; they mix the root with niter and tragacanth for cold sores. They use this and other blackberry species to poultice with hollyhock or mallow for cuts and infections. This species is used by the Lebanese as is Rubus collinus, for colds, diarrhea, dropsy, dysmenorrhea, and piles. The fruit sherbet is used for colds and flu. Dried leaves are powdered or fresh leaves are pounded and worked into mastic for hemorrhoids.

BLUE MALLOW – (MALVA SYLVESTRIS)
...Who cut up mallows by the bushes...Job 30

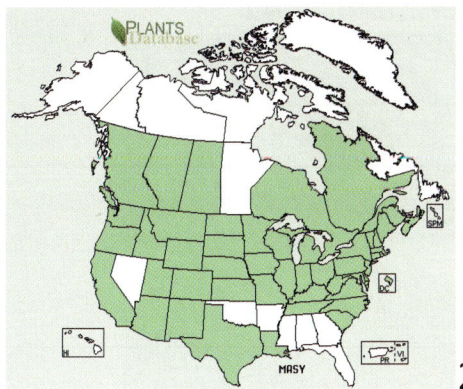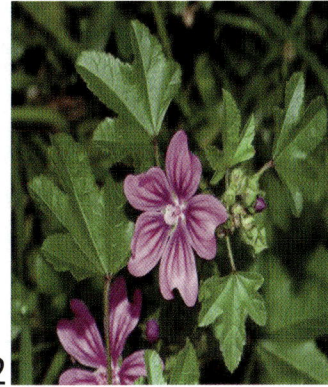

Some authors argue for Malva, others for Atriplex, for the mallow of the Bible. Both are edible. Malva is often used as a pot herb; the fruit and leaves edible. Flowers are collected and exported from Iran as medicinal. Seeds are also edible. In old times, flowers were strewn before peasants' doors and woven into garlands. The flower tincture is a delicate test for alkali.

Unani regard the plant as cooling, febrifuge, and mucilaginous, and endorse it for belpharitis, inflammation, jaundice, scorpion sting, sore throat, splenomegaly, strangury and urinary discharge. It is employed as an emollient cluster in tenesmus. The leaves and/or the flowers (known as foliae malva or flos malvae) are used as a gargle and mouthwash in Palestine. Leaves of Malva parviflora are sometimes pounded into a poultice for scorpion stings in Egypt. Europeans use the infusion for colds, coughs, gravel, and strangury.

Box – (*Buxus Longifolia*)
...I will set in the desert the fir tree, and the pine, and the box tree together...Isaiah 41

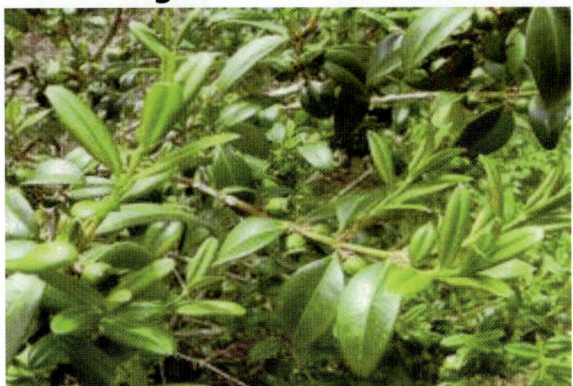

The wood, hard and taking a fine polish, is valued wherever a hard wood is needed, for carvings, combs, mathematical instruments, spoons and turnery, etc. It was cultivated by the Romans for the hard wood, which they inlaid with ivory for cabinet work and jewel caskets. Some authors consider this only a variant of the Europen box, Buxus sempervirens, leaves and bark of which were once promoted as a stimulant of hair growth. The European Box was said to be used, both as a substitute for hop, and as a green manure for hop. Boiled with lye it was supposed to tint the hair auburn. It is prized in the Holy Land as an ornamental evergreen. The hard and durable wood was formerly used for tablets which were covered with wax and used for writing. It is used by the wood engraver, the turner, etc.

Oil from the wood is used as a cancer treatment in Belgium. It contains the alkaloid cycloprotobuxine, which shows anticancer activity in PSI 45 and Wilms tumor systems. The leaves are sometimes used to adulterate uva ursi. The wood is considered diaphoretic and is given in decoction as an alternative for rheumatism and secondary syphilis. It is used as a substitute for guaiacum in treating venereal diseases where sudorifics are advisable. It is narcotic and sedative in full doses, emeto cathartic; possibly fatally so, and convulsant in overdoses. Tincture was once used for leprosy and malaria. Volatile oil from the wood is used for epilepsy, hemorrhoids, and toothaches. The leaves are alterative, cathartic, sudorific, and vermifuge. Powdered leaves have been applied to botworms in horses; though the mixture is poisonous, it is said to improve the horse's coat.

BROADBEAN – (VICIA FABA)
...and flour, and parched corn, and beans...II Samuel 17

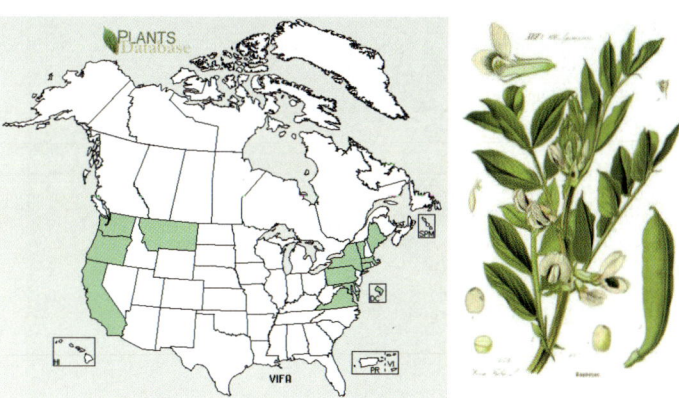

So ancient is this vegetable that it is recorded by Pliny. Even today, broadbeans are cultivated in Biblical countries, and their meal is made into bread today as in Biblical days. They are boiled and eaten also. Elsewhere they are cultivated as a vegetable and used green or dried, fresh or canned, and for stock feed. Broadbean has been considered as a meat extender or substitute and as a skim milk substitute. It is sometimes grown for green manure, but more generally for stock feed. Large seeds are used as a vegetable and frequently grown as a home garden crop, and for canning. Roasted seeds are eaten like peanuts in India. Beans are fed to horses and the stalks are given to camels. In ancient days beans were used in collecting votes from the people; a white bean signifying approval of the measure proposed; a black one, condemnation. Magistrates were elected by casting beans.

Said to be antidotal, aphrodisiac, cyanogenetic, diuretic, estrogenic, expectorant, stomachic, and tonic, faba fean is a folk remedy for chest, pneumonia, sclerosis, stomatitis, swellings, tumors, viscera, and warts. Inhalation of the pollen or ingestion of the seeds may cause favism, a severe hemolytic anemia, perhaps causing collapse. It is an inherited enzymatic deficiency occasional among Mediterranean people (Greek, Italian, Semitics). Injected intravenously in rabbits, broadbean extracts have produced hemoglobinuria and death. An ethanol ether extract of broadbeans has estrogenic activity; 50 milligrams stimulates the nonpregnant uterus at dioestrus. It is a folk remedy for such cancerous maladies as calluses, cancer of the breast, corns, felons, indurations of the breasts, heels, liver, spleen, and stomach; tumors of the bladder, breasts, eye, eyelids, genitals, glands, parotids, penis, and testicles; warts, and wens. In Iran, the shoots are said to be efficacious in rousing a drunkard from stupor. North Africans take two grilled beans in the morning for stomach distress; they also use them for hepatic and nephritic pain.

The fruit contains the following minerals:
Calcium	Iodine	Potassium
Chlorine	Magnesium	Sodium
Copper	Nitrogen	Sulfur

The seed contains the following minerals:
Calcium	Magnesium	Potassium
Iron	Nitrogen	Sodium

The seed contains the following amino acids:
Alanine	Isoleucine	Proline	Valine
Arginine	Leucine	Serine	
Glutamate	Lysine	Threonine	
Glycine	Methionine	Tryptophan	
Histidine	Phenylalanine	Tyrosine	

Hillman Health Food Store call 855-Amish-Dr (855-264-7437) www.emineral.info Vitamins and Minerals for Better Living

Brown Juniper – (*Juniperus Oxycedrus*)
...for he shall be like the heath in the desert...Jeremiah 17

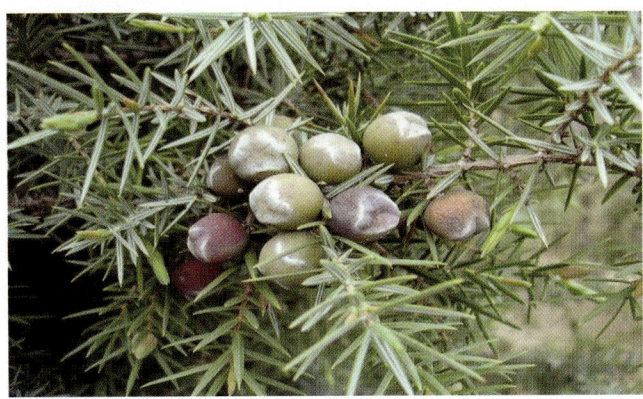

The shrubby form of cade juniper is valued as a forest understory, preventing erosion on steep mountainsides. Because of its spininess, it protects tree seedlings from being devoured by grazing animals. The refined oil is prized in men's fragrances to which it gives a woody or smoky leathery character; also in soap and other toiletries. It is also employed in food manufacturing to impart a smoky flavor to unsmoked fish and meat products. Oil distilled from the fruits is sometimes sold deceptively as juniper berry oil. Cade oil is used in antiseptic soaps. Rectified cade oil is used as a fragrance component in creams, detergents, lotions, perfumes, and soaps.

It is regarded as antiseptic, contraceptive, diuretic, parasiticidal, stimulant, vermifuge, and vulnerary, the cade cedar finds it way into folk remedies for alopecia, cancer, eczema, favus, leprosy, ophthalmia, pediculosis, psoriasis, scabies, and other skin ailments, sores, and toothaches. It is a folk remedy for cancer, tumors and malignant ulcers. In Palestine, cade yields the dark brown tar (cade oil) used for healing skin ailment.

Cade oil was once employed to treat corneal opacities, to allay pain in dental cavities, to kill head lice and their eggs, for snakebite and was applied to the penis before intercourse as a contraceptive. It was administered internally and externally as a remedy for leprosy. In modern Europe, refined cade oil is taken internally as a vermifuge three to five drops in a little water, followed by a weak purgative. It is applied sparingly to old wounds and ulcers to promote healing.

Cade oil has a long history for treating parasitic skin diseases of animals. Its application to similar human afflictions, especially eczema, psoriasis and pruritic dermatosis, is more recent. It has been reported to be antipruritic, antiseptic and keratolytic properties in cade oil. Cade oil is irritant and not recommended for internal use in the United States. Crushed berries are applied as an antiseptic to wounds. Steeped in oil, the berries are used in Lebanon for bladder and kidney ailments, in alcohol as a carminative and stomachic, in water for jaundice and other liver ailments. North Africans consider the fruits a diuretic, stimulant and vermifuge.

BRUTIAN PINE – (*PINUS BRUTIA*)

...Go forth unto the mount, and fetch olive branches, and pine branches and myrtle branches, and palm branches, and branches of thick trees, to make booths...Nehemiah 8

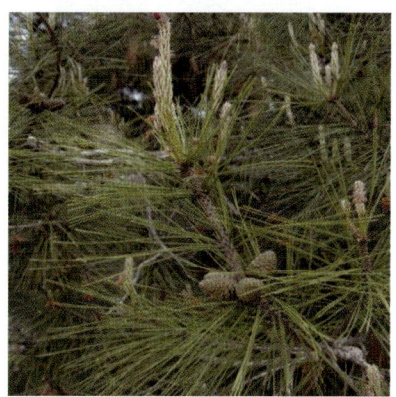

After Nehemiah the word pine is said not to reoccur in the Bible, but about 500 years later it is mentioned by Josephus, who says Solomon had pine wood brought in ships from Ophir which was used for pillars and support to the King's temple and palace, partly for musical instruments, e.g. cymbals, harps, and psalteries, for the glorification of God by the Levites. Whether or not Pinus brutia is properly identified as the Biblical pine branch, the turpentine was doubtless used for medicine like other turpentines. A substance known as burasu was the most common drug in tlte herbals of ancient Assyria. Prepared by soaking pinewood in water, it was applied externally to muscles and ligaments as an embrocation. Internally it was taken for kidney or liver ailments.

BUTCHER'S BROOM – (*RUSCUS ACULEATUS*)
...And there shall be no more a pricking brier unto the house of Israel...Ezekiel 28

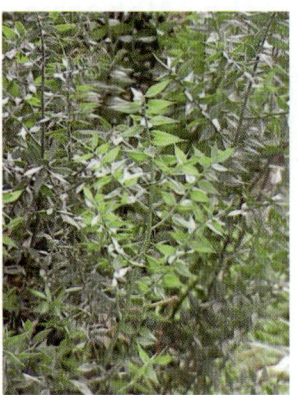

Butcher's Broom is sometimes grown as a spiny ornamental hedge. Ruscogenin, first isolated from Ruscus aculeatus, is identical with Sapogenin B, which could be used as a starter material for steroids. The young shoots of Butcher's Broom have often been eaten like those of Asparagus. Matured branches were in the past bound up and sold as brooms.

In Lebanon, the rhizome is sliced and dried, and decocted for catarrh, diuresis, dropsy, jaundice, kidney trouble and respiratory difficulties. The root, considered aperient, deobstruent, diaphoretic, and diuretic, is used for nephritis and urinary obstructions. It is also suggested for scrofulous tumors. Boughs have been employed in self flagellation for chilblains. The decoction, sweetened with honey, is suggested for dyspnea, being expectorant. Boulos reports that the leaf infusion is febrifuge.

The root contains the following minerals:

Aluminum	Magnesium	Silica
Calcium	Manganese	Sodium
Chromium	Nitrogen	Tin
Copper	Potassium	
Iron	Selenium	

The root contains the mineral tin.

CAMEL THORN – (ALHAGI CAMELORUM)
...we have sent you money to buy burnt-offerings, and sin offerings, and incense, and prepare ye manna...Baruch 1

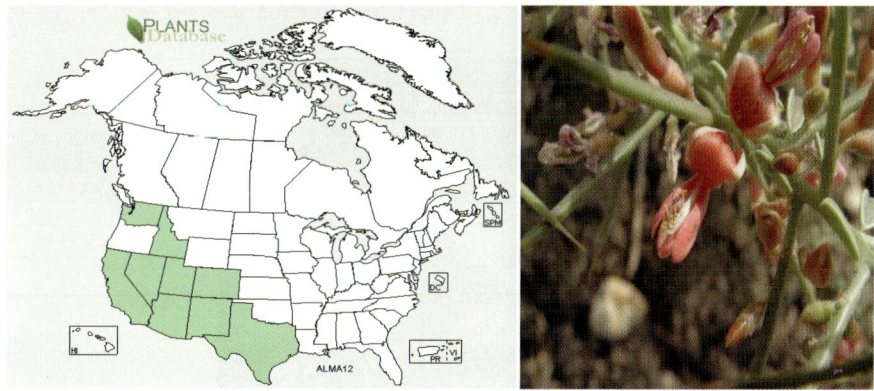

Since the Baruch manna was for sale, it was probably the resinous gum from some tree of the Levant. During the heat of the day, a sweet gummy substance oozes from the leaves and stems. This hardens upon contact with the air and is then collected by shaking over drop cloths. The sugary secretion (manna) obtained is edible, occuring in small round grains, consisting mostly of sugar. The plant is given as fodder to camels. The twigs are much used in making screens (tatties).

Regarded as antibilious, demulcent, expectorant, and laxative, camel thorn is a folk remedy for the chest, for polyps, and for tumors, especially of the abdomen and glands. In Iran, the white grains of manna are administered as a laxative and expectorant. Ayurvedics, considering the plant diuretic, laxative, refrigerant, and tonic, use it for bad appetite, brain ailments, bronchitis, epistaxis, leprosy, and obesity. Unani consider the manna as aperient, aphrodisiac, cholagogue, depurative, diuretic, and expectorant, using it for asthma, nausea, piles and smallpox eruptions. They use oil from the leaf for rheumatism. Regarding the whole plant as alexiteric, aperient, attenuate, and suppurative, they use it for opacities of the cornea and hemicrania. In the Konkan, the plant is smoked with jimsonweed, tobacco, and ajwan seeds for asthma. In Ormara, the root decoction is used to bathe abscesses and swellings.

CAPER – (CAPPARIS SPINOSA)
...Fears shall be in the way, and the almond tree shall flourish, and the grasshopper shall be a burden, and desire shall fail: because man goeth to his long home...Ecclesiasters 12

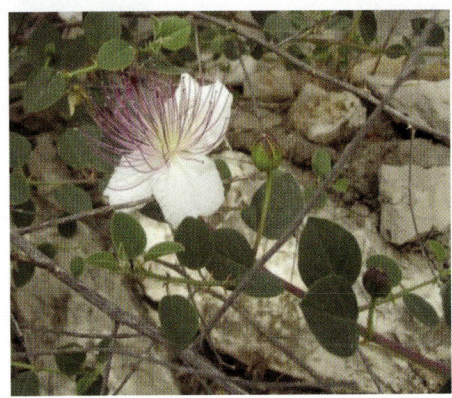

The young pickled buds of the caper give the "desire" or relish to food. Today in the Mediterranean islands they are gathered and steeped in vinegar for an appetizer. Caper bush is cultivated for its flower buds, used as a condiment in cooking and for flavoring in canapes, gravies, salads, and sauces, after being cooked and pickled. For pickling, one kilo of buds is steeped in one kilo of brine vinegar for a month. The sprouts are sometimes eaten like asparagus, as well as the buds and shoots. Pickled fruits are eaten in the Punjab and Arabia and also grown for the large ornamental white and purple flowers.

The root and its bark, prepared variously (malagmas, cataplasms, drunk with wine or vinegar, etc.), is a folk remedy for indurations (of the bladder, kidney, liver, spleen, and uterus) and tumors in general, (axilla, head, groin, liver, neck), and warts. Medicinally, root bark is alterative, analgesic, anthelmintic, aperient, aphrodisiac, astringent, diuretic, emmenagogue, expectorant, stimulant and tonic, and is used in rheumatism, scurvy, enlarged spleen, sclerosis (spleen), tubercular glands, and toothache. Unani use the juice to kill worms; they consider the root bark anthelmintic, aperient, analgesic, emmenagogue and expectorant and use it in adenopathy, rheumatism, splenomegaly, paralysis, and toothache. Broken leaves are used as a poultice in gout. Tender stems are used for dysentery. The caper is a stimulant, exciting both hunger and thirst and thus strengthening the appetite which becomes a bit sluggish. Bedouins are said to use caper with Teucrium pilosum as an inhalant for colds. They boil the ground leaves in water and inhale the vapors for headache. For arthritic like pains of the back, joints, and limbs, the Bedouins boil the ground leaves in water, and poultice them, wrap them in a thin cloth, and then apply them to the ache, even as they sleep. Barren women are covered with a mixture of ground leaves of Capparis and Tamarix to inhale the vapors and sweat to correct their barrenness. Lebanese boil the root and plant for dengue, malaria and Malta fever, Iranians for intermittent fever and rheumatism. Lebanese regard the roots as specific for malaria or splenomegaly following malaria. Algerians boil the whole plant in oil as a puerperal hydragogue. Crushed seeds have been suggested for dysmenorrhea, female sterility, ganglions, scrofula and ulcers. The capers themselves have been suggested for arteriosclerosis, chills, ophthalmia and sciatica, especially in North Africa. The fruits are considered antiscorbutic and used for colds, dropsy and sciatica.

CAROB – (CERATONIA SILIQUA)
...John had his raiment of camel's hair, and a leathern girdle about his loins; and his meat was locusts and wild honey...Matthew 3

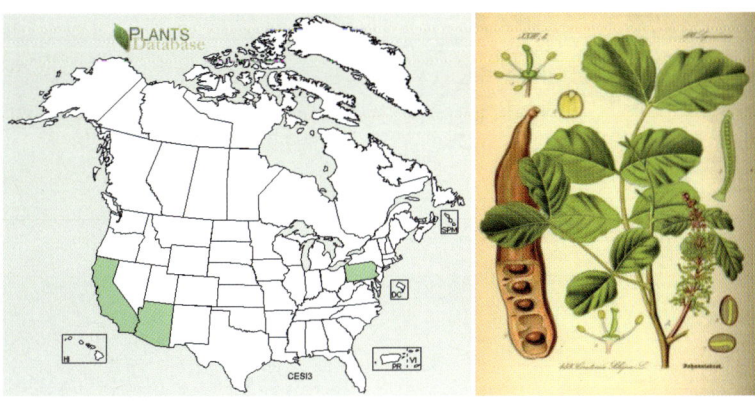

The fruit of the carob tree, a source of food for the poor man in Jewish folklore, also appears in the Christian tradition as "St. John's Bread," eaten by St. John the Baptist in the wilderness. The locust fruit is spread out and dried as food that is sustaining for cattle as well as for people. In Palestine, a molasses named dibs is prepared from the ripe fruits. The seeds are said to be the ancient and original weight used by goldsmiths and instituted from early times as carat weight. Each harvest, one carob tree may carry eight hundred pounds of husks. Carob is cultivated for its fruit and seeds, both high in sugar and calcium and low in protein and fats. In Cyprus a brittle candy known as "pasteli" is made from the pods. It is used in "health foods" as a chocolate substitute. Roast seeds have been used as a coffee substitute. Alcoholic beverages have been made from infusions of the pod. Carob is also used in textile printing, synthetic resins, insecticides, and fungicides. American imports are mostly used in tobacco flavorings and cosmetics.

The pod is used as an anticatarrhal, demulcent, and resolvent. In southern Europe, the pods are used for asthma and cough. The leaf is astringent. Various portions of the plant are said to be used as antitussive, astringent, pectoral, and purgative. The pods contain gallic acid, a reported antitumor compound. The seeds contain tannins. Perhaps it should come as no surprise that carob has a folk reputation against cancer (specifically verruca and indurations).

The seed contain the following amino acids:

Alanine	Isoleucine	Proline
Arginine	Leucine	Serine
Glutamate	Lysine	Threonine
Glycine	Methionine	Tyrosine
Histidine	Phenylalanine	Valine

Castor Bean – (*Ricinus Communis*)
...And the Lord God prepared a gourd, and made it to come up over Jonah, that it might be a shadow over his head...Jonah 4

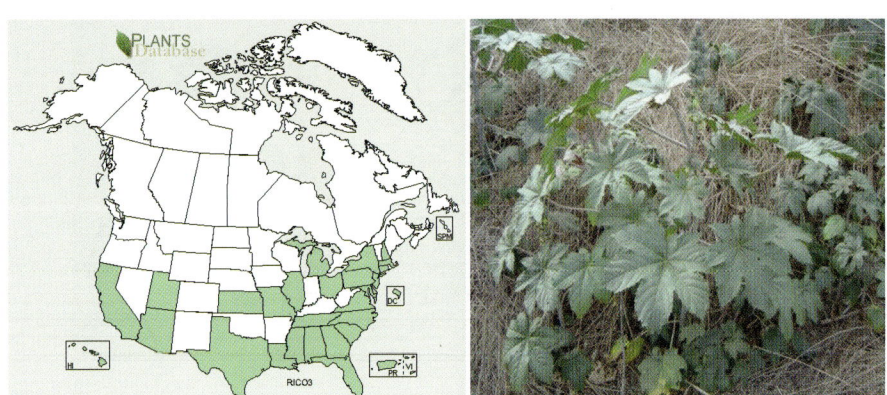

The huge leaves of this plant are excellently adapted for producing ample shade when growing alongside a bower, booth, or hut or overhanging a bench. Castor bean is cultivated for the seeds which yield a fast drying, non-yellowing oil, used mainly in industry and medicines. The oil was extensively used by the Hebrews, being one of the five oils which rabbinical tradition sanctions for such use. Oil used in coating fabrics and other protective coverings, in the manufacture of high grade lubricants, transparent typewriter and printing inks, in textile dying (when converted into sulfonated castor oil or turkey red oil, for dying cotton fabrics with alizarine), in leather preservation, and in the production of "Rilson," a polyamide nylon-type fiber. Dehydrated oil is an excellent drying agent which compares favorably with tung oil and is used in paints and varnishes. Hydrogenated oil is utilized in the manufacture of waxes, polishes, carbon paper, candles and crayons. "Blown Oil" is used for grinding lacquer paste colors, and when hydrogenated and sulfonated it is used for preparation of ointments. South Africans mix castor oil with kerosene as a culicide; the oil prevents tabanid flies from attacking camels. Castor oil pomace, the residue after crushing, is used as a high nitrogen fertilizer. The pomace is said to induce asthma among individuals who inhale it. Although it is highly toxic due to the ricin, a method of detoxicating the meal has now been found, so that it can safely be fed to livestock. The stems are made into paper and wallboard.

Neither the ancient Hebrews nor modern inhabitants of Palestine and Syria use it for medicine. But the Lebanese used the leaves and crushed beans externally as a dressing, not internally as a purgative. They applied the crushed seed to abscesses and cancerous swellings. Castor oil was applied to bunions. Today, Egyptian farmers poultice fresh leaves to cure boils. In Algeria, castor oil with rabbit blood was used as a contraceptive. Considered anodyne, antidote, aperient, bactericide, cathartic, culicide, cyanogenetic, discutient, emetic, emmenagogue, emollient, expectorant, insecticide, lactagogue, larvicidal, laxative, POISON, purgative, tonic, and vermifuge, castor or castoroil is a dangerous ingredient in folk remedies for abscess, anasarca, arthritis, asthma, boils, burns, cancer, carbuncles, catarrh, chancre, cholera, cold, colic, convulsions, corns, craw craw, deafness, delirium, dermatitits, diarrhea, dogbite, dropsy, epilepsy, erysipelas, fever, flu, gout, guineaworm, headache, inflammation, moles, myalgia, nerves, osteomyelitis, palsy, parturition, piles, prolapse, puerperium, rash, rheumatism, scald, scrofula, seborrhea, skin, sores, stomachache, strabismus, swellings, toothaches, tuberculosis, tumors, ulcers, urethritis, uteritis, venereal disease, warts, whitlows, and wounds. The oil and seed have been used as folk remedies for: warts, cold tumors, indurations of the abdominal organs, whitlows, lacteal tumors, indurations of the mammary gland, corns, and moles, etc. Castor oil is cathartic and has labor inducing properties.

Ricinoleic acid has served in contraceptive jellies. Ricin, a toxic protein in the seeds, acts as a blood coagulant. Oil used externally for dermatitis and eye ailments. Seeds, which yield 45 to 50% of a fixed oil, also contain the alkaloids ricinine and toxalbumin ricin, and considered purgative, counter irritant in scorpion sting and fish poison. Nigerians burn the stem with Calotropis for chancre. Leaves applied to the head to relieve headache and as a poultice for boils; they are heated and applied to gout, rheumatism, and swellings. The juice is dangerously ingested to cure deafness resulting from cold and to rub stiffness out of joints. South Africans use the root for toothache. Ayurvedics use the root for ascites, asthma, bronchitis, eructation, fever, inflammation, leprosy, and diseases of the head, glands and rectum. They use the leaves for earache, nightblindness, strangury and worms, the flowers for anal troubles, glandular tumors, and vaginalgia, the fruit for hepatosis, pain, splenosis, and tumors, the seed oil for ascites, backache, convulsions, elephantiasis, fever, inflammation, leprosy, lumbago, tumors and typhoid. Additionally, they use the rootbark for skin ailments, the leaves for oligolactea, burns; the seeds and/or seed oil for amenorrhea, asthma, ascites, boils, dropsy, hepatosis, lumbago, pain, paralysis, piles, rheumatism and ringworm. Zulus administer the leaves for stomachache, administered orally or rectaliy. In Guiana the leaves are applied to the breast to augment the secretion of milk.

CATTAIL – (TYPHA AUSTRALIS)
...And they smote him on the head with a reed...Mark 15

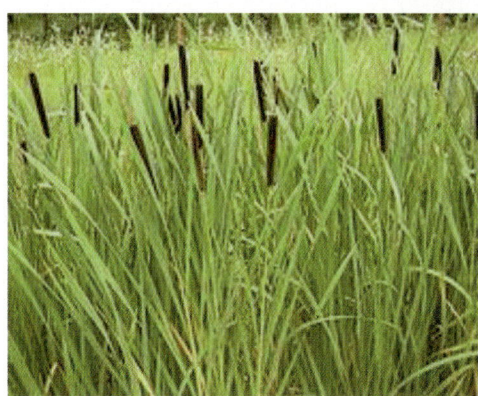

Many old paintings depicting Jesus' mock trial picture him with the cattail in his hand as a sceptre. Young shoots, inflorescence, and rhizomes are eaten in various ways. Flowers and anthers are made into a sweetmeat. The sweet and soft marrow of the immature spike is considered a delicacy. The leaves are plaited into such articles as ropes, winnowing-trays, mats, and also are employed as caulking. The silky florets of spikes are used for stuffing and tinder. Ashes are sometimes used as a salt substitute.

Considered astringent, cyanogenic, diuretic, and hemostat, this cattail is suggested as a folk remedy for epilepsy, madness, tumors, and wounds. A flavonol glucoside, yielding quercetin on hydrolysis, has been reported in the plant. The pollen was used during emergency as an absorbent in surgery.

CEDAR OF LEBANON – (*CEDRUS LIBANI*)

...let fire come out of the bramble, and devour the cedars of Lebanon...

Judges 9

Behold...a cedar in Lebanon with fair branches...Ezekiel 31

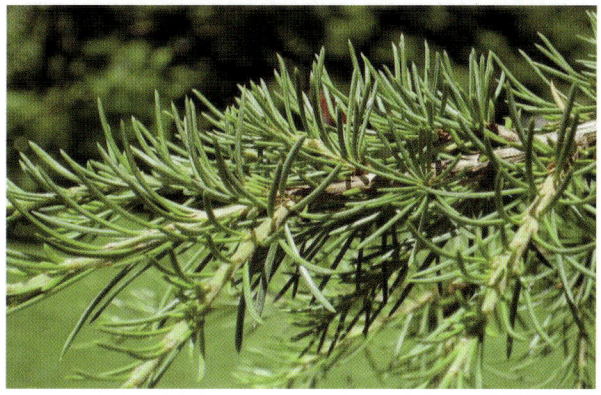

Cedar of Lebanon grows wild in Turkey, Lebanon, and Syria, but cultivated in England, France, and the U.S. It exudes a gum or balsam which makes the wood fragrant. Wood is particularly adaptable for building; it does not quickly decay, nor is it eaten by insects. Lebanese believe that the tree purifies the air. No doubt it does!

Medicinally the plant is considered diuretic and insecticidal, and it has worked its way into folk remedies for burns, cancer, indurations of the limbs and tumors. The pitch is used for infections, especially a deep infectious little boil growing under the skin. The Lebanese believe the smoke helps chest difficulties suggestive of asthma. It has been suggested for blenorrhagia, bronchitis, phthisis and skin eruptions.

CEYLON CINNAMON – (CINNAMOMUM VERUM)

...And the merchants of the earth shall weep and mourn over her; for no man buyeth their...cinnamon, and odours, and ointments...

Revelation 18

...Take thou also unto thee principal spices...of sweet cinnamon...

Exodus 30

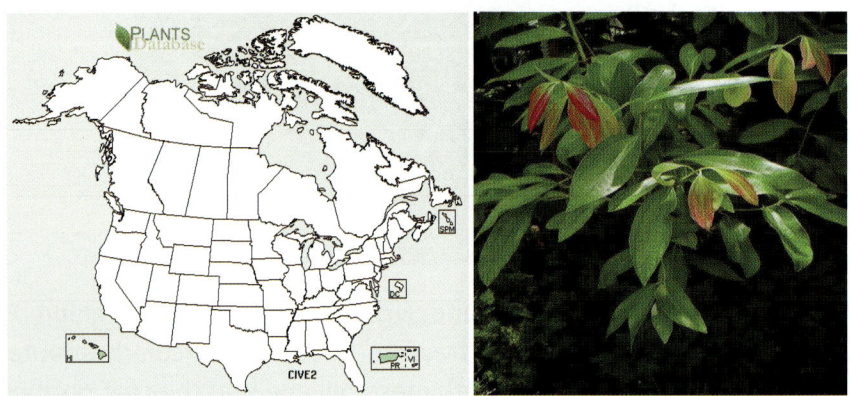

Cinnamon bark constitutes an important condiment used in food, incenses, perfumes, and dentifrices. Think of cinnamon as a flavor, but in Biblical times, spices were used to prepare incense and holy oils used in religious rites, in medicines, and as perfumes. In Proverbs 7, *the clever woman ensnared her young man by decorating her room with tapestry and carvings*, and fine linen from Egypt, and perfumed it with aloes, cinnamon, and myrrh. A fat procured by boiling the fruits was used by the Portuguese for making candles. Cinnamon bark oil, distilled from chips and bark of inferior quality, is used in foods, perfumes, soaps, cordials, and in drug and dental preparations. Cinnamon leaves, like laurel leaves, were woven into decorative wreaths for Roman temples. Cinnamon leaf oil, distilled from dried green leaves, is a powerful germicide, and is also used in perfumes, spices, and in the sythesis of vanillin. Cinnamon was a major ingredient in the holy oil which Moses was ordered to use in the Tabernacle to anoint the sacred vessels and the persons of the officiating priests.

Regarded as antiseptic, astringent, balsamic, carminative, diaphoretic, febrifuge, fungicide, germicide, stimulant and stomachic, cinnamon is used in folk treatments for amenorrhea, arthritis, asthma, bronchitis, cholera, cough, diarrhea, dysentery, dyspepsia, female ailments, fever, fistula, heart, kidney, lumbago, lungs, metrorrhagia, nausea, phthisis, proctosis, prolapse, psoriasis, renitis, spasms, vaginitis, warts, and wens. It was used in massive doses with success in the treatment of cancer. It is also regarded as a folk remedy for cancer (especially of the rectum, breast, gums, mouth, stomach, and uterus), indurations (of spleen, breast, uterus, liver and stomach), and tumors (especially of the abdomen, liver, and sinews), cinnamon contains the antitumor agent benzaldehyde. The Lebanese used the cinnamon as a stimulant, for colds, rheumatism, halitosis, and to check slobbering in young and elderly people. Mothers are given hot cinnamon tea, with ginger and caraway "to prevent blood clotting which can kill the mother." It is also used for chills, menstrual cramps, and to loosen coughs. Cinnamon is used as a stimulant of the uterine muscular fiber in menorrhagia and in tedious labor due to defective uterine contractions.

Ayurvedics consider the bark aphrodisiac and tonic, and use it for biliousness, bronchitis, diarrhea, itch, parched mouth, worms and cardiac, rectal, and urinary diseases. They use the oil for "eructations," flatulence, loss of appetite, nausea, and toothache. On the other hand, the Unani consider the oil carminative, emmeagogue and tonic to the liver, and use it for abdominal pains, bronchitis, headcolds and inflammation. They consider the bark alexiteric, aphrodisiac, carminative, expectorant, sialogogue and tonic, using it for flatulence, headache, hiccup, hydrocele, liver ailments, piles and scorpion stings.

Chicory – (Cichorium Intybus)
...And they shall eat the flesh in that night, roast with fire, and unleavened bread; and with bitter herbs they shall eat it...Exodus 12

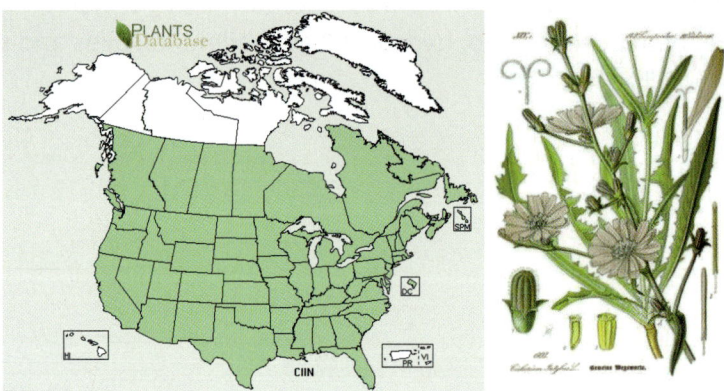

Chicory, cultivated since ancient times for its leaves, is used for salads. It is usually blanched by covering with litter to make it less bitter. Whole or shredded leaves are served with oil and vinegar as salads; blanched hearts serve as a vegetable. Young plants are satisfactory for fodder, but older plants may embitter the milk. Turning black, the leaves render hay less marketable. Root chicory, established in Europe during the Napoleonic blockade, is cultivated for roots used as a coffee substitute. When blended with ground coffee, they enhance the flavor and aroma of the brew. Roots are used in seasoning soups, sauces, and gravies, and to impart a rich deep color.

Regarded as alexiteric, aperient, cholagogue, demulcent, depurative, diuretic, emmenagogue, laxative, refrigerant, sedative, stomachic, sudorific and tonic, chicory is a folk application for asthma, biliousness, cancer, catarrh, consumption, diarrhea, dysmenorrhea, dyspepsia, eyes, fever, gall, hemorrhoids, inflammation, jaundice, liver, lumbago, lungs, nausea, ophthalmia, sclerosis, spleen, typhoid and warts. The juice is a folk remedy for tumors and cancer of the liver, stomach, and uterus. Powdered seed are applied for indurations of the spleen. The leaf, boiled with honey, is used as a gargle for cancer of the mouth. Chicory root is used for cancer of the breast, face and mouth. The chicory was regarded as an aphrodisiac and its seeds were used in love potions. Some Lebanese peasants also consider the plant aphrodisiac; others consider the fresh leaves, as a salad, depurative and tonic; the juice from macerated leaves is sedative and soothing; the root is calmative and believed to overcome the stimulus of coffee. Egyptians value the root for tachycardia. In Iran, chicory, like endive, is used as a resolvent and cooling medicine in bilious attacks, sometimes mixed with Cordia, Nymphaea, and Viola. Considering the plant alexiteric, astringent, depurative, emmenagogue, tonic, the Unani use the wild bitter type for asthma, biliousness, and inflammation.

The root contains the following minerals:

Boron	Magnesium	Sodium
Calcium	Nitrogen	
Iron	Potassium	

The leaf contains the following minerals:

Calcium	Magnesium	Potassium
Iron	Nitrogen	Sodium

The leaf contains the following amino acids:

Arginine	Lysine	Tryptophan
Histidine	Methionine	Valine
Isoleucine	Phenylalanine	
Leucine	Threonine	

The bark contains the following minerals:

Bromine	Copper	Manganese
Calcium	Iodine	Nitrogen
Chlorine	Iron	Potassium
Chromium	Magnesium	Rubidium

COCKLEBUR – (XANTHIUM SPINOSUM)
...And thorns shall come up in her palaces...Isaiah 34

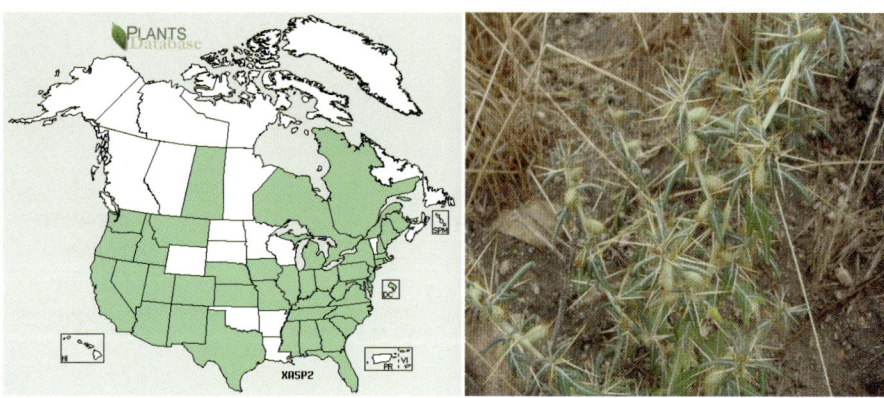

Clotbur is reported to be used against arthralgia, diabetes, hydrophobia, malaria, rabies, and intermittent fevers. It has a diuretic, antiperiodic, styptic, and sudorific action. Clotbur is used for cancer (especially of the liver) and tumors. The burs are prescribed for diarrhea. In Lebanon, the leaf infusion is used for dyspepsia, the strong tea for ulcers, both internal and external. Lebanese fed crushed seeds (perhaps dangerous) to the children to "make their bones and blood strong." Powdered fruits were applied to boils. Lebanese regarded the root as depurative and tonic, highly regarded for rabies. The young plants are reported to cause poisoning in cattle and horses. Choline is believed to be the toxic principle. The dried fruit and the juice of the fruit bearing plant contain an unidentified alkaloid, which has an intense pharmacological action on the central nervous system. They also contain a notable quantity of formic acid (antiseptic).

COMMON REED – (*PHRAGMITES AUSTRALIS*)
...I will not with ink and pen write unto thee...III John 13

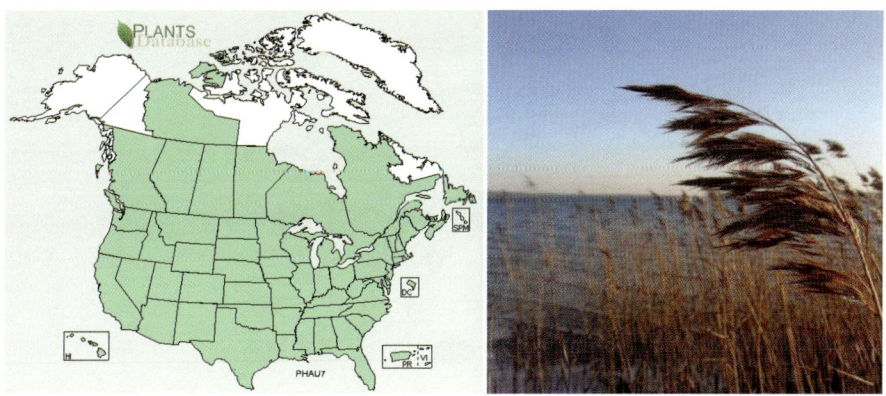

Common reed provides high quality warm season forage and is readily eaten by cattle and horses. However, it becomes tough and unpalatable after maturity. Animals grazing this grass during the winter should be fed a protein concentrate. Extensively used in Mediterranean region and elsewhere for building dwellings, lattices, fences, arrows by Indians, and for weaving mats and carrying nets. Young shoots are sometimes used as a vegetable. In Japan, young shoots are cooked like bamboo sprouts. The stalks ooze a manna-like gum which is eaten. The rhizomes and roots also serve as emergency food. In Russia they are harvested and processed into starch. A multicolored form is used as an ornamental grass. The reed is useful in the manufacture of pulps for rayon and paper. It is also useful in the production of homogeneous boards of good strength. It can be processed into a fine fibrous material suitable as a filling material in upholstery. Flowering stalks yield a fiber suitable for rope making. It is also used for thatching and for making partitions, fences, coarse mats, baskets, sandals, etc. Panicles are used for baking brooms and for decoration. Pens for writing on parchment were cut and fashioned from this reed, and the stems were used as a linear measuring device. Bedouins use the stem to make flutes. Chinese commonly use the stem for fuel.

Said to be alexiteric, diaphoretic, diuretic, emetic, refrigerant, sialogogue, and stomachic, the reed is listed in folk remedies for abscesses, arthritis, bronchitis, cancer, cholera, condylomata, diabetes, dropsy, dysuria, fever, flux, gout, hematuria, hemorrhage, hiccups, indurations, jaundice, leukemia, lungs, mammary carcinoma, measles, nausea, rheumatism, sores, sore throat, stomach, sunstroke, thirst, and typhoid. Decoction of the rhizome is taken for earache and toothache. In China it is used as a remedy for hiccups and poisoning from eating stale seafood. In the Orient, a packing of reeds is used as a splint for fractures. Cape Africans apply the powdered seed to burns. Africans use the sugary exudate for chest pain and pneumonia.

CORIANDER – (*CORIANDRUM SATIVUM*)
...And the manna was as coriander seed...Numbers 11

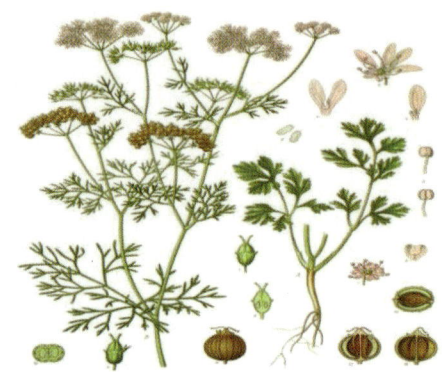

Coriander seeds, size of a peppercorn, have a sharp though pleasant aroma. Arabs find it a wholesome spice, as do the Egyptians and Indians, who add it to their meat. Bread in the east is flavored with coriander; confectioners in Europe add it to baked cakes and sweetmeats. The plant was used as early as 1550 B.C. for culinary and medicinal purposes. It was one of the drugs employed by Hippocrates ca 400 B.C. Coriander is cultivated primarily as a spice and drug source. Dried fruits, called coriander seed, are fragrant combining the taste of lemon peel and sage. It is used to flavor pastries, cookies, buns, processed meats (such as sausage, bologna, and frankfurters), pickling spice, and curry powder. Coriander seed is available whole or ground. Whole seed may be sugar coated for a confection, or may be used to flavor liqueurs, such as gin and vermouth; also used in perfumes and tobacco products, and in the cocoa, chocolate and cordial industries. Seeds contain an essential oil (0.51 percent), extracted by steam distillation, used for flavoring and in medicine. In the USSR, the essential oil is used as a source of linalol, which is used as a starting material for other chemurgics. Young plants used in salads as a vegetable and in chutneys, sauces, soups, and curries. In Ethiopia, the leaves are added as an aromatic to bread, spiced sauces, and tea. Extracted seed cake is used as fodder. In the Philippines, the leaves are eaten raw with native dishes and used to flavor soups.

Coriander is a folk remedy for cancer (especially of the uterus), condylomata, indurations of limbs and spleen, kernels, tumors of the adbomen and sinews, and wens. It is said to be alexiteric, apertif, aphrodisiac, carminative, digestive, diuretic, emmenagogue, pectoral, refrigerant, sedative, stimulant, stomachic, and tonic, coriander is reported to be good for abdominal tumors, arthritis, bad appetite, bilious ailments, cancer, catarrh, colic, condylomata, cramps, dyspepsia, dysentery, erotomania, erysipelas, erythema, fever, flatulence, flux, giddiness, halitosis, headache, heart, hernia, hysteria, indigestion, induration of the spleen, intoxication, kernels, measles, nausea, nervousness, neuralgia, piles, ptomaine, rheumatism, schlerosis, scrofula, snakebite, spasms, splenitis, stomachache, syphilis, toothache, tumors, ulcers, venereal diseases, warts and wens. Pills made from the seed are said to be folk remedies for abdominal tumors. A plaster or unguent made from the juice is said to remedy hot tumors, wens, and kernels. The herb, boiled with meal, is also said to help "hot tumors." Iranians smoke the fruits for toothache. Ethiopians chew the leaves for colic and stomachache.

The seed decoction is taken as a medical stimulant or, in excess, as a narcotic anodyne. Iranians use the leaf too for headache. Coriander was used in love potions, its use as an aphrodisiac. Ayurvedics recommend it for dysentery. Ayurvedics also consider the plant aphrodisiac, apertif, anthelmintic, antipyretic, diuretic, laxative, refrigerant, stimulant, stomachic, using it for biliousness, bronchitis, dysentery, fever, nausea, and thirst. Unani use the leaves, considered analgesic and hypnotic, for bleeding gums, eye pains, gleet, hiccup, inflammation, jaundice, piles, scabies, stomatitis, toothache and tubercular glands. They used the seed to prevent bronchitis and coryza, for biliousness, dyspepsia, headache, syphilis, and ulcers on the penis. They too consider the seed aphrodisiac, and tonic to the brain, heart and liver.

CORN COCKLE – (AGROSTEMMA GITHAGO)
...If my land cry against me...Let thistles grow instead of wheat, and cockle instead of barley...Job 31

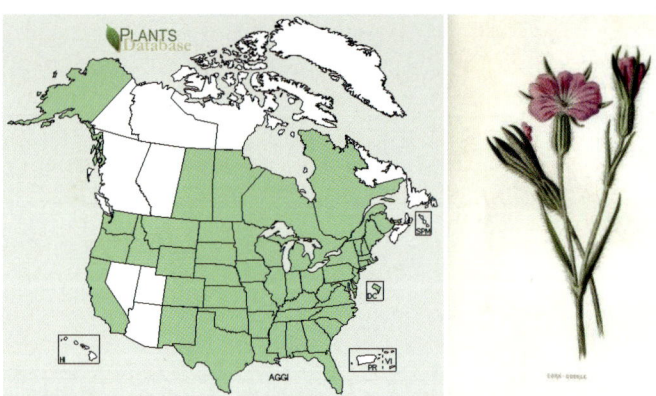

Rarely encouraged for the small but attractive flower, corn cockle is more often regarded as a weed. It is regarded as diuretic, emmenagogue, expectorant, POISON, and vermifuge, and cockle has been used to treat cancer, dropsy, and jaundice. Homeopathically, the seeds are used in gastritis and paralysis. It is a noxious weed, growing in cereal field, whose seeds are quite poisonous if ground up with the cereal. Cockle, especially the seeds, has been used in Europe for cancers, hard tumors, warts, and apostemes or hard swellings in the uterus.

COSTUS OIL – (*SAUSSUREA LAPPA*)
...All thy garments smell of myrrh, and aloes, and cassia...Psalm 45

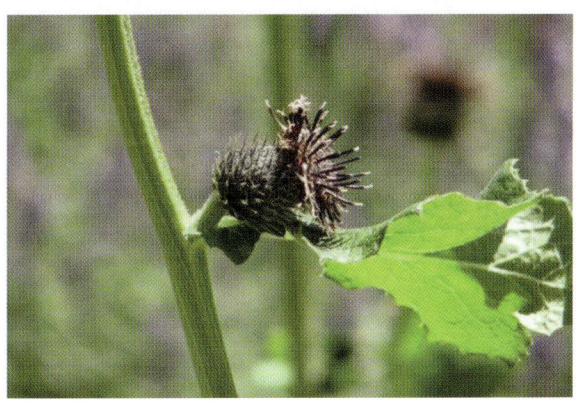

Cassia was the Indian orris, widely used in perfumes and incenses. Though noted as an aphrodisiac, its chief use is as a perfume. In China and India it serves as incense in temples. The essential oil is valued in perfumery and cosmetics. The essential oil has strong antiseptic and disinfectant properties especially against streptococcus and staphylococcus. The root owes its insecticidal property to its essential oil content. Roots are employed in Kashmir as insecticide to protect shawls and woolen fabrics. A process for treating costus roots or inulin obtained from them for the production of fructose has been reported. Dried stems of the plant are used as fodder in winter.

Considered anodyne, antiseptic, aphrodisiac, bactericide, carminative, digestive, diuretic, expectorant, fungicide, insecticide, spasmolytic, stimulant, stomachic, tonic, and vermicide, costus is used for asthma, bronchitis, cancer, candidiasis, cholera, cough, diarrhea, dysentery, dyspepsia, fever, hypotension, nausea, parturition, skin, smallpox, spasm, stomachache, tumor, and tympanites. The root is sometimes smoked as an opium substitute. It has been used in coughs and asthma. An alcoholic extract of the root containing both the essential oil and the alkaloid has been found very useful in the treatment of bronchial asthma. The root is used for cancer, indurations of the liver and spleen, and tumors, especially of the abdomen. It is useful for chronic bronchitis and asthma. Inhalation of the smoke of the powdered drug produces a marked depression of the cerebral nervous system. Drug containing the alkaloid saussurine and the essential oil is effective in controlling paroxysms of bronchial asthma and useful in persistent hiccup. In Iran and vicinity, costus root is prescribed externally and internally for various complaints, and is taken locally to ward off the effects of animal and snake bites.

Cotton – (Gossypium Herbaceum)
...There were white cotton curtains and blue hanging caught up with cords of fine linen...Esther 1

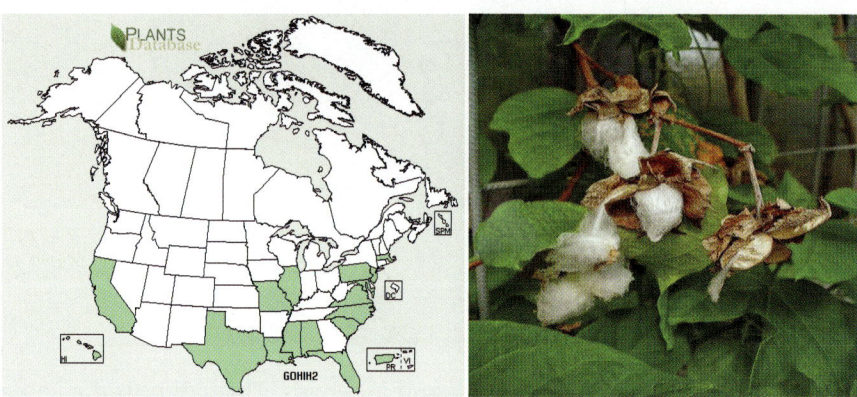

Mentioned only once in the Holy scriptures, cotton was used as clothing in which the Egyptian mummies were wrapped. Plants cultivated as an annual for the fiber among the seeds that furnish Asiatic or Levant cotton. Seeds used for extraction of oil, used for cooking, soapmaking, and other domestic purposes. Oil cake was used as fertilizer and fodder.

Considered abortifacient, antiseptic, aphrodisiac, demulcent, emmenagogue, emollient, expectorant, hemostat, iactagogue, laxative, nervine, oxytocic, vasoconstrictor, and vulnerary, cotton is a folk "remedy" for dysentery, fever, fibroma of the uterus, headache, hemorrhage, leprosy, malaria, parturition, pharyngitis, polyps, scabies, scorpion stings, snakebite, sores, and tumors. The seed or root is used for cancer, uterine fibromas, and nasal polyps. In South America, the root decoction is drunk by females as a contraceptive, the seed taken as a lactagogue or breast enlarger. Africans take the leaf decoction for dysentery and headache. The oilseed cake contains ca. 4% glutamic acid. In its free state L. glutamic acid is used to treat mental deficiencies in infants and adolescents. In the United States, early southerners are said to have used cottonseed for malaria with good results.

Ayurvedics regard the flowers as antibilious, antihallucinogenic, lactogogue, refrigerant and tonic, the leaves they use for ear trouble, anemia and oliguria, regarding the seeds as aphrodisiac and lactogogue. They use the plant for snakebite, scorpion stings, skin ailments and uterine discharges. Unani regard the seeds as an aphrodisiac, expectorant, and laxative, using them for orchitis; they poultice the flowers on burns, scabies, and scalds, and use them in syrup for hypochondria, and insanity; the leaves they take internally for dysentery, externally for gout; flowers are also used as analgesic for burning eyes and inflammation. Roots of the plant were used by Lebanese for malaria and Malta fever. Lebanese men suffering impotency use the decoction cautiously, while the women use it as an emmenagogue and lactagogue. Finally, strong repeated applications are said to reduce tumors.

CROWN OF THORNS – (*PALIURUS SPINA*)
...And when they had platted a crown of thorns...Matthew 27

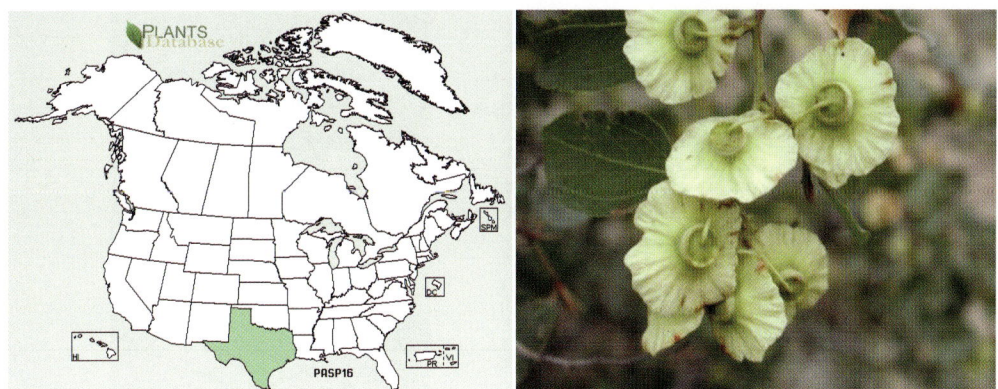

There are two Rhamnaceous crown of thorns, one in the genus paliurus, the other is ziziphus. Paliurus has a dry flattened fruit with a winglike margin; ziziphus has a fleshy globular fruit. In Palestine, the plant was used as an anticathartic, astringent, diuretic, and tonic.

Cucumber – (*Cucumis Sativus*)
...as a lodge in the garden of cucumbers, as a besieged city...Isaiah 1

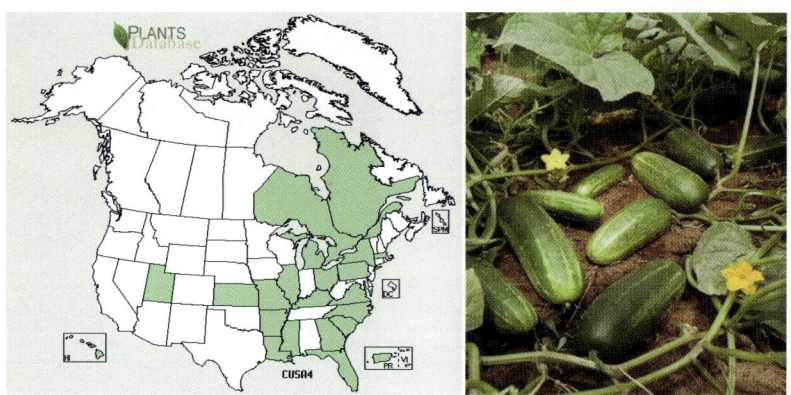

Most famous perhaps as a vegetable, less famous as a soup ingredient and cosmetic, the cucumber needs little introduction. Young leaves are eaten raw or steamed in Malaya. Cucumber soap is said to be especially beneficial for windburn. Cucumber juice is said to kill cockroaches, repelling fish moths and wood lice. Even the strewing of the green peel on the floor at night "is effective."

Iranians use the seed for typhoid. The plant is used in Ayurvedic and Unani medicine just like the melon. The fruit is regarded as cooling and diuretic. Cucumber soup has been prescribed for urine retention. In Indochina, candied cucumbers are prescribed for children's dysentery. In Indonesia, the fruit or its juice is suggested for gallstones and sprue. In Korea, cucumber salve is used for burns, scalds, and skin disorders. Leafjuice is used as a children's emetic. The diuretic root decoction is a treatment for beri beri. The proteolytic enzymes reported in cucumber may provide a rational backdrop to its use cosmetically to remove facial blemishes. In Lebanon the sap that oozes from the scraped cucumber skin is mixed with yoghurt to treat cold sores. Lebanese believe that cucumbers prevent colds. A favorite Lebanese salad; laban, cucumbers and yoghurt, is also used to soften skin, dispel acne, smooth rash, and heal sunburn. In Madagascar the fruit is used as an anthelmintic, a use showing up in many cultures.

Cumin – (*Cuminum Cyminum*)
...for ye pay tithe of mint and anise and cummin...Matthew 23

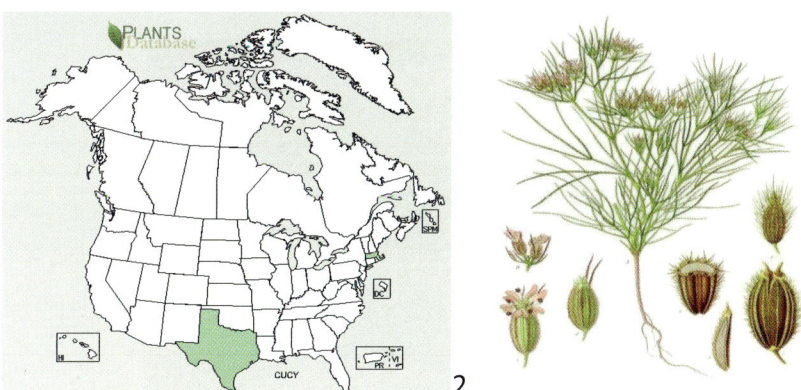

Used as a spice, cumin is crushed and mixed with bread and added to the meat pot. In Biblical times, cumin was used with fish and meat, especially stews. Egyptian cooks sprinkled the seeds on bread and cakes. Today the seeds flavor breads, cheeses, chutney, meat, pickles, rice, sauerkraut, sausage and soups. The essential oil is used in liqueurs and perfumes.

Said to be antispasmodic, astringent, carminative, digestive, em menagogue, lactagogue, stimulant, stomachic, sudorific, and tonic, cumin has been suggested as a folk remedy for chills, cold, colic, cough, corns, diarrhea, dyspepsia, flu, headache, heart, hysteria, puerperium, spasm, stomachache, tumors, veneral warts, and whitlow. Hartwell cites cumin as a folk treatment for scleroses of the liver, spleen, and uterus, and tumors of the abdomen, ears, fauces, feet, liver, parotid, spleen, testicles, and uvula. Oil of cumin is bactericidal and larvicidal. Cumin has some antioxidant properties. The essential oil is somewhat anesthetic.

In Biblical times, cumin was used as a medicine and an appetite stimulant. Ethiopians apply the pounded leaves to skin disorders. Unani use the fruit for asthma, boils, corneal opacities, epistaxis, gonorrhea, hemoptysis, hiccup, inflammation, scabies, splenomegaly, styes and ulcers, considering it abortifacient, astringent, carminative, emmenagogue, and vulnerary. Ayurvedics add aphrodisiac, anthelmintic, and alexipharmic to the list of fruit virtues, using it for belching, biliousness, consumption, dysentery, eye diseases, fever, leprosy, leucoderma, scorpion stings, and tumors. Arabs consider oil of cumin as an aphrodisiac, mixed with honey and pimenta and taken three times a day. In ancient Assyria, cumin was prescribed with garlic for constipation and gas. Lebanese use the seed oil, sometimes with orange flower water, for cramps, syncope, and tachycardia. In Iran the seeds are prescribed for the pain following childbirth. North Africans poultice the seeds on the nape of the neck for mumps.

The fruit contains the following minerals:

Boron	Manganese
Calcium	Nickel
Chromium	Nitrogen
Cobalt	Potassium
Copper	Sodium
Iron	Zinc

Hillman Health Food Store call 855-Amish-Dr (855-264-7437) www.emineral.info Vitamins and Minerals for Better Living

CYPRUS TURPENTINE – (PISTACIA TEREBINTHUS)
...As the turpentine tree I stretched out my branches...Ecclesiasticus 24

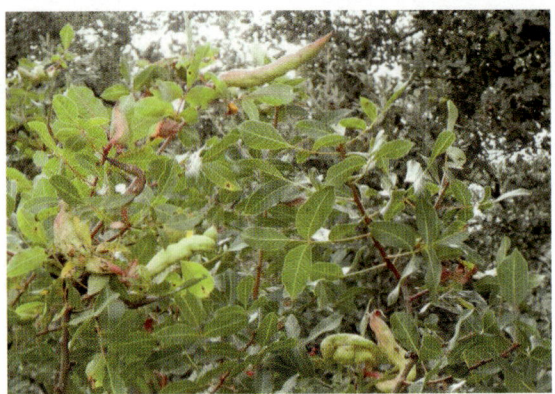

The teil is a tree of spreading habit, with a thick trunk. The wood is hard and white. Its foliage is dense enough to cast a heavy shade on the deserts heated in the sun. When the bark is cut, Chian turpentine flows out: this has an agreeable perfume, not unlike jessamine, and is mild to the taste. Exposure to the air solidifies it to a transparent gum. This Gilead turpentine probably formed part of the spicery carried into Egypt from Gilead by the Ishmaelites as mentioned in Genesis 37:25. Bark and leaves a source of tannin. The astringent leaves are also used for dyeing. The gum is used to sweeten the breath, e.g. in Tehran.

Few resins have a greater "repertoire" in anticancer folklore than this plant, used for ascites, calluses, cancers (of the breast, face, lip, liver, medullary, pylorus, rectum, spleen, testicle, tongue, uterus, vagina), carcinoma, corn, cysts, epithelioma, excrescences, fungoids, inflammation, melanosis, polyps, sclerosis (breast, liver), skin ailments, and tumors (especially of the spleen). With tannins, sitosterol, and shikimic acid reported, perhaps this cancer "repertoire" is justified. Leaves are used as an emmenagogue and for albuminuria and diarrhea. Lebanese infuse the leaves for diarrhea and fever.

DANDELION – (TARAXACUM OFFICINALE)
...eat it with unleavened bread and bitter herbs...Numbers 9

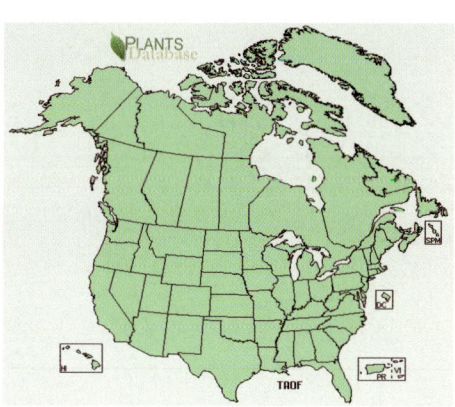 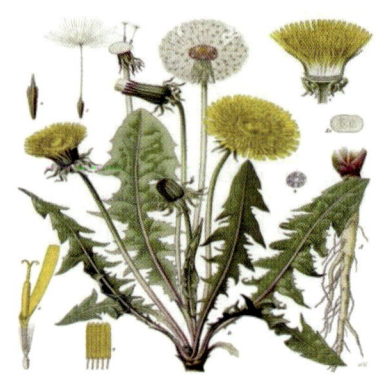

Probably the children of Israel learned to eat bitter herbs from the Egyptians. Ancient Egyptians used to place the green herbs on the table, mixed with mustard, and then dunked their bread in the mixture. Cichorium endivia, cichorium intybus, lactuca sativa, nasturtium officinale, rumex acetosella, and Taraxacum officinale were among the green herbs of the Bible. Dandelion is sometimes eaten raw in salads, but often blanched like endive and used as a green; frequently cooked with salt pork or bacon to enhance the flavor. The roots are sometimes pickled. Flowers are used to make a wine. Ground roasted roots are used for dandelion coffee, and sometimes mixed with real coffee. Dried leaves are an ingredient in many digestive or diet drinks and herb beers. Birds like the seeds and pigs devour the whole plant. Goats eat the leaves, but sheep, cattle, and horses do not care for it. Dandelion has also been used as a source of latex.

Said to be alterative, aperient, apertif, bactericidal, cholagogue, depurative, diuretic, intoxicant, lactagogue, laxative, stimulant, stomachic, and tonic, dandelion finds a place in many folk remedies, for abscesses, ague, anemia, arthritis, bad appetite, bilious afflictions, blood, bronchitis, bruises, cancer, caries, catarrh, conjunctivitis, consumption, diabetes, dropsy, dyspepsia, eczema, fever, gallbladder, gallstones, gonorrhea, gout, gravel, heart, heartburn, hemorrhoids, hepatitis, hypochondria, inappetence, indigestion, indurations, insomnia, jaundice, kidney, liver, malaria, nephritis, nerves, piles, rheumatism, scirrhus, sclerosis, scurvy, scrofula, skin, snakebite, splenitis, stones, swelling, tumors, urinary ailments, warts, and wounds. Indurations of the glands, liver, mesentery and spleen, and cancer of the bladder, bowel and breast may be treated. The leaves have a higher Vitamin A content (14,000 IU/100g) than carrots (11,000 IU/100g). Dandelion has demonstrated hypoglycemic activity in animals. Dandelion extracts are used in antismoking compounds. Species of dandelion have been used in China for breast cancer for over 1,000 years. Widely distributed, beta sitosterol has shown several types of anti-tumor activity. Roots have been used medicinally as a simple bitter and mild laxative. Roots, considered aperient, diuretic, and tonic, are used for chronic disorders of kidney and liver, for gallstones, piles, and warts. Lebanese extract the root in wine as a laxative or purgative, depending on the strength.

The leaf contains the following minerals:

Boron	Chromium	Magnesium
Bromine	Copper	Nickel
Calcium	Iodine	Potassium
Chlorine	Iron	Sodium

Hillman Health Food Store call 855-Amish-Dr (855-264-7437) www.emineral.info Vitamins and Minerals for Better Living

The root contains the following minerals:

Aluminum	Magnesium	Silica
Calcium	Manganese	Sodium
Chromium	Nickel	Tin
Cobalt	Potassium	Zinc
Iron	Selenium	

The plant contains the following minerals:

Calcium	Nickel	Sulfur
Manganese	Rubidium	Titanium
Molybdenum	Strontium	

The fruit contains the following minerals:

Aluminum	Boron

The leaf contains glutamate.

DARNEL – (LOLIUM TEMULENTUM)
...But while men slept, his enemy came and sowed tares among the wheat...Matthew 13

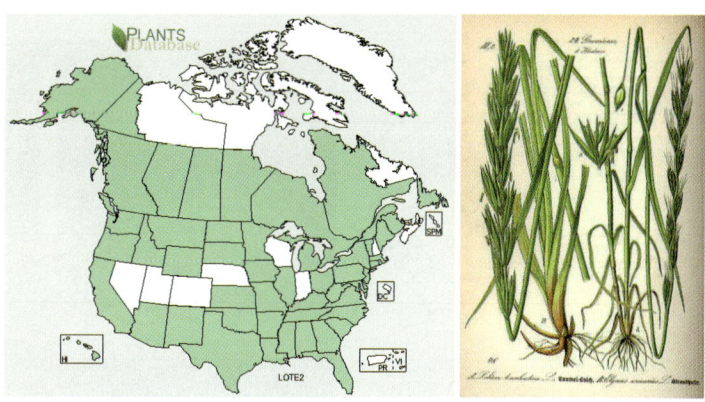

Darnel affords a nutritive feed for livestock, but animals should not be allowed to graze after the seeds set. Human deaths are attributed to eating the infected seed, ground up with wheat. It serves as chicken and pigeon feed, but even this is discouraged.

Regarded as anodyne, narcotic, POISON, the tare is a folk remedy for gangrene, headache, meningitis, neuralgia, rheumatism, and sciatica. It has quite a reputation for "cancer remedies." Moroccans use the plant decoction for hemorrhage and urinary incontinence. Used for cancer, indurations, kernels, "knots," putrid flesh, scirrhus (liver and spleen), tumors and wens. According to homeopath, it is used for St. Vitus' dance and idiocy, having been dropped by the allopaths. Boulos cites homeopathic usage of the seeds for arthritis, epistaxis, intestinal cramps, nausea, neuralgia, rheumatism and trembling limbs.

In Lebanon, where the plant is commonly known to be the tares of the Bible, and where the danger of ergotism is well known, the Lebanese hint that there is a mystic cult "in the mountains" which infuses the grass or soaks the seeds to extract the ergot which is then used to induce religious ecstasy. Lebanese women made a tea of the whole grass for children with colic. Adults used the ground seed for blood poisoning, leprosy, migraine, rheumatism and toothache. Seed meal has been used as a poultice in skin diseases and taken internally during menopause. Finally, the poultice is said to bring out splinters and broken bones.

DATE PALM – (PHOENIX DACTYLIFERA)
...and brought them to Jericho, the city of palm trees...
II Chronicles 28

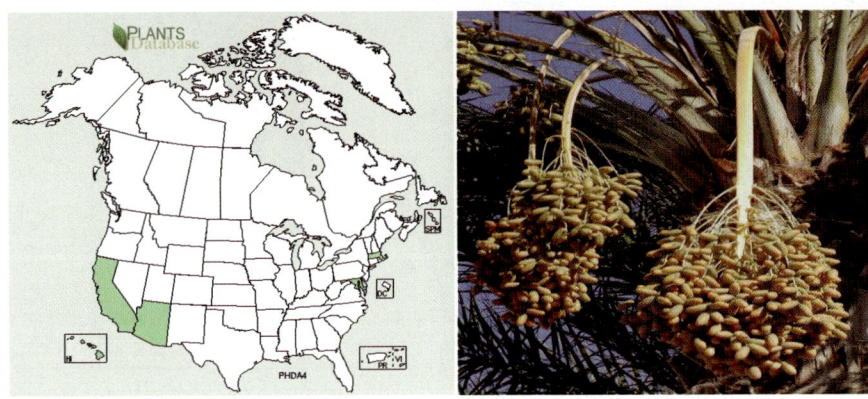

Date palm "was from earliest times associated with Palestine, and was the symbol on its coinage." The Psalmist says, "The righteous shall flourish like the palm tree." To those who inhabited Palestine, the illustration would lead them to contemplate the straight and erect growth of the tree, its unbranched and unencumbered stem, and the beauteous crown of leaves at its summit. It would also recall to their minds that the palm flourished in the desert, and that its presence there always indicated moisture. Arabs says, "Its head should be in fire (sunshine) and its feet in water." Mats are woven from the leaves, while the fibers provide thread and rigging for boats. There is sap in the palm tree which, after fermentation, is used as liquor. This may be some of the strong drink or wine of the Bible. Still Hausa add dates with hot peppers to native beer to make it less intoxicating. The Arabs say that there are as many uses for dates as there are days in the year.

Date palm is cultivated primarily for fruit, eaten fresh, or dried. It is thought of as a high energy food or having high sugar content, as well as a good source of iron and potassium. Balfour recounts that 95% of the people of Fezzan survive on dates for nine months of the year, 100% of the doors are made from date timber, and most huts are thatched with leaves. Fruits are often preserved by drying or pressing them together into large cakes. Other products include date "honey" (bees are mentioned only four times in the Bible, while "honey" is mentioned 49 times), made from juice of fresh fruit; date sugar; date sap, often made into a fermented beverage; date palm flour, made from pith of tree; oil from seeds; the kernels are ground up or soaked in water for days and used for animal food; seeds are also strung as beads; both wine and honey are derived from the date. In medieval days, the palm was thought to prevent sunstroke, avert lightening, cure fevers, and drive away mice and fleas.

Nigerians feed dates with bran and Sterculia to immature young heifers to make them more prolific. In the Holy Land, the large leaves are still used to cover the roofs and sides of houses and to solidify reed fences. Mats, baskets, even dishes are made from them. Small leaves are used as dusters and the trunks for timber. Rope is made from the integument in the crown.

Regarded as aphrodisiac, contraceptive, demulcent, diuretic, emollient, estrogenic, expectorant, laxative, pectoral, purgative, refrigerant, the date is listed in folk remedies for ague, anemia, asthma, bronchitis, cancer, catarrh, chest, condylomata, cough, diarrhea, eyes, fatigue, fever, flu, gonorrhea, indurations, longevity, piles, pterygia, splenitis, sterility, stomachache, thirst, toothache, tuberculosis, urogenital ailments, vaginitis, virility, warts and whitlows. Medicinally, fresh juice is cooling and laxative; gum useful in treatment of diarrhea and diseases of genitourinary system; fruit is demulcent, expectorant, anti scorbutic, nutrient, laxative, aphrodisiac, and is prescribed in asthma, chest complaints and cough, fever and gonorrhea.

Cancers, indurations or tumors of the abdomen, gum, liver, mouth, parotids, spleen, stomach, testicle, throat, uterus, and viscera can be treated. A plaster of the nuts or of the bark is a folk remedy for whitlows, hardnesses and scirrhi. The nut cataplasm is said to help testicle tumors. The fruit, prepared in various manners, is said to remedy cancer of the stomach and uterus, abdominal tumors, hardnesses of the liver and spleen, and ulcerated and non ulcerated cancers. Unripe fruits are used as an astringent for hemorrhoids by the Arabs. Lebanese believe the sugar from the fruits helps hepatitis. They applied powdered seeds or directed the smoke onto any affliction. Algerians smoke the seed powder for fever. Dates were used, with other ingredients, in vaginal pessaries by North Africans to enhance fertility. Ashes of the seeds used in ophthalmic collyria.

The fruit contains the following minerals:

Aluminum	Iodine	Potassium
Boron	Iron	Silica
Calcium	Magnesium	Sodium
Chlorine	Manganese	Sulfur
Copper	Nitrogen	Zinc

The fruit contains the following amino acids:

Alanine	Leucine	Threonine
Arginine	Lysine	Tryptophan
Glutamate	Methionine	Tyrosine
Glycine	Phenylalanine	Valine
Histidine	Proline	
Isoleucine	Serine	

The seeds contain the following minerals:

Aluminum	Iron	Potassium
Calcium	Manganese	Sodium
Copper	Nitrogen	Zinc

Hillman Health Food Store call 855-Amish-Dr (855-264-7437) www.emineral.info Vitamins and Minerals for Better Living

DATE-PLUM – (DIOSPYROS EBENUM)
...they brought thee for a present horns of ivory and ebony...
Ezekiel 27

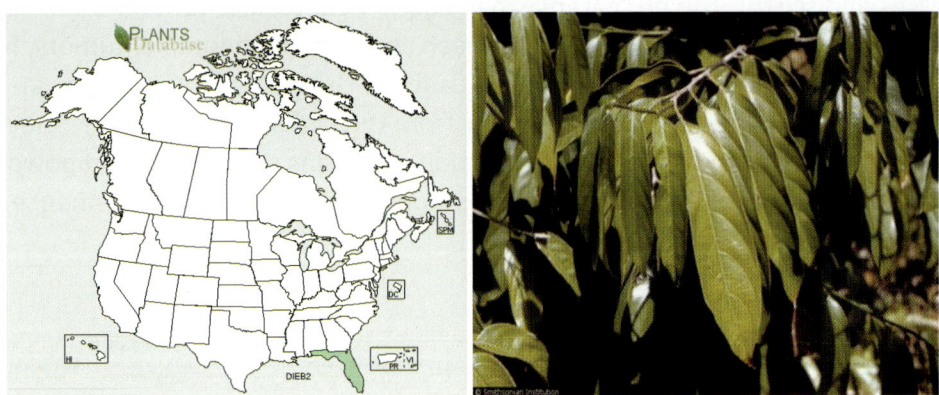

The heartwood of several tropical species is the source of ebony. It is a hard black wood used for piano keys. Ebony was used, of old as it is today, frequently inlaid with ivory. It is thought that 200 logs of ebony presented to the Kings of Persia every year by the Ethiopians were originally from India or Sri Lanka. The royal throne of Pluto, King of the mythical underworld, was made of ebony, as were carvings of many Egyptian gods and goddesses, especially those of Darkness, Night and Sorrow. The plant is astringent, attenuant and lithontryptic. It has been used also for such skin ailments as itch, leprosy, and ringworm, as well as cancerous excrescences.

Desert Date – (Balanites Aegyptiaca)
...Is there no balm in Gilead; is there no physician there?...Jeremiah 8

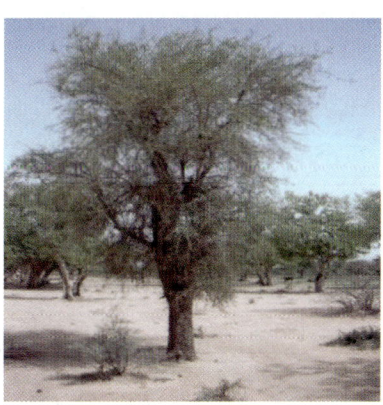

Monks of Jericho regard balanites as the balm. They prepare an oily gum from the fruit which is sold in tin cases to travelers as the balm of Gilead. Both Balanites and Pistacia are common in Palestine and both are called balm. A desert-loving plant, Balanites is also revered by the Mohammedans in western India. The wood is used for axes, cudgels, Mohammedan writing boards, mortars and pestles, walking sticks, and wooden bowls. Since it gives little smoke, it is a favorite firewood for burning indoors. Spiny branches are used to pen up animals. The bark yields a strong fiber. The fruit is fermented to make an intoxicating beverage. In West Africa and Chad the seed is used for making breadstuffs and soups, whole the leaf is used as a vegetable, the pericarp crushed and eaten. Flowers are eaten in soups in West Africa. The oil which constitutes 40% of the fruit is comestible and used to make soap. African Arabs use the fruit as a detergent, and the bark to poison fish. The active principle, probably a saponin, is lethal to cercaria, fish, miracidia, mollusks and tadpoles.

Fruits are pounded and boiled to extract the medicinal vulnerary oil. The oil was poured over open wounds and apparently acted as an antiseptic and protective covering against secondary infections. One Turkish surgeon regarded this as one of the best stomachics, a most excellent remedy for curing wounds. In Ethiopia the bark is used as an antiseptic, the leaf to dress wounds, and the fruit as an anthelmintic laxative. In Palestine, the oil is said to be used in folk medicine. Ghanans used the leaves as a vermifuge while Libyans use them to clean malignant wounds. Powdered root bark is used for herpes zoster while the root extracts are suggested for malaria. Ghanans use the bark from the stem in fumigation to heal the wounds of circumcision. Nigerians consider it abortifacient. The oil from the fruits is applied to aching bones and swollen rheumatic joints by the Lebanese. Extracts of the root have proven slightly effective in experimental malaria. Bark has been used in treating syphilis. In Chad the plant is used as a fumigant in liver disease, the seed as a febrifuge and the fruit for colds. Ugandans use the oil for sleeping sickness, but the efficacy is questioned. Ayurvedics apply the fruit oil to ulcers, the fruit for other skin ailment and rat bites, regarding the fruit as alexipharmic, alterative, analgesic, anthelmintic, antidysenteric. Finally, Unanis use the fruit also for boils and leucoderma.

DILL – (ANETHUM GRAVEOLENS)
...Woe unto you, scribes and Pharisees, hypocrites! For ye pay tithe of mint and anise and cummin...Matthew 23

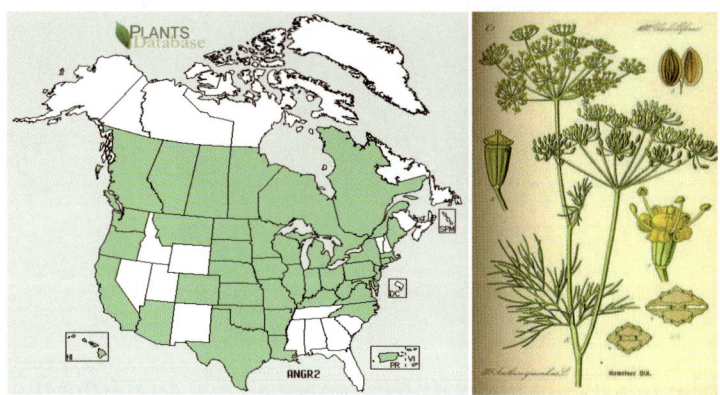

Dill was grown by the ancient Greeks and Romans. The Talmud records that its seeds, stems, and leaves were subject to tithe. Today in India, dill is a universal medicine. Dill is more characteristically a plant of oriental cultivation than anise. Dill is used primarily as a condiment. Dried fruits (seeds) are used in pickles, soups, spiced beets, fish, and fish sauces, with eggs and in potato salads. Roasted fruits have served as coffee substitute. Hot extracts of the fruit are used to make jams and liqueurs, the dill oil in other liqueurs. Fresh leaves are used in salads, with cottage cheese, cream cheese, steaks, chops, avocado, cauliflower, green beans, squash, tomatoes, tomato soup, zucchini, and shrimp. Dried leaves, known as dill weed, are also used to season various foods. Ethiopians use tender plant parts, dried fruits and flowers in flavorings, especially alcoholic beverages. Oil from the seed is used chiefly as a scent in soaps and perfumes, and in the pickle industry. Weed oil, from the aboveground parts of the plant, is used in the food industry because of its characteristic dill herb smell and flavor. The essential oil has shown inhibitory effects on various organisms, like Bacillus anthracis.

Said to be anodyne, apertif, balsamic, calmative, carminative, detersive, diaphoretic, digestive, diuretic, lactagogue, laxative, narcotic, psychedelic, resolvent, sedative, stimulant, and stomachic. Dill is one folk remedy for anemia, bad appetite, bad breath, bruises, colic, condylomata, cough, cramps, dropsy, flatulence, halitosis, hangover, hiccoughs, indigestion, insomnia, jaundice, nerves, sclerosis, scurvy, sores, spasm, stomachache, swellings, and tumors. Hartwell also mentions dill as a folk remedy for cancerous conditions like: apostemes, indurations of the liver, spleen, and stomach, tumors of the abdomen, anus, liver, mouth, and throat, and uterine fibroids. Ayurvedics use the seed for abdominal pain, biliousness, eye ailments, fever, ulcers and uterine pains. Unani use it for bladder ailments, cold, dysentery, earache, gleet, griping, hiccough, liver ailments, piles, splenitis and syphilis, considering it alexiteric, carminative, diuretic, emmenagogue, laxative, stomachic, suppurative and vulnerary. In Ethiopia, the plant is used for gonorrhea, parturition and stomachache. The leaves are boiled in coffee or tea, or chewed as a diuretic in gonorrhea and as a laxative in stomachache. Ethiopians use the fruit for cough, headache, stomachache, and urine retention. All these uses are shared with fennel there. In Lebanon, dill tea is used interchangeably or together with Pimpinella for colic in babies. Drops of dill oil are taken for dyspepsia, and sometimes the oil is mixed with charcoal, starch and tragacanth, or other gums like acacia, to make a digestive pill.

Dill fruit has the following minerals:

Calcium	Magnesium	Potassium
Copper	Manganese	Sodium
Iron	Nitrogen	Zinc

The dill plant contains the following minerals:

Aluminum	Fluorine	Potassium
Boron	Iron	Rubidium
Bromine	Magnesium	Selenium
Calcium	Manganese	Silica
Chromium	Molybdenum	Sodium
Cobalt	Nickel	Sulfur
Copper	Nitrogen	Zinc

The seed is high in boron.

The following amino acids are found in dill fruit:

Arginine	Leucine	Phenylalanine
Histidine	Lysine	Threonine
Isoleucine	Methionine	Valine

Dyer's Oak – (Quercus Aegilops)
...and as an oak, whose substance is in them, when they cast their leaves...Isaiah 6

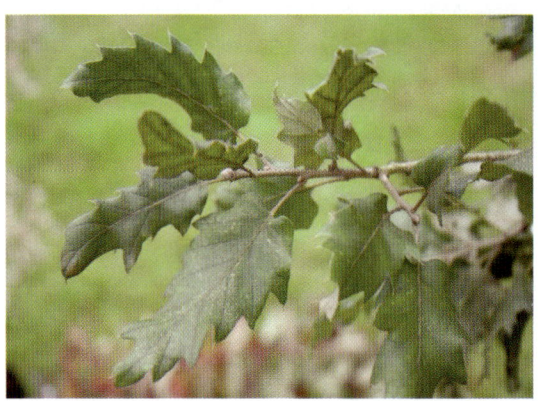

In Tyre, oak was used for making oars (Ezekiel 27). In olden times persons were sometimes buried in oak shade. The tree grows to handsome proportions. The acorn it bears is very large. An insect attacks the bark of the tree and results in galls or swellings that contain gallic acid and tannin from which writing ink is made. A strong black dye of commercial value is derived from the acorn cups. Swine are fed acorns, and in Algeria and Greece the poor eat them too. Dyer's oak is a European folk medicine for malignancy. A thick liquid made from the bark is used on burns in Lebanon.

EAGLEWOOD – (AQUILLARIA AGALLOCHA)
...*All thy garments smell of myrrh, and aloes...Psalm 45*

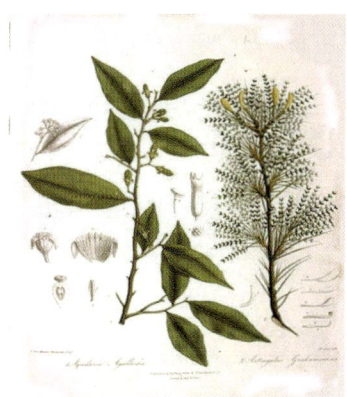

Eaglewood is the aloe of the Old Testament; that of the New Testament is generally regarded as a true aloe. The darker wood, especially when partially diseased and decayed, is highly valued in perfumery, as incense, and for fumigation. The treasured unhealthy wood is so much more valuable than the healthy, that the healthy tree is usually destroyed in search for patches of unhealthy wood. Known as agar, it is powdered and used to prevent or repel fleas and lice. The soft and fragrant inner wood was molded and used as a setting for precious stones. It was worth its weight in gold to the ancients. In the East, this aloe is the only tree believed to have descended to man from the Garden of Eden, all others being lost. According to legend, Adam brought away from the garden one of its shoots, transplanted it in the land where he settled, and all other aloes have sprung from this shoot. To this day it is called shoot of Paradise and Paradise wood. The bark was beaten to make a primitive cloth in Malaya. Annamese make a paper substitute from the bark, having presented 30,000 rolls of aloe paper to a Chinese emperor in A.D. 284.

Regarded as anodyne, aphrodisiac, carminative, cordial, diuretic, stimulant, stomachic, and tonic, agar is a folk remedy for abdominal pains, asthma, cancer (especially cancer of the thyroid), chest, colic, congestion, diarrhea, fever, gastralgia, gout, hiccups, kidney, malaria, nausea, paralysis, rheumatism, skin ailments, and tumors (especially of the abdomen and lung. It's used for cancer, indurations (of the liver and stomach), putrid flesh, and tumors of the abdomen. Sanskrit literature advises that an aloes preparation was burned as an anodyne fumigation for surgical wounds. In Malaya, the root is recommended for dropsy and the leaves are used if the roots fail. The wood enters decoctions drunk by females during pregnancy, following childbirth, and for other female ailments. Ayurvedics use the wood for ear and eye ailments, asthma, hiccup, and leucoderma and skin trouble. Unani use it for asthma, bronchitis, diarrhea, enteritis, gastritis, hepatitis, nausea, and to stabilize the fetus in the uterus. The smoke from burning wood is used for palsy and vertigo.

EBONY PERSIMMON – (*DIOSPYROS MELANOXYLUM*)
...they brought thee for a present horns of ivory and ebony...
Ezekiel 27

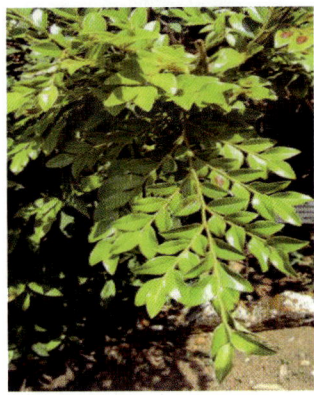

Probably most famed as a source of ebony, this species is also the source of an edible fruit and a cigarette wrapper. Indian bidis are frequently wrapped in the leaves from coppice shoots of this fine fuel species. Bidis, the popular cigarettes of India's working class are made by wrapping tobacco (or herbs) in a specially prepared leaf. The other raw materials are tobacco and cotton thread. Quality bidi leaves are plucked after they have turned from crimson to green and become leathery in texture. Softness, pliability and absence of pubescense are the three qualities conditioning selection of bidi leaves.

Charak, the great historical Hindu physician, correctly classified this tanniniferous species under astringents. Another famed Indian physician suggested that it was benefitical for ulcers, uterine and vaginal disorders. The bark is burnt in Central India to treat smallpox. The fruits are regarded as astringent and refrigerant. The Hindu pharmacopoeia considers the seeds intoxicating yet prescribe them for heart palpitations, mental disorders, and nervous breakdowns. The leaves are said to be carminative, diuretic, laxative and styptic. The dried flowers are used in urinary, blood, and skin disorders. The astringent bark is used for diarrhea and dyspepsia and the diluted extract as a collyrium. In India, magical properties are also attributed to the ebony; in procuring obedient servants, deciding the water level in the soil, and in breaking an exceptionally hard rock. Indian Hakims apply powdered bark to corneal ulcers, and suggests its internal use for black pepper dysentery. According to Kirtikar and Basu, the Unani use the leaves for burns, epistaxis, ophthalmia, scabies, trichiasis, tubercular glands and wens, the flowers for anemia, leucorrhea, nightblindness, scabies, splenitis and urinary discharges.

Egyptian Marjoram – (*Origanum Maru*)
...Purge me with hyssop, and I shall be clean...Psalm 51

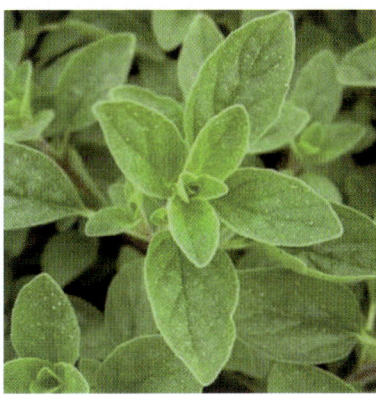

The hyssop of the Old Testament is most probably Origanum maru, the Syrian marjoram or the Egyptian marjoram, while the hyssop of the Crucifixion is sorghum. The common kind of marjoram (O. vulgare), so well known in gardens, grows only to the north of the Biblical settings, but the allied species (O. maru) abounds through the central hills. The uses of the Syrian marjoram, if in fact it is specifically distinct, are not expected to differ from those of the true marjoram. An aromatic substance is obtained from the crushed and dried leaves. The "hyssop" of the Scriptures was used to sprinkle the door posts of the Israelites in Egypt with the blood of the paschal lamb so that the angel of death would pass by that house. It was employed in the purification of lepers and leprous houses, suggesting the psalmists purge.

Origanum maru has a folk reputation for tumors of the uterus, flbroids, and polyps, but probably shares other medicinal attributes with Origanum vulgare, viz. anodyne, anthelmintic, antiseptic, carminative, choleretic, decongestant, diaphoretic, digestive, diuretic, emmenagogue, expectorant, fungicidal, nervine, pectoral, purgative, rubefacient, sedative, spasmolytic, stimulant, stomachic, stupefacient, sudorific, and tonic properties. Whether it contains the anticancer agent, ursolic acid, found in Origanum vulgare, has not been shown. The flowers are said to be antispasmodic, emmenagogue, stimulant and sudorific and are used for paralysis and skin ailments. Seeds are regarded as a diuretic and a laxative. In Lebanon tea of Origanum maru is used for children's colds and colic; macerated leaves are applied to rheumatic swellings and sprains.

ENDIVE – (CICHORIUM ENDIVIA)
...eat it with unleavened bread and bitter herbs...Numbers 9

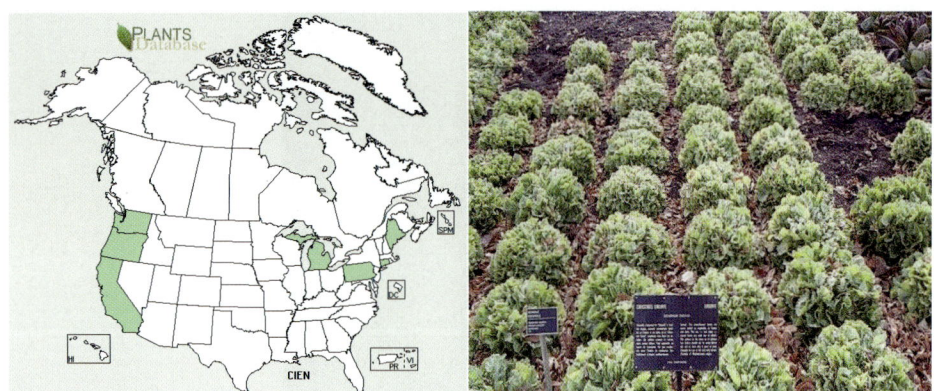

Many regard endive as the bitter herb of Moses. The Jews of Alexandria, who translated the Pentateuch, would have known which herbs were eaten with the Paschal lamb. Fresh leaves have a bitter smell, but full grown blanched leaves are pleasant. For blanching, the outer leaves are tied up in the form of a cone, or a big flower pot is placed over each plant to cut off the light. Blanching is complete in about three weeks. Seeds are used in sherberts.

Regarded as antibilious, carminative, demulcent, diuretic, laxative, refrigerant, resolvent, and tonic, endive is useful for dyspepsia and fevers. The fruit is used for fever, headache and jaundice. The latex is used for cancer of the uterus, tumors of the liver and spleen and throat, and indurations of the spleen. The endive, used by the Lebanese as a salad and vegetable, and to increase flow of bile, is used medicinally like chicory. They also have dwarf chicory which the peasants use for dropsy, gout, and warts. The root is used for dyspepsia.

The leaf contains the following minerals:

Aluminum	Lithium	Selenium
Boron	Magnesium	Silver
Calcium	Manganese	Sodium
Chromium	Molybdenum	Titanium
Cobalt	Nickel	Zinc
Copper	Nitrogen	
Iron	Potassium	

The shoots contain the following minerals:

Strontium	Sulfur	

The leaf contains the following amino acids:

Alanine	Leucine	Threonine
Arginine	Lysine	Tyrosine
Glutamate	Methionine	Tryptophan
Glycine	Phenylalanine	Valine
Histidine	Proline	
Isoleucine	Serine	

English Walnut – (*Juglans Regia*)

...I went down into the garden of nuts to see the fruits of the valley, and to see whether the vine flourished, and the pomegranates budded...

Song of Solomon 6

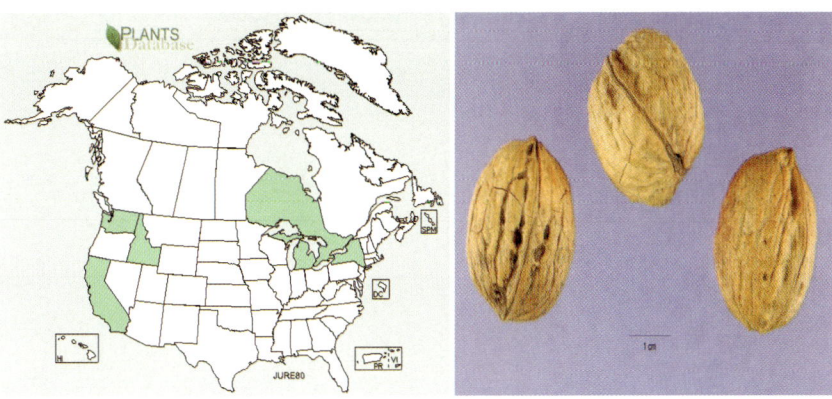

One of King Solomon's most valuable fruit trees was the walnut, a handsome tree with smooth gray bark and fresh green leaves. Walnuts were widely cultivated in Biblical times for the nuts and timber. Greeks and Romans regarded walnuts as symbols of fecundity, and scattered walnuts about at weddings. The heavy green rind encasing the nut is steeped in boiling water to produce a brown dye. In Jesus' time, walnut trees grew on the shores of the Sea of Galilee. His seamless coat was a rich brown, the dye said to have been made from walnut leaves and nuts. Walnuts are also used to tint gray hair black. In Algeria, the leaf decoction is used as a shampoo "against fall of hair."

Today the walnut is principally valued as an orchard tree for commercial nut production. Nuts are consumed fresh, roasted, or salted, and are used in candies, pastries, and flavorings. Ground nut shells are used as adulterant of spices. Crushed leaves or a decoction are used as insect repellant and as a tea. The outer fleshy part of fruit is very rich in Vitamin C and produces a yellow dye. Fruits, when dry pressed, yield valuable oil used in paints and soaps. When the fruit is cold pressed, it yields light yellow edible oil which is used in foods as flavoring. A decoction of leaves, bark, and husks are used with alum for staining wool brown. The wood is hard, durable, close grained, heavy, and used for furniture and gun stocks. The tree is often grown as ornamental.

Orientals use the kernels for laryngeal and lung disorder, and mix them with almond and ginseng for chronic cough and the oil is used for skin ailments. Lebanese think the nut increases fertility. The leaves, bark, and hulls are an alternative, astringent and a laxative. Leaf infusion is considered antidiabetic, antiscrofulous, astringent and tonic. The oil from old nuts, gone rancid, was applied to old ulcers. Husks of the nuts were used by the Lebanese as an anodyne. Algerians burned the shells in sugar for headache. Other North Africans inhaled the smoke of burning shells for coryza and influenza. The bark is used to cleanse and whiten the teeth, to redden the gums and lips, and to alleviate gingivitis, halitosis and pyorrhea. Regarded as alterative, anodyne, anthelmintic, astringent, bactericidal, cholagogue, depurative, detergent, digestive, diuretic, hemostat, insecticidal, laxative, lithontryptic, stimulant, tonic, and vermifuge, walnut is a folk remedy for anthrax, aphtha, backache, caligo, carbuncle, carcinomata, chancre, colic, condylomata, conjunctivitis, corns, cough, dysentery, eczema, egilops, favus, gangrene, heartburn, impotence, inflammation, legs, leucorrhea, lungs, rejuvenation, renitis, rheumatism, scrofula, skin, swellings, syphilis, toes, warts, whitlows, and worms. Walnut is a folk "remedy" for cancer of the intestine, lip and stomach; scleroses of the liver and uterus; tumors of the breast, fauces, gullet, kidney, stomach, and throat.

Hillman Health Food Store call 855-Amish-Dr (855-264-7437) www.emineral.info Vitamins and Minerals for Better Living

With such an anticancer folk history, it is interesting to note that walnut contains the antitumor compound, juglone, a compound with some pesticidal and weedicidal attributes as well. Chinese use the leaves and powdered hull as an astringent and as a depurative in syphilis. The decoction is used externally in phylctenular conjunctivitis. In Ayurvedic medicine, walnut is anodyne, aphrodisiac, cardiotonic, carminative, expectorant, and used for bronchitis, bruises, piles, rabies, ringworm and watery eye in Unani.

EUPHRATES ASPEN – (*POPULUS EUPHRATICA*)
...We hanged our harps upon the willows in the midst thereof...
Psalm 137

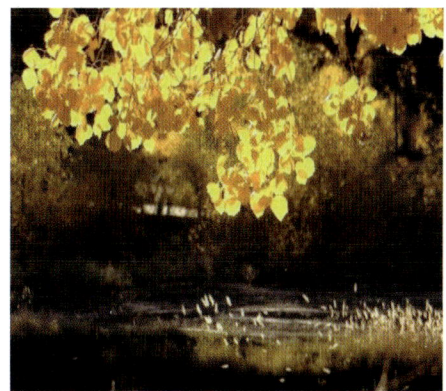

The willows, on which the Jews hung their harps as they wept at the thought of suffering Zion, are now believed to be Euphrates aspens. Some versions of the Bible even say poplars instead of willow. Early Christian legendry assumed Jesus' cross was made of aspen wood. Aspen trees everywhere shuddered when nails were driven into the wood and have trembled ever since. Judas was said to have hanged himself on Populus, or Cercis, or Ficus, or Pistacia. This is a fast-growing producer of soft timber, suitable for some kinds of carpentry. In Palestine, the resin from the bark was used in popular medicine.

Hillman Health Food Store call 855-Amish-Dr (855-264-7437) www.emineral.info Vitamins and Minerals for Better Living

European Box Thorn – (*Lycium Europaeum*)
...let fire come out of the bramble, and devour the cedars of Lebanon...
Judges 9

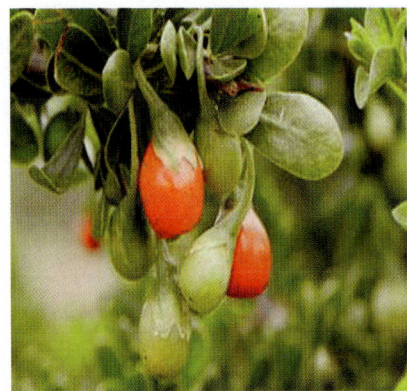

The berries of the box thorn are eaten; they contain ascorbic acid; oxidases and peroxidases are present. The plant is browsed by camels and goats.

It is a folk remedy for spasms and tumors, and sclerosis of the liver and spleen. Because of the high content of solanine, Arabs and Bedouins used the plants as an anti-inflammatory and agent in cataplasms. The branches are used in constructing wattled frames for walls, and frequently used for hedges.

European Rock Rose – (*Cistus Creticus*)
...a company of Ishmaelites came from Gilead with their camels bearing spicery and balm and myrrh...Genesis 37

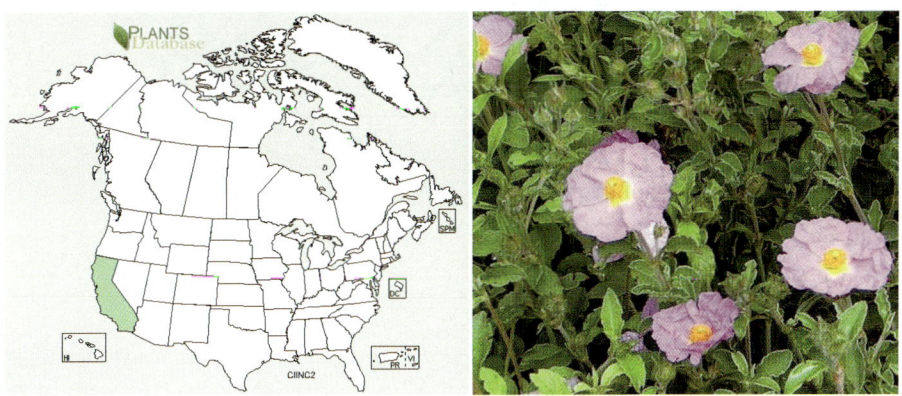

European rock rose is a source of an aromatic gum similar to the ladanum of commerce. It has a viscid gummy exudate with a fragrant odor and bitter taste. In early time ladanum was collected by herdsmen who combed it with the fleeces of their flock. The gum was once used extensively in medicine. Myrrh, perhaps this species, perhaps commiphorn myrra, was dissolved in beer for dyspnea. It was also used internally in catheters, enernas, and suppositories. Anderson says that ladanum was used to prepare plasters and wound dressings. It was valued as a stimulant, expectorant and emmenagogue. It has been used in catarrh and dysentery. Ladanum was also used for asthma and he reports its use also for "characteristic" female diseases.

FENUGREEK – (*TRIGONELLA FOENUM*)
...We remember the fish...and the leeks...Numbers 11

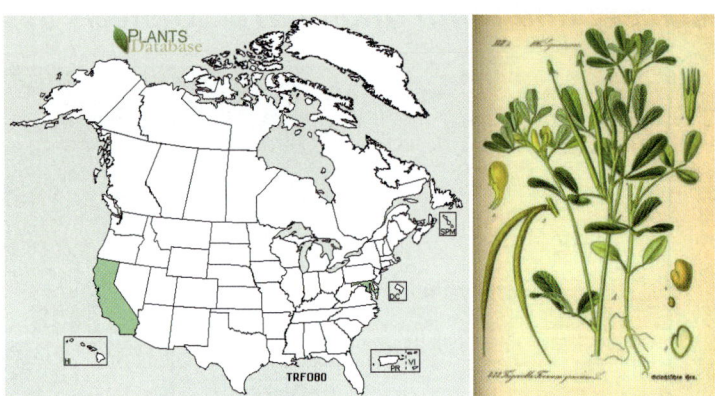

Some scholars consider the fenugreek more likely than Allium porrum to be the leek of the Bible. In India, the seeds are used as a condiment and in perfumery. Europeans add them to hay, especially old hay, to make it more appealing to the animals. Seeds are used as an adulterant in or substitute for coffee. They are also the source of a yellow dye. Fenugreek also has wide use in the Middle and Near East today. Fenugreek is almost as popular in Lebanon today as the peanut is in America as a snack. In Beirut, they make a mush from the green seed after soaking, forming a fenugreek "milkshake." The "milkshake" is prescribed in Lebanon for hypertension.

In the Middle East, fenugreek is often believed to be both preventive and panacea. At a Lebanese clinic, patients reported using it as a poultice, and for diabetes, dyspepsia, and fever and heart trouble. The root is more often used than the herb for pain and rheumatism. A fenugreek diet was reported (by only one informant) to speed the healing of broken bones, and to help convalescents, especially those suffering from chest inflammations, and recovering from typhoid. The mucilaginous seeds, emollient, tonic, and vermifugal, are used for chapped lips, oral ulcers, and stomach irritation. Crushed leaves were taken for dyspepsia. The seeds were used for alactia, diarrhea, dyspepsia, fistula, glands, gout, neuralgia, rheumatism, sciatica, skin, sores, stomachache, tumors and wounds. Containing up to 40% mucilage, the seeds are used in ointments and poultices. The plant is also suggested to be an aphrodisiac, astringent, carminative, demulcent, diuretic, emmenagogue, emollient, expectorant, lactogogue, restorative and tonic. Iranians infuse the seed for menorrhagia.

The leaf contains the following minerals:

Calcium	Copper
Chlorine	Sodium

The seed contains the following minerals:

Aluminum	Copper	Selenium
Calcium	Iron	Silver
Chlorine	Magnesium	Sodium
Chromium	Manganese	Tin
Cobalt	Nitrogen	Zinc

The seed contains the following amino acids:

Alanine	Leucine	Threonine
Arginine	Lysine	Tryptophan
Glutamate	Methionine	Tyrosine
Glycine	Phenylalanine	Valine
Histidine	Proline	
Isoleucine	Serine	

The plant contains sulfur and the leaf contains methionine.

FIELD MUSTARD – (*SINAPIS ARVENSIS*)
...it was all grown over with thorns, and nettles had covered the face...
Proverbs 24

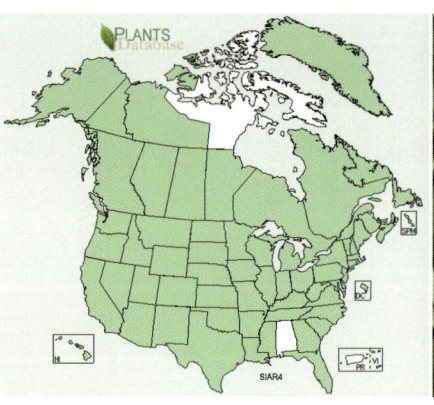
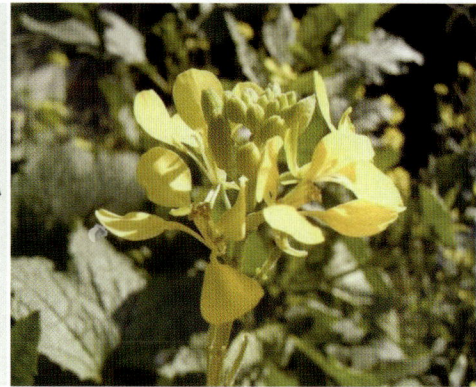

Field mustard is a notorious invader of grainfields and can be viewed as friend or foe. Zohary in the Flora of Palestine describes it as one of the most noxious weeds in the area. Seeds make a good mustard substitute and yield good illuminating oil. In Ireland and Sweden, it is boiled as a potherb. Surprisingly it is eaten by cattle, especially sheep. An old folk remedy for throat tumors, field mustard is milder than but similar to black and white mustards in medicinal applications. The plant is thought to have emollient and sedative, even narcotic properties.

The plant contains the following minerals:

Calcium	Iron	Potassium
Chlorine	Magnesium	Sodium
Cobalt	Manganese	Sulfur
Copper	Nitrogen	

The plant contains the following amino acids:

Isoleucine	Lysine	Proline
Leucine	Phenylalanine	

The seed contains the following amino acids:

Arginine	Serine	Threonine
Glutamate	Lysine	Tryptophan
Glycine	Methionine	Valine
Histidine	Phenylalanine	
Isoleucine	Proline	

The seed contains the following minerals:

Boron	Magnesium	Sodium
Calcium	Manganese	Sulfur
Chlorine	Nickel	Zinc
Copper	Nitrogen	
Iron	Potassium	

The shoot contains the amino acid proline.

FIG TREE – (FICUS CARICA)
...And Isaiah said, Take a lump of figs. And they took and laid it on the boil, and he recovered...II Kings 20

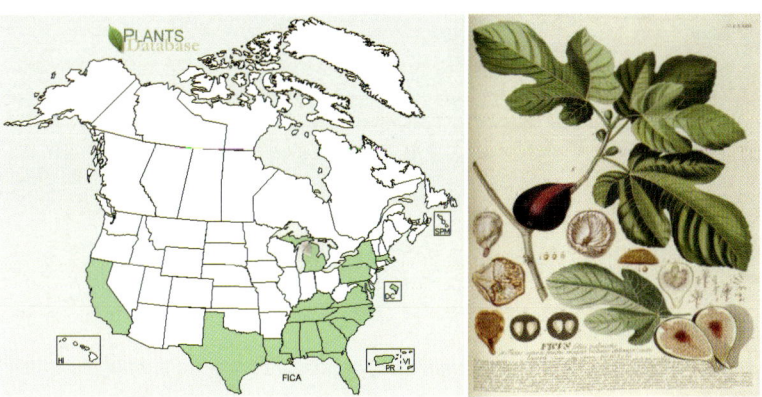

The leaves of the fig, the first fruit recorded in the Bible, were used to make a covering for Adam and Eve. To sit under one's own vine and fig tree was the Jewish concept of peace and prosperity as indicated in I Kings 4:25. Figs are eaten fresh or dried and threaded on long strings. "Cakes of Figs" are mentioned in I Samuel 25:18 and these were also for travel. Fig leaves are still sewn together and used as wrappings for fresh fruit. To Egyptians the fig represented the Tree of Life. Some suggest that the fig was the forbidden fruit of the Garden of Eden. The fruit is said to be poisonous when green, the poison being replaced by sugar in ripening.

Regarded as aperient, demulcent, digestive, disinfectant, diuretic, emollient, expectorant, laxative, pectoral, restorative, stomachic, and vermifuge. Figs find their way into folk medicines for abscess, asthma, boils, cancer, carbuncles, catarrh, condylomata, corns, cough, diptheria, flu, gingivitis, inflammation, measles, pertussis, piles, pimples, polyps, scrofula, sorethroat, tumors, warts, and worms. K.P. Hong, in the Jerusalem Post (Nov. 14, 1979), recalls that a Japanese bacteriologist, Dr. Kochi, reported "permanent cures" (no further cancer cell divisions were seen). "Malignant tumours are changed into foreign matter and cease growing." It is a small wonder the fig has such an anecdotal repertoire for cancer remedies. The fig is a treatment for cancer of the gums and uterus, calluses, condylomata, corns, exacerbations, excrescences of the eyelids, vulva or uterus, fibroids, impostumes, moles, myrmecia, neoplasms, polyps, scleroses of the cervix, kidney, limbs, liver, sinews, spleen, stomach, testicles, and uterus; thymi; tumors of the abdomen, bladder, fauces, feet, glands, liver, neck, parotid, uterus, and wind pipe; warts and wens. Ayruvedics use the fruit for epistaxis, leprosy and diseases of the blood and head. Unani use the root for leucoderma and ringworm, the alexiteric, aphrodisiac, lithontryptic, purgative, tonic, fruit for alopecia, chest pains, hepatosis, fever, inflammations, paralysis, piles, splenosis and thirst. They regard the milky juice as diuretic, expectorant, yet dangerous to the eyes. Contrarily, North Africans rub red and painful conjunctiva with the leaves, then bathing them in a rose water infusion of almonds. Africans use the fresh root in a lotion for thrush. Chinese apply the leaves to hemorrhoids.

The fruit contains the following minerals:

Boron	Magnesium	Sodium
Calcium	Manganese	Zinc
Copper	Nitrogen	
Iron	Potassium	

The fruit contains the following amino acids:

Alanine	Leucine	Threonine
Arginine	Lysine	Tyrosine
Glutamate	Methionine	Tryptophan
Glycine	Phenylalanine	Valine
Histidine	Proline	
Isoleucine	Serine	

The leaf contains calcium.

FLAX – (*LINUM USITATISSIMUM*)
...And he took it down, and wrapped it in linen...Luke 23

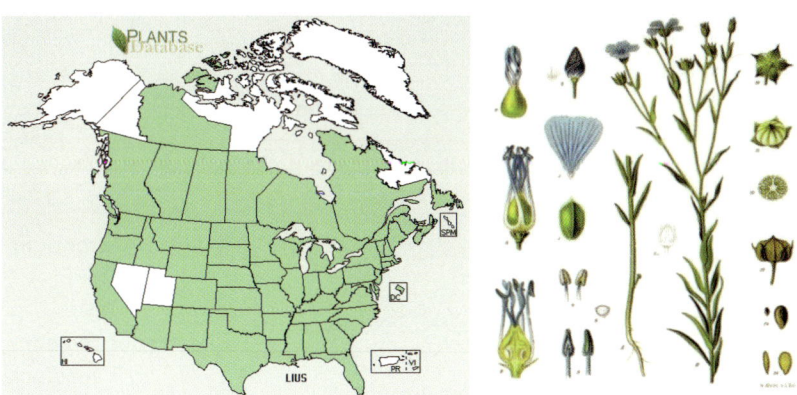

The flax plant is commonly used to make linen, the most ancient of all textile fibers. Linen is the most important product made from the fiber of the flax plant. Flax fibers are soft, lustrous, and flexible, although not so flexible or elastic as those of cotton or wool. Seeds contain 24% protein, and are also the source of linseed oil. In some countries it is also used as edible oil and in soap manufacture. Linseed is often employed with other seeds as food for small birds.

It is considered anodyne, astringent, cyanogenetic, demulcent, diuretic, emollient, expectorant, laxative, suppurative and vulnerary. In Ethiopia, the seeds are used for amebic dysentery. Linum finds its way into folk remedies for boils, bronchitis, burns, cancer, carbuncles, cold, conjunctivitis, corns, coughs, cystitis, diarrhea, gallstones, gonorrhea, gravel, hepatitis, inflammation, intoxication, labor, rheumatism, scalds, sclerosis, sores, spasms, swellings, and tumors. Since linen has long anticancer folk history, it is interesting to see that Linum contains the anticancer agents 3'-demethylpodophyllotoxin podophylotoxin and beta sitosterol. Glutamic acid is used to treat adolescent mental deficiencies. Seeds are considered emollient, demulcent, pectoral, diuretic, and astringent. Crushed seeds make a good poultice (for colds, pleurisy, etc.), either alone or with mustard; lobelia or hollyhock seed added to the poultice for boils. Sometimes seeds are roasted and used in a poultice. Hot seeds are applied to abscesses and rheumatism and sometimes employed as an addition to cough medicines. Linseed tea is used for colds, coughs, and irritation of the urinary tract (when honey and lemon juice may be added). With lemon, it is used in Lebanon for cystitis, gallstones, gravel, hepatitis, and kidney stones. Internally, the oil is given as a laxative. Linseed oil mixed with equal quantity of lime water, known as carron oil, is an excellent application for burns and scalds. Oil mixed with honey is used as a cosmetic for removing spots from the face.

In veterinary medicine, oil is used as a purgative for sheep and horses, and a jelly formed by boiling seeds is used as a purgative for sheep and horses, and a jelly formed by boiling seeds is often given to calves. Flax is a folk remedy for such cancerous conditions as apostemes, cancer of the breast, and mouth; condylomata, indurations of the breast, cervix, limbs, liver, spleen, stomach, testicles, uterus, and viscera; sycosis; tumors of the abdomen, fauces, feet, glands, intestines, neck, parotids, testicles, uterus, and uvula; warts and whitlows.

Ayurvedics use the leaves for asthma and cough, the seeds (considered harmful to the eyes and leading to impotency) for backache, biliousness, consumption, inflammation, leprosy, ulcers and urinary discharges. Unani use the oil from the seed also for "bad blood," internal wound, and ringworm; the burnt bark for wounds as a styptic. They use the bark and leaves for gonorrhea; the seeds, considered aphrodisiac, diuretic, emmenagogue, and lactagogue, for cough and kidney ailments.

The hay contains the following minerals:

Calcium	Manganese	Potassium
Magnesium	Nitrogen	

The plant has the following amino acids:

Isoleucine	Lysine

The seed contains the following minerals:

Calcium	Manganese	Strontium
Chlorine	Molybdenum	Sulfur
Chromium	Nickel	Tin
Cobalt	Nitrogen	Titanium
Iron	Potassium	Vanadium
Lithium	Silver	Zinc
Magnesium	Sodium	

The seed contains the following amino acids:

Alanine	Leucine	Threonine
Arginine	Methionine	Tyrosine
Glutamate	Phenylalanine	Tryptophan
Glycine	Proline	Valin
Histidine	Serine	

FRANKINCENSE – (BOSWELLIA CARTERI)
...Spikenard and saffron; calamus and cinnamon, with all trees of frankincense; myrrh and aloes, with all the chief spices...

Song of Solomon 4

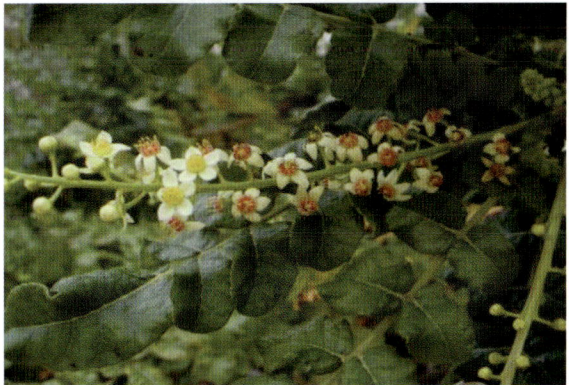

Frankincense is mentioned 22 times in the Bible, 16 times as an item of worship, three times as a product of the garden of Solomon, twice as a tribute of honor, and only once as an item of merchandise. It is chiefly used in incense as a perfume, especially in Catholic ceremonies. Recent authorities maintain that the "incense" used in the service of the Tabernacle was a mixture, in definite proportions of frankincense, galbanum (Ferula galbaniflua), onycha (Styrax benzoin), and stacte (Styrax officinalis), and the use of any incense not composed of these four ingredients in the proper proportions was strictly forbidden. Frankincense was highly regarded by Egyptians for embalming and fumigating. The gum is used as a masticatory, to clean the mouth. Oil of olibanum is used in high grade perfumes, especially for oriental and floral types. It was once used as a depilatory. Resin is imported into Lebanon, primarily as incense, but secondarily as a cosmetic and medicine.

Regarded as alterative, astringent, carminative, diuretic, expectorant, fumigant, sedative, stimulant and tonic, frankincense has quite an anecdotal repertoire. The resin is applied to various cancers and tumors, of the anus, breasts, eyes, teats, testicles, penis, etc., and calluses, carbuncles, corns, polyps, and indurations of the spleen. Also, the resin is used for bilharzia, dysentery, fever, gonorrhea, spermatorrhea, swellings and syphilis. It is used in the orient for leprosy and rheumatism. Pliny mentioned this as an antidote for hemlock. It's used against urogenital ailments in China. Vapors inhaled are said to alleviate bronchitis and laryngitis. The exudate of the bark is used as a tonic and diuretic in East Africa. Swahili use the gum as a diuretic. A dose of 35 grains is said to improve the memory. In Tanganyika the resin is boiled with sesame oil and taken daily for bilharzia. A decoction with cardamoms is taken for stomachaches. East Africans use the resinous exudate to treat syphilis and Asian Indians use it for nervous disorders and rheumatism.

GALBANUM – (FERULA GALBANIFLUA)
...Moses, take unto thee sweet spices, stacte, and onycha, and galbanum...Exodus 30

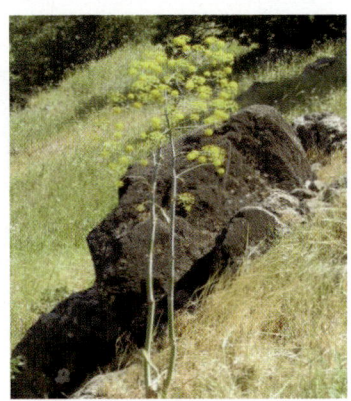

Galbanum was an ingredient in the incense burned at the golden altar in the Holy Place. It is a fetid yellowish gum resin, containing a chemical substance called umbelliferone. The gum is collected by cutting the young stem a few inches above the ground. A milky juice flows out and soon hardens. Today it is used in the making of varnish. Galbanum oils and resinoids are used as fragrance components in lotions, perfumes, and soaps. They are also used as flavor components in many foods, including non-alcoholic beverages, baked goods, candies, condiments, gelatins, puddings, relishes; the oil is used in meats and gravies. More recently, galbanum's popularity has increased because of the "herbaceous-green" odored personal care products that have appeared on the market. Extracts of galbanum have preservative and antimicrobial properties. Aqueous, hydroalcoholic and chloroform extracts are all antiseptic.

Regarded as antispasmodic, carminative, expectorant, stimulant, stomachic, and uterotonic, galbanum is used for allergies, bronchitis, cancer, colds, colic, hysteria, indurations (breast, gums, liver, spleen, stomach, and viscera), inflammations, nerves, polyps, spasms, swellings, and tumors (of the abdomen, liver, parotid, spleen, stomach, and testicles). Galbanum was applied externally to soothe chilblains and cleanse the aural canal where discharges were evident. Internally it was popular for dyspepsia, and was plugged into tooth cavities, to stop decay. Resin lumps are worked into some emollient, like olive oil, to dress lesions. It is used internally to calm nerves and reduce allergic swellings.

GARDEN RUE – (RUTA GRAVEOLENS)
...But woe unto you, Pharisees! For ye tithe mint and rue and all manner of herbs...Luke 11

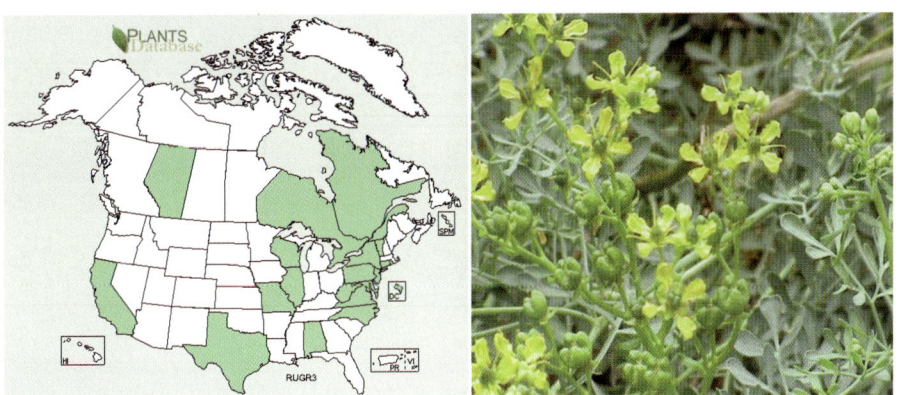

Rue, mentioned only once in the Bible, is a valuable herb. Pliny mentions honeyed wine flavored with rue, as well as eighty-four remedies containing rue. Fresh or dried leaves are used sparingly to season such foods as cheese, vegetable juice, salads, stews, and vegetables. In Ethiopia, the fruits are ground up in a capsicum sauce. Ethiopians make a cheese adding the washed leaves to sour milk. The leaves are infused with coffee leaves to make an Ethiopian beverage. Arabs add rue to water or chew the leaves to prevent the ill effects of water drunk from strange places. Eaten in Italian salads, it is said to preserve the eyesight.

The herb itself shows up in baked goods, candy, frozen dairy desserts, and nonalcoholic beverages. Fresh herbs contain about 0.06% of a volatile oil, for flavoring, as an aromatic in perfumes, in soaps and toilet preparations. Rue water, sprinkled about the house, was supposed to kill fleas, and still believed to repel insects. The rule alkaloid, arborinine, has anti-inflammatory and antihistaminic properties. Rutin, first isolated from rue, is best known for its ability to decrease capillary permeability and fragility. It is also said to be a cancer preventive, i.e. inhibiting tumor formation on mouse skin by the carcinogen benzopyrene, and protective against irradiation damage. Rutin is also useful to counteract edema, atherogenesis, thrombogenesis, inflammation, spasms, and hypertension. It was once official in the U.S. for arteriosclerosis, hypertension, diabetes, and allergic manifestations. It is suggested that it may be useful for stroke prevention. TOXIC, the essential oil can cause death.

Warm fomentations of the oil are folk rememdies for liver indurations. The leaf is said to remedy scirrhus and scleroma of the uterus, cancer of the mouth, tumors, and warts. The seed is said to remedy warts and tumors. This herb is used medicinally as bitters, an aromatic stimulant, antispasmodic, and emmenagogue, in suppression of the menses, for gas pains and colic, epilepsy, hysteria and amenorrhea. In Indochina, the herb is prescribed for dropsy, neuralgia, rheumatism, syncope, and tetanus with the caveat that it should not be given to pregnant or weak people. The juice can be dropped into the ear for an earache. Rue was supposed to heal the stings of bees, scorpions and wasps and snakebites and to prevent dizziness, dumbness, epilepsy, evil eye, eye inflarnmations, and insanity. For many centuries it was thought to prevent contagion and germs. Lebanese used for colds and colic, as well as arthritis, bruises, rheumatism and sciatica. Algerians mixed the powdered seeds with honey for spleen ailments, and use the leaves for fever, fumigation, and syphilis. Rue was also used by Syrians for melanodermic lotions and for mumps. In Iran, rue is mixed with mast and applied to relieve itch. Unani, who believe the plant increases mental activity, consider it abortifacient, anaphrodisiac, digestive, a diuretic and emmenagogue, and use it for gleet and other urinary discharges. Punjabis use the leaves for rheumatic pain.

Hillman Health Food Store call 855-Amish-Dr (855-264-7437) www.emineral.info Vitamins and Minerals for Better Living

GARLIC – (ALLIUM SATIVUM)
...We remember the fish...and the onions, and the garlick...Numbers 11

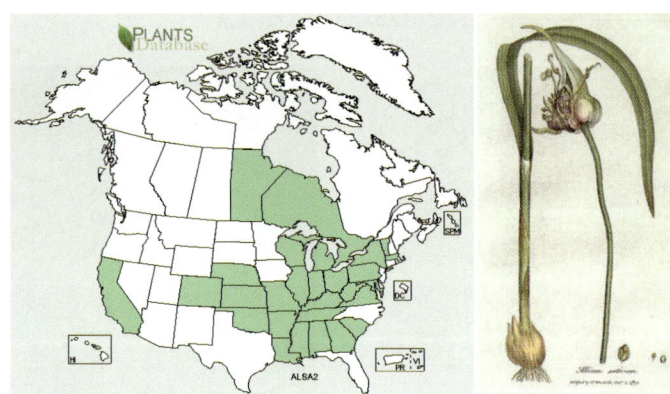

Garlic is cultivated for the underground bulb which has a strong flavor and pungent odor. It is used fresh, dried or powdered as a seasoning, rather than as a vegetable. For most purposes it should be crushed very finely and used in moderation. If fried in fat or oil too hot, it develops an acrid flavor. Bulbs yield 0.6 - 0.1% of an essential oil containing allyl propyl disulphide, diallyl disulphide and two other sulfur compounds, allicin and allisatin. Hippocrates prescribed eating garlic as treatment for uterine tumors. The Bower manuscript, dating about AD 450 in India, recommended garlic for abdominal tumors. The NCI files report that cancer incidence in France is supposedly lowest where garlic consumption is greatest, that garlic eaters in Bulgaria do not have cancer, and that a physician in Victoria, British Columbia, related that he has successfully treated malignancies by prescribing garlic eating.

Garlic extracts contain a powerful bactericide, allyl thiosulfinic allyl ester or allicin, formed by the interaction of a garlic enzyme alliinase and the substrate S ethyl L cysteine sulfoxide. When enzymes or substrate was inoculated into mice with sarcoma, all the animals died within 16 days; when the enzyme was allowed to react with substrate, followed by administration to the tumor bearing animals, no tumor growth occurred and the animals remained alive during a six month observation period. Recent Italian studies suggest that feeding garlic to pigs instead of zinc bacitracin is better because its antibiotic activity is as great while it stimulates growth without affecting the organoleptic qualities of the pork.

It is said to be alexiteric, amebicidal, antiseptic, ascaricidal, bactericide, carminative, cholagogue, demulcent, diaphoretic, digestive, diuretic, emmemagogue, expectorant, rubefacient, sedative, stimulant, stomachic, tonic, and vermifuge. In fact, garlic is one of the most versatile of folk medicines. Also, it is said to be useful in alopecia, angina, anthrax, arteriosclerosis, arthritis, asthma, baldness, bilious ailments, bronchitis, bronchiectasis, bugbite, burns, calluses, cancer, catarrh, cholera, cold, colic, consumption, corns, coughs, cramps, dandruff, diabetes, diarrhea, diptheria, dropsy, dysentery, dysmenorrhea, dyspepsia, earache, eczema, egilops, epil

epsy, felons, fever, flatulence, gallbladder, gangrene, gastroenteritis, heart, hematuria, hepatitis, hoarseness, hypertension, hypotension, hysteria, indigestion, itch, jaundice, leprosy, leukemia, lungs, lupus, malaria, melancholy, neurosis, oliguria, paratyphoid, parturition, phthisis, piles, pinworms, plague, polyps, prostatitis, rabies, rheumatism, ringworm, scabies, sclerosis, scrofula, senescence, sinusitis, skin, smallpox, snakebite, sores, spasms, splenitis, stings, stomach, stomachache, stones, sunstroke, thirst, thrush, tinea, toothache, trichomoniasis, tuber culosis, tumors, typhoid, ulcers, vaginitis, warts, wens, whitlow, whooping cough, worms, and wounds. Extracts of garlic have shown marked larvicidal activity. It is believed by some to be a cancer preventative. Its reputed action in alleviating problems caused by putrefactive intestinal bacteria might be useful in preventing cancer of the colon. Garlic is rather highly regarded for lowering blood pressure and counteracting arteriosclerosis.

Among cancerous ailments, as treated by garlic in home remedies are: cancer of the skin, uterus, fibroids, and neoplasms, sclerosis of the uterus, seed warts, tumor of the abdomen, bladder, glands, and uterus. Inhalations of the stalk are said to be a folk rememdy for uterine tumors, fibroids, polyps and neoplasms. A poultice of the bulb is said to help tumors (bladder, uterus) and an ointment of the root is said to remedy cold tumors and corns. An ointment of the juice is said to correct hard swellings and skin cancer. It contains the antibiotic and antifungal allicin and has shown antitumor activity. Without citing all the evidence, M. Walker says that garlic is successful in treatment of anemia, arthritis, asthma, colds, cough, diabetes, diptheria, dysentery, gas, gastrointestinal disorder, hypotension, hypertension, intenstinal putrefaction, intestinal worms, pneumonia, tuberculosis, typhus, and whooping cough. Recent studies document the fungicidal activity of garlic extracts against Candida albicans, show that low concentrations of garlic extract are both lethal and inhibitory to numerous strains of Cvyptococcus neoformans, and document a hypocholesterolaemic effect. Garlic is considered an aphrodisiac, carminative, diaphoretic, diuretic, expectorant, stimulant, and stomachic. It is used in cough, fevers, and intermittent fever. The juice is rubefacient, mixed with oil; it is useful for curing skin diseases, ulcers, wounds, insect bites, and as eardrops for earache. As an expectorant, it is useful as a potent remedial agent in the treatment of TB. As an anthelmintic for tapeworms, garlic is eaten along with prescribed medicine. It acts as an anodyne in headaches, earaches and rheumatic pains. Oil of garlic is used for flavorings and medicinal uses, being known for these purposes by the ancient Hindus. Lebanese believe that eating garlic freely prevents infection, malaria and typhoid, and cures tuberculosis, mitigates stroke, and reduces blood clots, promoting virility all the while. Seeds are sold in Iranian bazzars for use as a demulcent, purgative and stimulant especially in cases of typhoid fever.

The bulb contains the following minerals:

Aluminum	Iodine	Selenium
Boron	Iron	Silica
Calcium	Magnesium	Sodium
Chromium	Manganese	Tellurium
Cobalt	Nickel	Tin
Copper	Nitrogen	Zinc
Germanium	Potassium	

The flower contains the following minerals:

Calcium	Iron	Nitrogen

The leaf and stems contains the following minerals:

Calcium	Nitrogen	Sodium
Iron	Potassium	

The following amino acids are contained in garlic:

Alanine	Isoleucine	Proline
Arginine	Leucine	Serine
Glutamate	Lysine	Threonine
Glycine	Methionine	Tryptophan
Histidine	Phenylalanine	Tyrosine

GIANT REED – (ARUNDO DONAX)
...A reed shaken with the wind...Matthew 11

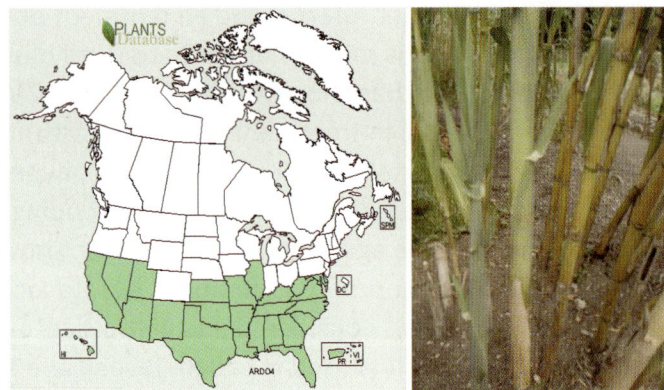

Although believed by Egyptians to be a Syrian plant introduced to Egypt, the reed has not been observed as a truly wild plant or seedling. It is cultivated in different parts of the country, along water courses, but above the water level. Even around big lakes, it seems to be exclusively propagated by root divisions, usually by the fishermen who use the reeds. Stems serve as support for vines and similar climbing plants, and for making trellises and the like for climbing cultivated plants. In Egypt, the reeds are also used for fencing and roofing. Reeds are also used as measuring rods, walking sticks, arrowshafts, fishing poles, musical instruments (e.g. clarinets and bagpipes in Europe), baskets, and mats. Romans used such reeds for pens. It makes a good quality of paper; in Italy the plant is used in the making of rayon. Mulitcolored and glaucous leaved varieties are used as ornamentals. Because of rather high yields from natural stands, the cane has been suggested for biomass for energy.

The rhizone has diuretic and sudorific properties and is used for dropsy and to reduce the flow of milk. The root or rhizome, boiled in wine with honey, has been used for cancer. This or other species of Arundo is also reported to be used for condylomata and indurations of the breast, syphilis, and both hypo and hypertension. In Egypt, the folk medicinal uses of Arundo were seemingly interchangeable with those of Phragmites, i.e. diaphoretic and diuretic.

The reed plant has the minerals:

Calcium   Nitrogen   Potassium

Glasswort – (Salicornia Europaea)
...for he is like a refiner's fire, and like fullers' soap...Malachi 3

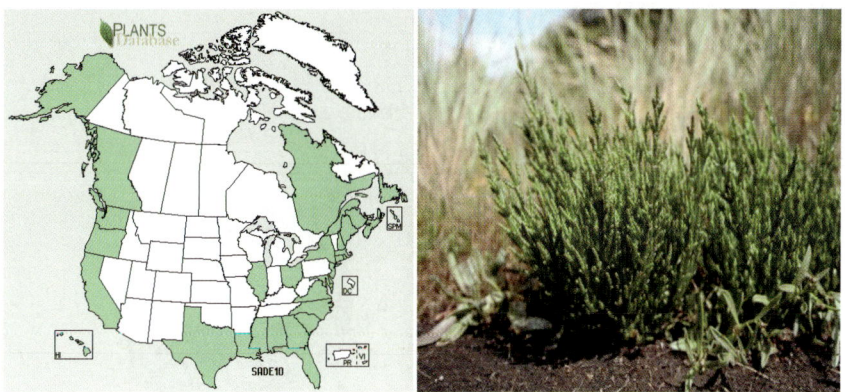

There are references in the Bible to the use of Glasswort for soap and for glass. The potash, or alkaline salts, used in Biblical "sope making" were derived from the ashes of glassworts and other species. The potash was then mixed with olive oil. Some ethnic groups eat the glassworts sparingly as potherbs or salad. In Palestine, the fleshy stems are eaten. This and other species of glasswort, called kelpwort and samphire, are used as folk remedies for tumors and superfluous flesh.

GLASSWORT – (SALSOLA KALI)
...For though thou wash thee with nitre, and take thee much soap...Jeremiah 2

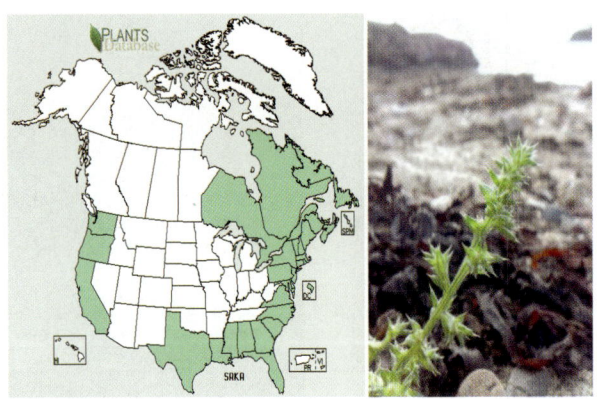

The alkaline salts used in soap making during Biblical times were obtained by burning the plants of the saltwort, salsola kali being the most common of twenty kinds of saltwort in the Holy Land. Soap was made by mixing such ashes with olive, instead of animal fat. Glass is also made therefrom, because of the high alkali content. Young shoots are sometimes eaten as potherbs, but it is said to be toxic. Still camels, goats, and horses are said to graze it. It is suggested as cathartic, diuretic, emmenagogue, POISON, stimulant and vermifuge. The saltwort is used for dropsy. This is a folk remedy for that cancerous condition known as superfluous flesh. The same ashes used for soap are used as a therapeutic dressing, antiseptic, and cleansing in the Dutch East Indies.

GOPHER WOOD – (*CUPRESSUS SEMPERVIRENS*)
...He heweth him down cedars, and taketh the cypress and the oak...Isaiah 44

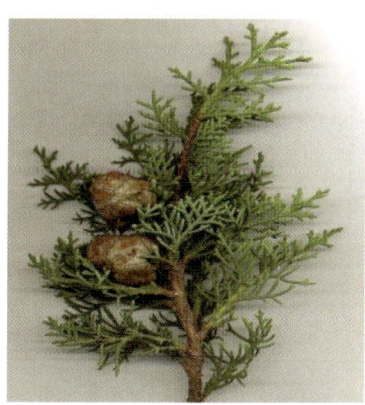

An important Biblical timber tree, gopher wood was used by the Egyptians for coffins in olden times, in Greece, more recently. Doors of St. Peter's in Rome, made of cypress, showed no sign of decay after 1200 years. The gates of Constantinople, which stood more than a thousand years, were made of it. The wood was used for house building, ship building (even the ark), and musical instruments. David and all the house of Israel played on musical instruments of cypress. Oil of cypress is a valuable perfumery item, providing ambergris and labdanum like odors. It is planted for decoration in parks and cemeteries. The Island of Cyprus, where the tree was worshipped, was named for the cypress.

Regarded as antiseptic, astringent, diuretic, expectorant, pectoral, styptic, sudorific, vasoconstrictor, vermifuge, and vulnerary, cypress is used in folk remedies for cough, diabetes, dyspepsia, flu, metrorrhagia, myofibroma, pertussis, piles, polyps, preventitive (abortion), prolapse, rheumatism, sclerosis, swellings, warts, and worms. Cypress is a folk remedy for cancer or tumors of the eyes, nose, breast, tests, uterus, and indurations of the liver, spleen, stomach, and testicles. In Palestine, the oil derived from the leaves was used for whooping cough. Lebanese use it for cough, dyspepsia, hiccup, inflammation, and ulcers. The berries serve in a cough syrup and mashed berries are applied to lesions. Algerians ate stewed fruits for dyspepsia. In India, the fruits are described as "an aromatic stimulant" in piles. The cones have been used for bronchitis, cough, diarrhea, enuresis, fefer, hemmorhage and hemorrhoids.

GRECIAN JUNIPER – (JUNIPERUS EXCELSA)
...Send me also cedar trees, fir trees, and algum trees, out of Lebanon...II Chronicles 2

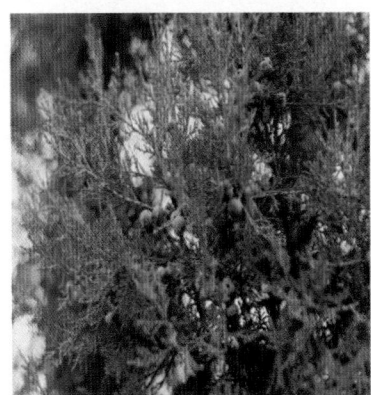

In Biblical times, as today, the plant is esteemed as a timber source. Assuming that juniperus excetsa and J. procera bochst are synonyms, the fruits are eaten by animals and birds. The leaf extract (cold aqueous) is active against Mycobacterium tuberculosis. Podophyllotoxin, present in juniper leaves, is an antibiotic, antitumor compound. Cedrol, the most important component of the cedar wood oil, is used in microscopy, perfumery, and soaps. In funerals in Ethiopia the corpse is often strewn with the twigs, before the grave is filled. The timber is used in church construction, and the trees, sacred in Ethiopia, are planted about cemeteries and churches. In Lebanon, this is claimed to be the best source of cade oil. Leaves are used as incense in Khorasan.

The fruit decoction is emmenagogue and sudorific. The stimulant resin is used against ulcers. Fruiting branches are burned as a fumigant for rheumatic pains. Twigs and buds are ground up to treat intestinal worms. Powdered leaves are applied to wounds, in animals and humans. The fruits, mixed with those of other species, are employed against headaches. Mixed with honey, the resin is used for liver ailments. Elsewhere the oil has been employed to induce abortion. In Lebanon, it is used in liniments and salves, in cough and liver medicines, and in pills and suppositories. In Iran the fruits are considered diuretic and emmenagogue; they are used for dyspepsia.

HEMLOCK – (CONIUM MACULATUM)
...judgment springeth up as hemlock in the furrows of the field...
Hosea 10
...for ye have turned judgment into gall, and the fruit of righteousness into hemlock...Amos 6

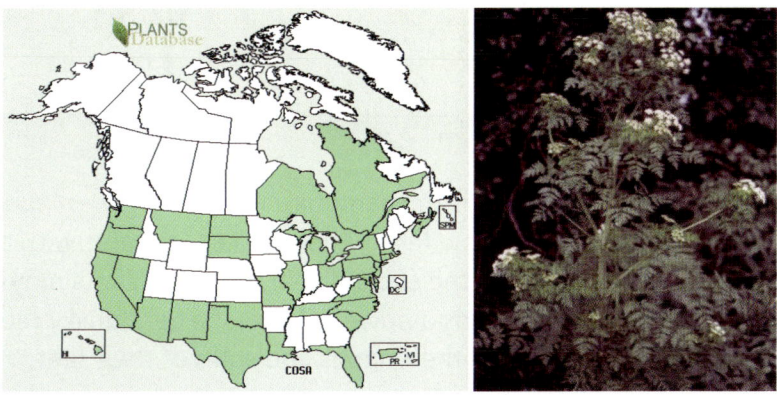

Hemlock, the poison which Socrates took, is too dangerous for herbal administration by the uninitiated. It is sometimes used as an antidote to strychnine, and to the poisons of rabies and tetanus. The Biblical hemlock to conium, truly a dangerous medicinal plant, relates it to a more innocuous herb, closer to wormwood.

The plant is poisonous; dried unripe fruits contain the alkaloid coniine, and have been used as antispasmodic and sedative. Greek and Arab physicians used hemlock for hydrophobia, indolent tumors, pain, scrofula and swelling in the joints, skin affections, and it was often poulticed onto ulcers and cancers. Avicennia raise it as a cure for breast tumors. Millspaugh related that 26 or 46 cases of cancer were ameliorated by Conium. Plants used against cancer suspect that hemlock is used for cacoethes, cancer of the breast, intestine, nose, parotids, skin, sternum and uterus; car cinoma; indurations of the breast, glands, liver, and viscera; scirrhus of the breast, liver, pancreas, and spleen; tumors of the breast, ganglia, liver, mammae, mesentery, neck, penis, scrotum, and testicles; ulcers, and wens. In Lebanon, the cancer "specialist" uses hemlock in his medications and adds "exact information must be withheld, both to safeguard his economic independence and freedom from interference by recognized medicine and the law."

HENNA – (LAWSONIA INERMIS)
...My beloved is unto me as a cluster of camphire in the vineyards...Song of Solomon 1

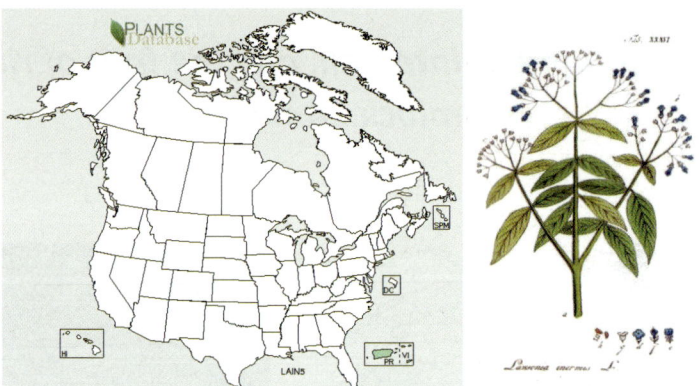

One of the earliest known spices and perfumes is the camphire or henna flower lauded by King Solomon for its fragrance. The young leaves, dried and powdered, then soaked in water with a little lime juice, constitute the dye. Leaves may be harvested in the second year, and the plants may live 15 years. Henna is valued, especially by women of Egypt, for it yields a powerful dye of a dark dusky red, rather like iron rust in color. The women use it to stain the palms of their hands and soles of their feet.

Mummies entombed for three thousand years still retain the dye used on their nails. In India and Pakistan henna is widely used by both men and women for coloring nails, fingers, hands, and hair. Hair is dyed a brownish chestnut shade which turns black in conjunction with indigo. To dye the hair, an infusion of dried leaves to which has been added a little lime juice is used. Menna leaves dye fingers, nails, hands, and feet a dull orange. A deep red color may be obtained when henna is mixed with catechu. Infusion of leaves also used for dyeing cotton fabrics is a light reddish brown. Wool and silk may also be dyed by henna. The leaves are also used in making of perfumed oils and as a tanning agent. The rose-scented flowers, attractive to bees, gives an essential oil (mehndi oil) long used in Indian perfumery. The plants are grown as hedge plants throughout India. The wood is used to make tool handles, tent peg, and other articles. Gallic acid from the leaves inhibits Streptococcus aureus slightly.

Regarded as alterative, anthelmintic, astringent, bactericidal, collyrium, deodorant, emmenagogue, fungicidal, sedative and vulnerary, henna is included in old folk remedies for boils, bronchitis, bruises, burns, calculus, candidiasis, condylomata, headache, herpes, hysteria, inflammation, jaundice, leprosy, myalgia, polyps, rheumatism, skin, sores, sorethroat, splenomegaly, spermatorrhea, stomachache, syphilis, stomatitis, tumors, unterine fibroids and whitlow. Fruit oil is a folk remedy for indurations of the liver and diaphragm. The ointment made from the oil is said to remedy indurations. Chewing the leaf is said to remedy tumors of the mouth. Poultices of the leaf are said to help various types of tumors. The plant contains gallic acid which is a demonstrated antitumor compound. In Malaysia, the leaf decoction is used after childbirth, and for stomach disorders and venereal disease. Mixed with the poisonous plumbago, it is said to be abortifacient. Henna powder can be sprinkled onto rheumatic pains and the leaf is pasted onto herpes in Java. Cambodians drink a root decoction as a diuretic. Bark is given in jaundice, and enlargement of the spleen, and as alterative in skin diseases and leprosy. Henna leaves are used as prophylactic against skin disease. The powdered seed is said to be cerebral stimulant. Decoction of leaves used as astringent gargle in sore throat. Oil and essence is rubbed over the body to keep it cool. The flowers are refrigerant and soporific and the fruit is said to be emmenagogue. The leaves act as an antiperspirant and are said to be used for jaundice, leprosy, and scurfy affections. Root decoction is used for blennorhea, boils, and bronchitis and eye diseases. A tea made of the leaves is said to prevent obesity.

In Merjayoun the leaf infusion is used for fever and hypertension. In the Antilebanon, powdered leaves and flowers are used in salves; the seeds are ground and applied to itch. Algerians apply the powdered leaves on abscesses and cautery, adding juniper resin in cases of dropsy. Near Iran, henna is applied externally for blind boils, leprosy, and skin diseases. It is painted on pubic regions for stoppage of the bladder. Ayurvedics use the seeds for bowel ailments fever and insanity, the leaves, considered emetic and expectorant, for leucoderma. Unani use the vulnerary flowers for headache, the leaves for amenorrhea, boils, bronchitis, baldness, headache, hemicrania, lumbago, ophthalmia, scabies, splenitis, stomatitis, syphilitic sores and ulcers. They also consider the seed to be tonic to the brain. The leaves contain the antibiotic oxynapthoquinone called lawsone.

HOLLY OAK – (*QUERCUS ILEX*)
...and she was buried beneath Bethel under an oak...Genesis 35

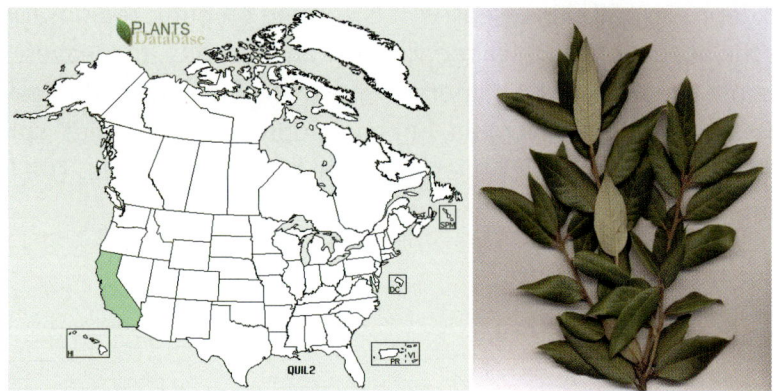

When seasoned, the holly oak wood works well and takes a fine polish. It is used for agricultural tools and joinery. Coppicing readily, it yields good fuel and charcoal. The leaves are lopped for fodder, the spiney branches used for fencing. The acorns are eaten and are said to be the most edible of all acorns. They have been used as sources of industrial alcohol. Regarded as astringent, diuretic and stimulant, the holly oak has been used in folk remedies for cacoethes, cancers (of the intestines, liver, stomach), fevers, and tumors.

HORSEMINT – (MENTHA LONGIFOLIA)
...for ye tithe mint and rue and all manner of herbs...Luke 11

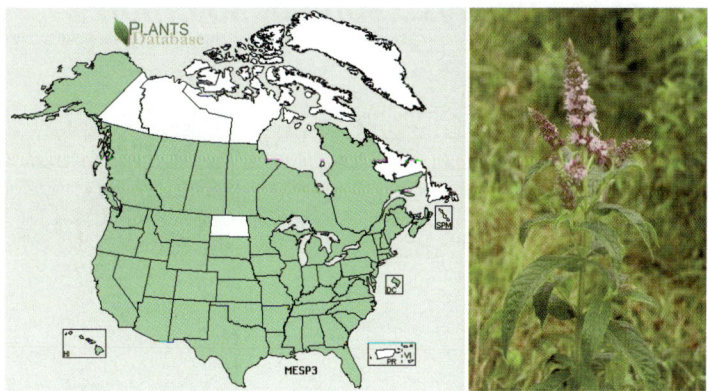

In Matthew and in Luke, the lesser herbs are mentioned. Jews were entirely scrupulous in paying the tithe, or tenth, demanded of them. Jews served mint with their meat dishes, especially at the Spring Feast of the Paschal Lamb. The ancient Hebrews, Greeks, and Romans used it; a writing from A.D. 37 states that mint was mentioned often in cooking recipes. Jews strewed synagogue floors with mint so that its perfume scented the place at each footfall. The plant is eaten in chutney. Steam distillation of dried leaves and flowering tops of the plant from Kashmir gave 1.2% of pale yellow oil with a minty odor. The oil can be used as a substitute for imported peppermint oil for flavoring confectionery. Grieve equates it more with spearmint oil.

Regarded as anodyne, antiseptic, astringent, carminative, stimulant, and stomachic, horsemint is used in folk remedies, often as an herbal tea, for apoplexy, chest, colds, fever, headache, indurations, rheumatism, and sclerosis. Pliny gave 41 remedies in which mint was considered efficacious. At one time apparently, England had concluded that mint juice mixed with vinegar stirred up venery and bodily lust. Egyptian farmers regard the flowering tops and leaves for making a carminative tea. Finally, the plant is added to hot baths for skin ailments.

Hyacinth – (*Hyacinthus Orientalis*)
...I am the rose of Sharon, and the lily of the valleys...Song of Solomon 2

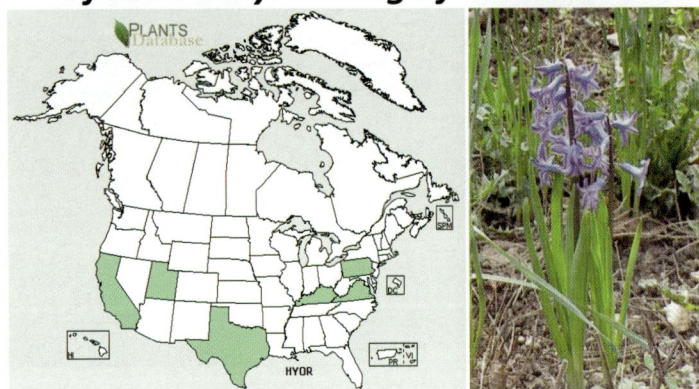

A handsome ornamental, regarded as the Biblical lily of the valley by some, the hyacinth has also been a source of perfume, once extracted from the flowers in France and Holland. Roots (bulbs) are used locally and in teas for venereal disease in Lebanon. The seeds are used for dysuria and jaundice. Roots of the related hyacinthus nonscriptus are used for leucorrhea; dried and powdered they are used as a styptic. The essential oil contains the antitumor compound benzaldehyde.

Ivy – (Hedera Helix)
...they were compelled to go in procession to Baccus carrying ivy...
II Maccabees 6

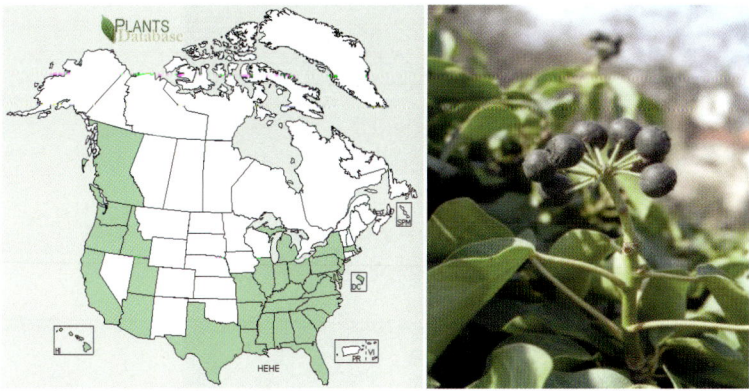

Ivy is planted as an ornamental evergreen vine. In olden days, the leaves formed the poet's crown, as well as the wreath of Bacchus, to whom the plant was dedicated. Ivy was once bound around the brow to prevent intoxication; hence a garland of ivy was hung outside olden roadhouses to indicate that wine was sold therein. Greek priests presented a wreath of ivy to newly-married persons, symbolizing fidelity.

Sheep and deer will eat the leaves in winter, though cows often will not. Leaves boiled with soda are said to be suitable for washing clothes. Young twigs are a source of yellow and brown dye. Hardwood can be used as a boxwood substitute in engraving. Recently extract of ivy has found its way into a French massage cream and soap. In Palestine, the fruit is said to be toxic to children.

Regarded as antiseptic, astringent, cathartic, contraceptive, diaphoretic, emetic, emmenagogue, laxative, pediculicide, purgative, stimulant, sudorific, vasoconstrictor, vasodilator, and vermifuge, ivy is used for rheumatism, sclerosis, scrofula, toothache, etc. The leaf is used for cacoethes, calluses, cancer, cancromas, chironies, corns, warts, and wens; the juice for cancer or polyps of the nose. South African whites apply the vinegar steeped leaves to cancerous growths and corns. The plant is also used for various indurations and cancers (lymph, mammaries, and uterus). Ivy leaves were once bruised, gently boiled in wine, and drunk to alleviate intoxication by wine. Flowers, decocted in wine, were used for dysentery. The plant is said to have been used as an emetic and narcotic in at least three continents. Yellow berries used for jaundice and hemoptysis. Infusion of the fruits is used for rheumatism.

In the Mediterranean, ingestion of one gram powdered fruit is said to result in sterility. The resinous exudate from old stems is placed in hollow teeth to alleviate toothache, and is also used as an aphrodisiac, stimulant and emmenagogue. The leaf has been applied to destroy vermin, e.g. head lice. It reportedly has a slight antimalarial activity.

JERICHO ROSE – (ANASTATICA HIEROCHUNTICA)
...O my God, make them like a wheel; as the stubble before the wind...
Psalm 83

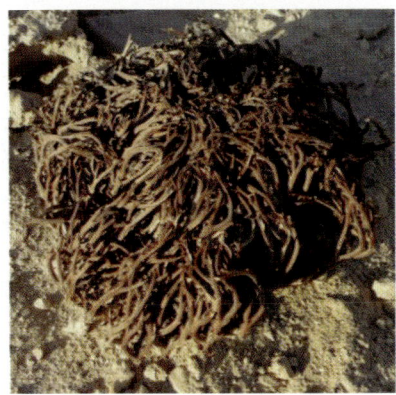

A typical tumbleweed and resurrection plant, anastatica is the most probable identification for the "wheel" of Psalm 83. This may be the true rose of Jericho. Fruiting branches are hygroscopic and expand as a curio into the "Jericho rose" when placed in water, even if the tumbleweed is several years old.

Anastatica is sold in the Egyptian drug market as "Kaff Mariam." It is sold in folk drug shops in Qatar and other countries of the Arabian Peninsula, especially for use by parturient women. The plant is soaked in water and, when it has unfurled, the water is drunk by the expectant mother, perhaps in hopes that the offspring will fill out as readily as the Jericho rose, held to be a symbol of resurrection. Around Rabat, the infusion is also used for colds and epilepsy.

JUDAS TREE – (CERCIS SILIQUASTRUM)

...And he cast down the pieces of silver in the temple, and departed, and went and hanged himself...Matthew 27

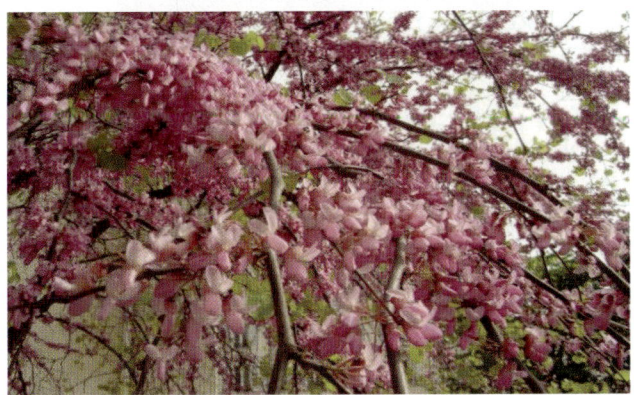

The Judas tree is said to be what Judas hung himself from, causing the tree to blush or burn in shame because Judas selected it. However, in modern times it is called a burning bush. As medicine, it is used in eye ailments and headaches.

JUDEAN SAGE – (SALVIA JUDAICA)
...And he made the candlestick of pure gold...Exodus 37

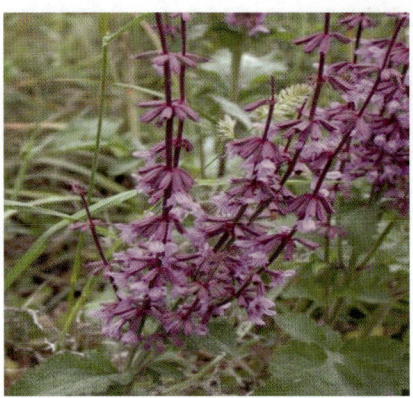

The seven-branched candlestick, a traditional Jewish symbol, had its origin in the branched inflorescence of this lowly sage growing in the uplands of Palestine. On each branch of the plant's inflorescence are whorls of buds which probably inspired the artist to put the knobs on the Biblical golden candlestick. In all probability, this is used medicinally like many of the other mints of the Holy Land.

JUNIPER – (CYNOMORIUM COCCINEUM)
...Who cut up mallows by the bushes, and juniper roots for their meat...Job 30

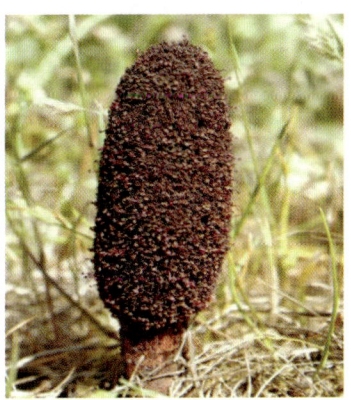

Since this parasite is edible and juniper (broom) roots are not very edible, it is suggested that cynomorium constitutes the juniper roots of Job. It was frequently eaten in times of scarcity, e.g. on the Canary Islands. In Qatar, where given the Arabic name tarthuth, natives eat it. In Northern Africa, the roots are pulverized and used as a spice.

On Malta, where it was once considered endemic it was so highly prized for its supposed medicinal help in dysentery that military sentinel were posted around places where it occurred. Chinese regard the herb as a folk remedy for the back, kidney, and knees and prescribe it for constipation, impotency and sterility. In some cultures it is considered an aphrodisiac for males (suspected to increase the sperm count); in others, for females. Bedouins either peel the root and eat it or grind it and make a sweetened tea for colic. North Africans mix powdered plants with butter for biliary obstructions.

Kashmir Willow – (Salix Fragilis)
...the willows of the brook compass him about...Job 40

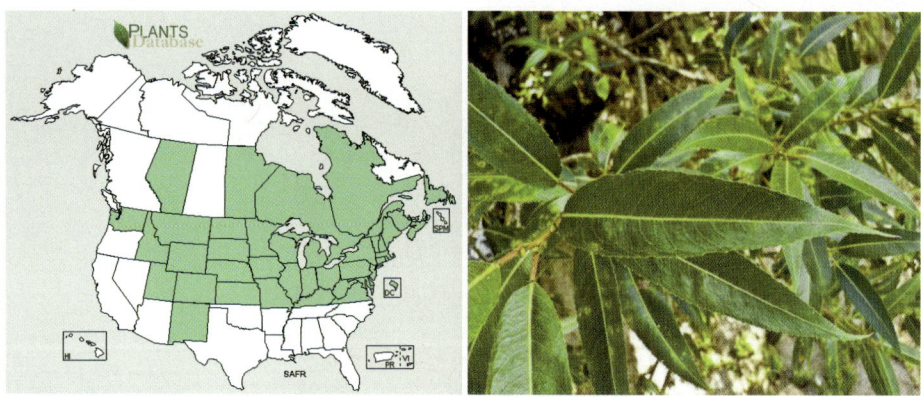

The Kashmir willow tree is cultivated in fuel plantations on swampy ground in India. The wood, soft, light and even grained, is said to be more durable than other willows and is suitable for cricket bats. It is also employed in match industry and as a fuel. The charcoal from the wood is used for gunpowder. In Iran the tree is reported to yield a sweet exudation. Twigs are employed for basketry.

This sedative willow is used for colds, fever, malaria, rheumatism, sedative, and tumors. The salicin, contaitied in the bark, is slightly bitter, antirheumatic, and atitiperiodic, and is the rationale behind treating cold, fever, and malaria. This is the herbalist's aspirin. Tannin and gallic acid might explain the anticancer activity.This species has a saccharine manna-like secretion, recommended for Herpes labialis or thrush.

KERMES OAK – (QUERCUS COCCIFERA)
...And he shall take to cleanse the house two birds, and cedar wood, and scarlet, and hyssop...Leviticus 14

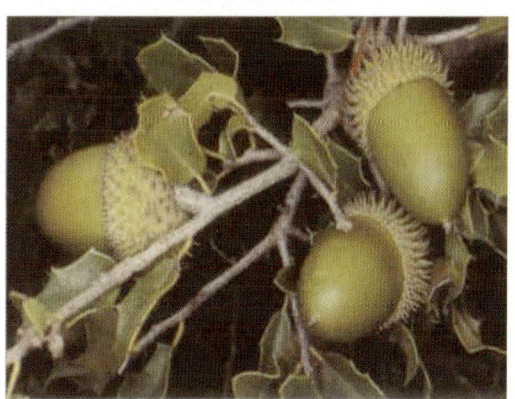

The oak from which the scarlet of the Old Testament was derived is a large evergreen shrub, growing ten to twenty feet high. Its young shoots are covered with white, soft down which is the breeding ground of the kermes insect, Chermes ilicis (Coccus ilicis). These creatures yield a beautiful scarlet dye remarkable for its richness and lasting quality. The scarlet was known commercially as "grain" and "scarlet grain." When the bark of this kermes oak is steeped in boiling water, it yields a black dye, once used to dye hair. The Dyers Company of England selected three sprigs of this plant for their heraldic crest, which was granted by charter in 1420 and is still used by the company in the city of London. This has been cited as a folk remedy for tumors. Lebanese walk miles to get twigs and leaves of this tree to bathe feverish and sickly children. Powdered galls are mixed with honey to treat sores and wounds.

LENTIL – (LENS CULINARIS)
...Then Jacob gave Esau bread and pottage of lentiles; and he did eat...
Genesis 25

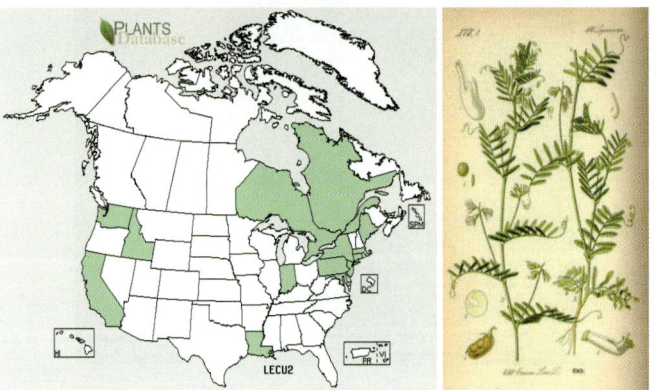

Some people think it was the food that made Daniel wise. Lentil is cultivated for its nutritious seed, considered one of the most nutritious of pulses. Split seeds are used in soups; flour is used mixed with cereals, in cakes and as a food for invalids and infants.

In Biblical times, as today, a breadstuff was made from lentils and barley. Lentils have been found in Syria prior to 5000 BC, in Iran before 5000 BC, and in Greece (with barley and wheat) earlier than 5000 BC. Along parts of the Nile, it is the only breadstuff. Lentils are used as a meat substitute in many countries. Young pods are used as a vegetable in India. Husks, dried leaves and stems, and bran fed to livestock. Seeds are a source of commercial starch for textile and printing industries. Green plants are used as green manure.

Lentils are supposed to remedy constipation, scurvy, ulcers, and other intestinal afflictions. In Ethiopia, e.g. the seeds are used for dysentery. In India, lentils are poulticed onto the ulcers that follow smallpox and other slow healing sores. Lebanese believe lentils are good for the anemia that follows dysentery. Lebanese use hot lentil soup with or without onions, as a poultice for sores. In Iraq, ground lentils are used to ease delivery. Seeds, often in cataplasms, are used for apostemes, cancers, condylomata, indurations, scirrhus, tumors, and warts (of the abdomen, anus, breast, ear, eye, face, fauces, feet, genitals, gums, intestines, parotids, rectum, etc.).

Ayurvedics use the seed for biliousness, dysentery, eye ailments, heart ailments, skin diseases, strangury, and tumors. Unani use them for breast inflammation, blood ailments, bronchitis, chest ailments, eye disorders and stomatitis. In Germany, lentil soup is used to facilitate the eruption in smallpox, and to poultice onto the ulcers following smallpox.

LETTUCE – (LACTUCA SATIVA)
...eat it with unleavened bread and bitter herbs...Numbers 9

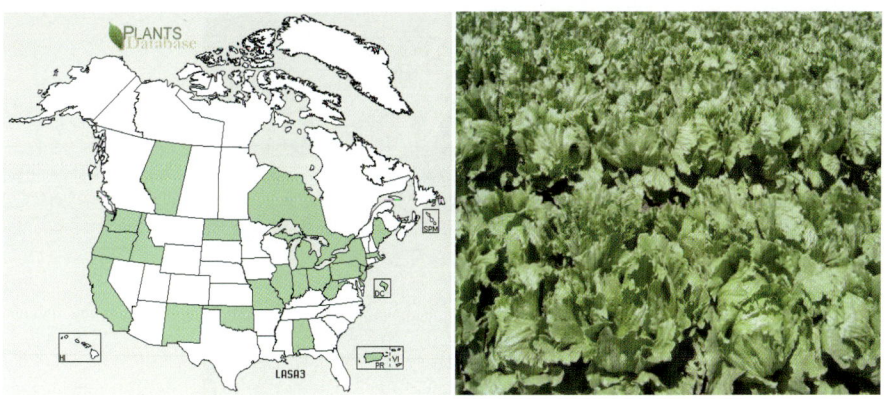

Lettuce is the most popular of the salad vegetables, yet one of the bitter herbs of the Bible. Leaves, produced in heads, are used raw in or under salads, eaten braised or wilted, or used in soups with broth, with boullion cubes or spices. In the stem lettuce variety, the young stems are peeled and cooked, but not the coarse unpalatable leaves.

Considered by some as alexiteric, anaphrodisiac, anodyne, antispasmodic, cardiac, carminative, demulcent, diaphoretic, diuretic, emollient, hypnotic, lactagogue, narcotic, parasiticide, psychdelic, purgative, refrigerant and sedative, lettuce has been recommended as a folk remedy for asthma, bronchitis, bubo, burns, cough, dysmenorrhea, fever, hyperglycemia, insomnia, neuralgia, palpitations, pertussis, sclerosis, sores, spasms, swelling, tuberculosis, tumors, typhoid, and urogenital ailments. Folk remedies use it for cancers of the breast, face, tongue, and uterus, cancerous ulcers and tumors. Bolted lettuce, eaten as a vegetable in some quantity, has been known to cause coma. Lebanese druggists keep powdered lettuce seed to calm feverish patients, and to deter boys from excessive masturbation. Lebanese occasionally apply wilted lettuce to dress abrasions, swellings and wounds. Lettuce is poulticed onto ulcers. Lettuce seeds, "by relaxing the genital organs...diminish the spermatic secretions." Apparently, quite the opposite opinion was held in ancient Egypt, where, according to Boulos, lettuce was a symbol of fertility. In homeopathy the whole plant is used in treatment of impotence.

The leaf contains the following minerals:

- Aluminum
- Boron
- Bromine
- Calcium
- Chlorine
- Chromium
- Cobalt
- Copper
- Fluorine
- Gallium
- Iron
- Lithium
- Magnesium
- Manganese
- Molybdenum
- Nickel
- Nitrogen
- Potassium
- Selenium
- Silica
- Silver
- Sodium
- Strontium
- Sulfur
- Titanium
- Vanadium
- Yttrium
- Zinc

The leaf contains the following amino acids:

- Alanine
- Arginine
- Glutamate
- Glycine
- Histidine
- Isoleucine
- Leucine
- Lysine
- Methionine
- Phenylalanine
- Proline
- Serine
- Threonine
- Tyrosine
- Tryptophan
- Valine

Hillman Health Food Store call 855-Amish-Dr (855-264-7437) www.emineral.info Vitamins and Minerals for Better Living

LOVEAPPLE – (MANDRAGORA OFFICINARUM)
...The mandrakes give a smell...Song of Solomon 7

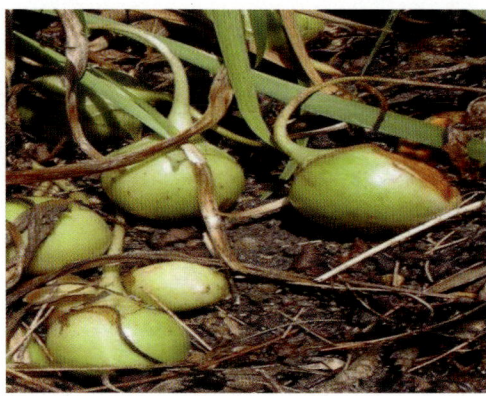

As indicated in the story of Leah and Rachel, mandrake (loveapple) was thought to induce fertility. Arabs called it "devil's apples" because of its supposed powers to excite voluptuousness. When ripe, it is a yellow plum like fruit. The flavor is sickeningly sweet, though rather insipid. Eaten in quantity, they produce dizziness, and may even stimulate men and women to insanity. It is also thought to stimulate conception and has a long fame for use in love potions and incantations.

The mandrake has a large root that is dark brown and rugged and resembles the human body. From early times it has been an object of superstition. Jews considered the mandrake a charm against evil spirits. Others believed that mischief-making elves would find its strange odor unbearable. According to Temple, Josephus related that Jews tied a dog to the plant to pull it out of the ground, as it would kill a man to touch it so fresh, without certain precautions; the mandrake shrieked, the dog died, rendering the root harmless thereafter. Once esteemed for its medicinal and narcotic properties, mandrake still may have orgiastic and magical applications among cults involving the sexes and has been used as an aphrodisiac.

Poisonous, containing several dangerous hallucinogenic alkaloids, mandrake is however regarded as anesthetic, aphrodisiac, cathartic, cholagogue, emetic, hypnotic, mydriatic, narcotic, nervine, purgative, refrigerant, sedative, and stimulant. Fresh roots were once used for procuring sleep in continued pain, convulsions, rheumatic pain, and scrofulous tumors. Crushed leaves and boiled roots used to treat tumors. Boiled in milk, the roots were poulticed onto indolent ulcers. Mixed with brandy, the root is used for chronic rheumatism. Other conditions treated are asthma, arthritis, colic, coughs, hayfever, hepatitis, schizophrenia and sclerosis. Atropine is anticholinergic, both central and peripheral. It tends to reduce secretions (gastric, intestinal, nasal, saliva, sweat, teats), decrease gastric and intestinal motility, and increase heart rate. It also causes pupil dilation, increase in intraocular pressure and photophobia.

Madonna Lily – (Lilium Candidum)
...to feed in the gardens, and to gather lilies...Song of Solomon 6

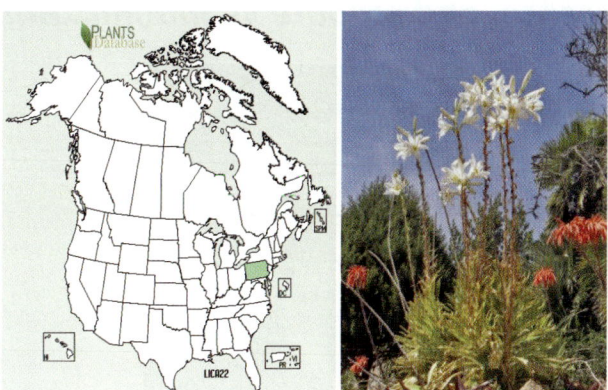

The lily has been found doubtfully wild all over the Mediterranean basin from France to the hills of Syria, suggesting the Roman Empire. In perfumery, the absolute of lily may be used with great advantage in high grade compositions of floral as well as oriental type. It is an excellent fixative.

It is considered astringent, demulcent, diuretic, emollient, expectorant, stimulant, and sudorific. The Madonna lily is a folk remedy for calluses, corns, dropsy, epilepsy, inflammation, nausea, skin, sore, spasm, and tumors. Madonna lily is also a folk "remedy" for cancer of the breast, lungs, ribs, and of the uterus; corns, indurations of the liver, spleen, uterus, and viscera; neoplasms, polyps; tumors of the breast, ear, neck, scrotum, testicles, throat, and uterus; and warts. A decoction of the bulbs in milk or water is taken for dropsy; a poultice is used as an external application for tumors, ulcers and skin inflammations. The fresh flowering part is used in homeopathy as an antispasmodic; the pollen is used against epilepsy. In Lebanon the cooked roots are used for everything from corns to epilepsy.

MANNA ASH – (FRAXINUS ORNUS)
…Behold, we have sent you money to buy burnt offerings, and sin offerings, and incense, and prepare ye manna…Baruch 1

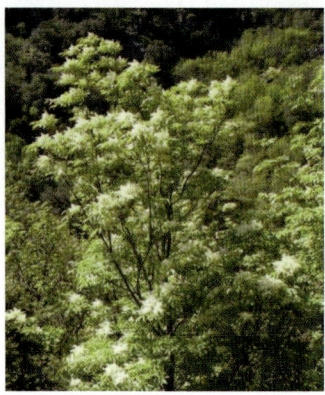

There may be three distinct types of manna in the Bible. The more familiar is the first type.

(1) Secured by purchase and trade, consisting of the gummy exudate of either fraxinus ornus, Alhagi maurorum, and Taniarix mannzjera, possibly Acacia raddiana, Anabasis setzfera, Astragalus echinus, Capparis cartitaginea, Capparis spinosa, Gomphocarpus sinaicus, Hammada salicornica, and Pyrethrum santolinoides.

(2) Grew up during the night when the ground was moist, but which "*withered away*" and "*stank*" when the heat of the sun fell upon it (Exodus 16). The tiny blue-green algae can grow with unbelievable rapidity during the night. Soft and gelatinous, these algal growths disappear the next morning when the sun evaporates the dew, only to reappear the next night when there is abundant dew.

Botanists tend to suspect lichens of the genus lecanora, which after periods of drought dry up, curl up, break loose from the ground and are transported by the wind. Ca. 1889 a shower of such lichens fell into Iran during a great famine. Not mentioning the Iranian shower of manna. It has been noted that the manna obtained from Fraxinus can be secured either as flakes ("flake manna") or fragments ("common manna") or as a viscid mass ("fat manna"). A good tree can yield a pound or more per season. Annual production in Sicily, where manna was once produced commercially, has been around 750 tons.

Manna is described as a gentle laxative, demulcent and expectorant. Manna was chiefly used as a children's laxative or to disguise other medicines. In 1906, Dr. Steinberg is said to have recommended dulcinol, a mixture of manna and common salt as a sweetening agent in diabetes. It is also used as an aperient, debility, purgative, restorative and tonic. The leaves of the manna ash contain, in addition to aesculetin, cichoriin, ornol, and sedoheptulose, two marginal antitumor compounds, ursolic acid and rutin. Aesuletin and aesculin are anti inflammatory. Manna from Fraxinus contains glucose, levulose, manneotetrose, mannite, manninotriose and resin. Ash was recommended by Lebanese for diarrhea and malaria and the bark flakes for fever. Algerians powdered the seeds in olive oil and honey for gonorrhea.

MASTIC – (*PISTACIA LENTISCUS*)
…Who answered, under a mastick tree…Susanna 51

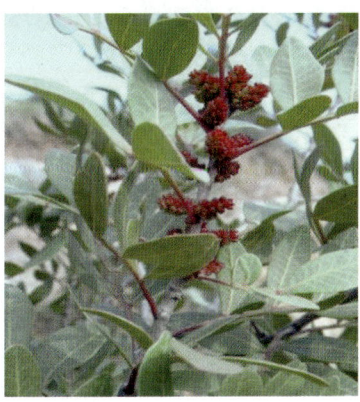

Mastic is cultivated primarily for the resin and used as a masticatory and a medicine. Women living in harems use the resin obtained from the bark by incision. They chew it to sweeten their breath. It is also used to harden gums and alleviate toothache and is used for filling dental caries. Eastern children buy this for a chewing gum. It is also used in cosmetics and depilatory creams as well as in the making of confectionary, liqueurs, and varnishes. Poorer grades are used for varnish, used for coating metals and paintings, for lithography for retouching negatives. Egyptians used mastic as an embalming agent. Sometimes used in incense; oil of mastic used in cosmetics. Greeks made a liqueur, mastiche, flavoring the mastic with grape skins. Syrians also make a mastic beverage. The wood and leaves burn green; when burned, both the fruit and wood give out a pleasant aroma. The oil expressed from the berries is used by the Arabs for both food and illumination. The twigs are used in basketry.

The best grades of mastic, yellowish white translucent tears, are medicinally employed as an aromatic astringent. Frequently cited in the cancer folklore, the resin or juice from mastic is used for indurations or tumors of the anus, breast, liver, parotid, spleen, stomach, testicles, throat, and uterus. It is used for diarrhea in children. Regarded as analgesic, antitussive, aperitive, aphrodisiac, astringent, carminative, diuretic, expectorant, hemostatic, stimulant to the mucous membranes, stomachic and sudorific, mastic finds a way into folk remedies for apostemes, boils, cancer, canker, carbuncle, cardiodynia, condyloma, debility, excrescences, gingivitis, halitosis, leucorrhea, mastitis, phymata, sclerosis, stomach and tumors. Lebanese dissolve the resin in alcohol adding lemon juice, for gall bladder and liver trouble. Algerians use the root decoction for cough. Finally, the oil obtained by hot extraction of the nuts is used for itch and rheumatism.

MILK THISTLE – (SILYBUM MARIANUM)
...Thorns also and thistles shall it bring forth to thee; and thou shalt eat the herb of the field...Genesis 3

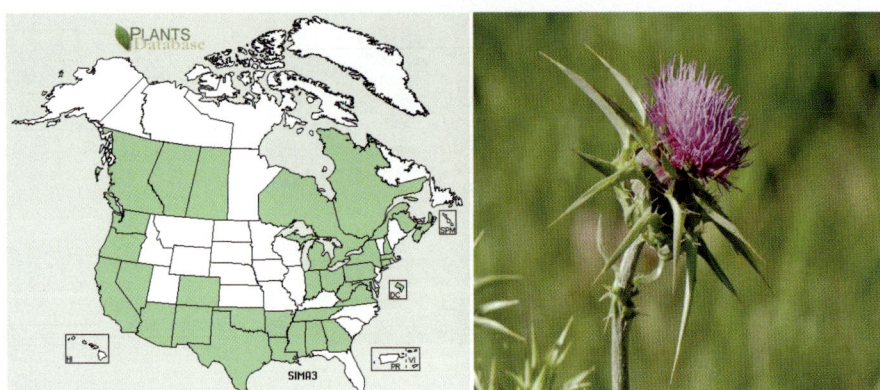

The stalks, like those of most thistles, are said to be quite edible and nutritious. Still they are reported to have caused fatalities in cattle. The young leaves are often eaten as salad ingredients. The roots also are eaten like salsify. Birds like the seeds, which might also serve as a famine food for humans. The heads were once eaten like artichoke. The seeds have served as coffee substitutes, and the seed cake is used for cattle fodder, the seed oil being used for food or lubrication.

Considered alterative, aperient, cholagogue, demulcent, depurative, emmenagogue, expectorant, hemostat, lactogogue, purgative, stimulant, sudorific, and tonic, the milk thistle is said to be a remedy for anthrax, asthma, calculus, cancer (breast, nose), catarrh, chest, dropsy, fever, gallbladder, hemoptysis, hepatitis, hydrophobia, jaundice, leucorrhea, malaria, melancholy, piles, plague, pleurisy, spasm, spleen, and uteritis. Lebanese believe the flower infusion is an alterative, refrigerant and tonic. Boiled in vinegar, the leaves are used as skin ailments and tonics. The astringent vulnerary root is used for hemorrhoids and worms. Lebanese used the seed infusion for stones of the gall bladder and liver, and as a hydragogue, lactogogue, litholytic, stimulant and tonic. Seeds, used in liver diseases, contain the active flavolignans called silybin, silychrystin, and silydianin, collectively called silymarin. Silymarin has antihepatotoxin activity or it has protective action on the liver. The seed tincture is also used for cough, peritonitis, pulmonitis (or bronchitis), uteral congestion and varicose veins. Milk thistle contains selenium which is used to detoxify the liver.

The plant contains the following minerals:

Aluminum	Magnesium	Potassium
Calcium	Manganese	Silica
Chromium	Nitrogen	Sodium
Cobalt	Potassium	Tin
Iron	Selenium	Zinc

MILLET – (*PANICUM MIlIACEUM*)

...Take thou also unto thee wheat, and barley, and beans, and lentiles, and millet, and fitches, and put them in one vessel, and make thee bread thereof...Ezekiel 4

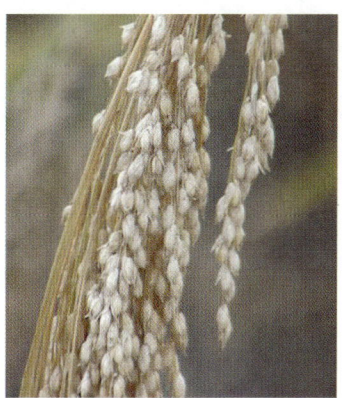

Ezekiel is said to have received an order from God to make bread with wheat, barley, beans, lentils, and pannag (millet). The mixture was moistened with camel's milk, oil, or butter. It was the main food that the common people ate. Proso millet is grown mainly in the United States as a grain crop, but may occasionally be grown for forage, but as forage the stems are coarse, hairy and unpalatable. As a human food in Old World countries, millet is used as a meal for making baked foods, as a paste from pounded wet seeds, or as a boiled gruel. The grain is eaten readily by livestock, mainly hogs, cattle, and poultry, but not suited for horses. It is also grown for commercial bird feeds. It should be ground for livestock feed, equal to or superior in food value to oats. In Eastern Europe, Balkans, Caucasus, and Asia, it is used to make an alcoholic beverage.

Some writers suggest that pannag may be etymologically related to the Greek "panexia," meaning a universal medicine or panacea, considered by Greek physicians as a cure for many human ailments. Considered demulcent, diuretic, pectoral and refrigerant, millet is used in folk remedies for abscesses, boils, edema, fevers, fluxes, gonorrhea, hematuria, labor, pyrosis, sores, and venereal disease. A paste from the seed is said to be a folk remedy for breast cancer. The seeds are chewed and the juice applied to children's sores.

MULBERRY FIG – (*FICUS SYCOMORUS*)
...I was an herdman, and a gatherer of sycomore fruit...Amos 7

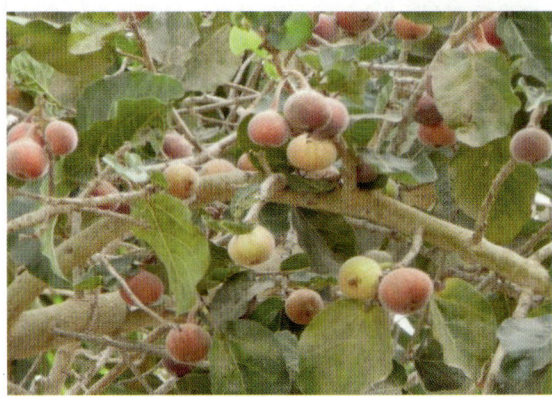

The sycomore that Zacchaeus climbed to see Jesus pass is a curious tree combining the characteristics of fig and mulberry. The yellowish fruit smells like an ordinary fig, but is inferior in taste. This porous, though very enduring wood was used for temples and auditoriums. It was also used for fashioning mummy chests or coffins which were found in perfect condition after more than three thousand years. In Africa, Masai use twigs in fire making. The latex is used to coagulate milk. It grows apparently quite rapidly and might be considered as a biomass candidate. The milky latex is said to contain rubber.

In Biblical Land, it is often planted as a shade tree. This is the shade reported to have embraced the Virgin Mary. At Marhave is a large sycamore or Pharaoh's fig; it is very old but bears fruit each year. They say that upon the Virgin passing by that way with her son Jesus and being pursued by the people, this fig tree opened to receive her and closed her in again, until the people had passed by and then opened again. The tree is still shown to travelers.

The latex was used for burns, cancer, indurations (of the limbs and spleen), tumors (especially of the fauces) and warts. The latex probably contains the proteolytic ficin. Fruits and leaves are fed to cows to increase the flow of milk especially in arid areas. The bark and/or latex are used for chest ailments, cough, diarrhea, inflammation, scrofula and sore throat. In Ethiopia, the root is used as a prophylactic against typhoid. Lebanese apply the latex to shallow abrasions and skin infections to ward off tetanus. They used the bark decoction for blood poisoning. Dioscorides recommended the fruit as an antivenom, for cirrhosis, melancholy, slow healing wounds, and stomach trouble. In East Africa, the Masai use the bark for diarrhea. East Africans use the bark for sore throat.

MUSKMELON – (CUCUMIS MELO)
...We remember the fish, which we did eat in Egypt freely; the cucumbers, and the melons...Numbers 11

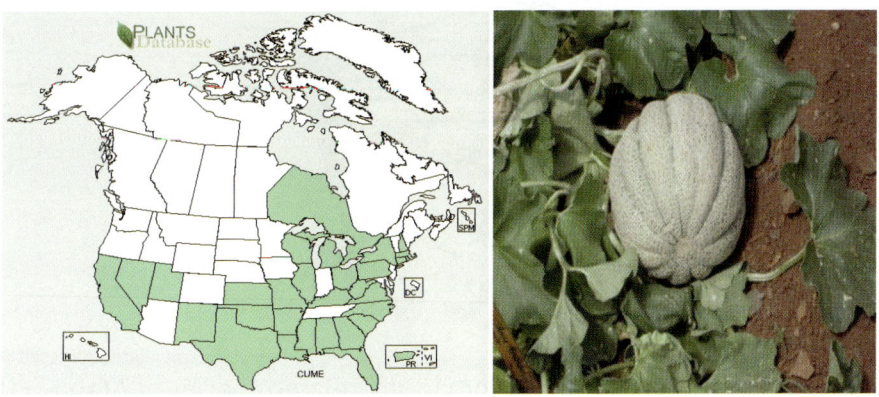

Some think the Biblical melon was this, others think watermelon. Both are cultivated as pleasantly juicy fruits in a dry country. Muskmelon is a fruit that is eaten fresh out of rind after the removal of seeds, as dessert and sometimes with sugar or powdered ginger. Fruits of some cultivars used it for preserves or as vegetables. The seeds are edible and yield edible oil. Lebanese believe it repels bedbugs.

Considered antivinous, demulcent, digestive, diuretic, emetic, emmenagogue, refrigerant, stomachic, taenifuge, and vermifuge, melons have been suggested for anasarca, bruises, cancer, cold, coryza, cough, diabetes, dyspepsia, dysuria, eczema, extravasation, gonorrhea, jaundice, menorrhagia, micturition, oliguria, polyps, stomatitis, and tumors. Some think it can help prevent sunstroke. The fruit is used as a lotion for eczema, and for removing tan and freckles. The rind is said to help tumors of the stomach and cancer of the uterus. The root, boiled with pine wood, is said to be a cure for stomach, bladder, and uterine cancers. Dietary use of the pulp or the seeds is believed by some to help tumors (especially of the bladder, liver and stomach). Seeds have been recommended for stomach cancer, and purulent ailments of the digestive tract. After oil extraction, the seeds are suggested for menorrhagia. Flowers are emetic (but the stalks are antiemetic); powdered buds are used for jaundice and nasal ulcers. The fruit is stomachic, seeds bechic and digestive. Weaning Lebanese mothers rub the pulp on their breast and give it to their children to suck. Chinese are said to use the peduncles for anasarca and dyspepsia. In North Africa the fruiting peduncle is regarded as emetic and expectorant. In Unani medicine, the seeds are regarded as diuretic, lachrymatory, and tonic and are used in ophthalmia, liver and kidney troubles, bronchitis, burning of the throat, chronic fever and thirst. In Ayurvedic medicine, the fruit is regarded as aphrodisiac, diuretic, laxative and tonic. It is used for ascites, biliousness, fatigue and insanity.

The fruit contains the following minerals:

Aluminum	Lithium	Selenium
Boron	Magnesium	Silver
Calcium	Manganese	Sodium
Chromium	Molybdenum	Strontium
Cobalt	Nickel	Sulfur
Copper	Nitrogen	Titanium
Iron	Potassium	Zinc

Hillman Health Food Store call 855-Amish-Dr (855-264-7437) www.emineral.info Vitamins and Minerals for Better Living

Myrrh – (Commiphora Myrrha)
...six months with oil of myrrh, and six months with sweet odours, and with other things for the purifying of women...Esther 2

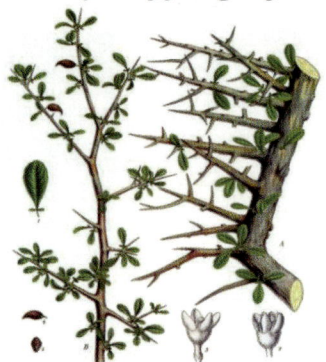

Much of the myrrh of commerce comes from this or closely-related species of Arabia, Ethiopia, and Somalia. It is highly regarded in the Orient as an aromatic substance, perfume, and medicine. Ancient Egyptians burned it in their temples and used it for embalming. There is even a term "myrrophore" applied to the women who bore spices to the sepulcher of Jesus with aloes, cassia, and cinnamon; it was an ingredient of the holy oil and a domestic perfume. Some authorities maintain that the Biblical myrrh was in reality a mixture of myrrh and ladanum. Myrrh was burned as incense for the sun god at Heliopolis at noon. Persian Kings wore it in their crowns. Myrrh and frankincense were even burned during the reign of King George III. One old legend says that Myrrha, daughter of the King of Cyprus, became unnaturally obsessed with her father, who exiled her to the Arabian Desert, where the gods transformed her into the myrrh tree "in which guise she remains, weeping tears perfumed of repentance." The gum makes good mucilage and the insoluble residue from the tincture can be used as glue.

Bitter and pungent, the myrrh was esteemed by Orientals as an astringent tonic, internally, and as a cleansing agent, externally. In Algeria, myrrh is used to dress suppurations. Myrrh is a direct emmenagogue, a tonic in dyspepsia, an expectorant in the absence of feverish symptoms, a stimulant to mucous tissues, a stomachic carminative, exciting appetite and the flow of gastric juice, and an astringent wash. It is used in chronic catarrh, phthisis pulmonalis, chlorosis, and in amenorrhea is often combined with aloes and iron. As a wash it is good for spongy gums, ulcerated throat and aphthous stomatitis, and the tincture is also applied to foul and indolent ulcers. It has been found helpful in bronchorrhea and leucorrhea. It has been used as a vermifuge.

MYRTLE – (MYRTUS COMMUNIS)
...I will plant in the wilderness the cedar, the shittah tree, and the myrtle, and the oil tree...Isaiah 41

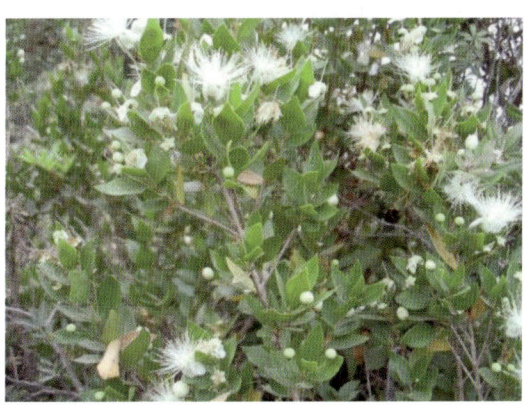

Jews collect myrtle to adorn their sheds and booths at the Feast of Tabernacles. Purplish black berries known as mursins have medicinal value and are also edible. In Italy the leaves are used as a spice; in Syria all parts of the plant are dried for perfume. Around Rabat they mix the leaves with shampoo, believed to darken the hair. It is still used today by the Jews at the Feast of the Tabernacles, when it is procurable. Sprigs with three leaves in a whorl (which are not common) are especially esteemed. It is referred to chiefly as a symbol of divine generosity. Greeks consider it a symbol of love and immortality, and used it for crowning their priests, heros, and outstanding men. It is emblematic of peace and joy in the Bible. To ancient Jews it was symbolic not only of peace, but also of justice. In the bazaar of Jerusalem and Damascus, the flowers, leaves and fruits are sold for making perfume. Arabs say that myrtle is one of the three plants taken from the Garden of Eden, because of its fragrance.

Turkish and Russian leather is tanned with the bark and roots, imparting a distinctive odor. Originally sacred also to Venus, to whom it was a symbol of sensual love and passion. It is placed on Bohemian caskets as a symbol of immortality. Myrde has been grown since ancient times for the fragrant, aromatic flowers, leaves and bark. The leaves are used for massage to work up a glowing skin. A fragrant oil that is obtained from these is used in perfumery. The oil is also used in toilet waters. Green and dried fruits are sometimes used as a condiment. The wood is very hard and of interesting texture and grain. Plants are often ground for ornament, as it makes a nice evergreen hedge in appropriate Mediterranean climate.

Regarded as antiseptic, antispasmodic, astringent, carminative, cordial, parasiticide, pectoral, rubefacient, sedative, stimulant, stomachic, tonic, and vermifugal, myrtle is an ingredient in folk remedies for aphthae, bladder, brain, bronchitis, cacoethes, chest, collyrium, condylomata, cystitis, diarrhea, dysentery, dyspepsia, eczema, epilepsy, fever, figs, headache, hemorrhage, hepatitis, leucorrhea, lung, phthisis, polyps, prolapse, pyelitis, rheumatism, sores, stomach, ulcers, urogenital problems, uterus, whitlows and wounds. The plant contains antibacterial phenols. Medicinally, an infusion or tincture of leaves is given for prolapsus and leucorrhoea, and for washing incisions and joints. Also, it is used to check night sweats of phthisis and for all types of pulmonary disorders.

Lebanese consider the plant binding and diuretic, believing it holds loose things in place, the bowels, the emotions, or the teeth. The leaf, in various forms, is a folk treatment for condylomata, whitlows, warts, figs, parotid tumors, cancer of the gums, ulcerated cancers, and polyps. Iranians make a hot poultice for boils from the plant. The oil, in plasters or unguents is said to help indurations of the breast, condyloma of the genitals, and cancer. The berries and seed are said to cure tumors and uterine fibroids. Unani direct smoke from the leaves onto hemorrhoids and use the fruit for bronchitis, headache, and menorrhagia.

Hillman Health Food Store call 855-Amish-Dr (855-264-7437) www.emineral.info Vitamins and Minerals for Better Living

They consider the fruits useful for the blood, brain, hair, and heart. Algerians recommend the leafy infusion for asthma. North Africans use the dry flower buds for smallpox.

Narcissus – (Narcissus Tazetta)

...The wilderness and the solitary place shall be glad for them; and the desert shall rejoice, and blossom as the rose...Isaiah 35

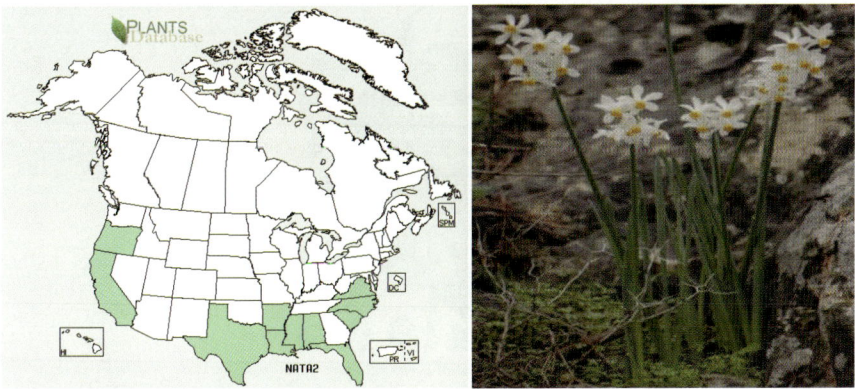

Widely cultivated as a beautiful ornamental, this narcissus also has very aromatic flowers. In the Holy Land this narcissus is a dazzling golden yellow, a color not seen in cooler climates. It grows wild in the desert from the Mediterranean Sea to the center of Palestine, near Joppa, and in January the land is a profusion of color. Palestinians still delight in the arrowy fragrance of this "Rose of Sharon" and carry the blossoms with them onto the streets and into their houses. From the flowers is extracted an essential oil, the absolute of which is a valuable adjunct in high grade French perfume. It blends well with jasmine perfume. The plant holds a deserved place among oriental medicinals. Bulbs are imported into Bombay, dried, sliced, and sold as a substitute for bitter hermodactyls. The root extract in olive oil is a skin lotion, in vinegar a shampoo rinse, in brandy an aphrodisiac "to be treated with the greatest caution."

Regarded as absorbent, analgesic, antiphlogistic, demulcent, diuretic, emetic, POISON, and purgative, this species has found its way into folk remedies for abscesses, boils, cancer (especially of the breast), gynecopathy, mastitis, sclerosis (especially of the uterus), swellings, and tumors (especially of the ear). The anticancer folklore is interesting in view of the fact that the narcissus has shown genuine antitumor activity, perhaps due to the presence of antitumor compounds lycorine and benzaldehyde.

Narcissus has been suspected of giving off an evil emanation, producing dullness of the intellect, insanity, and even death. Bulbs used as a demulcent bolus to carry bones out of the esophagus, juice of the bulb used for eye ailments. Dried flowers are used for female fevers. In Lebanon boiling water is poured over the flowers, and steeped for two or three minutes as a stomach tonic. The dangerous roots are used for epilepsy and fits, but sometimes the spasms are worsened by the bulbs.

Hillman Health Food Store call 855-Amish-Dr (855-264-7437) www.emineral.info Vitamins and Minerals for Better Living

NETTLES – (ACANTHUS SYRIACUSS)
...Among the bushes they brayed; under the nettles they gathered together...Job 30

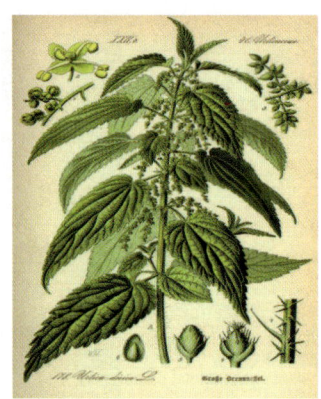

Since time immemorial, nettle leaves of this species have served as models for scroll decorations in art. Most authors regard acanthus spinosus L. as the model and the Biblical species, but the Holy Land variety has been identified as acanthus syriacus. Acanthus spinosus is listed as an astringent and diuretic.

OLIVE – (OLEA EUROPEA)
...His branches shall spread, and his beauty shall be as the olive tree...Hosea 14

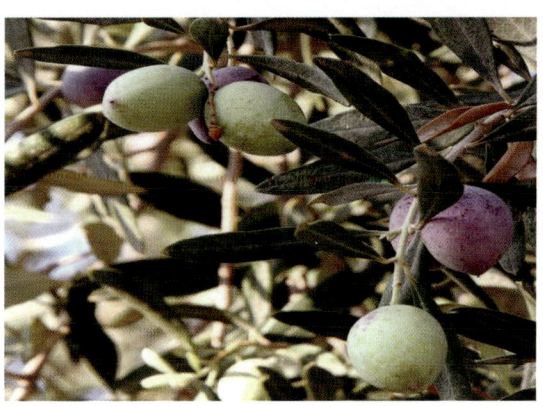

The olive, one of the most valuable of Hebrew trees, is one of the most frequently mentioned medicinal plants of the Bible. Passages where the word anoint appears usually means with olive oil. One scholar has said that no tree is more closely associated with the history of man and development of civilization than the olive. An Arabic proverb has it that gardens are folly while olives are kings. The olive tree is cultivated primarily for the oil extracted by crushing its fruit, consuming about 90% of the world production. The remainder provides the various preparations of table olives, the black olives being treated in brine solution for 3 to 9 months and the green produced by lactic acid fermentation. Olive oil is used for cooking and as a salad oil. Olive oil is also used for canning sardines and other fish. It's also used as illuminating oil, for anointing, and for medicinal and cosmetic uses. Olive oil was the base of the perfumed ointments sold in classic Athens and Rome. It is also used in the textile industry in wool combing. Olive pomace, the residue after milling, is used in animal feeds. The stones (seeds) are used in the making of molded products and plastics. The bitter glucoside, oleuropein, of green olives is usually neutralized with lye or caustic soda before pickling. In Italy, an olive branch is hung over the door to keep out evil spirits.

Suggested as antiseptic, aperient, astringent, cholagogue, demulcent, diuretic, emollient, hypotensive, laxative, sedative, tonic, the olive is encountered in folk remedies for cancer, chills, diarrhea, ear ache, fever, heinoptysis, hypertension, malaria, scofula, toothache, tumors, and wounds. Iranians use the leaf decoction for cough. Olive is cited in folk remedies for such cancerous conditions as acrochordons, cancer of the breasts, gums, and stomach; condylomata; figs; polyps; scleroses of the liver, spleen, stomach, and uterus; tumors of the ear, fingers, neck, stomach, and warts. Olive contains the antitumor compound sitosterol-d glucoside. The leaf, pounded with wine, is a folk remedy for condylomata, or if used in a cataplasm, is said to cure tumors. The fruit decoction is said to help cancer of the mouth. The flower, used in a poultice or cataplasm is said to remedy condylomata, acrochordons, warts, figs, and syka.

The salve from the juice is said to cure indurations. The oil, in any number of forms, is said to cure cancer and is applied as an emollient to dermatitis and swellings. The oil is considered a panacea in the orient, for example, Lebanon, where it is used for burns, colds, constipation, lesions, stomachache, sore throat and sunburn. Olive oil is recommended in diets for patients recovering from heart attacks with other oils rigidly excluded from the diets. Algerians chew the leaves for toothaches and oral sores caused by excess tobacco. Algerians also used it for baldness, cough, earache, fractures, gonorrhea, hemorrhage, hernia, impotence, liver congestion, skin diseases, sprains and stones. The bark has had "a great reputation as a substitute for cinchona." North Africans use the wood decoction for aphtha and stomatitis. Boulos reports that the leaves and/or their extracts are antibacterial, antidiabetic, cholagogue, diuretic, hypoglycemic, hypotensive, as well as pectoral.

The fruit contains the following minerals:

Boron	Iron	Potassium
Calcium	Nitrogen	Sodium

The leaf contains the following minerals:

Calcium   Nitrogen

ONION – (ALLIUM CEPA)
...We remember the fish, which we did eat in Egypt...the leeks, and the onions...Numbers 11

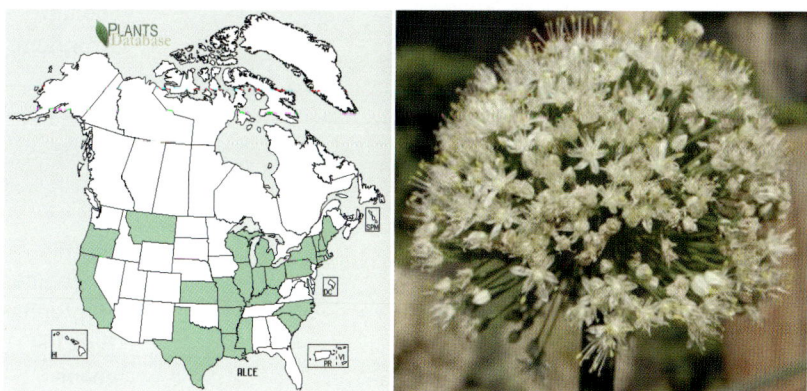

Onions are generally produced as green or dry onions. Green onions are eaten raw with meats, fish, and cheese or as a vegetable, or chopped and added to cottage cheese, or cooked. Dry onions may be served as a vegetable dish, or to flavor meat, fish and poultry dishes. They are good raw, boiled, baked, creamed, broiled, fried, french fried, roasted or pickled, and in soups, stews, dressings, or salads. Onion is used widely with other ingredients for innumerable dishes.

Although widely used in Biblical times, the onion is only mentioned once, in Numbers 11. Like garlic, the onion is highly regarded as an antiseptic, apertif, aphrodisiac, bactericide, carminative, diaphoretic, digestive, diuretic, expectorant, pectoral, sedative, soporific (yet stimulant)), stomachic, suppurative, tonic, and vermifuge. Among other ailments, it is often recommended for abscesses, albuminuria, alopecia, anasarca, angina, arteriosclerosis, bilious ailments, bladder ailments, bleeding, breast cancer, Bright's disease, bronchitis, bubo, burns, cancer, cataracts, catarrh, chest, chilblains, cholera, cold, colic, consumption, corns, cough, diabetes, diarrhea, diptheria, dropsy, dysentery, earache, edema, epilepsy, erysipelas, eyes, felons, fever, flatulence, flu, fracture, freckles, gallbladder, gangrene, gout, gravel, hangover, headache, heart, heartburn, hepatitis, hoarseness, hydropsy, hyperglycemia, hypertension, impotency, indurations, inflammation, liver cancer, paralysis, piles, rabies, rectum cancer, rheumatism, scarlatina, sciatica, stones, syphilis, tuberculosis, tumor, urogenitary problems, uterine cancer, venereal disease, warts, whitlows, whooping cough, worms, and wounds. Allicin, a compound found in garlic and onion, is antiseptic, hyperglycemic, hypocholesterolemic, insecticidal, and larvicidal. Arresting putrefaction and fermentation processes in the gastrointestinal tract, onion might help prevent cancer of the lower gut. Widely distributed, beta sitosterol has shown several types of antitumor activity. Rutin, isolated from onion, is said to be antiatherogenic, antiedemic, anti-inflammatory, antispasmodic, antithrombogenic, hypotensive, and is said to prevent cancer as well as protect against x radiation. Roasted onion has been applied to tumors. The seed, with honey, is a folk remedy for warts. The juice is said to help cancers of the breast and rectum. The bulb, prepared in various manners, is said to help indurated glands and tumors. Reputed to be hypotensive, onions have recently been shown to contain the antihypertensive agent prostaglandin A1. Lebanese believe that onions prevent typhoid, and alleviate or cure colds, dyspepsia, jaundice and nephritis. They apply onion juice to abscesses, boils, earache, eyeache, rhinitis, and sinusitis. Onion seeds are sold in Iran and Iraq as demulcent stimulants. Boiled with sugar and almond oil, they are given as a purgative during typhoid fever.

Hillman Health Food Store call 855-Amish-Dr (855-264-7437) www.emineral.info Vitamins and Minerals for Better Living

Onions contains the following minerals:

Aluminum	Iron	Rubidium
Boron	Lithium	Selenium
Bromine	Magnesium	Silica
Calcium	Manganese	Silver
Chromium	Molybdenum	Sodium
Cobalt	Nickel	Strontium
Copper	Nitrogen	Sulfur
Fluorine	Potassium	

Onions contains the following amino acids:

Alanine	Leucine	Serine
Arginine	Lysine	Threonine
Glycine	Methionine	Tryptophan
Histidine	Phenylalanine	Tyrosine
Isoleucine	Proline	Valine

ONYCHA – (STYRAX BENZOIN)
...Take unto thee sweet spices, stacte, and onycha...Exodus 30

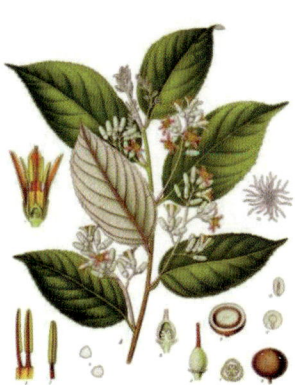

The Biblical onycha may have been the gum resin known today as benzoin. Others believe it was Commiphora. Even today benzoin is burned as incense in churches. Benzoin has been added to cigarettes. Benzoin adds the gloss to chocolate eggs, the turbidity to syrups, and some of the flavor to baked goods, candies, chewing gums, gelatins, ice creams, puddings, and soft drinks. Benzoin is valued as an antioxidant and antiseptic. Benzoin also enters cosmetics, colognes, lotions, perfumes, and toiletries.

Internally benzoin is considered carminative, diuretic and expectorant and is used, as an inhalator, for bronchitis or laryngitis. "Virgin's milk," the milky alcoholic solution of benzoin, diluted with water, has been employed in feminine hygiene, and is applied to cracked nipples. In Malaya, benzoin was applied to circumcision wounds, ringworm, shingles, skin affliction, and sore feet.

PALESTINE BUCKTHORN – (RHAMNUS PALAESTINA)
...Whoso breaketh a hedge, a serpent shall bite him...Ecclesiastes 10

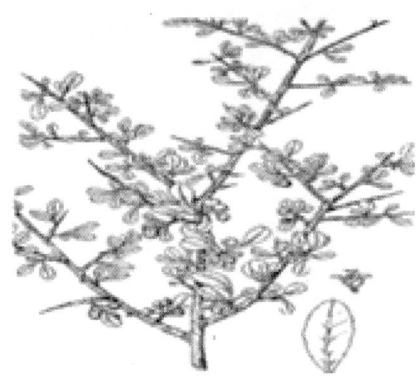

Like so many other thorny shrubs of the Bible, this one has been used as a fence to exclude grazing animals from gardens and orchards. The Palestine buckthorn probably shares cathartic properties with other medicinal species of the genus.

PAPYRUS – (CYPERUS PAPYRUS)
...Can the rush grow up without mire? Can the flag grow without water...Job 8

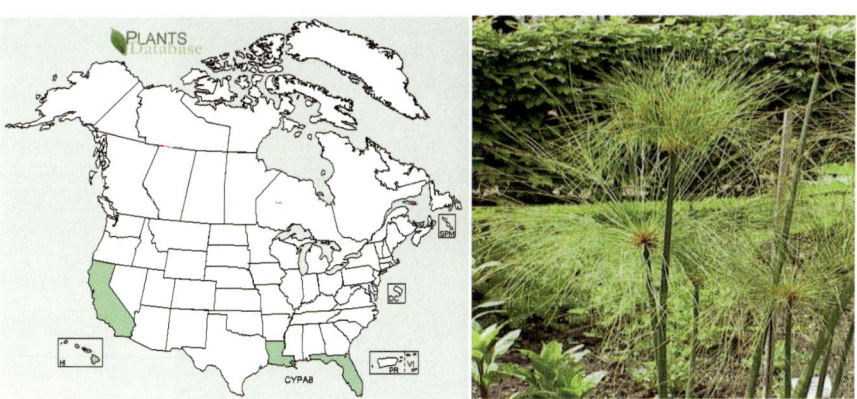

Very important in ancient Egypt (as early as 2400 B.C.), papyrus was used for food, medicine, fiber, fuel, and shelter. Egyptians have used papyrus additionally for formal bouquets, funeral garlands, boats, cordage, fans, sandals, matting, corkage, boxes, and paper. It was one of the favorite plants of ancient Egypt. The pith of papyrus was recommended for food, while the starchy rhizomes and lowermost parts of the stem were cut off and consumed raw, boiled, or roasted. They were also chewn, sucked, and spit out, much as sugar cane is done today. Papyrus was also a favorite ornament in ancient art and craft.

Papyrus stems were used for caulking seams in wooden ships. Papyrus mats are used for making fences and huts. For paper, the ancients stripped the fibrous coverings off the stem, and slit the inner pith into waferlike strips. Laid side by side, with others placed crosswise on top, the strips were dampened, pressed with glue which cemented them together, and dried into a sheet. Moses was laid in a cradle woven from the bulrushes of papyrus growing in the rivers of lower Egypt. Among these same bulrushes the ark was placed, to be discovered by Pharaoh's daughter who brought Moses up as her son. Papyrus provided the earliest known material for the making of paper, which gets its name from the plant. The writing material of the old Egyptians was made of the stem pith, laid flat and glued together. Then the whole mass was pressed under heavy weights, and when dry, it was ready to be written on. The first paint brushes were fashioned from this reed by fraying stalk ends. In the treeless valley of the Nile, the rhizome was valued for fuel.

Hillman Health Food Store call 855-Amish-Dr (855-264-7437) www.emineral.info Vitamins and Minerals for Better Living

PHOENICIAN ROSE – (*ROSA PHOENICIA*)
...whereup they grew roses and lilies...II Esdras 2

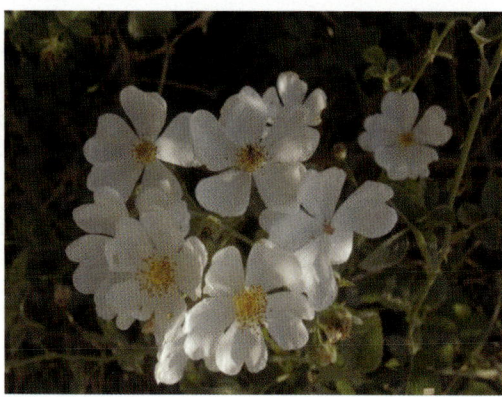

In the Wisdom of Solomon 2:8 there is talk of crowning oneself with rosebuds. Crowning oneself with rosebud at a feast is a purely Greek custom borrowed by the Romans. A century or so later, Egyptians were growing roses under glass to send to Rome for banquets. While rose in the Bible may mean many species (Cistus, Hibiscus, Nerium, Rosa), it is concluded that they meant Rosa in the Wisdom of Solomon. Petals of some species of rose are used to make sandwiches. The rose hips and petals of this species, probably also rich in vitamins, might serve medicinally in the stead of other species.

PISTACHIO NUT – (PISTICIA VERA)
...carry down the man a present, a little balm, and a little honey, spices, and myrrh, nuts and almonds...Genesis 43

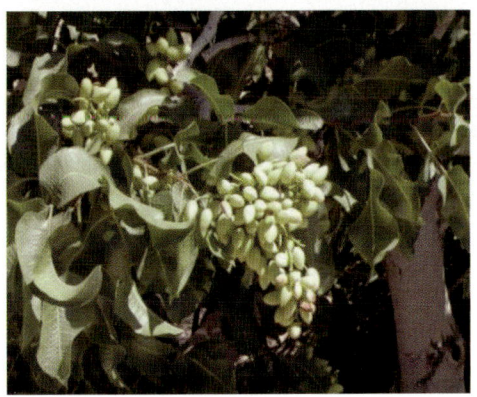

Most commentators agree that the "nuts" of Jacob were pistachio nuts. Pista kernels have a delicious nutty flavor and are used as ingredients of sweetmeats, confectionery, and ice creams. Pista is also eaten as a dessert; salted and roasted, it is much relished. It is considered to be digestive, sedative and tonic. Fruit husks are reported to be made into marmalade in Iran; they are also used as fertilizer. They are imported to India as a dyeing and tanning agent. Pistacio kernels yield ca. 50% of a low melting fatty oil used to a small extent in confectionery as spice oil and in medicine. The leaves of P. Vera bear small irregularly spheroid galls (Bokhara galls) which have been reported to be imported into India for dyeing and tanning purposes.

Considered anodyne, and decoagulant, the pistachio is used for abdominal ailments, abscesses, amenorrhea, bruises, chest ailments, circulation, dysentery, gynecopathy, pruritus, rheumatism, sclerosis of the liver, sores, and trauma. Algerians used the powdered root in oil for children's cough. Iranians infused the fruits' outer husks for dysentery. Lebanese used the leaves as compresses, believing the nuts enhanced fertility and virility.

The fruit contains the following minerals:

Aluminum	Iron	Silica
Boron	Magnesium	Sodium
Calcium	Manganese	Sulfur
Copper	Nitrogen	Zinc
Iodine	Potassium	

The seed contains the following minerals:

Aluminum	Iron	Potassium
Calcium	Manganese	Sodium
Copper	Nitrogen	Zinc

The fruit contains the following amino acids:

Alanine	Leucine	Threonine
Arginine	Lysine	Tryptophan
Glutamate	Methionine	Tyrosine
Glycine	Phenylalanine	Valine
Histidine	Proline	
Isoleucine	Serine	

Hillman Health Food Store call 855-Amish-Dr (855-264-7437) www.emineral.info Vitamins and Minerals for Better Living

PLANE TREE – (*PLATANUS ORIENTALIS*)
...And Jacob took him rods of green poplar, and of the hazel and chestnut tree...Genesis 30

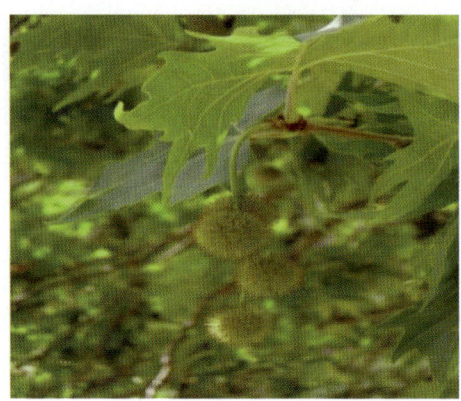

Commonly cultivated and highly valued as an ornamental tree, in the Orient, the "chestnut" is said to be the tree under which Socrates enthralled his students. It has a short trunk and a roundish spreading crown and is mostly grown for shade in parks and on roadsides. Seldom felled, it is allowed to grow to large dimensions. The wood is white, tinged with yellow or red; heartwood not distinct. The wood is also fine grained and moderately hard and heavy, but strong. It warps during seasoning and is durable only under cover. It is easy to saw and presents a decorative figure when quarter sawn. It can be finished to a smooth surface which takes a beautiful polish. In Kashmir, the wood is mostly used for small boxes, trays, and similar articles which are lacquered and painted. In West Asia and Europe, it is used for cabinet making, furniture, veneers, carving, coach building, and general turnery and for wood pulp. It has been reported to be suitable for boot lasts.

Considered cyanogenic, tonic and vulnerary, the plane tree is used for cancer, carcinomata, diarrhea, dysentery, ophthalmia, rheumatism, scurvy, and inflammatory tumors. The bark possesses antiscorbutic and antirheumatic properties. Boiled in vinegar, it is given for hernia and toothache. Bruised fresh leaves are applied in ophthalmia. Unani used the bark for animal bites and leucoderma, the fruits and leaves for lacrymation, leucoderma, ophthalmia, toothache and wounds, and disorders of the kidney, lungs, throat and voice.

POMEGRANATE – (PUNICA GRANATUM)
...I would cause thee to drink of spiced wine of the juice of my pomegranate...Song of Solomon 8

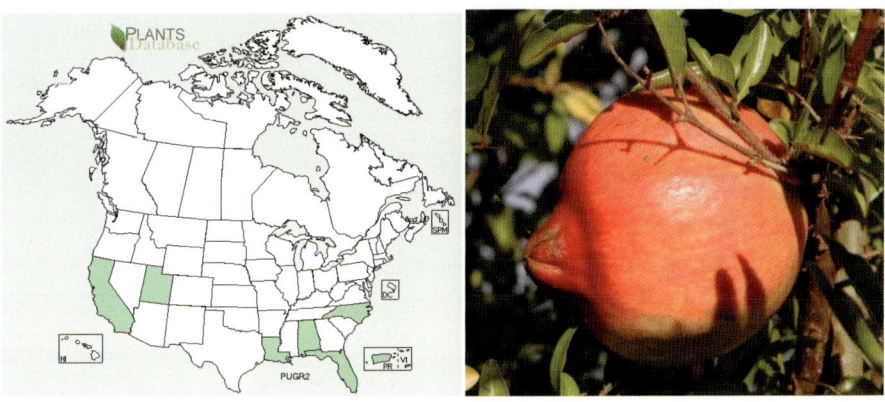

Pomegranate literally means "apple with grains," the reference being to the many clear ruby-colored seeds, covered with a thin skin and full of juice, found in each fruit. Syrup made from the seeds is known as grenadine. The first sherbet was a preparation of pomegranate juice mixed with snow. Apothecaries use the blossoms, known as balausts, in the preparation of an astringent medicine used in treating dysentery. The acid pulp surrounding the seeds is the edible portion of the fruit, used as a salad or table fruit, or made into beverages or jellies. In Syria and Iran the fruit is cut open, seeded, strewn with sugar, and sprinkled with rose water. Wine is made from the fruits, and seeds are used in syrups, preserves, gelatin desserts, icings, puddings, and sauces. Grenadine is a soft drink based on pomegranate, and grenadine syrup is used to flavor drinks. Rinds are used for tanning Morocco leather, giving it a yellow color. Flowers give a red dye. Plants make good ornamental hedge, especially in dry climates. Also, it is useful as a greenhouse potted plant and the cut flowers are longlasting in arrangements. Pomegranate is the national flower emblem of Spain. Wood, though scanty, is hard and can be used for small objects and for walking sticks. Flowers are used by some women to give a red color to the teeth, and rind is used in Polynesia to give shining black color to teeth. In some areas an unfading ink is made from the rind. The dried rind, called Malicorium, is sold in curved brittle fragments. In China, the pomegranate symbolizes fertility; women offer pomegranates to the goddess of mercy in the hope of being blessed with children. Boulos reports that the seed oil is estrogenic, perhaps providing a rationale for the Chinese beliefs.

Most important is the specificity of the rootbark for tapeworm. Considered anodyne, astringent, bactericide, cardiotonic, parasiticide, refrigerant, stimulant, stomachic, styptic, taenifuge, and vermifuge, the pomegranate appears in folk medicaments for amygdalitis, asthma, bilious afflictions, bronchitis, caked breasts, cancer, colic, conjunctivitis, cough, diarrhea, dysentery, dysmenorrhea, dyspepsia, epistaxis, fever, flux, gingivitis, halitosis, heart, hemorrhage, hemorrhoids, inflammation, leucorrhea, malaria, menorrhagia, metrorrhagia, nightsweats, oxyuriasis, paralysis, pimples, prolapse, rectitis, rectocele, sore throat, snakebite, spienomegaly, stomatitis, tapeworm, thirst, throat, tumors, and urogenital ailments. Ayurvedics use the fruit rind, appropriately enough, for diarrhea, dysentery and worms, the root for worms, the flowers for epistaxis, the bark and seeds for bronchitis, the ripe fruit, considered astringent, aphrodisiac and tonic, for biliousness, burning sensations, fever, heart disease, sore throat and stomatitis. Unani use the astringent bark for anal prolapse, colic and piles, the flowers for biliousness, liydrocele, nausea, sore eyes and sore throat, the green fruit for inflammation and keratitis, the ripe fruit for brain disorders, bronchitis, chest ailments, earache, scabies, sore eyes, sore throat, splenitis, and thirst, the seeds for biliousness, bowel ailments, hepatitis, liver ailments, nausea, and scabies. Leaf juices inhibit some viruses. The rind is a folk remedy for indurated tumors, excrescences of the fundament, corns, carcinoma of the mouth and anus, and wens. The leaf cataplasm is said to cure tumors. The juice, prepared in various manners, is said to remedy pterygia on the finger, nasal polyps, tumors of the fauces, etc. The fruit is said to cure various types of tumors. Small wonder, then, that it contains tannins, betulinic, gallic, and ursolic acids, all recognized experimental anti-tumor agents.

The fruit contains the following minerals:

Calcium	Iron	Potassium
Chlorine	Magnesium	Sodium
Copper	Nitrogen	Sulfur

POPPY SEED – (PAPAVER SOMNIFERUM)
...They gave him vinegar to drink mingled with gall: and when he had tasted thereof, he would not drink...Matthew 27

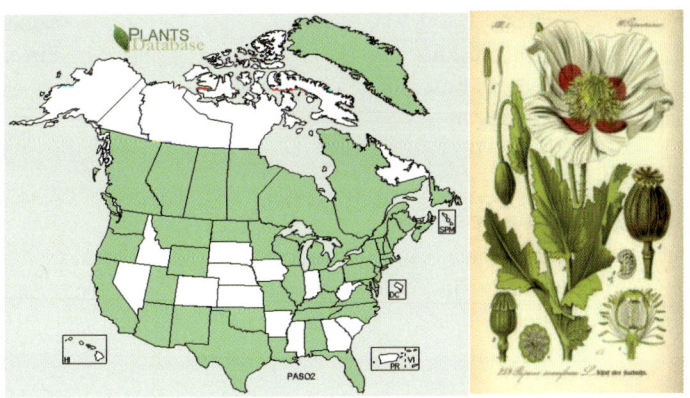

Researchers equate this gall with papaver somnzjerum while other researchers equate it with citrullus colocynthis, not even considering the opium poppy. The gall that was added to the vinegar and offered to Jesus was the juice of the opium poppy, a flower thriving in the Holy Land. The plant provides a narcotic that induces sleep, a sleep so heavy that the person becomes insensible. When the Roman soldiers at Golgatha took pity on their prisoner on the cross, they added this poppy juice to the potion of sour wine. Opium is the air-dried milky exudation obtained from excised unripe fruits. Its compounds are used in medicine as analgesic, anodyne, antispasmodic, hypnotic, narcotic, sedative, and as respiratory depressants and to relieve severe pain. Jewish authorities maintain that the plant and its stupefacience were well known among the Hebrews more than 2000 years ago. The Jerushalmi warns against opium eating. The seeds contain no opium, and are used extensively in baking and sprinkling on rolls and bread. The seeds are a source of a drying oil. Although the seeds contain no narcotic alkaloids, urinalysis following their ingestion may suggest the morphine or heroin addict urinalysis.

Regarded as analgesic, anodyne, antitussive, aphrodisiac, astringent, bactericidal, calmative, carminative, demulcent, emollient, expectorant, hemostat, hypotensive, hypnotic, narcotic, nervine, sedative, sudorific, and a tonic. Poppy has been used in folk remedies for asthma, bladder, bruises, cancer, catarrh, cold, colic, conjunctivitis, cough, diarrhea, dysentery, dysmemorrhea, enteritis, enterorrhagia, fever, flux, headache, hemicrania, hypertension, hypochondria, hysteria, inflammation, insomnia, leucorrhea, malaria, mania, melancholy, nausea, neuralgia, otitis, pertussis, prolapse, rectitis, rheumatism, snakebite, spasm, spermatorrhea, sprain, stomachache, swelling, toothache, tumor, ulcers, and warts. It has been mentioned opium as a remedy for such cancerous conditions as cancer of the skin, stomach, tongue, uterus, carcinoma of the breast, polyps of the ear, nose, and vagina; scleroses of the liver, spleen, and uterus; and tumors of the abdomen, bladder, eyes, fauces, liver, spleen, and uvula. The plant, boiled in oil, is said to aid indurations and tumors of the liver. The tincture of the plant is said to help cancerous ulcers. Smoking the plant is said to cure cancer of the tongue. The capsule decoction is said to cure uterine cancer. An injection of the seed decoction is also said to help uterine cancer. Egyptians claim to become more cheerful, talkative, and industrious following the eating of opium. When falling asleep, they have visions of "orchards and pleasure gardens embellished with many trees, herbs and various flowers." Lebanese used their opium wisely, to quiet excitable people, to relieve toothaches, headaches, incurable pain and for boils, coughs, dysentery, and itches. Algerians tamp opium into tooth cavities.

In Ayurvedic medicine, the seeds are considered aphrodisiac, constipating, and tonic, the fruit antitussive, binding, cooling, deliriant, excitant, and intoxicant, yet anaphrodisiac if freely indulged, the plant aphrodisiac, astringent, fattening, stimulant, tonic, and good for the complexion. In Unani medicine, the fruit is suggested as well for anemia, chest pains, dysentery, fever, but is correctly deemed hypnotic, narcotic and perhaps harmful to the brain.

The seed contains the following minerals:

Boron	Iodine	Potassium
Calcium	Iron	Sodium
Chromium	Magnesium	Zin
Cobalt	Manganese	
Copper	Nitrogen	

The seed contains the following amino acids:

Alanine	Histidine	Methionine	Threonine
Arginine	Isoleucine	Phenylalanine	Tryptophan
Glutamate	Leucine	Proline	Tyrosine
Glycine	Lysine	Serine	Valine

POPLAR – (POPULUS ALBA)
...and Jacob took him rods of green poplar...Genesis 30

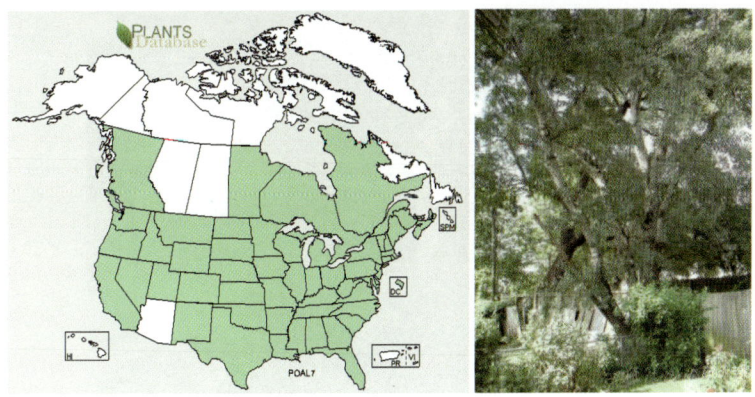

Water sprouts of populus alba are the most likely interpretation of Jacob's poplar rods. The young buds are covered with a resinous varnish with a balsamic aroma in the spring. Bruised buds produce a fragrant resin that may have been the incense burned by Ephraim in the groves of poplars. Because it casts a dense shade, white poplar has been extensively cultivated in the Holy Land. Bitten by a poisonous snake, Hercules found a mythical antidote in poplar leaves. The tonic bark is used for strangury and blood and skin diseases.

RED SAUNDERS – (*PTEROCARPUS SANTALINUS*)
...brought in from Ophir great plenty of almug trees...I Kings 10

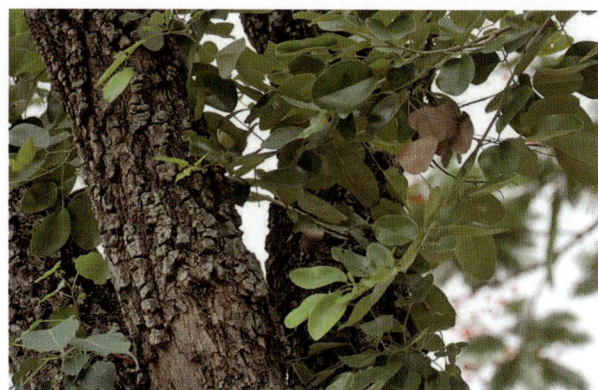

Most Biblical scholars believe the almug of Kings was the red sandalwood pterocarpus santalinus. Its wood is hard and heavy, red to garnet in color, takes a good polish, and would be well suited for Solomon's purposes. It is still used for lyres and other medical instruments. The wood is extremely hard and resistant to termites. Recently it has been more important as a dye wood, used for imprinting a red or pink color to calico, cotton or silk. Red sandalwood is well known in Europe as an ingredient of "French polish."

The astringent wood, usually powdered, is used as a cooling agent for boils, fevers, headache, inflammation, scorpion stings and swellings. It is said to be depurative, diuretic, and emetic. Following the doctrine of signatures, the red wood is considered a blood remedy, used for hemorrhages, suppurations, wounds and ulcers. In Indonesia, the natives consider it a secret remedy for poisoning. Chips of the wood are sold for use against dysentery in Tehran. Ayurvedics, regarding the wood as alexiteric, anthelmintic, aphrodisiac, and refrigerant, use it for biliousness, blood disorders, eye ailments, fever, mental aberrations and ulcers. Unani used the seeds for dysentery and urethral hemorrhage; they apply the wood externally for fever, headache, hemicrania, inflammation, neckache and toothache. Others in India use the wood, lathered up in water, to wash blepharitis and superficial excoriations of the genital organs.

ROMAN NETTLE – (URTICA PILULIFERA)
...the pleasant places for their silver, nettles shall possess them...Hosea 9

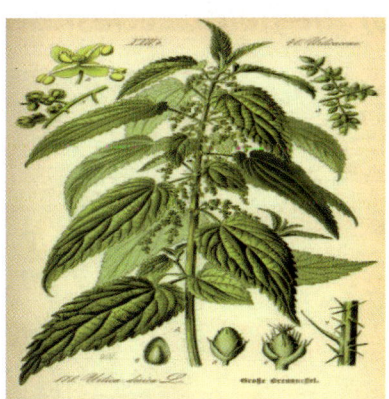

Young shoots of nettle were and are still eaten, but the sting of the Roman nettle is said to be more irritating than those of our American species. The Roman nettle was said to have been introduced into the United Kingdom by Caesar's troops, who, with thin clothing, unable to tolerate the cutting Brittish cold, flagellated their numb legs with nettle to make them burn.

According to the Wealth of India, Roman nettle was used as a substitute for Urtica dioica, which is reported to be a folk anodyne, astringent, bactericide, counterirritant, depurative, diuretic, emmenagogue, hemostat, stimulant, stomachic, tonic, and vermifuge, used for alopecia, asthma, ataxia, backache, bronchitis, bruise, burns, cacoethes, cancer, carcinomata, catarrh, cholecystitis, cholengytis, constipation, cough, dandruff, dropsy, dyspnea, epilepsy, epistaxis, gout, hematemesis, hemoptysis, hemorrhage, hepatitis, hyperglycermia, insanity, menorrhagia, palsy, paralysis, parturition, polyps, rheumatism, sciatica, shigellosis, snakebite, sores, sprains, tan trums, and tumors. Urtica pilulifera is a folk treatment for tumors of the ear, feet, lung, mouth, parotid, ribs, spleen, and stomach. Country folk stewed the nettle to cure almost any ailment. Wild nettles of this species may also have been included in the Passover herbs. In ancient times, the infusion was used to relieve the pains of arthritis and lumbago. North Africans take the juice of Urtica pilulifera with oil for sore joints, using the stinging hairs for hemorrhage and rheumatism. They regard the tops as depurative and diuretic, the seeds as anticholecystitic, anthlithic, aphrodisiac and diuretic.

ROSE – (NERIUM OLEANDER)
...Hearken unto me, ye holy child, and bud forth as a rose growing by the brook of the field...Ecclesiasticus 39

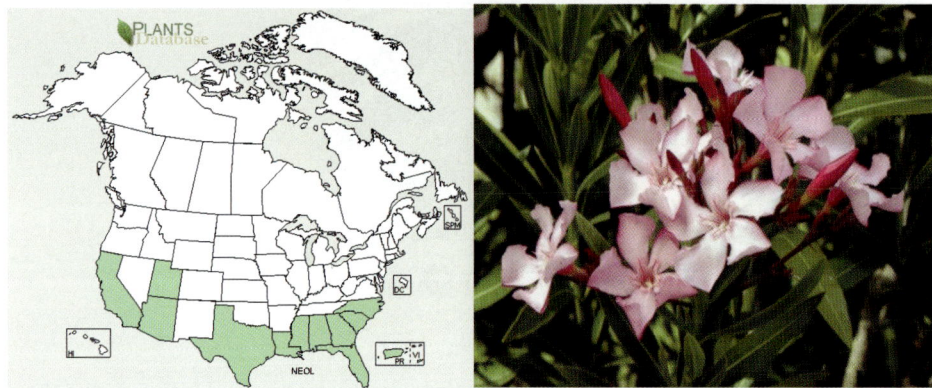

According to careful students of the Scriptures, the oleander is the "rose of the waterbrooks," the "rhododendron," or "rose tree" of the Greeks. To the Spanish it is known as "laurel" and is their favorite shrub for parks and gardens. As an evergreen summer favorite, it is termed "tough and attractive" and does well in almost any soil. In Greece, India, and Italy, it is a funeral plant. It is used to decorate Hindu temples. Palestinians secure from it a very active cardiac glucoside used in pharmacy. It is used as a rat poison in Europe. Honey from the flowers may even be poisonous.

It is widely planted as an ornamental in tropical and subtropical countries. It has been suggested that it is the "*willow of the brook*" of Leviticus used for constructing booths for the Feast of Tabernacles. It is also regarded as the Jericho rose, since on the eastern side of Jordan, the oleander becomes a tree 25 feet tall.

A very POISONOUS plant, regarded as cardiac, cardiotonic, cyanogenetic, diuretic, emetic, emmenagogue, insecticidal, insect repellant, parasiticide, purgative, sternutatory, stimulant and tonic, oleander finds its way into folk remedies for apostemes, asthma, atheroma, carcinomata, corns, dysmenorrhea, eczema, epilepsy, epitheliomas, eruptions, herpes, malaria, psoriasis, ringworm, scabies, skin, sore, tumors, and warts. With such a fabulous folk repertoire of anticancer activity, oleander will probably be found to contain more proven anticancer agents that just the rutin and ursolic acid reported from Nerium indicum. Leaves, flowers and stembark possess cardiotonic properties, especially oleandrin which is diuretic and stimulates the heart. In Ethiopia, the leaves are used for dressing skin diseases on head. The flavonal glycosides influence vascular permeability and possess diuretic properties.

The leaves are dangerously applied to cutaneous eruptions; the decoction is used to destroy maggots in wounds. In Lebanon, as perhaps elsewhere, informants contradict, consider it calming yet irritating, a cause yet a cure for sore eyes, a medicine yet a poison. Such contradictions fan the flames of homeopaths. Lebanese are said to use it to lower the blood pressure and pulse and stimulate the heart. Used externally, the leaf decoction reduces edema, whereas fresh macerated leaves are said to relieve itch. Root extracts are used for impetigo, leprosy, ringworm, and venereal diseases.

Russian Olive – (Elaeagnus Angustifolia)
...Go forth unto the mount, and fetch olive branches, and pine...Nehemiah 8

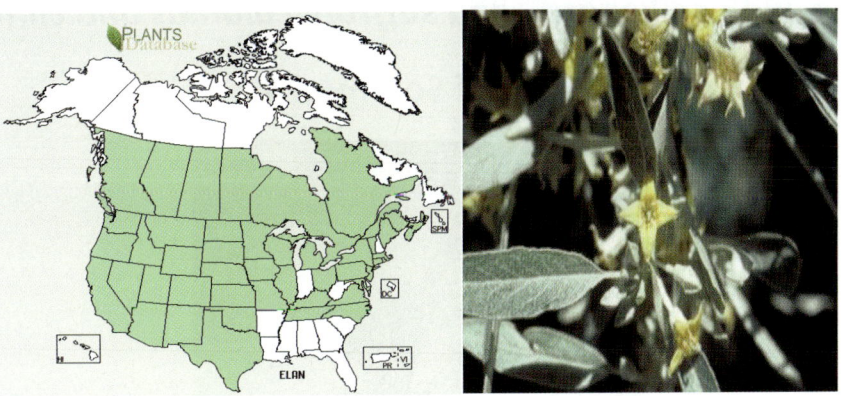

Planted in the wilderness, some of the Biblical oil or olive trees are concluded to be the Russian olive, a common shrub in Palestine. The fruit is small and insipid, or large and quite edible. I have eaten many of the astringent fruits as a boy in, Carolina, not realizing I might be sharing a culinary experience with the Children of Israel. The fruits, known as trebizond dates, are dried and powdered into an Arabian breadstuff. An intoxicant is distilled from the fruits. The hard, fine-grained wood is used for carving figurines. The leaves are used for fodder.

The oleaster yields inferior oil, used as a medicine, but not as a food. Spaniards use the flower juice for malignant fevers. The seed oil is used for bronchitis and catarrh. The oil is also used for burns, constipation and as an antiseptic in Lebanon. The leaves are astringent. Seeds have been used in homeopathy. Lebanese use all parts of the plant medicinally, including hot flowers compressed onto neuralgia and aching wounds. Persons near death are sometimes turned around by the flower infusion.

Hillman Health Food Store call 855-Amish-Dr (855-264-7437) www.emineral.info Vitamins and Minerals for Better Living

SAFFRON – (CROCUS SATIVUS)
...Thy plants are an orchard of pomegranates, with the pleasant fruits; camphire, with spikenard...and saffron; calamus and cinnamon...

Song of Solomon 4

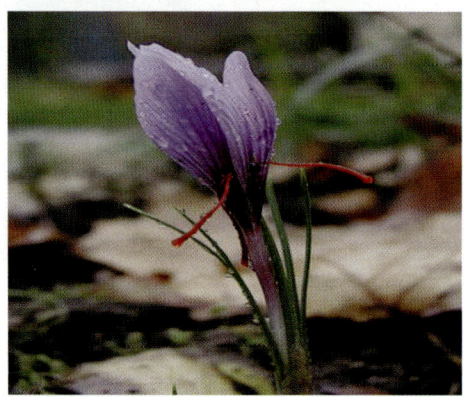

In Biblical times saffron was important to people of the East as a condiment and sweet perfume, the stigmas being particularly valued for their food coloring property. In India, they are used to add yellow shades to curry. Pliny records that the benches of the public theaters were strewn with saffron, and the costly petals were placed in small fountains to diffuse the scent into public halls. In Europe it is used as a flavoring and as a coloring ingredient, and druggists add it to medicines. Saffron is cultivated for the coloring dye obtained from the stigmas of the flowers; about 100,000 flowers yield 1 kg saffron. Dye used chiefly as a coloring agent and spice in cookery (especially Spanish), soups, stews, especially chicken dishes, and in confectionery to give color, flavor, and aroma. It is used in cosmetics for eyebrows and nail polishes, and as incense. Dioscorides mentions its use as a perfume; Harrison, its use as a mild deodorant. Dissolved in water it is used as an ink and is applied to foreheads on religious and ceremonial occasions.

Saffron is an extremely often cited folk remedy for various types of cancer, e.g. tumors of the abdomen, bladder, ear, eye, kidney, liver, neck, spleen, stomach, and tonsils, as well as cancers of the breast, mouth, stomach, and uterus, veneral condylomata, warts, etc. Saffron is used to promote eruption of measles, and in small doses is considered antihysteric, antispasmodic, aphrodisiac, carminative, diaphoretic, ecbolic, emmenagogue, expectorant, sedative, stimulant, and stomachic, but overdoses are narcotic, and saffron corns are toxic to young animals. Apoplexy and extravagant gaiety are possible after-effects. Saffron is not included in American and British pharmacopoeias, but some Indian medical formulae still include it. It is sometimes used to promote menstruation. In India, saffron is regarded for bladder, kidney, and liver ailments, also for cholera. Mixed with ghee, it is used for diabetes. Saffron oil is applied externally to uterine sores. Lebanese add a dozen pistils to a large cup of hot water for children coming down with chickenpox, measles, or mumps. The tea is considered antiseptic, antispasmodic, and tonic. Algerians and Gypsies use the saffron infusion as a collyrium.

The silk stigma style contains the following minerals:

| Copper | Manganese | Nitrogen |

SAIGON CINNAMON – (CINNAMONUM CASSIA)
...the Lord spake unto Moses, saying, Take thou also unto thee principal spices,... of cassia five hundred shekels...Exodus 30

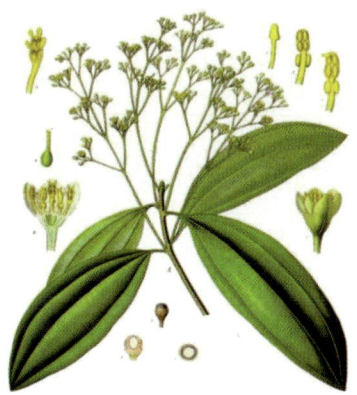

Moses and Solomon probably obtained cassia, through trade, from Sri Lanka. From the fruits distilled oil of cassia and oil of cinnamon is made. Dried green fruits are the cassia buds of commerce, which resemble cloves. Cassia bark is also an important spice. All parts of the plant possess an essence, cinnamic aldehyde, which may be distilled for export. Buds of the tree are used in place of cloves to season dishes.

Regarded as alexiteric, analgesic, antiseptic, aperient, astringent, bactericidal, balsamic, carminative, diaphoretic, febrifuge, fungicidal, lactafuge, sedative, stimulant, stomachic, tonic, and vermicidal, cassia is a folk "remedy" for colds, colic, condylomata, diarrhea, dysmenorrhea, dyspepsia, dysuria, fever, headache, hypertension, lumbago, menorrhagia, nausea, phymata, postpartum, snakebite, stomachache, vaginitis, and warts. The bark is prepared as a tea for excessive salivation, frequent in Iran. The leaves are taken internally for rheumatism. Consider the bark carminative, emmenagogue, and tonic, using it for headache, inflammation, piles and pregnancy. It is a folk treatment for cancers, indurations and tumors (of liver, spleen, stomach, bladder, uterus, womb, etc.). Cassia does contain the antitumor (and probably oncogenic) agents benzaldehyde, coumarins, and tannins. The bark is astringent and carminative, and the essential oil is antiseptic. The major component, cinnamaldehyde, is sedative, hypothermic, and antipyretic. The eugenol found in the oil from the bark (12.5%) has antiseptic, irritant, and local anesthetic properties, as well as weak tumor promoting activity on mouse skin. It enhances trypsin acticity in vitro.

SANDARAC – (TETRACLINIS ARTICULATA)
...and all thyine wood, and all manner vessels of ivory...Revelation 18

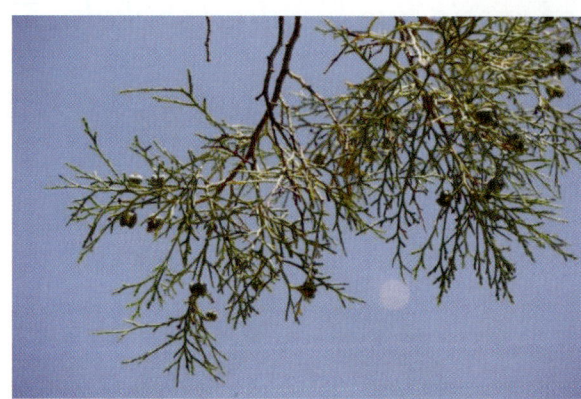

The thyine was the last vegetable mentioned by name in the Bible. Thyine wood was extensively employed by the ancients for cabinet work. It is said to be worth its weight in gold. The sandarac resin is still highly valued for varnish and incense. The tears of sandarac have been burned on Greek altars for ages. Thyine probably has many of the same uses as turpentine. The leaf decoction is abortifacient. Crushed leaves are applied to relieve migranes, neckache, and insolation.

Sea Purslane – (Atriplex Halimus)
...Who cut up mallows by the bushes, and juniper roots for their meat...Job 30

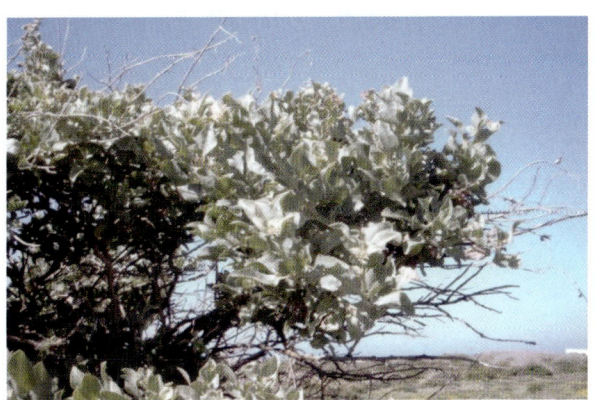

The purslane leaves and young shoots, like those of many chenopodiaceae, have served as a potherb. These "mallows" are commonly eaten by the poor between Aleppo and Jerusalem. In Flora Palaestine we read that it is rather a palatable browse shrub; the leaves are sometimes eaten by hungry shepherds; the salt content of the leaves increases with the aridtty of the habitat, which makes the plant less palatable, but more useful as a salt substitute. The ash is used in soap manufacture. The Israel Soil Conservation Service has been planting it near settlements in southern Israel to provide protein and mineral rich browse in drought years. King adds that it is a saline plant, something like spinach, eaten by Palestinian poor, "although it is a miserable diet." According to the Talmud, Jews working on the reconstruction of the Temple in 520-516 BC ate these mallows. A strong growing bush or shrub five feet or more tall, with gray foliage and inconspicuous flowers, mallows are cultivated in California for hedges and seaside plantings.

The closely related Atriplex rosea, which occurs in the Biblical area as well, has been a folk remedy for such cancerous conditions as corns, hard lumps and indurations. Bedouins apply powdered leaves of Atripltex halimus to sores and ulcers. Smoke from burning seed is used to treat skin ailments and sores. Lebanese doctors are said to extract anodynes, emetics, hynotics and purgatives from the plants. The seeds are in small doses emetic, in large doses poisonous. Ashes of the plant are taken for gastric acidity, the roots for dropsy.

Sea-Wrack – (Zostera Marina)
...the depth closed me round about, the weeds were wrapped about my head...Jonah 2

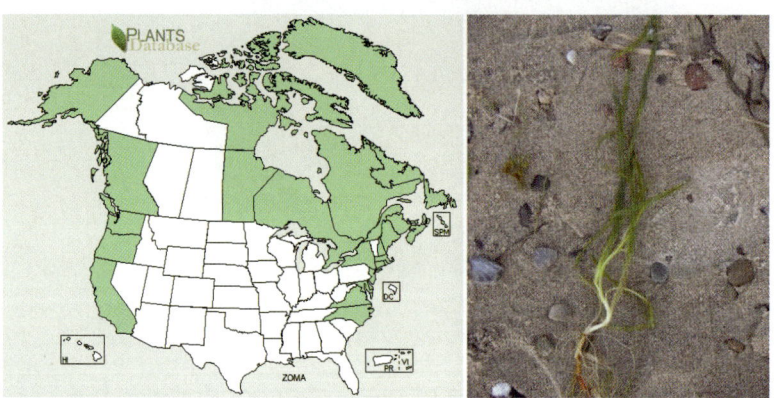

The grain derived from zostera marina is relatively bland and can be variously flavored. The grain is toasted, rewinnowed, and ground into flour. Cooked in water into a thick or thin gruel, the flour has a bland flavor. Traditionally it was combined with other food, usually sea turtle oil or honey in Baja California. The leaves may prove valuable as fodder, thatching, or packing material. The foliage is an important food for some sea turtles and water fowl. An important shallow water mud flat stabilizer, the plant helps to sustain the productivity of estuarine areas. Finally, the plant is used by the Seri Indians of Mexico for diarrhea.

SHEEP SORREL – (*RUMEX ACETOSELLA*)
...eat it with unleavened bread and bitter herbs...Numbers 9

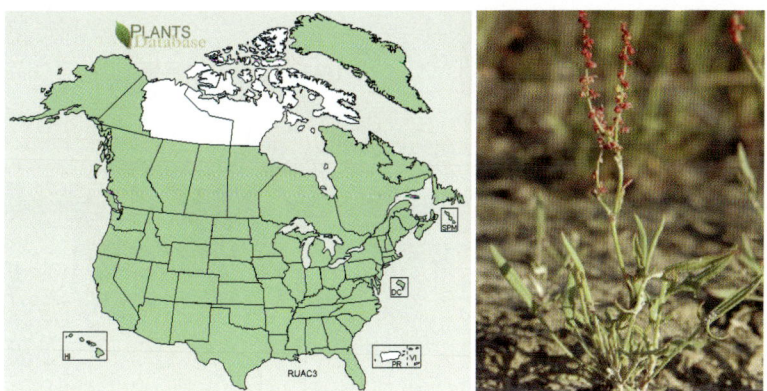

Young sorrel shoots are used for salads, but may produce oxalic acid poisoning. Fruits are used as poultry feed. They are, however, reported to be poisonous to horses and sheep. Regarded as depurative, diaphoretic, diuretic, POISON, purgative, refrigerant, styptic, and sudorific, sheep sorrel is used for cancer, dyspepsia, epithelioma, fever, jaundice, nephritis, scurvy, skin, tumor, warts, and wens.

Essiac tea, marketed as Flor Essence, is a blend of herbs promoted as an alternative treatment for cancer and other illnesses. As with many alternative remedies, the exact composition of essiac is unclear, but it reportedly contains burdock, Indian rhubarb, sheep sorrel, and slippery elm bark.

SHITTIM WOOD – (*ACACIA TORTILIS*)
...And I made an ark of shittim wood...Deuteronomy 10

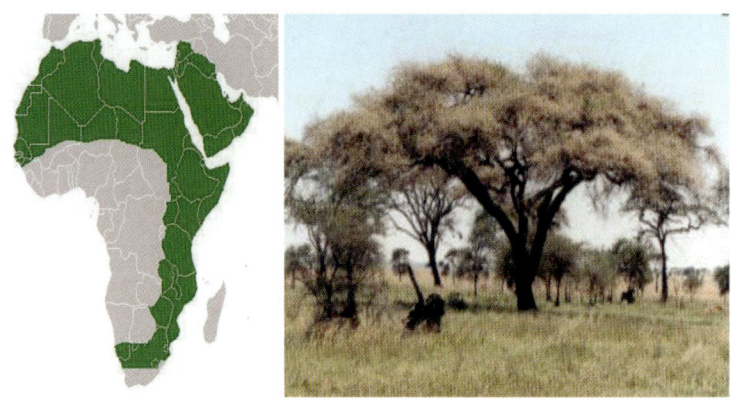

Most authorities agree that this species, or A. Seal, furnished the wood of the ark of the Tabernacle, since these are the only timber trees of any considerable size on the Arabian Desert. The wood is used for fence posts and for manufacturing small implements and articles. Pods, produced prolifically, fall to the ground and are devoured by wild herbivores and goats, sheep, and other domestic livestock. They provide sustenance for wildlife in East Africa's national parks and have 19% protein content. The foliage is also palatable. It is, for example, the major dry season (9 months) fodder for sheep and goats in the whole Sahara Sahelian belt in the Sudan. The thorny branches are used to pen cattle, goats, and sheep. Finally, roots and stems are made into spears, the flexible roots for frameworks.

Sodom Apple – (*Solanum Incanum*)
...and it shall burn and devour his thorns and his briers in one day...
Isaiah 10

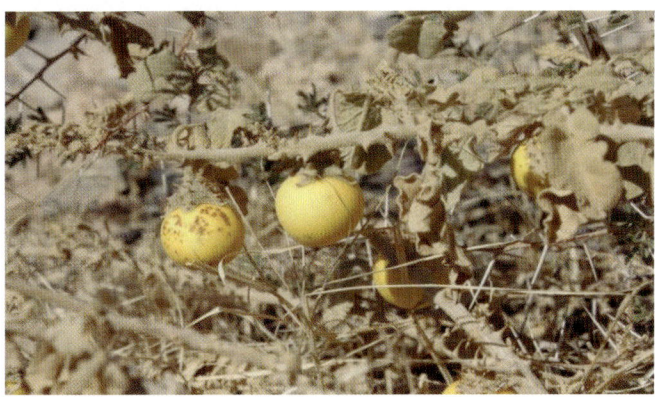

The fruits of the sodom apple are used as a rennet and immature fruits are used as a cooked vegetable in Africa. It is also a component of some arrow poisons and love philtres. Ethiopians use the fruits as a condiment in certain beverages. The leaves not used as a pot herb. A glyco alkaloid content up to 4.81% is found in some races, particularly the one cultivated by the Paniya tribe of Iritty, North Kerala. Bushmen use the fruit juice in arrow poison. The root and seed contain a rennet like enzyme.

Considered anodyne, antiseptic, CARCINOGENIC, piscicide, and POISON, the sodom apple is used in folk medicines for chest ailments, colic, cough, craw craw, gonorrhea, sore throat, syphilis, toothache, and tumors. A poultice or infusion of the fruit is said to be a folk remedy for external benign tumors. It is used as an oral contraceptive by women of the Paniya tribe, yet used by barren Nigerians as a fertility symbol. Plants are also used as a remedy for toothaches and for sore throats. A decoction is taken for chest troubles (pleurisy, pneumonia). The root is used as medicine for horses. It has a pretty good track record with cancer, with reported or reputed "cures" for carcinoma, epithelioma, and melanomata. Ethiopians use the leaf for bloat and epistaxis, the fruit for calculus, constipation, gonorrhea, itch, renitis, and wounds, the root for gonorrhea, and the ash for scabies. In Lesotho, the fruit is also used for sore throat and toothache. Zulu use the juice of the plant for ringworm. Europeans in South Africa use the fruit juice for dandruff. Tanganyikans use the root for abdominal pain, carbuncles, and hepatosis, the fruit for snakebite, the gall for earache.

Soft Rush – (*Juncus Effusus*)
...the reeds and the flags shall wither...Isaiah 19

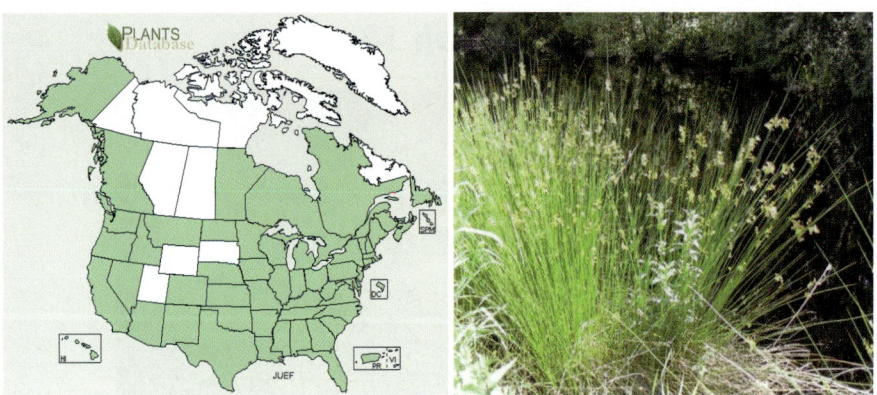

This may be the first among five candidates for the flags and rushes of Isaiah and Job, doubting that any of them are the nutritious river grass of Egypt. In China the pith is used for lamp wicks and mat making. Indians in California use the rush for domestic utensils and fodder. In China the pith, also depurative and diuretic, is used to keep fistulous sores open. The pith decoction is considered antilithic, discutient, and pectoral, the root diuretic. The pith is prescribed for insomnia, anuria, cough, dropsy, micturition, and sore throat. In South Africa, the herb is suspected of causing "vlei poisoning."

The pith contains the following minerals:

Calcium	Magnesium	Sodium
Copper	Manganese	Zinc
Iron	Potassium	

SORGHUM – (SORGHUM BICOLOR)
...they filled a spunge with vinegar, and put it upon hyssop, and put it to his mouth...John 19

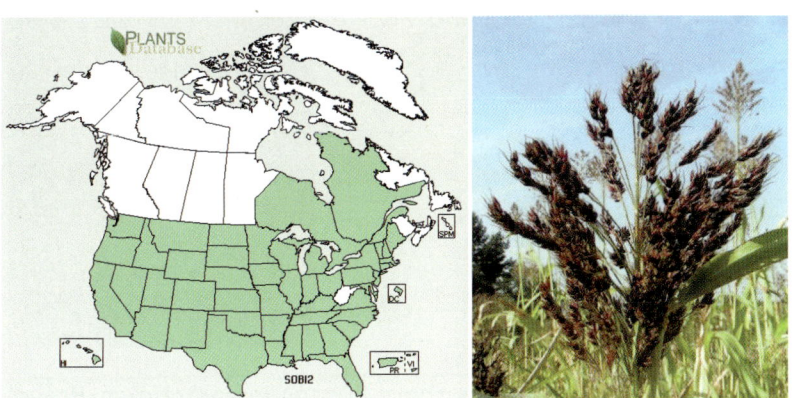

The last few moments of Christ's agony on the cross were relieved by moistening his lips with a sponge filled with sour wine. In Palestine hyssop is known as "Jerusalem corn," a main and nutritious part of the people's diet. The grains are gathered and ground for meal used in baking coarse bread. A single seed head is of such enormous size that one can supply a meal for a large family. Some students suggest that the "parched corn" Ruth received from Boaz was this grain. It is grown for grain, forage, syrup, and sugar. There are industrial uses for the stems and fibers and the stalks used as animal feed. Pearled grain is cooked like rice or ground into flour. Broomcorn is used for making brooms. Sorghums with large juicy stems are used in the making of syrup, sugar, or energy alcohol. Africans use sorghum stems for fencing and hut building, especially for the radiating bands of the conical roofs. They burn them for fuel, using the ashes for manure.

Regarded as antiabortive, cyanogenetic, demulcent, diuretic, emollient, sorghum is a folk remedy for burns, cancer, epilepsy, flu, flux, measles, renitis, stomachache, and urinary ailments. In Lebanon, the gruel is used for the debility due to long maladies like tuberculosis. Finally, hot sorghum was used by the Lebanese as a poultice.

Spelt – (*Triticum Spelta*)
...But the wheat and the rie were not smitten...Exodus 9

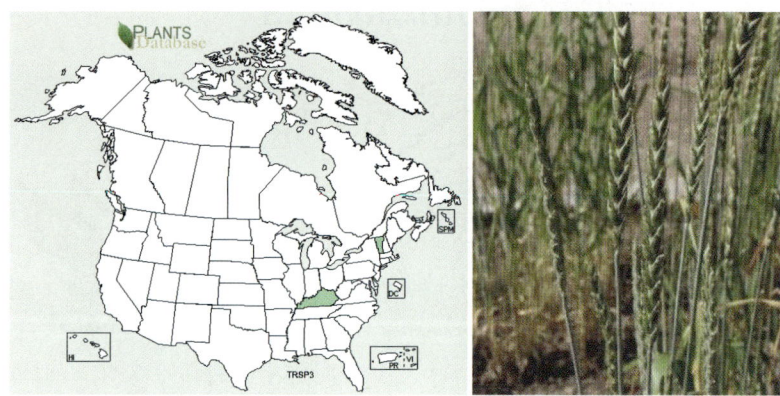

Spelt was the most common form of wheat in southern Europe in early times. Bread made from spelt is far inferior to the cakes of flour baked from wheat, but it will yield a crop from soil not rich enough to grow wheat. Grain was threshed by the staff or the flail or by an instrument with teeth that was drawn over the sheaves by oxen. Ancients preferred it to barley. Spelt once was a European "remedy" for the ailment known as egilops.

SPIKENARD – (NARDOSTACHYS JATAMANSI)
...Thy plants are an orchard of pomegranates, with pleasant fruits; camphire, with spikenard...Song of Solomon 4

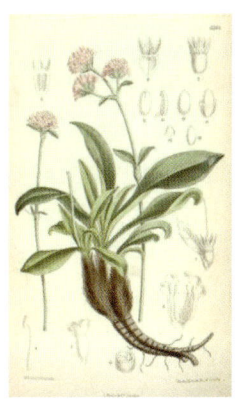

Spikenard is valued for its rhizomes used in India as a drug and also in perfumery. The drug Jatamansi or Nardus Root consists of short, thick, dark grey rhizomes crowned with reddish brown tufted fibrous remains of the petioles of radical leaves. The rhizome is used as an aromatic adjunct in the preparation of medicinal oils; it is reported to promote the growth of hair and also impart blackness.

Spikenard is suggested to be carminative, cordial, deobstruent, deodorant, emmenagogue, hypotensive, laxative, nervine, sedative, stimulant, stomachic, and tonic. Spikenard has been suggested as a help in arrythmia, bronchitis, cholera, chorea, colic, consumption, convulsions, cough, delirium, depression, dysentery, epilepsy, faintness, headache, hypertension, hysteria, madness, malaria, palpitations, parturition, sclerosis, skin, smallpox, sores, spasms, tachycardia, and tumors (especially of the abdomen). Spikenard has a folk reputation to help such cancerous ailments as cancer (especially of the bladder, kidney, liver, spleen, stomach and uterus), and tumors (especially of the abdomen, eye, larynx, liver, rectum, spleen, stomach, uterus, and vagina). The rhizome is considered tonic, stimulant, antispasmodic, diuretic, deobstruent, emmenagogue, hypotensive, stomachic, and laxative. An infusion of the rhizome is reported to be useful in epilepsy, hysteria, palpitation of heart and chorea. Finally, its tincture is given in intestinal colic and flatulence.

Spikenard oil possesses antiarrhythmic activity of possible therapeutic use in auricular flutter; it is less effective than quinidine, but less toxic. Jatamansone is more potent than the oil and is also more active than quinidine in ventricular tachycardia resulting from acute myocardial infarction; in experimentally induced arrhythmias it is as effective as quinidine except in the acetylcholine induced auricular fibrillation, in which it is considerably weaker. Jatamansone possesses sedative and anticonvulsant action as well. The oil exerts a hypotensive effect. In moderate doses it has a distinct depressant action on the central nervous system; and relaxes the skeletal and smooth muscles. Lethal doses cause deep narcosis and ultimately death within a few hours. The root extracts show sedative properties.

In Iran the root tea is used for cardiac and nervous disorders. Ayurvedics use the roots for bad complexion, biliousness, blood disorders, burning sensation, erysipelas, fever, leprosy, skin ailments, throat disorders and ulcers. Unani, considering the root aperitive, carminative, diuretic, emmenagogue, laxative, pectoral, stimulant, stomachic, and tonic, take it for chest pain, cough, gleet, kidney and lumbar problems, intestinal inflammation and wounds.

The rhizome contains the following mineral:

Calcium	Magnesium	Sodium
Copper	Manganese	Zinc
Iron	Potassium	

STACTE – (STYRAX OFFICINALIS)

...Take unto thee sweet spices, stacte, and onycha, and galbanum; these sweet spices with pure frankincense: of each shall there be a like weight: and thou shalt make it a perfume...Exodus 30

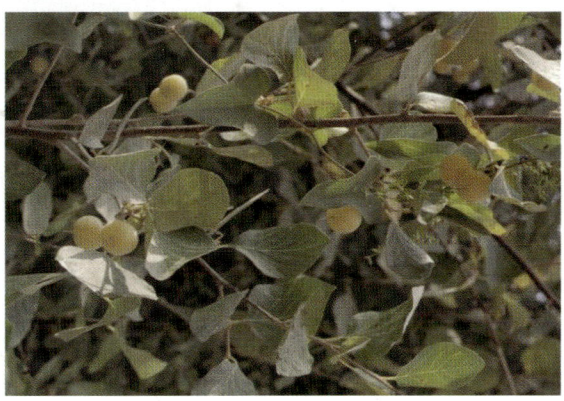

Stacte, a gum that exudes from trees, was a component of the perfume to be offered in the Holy Place. Incisions are made in the branches so that a resin will flow; this is gathered in reeds. After hardening, the stacte is scraped off in irregular compact masses, interspersed with small drops known as "tears." These contain resin and benzoic acid and will dissolve in wine. In early days in England, storax was used to perfume pomades. More recently the Roman Catholic Church uses it in incense.

Medicinal attributes against cancer and tumors to the storax, the plant probably shares many medicinal at tributes, real and imagined, with styrax benzoin, regarded as antiseptic, carminative, deodorant, disinfectant, diuretic, expectorant, insecticidal, stimulant and vulnerary, and used for arthritis, bronchitis, cancer, catarrh, colds, colic, cough, hysteria, sores, spermatorrhea, and wounds. Indurations of the liver, spleen, stomach, and uterus and tumors of the bladder and parotids can be treated. Combined with alcohol, it is used as an antiseptic and disinfectant. Diluted, it was used for venereal diseases.

STAR OF BETHLEHEM – (*ORNITHOGALUM UMBELLATUM*)
...and the fourth part of a cab of dove's dung for five pieces of silver...
II Kings 6

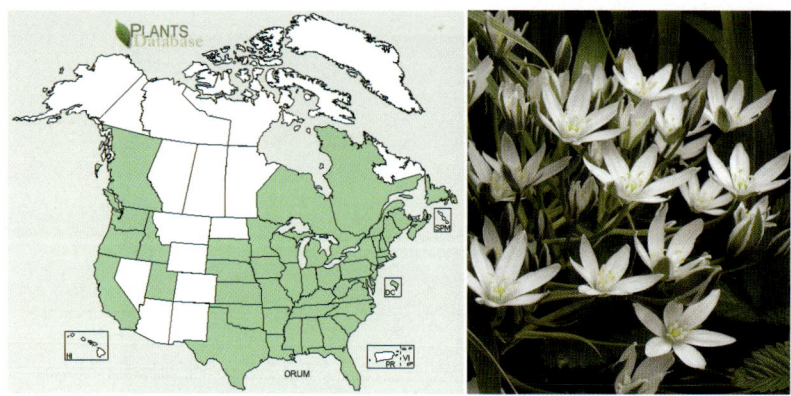

Bulbs were used for food in Syria. In Dioscorides' day, the bulbs were commonly gathered, ground into meal, and mixed with flour to make bread. Modern Italians in time of scarcity eat the bulb. Grazing animals avoid it, or, if they do eat of it, are poisoned...the bulbs are edible only after being thoroughly roasted or boiled. Egyptians and Syrians stored the bulbs for their pilgramages to Mecca. Edible Wild Plants of Eastern North America treats them as edible. Poisonous plants text reports that the bulbs have caused death in cattle in the U.S., although early reports of the gout medicine colchicine have been extricated from the credible literature. Lebanese used the bulb for lymphatic ailments and recommended them in diets for debility. Bulbs of other eastern species were used for cachexia, infections, parotitis, scabs, ulcers and wasting disease.

STAR THISTLE – (CENTAUREA CALCITRAPA)
...Thorns also and thistles shall it bring forth to thee...Genesis 3

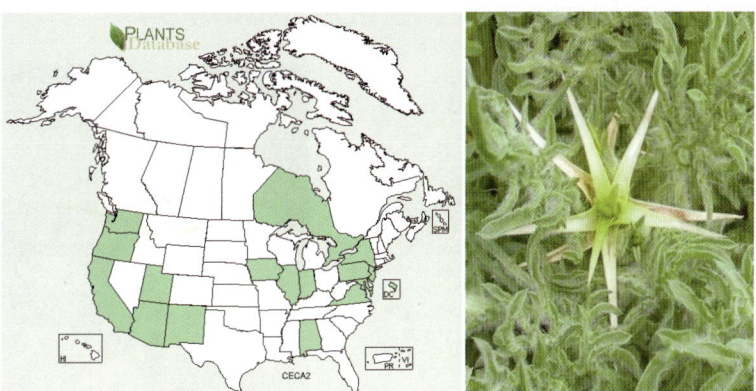

The worst of weeds and sometimes head high, thistles are said to make nutritious vegetables, potherbs, and depuratives. Many of these thistles, which grow from 10 to 15 feet high and briers, are decided ostructionists to travellers who leave the beaten track, and are consequently described as noxious thorny plants. Bedouins grind the seeds for food; they contain some oil.

Considered cholagogue, depurative, diuretic, emmenagogue, sudorific and tonic, this thistle has been suggested as a folk remedy for cancer, corns, fevers, fistula, gravel, jaundice, and stones. The powdered seeds are administered with wine for stones. Lebanese eat boiled stems for jaundice. In North Africa the seeds are considered anodyne, antilithic, febrifuge, and vulnerary. The whole plant is used for malaria and ophthalmia, the leaves for headache.

STINGING NETTLE – (URTICA DIOICA)
...And thorns shall come up in her palaces, nettles and brambles in the fortresses thereof...Isaiah 34

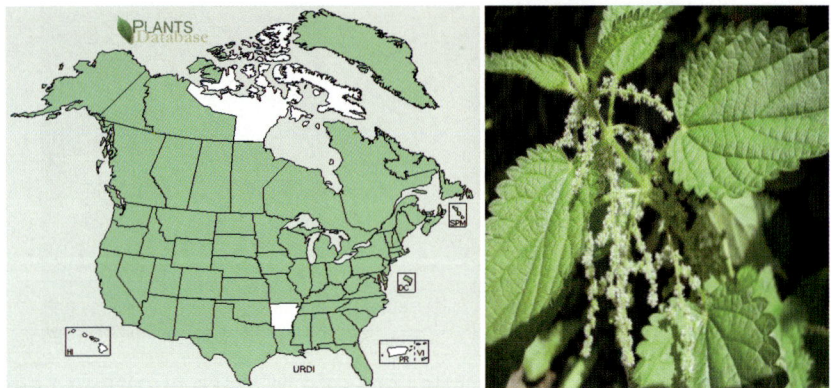

Young tops of the nettle, gathered when about 15 cm. high, can be used as a spring green vegetable, usually in the form of a puree, but their rather earthy flavor is not liked by some. In Scotland, nettles are combined with leeks or onions, broccoli or cabbage, and rice, boiled in a muslin bag and served with butter or gravy. Nettle beer and nettle tea are made by some people. Dried nettles can be fed to livestock and poultry, but few animals will eat the living plants. In Sweden and Russia, nettles are sometimes cultivated as a fodder plant. Alcoholic extracts of nettle, chamomile, thyme, and burdock have been used in hair and scalp preparations. In Russia, the nettle has been used for a green pigment in confectionary. Nettle fiber can be used for making textiles and paper, as has been done during war-time or when other fibers are not available. The fiber is similar to hemp or flax and can be used for fine or coarse materials.

Nettle is cited as a folk remedy for cacoethes, cancerous ulcers, carcinomata, endothelioma, epithelioma, polyps, sarcoma, and cancers, indurations and/or tumors of the breast, ear, face, feet, joints, liver, lungs, mouth, nostrils, parotids, ribs, spleen, stomach, and swellings of the womb, etc. In Algeria, nettles are powdered and mixed with powdered jasmine for gonorrhea. In Russia, the leaves are used in the preparation of, "Alochol" used for chronic hepatitis, cholengitis, cholecystitis, and habitual constipation. The roots and seed are prescribed as a vermifuge. Clinical experiments are said to have confirmed the utility of the herb as a hemostatic. It is also used in ague, anemia, asthma, bronchitis, catarrh, constipation, consumption, cough, diabetes, diarrhea, dropsy, dysentery, dysmenorrhea, dyspnea, epilepsy, epistaxis, gastritis, gout, gravel, headache, hemoptysis, jaundice, malaria, menorrhea, nephritis, neuralgia, palsy, paralysis, pertussis, piles, rheumatism, sciatica, and tuberculosis, and as a hair tonic. The roots are diuretic. Juice of the plants is used as an external irritant. Decoction of plant is anthelmintic, antiseptic, astringent, depurative, diuretic, emmenagogue, rubefacient, and vasoconstrictor. Homeopaths prescribe a tincture of the flowering plant for alactia, beestings, burns, colic, dysentery, erysipelas, erythema, gout, gravel, hemorrhage, intermittents, lactation, leucorrhea, and menorrhagia, phlegmasia, preventing calculus, renitis, rheumatism, sore throat, splenitis, uremia, urticaria, vertigo, whooping cough and worms.

The leaf contains the following minerals:

Aluminum	Iron	Selenium
Bromine	Magnesium	Silica
Boron	Manganese	Sodium
Calcium	Molybdenum	Sulfur
Chlorine	Nickel	Tin
Chromium	Nitrogen	Zinc
Cobalt	Potassium	
Copper	Rubidium	

SUGARCANE – (SACCHARUM OFFICINARUM)
...Thou has bought me no sweet cane with money...Isaiah 43

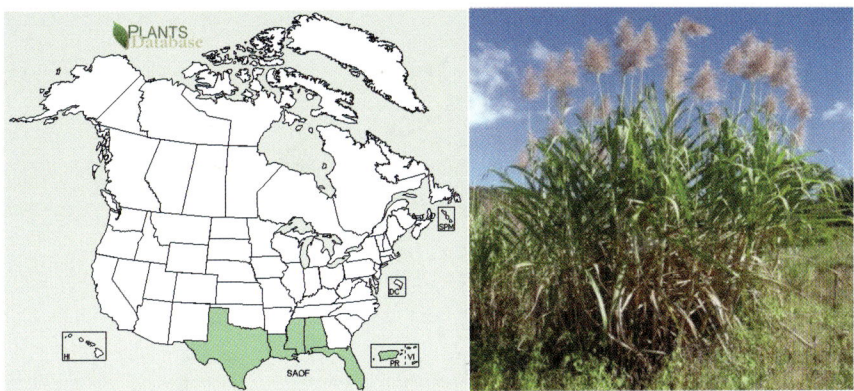

The sweet cane of Isaiah is probably our sugarcane of today. Although the Hebrews then probably knew not how to make sugar, they probably respected the cane for sweetening food and drinks and for chewing as a confection. Sugarcane is cultivated in all tropical and subtropical countries for sugar and sugar syrup. The residue, bagasse, is used in building materials, insulation against temperatures and sound, resins in phonograph records, mulch and litter, plastics, paper making, and in industrial chemicals. More recently, it has assumed importance as an energy source.

Regarded as antidotal, antiseptic, antivinous, aphrodisiac, bactericidal, cardiotonic, demulcent, diuretic, laxative, pectoral, piscicide, refrigerant and stomachic, sugarcane has been used for arthritis, bedsores, boils, cancer, catarrh, cold, cough, diarrhea, dysentery, eyes, fever, frambesia, gingivitis, hiccups, inflammations, laryngitis, opacity, pertussis, skin sore, sorethroat, spleen, tumor, ulcers and wounds. The whole plant is used as ghees, powders, bolmes and enemas for abdominal tumors. Powdered sugar is said to cure granulations and "proud flesh." A cane decoction is said to help tumors. Molasses has been suggested for cancer of the breast, mouth, rectum, stomach, tonsils, and uterus. Stems are a laxative, diuretic, cooling, and aphrodisiac; the decoction is used for abdominal and kidney complaints and smallpox. Root fibers are used for dysentery. Finally, the peel, mixed with the juice, is applied to hemorrhoids.

SWEET BAY – (LAURUS NOBILIS)
...I have seen the wicked in great power, and spreading himself like a green bay tree...Psalm 37

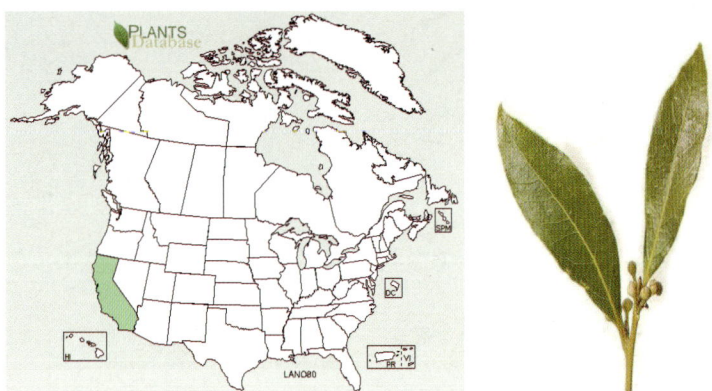

In Biblical times, the bay was symbolic of wealth and wickedness. The evergreen leaves, when broken, emit a sweet scent and furnish an extract used by the Orientals in making perfumed oil. In the ancient Olympic Games the victorious contestant was awarded a chaplet of bay leaves, placed on his brow. The Roman gold coin of 342 B.C. has a laurel wreath modeled on its surface. Dried bay leaves are used to flavor meats, fish, poultry, vegetables, soups, and stews, and are especially popular in French dishes; also as an ingredient in pickling spices and vinegars. The leaves were once used as a tea substitute. An essential oil, distilled from the leaves, is used for flavoring food products, such as baked goods, confectionary, meats, sausages, and canned soups, and in perfumery. Oil replaces dried leaves to great advantage because it can be measured more precisely and provides more uniform results. The fat derived from the fruits has been used for soapmaking and veterinary medicine. Leaves twined into wreaths by ancient Greeks and Romans were used to crown their victors in sports and wars. The wood, resembling walnut, can be used for cabinetry.

Regarded as apertif, carminative, diuretic, emetic, emmenagogue, narcotic, nervine, stimulant, stomachic, sudorific, bay has found its way into folk remedies for amenorrhea, colic, condylomata, hysteria, impostumes, polyps, scleroses, spasms, and wens. Methyl eugenol, which constitutes 4% of bay oil, is narcotic and sedative in mice, producing sedation at low doses and reversible narcosis at higher doses. The essential oil has bactericidal and fungicidal properties. An ointment or unguent derived from the plant is said to remedy sclerosis of the spleen and liver and tumors of the uterus, spleen, parotid, testicles, liver and stomach.

The fruit, prepared in various manners, is said to remedy uterine fibroids, tuberosities of the face, scirrhus and scleroma of the uterus, scirrhus of the liver, indurations of the joints, spleen and liver, internal tumors, wens, and tumors of the eye. The leaves and fruits, said to possess aromatic, stimulant and narcotic properties, were once employed for amenorrhea, flatulent colic, cough and hysteria. In small doses, leaves can promote sweating, in large doses, they promote vomiting.

Bay oil is sometimes used as a liniment or anodyne for earache. In Lebanon the leaves and berries are extracted to a carminative liver and stomach tonic, tightly corked and steeped in brandy in the sun for several days. The residue, after subsequent distillation, is used as a liniment for rheumatism and sprains, the distillate as an emmenagogue. Lebanese mountaineers are said to use raw berries to induce abortion. Berries macerated in flour were poulticed onto dislocations.

The leaf contains the following minerals:

| Boron | Copper | Manganese |

Syrian Christ Thorn – (Ziziphus Spina)
...Do men gather grapes of thorns, or figs of thistles?... Matthew 7

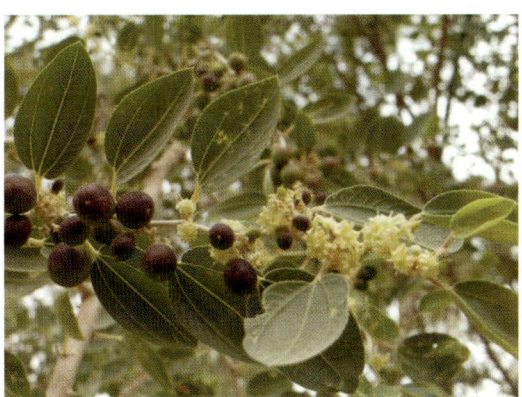

Planted as a hedge, this thorn is highly successful, for it forms an almost impenetrable fence. The Arabs revere the tree as sacred, planting it for shade. Arabs use it to keep goats and cattle off the fields. If, however, it is grown with crops, cattle will eat it as herbage. African wood is reddish, turning dark brown, fairly hard and heavy. Believed to be antproof, the wood is used in the roofs of mud houses. It has been suggested for cabinetry. The stems have been used for spear shafts in Africa and the seeds are used in necklaces. The tree is sometimes planted to stabilize sand dunes. Good liquor is also obtained from the fruit. Some think this is the thorn used to make Christ's cruel corona. The bark can be used as a source for tannin. Fruits, eaten by Arabs, have the taste of dried apples. If not grapes, the Arabs gathered apples of "thorns!"

Said to be anodyne, astringent, demulcent, depurative, emollient, laxative, pectoral, refrigerant, stomachic, and tonic, this thorn is said to be used for toothaches and tumors, even as mouthwash. Lebanese believe that all parts of the plant are medicinal; the powdered seeds are used with lemon juice for liver complaints, the flower infusion is used as an eyewash and febrifuge. Also, the boiled bark is used for venereal disease, the cathartic raw root juice is used for arthritis and rheumatism and the fruits for bronchitis, coughs and tuberculosis. Africans apply the leaves to sores and skin ailments. North Africans use the wood ash, with vinegar, for snakebite. Bedouins poultice the leaves onto swollen eyes when retiring. They also poultice them onto abscesses and furuncles. The fruit infusion, considered emollient and laxative, is used for fever and measles. Perhaps the antitumor activity may be attributed to the presence of beta sitosterol, a proven antitumor agent.

TAMARISK – (TAMARIX APHYLLA)
...And Abraham planted a grove of Beer-sheba...Genesis 21

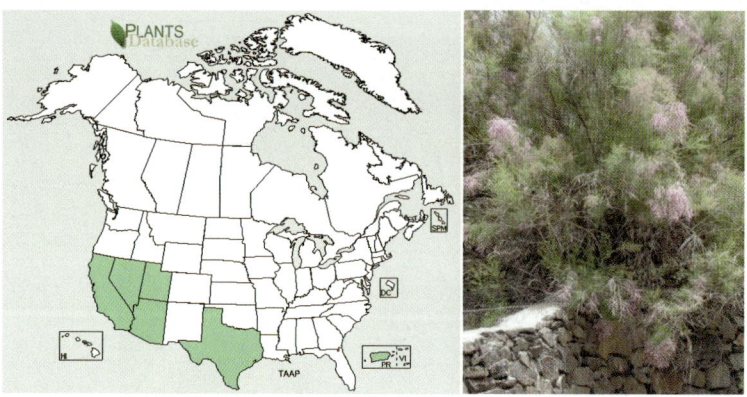

Larger tamarisks are valued for their wood in a region where wood is scarce. The wood is used for construction and, partly burned, for charcoal. The wood is used to make bowls for milking Bedouin camels and in making plows. This species is widely grown as a shade and afforestation tree, especially in desert regions. The bark has been used in tanning and as a mordant in dyeing.

Shoots of some species are used to correct scabies in camels in Ethiopia. Bedouins roast the bark to use in collyrium for scratched eyes. Leaves of Tamarix are mixed with those of Capparis, ground, boiled in water, and used to cover a barren woman, who inhales the vapors of the sweat bath, hoping to cure her infertility. Galls of tamarix aphylla are employed as astringent. The astringent, bitter bark is powdered and mixed with oil, etc., as an aphrodisiac, and for application of eczema capitis and other diseases. North Africans use the wood for psoriasis and syphilis. They use the foliar decoction for splenic edema, and, mixed with ginger for uterosis; the bark they boil in water and vinegar to fabricate a pediculicide.

THORN BUSH – (ACACIA NILOTICA)
...The Lord appeared unto him in a flame of fire out of the midst of a bush...Exodus 3

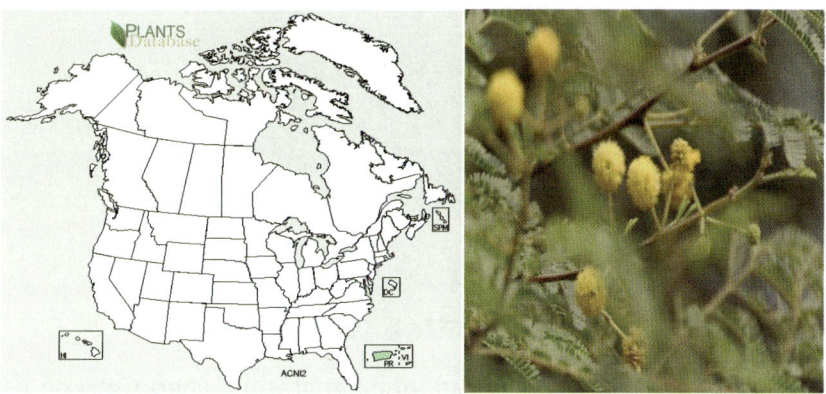

The thorn bush seed was used to tan and dye leather black. The young branches were used as toothbrushes or chew sticks. Chewing the gum or bark would help in healing cancer or tumors of the ear, and eye. It also helped colds, fevers, diarrhea, and bleeding.

Young pods produce a very pale tint in leather, notably goat hides (Kano leather). Pods were used by the ancient Egyptians. Wood was used for boats, farm implements, furniture, housebeams, panellins, and statues. Tender pods and shoots are used as vegetable and as forage for camels, sheep, and goats, especially in Sudan, where it's said to improve milk from these animals. The seeds are a valuable cattle food and oasted seed kernels, sometimes used for flavoring.

Hillman Health Food Store call 855-Amish-Dr (855-264-7437) www.emineral.info Vitamins and Minerals for Better Living

TRAGACANTH – (ASTRAGALUS GUMMIFER)
...I have gathered my myrrh with my spice...Song of Solomon 5

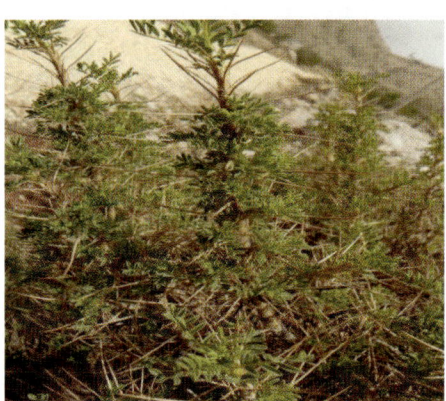

Perhaps man first used tragacanth as a survival food. Ants, goats, and sheep appear to relish the sweeter gums. Tragacanth gum is one of the oldest natural emulsifiers known to man. It is extensively used in vaginal jellies and creams, low calorie syrups, toothpastes and hand lotions. The gum is used in salad dressings, sauces, ice creams, confections, syrups, milk powder stabilizers, citrus oil emulsions, and cheeses. Importance of the wood as fuel might jeopardize many natural stands. In Iran (the source of the best tragacanth) it is largely used in medicine and confectionary.

Mucilaginous, demulcent, diuretic, emollient, and laxative; tragacanth is occasionally used as a remedy for burns, cough or diarrhea. Aphrodisiac qualities are ascribed to the gum. Species of the difficult Astragalus genus with common names suggesting tragacanth have been used for nasal polyps, superflous flesh, chronic indurations of the liver, non ulcerated cancers, and tumors of the eye, fauces, and liver. Leung cites a source noting that tragacanth strongly inhibits cancer cells. Lebanese dry and powder the gum to sprinkle on cuts and wounds.

VETIVER – (*VETIVERIA ZIZANIOIDES*)
...bright iron, cassia, and calamus, were in thy market...Ezekiel 27

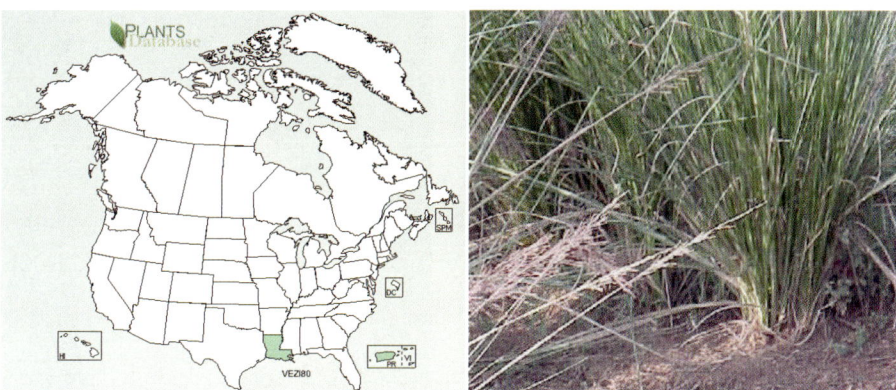

Whether this has been correctly identified the calamus with vetiver, an association not ventured by any of my major sources, the calamus of the Bible was apparently an aromatic plant like vetiver, imported from afar. It with the obscure binomial Andropogon aromaticus Roxb., which some authors have equated with vetiveria, others with andropogon (Cymbopogon) schoenanthus L, one of the "lemon grass" assemblage; they also suggested Andropogon muricatus, now considered a synonym of vetiver. Suggestions that it might be the calamus of today have generally been rejected. Acorus calamus did not apparently occur in Biblical Palestine and was less likely to have been imported than the lemon grass or vetiver, to either of which the alternative translation sweet cane seems more appropriate. In Hispaniola, the plant is cultivated as a medicinal and aromatic tea material. It serves for making awnings, bags, baskets, fans, mats, pillows, sachets, screens, and sunshades, and is used for thatch in Haiti. Young leaves, not being too aromatic, may serve as fodder.

Regarded as alexiteric, carminative, detersive, diaphoretic, diuretic, emmenagogue, excitant, expectorant, parasiticidal, refrigerant, stimulant, stomacliic, sudorific, tonic and vermifuge, vetiver has been suggested as a folk medicine, usually as a tea, like lemon grass tea, for boils, burns, colic, epilepsy, fever, flu, hepatitis, lumbago, malaria, nausea, pleurisy, rheumatism, snakebite, sores, spasms, sprains, stomatitis, swellings, tumors of the abdomen, worms and yellow fever. In Mauritius, the root (which contains a resinous material) is used as abortifacient. In the Philippines a decoction of the roots is taken as a tonic bath and ingested to dissolve stones.

VINE GRAPE – (VITIS VINIFERA)
…But they shall sit every man under his vine and under his fig tree… Micah 4

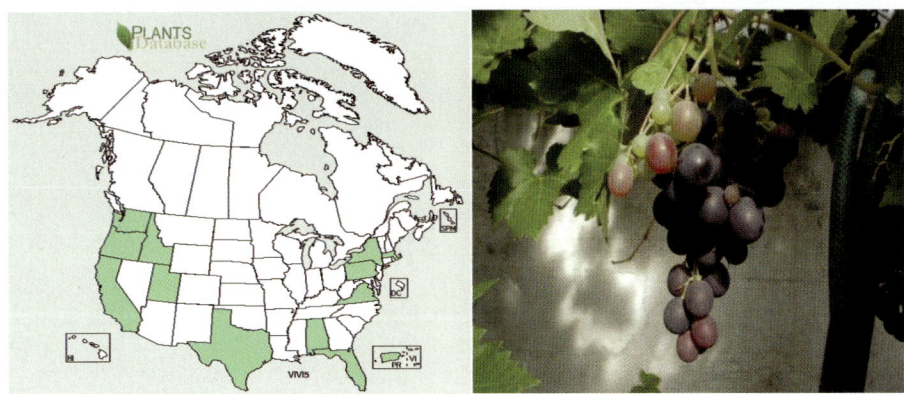

Vine grape is cultured for fruit, eaten fresh, or processed into wine, raisins, juice, with some cultivars adapted for the canning industry. Even Noah planted the grape after the flood and made wine from it. Grape seeds contain 6 to 20% oil, used for edible purposes, soaps, and as a linseed substitute. The leaves of this and other species are eaten in other cultures.

The sap of young branches is used as a remedy for skin diseases. The leaves are astringent and used in diarrhea. The juice of unripe fruit is astringent and used in throat infections. Regarded as apertif, astringent, demulcent, diuretic, expectorant, hemostat, laxative, lithontryptic, refrigerant, restorative, stomachic, and tonic, the grape is a folk treatment for cachexia, cancer, cholera, consumption, diarrhea, dropsy, heart, hoarseness, kidney, nausea, ophthalmia, seasickness, skin, smallpox, sore throat, thirst, tuberculosis, and warts. Grapes figure into several anticancer "remedies:" cancer, condylomata, corns, fibroids, impostumes, moles, neoplasms, polyps, scirrhus, sclerosis of the liver, testicles, and uterus; tumors of the ear, fauces, neck, testicles, throat, tonsils, uterus, and uvula; and warts. In the Trensvaal, grape syrup is used for diphtheria. Lebanese have a grape "cure" for fever, liver, nervousness, smallpox, and tuberculosis.

Small young leaves and/or tendrils are fed to infants to prevent scurvy and iron deficiency. The seeds and roots are ground for an anemia treatment, as is wine itself. The expressed leaf juice is applied to various skin conditions, including "cancer." Wine or its distillate is used by Lebanese for cramps, stomachaches, toothaches, or for any pain. More recent headlines in the U.S. proclaim that red wine (perhaps due to tannin) show some viricidal activity against herpes, more so than white wine. Ayurvedics regard the fruits, especially the black fruits, as an aphrodisiac, diuretic, laxative, purgative and refrigerant, and use them for asthma, biliousness, blood disorders, burning, eye ailment, fever, hangover, jaundice, sore throat, and strangury. Unani use the leaves, or their juice, for bleeding at the mouth, headache, nausea, piles, scabies, splenitis, and syphilis, the ashes of the stem for arthritis, bladder stones, orchitis and piles, the fruit for fever, the seed ash for inflammation. They consider the seeds astringent, the fruit as depurative, digestive, expectorant, and stomachic.

The fruit contains the following minerals:

Aluminum	Fluorine	Nitrogen
Boron	Iron	Potassium
Bromine	Lithium	Rubidium
Calcium	Magnesium	Selenium
Chromium	Manganese	Silica
Cobalt	Molybdenum	Silver
Copper	Nickel	Sodium

Strontium
Sulfur

Titanium
Zinc

The stem contains the following minerals:

Aluminum	Chlorine	Silica
Calcium	Magnesium	Sodium
Chromium	Manganese	Tin
Cobalt	Potassium	Zinc
Copper	Selenium	

The fruit contains the following amino acids:

Alanine	Leucine	Threonine
Arginine	Lysine	Tryptophan
Glutamate	Methionine	Tyrosine
Glycine	Phenylalanine	Valine
Histidine	Proline	
Isoleucine	Serine	

VINE OF SODOM – (*SOLANUM SODOMEUM*)
...For their vine is the vine of Sodom, and of the fields of Gomorrah...
Deuteronomy 32

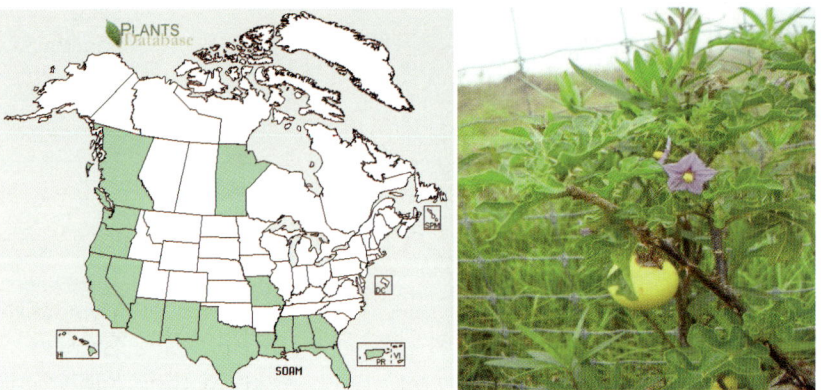

A useless weed in the past, this plant might be investigated as a source of steroids. Bad spiny weeds like this might be reduced in whole plant utilization schemes, producing energy in the process.

This diuretic but poisonous plant has been used for cystitis and tumors, cancers and excrescences of the anus. In Africa, the Xhosa apply the fruit or root juice to skin ailments. Tonga hold the fruit onto an aching tooth. Zulu use the root bark for barrenness and impotency. South Africans apply the fruit for ringworm in cattle and horse. Manyika chew the root and spit the juice onto the wound as a vulnerary.

WATER LILY – (NYMPHAEA ALBA)
...And upon the top of the pillars was lily work...I Kings 7

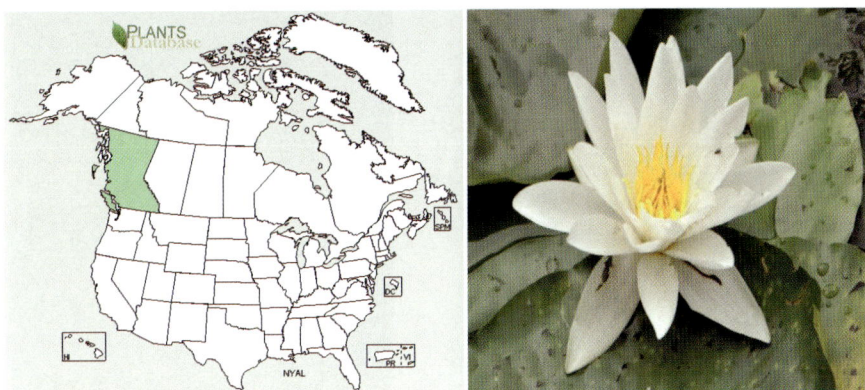

Numerous sculptured representations in ancient Egyptian tombs show their concern with water lilies, probably N. Alba or N. Lotus. The seeds, roots, and stalks are common foodstuffs in Egypt. The seeds are ground into flour for bread or are roasted and eaten like a nut. Rhizomes are boiled before consumption. The flowers are still admired by Egyptians, whose belles often wear them in their headdress. The flower was sacred to Egyptians more than 4000 years ago. Water lilies prevail in such distant cultures as Mexico, Japan, India, and China. Even ancient Greeks had a legend that a beautiful nympli, deserted by Hercules, flung herself into the Nile to be transformed into a white lotus. It is the national flower of Thailand. Some suspect water lilies of being narcotic. Rhizomes are used for tanning. There was in Homer's Odyssey a mythical nation where the people subsisted wholly on lotus and live in dreamy indolence induced by the diet.

Regarded as an aphrodisiac, astringent, diaphoretic, hemostat, narcotic, and sedative, this species has reportedly served as a folk remedy for cancer, diarrhea, spasms, and tumors (of the testes e.g.). The alkaloid nymphaeine is present in all parts of the plant, except the seeds. Toxic to frogs, it produces tetanus-like symptoms. Alcoholic extracts of the rhizome (containing the alkaloid) are mildly sedative and spasmolytic; they do not significantly depress the heart; in large doses, they paralyze the medulla.

WATERCRESS – (NASTURTIUM OFFICINALE)
...Eat it with unleavened bread and bitter herbs...Numbers 9

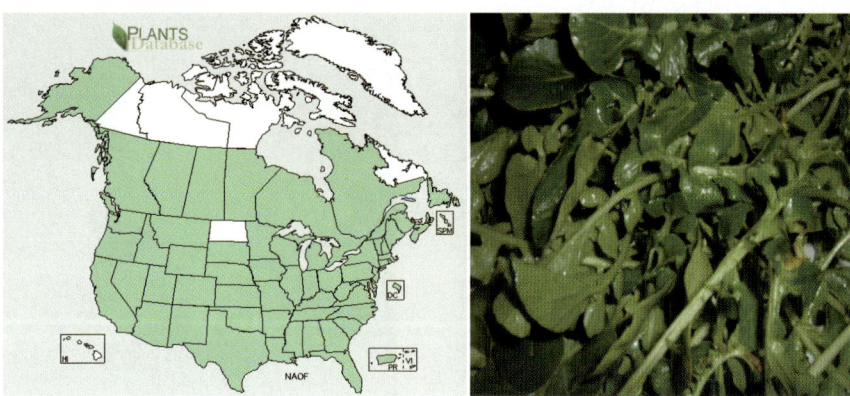

Watercress is one of the bitter herbs of the Passover (with chicory, endive, and lettuce). Watercress is grown for the pungent leaves and young stems, and is used widely for garnishing meats, salads, and other dishes, even biscuits. The plants are fairly high in vitamins, minerals, and protein. The leaves are eaten by ducks, muskrats, and deer and serve as shelter for small aquatic animal life. The pungent flavor is due to gluconasturtin.

Considered abortifacient, apertif, aphrodisiac, bactericide, cicatrizant, cyanogenetic, depurative, diuretic, emmenagogue, expectorant, laxative, restorative, stimulant and vermifuge, watercress is used for alopecia, anthrax, asthma, boils, bronchitis, cancer, catarrh, cough, earache, eczema, fever, flu, goiter, headcold, heart, impetigo, kidneys, leprosy, liver, nose, pertussis, polyps, scabies, sciatica, scrofula, scurvy, snakebite, sores, stomach, strangury, throat, tuberculosis, tumors, warts, and worms. It is used as a blood cleanser and for kidney ailments and tuberculosis. Lebanese use the seeds as alterative and depurative. As a salad, it is said to promote the appetite. Bruised leaves are said to free the face of blemishes, blotches and spots. Lebanese apply macerated leaves with yoghurt to acne. The juice, mixed with egg whites, is said to help carcinoma. Made into snuff it is a "cure" for polyps. Cress in vinegar is one remedy for anthrax. In Africa, chopped watercress, covered with honey overnight, is a cough syrup with vitamin C. In Western Europe, it is said to be ecbolic in large doses and to assist menstruation in smaller doses. It is believed to interfere with implantation of the ovum or gestation. In small quantities, it is thought to act as an oral contraceptive and produce temporary sterility. Stuffing the pillow with the leaves is supposed to induce sleep. In China, the plant is used for asthma. The plant is said to be an antidote to nicotine poisoning and also to be useful in strangury and goiter. The antibacterial juice is used for asthma, dry throat, headcold, and tuberculosis.

The herb contains the following minerals:

Calcium	Magnesium	Potassium
Iron	Nitrogen	Sodium

The plant contains the following minerals:

Copper	Manganese	Zinc

The herb contains the following amino acids:

- Alanine
- Arginine
- Glutamate
- Glycine
- Histidine
- Isoleucine
- Leucine
- Lysine
- Methionine
- Phenylalanine
- Proline
- Serine
- Threonine
- Tyrosine
- Tryptophan
- Valine

Hillman Health Food Store call 855-Amish-Dr (855-264-7437) www.emineral.info Vitamins and Minerals for Better Living

WATERMELON – (CITRULLUS LANATUS)
...We remember the fish, which we did we eat in Egypt freely; the cucumbers, and the melons...Numbers 11

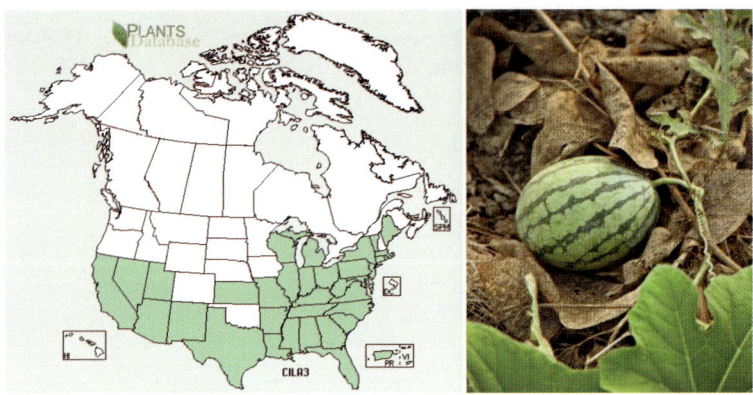

There is doubt as to whether the melon, mentioned in the Bible only once (Numbers 11), was the watermelon or the muskmelon (cucumis melo) for which the children of Israel longed in the Sinai. The watermelon has been cultivated in Egypt since time immemorial, serving for food, drink, and medicine. Seeds are also roasted and salted as a popular Egyptian side dish. The seed oil is used for salads and cooking. Slightly roasted, the seeds are used as a peanut and coffee substitute. In the semi desert areas the fruits are used as a source of water. In parts of Iran and Iraq, for two months of the year, the watermelon with a little bread is the people's food.

Regarded as antiseptic, demulcent, digestive, diuretic, laxative, pectoral, and repellant, the watermelon is used in folk remedy for alcoholism, aphtha, calculus, cancer, catarrh, diabetes, dropsy, hepatic congestion, hypertension, malaria, nephritis, renitis, stomatitis, strangury, and urogenital ailments. Lebanese use the plant to lower fevers and flush the kidneys. The juice of the root has been used to check bleeding following abortion. The leaf decoction is used for fever, the fruit juice an antiseptic in typhus fever. Tonkinese used the pericarp for diarrhea. In many different cultures, the seeds are prescribed for urinary ailments, like cystitis and gonorrhea. Africa's Yoruba boil the diced fruit with onion and other roots for gonorrhea and leucorrhea. In China, the rind is powdered and ashed and applied to aphthous sore mouth. Crude seed extract lowers the blood pressure. Ayurvedics consider the green fruit astringent, aphrodisiac, and refrigerant, the leaves hematinic. Unani consider the fruits depurative, diuretic, expectorant and stomachic, and use them for itch, scabies, and sore eyes. They consider the seed a stimulant to the brain. In Guyana the pulp is used "as a cooling enema." The so-called Four Greater Cold Seeds of the old materia medica were those of watermelon, pumpkin, gourd, and cucumber. They were bruised and rubbed up with water to form an emulsion used for catarrh, dyspepsia, fever and urinary disorders. It seems probably that they would have functioned, at least in the last named capacity, as a vermifuge.

The fruit contains the following minerals:

Boron	Magnesium	Sodium
Calcium	Manganese	Zinc
Copper	Nitrogen	
Iron	Potassium	

The fruit contains the following amino acids:

Alanine	Leucine	Threonine
Arginine	Lysine	Tyrosine
Glutamate	Methionine	Tryptophan
Glycine	Phenylalanine	Valine
Histidine	Proline	
Isoleucine	Serine	

The seeds contain the following minerals:

Calcium	Iron	Nitrogen

The seeds contain the following amino acids:

Alanine	Leucine	Serine
Arginine	Lysine	Threonine
Glutamate	Methionine	Tyrosine
Histidine	Phenylalanine	Valine
Isoleucine	Proline	

WEEPING WILLOW – (SALIX BABYLONICA)
...We hanged our harps upon the willows in the midst thereof...
Psalm 137

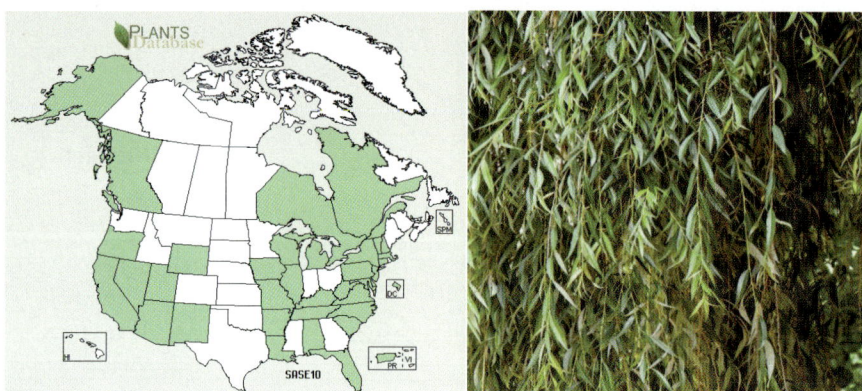

Several authors think the willow of Psalm 137 is salix babylonica, also identified with the legend that hanging the harps on the once erect branches caused them to droop, forever and ever. It is used as a honey plant in Palestine. The young shoot is valuable as stock food in spring. Bark, containing 6.2 to 7.8% tannin, has been used for tanning. Young leaves and branches are used in popular medicine in Palestine. In India, the leaves and bark are considered tonic and used in intermittent and remittent fever. The catkin and young twig have been used internally for slow continuous fever and externally as an application to sores. An infusion of the leaf is considered useful in rheumatism.

WHEAT CORN – (*TRITICUM AESTIVUM*)

...and he slept and dreamed the second time: and, behold, seven ears of corn came up one stalk, rank and good...Genesis 41

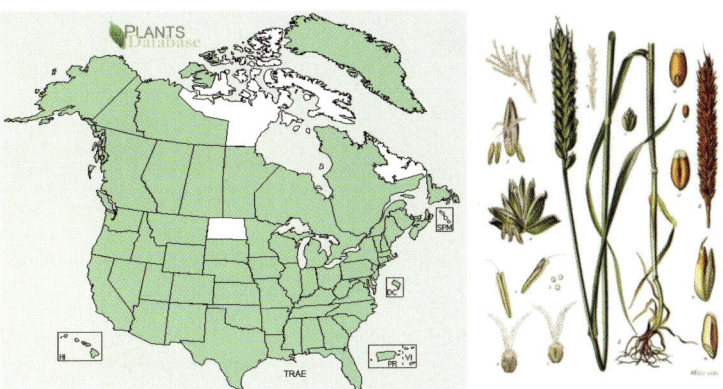

The Biblical term "corn" is synonymous with grain; it does not refer to Indian maize, but usually to wheat, the most common cereal. Corn in those days often included a mixture peas, beans, lentils, cumin, barley, millet, and spelt. Egypt was the chief storehouse of the Roman Empire.

Regarded as antibilious, antivinous, demulcent, discutient, emollient, laxative, restorative, sedative, and vulnerary, wheat is reported as a folk remedy for burns, cancer, diarrhea, dysentery, ecchymosis, epistaxis, fever, flux, gravel, hematuria, hemotysis, hemorrhage, incontinence, leprosy, leucorrhea, menorrhagia, neurasthenia, nightsweat, scalds, skin, smallpox, sunstroke, swellings, tuberculosis, tumors, warts, and wounds. Algerians use flour for diarrhea, fractures, metrorrhagia, and syphilis, the bran for scorpion stings. Lebanese recommend the bran for bones, constipation, antiseptic dressing, claiming that they had "empirical penicillin."

WHITE BROOM – (RETAMA RAETAM)
...Went a day's journey into the wilderness, and came and sat down under a juniper tree...I Kings 19

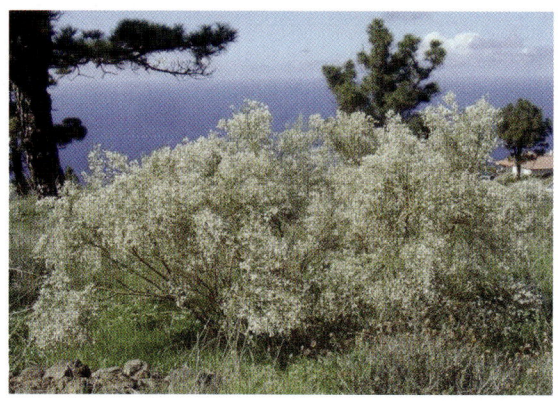

Bedouins have a saying indicating the importance of plants "by the life of the plant and our worshipped Lord." Small wonder that they prohibit the chopping down of desert shrubs such as acacia, pistacia, and retama. In some places retama is the only shade-casting tree on the desert. The bush makes the finest charcoal, which burns with intense heat, and the Arabs maintain that it holds its heat for a whole year. As a fuel it is unsurpassed in the East, and in the Cairo market fetches a much higher price than any other kind. The expressions "*coals of Juniper*" used in Psalm 120, "burning coals," "live brown coals," "coals of broom," and "coals that lay waste" in Biblical books indicate the popularity of the wood for charcoal.

One legend suggests that when Jesus was praying in Gethsemane he was disturbed by the cracking of the broom in the breeze. When finally led off by the soldiers he said to the broom: "May you always burn with as much noise as you are making now." Another legend has it that the crackling of broom plants among which they hid almost revealed Mary and baby Jesus to Herod's soldiers. The branches are used in homes of the Holy Land for coarse cords. At weddings and other ceremonies, the Bedouins fasten sprigs of green plants like retama to the entrance of the tent. Green, the color of live plants, is a symbol of life and vitality. The roots are used to insulate the handles to Bedouin coffee pots. Bedouins use the plant to make pins that fasten their roof to the outer curtain. Bedouins also use the plant as pins for their camel saddles.

The plant is ecbolic, POISON, purgative, and vermifuge. In the Flora Palaestina it is said that the branches are used in preparing a wash for the eyes. Bedouins ground the branches and green leaves over live coals until hot, placed them in a thin cloth, and applied them to arthritic aches, repeating this process as often as the patient could take it. The leaves are ground, powdered and applied to wounds by the Bedouins. Finally, the roots are used against diarrhea and the branches for fever and wounds.

WHITE WHISTLING WOOD – (ACACIA SEYAL)
...I will plant in the wilderness...the shittah tree...Isaiah 41

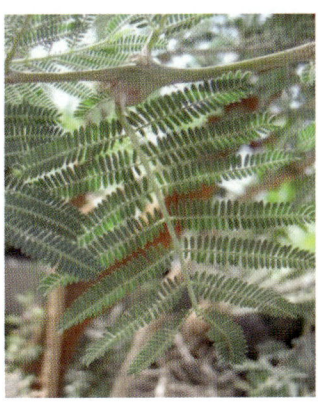

Noah used wood from the shittin tree, also known as shittah. Its use was to make beams and timber for the ark. The gum is said to be edible. The leaves are important for forage and the wood for fuel where the trees are abundant. In parts of Africa the tree is important for livestock, natives driving their animals to where it is common and lopping off branches for them, both leaves and young pods being eaten. The pods are sold, especially for fattening sheep. The slightly acid gum is believed to be somewhat aphrodisiac. The bark decoction is used for dysentery and leprosy. Tanganyikans use the bark as a stimulant in tropical Africa. The gum is used as emollient and astringent for colds, diarrhea, hemorrhage and ophthalmia. Mixed with Acacia sieberana DC it is used for intestinal ailments on the Ivory Coast. The wood is used as a fumigant for rheumatic pains and to protect puerperal mothers from colds and fevers. Eating the gum is supposed to afford some protection against bronchitis and rheumatism.

WILD GRAPE – (*VITIS ORIENTALIS*)
...and he looked that it should bring forth grapes, and it brought forth wild grapes...Isaiah 5

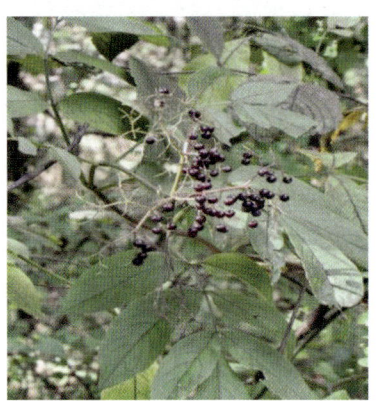

A wild grape has small acid fruits, with very little juice. Because the Biblical reference comparing the rebellious people of Israel to "wild grapes" and "the degenerate plant of a strange vine," it is concluded that it referred to the wild fox grape of Palestine and Syria. Probably this species could be substituted for the cultivated grape, and its folk medicinal applications. As medicine, we know that in modern times grapes are a source of resveratrol.

WILLOW – (SALIX ALBA)
...And they shall spring up as among the grass, as willows by the water courses...Isaiah 44

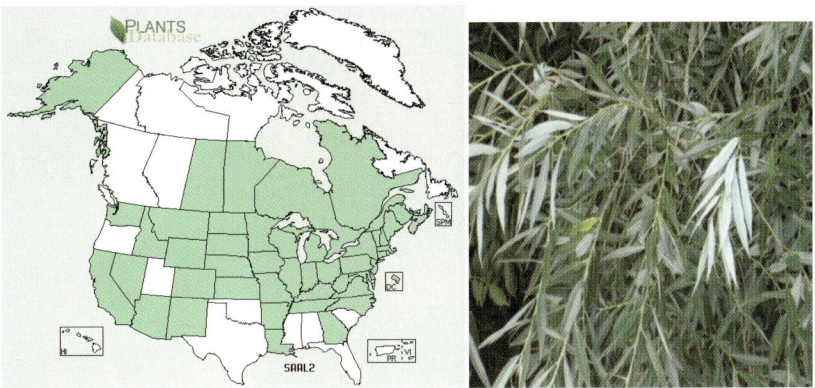

Willows are handsome fast-growing trees, useful for holding banks against flooding. The wood can be used for fuel, and some willows have been recommended as energy sources. Slender willow twigs, or withes, are used in wicker work. Salicene, a bitter principle extracted from the bark of young willow shoots, makes a good substitute for quinine. Willow branches were used by the Jews in some of their religious rites and ceremonies.

Regarded as antiperiodic, antiseptic, astringent, tonic, and vermifuge, the white willow is used in folk remedies for calluses, corns, debility, diarrhea, dysentery, dysmenorrhea, dyspepsia, fever, gout, hemotysis, malaria, rheumatism, tumors, and warts. Lebanese recognize the aspirin like quality of the bark decoction, using it for colds, grippe and pain, and a strong decoction for venereal disease. Even "transplanted" to America, the Lebanese used the bark of the American species for colds, flu, headache, pains, and rheumatism.

The bark contains the following minerals:

Aluminum	Magnesium	Potassium
Calcium	Manganese	Silica
Chromium	Nitrogen	Sodium
Cobalt	Potassium	Tin
Iron	Selenium	Zinc

WINDFLOWER – (ANEMONE CORONARIA)
...Consider the lilies of the field, how they grow; they toil not, neither do they spin: and yet I say unto you, That even Solomon in all his glory was not arrayed like one of these...Matthew 6

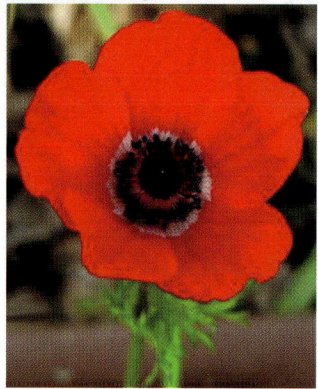

The windflower is quite a spectacular ornamental wild flower "abundant on the Mount of Olives today, as it doubtless also was in Jesus' day." A flower of ancient romance, the anemone was supposed to have sprung from the tears of Venus pining for Adonis: where a tear dropped, the windflower grew. It is introduced elsewhere as an ornamental. Today this is the most common anemone in the florist's trade. Magicians gathered them in his day as a remedy against disease, tying the flowers round the neck or arm of the patient as a charm to cure all illness. In Arabic folk medicine, the flowers were once used for tumors of the stomach. According to Philips, Lebanese used the juice to cleanse the nose as well as ulcers, and chewed the root for tuberculosis. They figured the plant could cure leprosy and the infusion could cure malaria.

WORMWOOD – (ARTEMISIA HERBA)
...But her end is bitter as wormwood, sharp as a two-edged sword...Proverbs 5

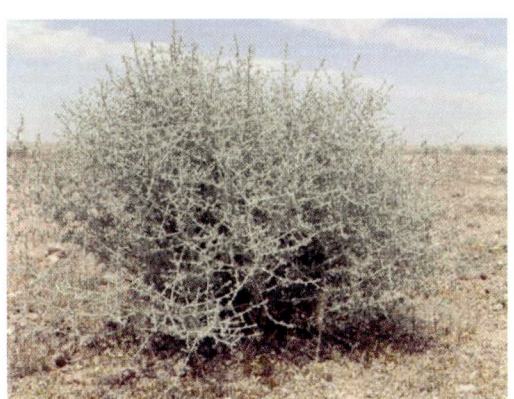

Artemisia herba alba was common in Palestine and A. Judaica in the Sinai, but one or the other of these species is probably the Biblical wormwood. Bedouins sell both species in the Cairo market. Herba alba is used in native perfumery. The drink absinthe is made from a similar species, and thousands of gallons were once consumed annually especially in France. It first produces activity and pleasant sensations and inspires the mind with grandiose ideas, illustrating the Biblical phrase, *"he hath made me drunken with wormwood."* Bedouins believe that the fumes emanating from the burning leaves will keep away the cosmopolitan evil eye. They use dry wooly galls from the plants for tinder to ignite with flint stone. Nile valley farmers fumigate their poultry with the smoke of the burning leaves, and hang out the herb as a snake repellent. Camels which graze on the plant are said to be spared certain skin diseases. Tea made from dried leaves is used for gastrointestinal cramps.

The flowers and leaves are febrifuge and hemostat, and used to calm cough, emotions, headache, nerves, ophthalmia and stomach. The diuretic vulnerary powdered plant is infused for bronchitis and rheumatism. Bedouins place the leaves inside the nostrils as a nasal decongestant when one has a cold. For cough they drink the leaf tea, in water or milk. For cough, they also grind the leaves and stem, strain it and then mix the juice with tepid water and sugar and drink. Newborn Bedouins are induced to breathe the incense of the burning leaves to insure their good health.

The leaves of artemisia herba alba are used as a Palestinian folk remedy for toothache. Artemisia judtica has been cited as an Arabic folk remedy for indurations of the uterus. In Egypt the plant is believed to be specific against tapeworms. Bedouins eat the seeds or make a herbage tea for colic.

Toxicity of the herb is explained in the Goodspeed version of the Bible, *"Then the third angel blew his trumpet, and there fell from the sky a great star blazing like a torch, and it fell upon one third of the streams of water. The star is called Absinthus, that is, wormwood. Then one third of the waters turned to wormwood, and numbers of people died of the waters, for they had turned bitter."*

Wormwood plant contains these minerals:

Calcium	Magnesium	Sodium
Copper	Nitrogen	Zinc
Iron	Potassium	

YELLOW FLAG – (IRIS PSEUDOACORUS)
...he shall grow as the lily, and cast forth his roots as Lebanon...
Hosea 14

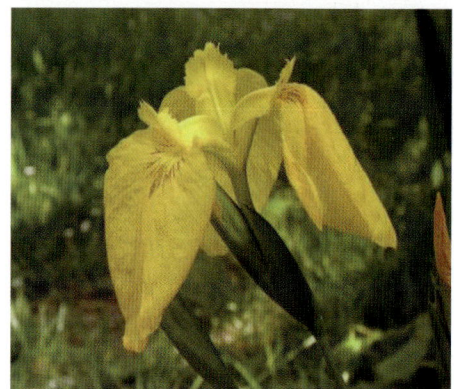

One of the most handsome wildflowers of Europe, the yellow flag has been equated with the lily of Hosea. The roots were once used like orris to scent linen closets. They are used also as a source of tannin and blue and black dyes. The flowers offer a yellow dye. Seeds have been used as a coffee substitute. Powdered root was once used as a snuff and as a breath freshener. The rhizome was once widely used as a cathartic. Its infusion was used for diarrhea, dysmenorrhea and leucorrhea. The vulnerary juice extraced from the roots was used for cholera, cough, convulsion, dropsy, jaundice, snakebite, splenitis and toothache. Boiled root has been applied to contusions. The oil extracted from the root or flower was used for arthritis, cramps, and myalgia. The plant has quite a folk anticancer repertoire, used for cacoethes, cancer (especially of the gums), condylomata, and polyps, scleroses of the liver and spleen, and tumors of the spleen. The essential oil has been used for cancer. Seeds were used as a carminative for flatulence. Old herbals suggested the root for rabies. North Africans boil the fragmented rhizomes (one of Morocco's favorite alexiterics) for rheumatism and sciatica. Rhizome also used for hypothermia and liver ailments.

Common Herbs

Aikal Skullcaps - (*Scutellaria Lateriflora*)

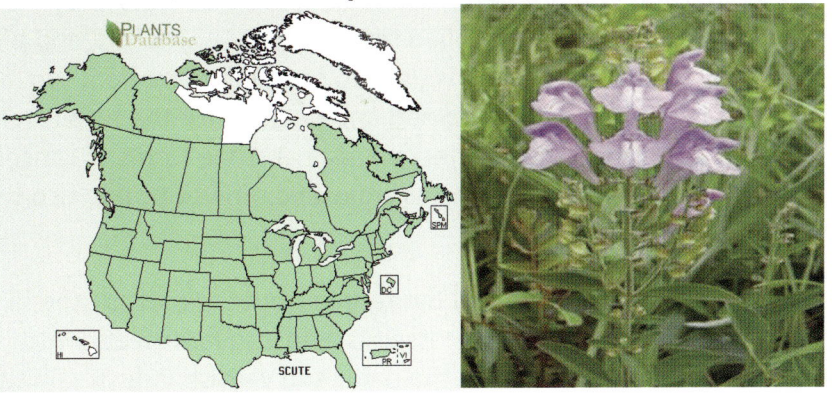

Skullcap is a native North American perennial herb. It can be found growing in rich woods, thickets, bluff and along roadsides in wet ditches. Flowers bloom from May to August. Gather above ground parts in the summer as flowers bloom and then dry and store them for later herb use.

Skullcap is a powerful medicinal herb used in alternative medicine for anti-inflammatory, spasms and a strong tonic. Skullcap is used in the treatment of a wide range of nervous conditions including epilepsy, insomnia, hysteria, and anxiety. It should not be given to pregnant women since it can induce a miscarriage. The infusion is also used for throat infections and nervous headaches without any unpleasant symptoms following. Skullcap is currently being used as an alternative medicine to treat attention deficit hyperactivity disorder and a number of nerve disorders.

Skullcap has been linked to liver damage, though it is suspected that the source of damage was actually from Germander being substituted for skullcap. Use it in moderation and avoid if you have liver problems. It should be used with some caution since in cases of overdose it causes silliness, stupor, confusion, and twitching. It was once believed of use in the treatment of rabies and schizophrenia.

The following minerals are in baikal skullcap's roots:

Calcium	Iron	Manganese	Sodium
Copper	Magnesium	Potassium	Zinc

Albizia – (*Albizia Lebbeck*)

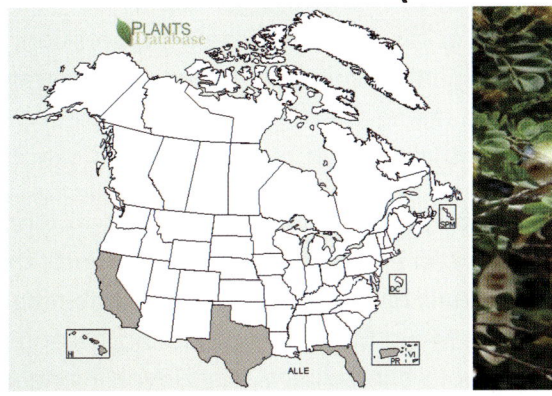 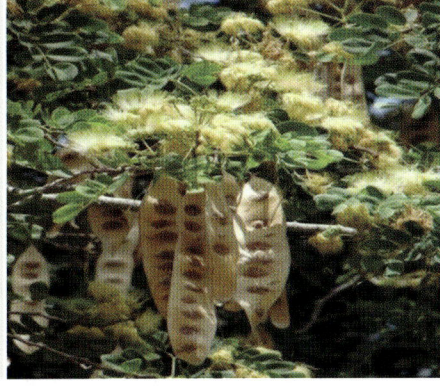

Albizia lebbeck trees grow generously in the Punjab province of Pakistan. The flowers, fruit, bark, leaves, and roots are all used in medicine. The seeds contain crude protein, calcium, phosphorous, iron, B_3, and ascorbic acid (vitamin C) and most of the essential amino acids. There are saponins in the seeds, but no harmful effects have been reported when the seeds have been eaten, as long as they are eaten in moderation; too many will induce vomiting.

A paste of the leaves is used to treat skin problems and to improve skin texture by making it smoother. Paste preparations from parts of the plant are applied to insect stings, wounds, and bites, and it is also said to be good to promote healthy gums and teeth. It is used to treat inflammation, too, and a powder from the different parts of the tree is said to purify the blood and be good for the respiratory system and to treat allergies. The ethanol extract of the pod is effective against some forms of cancer. Parts of the tree are also used to treat eye problems, impotence and as a diuretic. However, it is also thought that the seeds can cause infertility.

Saponins from the tree are used to make soap and the tannin from the bark is used in the tanning process. Bees love the nectar from the flowers, and the tree itself is a host to lac insects which leave a residue on the tree. This residue can be collected and used in the paint and varnish industry. In this way, it is similar to the banyan tree.

Modern medical trials have shown that Albizia lebbeck has "remarkable anti-inflammatory activity supporting the folkloric usage of this plant to treat various inflammatory diseases" (Babu N.P. et al).

The seeds contain:
Calcium   Phosphorous   Iron

ANDROGRAPHIS – (ANDROGRAPHIS PANICULATA)

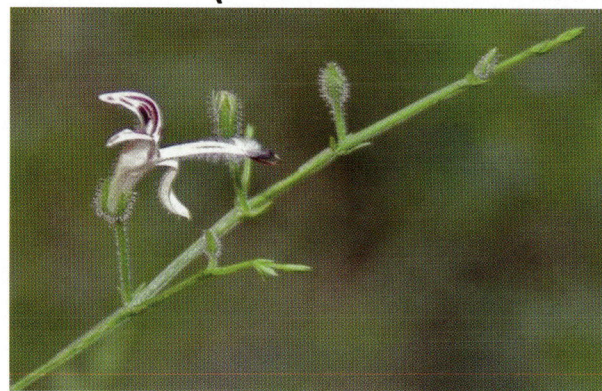

Andrographis paniculata is a plant that is native to parts of Asia and is commonly used as a medicinal herb for its flowers and leaves. If you have a common cold or flu, immune system suppression, gastrointestinal problems, viral hepatitis, malaria, dysentery, or certain infections, you can take andrographis to help ease your symptoms. Always consult your physician before taking andrographis or any other herbal remedy, because they can cause certain side effects and potentially interact with some medications.

Taking andrographis may help to reduce the severity of your symptoms from the common cold. Several double-blind studies have revealed that andrographis can ease cold symptoms, reports the University of Michigan Health System. Some double-blind clinical trials have also found that combining andrographis with Siberian ginseng may lessen cold symptoms. The Mayo Clinic notes that andrographis extract has shown antiviral activities. A 2004 review of seven double-blind clinical trials involving nearly 900 participants found that andrographis extract was indeed more effective than placebo in treating the symptoms associated with acute respiratory infections, including the common cold and flu, says the University of Pittsburgh Medical Center. Another study found that a particular andrographis concoction taken at a dosage of 6 grams daily for one week was as equally effective as acetaminophen in reducing fever and sore throat. Further, andrographis may also actually act to prevent the common cold. The University of Pittsburgh cites a double-blind study of 107 young adults found taking 100 milligrams of andrographis daily increased the participants' resistance to catching colds. After three months, only 16 andrographis users contracted colds, compared with 33 from the placebo group.

Andrographis paniculata is an effective herbal remedy for boosting your immune system. Some preliminary scientific evidence indicates that andrographis may stimulate the immune response and support the immune system, notes the University of Pittsburgh Medical Center. Andrographis contains constituents called andrographolides, which are responsible for this immune system stimulation, explains the University of Michigan Health System.

Andrographis's immunity-boosting constituents may also help to fight certain infections. In addition to its antiviral effects, andrographis may have antioxidant, an antibacterial, anti-malarial and anti-inflammatory activity, the Mayo Clinic says. One uncontrolled study found that andrographolide, the important constituent of andrographis, boosted CD4 lymphocyte counts and reduced the viral load in people with HIV infections, says the University of Michigan Health System. Other evidence indicates that andrographis can help to support antibiotic medications to treat dysentery and may help to treat chronic viral hepatitis. Andrographis extract taken orally can also treat snake bites by neutralizing the venom, the Mayo Clinic notes.

The andrographolides contained in andrographis may also help to treat certain gastrointestinal problems by stimulating the secretion of bile, notes the University of Michigan Health System. Andrographis has been used in traditional herbal medicine throughout China and India to treat digestive problems, and you may find the herb helpful in easing indigestion. The University of Pittsburgh Medical Center reports andrographis may act to stimulate gallbladder contractions. This and other actions may help to protect the liver from harmful toxins, according to preliminary medical studies.

ANISE - (*PIMPINELLA ANISUM*)

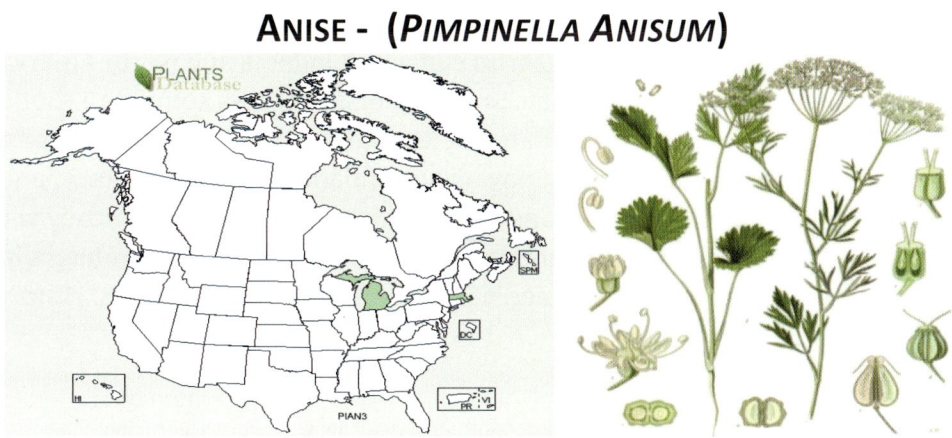

Anise is an annual and an herb.

The plant part used is the seed, in the form of extracted essential oil.

Anise has a sweet flavor and is considered a very good herbal remedy. It is considered an excellent tonic helpful in solving various digestive problems like bloating, nausea, and indigestion. Anise is used in treating breathing conditions, asthma, and whooping cough. Externally, it is used as a chest rub in treatments of breathing and lung disorders.

Hillman Health Food Store call 855-Amish-Dr (855-264-7437) www.emineral.info Vitamins and Minerals for Better Living

ARNICA - (ARNICA MONTANA)

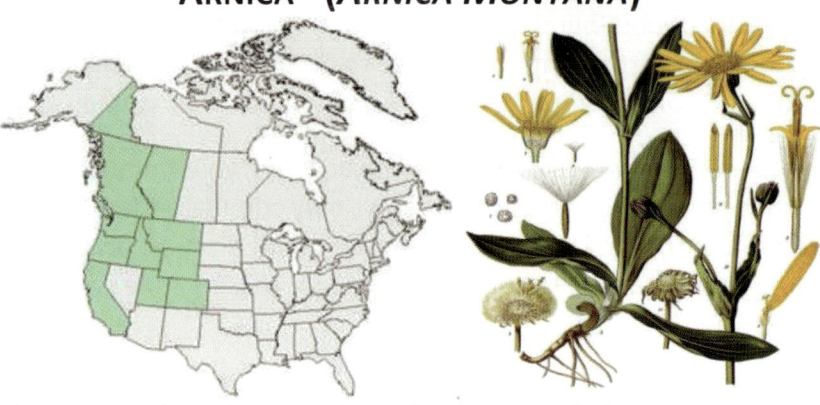

Used topically, arnica has various benefits. Used as a linoment and ointment preparation for bruises, sprains, and strains. Made into a gel, arnica has shown useful in treatment of hand arthritis, wound healing, inflammations caused by insect bites, swelling caused by fractures, and muscle aches.

ASHWAGANDHA, WITHANIA – (WITHANIA SOMNIFERA)

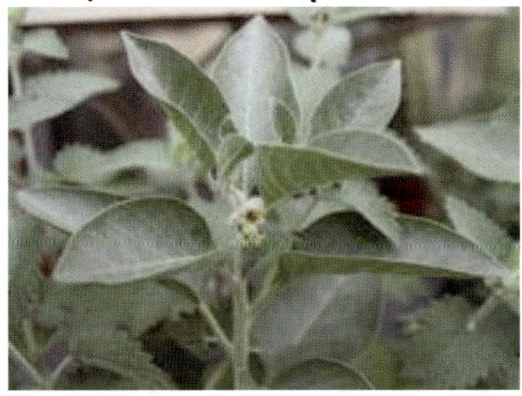

Withania somnifera, known as ashwagandha, is a shrub cultivated in India and North America whose roots have been used for thousands of years by Ayurvedic practitioners. Withania somnifera root contains flavonoids and many active ingredients of the withanolide class. Several studies over the past few years have looked into the role of withania somnifera in having anti-inflammatory, anti-tumor, anti-stress, and antioxidant, mind-boosting, immune-enhancing, and rejuvenating properties. Historically withania somnifera root has also been noted to have sex-enhancing properties. Withania somnifera has been an important herb in the Ayurvedic and indigenous medical systems for over 3000 years. Historically, the plant has been used for these conditions -

Adaptogen for patients with nervous exhaustion	Asthma	Insomnia
Anti-inflammatory agent	Cognitive and neurological disorders	Liver tonic
Anxiety	Immune stimulant in patients with low white blood cell counts	Parkinson's disease
Aphrodisiac	Inflammation	Senile dementia
		Ulcers

Ashwagandha herb and root extract health benefit and use for stress reduction, anxiety treatment and relaxation. Withania somnifera is widely considered as the Indian ginseng. In Ayurveda, it is classified as a rasayana (rejuvenation) and expected to promote physical and mental health, rejuvenate the body in debilitated conditions and increase longevity.

ASTRAGALUS - (ASTRAGALUS MEMBRANACEUS)

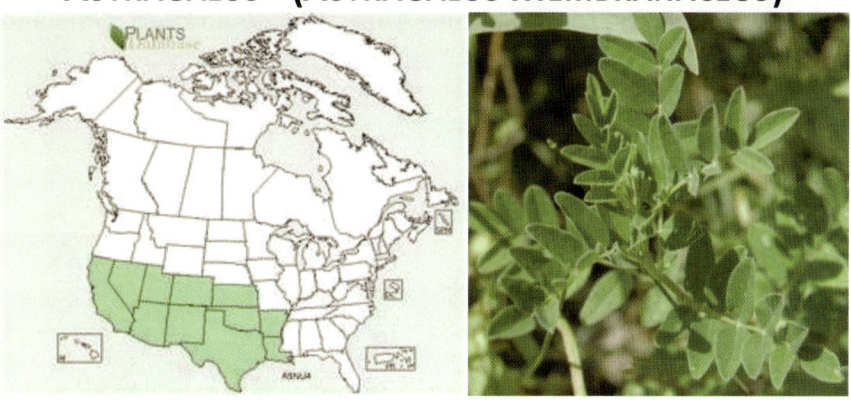

Astragalus is a perennial herb that grows to about 1 meter high. 4-7 year-old plant roots are dried from plants collected in the spring before leaves appear or in autumn after they have fallen. After the root is dug up, the crown and rootlets are removed along with dirt and usually sun dried. The most commonly used forms are from raw astragalus (dried root). Cured (honey-treated) astragalus is produced by frying the sliced root with honey (from 25–30 parts to 100 parts of root) over medium heat until no longer sticky to touch.

Astragalus is used for the common cold, lung infections, allergies, and to strengthen and boost the immune system. It is also used for tiredness, kidney disease, diabetes, and high blood pressure.

Some people use astragalus as a general tonic to protect the liver and to fight bacteria and viruses.

AVOCADO - (PERSEA AMERICANA)

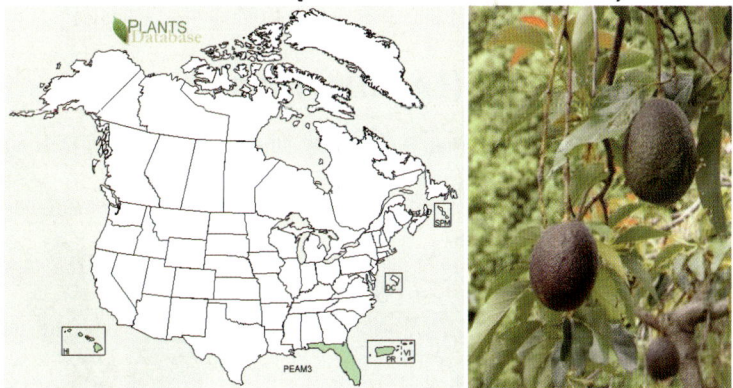

An avocado is a fruit and not a vegetable! It is actually a member of the berry family.
It is primarily used as a vegetable, yet it contains enough fat to pass as a meat substitute in sandwiches and other dishes. In some respects, an avocado is a tropical fruit akin to a banana, but its oily content and nutty flavor remind one of an olive.

The avocado is grown in warmer North American states like California and Florida, including the most popular variety, hass, which is often misspelled as haas in California. A variety of avocado grown in Florida is called a fuerte; it has a watery texture and lower fat content.

The avocado pit is mildly toxic, so it should be removed and discarded out of all animals' reach.

Avocados are taken by mouth to treat osteoarthritis. Its oils have been used topically to treat wound, infections, and arthritis. It is also used to promote hair growth. The seeds, leaves, and bark have been used for dysentery, diarrhea, and used in topical creams for regular skin care. Historically, the Amazonian natives used avocado to treat gout. The Mayan people believed it could keep joints and muscles in good condition, avoiding arthritis and rheumatism.

BASIL - (OCIMUM BASILICUM)

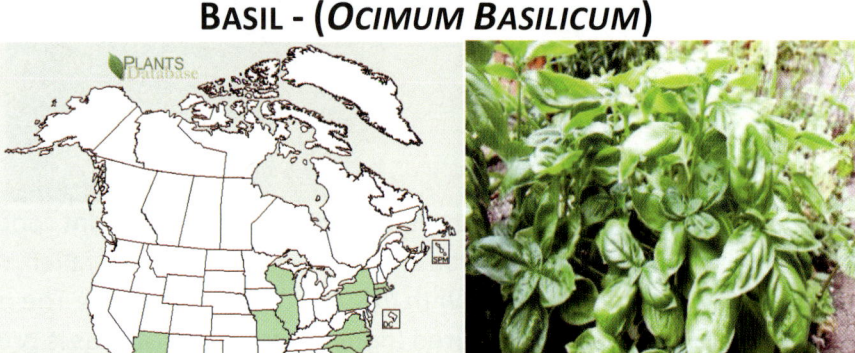

Basil is a low-growing annual plant. It has a square, slightly hairy stem and ovate with slightly toothed leaves. Leaves vary in color from bright green to dark purple. Flowers also vary in color: white, pink, or red. They appear along the leaf axils during August and September. A useful component is Camphor from the seeds.

Basil has many uses. It is considered antibacterial, antifungal, antispasmodic, a digestive aid and helpful with headaches and sore throat. Also, chewing the leaves on a daily basis fights against stress, ulcers, and mouth infection.

BAY - (LAURUS NOBILIS)

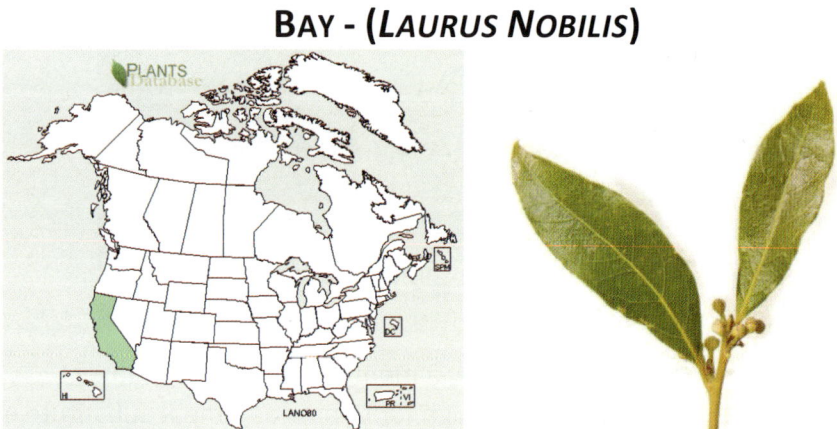

The bay plant's leaves, berries, and oil have a dulling effect on the system. Except as a stimulant in veterinary practice, the leaves and fruit are very rarely used internally. Oil of bay is used externally for sprains, bruises, and sometimes dropped into the ears to relieve pain. The leaves, powder, or soaked berries were taken as tea to remove obstructions and to create appetite.

BEARBERRY - (ARCTOSTAPHYLOS UVA-URSI)

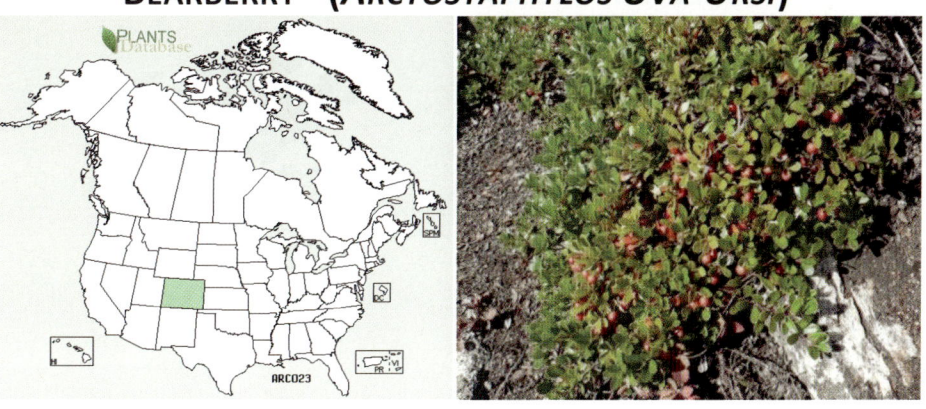

Most regions in the northern atmospheres up to the Arctic borderlands have naturalized populations of this plant, though the bearberry shrub was originally native to continental Europe.

Bearberry is a small groundcover shrub. Leaves are evergreen and leathery, alternately arranged on the stems. Stems can be red if the plant grows in full sun and green if it grows in shady areas. Flowering occurs in May. The only part used are its leaves.

Bearberry is considered to be an antiseptic and skin cleaner. It is also considered as an aide in getting rid of water weight and as a nerve tonic. It has been used in treatment of arthritis, bladder infections, lung conditions, diabetes, gallstones, hemorrhoids, kidney stones, infections, rheumatism, and vaginal disorders. It can be very effective against urinary tract infections and complaints. Some studies suggest that bearberry could also be effective against certain yeast (particularly Candida species).

BEGGAR'S LICE - (DESMODIUM STYRACIFOLIUM)

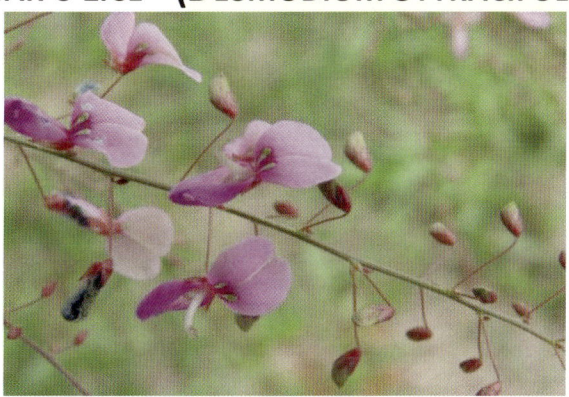

The beggar plant has both male and female organs. The organs are pollinated by insects and can fix nitrogen. The plant prefers light (sandy), medium (loamy), and heavy (clay) soils. It prefers partial sun, moderately dry conditions, and a sandy or rocky soil. The whole plant is diuretic. Beggar is used in the treatment of gallstones, gonorrhea, hepatitis, and urinary tract stones.

BILBERRY - (VACCINIUM MYRTILLUS)

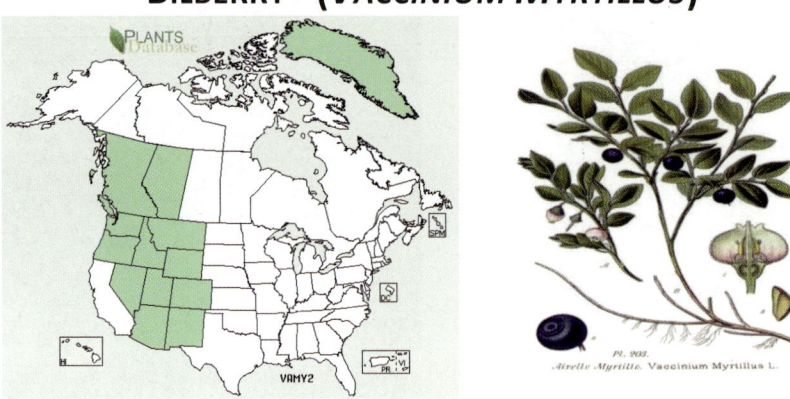

Bilberry is a low-growing perennial, small shrub with leathery, red leaves, and wax-like flowers. Bilberry flowers from April to June. The fruits are little black berries that are round, with a flat top.

The parts of this plant that are used are the ripe fruit and fresh or dried leaves. Bilberries are rich in sugar, flavonoids, vitamins A and C, antioxidants. Medicinal use: Bilberry has been used as an herbal remedy for centuries, all around the globe. Tea made from the leaves is primarily an excellent antiseptic for the urinary tract and has similar effects as Uva ursi. Taken for a prolonged period, it can be helpful in treatment of diabetes. The fruits are useful in the treatment of diarrhea, dysentery, and high blood pressure. Distilled water made from the leaves makes excellent eyewash and is helpful in cases of poor vision and night blindness. Bilberry tea is also used to treat stomach problems and can relieve mild swelling due to a cold.

BISHOP'S WEED - (AEGOPODIUM PODAGRARIA)

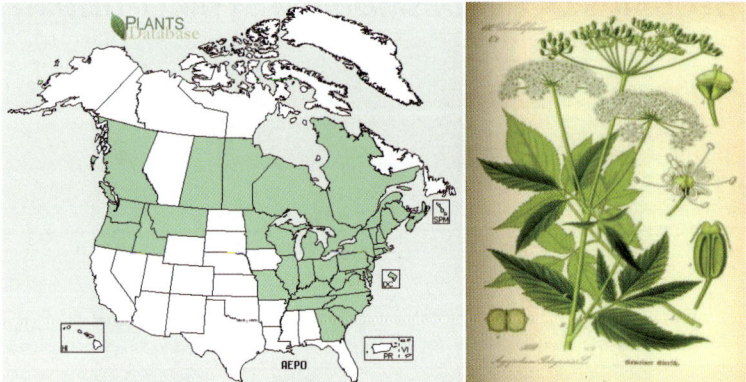

Goutweed has many tasty relatives, such as carrot, parsnip, or fennel. However, there are also some very poisonous members in this family–like the deadly water hemlock. Therefore, if you intend to pick ANY for food, make sure you are certain you have identified them correctly. Goutweed itself does not look much like water hemlock; it is just related to it. More dangerous for people in the United States is the similarity of its leaves with those of poison ivy. Like those of poison ivy, its leaves also sprout in threes and have a similar size and shape. One distinguishing feature–Goutweed will NEVER grow as a vine like poison ivy does.

As the name suggests, goutweed was once used to reduce the pain of gout. Nowadays goutweed is a useful herb for digestion and speed up weight loss as a water weight reducer. It is a good source of vitamins C and A, iron, manganese, copper, as well as trace minerals such as boron and titanium.

BITTER GOURD - (MOMORDICA CHARANTIA)

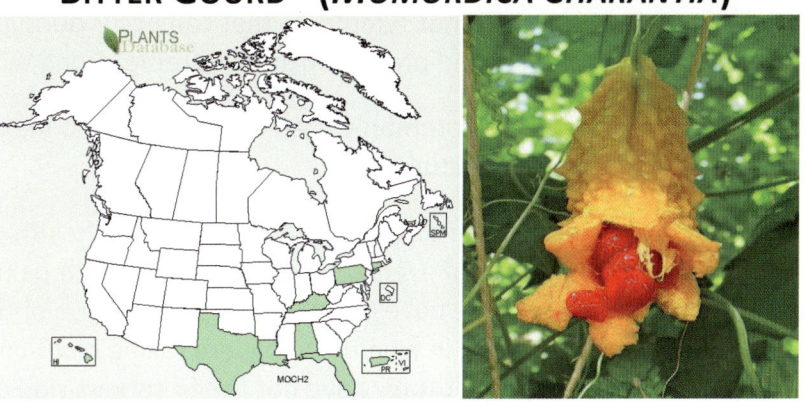

The bitter gourd is specifically used as a folk medicine for diabetes. Research has shown that it contains an insulin-like property that works like a "plant-insulin," which has been found to lower the blood and urine sugar levels. It should be included in the diet of the diabetic. For better results, the diabetic should take the juice of about four or five fruits every morning on an empty stomach. The seeds of bitter gourd can be added to food in the powdered form.

A majority of diabetics usually suffer from malnutrition as they are usually under-nourished. Bitter gourd, being rich in all the essential vitamins and minerals, especially vitamins A, B_1, B_2, C, and iron, can with regular use prevent many complications such as hypertension, eye complications, neuritis and defective digestion of carbohydrates. It also helps the body's resistance against infection.

Bitter gourd helps in the treatment of blood disorders like blood boils, scabies, itching, psoriasis, ringworm, and other fungal diseases. A cupful of fresh juice of bitter gourd mixed with a teaspoonful of lime juice should be taken, sip by sip, on an empty stomach daily for four to six months in these conditions. Its regular use in endemic regions of leprosy acts as a preventive medicine.

The plant's roots have been used in folk medicine for breathing disorders. A teaspoonful of the root paste mixed with an equal amount of honey or basil leaf juice, given once every night for a month, acts as an excellent medicine for asthma, bronchitis, colds, and rhinitis. Leaf juice is beneficial in the treatment of alcoholism. It is an antidote for alcohol intoxication and useful in liver damage due to alcoholism. Fresh juice of bitter gourd leaves is also an effective medicine in early stages of cholera and other types of diarrhea during summer. Two teaspoonfuls of this juice mixed with equal quantities of white onion juice and a teaspoonful of lime juice should be given in these conditions.

BLACK COHOSH - (ACTAEA RACEMOSA L. VAR. RACEMOSA AKA BLACK BUGBANE)

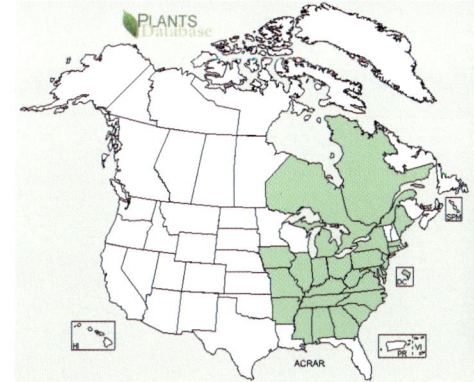
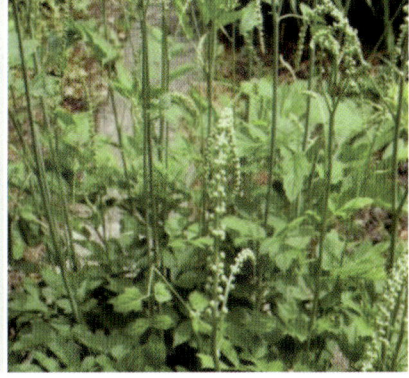

Black cohosh has been used for rheumatism, arthritis, and muscle pain, but has been used worldwide for hot flashes, night sweats, vaginal dryness, and other symptoms that can occur during menopause. Black cohosh has also been used for menstrual cycle and premenstrual syndrome, along with inducing labor.

Black cohosh underground stems and roots are commonly used fresh or dried to make strong teas, capsules, solid extracts used in pills, or liquid (tinctures).

Experts suggest women should discontinue use of black cohosh and consult a health care practitioner if they have a liver disorder or develop symptoms of liver trouble, such as stomach pain, headache, rash, dark urine, or yellowing of the skin or eyes. There have been several case reports of hepatitis (inflammation of the liver), as well as liver failure in women who were taking black cohosh. In general, clinical trials of black cohosh for menopausal symptoms have not found serious side effects.

BLACK HAW - (*VIBURNUM PRUNIFOLIUM*)

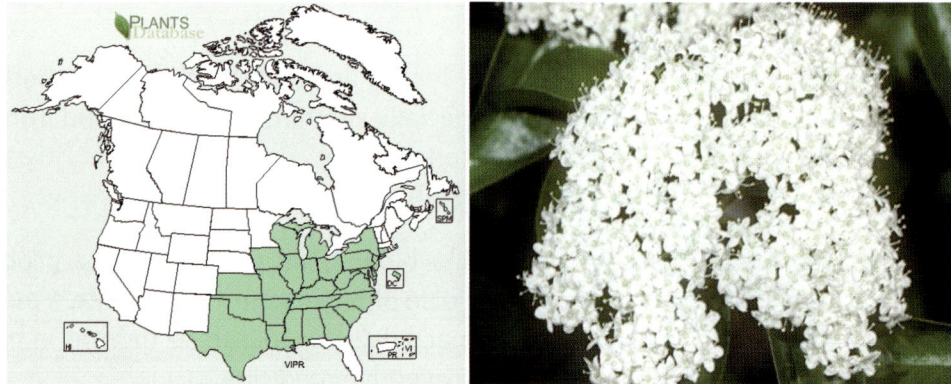

Black haw has been beneficial in all nervous complaints and successfully for cramps and spasms of all kinds. Black haw has also been used for convulsions, fits, lockjaw, rapid heartbeat, heart disease, and joint stiffness. In addition, black haw is a powerful relaxant of the uterus and is used for false labor pains as well as in threatened miscarriage.

Black haw's relaxing and sedative actions are used in reducing blood pressure and treatment of asthma. Traditional use of black haw is for uterine irritability, threatened abortion, uterine colic, lower back and bearing-down pains, cramp-like menstrual pain, and painful contractions of the pelvic tissues, after-pains, and false pains of pregnancy.

Other uses are as an analgesic, skin cleaner, and sedative. It also addresses water weight, nerve, and liver ailments. Extracts used from the whole bark have been shown to have an effect on the central nervous system.

Tinctures of the root bark have been used to alleviate pain after childbirth and to arrest bleeding.

BLACK HOREHOUND - (BALLOTA NIGRA)

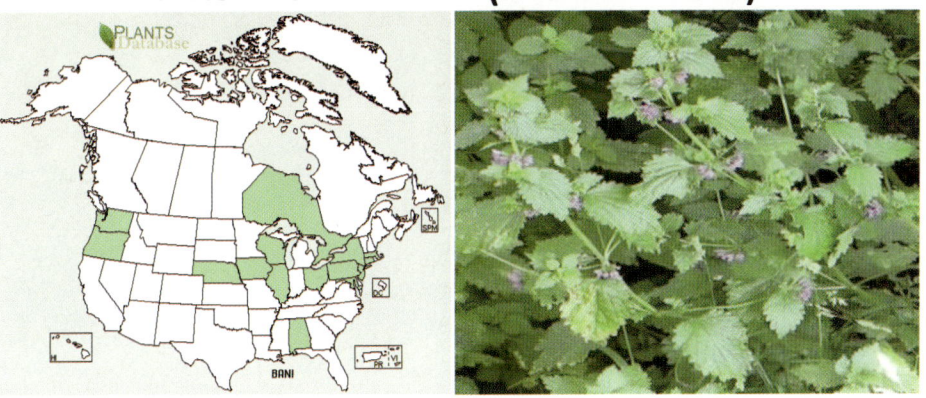

The herb should be gathered just as it begins to bloom in July and use the dried flowered parts. For the remaining of the summer it blooms from June to October.

Black horehound is an excellent remedy for the settling of nausea and vomiting because of nerves. It may be used for motion sickness if the nausea is inner ear related. This herb will also help with vomiting from pregnancy; it also works as a nerve tonic, skin cleaner, and loosens coughs. Black horehound has a terrible ordor that is rejected by cattle and they will not eat it. It is used for spasms and as a stimulant when made into a liquid extract.

BLACK NIGHTSHADE - (SOLANUM NIGRUM)

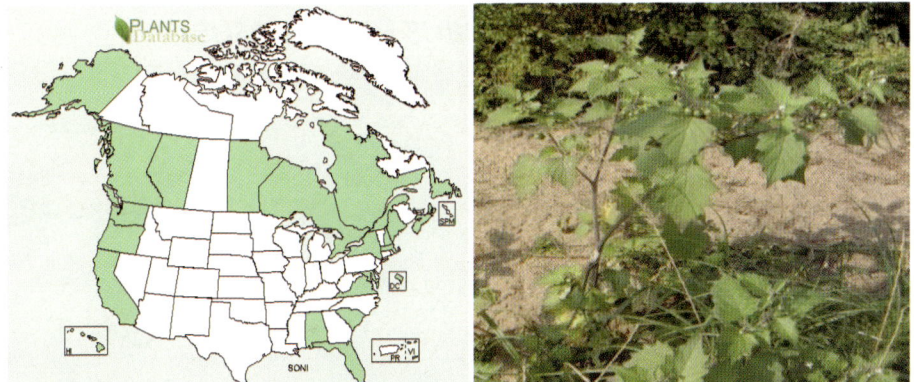

Flowers of the nightshade are arranged in clusters at the end of stalks springing from the main stems between the leaves. They are small and white but turn into small white round berries that are green at first but black when ripe. The plant flowers and fruits freely, and in the autumn the black berries are very noticeable; they have, when mature, a very polished surface.

The whole plant flowers and the fruit and leaves can be used when gathered in early autumn.

This species has the reputation of being very poisonous. The berries are poisonous to children, but adults can eat them when ripe. No green part of the plant is to be eaten because that is when it is poisonous.

It can be used as medicine; in small doses for external use, it relieves pain and swelling. It can be applied to burns and ulcers and the juice can be placed on an infected area of ringworm.

BLACK WALNUT - (JUGLANS NIGRA)

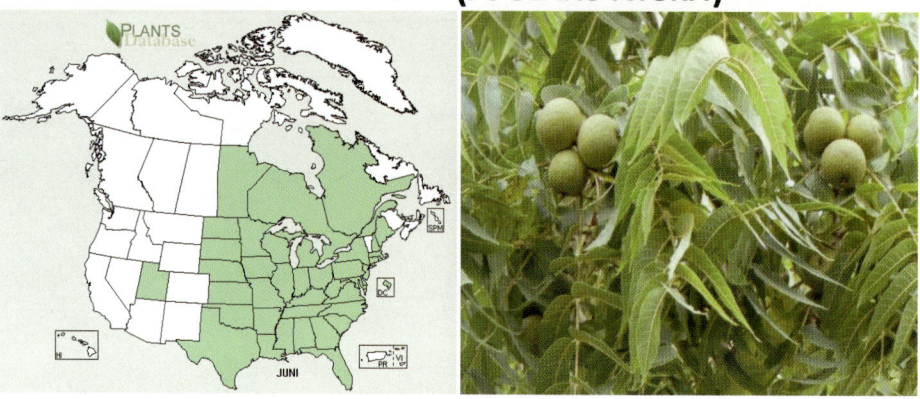

The tree grows to a height of 40 to 60 feet, with a large spreading top and a thick, massive stem. Black walnut can be 23 feet around and some have lived to be 300 years old.

The bark and leaves can be used for a laxative, skin cleaner, and laundry soap as well as for skin troubles. In healing ulcers, use one ounce of dried bark or leaves (slightly more of the fresh leaves) to one pint of boiling water. Allow to stand for six hours, and strain. It is to be taken in one-cup doses, three times a day. Use the same infusion at the same times for an outward application. Ulcers may also be cured with sugar, well saturated with a strong solution of walnut leaves. When green and unripe, the nut can kill worms of the intestine. The fruit, when young and unripe, makes a wholesome pickle. The vinegar in which the green fruit has been pickled can be used as a gargle for sore throats.

BLACKBERRY - (RUBUS FRUCTICOSUS)

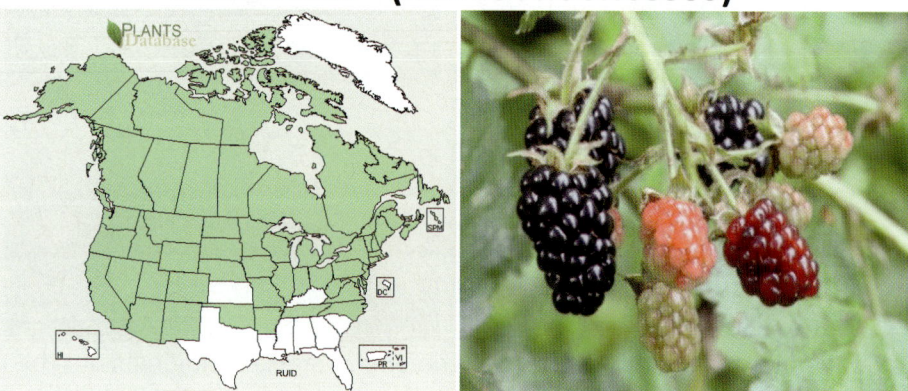

The bark of the root and the leaves contain tannin and have long been used as a skin cleanser, tonic, and is good for diarrhea. The fruit contains malic acid, citric acids, and pectin. The bark should be peeled off the root and dried by artificial heat or in strong sun. One ounce, boiled in 1½ pints water or milk, down to a pint, makes a good tonic. Half a teacupful should be taken every hour or two for diarrhea. One ounce of the bruised root, likewise boiled in water, may also be used, the dose being larger, however. The same dose is said to be useful against whooping cough.

BLOODROOT - (SANGUINARIA CANDENSIS)

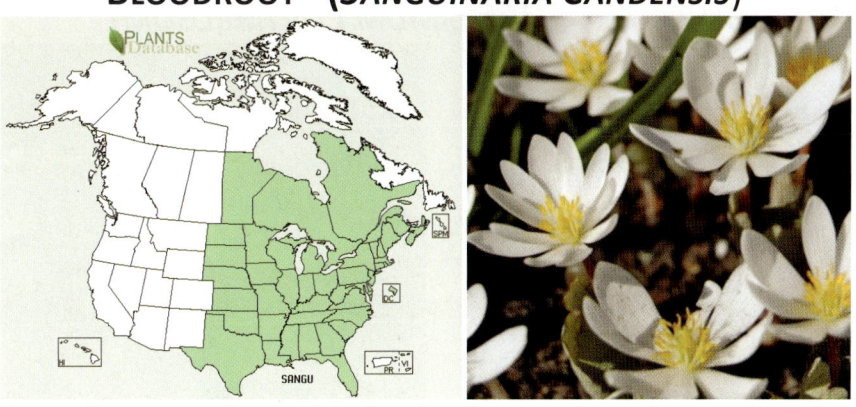

Bloodroot is one of the earliest, most beautiful of spring flowers. It produces only a single leaf and a lovely white flower about 6 inches high. When the leaf first appears, it is wrapped round the flower bud and is grey-green in color, covered with a downy bloom. The root is collected in the autumn, after leaves die down. It must be stored in a dry place or it quickly deteriorates.

Bloodroot tonic is for asthma, bronchitis heart, alcoholism, rapid heartbeat, and croup. The taste is so nasty that it may cause coughing. In toxic doses, it can cause stomach pain, thirst, vomiting, fainting, and dimmed eyesight.

BLUE COHOSH - (CAULOPHYLLUM THALICTROIDES)

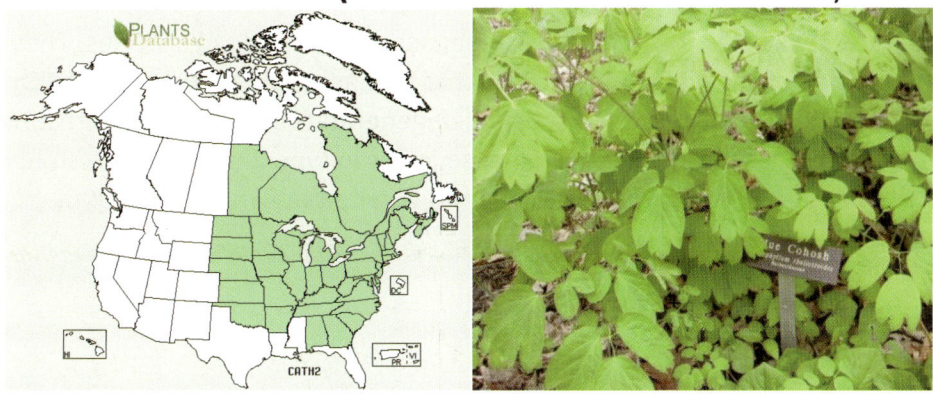

Blue cohosh is a perennial plant growing in low, rich, moist soil in swamps and near running streams. It has smooth bark and bears a tiny, panicle of yellowish green flowers in May and June, one or two seeds about the size of a large pea, which ripen in August. The seeds are sometimes roasted and boiled in water and given as a decoction resembling coffee. The berries are dry and mawkish; the root is a hard, thick, irregular, knotty and can grow up to 8 inches long. Externally it is yellowy brown and internally it is whitish to yellow, with a central pith running longitudinally. The taste is sweetish-bitter with a slightly (pungent) fragrant odor; yields its properties to alcohol, water, or glycerin.

Medicinal action and uses are for spasms and as a diuretic. It is said to be successfully used in chronic cases of rheumatism, epilepsy, hysteria, uterine inflammation. It is preferable to expediting newborn delivery, where delay results from debility, fatigue, or want of uterine and nervous energy.

The following minerals are to be found in blue cohosh roots:

Magnesium	Potassium	Sodium
Manganese	Selenium	Tin
Nitrogen	Silica	Zin

BLUEBERRY - (*VACCINIUM CORYMBOSUM*)

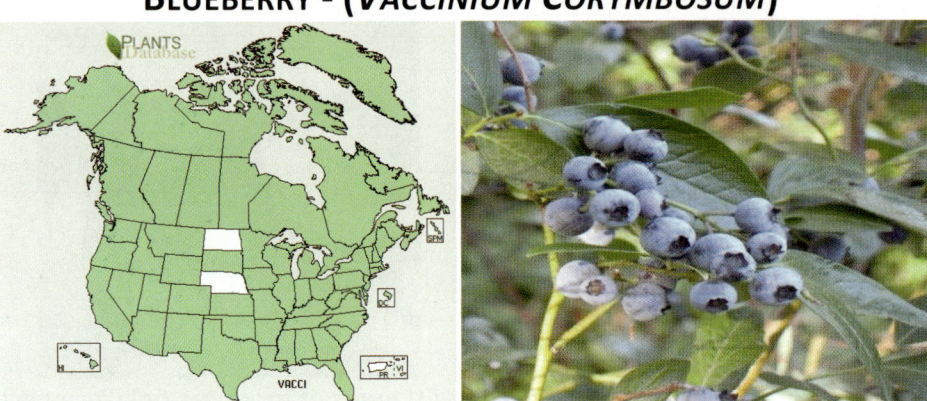

Different species are classified according to their growth habit as high-bush and low-bush berries.

High-bush blueberries (vaccinium corymbosum) are erect shrubs with many stems. It grows 10-12 feet tall on cultivated farms and bears clusters of small, cream-white flowers during spring, which subsequently convert to fruits after about 2 months. Wild, high bush blueberry is found on edges of marshes, lakes, ponds, and streams. Rabbit eye blueberry (vaccinium virgatum) are medium-sized shrubs, grown naturally in south eastern parts of USA.

Low-bush blueberry (vaccinium angustifolium) is short; the erect plant grows one to two feet in height, spreading by underground roots. They grow in a two-year cycle crop and are either mowed down or burnt to allow new shoots to appear only during next season.

Blueberries are very low in calories. 100 grams fresh berries provide only 57 calories. They are full of fiber, minerals, vitamins, and one of the highest in antioxidants that are needed for good health and wellness. Blueberries also protect the body from cancers, aging, degenerative diseases, and infections. Blueberries help lower blood sugar levels and control blood glucose levels in type 2 diabetes. Fresh berries contain small amounts of vitamin C, vitamin A, vitamin E, vitamin B_3, vitamin B_6, and vitamin B_9.

Minerals in blueberries are:

| Copper | Manganese | Zinc |
| Iron | Potassium | |

BORAGE - (*BORAGO OFFICINALIS*)

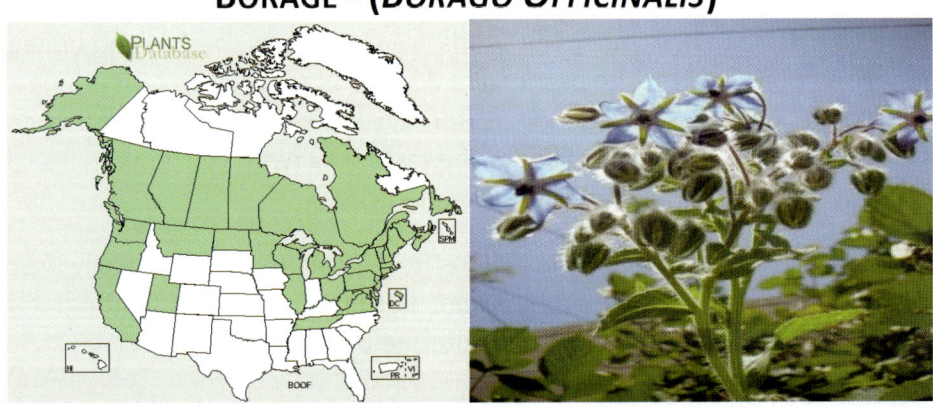

Borage is native to Syria, is natural throughout Europe, Africa, and South America, and is grown on sandy soil.

An annual plant deep green in color, it has branched, round stems and star-shaped bright blue flowers with cone-like formation. The leaves and flowers are all that is used.

Borage is a strong diuretic. Externally, relief can be obtained from the leaves made into a poultice for swellings. Internally, it has been widely used for fevers and heart disorders. The flowers and leaves are helpful in easing the symptoms of coughs and in treatment of diarrhea.

BROOM WEED - (AMPHIACHYRIS DRACUNCULOIDES)

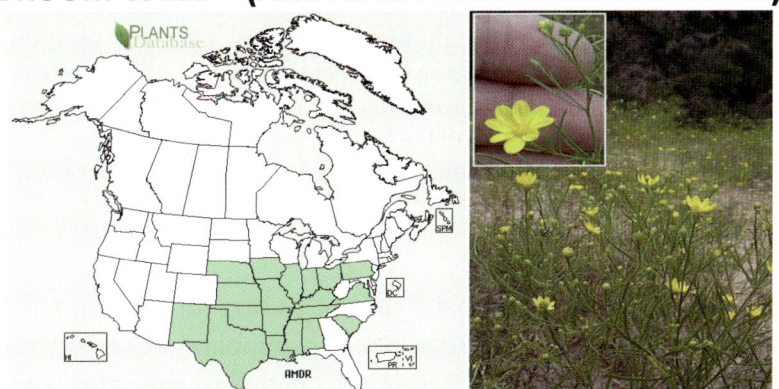

Sida acuta is a common weed in Florida. Some people refer to it as broom weed. Do you have little tiny yellow flowers in your lawn? Look at them closely; they might be broom weed.

It is also the host plant for Checkered Skipper Butterflies. According to Butterflies and Moths of North America, both the Tropical Checkered Skipper Butterfly, and the Common Checkered Skipper Butterfly are in Palm Beach County, Florida, and only the Tropical Checkered Skipper Butterfly is in Broward County, Florida.

BUCHU – (BAROSMA BETULINA)

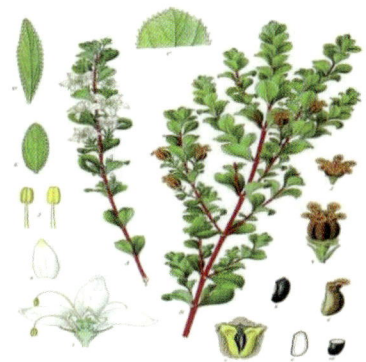

In 1909 Felter and Lloyd had this to say of buchu: "The plants yielding buchu are indigenous to Southern Africa, occupying a limited extent of territory." According to Burchell they are odoriferous, and are, when powdered, used by the Hottentots under the bame of bookoo or buku, for anointing their bodies. They likewise prepare a buchu brandy by distilling the leaves with wine, which they employ as an efficient remedy in all affections of the stomach, bowels, and bladder. They also apply a decoction of the leaves to wounds. Buchu is said to have been introduced into medicine by a London drug firm (Reece & Co., in 1821), to whom a supply had been sent by Cape Colonists, who learned its uses from the Hottentots. Buchu was first used by the tribes in South Africa as a general tonic and specifically for urinary tract infections. In time the South African Colonials came to know it and they too used it for general health purposes and in urinary tract infections. To this day, it is one of herbalists' favorites when urinary tract infections are causing a problem.

Buchu, in a few short words: Urinary tract infection miracle plant!

Uses: Contains oils that kill bacteria hanging out in the urinary tract: urethritis and cystitis. Every time you drink a cup of buchu tea, bacteria-killing oils pass through the urinary tract.

Buchu is useful in:

Antispasmodic
Chronic rheumatism
Cutaneous affections
Diuretic
Dropsy
Dyspepsia

In catarrh of the urinary bladder, and incontinence connected with diseased prostate
In irritation of the bladder and urethra attending gravel
Stimulant

Tonic
Useful in all diseases of the urinary organs

Urinary tract infections have always been a problem for the medical profession and this was the case in the last century. When buchu became known it was instantly popular because it very quickly cleared a urinary tract infection. In fact, it was so popular it became a highly sought after commodity. Reece and Company, London, 1821, first imported it and introduced it to pharmacy and to the medical profession, where, as well as in private formulae and domestic practice, it has ever since enjoyed more or less notoriety. Perhaps no "patent" American medicine has ever enjoyed greater notoriety than, about 1860, did the decoction of the leaves under the term "Hembold's Buchu," which, a weak alcoholic decoction, commanded one dollar for a six-ounce vial, and sold in large amounts. During the movement of this preparation the medical profession of America, probably inspired by the press comments, prescribed buchu very freely. It is still in demand and is still favored as a constituent of remedies.

One of the nice things about buchu is that it has a pleasant taste. Unlike some herbal remedies, buchu is a pleasure to use. The oils that give buchu its very pleasing black currant taste are also responsible for its ability to kill bacteria in the urinary tract. The oils are absorbed by the stomach and excreted by the kidneys into the bladder. As the oils pass through the bladder and urethra, they kill bacteria as they go. Science has revealed that buchu is a urinary tract disinfectant of the truest sort.

The issue with urinary tract infections is that they tend to be chronic in nature. One urinary tract infection clears just in time for another urinary tract infection to begin. This is not a coincidence. The first infection weakens the urinary tract and makes it easier for bacteria to move in and cause the second urinary tract infection. The third infection makes it even easier for the fourth and so on. One urinary tract infection makes the urinary tract vulnerable to infection. The term "sitting duck" comes to mind. It is important to interrupt the cycle of urinary tract infections. Many herbalists use a two-pronged approach to accomplish this. First, they advocate the use of an immune stimulant like Echinacea or Maitake. A fired-up immune system is much better able to police the urinary tract for bacteria and kill them if they run into any. So the first thing to do is to get the immune system marching double time in a war against bacteria. The second thing to do is to regularly use bacteria killing buchu. Every time you drink a cup of buchu tea, bacteria-killing oils pass through the urinary tract. As the oil passes through, it kills bacteria. This benifit has effectively ended the cycle of urinary tract infections for more than one long-time sufferer. By the by, buchu sometimes gives the urine a distinct black currant scent! We would not like anyone to be caught unawares.

A practitioner's opinion: It should be used long term to clear infection. Buchu is used to disinfect the urinary tract during infections of the bladder (cystitis), urethra (urethritis), prostate (prostatitis), or kidney (pyelonephritis). It is also used to treat sexually-transmitted diseases.

BUGLEWEED (AKA- GYPSYWORT)- (*LYCOPUS EUROPAEUS*)

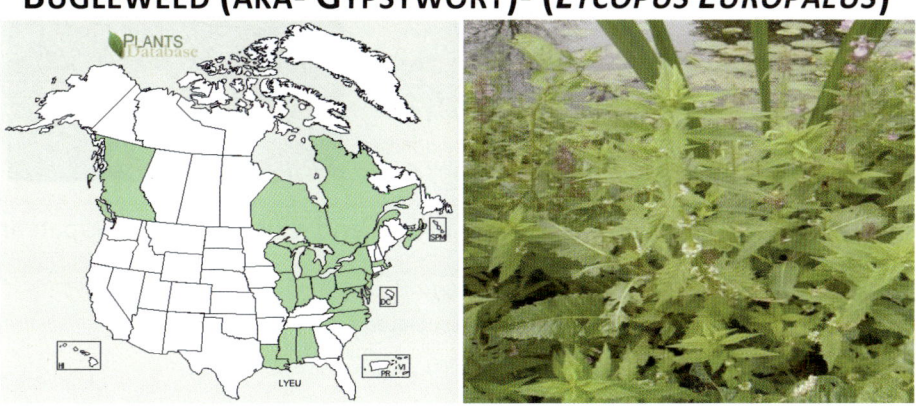

Gypsywort is an herbal plant that but has no culinary purposes at all but rather is used for industrial and medicinal purposes. This plant originated in Europe and Northwest Asia. Gypsywort's most important properties come from the stem and the leaves. These were used for the astringents, sedatives, anxiety, tuberculosis, and heart palpitations. Industrially, Gypsywort was extremely beneficial in making a permanent black dye. Oddly enough that is how it got its name; the Gypsies were said to have stained their skin with this black dye-like substance so they would resemble Africans or Egyptians while they were performing. The fresh or dried flowering herb is astringent and sedative. It inhibits iodine conversion in the thyroid gland and is used in the treatment of hyperthyroidism and related disorders. The whole plant is used as follows:

Astringent	Excessive menstruation	Mild sedative
Bleeding from the lungs and consumption	Hyperthyroidism	Strengthens heart contractions
	Hypoglycaemic	
Coughs	Mild narcotic	

The leaves are applied as a poultice to cleanse foul wounds. This remedy should not be prescribed for pregnant women or patients with hypothyroidism. The plant is harvested as flowering begins and can be use fresh or dried, in an infusion or as a tincture.

BUPLEURUM – (BUPLEURUM FALCATUM)

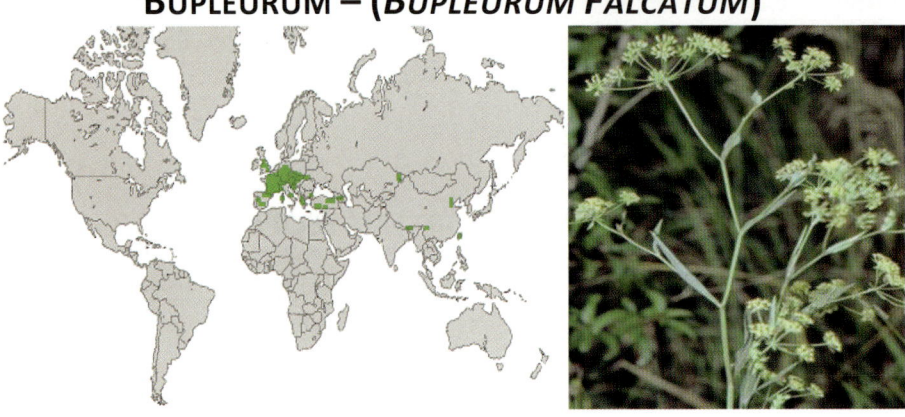

Bupleurum has been widely used for over 2,000 years in Asia and is used today in Japan and China for:

- Cirrhosis
- Deafness
- Diabetes
- Dizziness
- Hepatitis
- Other conditions associated with inflammation
- Vomiting
- Wounds

Clinical studies have suggested that this combination may be effective in the treatment of hepatitis B and in the prevention of hepatocellular carcinoma. The mixture has also shown some promise as a liver-protecting agent and as an adjuvant in the treatment of HIV infection.

BURDOCK - (ARCTIUM LAPPA)

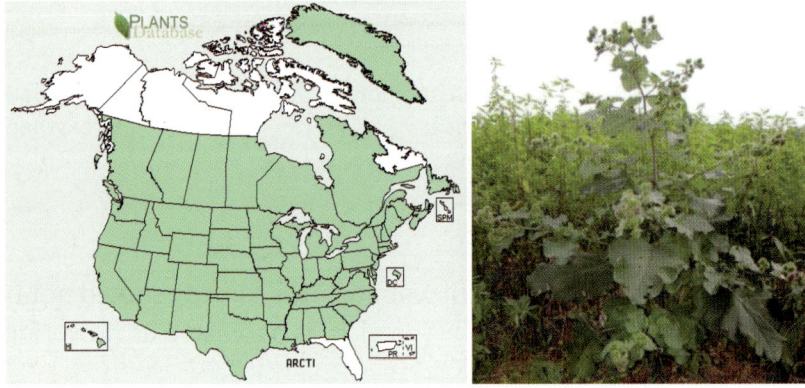

Highly adaptable, burdock can be found in fields, pastures, and along roadsides on recently disturbed soils. Seeds are brownish-green and wrinkled.

A biennial plant, it has a single stem divided at the top and large, dark-green leaves. Leaves are coarse, emerging from a long taproot. Lower ones are usually heart-shaped. Flowers appear in the second year, in July. They are purple, rounded with hooked spines.

The dried root from plants of the first year's growth along with leaves, fruits, and seeds can be used.

Traditionally, burdock has been used for all sorts of ailments. Folk medicine considered burdock to be an excellent blood cleaner and diuretic. It was also used for various skin conditions like acne, psoriasis, and eczema. Burdock root extract also shows mild antibiotic and laxative characteristics. Burdock seeds are used like tea in treatment of sore throat, tonsillitis, colds, and coughs. Burdock root oil extract (Bur oil) is used for scalp conditions (dandruff and hair loss).

Pregnant or nursing women should avoid burdock. People who are dehydrated should not take burdock because the herb's diuretic effects may make dehydration worse. Sometimes burdock could cause allergic reactions.

The following minerals are to be found in the root:

Aluminum	Copper	Nitrogen
Calcium	Iron	Potassium
Chromium	Magnesium	Selenium
Cobalt	Manganese	

BURNET SAXIFRAGE - (*PIMPINELLA SAXIFRAGA*)

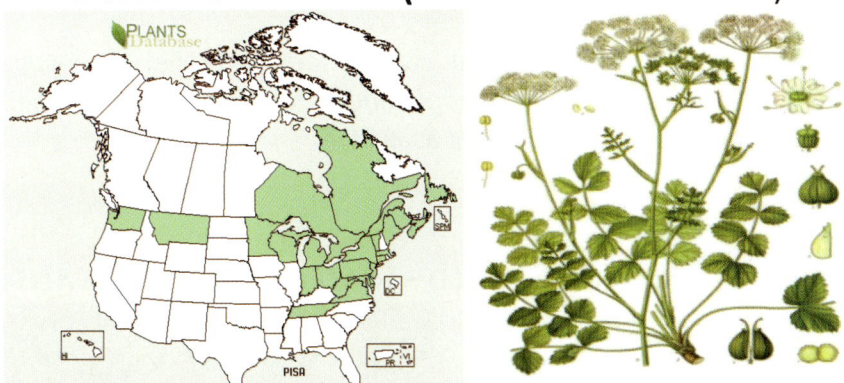

Burnet saxifrage grows well on dry ground of limestone, meadows, and hedgerows.

Burnet saxifrage is a perennial plant, its flower heads have crimson spots, flowers, and its leafstalks are reddish in color. It flowers from July to August. In addition, the whole herb is gathered and dried in July.

The plant is considered helpful in wounds. Internal use eases digestion and helps breathing problems. It's used in treatments of kidney and urinary diseases. The root is anti-inflammatory and when chewed fresh is effective for toothaches. Burnet also soothes coughs and symptoms of hoarseness and lung problems. Distilled water boiled with plant is used as an eye lotion.

BUTCHER'S BROOM - (RUSCUS ACULEATUS)

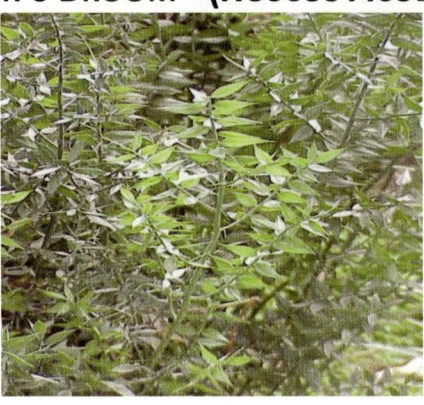

Butcher's broom is a low-growing, evergreen shrub. It has a thick root and tough, stem with false thorny leaves. Flowers are small and greenish-white in the early spring. Female flowers are followed by scarlet red berries. It grows in woods, waste, and bushy areas.

The root and stem are what is used for water weight, swollen feet, and relief of constipation. Topical use of butcher's broom is said to be helpful in treatment of varicose veins, also hemorrhoids that are varicose veins. In addition, butcher's broom has been used as a laxative.

CALENDULA AKA MARIGOLD - (CALENDULA OFFICINALIS)

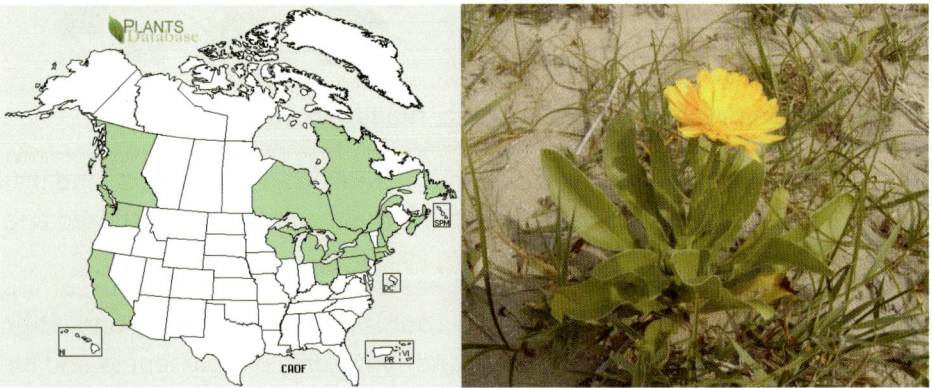

Marigold can be found in warm, temperate regions of the world. It prefers full sun and well-drained soil. Marigold is an annual plant having oblong, slightly toothed and hairy leaves that are pale-green in color. The flower is usually golden-yellow or orange with a thick flower head having a strong and unpleasant odor.

Marigold has anti-inflammatory, antiseptic, and antispasmodic properties. Used externally, it is an excellent healing agent and can be used to treat bruises, burns, wounds, rashes, sores, skin inflammations, and hemorrhoids. It can soothe pain and swellings after wasp or bee stings (just rub the affected part with marigold flowers). It can be an effective remedy against athlete's foot, candida, and ringworm. It is a beneficial herb for both internal and external ulcers. Used internally, marigold can help in cases of ulcers and various infections of mouth and throat. Used in form of a tea, it can improve digestion, soothe menstrual cramps, and help in cases of liver disorders, constipation, colitis, and menopause.

The leaf has been proven to high in the mineral calcium.

Californian Poppy – (Eschscholtzia Californica)

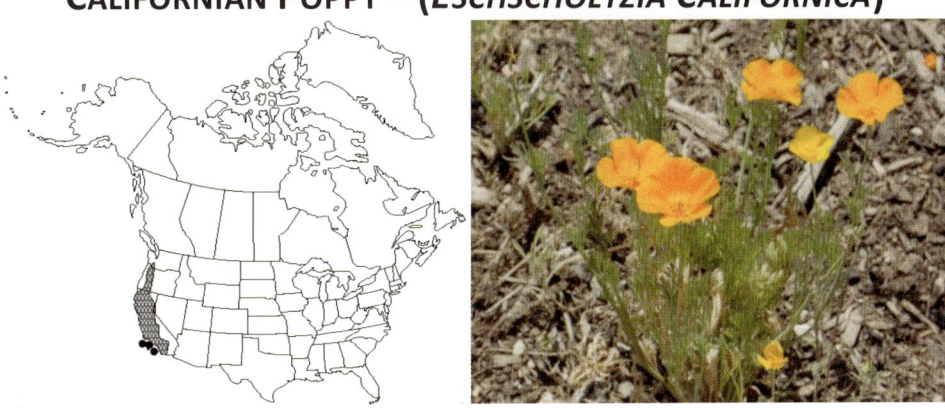

The Californian poppy is a bitter sedative herb that acts in these ways:

- As a diuretic
- Relieves pain
- Relaxes spasms
- Promotes perspiration
- Relaxes nervous tension and anxiety
- Helps insomnia
- Benefits incontinence (especially in children)

The whole plant is harvested when in flower and dried for use in tinctures and infusions. It is similar in its effect to the opium poppy (papaver somniferum) but is much milder in its action and does not depress the central nervous system. Another report says that it has a markedly different effect upon the central nervous system, that it is not a narcotic but tends to normalize psychological function. Its gently antispasmodic, sedative and analgesic actions make it a valuable herbal medicine for treating physical and psychological problems in children. It may also prove beneficial in attempts to overcome bedwetting, difficulty in sleeping, and nervous tension, and anxiety. An extract of the root is used as a wash on the breasts to suppress the flow of milk in lactating females.

Camu-Camu - (Myrciaria Dubia)

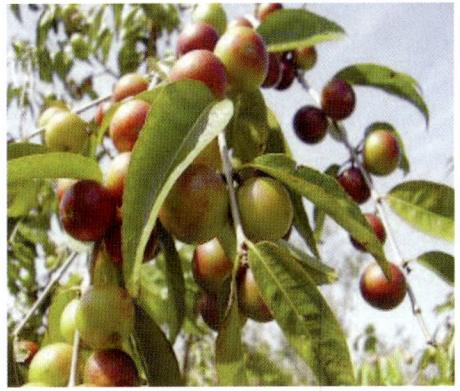

Camu-camu is the name of a bush which grows in the Amazonian rain forest of Peru. The camu-camu bush produces a fruit with the same name that contains powerful health benefits, including the amino acids serine, valine, and leucine, and more vitamin C than any other known plant in the world. The camu-camu fruit has a wide range health effects. Many people have stopped using large dosages of vitamin C because they find that camu-camu is energizing, mood lifting and highly effective in strengthening the immune system.

The camu-camu fruit is about the size of a large grape and has a purplish red skin with a yellow pulp. It grows wild and is harvested directly into a freezer boat, which travels down the river ways of the Amazon where the fruit is picked at the height of its ripeness and flash-frozen. It is then taken to a processing plant where it is thawed, peeled, liquefied, and spray dried. The resulting powder is a pale pink to yellow beige with very potent effects.

Although the number of milligrams of vitamin C, which camu-camu contains, is low compared to the milligrams in synthetically-derived vitamin C tablets, it has more natural vitamin C than any known plant on the planet. The effects on the human body are incomparable because of its food form with clinical evidence, suggesting that it is far more effective, milligram for milligram, than synthetic vitamin C (ascorbic acid).

CANKERROOT - (COPTIS TRIFOLIA)

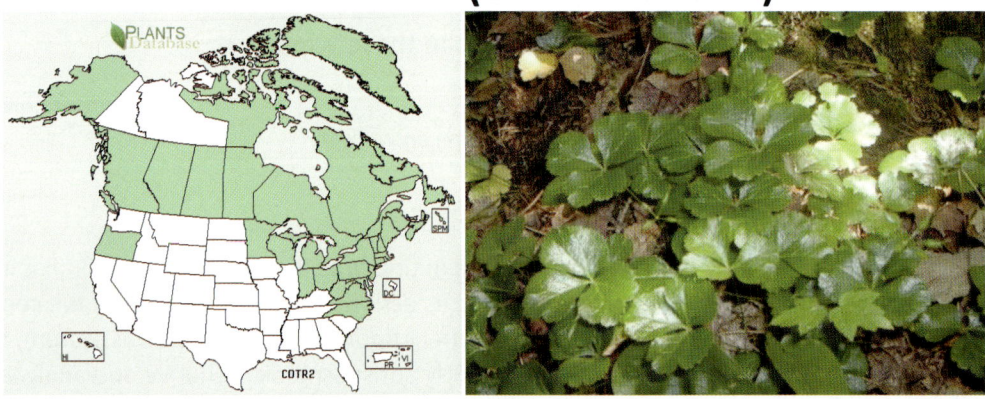

Cankerroot is a small, low-growing perennial plant. It has a slender, golden, creeping root and shiny evergreen leaves. The leaves end in a small, white flower. Each flower has 5-7 petals and many stamens. Flowering time is May to August. The fruit is an oblong capsule or pod-like. It is found in mossy, cool woods and swamps from Labrador south to Maryland and west to Minnesota, Iowa, and Tennessee. Also, found in Canada, Iceland, Siberia, and India.

Cankerroot is used to make bitter tonic for a sedative. Its main use has been as a wash or gargle for sores and ulcers in the mouth, jaundice, throat and even stomach. It has been a popular folk remedy for inflammations in the mouth and around the eyes. It is said to help people combat the craving for alcohol and is used in the treatment of alcoholism. In addition, it improves appetite and was given to children for thrush.

CAPERS - (CAPPARIS SPINOSA)

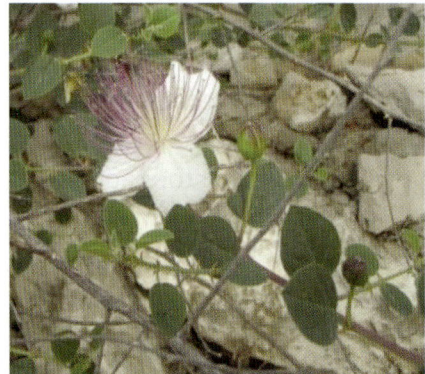

Capers are immature flower buds that have been pickled in vinegar or preserved in granular salt. Semi-mature fruits (caper berries) and young shoots with small leaves may be pickled for use as a condiment.

Capers have a sharp piquant flavor and add pungency, a peculiar aroma, and saltiness to comestibles such as pasta sauces, pizza, fish, meats, and salads. The flavor of apers may be described as being similar to that of mustard and black pepper. Capers make an important contribution to classic Mediterranean flavors that include: olives, anchovies, and artichokes. Tender young shoots including immature small leaves may also be eaten as a vegetable or pickled. More rarely, mature and semi-mature fruits are eaten as a cooked vegetable. Additionally, ash from burned caper roots has been used as a source of salt.

Capers are said to reduce bowel gas and relieve arthritic pain. Capers are recorded a stimulant and protector to improving liver function. Reported uses as a diuretics, kidney ailments, and tonics, infusions from caper root bark have been traditionally used for anemia, arthritis, and gout. Caper extracts and pulps have been used in cosmetics, but there has been reported skin rashes and sensitivity from their use.

CARDAMOM - (*ELLETARIA CARDAMOM*)

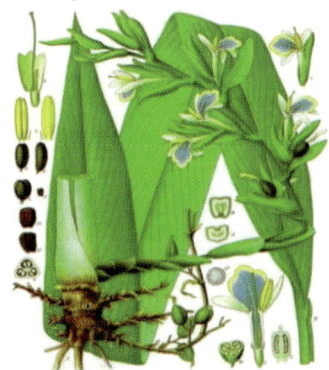

Cardamom plant, native to South Asia, is a perennial herb with a thick underground rhizome bearing stems above. Cardamom is cultivated in evergreen tropical forests under light shade conditions. The chemical constituents of cardamom are protein, fiber, starch, and vitamins A and C. It is used as a spice and traditional medicine in India, China, and Nepal.

Cardamom has a strong pungent smell with a cool taste, similar to mint. Due to its taste, it is popular in South Asia where it is chewed alone or with betel leaf. Cardamom is used to treat digestive disorders like dysentery, constipation, and stomach aches and shown useful in the treatment of congested lungs and pulmonary tuberculosis, inflammation of eyelids, throat troubles, and teeth and gum infections. Cardamom is also used to break up kidney and gallstones. From the research, it is used as an antidote for snake and scorpion venom in South Asia.

Carob - (Caroba Jacaranda Procera)

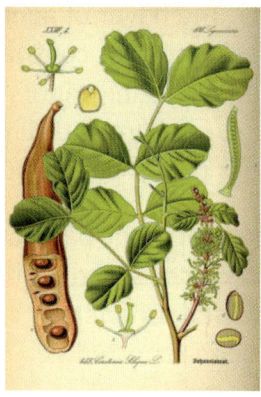

The caroba tree grows in Guiana and Brazil, attaining a height of 30 or 40 feet. The tree has many branches and a crown of beautiful deep-green foliage. The flowers are white, red, and showy, exhaling a honey-like perfume. The fruit is wood like with capsules that contain many seeds. The root of the tree is deep red externally and yellow-white internally. The bark of the tree is of an ash color.

As a medicine, it is used as a diuretic, used to treat syphilis and other venereal diseases. The soothing qualities of the herb have also helped epilepsy, as it has a sedative effect upon the nervous system.

Cascara – (Rhamnus Purshiana)

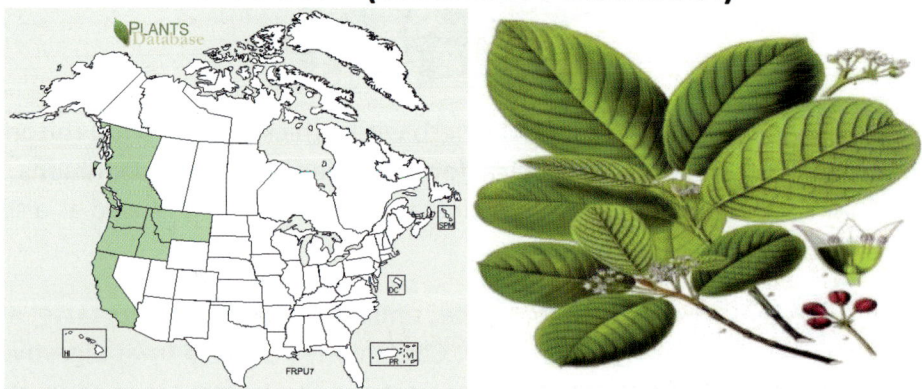

Cascara is obtained from the dried bark of rhamnus purshianus (rhamnaceae), both a medicinal and poisonous plant. It is found in Europe, western Asia, and in North America from northern Idaho to the Pacific coast in mountainous areas. In Spanish, "cascara sagrada" means "sacred bark," perhaps because this woody shrub has provided relief for several constipated individuals. Cascara has been used as a tree bark laxative by Native American tribes and Spanish and Mexican priests since the 1800s. The tree from which cascarilla is obtained is a native of the West Indies, and is found plentifully in the island of Eleutheria, from which it derives its name. It was, for a time, supposed to have been derived from the croton cascarilla, a small tree growing in the Bahamas, Haiti, Peru, and Paraguay, but this is now ascertained by botanists to have been an error. Cascarilla bark is imported from the Islands of Bahamas, Jamaica, etc.

Cascara possesses the following medical uses:

Arrest vomiting
Chronic diarrhoea
Convalescence from acute diseases
Dyspepsia
Flatulency
Purgative
Stimulant laxative for bowel cleansing

Stimulant and cathartic laxatives are the most commonly abused laxatives and have the potential for causing long-term damage.

CAT'S CLAW - (UNCARIA TOMENTOSA)

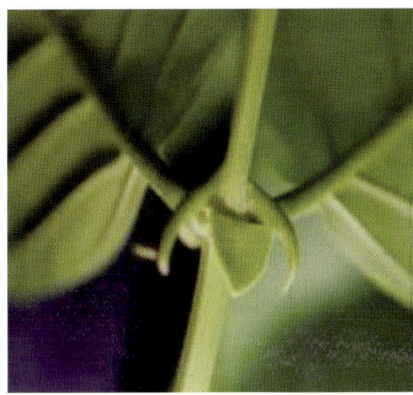

Cat's claw is a woody vine with hook-like thorns that look like claws of a cat. It has dark green leaves, opposite and compound, with small leaflets that grow into oval shaped leaves. Flowers are trumpet-shaped and bright yellow in color with airy clusters. Fruit is flat and linear, with oblong, winged seeds. Cat's claw is native to the tropical jungles of South and Central America.

Cat's claw has a rich history of medicine, using the inner bark and root. It was used by Native Americans in treatment of arthritis, digestive complaints, inflammations, wounds, stomach ulcers, and as a form of a birth control. Nowadays the plant is recognized by herbalists mainly due to its antioxidant, anti-inflammatory, anticancer and diuretic properties. The anti-inflammatory effects of cat's claw are very helpful in rheumatoid and osteoarthritis. The plant has a very beneficial influence on our immune system and is used in the treatments of various types of tumors, brain tumors, leukemia, cervical cancer, and melanoma, as well as an herbal supplement in HIV patients. Cat's claw could also be used in different sorts of infectious diseases including Lyme's disease, fevers, wounds, urinary tract infections, and internal hemorrhage.

CATNIP - (NEPETA CATARIA)

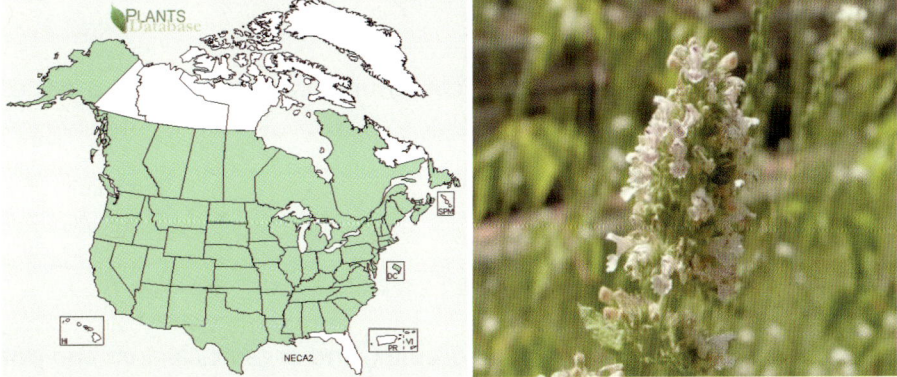

The root is perennial and sends up square, erect, branched stems, 2 to 3 feet high, which are very leafy and covered with a mealy down. The heart-shaped leaves are also covered with a soft, close down, especially on the under sides, which are quite white in color.

It has sedative properties that have a calming and effect. It is used in fevers, colds, headaches, eye inflammation, diarrhea, stomach aches, vomiting, chills, boils, and swellings. A drink of catnip sweetened with honey is taken for relieving coughs, colds, easing gas, spasm, colic, hemorrhoids, allergies, and considered good in treating attention deficit, hyperactivity disorder in children. The oil or a poultice of the leaves is administered for treating bruises, scalp irritations, sore breasts, tonsillitis, rheumatoid arthritis, and skin lesions.

CAYENNE – (CAPSICUM ANNUUM)

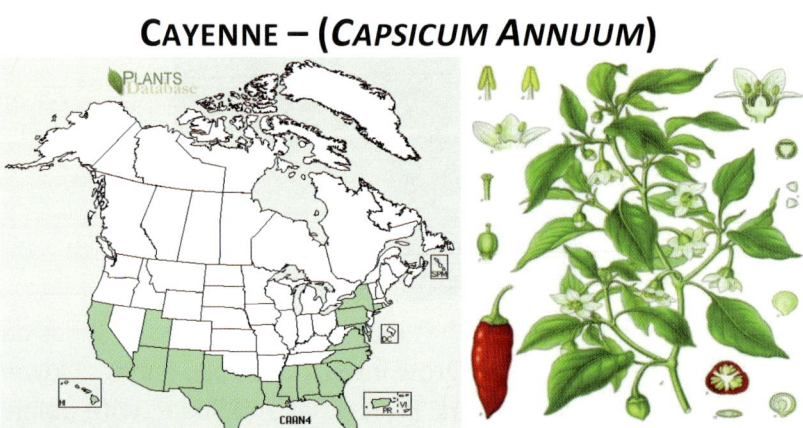

Cayenne or capsicum derives its name from a Greek term, "to bite," in reference to the hot pungent properties of the fruits and seeds. Cayenne pepper was introduced into Britain from India in 1548, and Gerard mentioned it as being cultivated in his time. The plant was described by Linnaeus under the name of C. frutescens proper. This species appeared in Miller's Garden Dictionary in 1771.

The Memorial Sloan-Kettering Cancer Center explains that capsicum is used to relieve pain, improve circulation, promote weight loss, and treat headaches and psoriasis. The FDA approved capsicum for postherapetic neuralgia management.

Cayenne is used for:

Arthritis	Menstrual cramps	Rheumatism
Colds	Muscle pain	Some types of herpes
Fevers	Neuralgia	Treat headaches
Increase appetite and sweating	Psoriasis	
Indigestion	Relieving gas and colic	

According to research, capsicum annum possesses a constituent called capsaicin and these properties apply to:

Analgesic alterative	Astringent	Stimulant
Antiseptic	Carminative	Stomachic
Antispasmodic	Hemostatic	

Capsicum annum is also rich in vitamins A, C, and B complex, and organic calcium and potassium as minerals. Capsicum is widely suggested as a heart stimulant and for its substantial antigenotoxic and anticarcinogenic effects, and as an important dietary phytochemical with potential chemopreventive activity. Capsicum annum has a strong effect upon the circulatory system, initially acting upon the heart and large arteries, followed by a stimulatory action upon the arterioles and the capillaries.

CELANDINE - (CHELIDONIUM MAJUS)

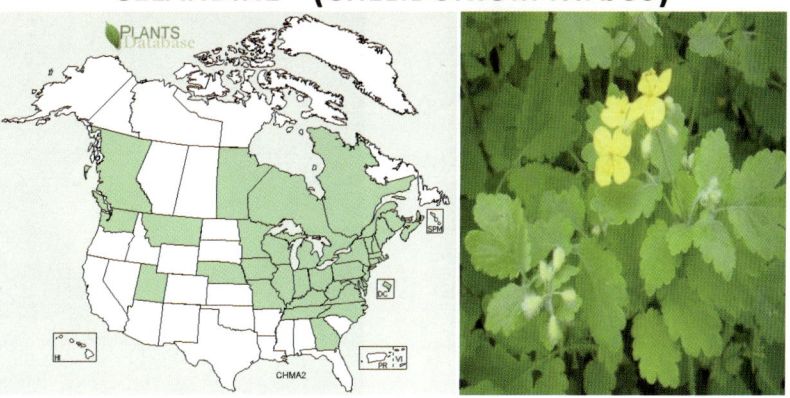

Greater celandine is native to Europe and western Asiaand is found on damp ground, hedgerows, and alongside walls.

A perennial plant, it has a fleshy orange taproot and an erect, hairy stem with a rosette of dark, basal green leaves. Flowers are bright yellow with four petals growing from the center clusters. Flowering starts in late spring, continuing throughout the summer. Seeds are pinhead size and black, borne in a long capsule.

The flowering parts and roots are considered a mild analgesic and sedative. Studies suggest that the plant could be very useful in relieving gallbladder spasms and can act as a gallbladder stimulator. Furthermore, Greater Celandine has shown to be very effective in calming abdominal pains and relieving symptoms of indigestion, abdominal cramps, and nausea. Finally, external use is very effective against warts and can be beneficial in small open wounds.

CELERY SEED - (APIUM GRAVEOLENS)

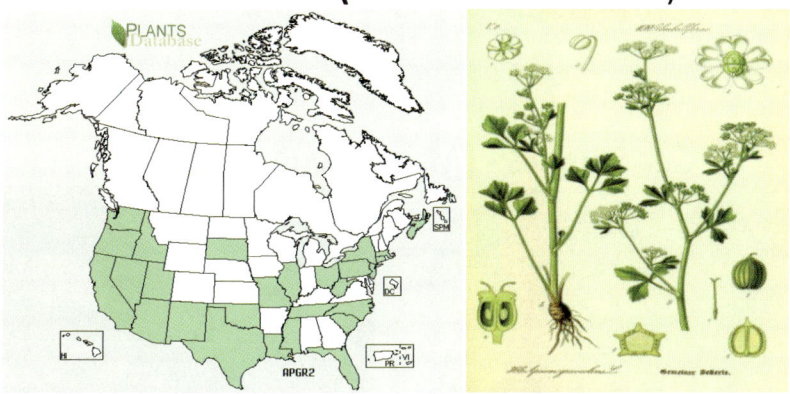

Celery seed is used primarily as a diuretic, meaning it increases urine output to help the body get rid of excess water. Sometimes it is used for treating arthritis, gout, reducing muscle spasms, calming nerves, and reducing inflammation. However, there are no scientific studies in people that show whether celery seed helps treat these conditions or any others. Studies do show celery seeds act as a mosquito repellent. A few animal studies suggest celery seed extracts may help lower blood pressure and cholesterol, as well as protect the liver from damaging substances such as the pain reliever.

Researchers have found people who eat a diet rich in lutein—found in celery, spinach, broccoli, lettuce, tomatoes, oranges, carrots, and greens—were less likely to develop colorectal cancer. However, celery was just one part of their diet. So no one knows whether it was celery, another food, or some combination of foods that lowered their risk of cancer.

CHAMOMILE - (MATRICARIA CHAMOMILLA)

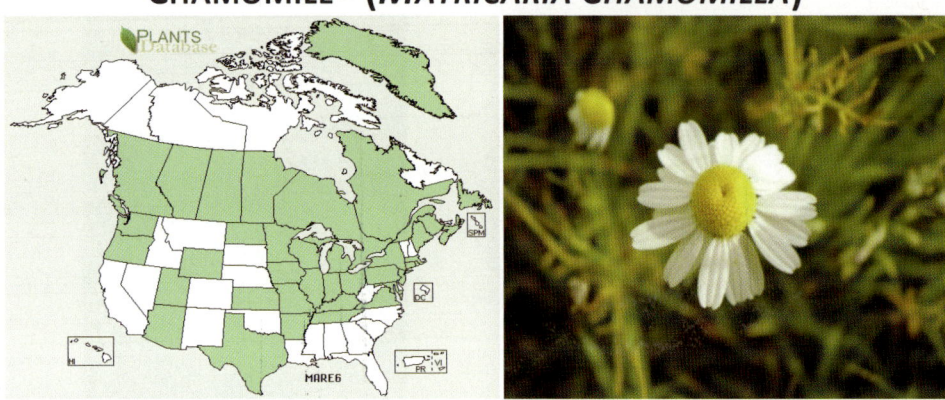

Chamomile is native to Europe. It grows best in clay, poor, and mountain soils. A low-growing annual plant, it has smooth, erect and hairy stems on leaves that are long and narrow. It has white flowers with a yellow center. Chamomile flowers from July to September with fruit that is small and dry.

Chamomile has been used for centuries with a variety of ailments, considered to have analgesic, anti-inflammatory and anti spasm relief. It has a strong scent. As a tonic, it is a laxative, a stomach aide (soothes and calms the stomach and is often recommended for various digestive problems; stomach pain and commonly used in treating ailments like, gas, colic, hernia and ulcer), and a sedative. Because of its calm, soothing effect it can be used for nerves and headaches, as well as anxiety and panic attacks. Chamomile tea is useful in easing menstrual pain, treating hay fever, asthma, and as a sleep aid. Used externally, it soothes the skin, helps in cases of various allergies, sore skin, and rash.

The following minerals can be found in the flower:

Aluminum	Magnesium	Silica
Calcium	Manganese	Sodium
Chromium	Nitrogen	Tin
Cobalt	Potassium	Zinc
Iron	Selenium	

CHAMOMILE - (MATRICARIA RECUTITA)

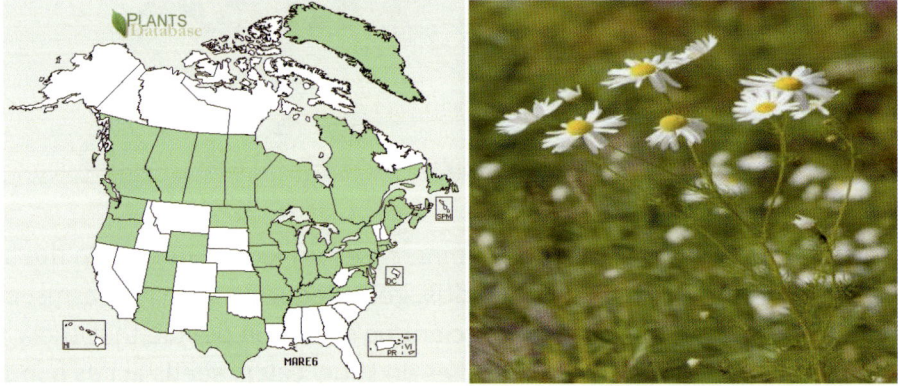

Drink chamomile tea on a regular basis in order to get the best effects and the following health benefits.

It has a relaxing, anti-inflammatory effect on the smooth muscles that line the digestive tract, beneficial to a wide range of gastrointestinal complaints, including heartburn, excessive gas, bloating in the intestines and inflammatory bowel disease. Drink chamomile tea twice a day. If you feel anxious, drink some chamomile tea. It is a natural stress reliever and will calm your nerves. Chamomile appears to have a mild sedating effect but, more importantly, it also calms the body, making it easier for the person taking it to fall asleep naturally. Chamomile tea can help relieve pain from migraine headache because of its anti-inflammatory effect and beneficial to those women suffering from menstrual cramps. Eyewashes made from the cooled tea may relieve the redness or irritation. For inflammations, prepare a fresh batch of tea daily and store it in a sterile container. (Label eye baths left and right, and use appropriately.) Chamomile tea used daily as a gargle or mouthwash can help heal mouth sores and prevent gum disease. Those dark circles under your eyes can disappear if you use chamomile. Dip tea bags into warm water, and then apply to your eyes.

Concentrated chamomile extracts are also added to creams and lotions or packaged as pills or tinctures.

Chamomile can help lighten your skin tone. Just bring two quarts of water to a boil with two chamomile tea bags in it. Then place your face above the steaming pot of tea. A bath in water mixed with chamomile tea works too. As a bath, it can be relaxing and provide relief for dry, irritated skin or sunburn. Add 10 drops of chamomile oil or several cups of chamomile tea to a cool bath and soak for half an hour or longer. Chamomile creams that you can buy in health-food shops, may relieve sunburn, as well as skin rashes such as eczema. Treat burns with chamomile creams or teas rather than greasy ointments. The latter contain oils that can trap the heat, slow healing, and increase the risk of infection. Creams, on the other hand, are made with a non-oily base. A dressing soaked in chamomile tea is also beneficial when applied to mild burns.

CHAPARRAL - (*LARREA DIVARICATA*)

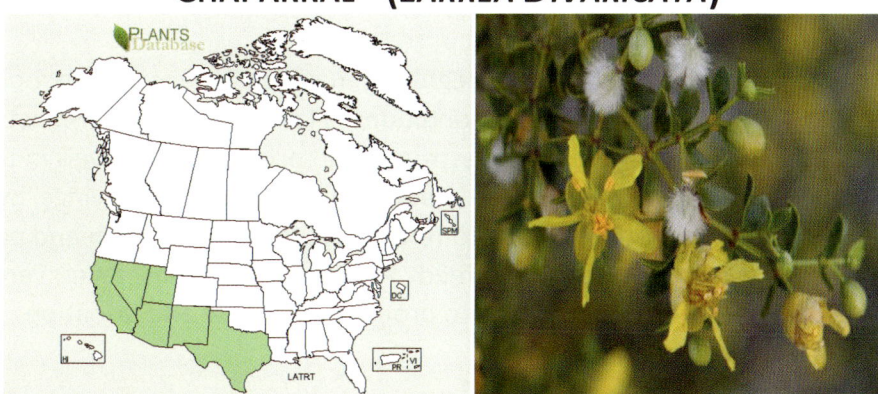

Chaparral's greatest ability is to move the lymphatic system, helping to draw toxic chemicals and harmful drugs out of the cells. Chaparral is a good blood purifier. It contains powerful antioxidants that protect against formation of tumors, cancer cells, over-exposure and against harmful effects of radiation. It has an anti-HIV activity, helps remove boils, abscesses, improves liver function, cleansing to the urinary system, and has a strong anti-inflammatory effect, is helpful against athlete's foot, nail fungus, ringworm, and vaginal yeast infections. It is applied to wounds as an antiseptic, to the scalp as a hair tonic, makes a good hair rinse, and reduces dandruff. A liniment made from chaparral or a bath made by soaking the leaves in water is used for rheumatism, also excellent for gout. It is used as remedy against poisonous bites including snakebites.

Note: Chaparral is very bitter and is usually mixed with other herbs or taken in tincture form.

Caution! Heavy users of drugs, including caffeine and alcohol, may experience headaches and nausea when using chaparral as a blood purifier. Always seek professional advice. People who have kidney or liver problems should consult a professional herbalist before using chaparral. Persons who have undergone chemotherapy or other type of drug therapies should seek an herbalist's advice before taking chaparral, because taking this herb may cause nausea or other types of side effects as it releases those substances from the tissues into the blood stream.

Chaste Berry - (Vitex Agnus-Castus)

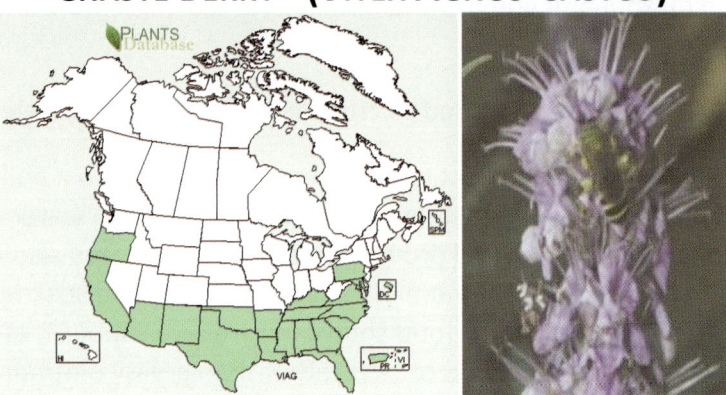

Chaste berry is a native to western Asia and Mediterranean region. The plant prefers full sun or partial shade and well-drained soil.

Chaste berry is a deciduous tree or large shrub. Its leaves are 5 to 7 fingerlike leaflets with slender spikes of violet-blue to deep purple flowers. Flowers are followed by a gray to purple fleshy fruit with four black seeds, similar to black pepper and flowers in early summer.

The leaves, flowers, berries are all used.

Chaste berry is mainly known as a female hormone regulator, having a balancing effect on female hormones and making it useful in a wide variety of conditions. Flavonoids found in chaste berry are now known to affect the pituitary gland, thus regulating estrogen and progesterone levels in the body. Chaste berry seeds can alleviate symptoms of PMS (such as abdominal bloating, mood swings, headaches, breast pain). It can also help in treating menopausal symptoms of irregular menstruation and polycystic ovarian syndrome. Additionally, chaste berry is used as a remedy for acne, headaches, fever, very helpful in cases of night sweats, hot flashes, and fatigue and is used to promote milk flow and urination.

Chickweed - (Stellaria Media)

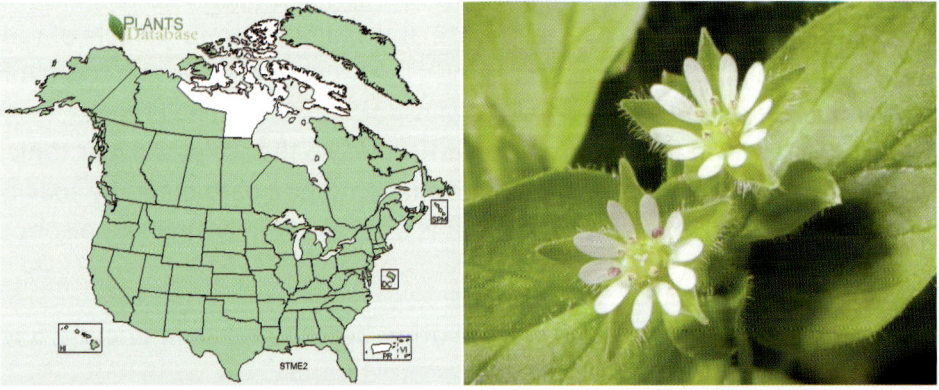

The whole herb is in the best condition for use when collected between May and July. Both the flower and root are used.

Best known for its soothing and healing quality, it has been used for centuries in relieving skin problems such as sores, rashes, and burns. Chickweed has been used traditionally as an external remedy for cuts, wounds, minor burns, abscesses, and skin irritations, especially such as itching, dryness, and irritation due to eczema or psoriasis. Taken internally as a tea or tincture, chickweed has a reputation for helping rheumatism and an infusion of the fresh or dried leaves added to bath water is thought to reduce inflammation caused by rheumatic pain. A poultice of the crushed leaves have been used traditionally to relieve any kind of red face rash and thought to be effective for fragile, superficial veins.

Taken internally in small quantities as a decoction, chickweed has been used for constipation, kidney complaints, quick relief of pain in the digestive system, cystitis and other related urinary tract inflammations. As a detoxification agent, chickweed is considered as effective as burdock root for its blood cleansing abilities. A decoction of the fresh flowering parts is a traditional treatment for relief from extreme physical fatigue and debilitation. Fresh chickweed is delicious and eaten in summer salads.

The medicinal actions of chickweed are anti-rheumatic, skin cleaner, calming effect, diuretic, lotion, and laxative. The benefits of chickweed may be due to its high nutritional value.

Chickweed has the following minerals:

Calcium	Potassium	Sodium
Iron	Phosphorus	Zinc
Magnesium	Selenium	
Manganese	Silica	

Chickweed has the following vitamins:

Vitamin A	Vitamin B_2	Vitamin C
Vitamin B_1	Vitamin B_3	Beta - carot

CHICORY - (CICHORIUM INTYBUS)

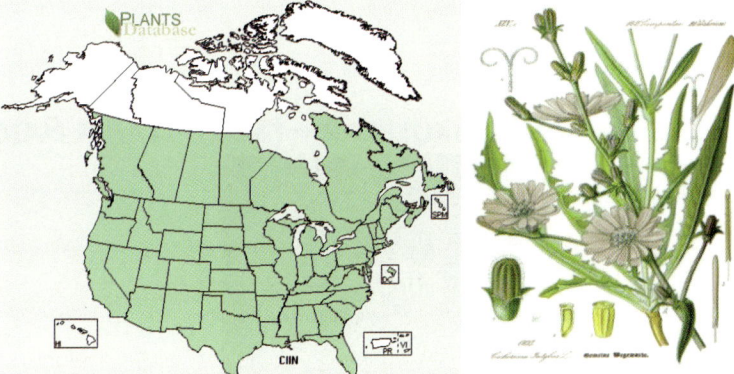

Chicory root is light yellow outside, white from within, containing milky, bitter juice, and is best used during autumn when it has the highest level of inulin. It has shiny leaves, coarsely-toothed near the bottom. The flowers are white to light blue and lavender and toothed at the ends. Flowering occurs from July to October. The root and whole herb are used during blooming period.

The whole plant, especially root, contains essential oils, which produce high toxicity to internal parasites. Chicory is used as a tonic in the treatment of gallstones, sinus problems, cuts, and bruises. Inulin, the dietary fiber found in chicory, is a helpful ingredient in treating diabetes and constipation. Chicory is often recommended for jaundice and spleen problems. The juice made of leaves and a tea made from the blooming plant help the release of gallstones, elimination of internal mucus and production of bile, they are also useful for intestinal problems: digestive difficulties, gastritis, and lack of appetite.

CHINESE ANGELICA - (ANGELICA SINENSIS)

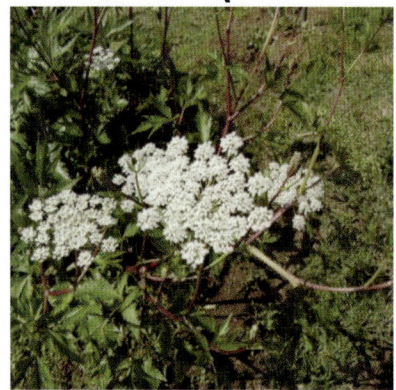

Chinese angelica is also called angelica root and dong quai. This herb is primarily used to relieve reproductive problems in females. In particular, treatment includes lowering menopausal symptoms, regulating cycles, and relieving menstrual cramps. There is no scientific evidence to support angelica's effectiveness in treating these problems, but angelica has been used in oriental medicine to treat these symptoms for centuries.

Oriental medicine often combines Chinese angelica root with various other herbs to provide treatment for conditions such as high blood pressure, arthritis, allergies, and asthma.

The following minerals can be found in Chinese angelica:

Silica	Sodium
Zinc	Tin

CHINESE SKULLCAP, BAICAL SKULLCAP – (SCUTELLARIA BAICALENSIS)

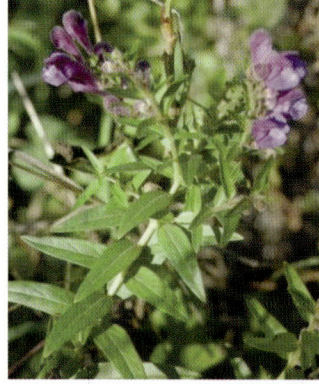

From at least the 2nd century, baical skullcap has had a central place in Chinese herbal medicine and is one of the main remedies for "hot and damp" conditions, such as dysentery and diarrhea. The root is used.

Scutellaria baicalensis seems to be a good:

Antiviral
Antibacterial
Antifungal
Anti-inflammatory

Both topical and oral preparations serve for reducing inflammation, inhibition of angiogenesis (the growth of the new blood vessels, which occurs during the spreading of cancerous tumors), and preventing ethanol-induced hyperlipidemia and histamine release from the mast cells.

All the scientists agree that flavonoids are the main chemicals which display beneficial effects in the human body. They are believed to possess anticancer abilities. The studies conducted by this time support this theory.

Baicalin is said to be the most powerful and promising flavonoid peculiar for this herb. The plant's root is a valuable herbal remedy against many diseases. Baicalin is believed to interfere with hormonal reactions and release of histamines and bile in the body; it stimulates gallbladder activity, inhibits inflammation, as well as suppresses the activity of leukaemia-derived T-cells and replication of viruses and bacteria.

Long history of use, herbalists' observations, and recently-conducted laboratory studies on animals support the claims that scutellaria baicalensis helps fight, lessen, or prevent such diseases as:

Allergies and asthma
Anxiety and stress
Cancer
Chronic fatigue syndrome
Diabetes and atherosclerosis
Ear infections
Headache and hangover
Heart attack
High cholesterol
Hypertension
Influenza
Periodontal disease
Pneumonia

Skullcap is a popular remedy among herbalists and those people who seek for disease elimination with natural means. Hopefully soon, scientific research will provide more information on the hidden power of the herb, its benefits, and what is even more important, on its practical use, dosage, and risks.

CHISO AKA BEEFSTEAK PLANT - (PERILLA FRUTESCENS)

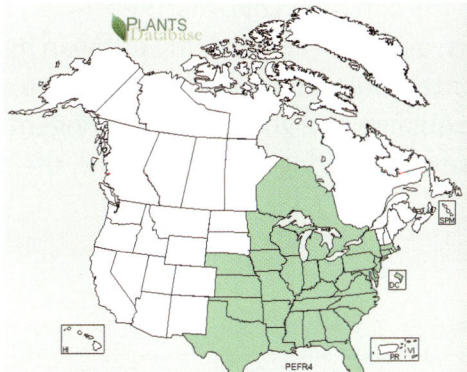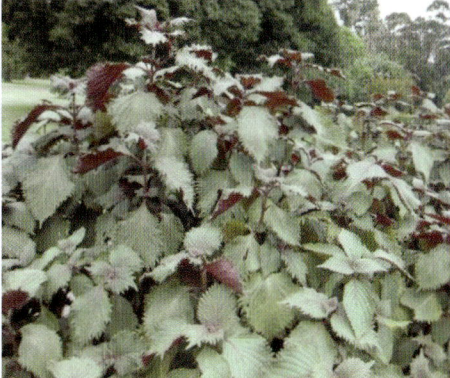

Chiso is a member of the mint family and has been used in Asian remedies for centuries. It is traditionally used as a natural remedy in China, Japan, India, and Vietnam. The popularity of the herb has grown in the West with increasing interest in health benefits for natural medicine.

Chiso's health benefits for the skin are part of its growing appeal. The leaves made into a tea contain anti-inflammatory, antioxidant, and allergy-fighting properties. It gives the immune system a boost and helps the skin look healthier by giving the complexion a radiant glow.

Chiso tea can be made iced or hot, depending on personal preference. The benefits provided to the skin are not only found in tea, but many different lotions, moisturizers, soaps, and salves contain chiso leaves or essential oils. Rich in vitamins and minerals that promote certain health benefits, the essential oils found in chiso are high in the omega-3 fatty acid ALA.

CINCHONA - (CINCHONA OFFICINALIS)

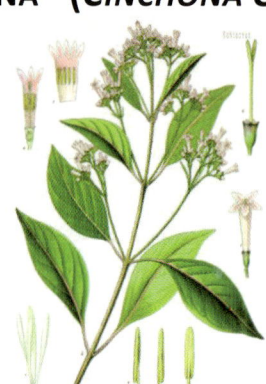

Cinchona is native to Amazon Rainforest vegetation and is renowned for its numerous health and therapeutic benefits. It is particularly found in the eastern slopes of the Andes Mountains. Cinchona is a tropical evergreen tree and shrub, with rather large opposite leaves and white or pink fragrant flowers arranged in clusters. Though its common name is quinine, not all species of cinchona can be used to produce quinine; in fact, many contain virtually no quinine at all. Apart from this, quinine is also found in the northern zone of the Andes, towards the eastern slopes of the central and western ranges. Because of its usefulness in curing diseases and ailments, the herb is now cultivated in many tropical areas for commercial purpose.

Quinine is an anti-fever agent and is used for the prevention and cure of malaria. Its bark is an important herbal medicine and is used as a tonic and a digestive stimulant for the cure of conditions like indigestion, gastro-intestinal disorders, and as an appetite stimulant. Certain forms of folk medicine in the southern zone of America use the herb for curing different types of cancer, like breast cancer, liver cancer, cancer of the spleen and other glands. Besides this, it is used for the common cold, diarrhea, fever, lumbago, malaria, pneumonia, sciatica, varicose veins, hangovers, and even typhoid. In European herbal medicine systems, quinine bark is used as an antispasmodic, a bitter tonic, and fever reducer, for treating irregular heartbeats, anemia, and leg cramps. Many people use quinine as a good throat astringent and its powdered form is often used in tooth powders because of its astringency. In general, the herb can be classified as an excellent analgesic.

CINNAMON - (CINNAMOMUM ZEYLANICUM)

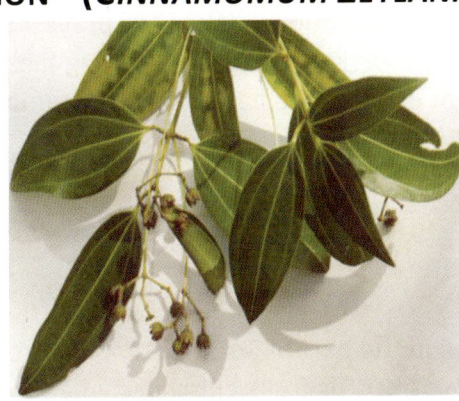

Cinnamon is traditionally used by many ancient cultures. It is indicated for a variety of ailments including gastrointestinal problems, urinary infections, and relieving symptoms of colds and flues. It also has remarkable anti-fungal and anti-bacterial properties. Some studies have shown that cinnamon helps people with diabetes metabolize sugar better.

True cinnamon, or cinnamomum zeylanicum, is the inner bark of a small evergreen tree native to Sri Lanka. It was used in ancient Egypt for embalming and to prevent spoiling of food. During the Bubonic Plague, sponges were soaked in cinnamon and cloves and placed in sick rooms. Cinnamon was the most sought after spice during explorations of the 15th and 16th centuries.

Cinnamon extracts have been used medically for intestinal problems and calming the stomach. It is useful in digestion, colic, grip, diarrhea, and nausea and vomiting. Also a carminative, an agent that helps break up intestinal gas traditionally used to combat diarrhea and morning sickness, infections and thrush (oral yeast infection), bacteria that causes stomach ulcers, and even head lice. It has an astringent action, stemming nosebleeds, heavy periods, and resolving diarrhea.

Cinnamon allows diabetics to use less insulin—helping control blood sugar levels.

In both India and Europe, cinnamon has been traditionally taken as a warming herb for "cold" conditions, often in combination with ginger. The herb stimulates circulation, especially to the fingers and toes and used for arthritis, a traditional remedy for aching muscles and symptoms of colds and flu.

CITRONELLA - (CYMBOPOGON NARDUS)

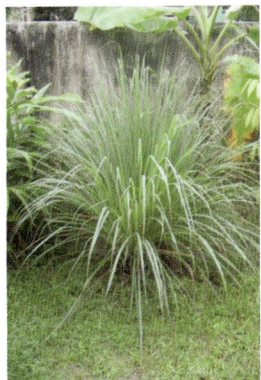

Citronella grass is a coarse, clumping tropical grass, with cane-like stems and its leaves are grayish green. It is often referred to as the "mosquito plant" because it naturally repels insects, so plant it near patios or along walkways to enjoy the fragrance.

Oil of citronella has been used for over 50 years as an insect and animal repellent. It is found in many familiar insect repellent products: candles, lotions, gels, and sprays. These products repel various insects, some of which are public health pests, such as mosquitoes, biting flies, and fleas. When used according to the label, citronella products are not expected to cause harm to humans, pets, or the environment.

CITRUS FRUITS

Citrus is believed to have originated in the part of Southeast Asia bordered by Northeastern India, and the Yunnan Province of China. Examples of citrus fruits cultivated in an ever-widening area since ancient times are oranges, lemons, grapefruit, and limes.

Citrus juice also has medical uses. Lemon juice is used to relieve bee stings. Oranges were historically used for their high content of vitamin C, which prevents scurvy. Scurvy is caused by vitamin C deficiency and can be prevented with 10 milligrams a day. An early sign of scurvy is fatigue, if ignored; later symptoms are bleeding and bruising easily. Citrus fruit juices, such as orange, lime, and lemons may be useful for lowering the risk factors for specific types of kidney stones. Lemons have the highest concentration of citrate of any citrus fruit, and daily consumption of lemonade has been shown to decrease the rate of stone formation.

Citrons

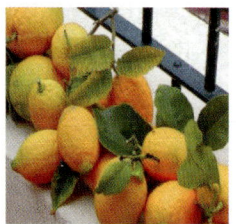

Key Lime - *(Citrus Aurantifolia)*

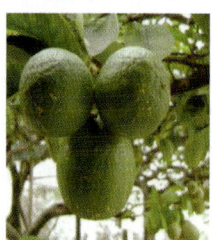

Pomelo - *(Citrus Maxima)*

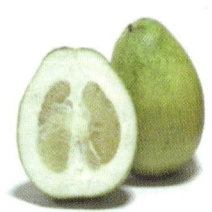

Citron, from India - *(Citrus Medica)*

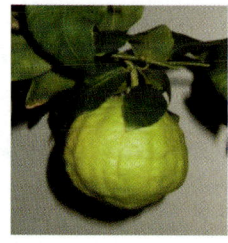

Mandarin orange, from China - China - *(Citrus Reticulata)*

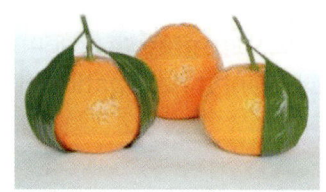

Trifoliate Orange, from Korea and adjacent *(Citrus Trifoliata)*

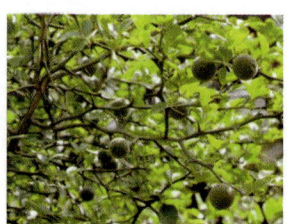

Australian limes

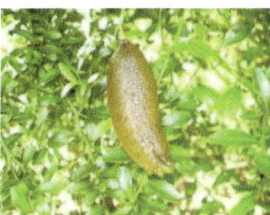

Finger Lime - (*Citrus Australasica*)

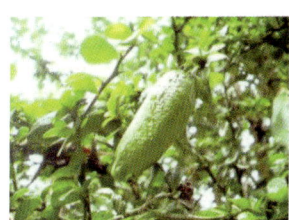

Australian Round Lime -

(*Citrus Australis*)

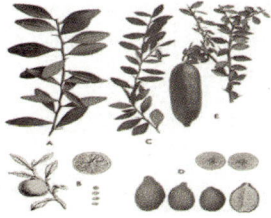

Desert Lime - (*Citrus Glauca*)

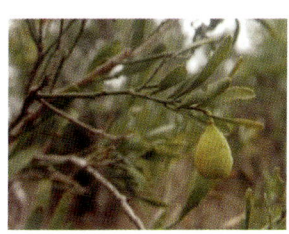

Kumquats

4-5 species from East Asia ranging into Southeast Asia

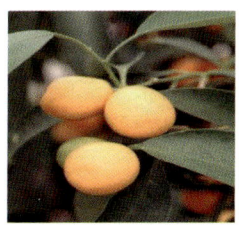

Limau Kadangsa, Limau Kedut Kera –

(*Citrus Halimii*) - Thailand and Malaya

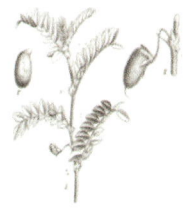

Indian Wild Orange

(**Citrus Indica**) - Indian subcontinent

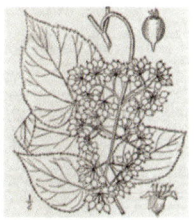

Citrus Macroptera

Indochina and Melanesia

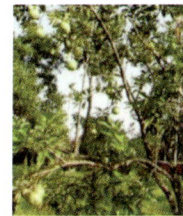

Chinese Angelica aka Dong Quai – (Angelica Sinensis)

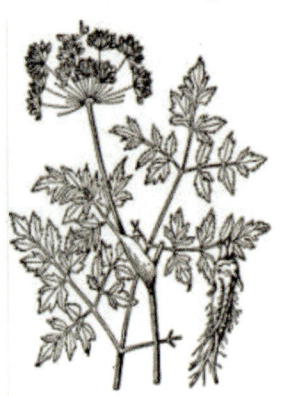

Chinese angelica has been used for thousands of years in traditional Chinese, Korean, and Japanese medicine. It remains one of the most popular plants in Chinese medicine, used primarily for health conditions in women. Dong quai is used for female disorders such as painful menstruation or pelvic pain, recovery from childbirth or illness, and fatigue/low vitality. It is also given for strengthening the blood, heart conditions, high blood pressure, inflammation, headache, infections, and nerve pain.

The following minerals can be found in Chinese Angelica:

Nitrogen	Silica	Zinc
Potassium	Sodium	
Selenium	Tin	

Cleavers – (Galium Aparine)

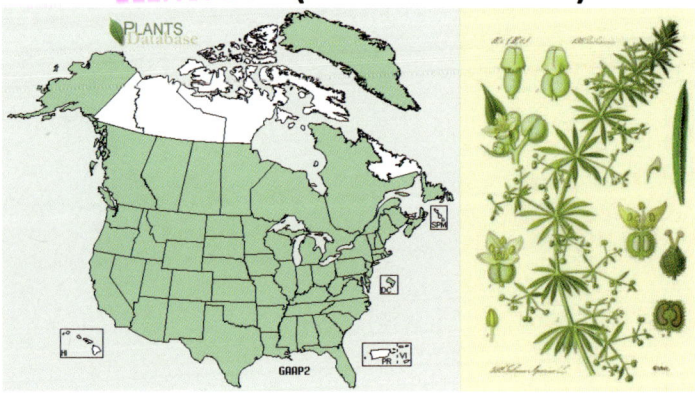

Cleavers (galium aparine) is a climbing plant native to North America, Europe, and Asia. It has been used to coagulate milk. According to some herbalists, cleavers is a good lymphatic and blood purifying tonic and is often used to treat swollen glands and skin eruptions caused by lymphatic congestion. It has also been recommended as a diuretic for chronic cystitis (inflamed bladder) and prostatitis (enlarged prostate), and has been used traditionally as a treatment for epilepsy. Herbalists have long regarded cleavers as a valuable lymphatic tonic and diuretic. The lymph system is the body's mechanism to wash tissues of toxins, passing them back into the bloodstream to be cleansed by the liver and kidneys. This cleansing action makes cleavers useful in treating conditions like psoriasis and arthritis, which benefit from purifying the blood. Cleavers is a reliable diuretic used to help clean gravel and urinary stones and to treat urinary infections. Externally, a tea made from cleavers can be used as a skin wash to improve the complexion and treat skin disorders, and heal cuts and scrapes. The tea can also be put to good use as a hair rinse to fight dandruff. Cleavers is a coffee relative, and the roasted seeds are used as a coffee substitute. The young leaves can be eaten like spinach.

Cleavers' side effects: Cleavers is considered a safe herb.

CLOVE - (SYZYGIUM AROMATICUM)

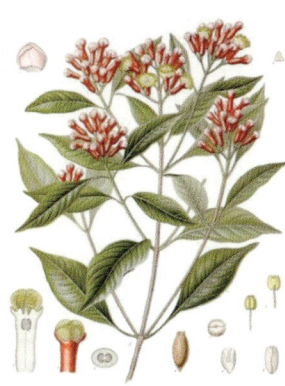

Cloves are used in Indian, Chinese, and western herbal dentistry where the essential oil is used as a painkiller applied to a cavity in a decayed tooth; it can relieve a toothache for dental emergencies. It also helps decrease infection in the teeth due to its antiseptic properties. Topical application over the stomach or abdomen are said to warm the digestive tract. Clove oil is used in various skin disorders like acne, pimples, severe burns, skin irritations and to reduce the sensitivity of skin. Cloves may be used internally as a tea and topically as oil for hypotonic muscles.

The following minerals can be found in cloves:

Aluminum	Iron	Potassium
Boron	Magnesium	Sodium
Calcium	Manganese	Strontium
Chromium	Nickel	Zinc
Cobalt	Nitrogen	

COCOA – (THEOBROMA CACAO)

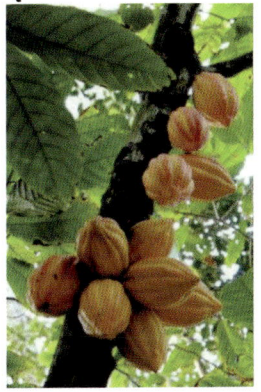

Cocoa comes from a small tree typically growing twenty to thirty feet in height and native to South America, but now cultivated in many hot climates around the globe, particularly in West Africa. The latest developments in chocolate research, published in the *Journal of the American Medical Association*, include two clinical studies suggesting that the chemicals found in cocoa have positive effects on vascular health. Additionally, chocolate, perhaps the world's favorite flavor contains chemicals like those found in grape seed and green tea that can help improve blood circulation, reduce blood pressure, and provide numerous other health benefits. Recent studies now confirm that flavonoids, such as those in cocoa, support heart health by decreasing oxidation of LDL cholesterol, decrease the body's inflammatory immune responses, improve the ability of arteries to dilate and inhibit that aggregation of platelets in the bloodstream. With today's additives, a chocolate bar is not the same as cocoa alone.

CODONOPSIS – (*CODONOPSIS PILOSULA*)

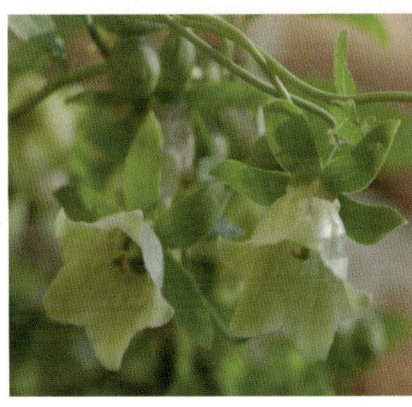

Codonopsis holds an important role in traditional Chinese and Japanese medicine as a remedy for chronic fatigue, or what is called "false fire syndrome" in China. Codonopsis was first described in the herbal tome Ben Jing Feng Yaun in 1695 C.E. as a lung cleanser. As a cooling herb, codonopsis is useful in any illness in which spleen deficiency of digestive energies is the underlying cause. It is also known to strengthen the digestive, respiratory, and immune systems. It has been called the "poor man's ginseng" as it has often been used as a ginseng substitute in herbal formulas when ginseng was too expensive or not available. Codonopsis has been used for centuries to treat appetite loss, diarrhea, and vomiting.

Laboratory studies suggest that codonopsis extracts act by reducing the secretion of pepsin in the stomach, and by slowing the rate at which the stomach passes food to the intestines. In animal studies, codonopsis can prevent the formation of peptic ulcers induced by stress. Codonopsis also eases asthma attacks by reducing the production of hormones that cause constriction of the bronchia passages. With the healing properties, this herb is especially useful for asthma or peptic ulcers that are compounded by loss of appetite, diarrhea, or vomiting. Codonopsis may also be used to assist recovery of cancer patients treated with radiation therapy.

COLEUS – (*COLEUS FORSKOHLII*)

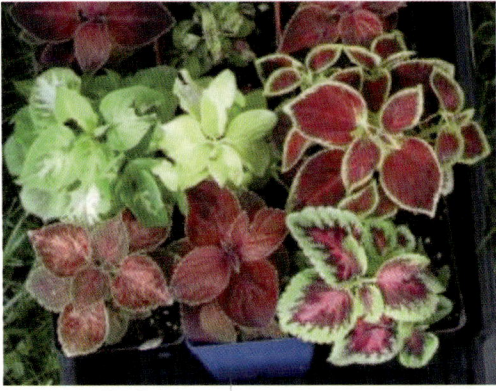

Coleus is a not a particularly remarkable plant to look at, yet is has a 3000-year history in Ayurvedic medicine and is mentioned in ancient Sanskrit texts as a tonic for healthy heart and lungs.

Today, coleus is not just an herb for cardiovascular ailments but is increasingly being used to assist weight loss by breaking down adipose tissue and preventing production of fatty tissue. In addition, coleus mildly stimulates the metabolism by increasing thyroid hormones and increases the secretion of insulin. Coleus forskohlii preparations used as eye drops are known to reduce eye pressure in glaucoma. Conditions such as hypothyroidism, eczema, and psoriasis are also improved by using coleus. It is a popular herb for angina and for the health of the hearth. Coleus increases stroke volume, which is the amount of blood pumped in each heart beat, and reduces the risk of blood clots; coleus lowers high blood pressure by acting to relax the arterial walls.

Indian and Chinese studies in the last two years have isolated a number of diterpenoids in the stem and leaves of coleus forskohlii with a focus on treatment of gastric cancer and preventing metastatic (secondary) cancers. These have been carried out on animal models with considerable success.

Care should be used when using coleus with any medication to control asthma or cardiac disease. It is essential to consult your health care professional when altering medications and to thoroughly investigate how medications may interact with each other. If you take blood pressure and heart medications such as beta-blockers, clonidine, hydralazine you should only take coleus under the guidance of a physician. Similarly, blood thinners including warfarin and heparin warrant coleus to be taken with caution under your physician's care.

COMFREY - (SYMPHYTUM OFFICINALE)

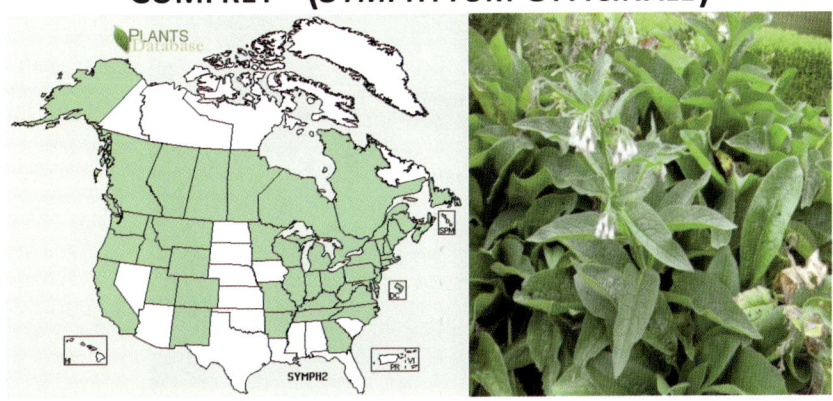

Comfrey leaves and roots also are used topically to treat:

- Arthritis
- Bone injuries
- Broken bones
- Cancer
- Circulation
- Diarrhea
- Expectorant
- Inflammation
- Sedative
- Sores
- Sprains
- Stimulant
- Swelling
- Wounds

Comfrey administration promotes an increase in bone density around titanium implants in the initial period of bone healing.

CORIANDER - (CORIANDRUM SATIVUM)

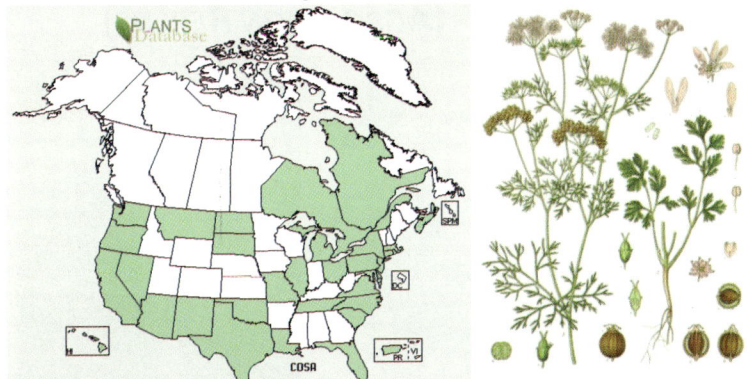

Coriander, like many spices, contains antioxidants, which can delay or prevent the spoilage of food seasoned with this spice. A study found both leaves and seeds to contain antioxidants, but the leaves were found to have a stronger effect. Coriander has been used as a folk medicine for the relief of anxiety and insomnia. In Iran, coriander seeds are used in traditional Indian medicine as a diuretic by boiling equal amounts of coriander seeds and cumin seeds, then cooling and consuming the resulting liquid. In traditional medicine, it is used as a calming aid and as a digestive aid. Coriander has been documented as a traditional treatment for diabetes. A study on mice found that coriander extract had both insulin-releasing and insulin-like activity. Coriander seeds were found in a study on rats to have a significant effect, resulting in lowering levels of total cholesterol.

Coriander juice (mixed with turmeric powder or mint juice) is used for acne, applied to the face in the manner of toner.

CORYDALIS – (CORYDALIS AMBIGUA)

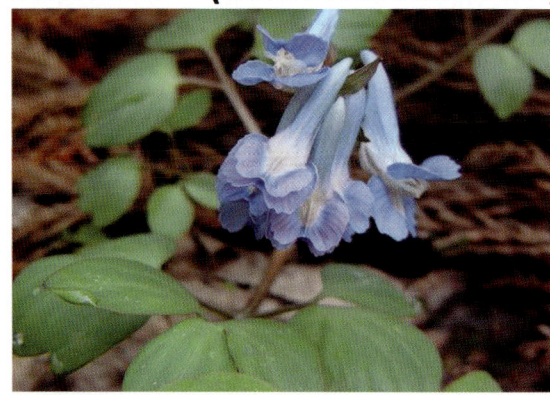

In Traditional Chinese Medicine, Yan Hu Suo has been used for thousands of years for its powerful analgesic properties. The root has a history of over a thousand years use in mitigating pain. This species was ranked 10th in a test of 250 potential antifertility drugs.

Corydalis' properties:

Analgesic	Blood stimulant	Hypnotic alterative
Anti-arrhythmic	Cardio-protector	Sedative
Antiperiodic	Contraceptive	Sedative
Antispasmodic	Deobstruent	Tonic
Astringent	Diuretic	
Bitter	Emmenagogue	

COUCHGRASS - (AGROPYRON REPENS)

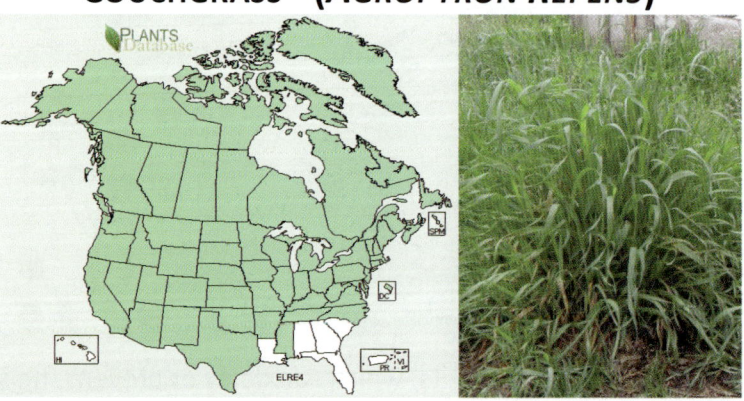

Couchgrass has been used in herbal medicine since the Classical Greek period. Sick dogs are known to dig up and eat the root, and medieval herbalists used it to treat inflamed bladders, painful urination, and water retention and it has antiseptic properties.

Couch grass is of considerable value as an herbal medicine, the roots being very useful in a wide range of kidney, liver, and urinary disorders. They have a gentle remedial effect, which is well tolerated by the body and has no side effects. This plant is also a favorite medicine of domestic cats and dogs, which will often eat quite large quantities of the leaves. Roots are harvested in the spring and can be dried for later use. A tea made from the roots is used in cases of urinary incompetence, as a worm expellant and is effective for urinary tract infections. It both protects the urinary tubules against infections, irritants and increases the volume of urine, thereby diluting it. Finally, externally it is applied as a wash to swollen limbs.

The following minerals can be found in couchgrass:

Silica
Sodium
Tin
Zinc

COUNTRY MALLOW - (SIDA CORDIFOLIA)

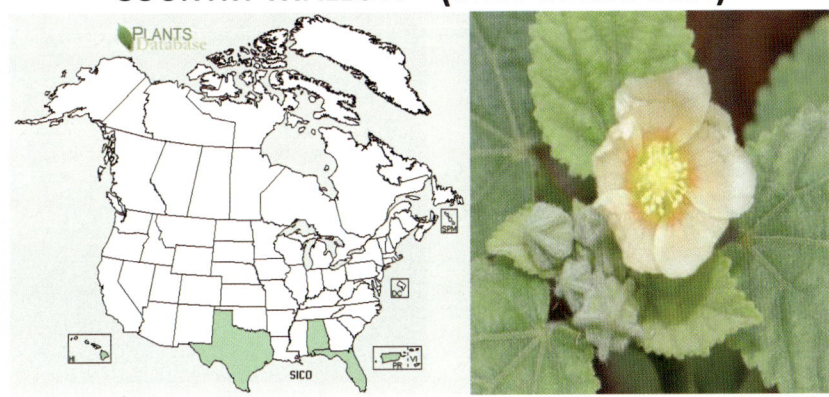

Country mallow has a long history of use particularly for medicinal properties and as a folk medicine in India for centuries. The plant is tonic, astringent, emollient, and useful in respiratory system related troubles. Bark is considered as cooling. It is useful in blood, throat, urinary system related troubles, piles, phthisis, insanity etc. The plant is analgesic, anti-inflammatory, and tonic. It affects the central nervous system and provides relief from anxiety. Its extract is consumed to reduce body weight. It tones the blood pressure and improves the cardiac irregularity and is useful in fever, fits, rheumatism, colic, and nervous disorders. The oils are used topically on sore muscles and joints in rheumatism and arthritis. Oil prepared from the decoction of root bark mixed with milk and sesame oil, finds application in diseases of the nervous system, and is very effective in curing facial paralysis and sciatica.

CRAMP BARK – (VIBURNUM OPULUS)

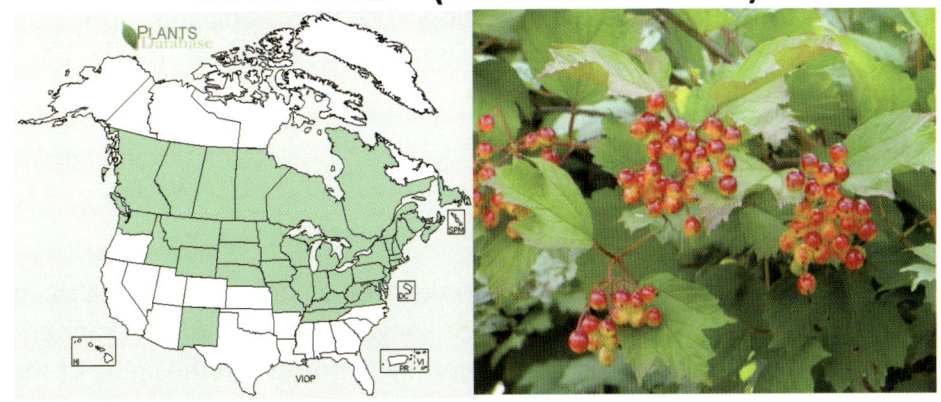

Common Herbs

One of the most common uses of viburnum opulus is for relieving menstrual cramps. Pains that begin in the lower back before moving around the loins to the abdomen are eased by the herb's antispasmodic action. Homeopathic practitioners suggest that it may be used by women who suffer miscarriages or early labor, and can even stop labor contractions. Scientists have isolated the chemical present in the bark that helps uterine contractions. They have determined that scopoletin, an anticoagulant, is the active ingredient that acts as a muscular sedative. This herb can help not only uterine cramps, but also the nervous tension, irritability, and depression that many women suffer during menopause. Since many synthetic medications for menopause have been shown to cause serious health problems, natural herbal remedies such as viburnum opulus are even more valuable.

CRANBERRY – (VACCINIUM MACROCARPON)

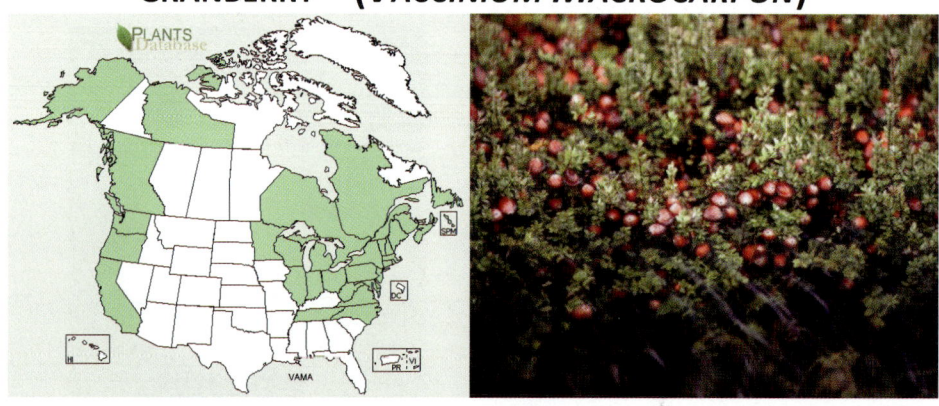

The cranberry is a native American fruit. Its native range extends in temperate climate zones from the East Coast to the Central U.S. and Canada and from Southern Canada in the north to the Appalachians in the south. Traditionally, cranberry has been used by herbalists to remove toxins from the blood and reduce the formation of kidney stones. One of the most popular uses for cranberries today is to help prevent urinary tract infections. Substances in cranberry juice called proanthocyanidins exihibit anti-adherence properties, which prevent the E. coli bacteria that cause most urinary tract infections from adhering to the wall of the bladder. There is also evidence that cranberry juice can help prevent plaque-forming bacteria from binding to the surface of one's teeth, reducing the incidence of cavities, gingivitis and gum disease. Women experience urinary tract infections with greater frequency during pregnancy. Given the evidence to support the use of cranberry for urinary tract infections (UTIs) and its safety profile, cranberry supplementation as fruit or fruit juice may be a valuable therapeutic choice in the treatment of UTIs during pregnancy.

Cranberries are a healthy source of antioxidants that support healthy aging and cardiovascular health. Cranberry extracts have also shown promise in the prevention of tooth decay. Historically, cranberry fruits and leaves were used for a variety of problems, such as:

Diabetes	Liver problems	Urinary disorders
Diarrhea	Stomach ailments	Wounds

Today most of the medicinal interest in cranberries is in the area on urinary tract health; indeed drinking cranberry juice at the first sign of a UTI is one of the best known home remedies. Cranberry juice helps flush out the urinary system by keeping bacteria from getting a foothold in the lining of the urinary tract. Cranberry juice has also been used infrequently in conjunction with antibiotics to treat chronic kidney inflammation.

CRATAEVA – (CRATAEVA NURVALA)

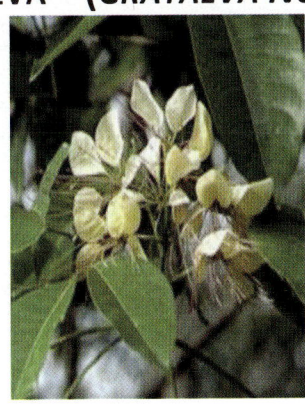

In Ayurveda, the bark of the crataeva has been traditionally used to heal kidney stones for more than 3,000 years. Presently, herbal medicine practitioners primarily use crataeva to treat kidney and prostate problems. The bark of the tree is particularly used to treat infections of the urinary tract, kidney stones as well as benign prostatic hypertrophy (BPH). Researches undertaken by scientists have demonstrated that this particular herb's actions support the cardiovascular system by properly maintaining the suppleness as well as openness of the arteries. In addition, it is believed that crataeva has beneficial uses either as an effective diuretic or a herb that slows down or hinders the formation of stones inside the organs. Both the barks as well as the leaves of the tree are extensively utilized for preparing herbal medications. Moreover, crataeva possesses these properties:

Anti-inflammatory
Antilithic
Bladder tonic

Demulcent (soothing or mollifying)
Diuretic

Lithontriptic (stone dissolving or destroying in the organs)
Tonic (stimulant) properties

CUBEB - (PIPER CUBEBA)

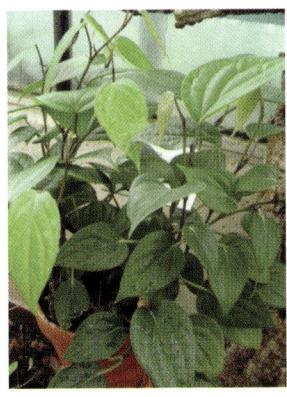

Cubeb berry is a spicy berry that is native to parts of the East Indies. It is often used in cooking as a ready substitute for the more familiar white or black peppers. Cubeb berry is also used for its fragrance in soaps and perfumes and as a flavoring in foods. As an herbal medicine, cubeb berry is considered a diuretic, expectorant, stimulant, antiseptic and shown to be effective easing symptoms of bronchitis and used for digestive ailments. The herb has often been associated with the reproductive system and has been used on prostate infections.

DAMIANA – (TURNERA DIFFUSA)

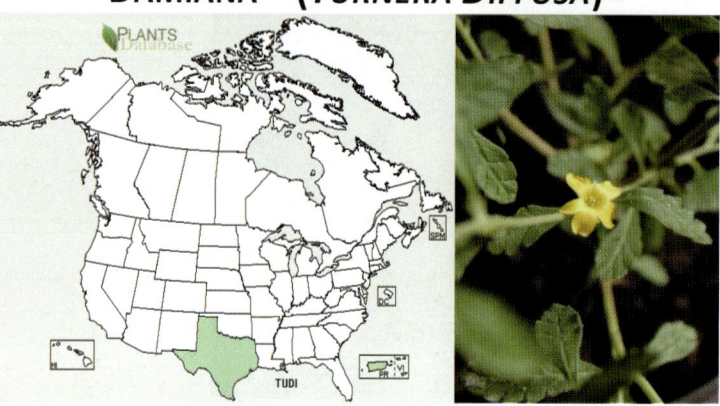

The first official record of damiana as an aphrodisiac comes from the Spanish missionary, Jesus Maria de Slavatierra, in his Chronica of 1699. After witnessing its use in northern Mexico, he bestowed the plant its current name either as a reference to Damian, the patron saint of pharmacists, or Peter Damiani, famous for fighting the immorality he saw among the clergy of the eleventh century.

An Austrian by the name of Josef August Schultes is credited as the first to write a formal botanical description of the plant early in the nineteenth century. Almost fifty years later, in 1874, the plant was first introduced to U.S. markets as an aphrodisiac. In the years immediately predating prohibition, Dr. John S. Pemberton, known as the inventor of Coca-Cola, even concocted a formula he called French Wine Coca, containing extracts of coca, cola, sweet wine, and damiana. By 1880 the plant had made its way across the Atlantic, where, as in Mexico and the U.S., it maintains a steady popularity as a "legal alternative" to marijuana and tobacco.

Damiana was recorded to be used as an aphrodisiac in the ancient Mayan civilization, as well as for "giddiness and loss of balance." A Spanish missionary first reported that the Mexican Indians made a drink from the damiana leaves, added sugar, and drank it for its supposed power to enhance lovemaking. Damiana has a long history of use in traditional herbal medicine throughout the world. It is thought to act as an:

Antidepressant   Cough-suppressant   Mild laxative
Aphrodisiac   Diuretic   Tonic

It has been used for such conditions as:
Anxiety   Debilitation   Menstrual irregularities
Bed-wetting   Depression   Sexual inadequacy
Constipation   Gastric Ulcers

In Mexico, the plant also is used for:
Asthma   Dyspepsia   Paralysis
Bronchitis   Headaches   Spermatorrhea
Diabetes   Nephrosis   Stomachache
Dysentery   Neurosis

Damiana first was recorded with aphrodisiac effects in scientific literature over 100 years ago. From 1888 to 1947 the damiana leaf and damiana elixirs were listed in the National Formulary in the United States. For more than a century damiana's use has been associated with improving sexual function in both males and females. Dr. James Balch reports in his book Prescription for Nutritional Healing that damiana "relieves headaches, controls bed-wetting, and stimulates muscular contractions of the intestinal tract. . . . " The leaves are used in Germany to relieve excess mental activity and nervous debility, and as a tonic for the hormonal and central nervous systems. E. F. Steinmetz states that in Holland, damiana is renowned for its sexual-enhancing qualities and its positive effects on the reproductive organs. The British Herbal Pharmacopoeia cites indications for the use of damiana for "anxiety neurosis with a predominant sexual factor, depression, nervous dyspepsia, atonic constipation, and coital inadequacy."

DRAGON'S BLOOD - (*DAEMONOROPS DRACO*)

Native to Indonesia and the Canary Islands, the dragon trees' ripe scaly fruit produces a resin that is used as dragon's blood. The resin is used externally as a wash to promote healing and stop bleeding. Internally it is used for chest pains, post-partum bleeding, internal traumas, and menstrual irregularities.

ECHINACEA - (*ECHINACEA ANGUSTIFOLIA*)

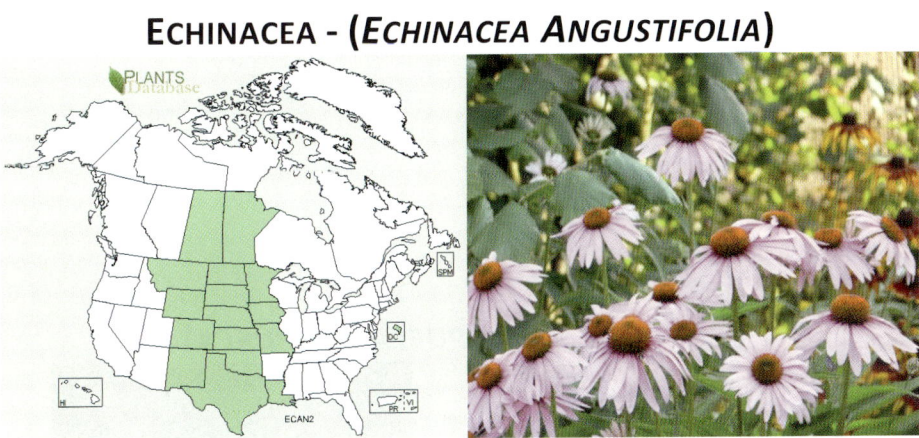

Echinacea is an herbaceous, perennial plant that is native to the plains of the American West and has been widely cultivated in Europe, where it is thought to be perhaps the most powerful natural antibiotic. The hairy plant bears narrow, lance-shaped leaves and long-stalked purple, rose, or white flowers with drooping petals. The two-foot tall plant may be found growing in barrens, prairies, and other dry, open places, thriving in rich, well-drained soil in full sun. The early American Colonists adopted echinacea as a home remedy for colds and flu, and the herb became popular in American herbal and traditional medicine. Today echinacea is the most widely used herb in the world.

Echinacea root is used for boosting immune systems, chronic fatigue syndrome, and malignant diseases. The leaves and aerial parts have no benefit. Word of the plant's healing properties traveled back to Europe, where it remains one of the most sought-after herbs and noted that German doctors prescribe echinacea as often as they prescribe antibiotics. There is now greatly renewed interest in the United States, because of the herb's positive effect on the immune system and the herb has achieved worldwide fame for its antiviral, antifungal, and antibacterial properties. Based upon recent scientific documentation, this North American plant will serve humanity well into the future.

Echinacea is believed to work by supporting the body's own efforts to crank-up the immune system to ward off disease and infection. As an herbal body cleanser, echinacea is now considered one of the most effective plant-based detoxicants in Western medicine for circulatory, lymphatic, and respiratory system support. It is reported to be an excellent herbal lymphatic tonic that facilitates the body's natural efforts to cleanse the system of toxic materials.

At the first sign of a cold, flu, fever, earache, or whenever antibiotic action is required, try some echinacea. It is said to support the body's natural efforts to ward off and fight infections, or at least diminish their length and severity. Daily use will not hinder the body's ability to use echinacea; it is best used daily to reduce all infections by 80%, thereby being a beneficial preventer of all kinds of sickness.

Echinacea is considered a fine herbal antiseptic and antibiotic that has a reputation for supporting the body in its fight against any type of infection, bacteria, viruses, and germs like no other; and it has been reported to be effective in cases of urinary tract infection, staph infection, recurring kidney infection, food poisoning, poisonous bites (snakes and insects), syphilis, diphtheria, and other putrid fevers. In Germany, it is used to fight bronchitis and abscesses. Other constituents include fatty acids, and essential oils.

Echinacea has the following minerals:

Calcium	Potassium	Sodium
Iron	Phosphorus	Zinc
Magnesium	Selenium	
Manganese	Silica	

Echinacea has the following vitamins:

Vitamin A	Vitamin B_2	Vitamin C
Vitamin B_1	Vitamin B_3	Beta - carotene

ECHINACEA - (*PURPUREA PURPUREA*)

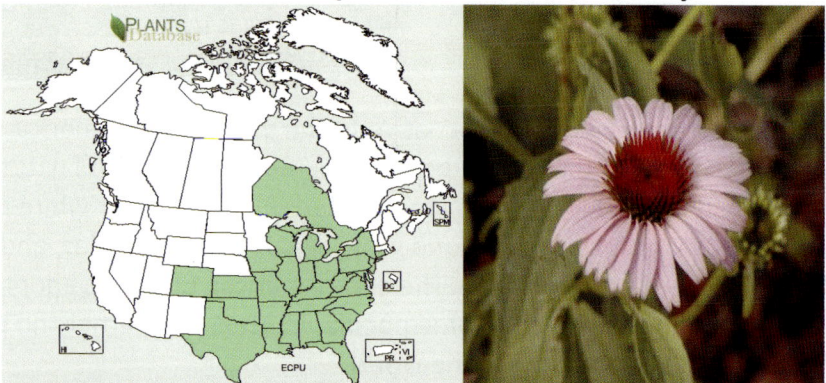

Echinacea, an extract from the coneflower, a very common plant in North America, is loved as a favorite botanical remedy among herbal and alternative medicine experts. The medicinal part of the plant is the rootstalk. Echinacea is growing in popularity because of recent media attention to its historic reputation of boosting the immune system in treating colds and flu and fighting infections. It has also been used to speed wound healing and reduce inflammation. Echinacea has a long history of use. For hundreds of years, the Plains Indians used it as an antiseptic, analgesic, and to treat poisonous insect and snakebites, toothaches, sore throat, wounds, and communicable diseases such as mumps, smallpox, and measles.

Early settlers then adopted the therapeutic uses of echinacea root, and it has been used as an herbal remedy in the United States ever since. In 1762, it was used as a treatment for saddle sores on horses. As stated earlier, daily use will not hinder the body's ability to use echinacea root; it is best used daily to reduce all infections by 80%, thereby being a beneficial preventer of all kinds of sickness.

Echinacea has the following minerals:

Calcium	Potassium	Sodium
Iron	Phosphorus	Zinc
Magnesium	Selenium	
Manganese	Silica	

Echinacea has the following vitamins:

Vitamin A	Vitamin B_2	Vitamin C
Vitamin B_1	Vitamin B_3	Beta - carotene

EGGPLANT - (SOLANUM MELONGENA)

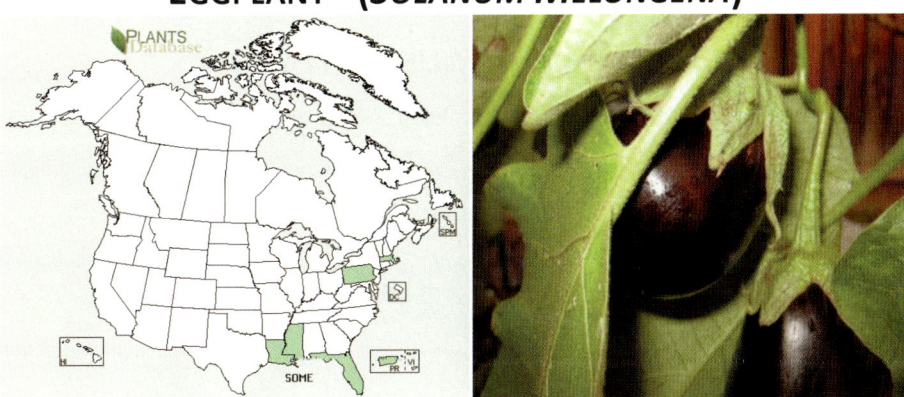

The part of the eggplant that is used is the roots. In the Philippines, eggplant roots are made into a decoction used internally as an antiasthmatic and general stimulant. The roots are also used in treatment of skin diseases.

ELDERBERRY - (SAMBUCUS NIGRA)

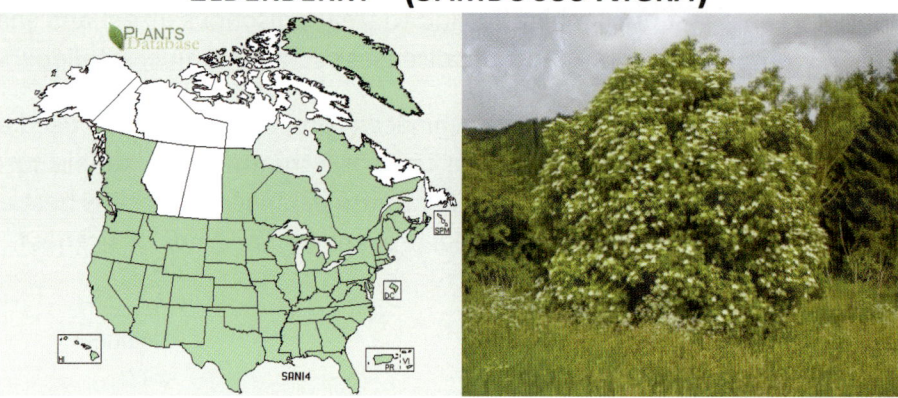

Traditionally used as a medicinal plant by many native peoples and herbalists alike, the stem, bark, leaves, flowers, fruits, and root extracts are used for bronchitis, cough, upper respiratory cold infections, and fever. A clinical trial published in 2004 showed reduction in time down and severity of flu-like symptoms for patients receiving elderberry syrup. Elderberry flowers are sold in Ukrainian and Russian drug stores for relief of congestion. The dried flowers are simmered for 15 minutes; the resulting flavorful aromatic tea is poured through a coffee filter. Some individuals find it better hot, others cold, and some may experience an allergic reaction. The flowers can be used to make an herbal tea as a remedy for inflammation caused by colds and fever.

ELECAMPANE - (INULA HELENIUM)

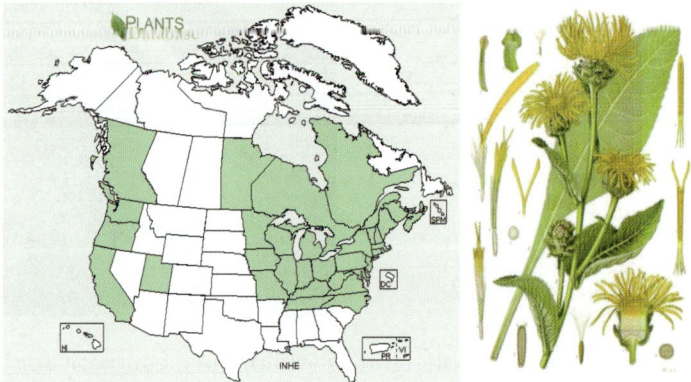

Elecampane was known to the ancient writers of agriculture and natural history, and even Roman poets wrote about it. The root is used both as a medicine and as a condiment, having a long history as a medicinal herb. A gently warming and tonic herb, it is especially effective in treating coughs, alcoholism, bronchitis, and many other complaints of the chest as well as disorders of the digestive system. A very safe herb to use, it is suitable for the old and the young. It is especially useful when the patient is debilitated. It cleanses toxins from the body, stimulating the immune and digestive systems, treating bacterial and fungal infections. The root is alterative, a skin cleaner, a bitter tonic, diuretic, loosens coughs and gentle stimulant and stomach aid. The roots should be at least 3 years old before use and best harvested in autumn and dried for later use. This remedy should not be prescribed for pregnant women. An extract of the plant is a powerful antiseptic and bactericide, particularly effective against the organism causing tuberculosis. The plant is sometimes recommended as an external wash for skin inflammations and varicose ulcers, but has been known to cause allergic reactions.

Traditionally, elecampane was used to treat:

Asthma	Common cold	Pneumonia
Bronchial coughs	Coughs	Pulmonary infections
Bronchitic asthma	Emphysema	Tracheal irritations
Catarrh	Irritations	Tuberculosis
Chronic bronchitis	Pertussis	

ELEUTHERO – (*ELEUTHEROCOCCUS SENTICOSUS*)

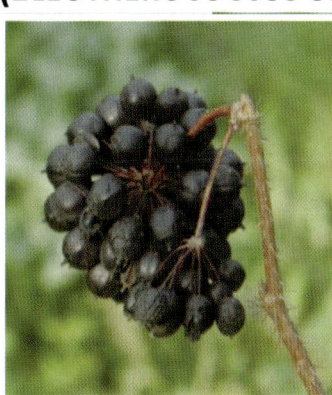

In ancient China, eleuthero was most commonly used in the form of a wine. Eleuthero is often colloquially referred to as Siberian Ginsengand and has a history of use in traditional Chinese medicine. Eleuthero was used by the Russian athletes during the late 1970s and early 1980s in preparation for the Olympic Games and by the Russian cosmonauts in the Russian space program in 1977. Eleuthero is used as a prophylactic and restorative tonic for enhancement of mental and physical capacities in cases of weakness, exhaustion and tiredness, and during convalescence.

Historical uses of Eleuthero:

Adjuvant treatment in cancer as Eleutherococcus enhances natural killer cells and T-helper cells

As a cardiovascular tonic, eleutherococcus has been shown to relieve angina symptoms, lower LDL cholesterol and triglyceride levels, relaxes the arteries relieving stress induced hypertension

Beneficial against effects from prolonged stress such as exhaustion, irritability, insomnia, and mild depression

Blood sugar regulation, reducing blood sugar in hyperglycaemia, and increasing it in hypoglycaemia

Can regulate stress-induced PMS symptoms, useful as a general tonic after childbirth, and is considered one of the best adaptogens for the menopause

Improves the body's resistance to environmental stress, and enhances physical and mental performance

Reduces swelling, treats difficult urination, oedema, poor circulation, coldness, and damp swelling of the legs

Regular use will reduce the incidence of colds and other common infectious diseases

Strengthens immune function

Supports recovery from acute or chronic diseases, trauma, and surgery

ENGLISH WALNUT - (*JUGLANS REGIA*)

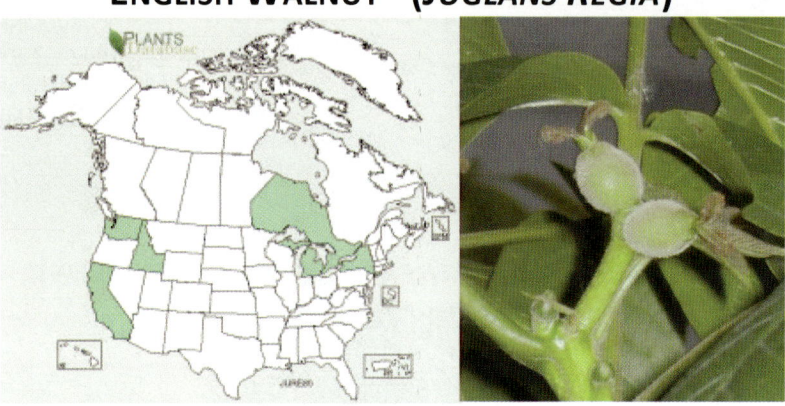

Walnuts have been found in prehistoric deposits in Europe dating from the Iron Age and are mentioned in Old Testament references to King Solomon's nut garden. Many legends have been associated with the walnut; the ancient Greeks and Romans regarded them as symbols of fertility. In the Middle Ages, walnuts were thought to ward off witchcraft, the evil eye, and epileptic fits because of the belief evil spirits lurked in the walnut branches.

Historically, walnut oil was prescribed for colic, to soothe intestines, relieve diarrhea, and hemorrhoids. Further folk uses include treating rickets, frostbite, glandular disturbances, and an astringent, tonic restorative, and disinfectant. Blisters, ulcers, itchy scalp/dandruff, sunburn, and perspiration are some of the conditions treated with various walnut preparations.

The inclusion of walnuts in the diet is recommended as a dietary source of polyunsaturated fatty acids and other nutrients. Walnuts have also been studied in metabolic syndrome with limited benefits. The effect of walnut extract in Alzheimer disease is being investigated.

EPHEDRA - (*EPHEDRA SINICA*)

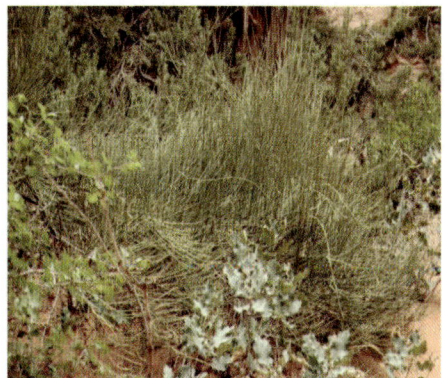

SPECIAL NOTE: THIS HERB HAS BEEN BANNED FOR USE IN SEVERAL COUNTRIES, INCLUDING THE UNITED STATES.

Ephedra is a very useful herb that the Chinese use to open the pores and promote perspiration, which can be helpful in treating chills, fever, and headache. It also controls wheezing and relaxes the muscles around the lungs, which explains its wide use as a treatment for asthma and cough. These components also stimulate the central nervous system. If you have high blood pressure, ephedra can be deadly.

It is possible for healthy people to safely use products containing ephedra when consumed in moderate amounts, and many people taking over-the-counter hay fever remedies do so with little or no trouble.

Unfortunately, ephedra is now sold as a stimulant and a weight-loss product for its metabolism-stimulating and appetite-suppressing properties. Many people who are overweight also have hypertension—just imagine how dangerous ephedra can be in these particular cases. That's not to say the herb doesn't work for weight loss too. In fact, it does, and the result is even more powerful when combined with green tea, due to the additional action of caffeine. The combination of these two types of stimulants can be especially powerful. Again, this should be done under the guidance of a professional with experience about safety and dosage. Asthma and weight loss are both complex, serious problems. You cannot treat them safely just by swallowing over-the-counter herbal pills.

EUCALYPTUS - (*EUCALYPTUS GLOBULUS*)

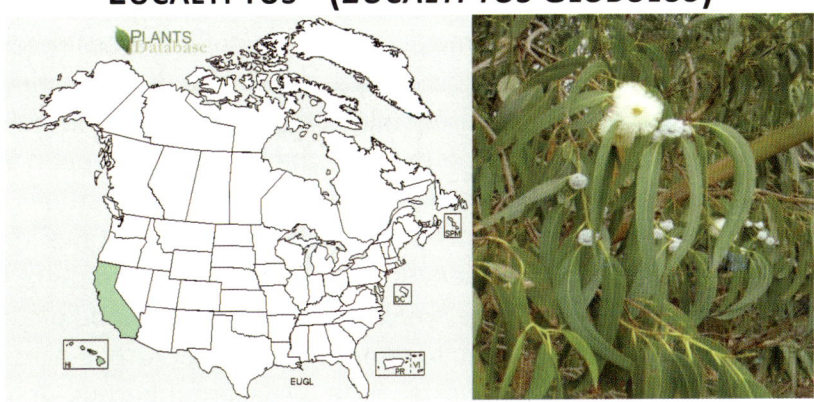

The eucalyptus tree is one of the largest trees in the world and can grow to heights well over 250 feet. There are hundreds of species, of which eucalyptus globulus is the most common, and all are native to Australia. Eucalyptus is considered to have the following properties: antibacterial, antifungal, antiseptic, antiviral, antispasmodic, astringent, circulatory stimulating, decongestant, disinfectant, and expectorant. The primary use of eucalyptus includes essential oils. The properties of the oils from different species vary slightly, but all are antiseptic. The number of ready-made preparations that contain eucalyptus oil is enormous. Every kind of product is represented, from pure oil through oil-containing ointments and rubs, to candies and syrups. The effect is convincing, and side effects from the tea or from any preparations are extremely rare. Eucalyptus oil is a strong antiseptic; lozenges from it are useful for lung diseases, colds, and sore throats. Its expectorant properties are useful in bronchitis and it can be used as a vapor bath or chest rub for asthma and other respiratory complaints. It is useful for burns, where it prevents infection. Externally, its antiseptic and deodorant qualities make it suitable for use on wounds and ulcers. Diluted in sunflower oil, it can be applied to cold sores or used as massage oil for painful joints. A cold extract made from the leaves is helpful for indigestion and for intermittent fever.

EUPHORBIA – (*EUPHORBIA HIRTA*)

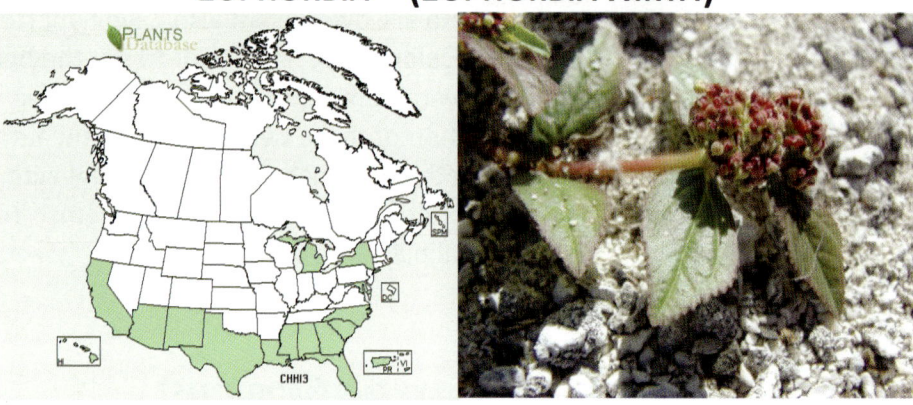

Euphorbia hirta, or asthma weed, has been used medicinally in various cultures for centuries. The entire plant can be used as a natural medicine whether it is collected during its dried, fruiting, or blooming stage. Each part of the plant is effective for treating different ailments. For example, the leaves can be used to treat skin disorders while the milky sap can be used to speed the healing of chapped or cracked lips. A decoction made from the flowers can aid in healing eye infections and inflammations, such as conjunctivitis or pinkeye. In the Philippines, euphorbia hirta is known as tawa-tawa and has long been the natural treatment of choice for dengue disease. Dengue fever is an infectious disease that is spread by mosquitoes in tropical areas. In addition to flu-like symptoms it causes the blood platelet count to drop, which can be fatal. Euphorbia hirta is administered to dengue victims because it increases the platelet count and speeds healing. Another name for euphorbia hirta is snakeroot because it is used to treat snakebite. Its antihelmintic properties help the body to expel worms and other parasites. Applying crushed leaves to a wound can stop bleeding, and it contains anti-inflammatory agents that speed the healing of pimples, wounds, and boils.

Medicinal properties of euphorbia:
- Antispasmodic
- Antiasthmatic
- Bronchiolytic sedative
- Expectorant

EVENING PRIMROSE - (*OENOTHERA BIENNIS*)

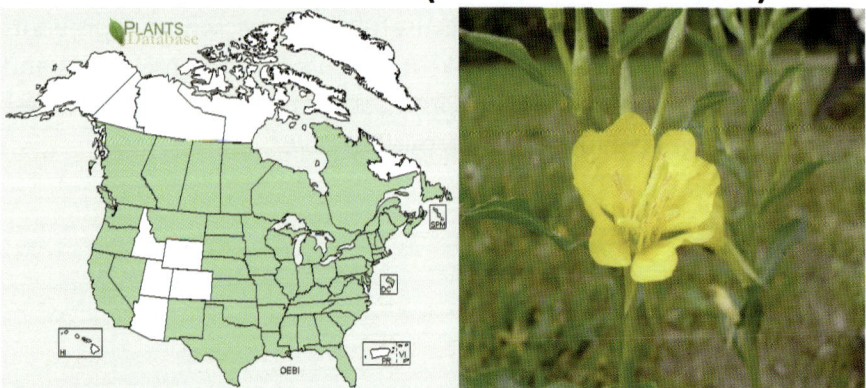

Evening primrose is a plant that grows in North America, but is now found in Europe, Asia, New Zealand, and Australia. The parts of this plant used medicinally are the seeds, leaves, oil of the seeds, and root. This plant is called "evening" primrose because its flowers open at night, so that nighttime insects can pollinate them.

Traditionally, evening primrose had been used as a soothing remedy for coughs associated with colds and had been used for mental depression, its effectiveness perhaps due to its stimulating effect on the liver, spleen, and digestive system. Evening primrose can also be made into an ointment, useful for rashes and other types of skin irritations. The entire plant is edible and has been used as a poultice for wounds.

To give them strength Native American people have rubbed the roots on muscles. Studies have indicated that about seven (7) - 500 milligram capsules of evening primrose oil daily, in conjunction with vitamins B_3, B_6, C, and zinc, can achieve remarkable results in the treatment of schizophrenia or premenstrual syndrome.

The following minerals can be found in Evening Primrose:

Boron	Iron	Potassium
Calcium	Magnesium	Sodium
Chromium	Manganese	Zinc
Cobalt	Nitrogen	

EYEBRIGHT – (*EUPHRASIA OFFICINALIS*)

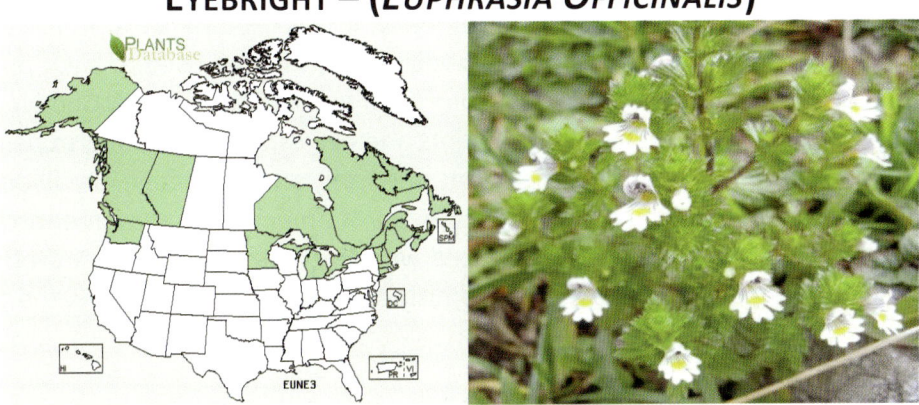

Eyebright's genus name, euphrasia, is derived from the Greek term "euphrosyne," the name of one of the three Graces who was distinguished for joy and mirth. Eyebright was used as early as the time of Theophrastus (Greek philosopher and biologist, student of Plato and Aristotle) and Dioscorides (Greek philosopher [circa AD 64] who authored a pharmacological account of plants), who prescribed infusions for topical applications in the treatment of eye infections. During the Middle Ages, eyebright was widely prescribed by medical practitioners as an eye medication, as a cure for "all evils of the eye."

In Europe, the herb eyebright has been used for centuries as a rinse, compress, or bath against eye infections and other eye-related irritations (a use reflected in many of its vernacular names). When taken by mouth, eyebright has been used to treat inflammation of nasal mucous membranes and sinusitis.

Eyebright is high in iridoid glycosides such as aucubin. In several laboratory studies, this constituent has been found to possess hepatoprotective (liver protecting) and antimicrobial activity. There is limited clinical research assessing the efficacy of eyebright in the treatment of conjunctivitis (pink eye), and the use of eyebright for other indications has not been studied in clinical trials.

Eyebright has anti-inflammatory, antibiotic, antioxidant and astringent properties. As its name suggests, eyebright is an excellent remedy for different sorts of eye problems. It can tighten the mucous membranes around the eyes, fighting free-radical damage, and can therefore be extremely helpful in cases of infectious and allergic reactions afflicting eyes. Disorders like conjunctivitis and blepharitis are easily reduced with eyebright. Its astringent properties are excellent for reduction of excessive mucus, associated with colds, sinusitis, problems with middle ear and upper respiratory conditions.

Safety: Some herbs could react with certain medications. Therefore it is advisable to contact your doctor/herbalist before consumption of any herb.

FALSE UNICORN – (CHAMAELIRIUM LUTEUM)

False unicorn is widely used as a woman's herb. Traditionally, it was used to prevent miscarriage and has a reputation for improving fertility. In Western herbal medicine, it has been used to treat pregnancy problems and ovarian cysts. It is also used as a balancing herb for the female reproductive system and has proved to be a beneficial remedy for menstrual problems and ovarian cysts; it can also be of help in the menopause. The root is adaptogen, diuretic, emetic, uterine tonic and vermifuge. Small doses of the dried and powdered root are used. It is employed in the treatment of amenorrhoea, dysmenorrhoea and leucorrhoea and also for a variety of ailments associated with the male and female reproductive organs. It should be used with caution since an excess causes vomiting. The root is harvested in the autumn and dried for later use.

FAVA BEAN - (VICIA FABA)

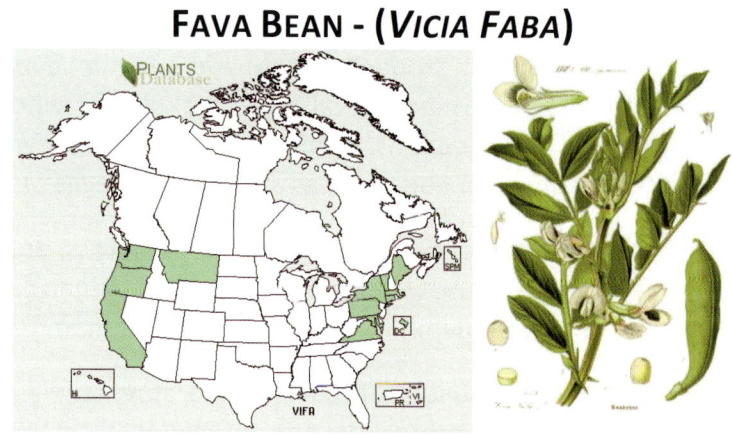

Fava beans can have both good and bad effects on people with Parkinson's disease.

Consult a qualified botanical prescriber before using fava beans and make sure all prescribing doctors know about adding them to your diet. The fava bean is very popular among all places in the world for its cooking uses. It is one of the most versatile bean species that ever been discovered. Some of its cooking uses include soups, salads, puree, fried beans, faba filling, chili beans, and dried faba beans. However, fava beans can also be beneficial to your health as it is rich in L-Dopa, which is proven effective to help curing or treating Parkinson's disease as well as hypertension or high blood pressure. However, fava beans can sometimes be harmful to your health or can cause unpleasant effects to your body. So when eating them be aware that they can also be harmful.

FENNEL - (FOENICULUM VULGARE)

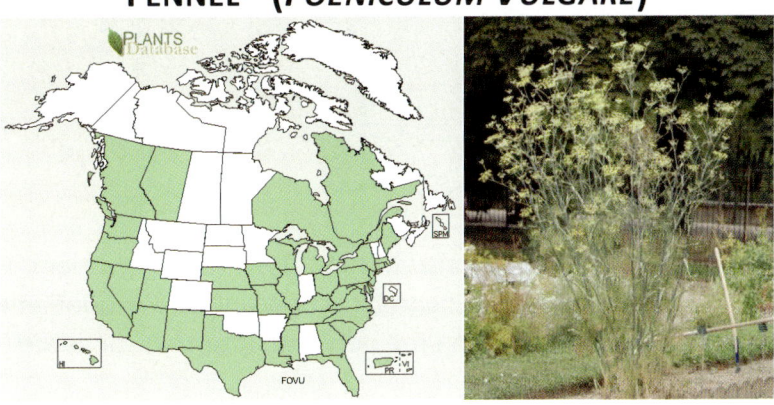

Fennel seed comes from the fennel plant, which was originally from Europe, where it is still grown today; however, it is cultivated in many parts of North America, Asia, and Egypt today. Ancient Greek athletes ate fennel seed so they would gain strength, but not weight and during the middle Ages, the seeds were chewed to put off hunger during fasting periods and during long church sermons. Eating the leaves has been a traditional tonic for the eyes, brain, and a means to improve memory. Fennel is used as a gas-relieving and gastrointestinal tract cramp-relieving agent. Fennel is also thought to possess diuretic (promoting urine production), pain reducing, fever-reducing, and anti-microbial actions. The seeds are used as a flavoring agent in many herbal medicines and to help disperse bowel gas. The seeds and roots are also said to help open obstructions of the liver, spleen, gall bladder and ease painful swellings. Fennel is believed to help relieve yellow jaundice, gout, and occasional cramps. Fennel seed was formerly considered an official drug in the United States and was listed for the treatment of indigestion.

The following minerals are in the fruit:
Silica   Sodium   Tin   Zinc

The following minerals are in the leaf:
Boron   Calcium

The following minerals are in the plant:
Iron   Nitrogen   Potassium

The following mineral is in the seed:
Alum

FENUGREEK - (TRIGONELLA FOENUM-GRAECUM)

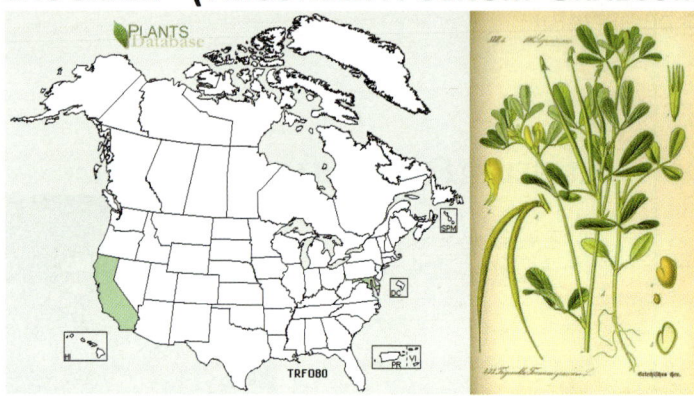

Fenugreek, one of the oldest medicinal plants, dates back to the ancient Egyptians, Greeks, and Romans who used it as a culinary and medicinal herb. Fenugreek actions include anti-inflammatory, emollient, expectorant, nutritive, soothing stimulant, acts on the nervous system to stimulate the appetite, tonic and tea.

Historically, fenugreek was used for a variety of health conditions including menopausal symptoms, digestive problems and for inducing childbirth. Today, it is used for diabetes, loss of appetite and to stimulate milk production in breastfeeding women. It is also applied to the skin to treat inflammation.

FEVERFEW - (TANACETUM PARTHENIUM)

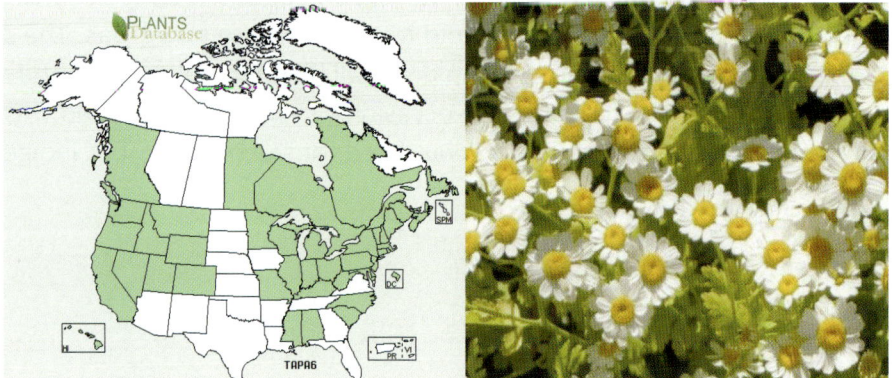

Feverfew is believed to aid digestion and lower blood pressure. A recent study indicates feverfew tea or fresh feverfew leaves on a sandwich everyday can reduce the frequency and severity of migraine headaches. Bees (and many other insects) dislike feverfew and will avoid an area where it is planted. Placed with roses and other ornamentals, feverfew can help repel damaging insects.

Feverfew is used mostly to treat and prevent certain headaches.

FORSYTHIA - (*FORSYTHIA SUSPENSA*)

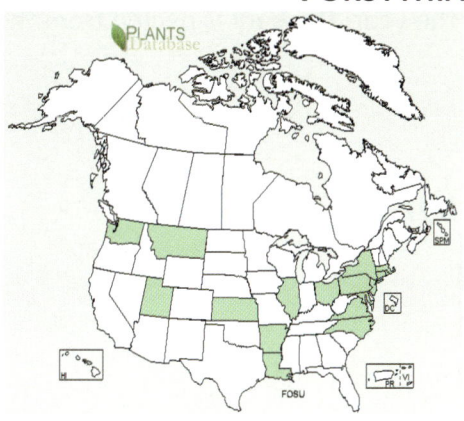
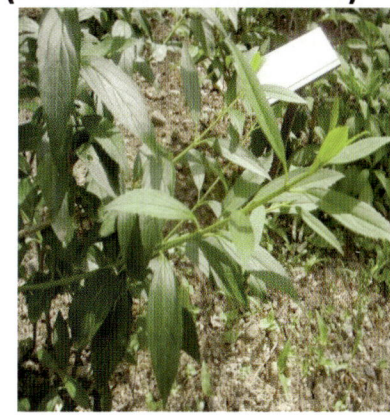

Forsythia has been used by Chinese herbalists for over 4,000 years and is considered one of the 50 fundamental herbs. A bitter-tasting herb with an antiseptic effect, it is chiefly used to treat boils, carbuncles, mumps and infected neck glands. The fruit contains vitamin P, stimulates the heart, nervous system, and gallbladder, and is used to strengthen capillaries. The fruit is harvested when fully ripe and is dried for use in extracts as an antidote, diuretic, laxative, and tonic. It is used internally in the treatment of acute infectious diseases such as mumps, tonsillitis, urinary tract infections, and allergic rashes. The flowers have a broad-spectrum antibacterial action. The root is used in the treatment of cancer, colds, fever, and jaundice.

FRINGE TREE – (*CHIONANTHUS VIRGINICA*)

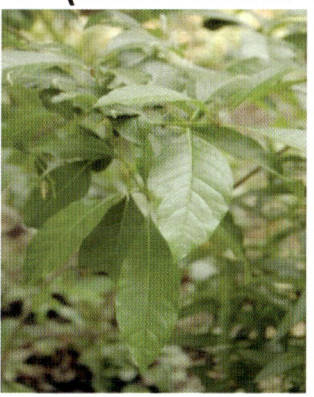

The fringe tree was commonly used by the North American Indians and European settlers alike to treat inflammations of the eyes, mouth, ulcers, and spongy gums.

In modern herbalism it is considered to be one of the most reliable remedies for disorders of the liver and gall bladder. The dried root bark is alterative, aperient, cholagogue, diuretic, febrifuge, and tonic. It is used in the treatment of gallbladder pain, gallstones, jaundice, and chronic weakness. A tincture of the bark was once widely used internally in the treatment of:

Bilious headache	Jaundice	Rheumatism
Gallstones	Liver	

The root bark also appears to strengthen function in the pancreas and spleen while anecdotal evidence indicates that it may substantially reduce sugar levels in the urine. Fringe tree also stimulates the appetite and digestion and is an excellent remedy for chronic illness, especially where the liver has been affected. A tea or a poultice can be made from the root bark for external use as a wash for wounds, inflammations, sores, infections etc. The roots can be harvested at any time of the year; the bark is peeled from them and is then dried for later use.

Gentian - (Gentiana Lutea)

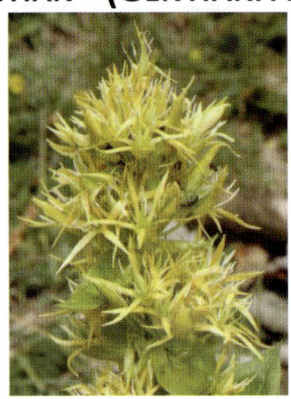

Gentian root has a long history of use as an herbal bitter in the treatment of digestive disorders and an ingredient of many medicines. It contains some of the most bitter compounds known and is used as a scientific basis for measuring bitterness. It is especially useful in states of exhaustion from chronic disease and in all cases of weakness of the digestive system and lack of appetite. It is one of the best strengtheners of the human system, stimulating the liver, gall bladder, digestive system and is an excellent tonic. The root is an anti-inflammatory, antiseptic, bitter tonic, and stomach aid. It is taken internally in treating liver complaints, indigestion, gastric infections, and anorexia. It should not be prescribed for patients with gas or ulcers. The root can be as thick as a person's arm. It has few branches it is harvested in autumn and dried for later use. It is quite likely that the roots of plants not having flowered are the richest in medicinal properties.

Ginger - (Zingiber Officinale)

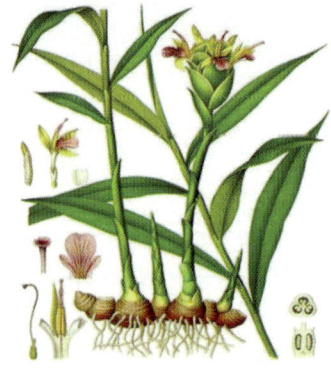

Ginger, an underground stem is a spice and used as a medicine. It can be used fresh, dried, and powdered or as a juice or oil. Ginger is commonly used to treat various types of "stomach problems," including motion sickness, morning sickness, colic, upset stomach, gas, diarrhea, nausea caused by cancer treatment, nausea and vomiting after surgery as well as loss of appetite. Other uses include treating upper respiratory tract infections, cough, and bronchitis. Fresh ginger is used for treating acute bacterial dysentery, baldness, malaria, poisonous snakebites, rheumatism, migraine headache, and toothaches. Dried ginger is used for chest pain, low back pain, and stomach pain. Some people pour the fresh juice on their skin to treat burns. The oil made from ginger is sometimes applied to the skin to relieve pain. In foods and beverages, ginger is used as a flavoring agent. In manufacturing, ginger is used as fragrance in soaps and cosmetics. One of ginger's chemicals is also used as an ingredient in laxative, anti-gas, and antacid medications.

The following minerals are in the rhizome of ginger:

Aluminum	Germanium	Selenium
Boron	Iron	Silica
Calcium	Magnesium	Sodium
Chromium	Manganese	Tin
Cobalt	Nickel	Zinc
Copper	Nitrogen	
Fluorine	Potassium	

GINKGO - (GINKGO BILOBA)

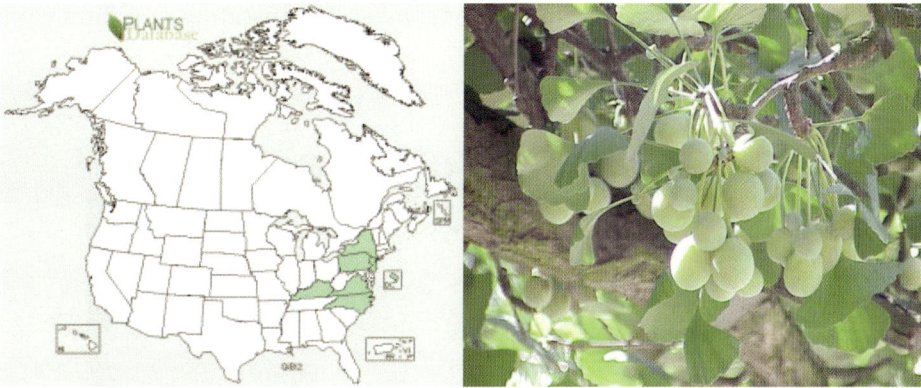

Ginkgo leaf extract has been used to treat a variety of ailments and conditions including asthma, bronchitis, fatigue, and tinnitus (ringing or roaring sounds in the ears). People use ginkgo leaf extracts hoping to improve memory (to treat or help prevent Alzheimer's disease and other types of dementia), to decrease intermittent leg pain caused by narrowing arteries, sexual dysfunction, multiple sclerosis, and other health conditions.

GINSENG - (PANAX GINSENG)

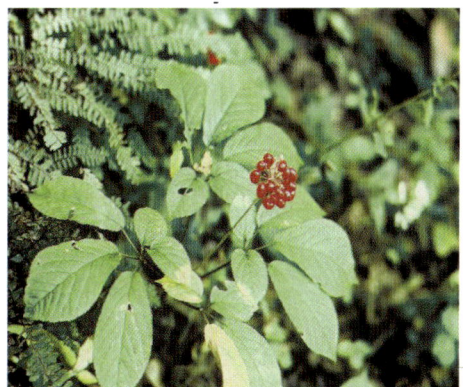

Panax ginseng root is used to make medicine. Do not confuse panax ginseng with American ginseng, Siberian ginseng, or panax. Panax ginseng is used for improved thinking, concentration, memory, work efficiency, physical stamina, and athletic endurance. Some people use panax ginseng to help them cope with stress and a general tonic for improving well-being.

Panax ginseng is also used for depression, anxiety, chronic fatigue syndrome (CFS), boosting the immune system, and fighting particular infections in a lung disease called cystic fibrosis. These infections are caused by a bacterium named Pseudomonas. Some people use panax ginseng to treat breast cancer, prevent ovarian cancer, liver cancer, lung cancer, and skin cancer. Other uses include treatment of anemia, diabetes, inflammation of the stomach lining and other intestinal problems, fever, hangover, asthma, bleeding disorders, loss of appetite, vomiting, fibromyalgia, sleeping problems (insomnia), nerve pain, joint pain, dizziness, headache, convulsions, disorders of pregnancy and childbirth, hot flashes due to menopause, and to slow the aging process.

In manufacturing, panax ginseng is used in making soaps, cosmetics, and flavoring in beverages. Used as a medicine for over two thousand years, today approximately 6 million Americans use it regularly. Be aware that panax ginseng products are not always what they claim. The contents of products labeled as containing panax ginseng vary greatly; many contain little or no panax ginseng. Panax ginseng interacts with many prescription drugs. Do not take panax ginseng without consulting you family physician.

GLOBE ARTICHOKE – (CYNARA SCOLYMUS)

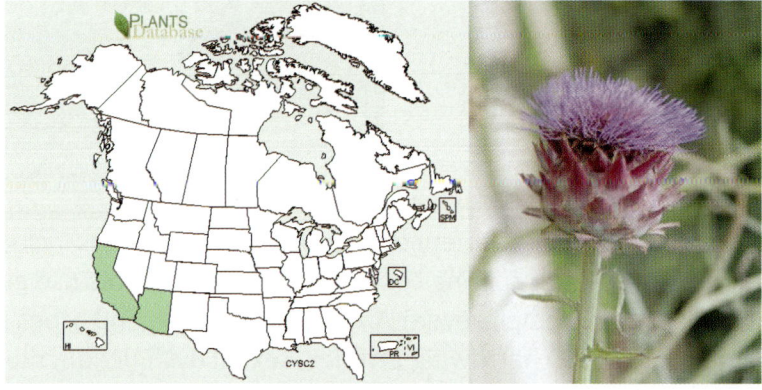

In the 1970s, European scientists first documented cynarin's ability to lower cholesterol in humans. Over the years, other researchers have continued to document artichoke's or cynarin's effect in this area. One of the more recent studies, published in 2000, was a double-blind, randomized, placebo-controlled study that used an artichoke leaf extract that was standardized to its cynarin content. For six weeks, 143 patients with high cholesterol were given the extract; at the end of the test, results showed a decrease of 10%-15% in total cholesterol, low density lipoprotein (LDL), and ratio of LDL to high-density lipoprotein (HDL) cholesterol. Scientists now report that the cholesterol-lowering effect of artichoke can be attributed to chemicals other than just cynarin, including several newly discovered ones. Artichoke has been used in traditional medicine for centuries as a specific liver and gallbladder remedy. In Brazilian herbal medicine systems, leaf preparations are used for:

Anemia	Fevers	Hypertension
Diabetes	Gout	Liver and gallbladder problems
Diarrhea (and elimination in general)	High cholesterol	Ulcers

In Europe, it is also used for liver and gallbladder disorders; in several countries, standardized herbal drugs are manufactured and sold as prescription drugs for high cholesterol and digestive and liver disorders. Other uses around the world include treatment for dyspepsia and chronic albuminuria. In France, a patent has been filed that describes an artichoke extract for treating liver disease, high cholesterol levels, and kidney insufficiency. In all herbal medicine systems where it is employed, artichoke is used to increase bile production in the liver, increase the flow of bile from the gallbladder, and to increase the contractive power of the bile duct. These bile actions are beneficial in many digestive, gallbladder, and liver disorders. Artichoke is also often used to mobilize fatty stores in the liver and detoxify it, and as a natural aid to lower cholesterol.

The main actions are as follows:

Cleanses blood	Lowers blood pressure	Supports gallbladder
Dries secretions	Reduces cholesterol	Supports heart
Increases urination	Stimulates bile	Supports liver

GOLDENROD - (OLIGONEURON SMALL)

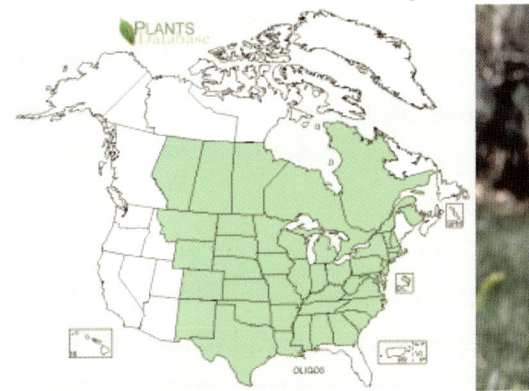
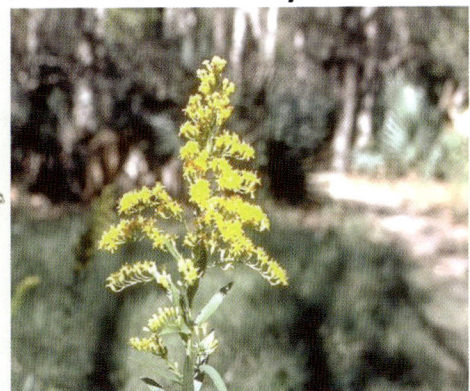

Goldenrod has been used for centuries as an external topical treatment to help speed the healing process for wounds and other skin ailments. While the traditional uses of goldenrod range from the treatment of hemorrhoids, asthma, gout, and tuberculosis, it has also been used as a diuretic, which means it increases the production of urine to remove excess fluid from the body.

Goldenrod is found growing throughout Europe, Asia, and North America. There are over 130 different species of goldenrod, as it can easily crossbreed with numerous other plant species. The plant is a perennial, growing up to 7 feet tall and identified by wooden stems highlighted by yellow flowers.

Even though there have not been highly detailed studies to determine the effectiveness of goldenrod, it is still commonly used by those searching for herbal remedies. Researchers have not determined the active ingredients within goldenrod; however, the University of Maryland states the compounds within goldenrod may feature powerful anti-inflammatory and diuretic properties. Because of this the University of Maryland Medical Center states goldenrod may help treat allergies, colds, kidney stones, and bladder inflammation. When used as a topical ointment it is suggested to be applied to the skin to treat eczema and wounds that are not opened.

GOLDENROD – (SOLIDAGO VIRGAUREA)

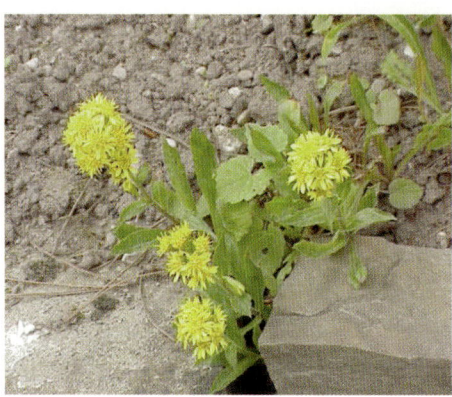

Historically, goldenrod has been used topically for wound healing. It has also been used as a diuretic (helps rid the body of excess fluid). The name solidago means to make whole. Traditionally, goldenrod has also been used to treat:

Allergies
Arthritis and gout
Asthma
Colds and flu
Diabetes
Diarrhea
Eczema (topically)
Enlargement of the liver
Gout

Hemorrhoids
Hot flushes
Inflammation of the bladder or urinary tract
Inflammation of the mouth and throat
Internal bleeding
Kidney and bladder infections
Kidney stones

Minor wounds (topically)
Nasal catarrh
Slow healing wounds
Tuberculosis
Urinary tract infections
Vaginal thrush
Whooping cough

No high quality studies have examined goldenrod's effect in humans. Goldenrod is often blamed for seasonal allergies, but it is another plant, ragweed, which blooms at the same time, that is usually responsible for allergic reactions.

GOLDENSEAL – (HYDRASTIS CANADENSIS)

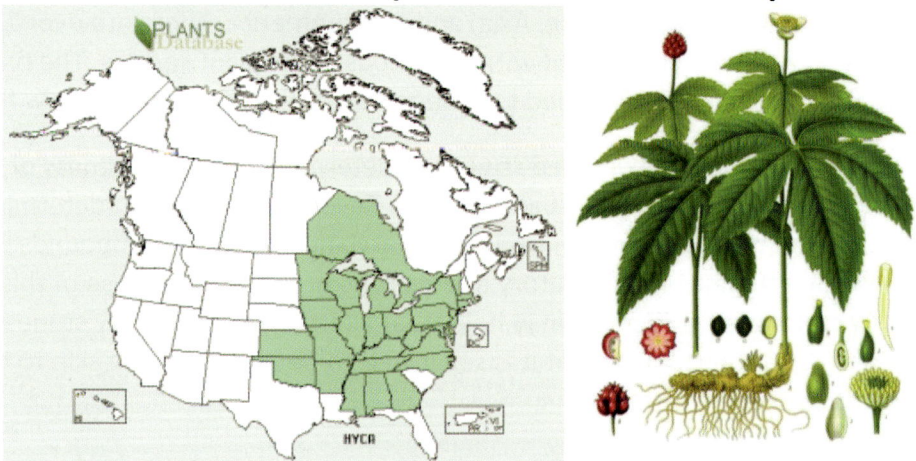

Goldenseal was originally introduced to early American settlers by Native American tribes, who used it primarily for skin problems, digestive disorders, and as a wash for sore eyes. It is now one of the most popular herbs in the United States, although there is little scientific evidence regarding its effects. Goldenseal is often combined with echinacea in cold remedies, but there is no evidence that it is effective.

Medicinal Uses and Indications:

1) Antibiotic or immune booster - Today, goldenseal is marketed as a tonic to aid digestion, sooth upset stomach, and as an antibacterial agent. It is considered a natural antibiotic and is most often combined with echinacea in preparations designed to strengthen the immune system. However, only one study found that goldenseal might help boost white blood cells (a measure of the infection-fighting ability of the immune system), and it wasn't well designed.

2) Upper respiratory problems - Goldenseal is often found in herbal remedies for hay fever (also called allergic rhinitis), colds, and the flu. However, there is no real evidence that it works in humans to treat upper respiratory infections or allergies. It may help ease a sore throat, which often accompanies cold or flu.

3) Minor wounds - Because goldenseal appears to have antiseptic properties in test tubes, it is sometimes used to disinfect cuts and scrapes.

4) Other problems:

Conjunctivitis
Mouthwashes for sore throats and canker sores
Sinusitis
Treat several skin, eye, and mucous membrane inflammatory and infectious conditions
Urinary tract infections

Pediatric - Goldenseal is not recommended for children unless under a doctor's supervision. Never give goldenseal to an infant. Adult - Besides being used orally, goldenseal is often mixed with water and other substances to create different topical washes, mouthwash, and even as a vaginal douche. Speak with a knowledgeable health care provider to determine the right dosage and form for you.

Precautions: Pregnant or breastfeeding women should not use goldenseal. Goldenseal can irritate the skin, mouth, throat, and vagina. It may also cause an increased sensitivity to sunlight. Goldenseal may interfere with the metabolism and effectiveness of certain medications. If you are taking prescription or over the counter medications be sure to ask your doctor before taking goldenseal.

The following minerals are in goldenseal:

Magnesium
Manganese
Nitrogen
Potassium
Selenium
Silica
Sodium
Tin
Zinc

Gotu Kola - (Centella Asiatica)

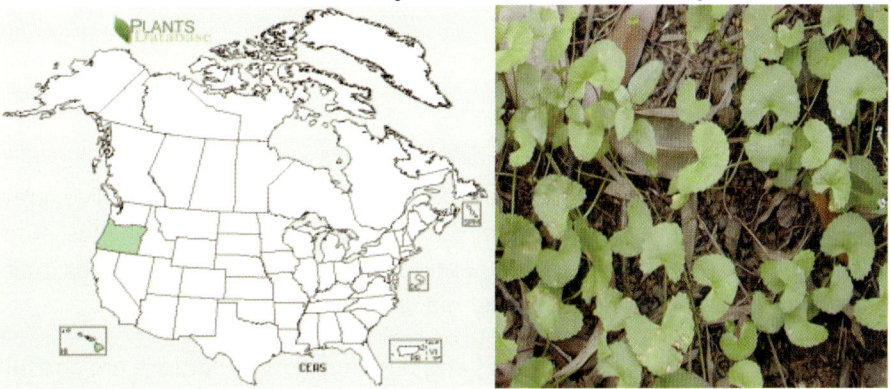

Gotu kola is recommended for nervous disorders, epilepsy, senility, and premature aging. As a brain tonic, it is said to aid intelligence, memory, combat stress, depression, increase libido, and improve reflexes. It strengthens the adrenal glands and cleanses the blood to treat skin impurities. It has also been indicated for chronic venous insufficiency, minor burns, scars, scleroderma, skin ulcers, varicose veins, wound healing, rheumatism, blood diseases, congestive heart failure, urinary tract infections, venereal diseases, hepatitis, and high blood pressure.

The leaf contains the following minerals:

Aluminum	Magnesium	Silica
Calcium	Manganese	Sodium
Chromium	Nitrogen	Tin
Cobalt	Potassium	Zinc
Iron	Selenium	

GREEN TEA – (CAMELLIA SINENSIS)

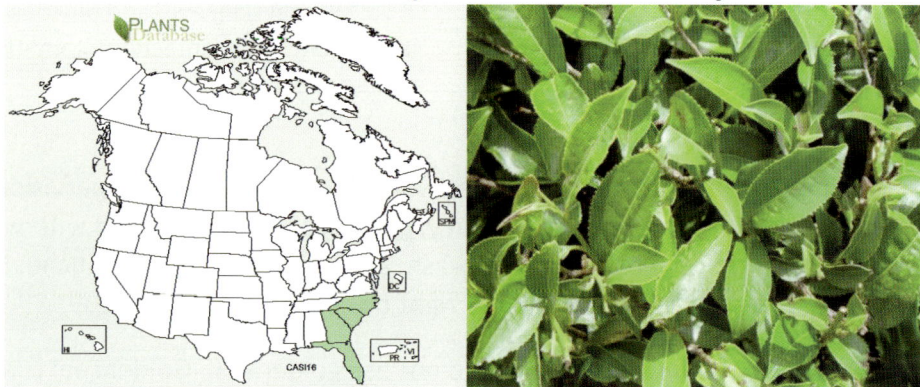

Green tea was a very recognized and utilized herb in traditional Chinese medicine. It was used in treatment of various pulmonary and cardiovascular disorders, including asthma, angina pectoris, peripheral vascular disease and coronary artery disease. Today, numerous studies suggest that green tea has enormous health benefits. It is a powerful antioxidant, and as such, it can help in prevention of atherosclerosis. It lowers the risk of heart disease, reducing the levels of cholesterol and triglycerides. Some studies also suggest that green tea could protect us against cancer, reduce inflammations associated with Crohn's disease and ulcerative colitis. Everyday consumption of green tea is also said to help control blood sugar levels in our body and acts as prevention against type 1 diabetes. Green tea leaves and extracts are effective against bacteria responsible for bad breath. It also protects the liver from the effects of toxic substances and can be used in weight loss diets.

Safety: Some herbs could react with certain medication. Therefore, it is advisable to contact your doctor/herbalist before consumption of any herb.

Indications

1) Cancer Prevention/Inhibition - Several studies have demonstrated green tea polyphenols' preventative and inhibitory effects against tumor formation and growth. While the studies are not conclusive, green tea polyphenols, particularly EGCG, may be effective in preventing cancer of the prostate, breast, esophagus, stomach, pancreas, and colon. There is also some evidence that green tea polyphenols may be chemopreventive or inhibitory toward lung, skin, and liver cancer, bladder and ovarian tumors, leukemia, and oral leukoplakia.

2) Green Tea Polyphenols - Many chronic disease states and inflammatory conditions are a result of oxidative stress and subsequent generation of free radicals. Some of these include heart disease (resulting from LDL oxidation), renal disease and failure, several types of cancer, skin exposure damage caused by ultraviolet (A and B) rays, as well as diseases associated with aging. Green tea polyphenols are potent free radical scavengers due to the hydroxyl groups in their chemical structure. The hydroxyl groups form complexes with free radicals and neutralize them, preventing the progression of the disease process.

3) Obesity/Weight Control - Recent studies on green tea's thermogenic properties have demonstrated a synergistic interaction between caffeine and catechin polyphenols that appears to prolong sympathetic stimulation of thermogenesis. A human study of green tea extract containing 90 mg EGCG taken three times daily concluded that men taking the extract burned 266 more calories per day than did those in the placebo group and that green tea extract's thermogenic effects may play a role in controlling obesity. Green tea polyphenols have also been shown to markedly inhibit digestive lipases in vitro, resulting in decreased lipolysis of triglycerides, which may translate to reduced fat digestion in humans.

4) Intestinal Dysbiosis and Infection - A small study in Japan demonstrated a special green tea catechin preparation (30.5% EGCG) was able to positively affect intestinal dysbiosis in nursing home patients by raising levels of Lactobacilli and Bifidobacteria while lowering levels of Enterobacteriaceae, Bacteroidaceae, and eubacteria. Levels of pathogenic bacterial metabolites were also decreased. An in vitro study also demonstrated green tea possesses antimicrobial activity against a variety of gram-positive and gram-negative pathogenic bacteria that cause cystitis, pyelonephritis, diarrhea, dental caries, pneumonia, and skin infections.

5) Other Applications - Sickle cell anemia is characterized by a population of "dense cells" that may trigger vasoocclusion and the painful sickle cell "crisis." One study demonstrated that 0.13 mg/mL green tea extract was capable of inhibiting dense-cell formation by 50 percent. Another potential therapeutic application of green tea is the treatment of psoriasis. The combination therapy of psoralens and ultraviolet A radiation is highly effective but has unfortunately been shown to substantially increase the risk for developing squamous cell carcinoma and melanoma. An in vitro study using human and mouse skin demonstrated that pre- and post treatment with green tea extract inhibited DNA damage induced by the psoralen/ultraviolet A radiation exposure.

GRINDELIA – (GRINDELIA CAMPORUM)

The plant known as the grindelia is commonly called the "gum plant" in North America. The Native American peoples utilized remedies made from the grindelia herb to treat bronchial problems as well as skin afflictions of all kinds, including allergic reactions to the poison ivy plant. The real effectiveness and medicinal value of this plant was not recognized by the orthodox practitioners of medicine in the US until the middle of the 19th century—after which it came into prominence as a major therapeutic and medicinal herb. Official recognition of the grindelia came with the introduction of the herb in the Pharmacopoeia of the United States from 1882 to about 1926. Modern herbalists still prescribe the herb as a major remedy in treating some types of disorders.

The remedy made from grindelia is considered to be valuable in dealing with cases of bronchial asthma. It is also effective in treating respiratory impediments caused by phlegm induced obstruction in the airways.

The grindelia is considered to posses strong anti-spasmodic as well as expectorant actions. The remedy made from the grindelia brings a relaxing effect on the muscles lining the smaller bronchial passages and helps in clearing congesting mucus in the respiratory passages on the pulmonary system. Additionally, he herbal grindelia remedy is also believed to desensitize the nerve endings found in the bronchial tree and in helping slow the heart beat rate-this action leads to easier breathing for the affected individual. Remedies made from the grindelia are also used in treating chronic bronchitis and disorders like emphysema. The herbal remedy effectively clears up the accumulated mucus in the throat and the nose of the person affected by respiratory illness. Problems and disorders such as whooping cough, hay fever, and cystitis have also been treated using the grindelia remedy. The speed of healing in the skin following physical irritation and burns is also boosted by topical application of a poultice made.

The use of the grindelia herb can produce some side effects, which is the reason for it being contraindicated for some patients affected by specific disorders in the kidney or the heart. Different parts of the grindelia plant have different properties, dried leaves and the flowering tops possess anti-spasmodic as well as anti-asthmatic effects. The compounds present in these parts of the herb also induce an anti-inflammatory action, as well as being expectorant and sedative in action. Grindelia is primarily used as an herbal treatment for bronchial catarrh, particularly if there is an asthmatic tendency evident in the person. Grindelia based active compounds are excreted via the kidneys, a side effect is that this excretion can at times induce signs of renal irritation in the person using the herb. The grindelia is also used as a topical remedy for the treatment of many disorders, including the treatment of burns, the treatment of poison ivy rash, the treatment of disorders such as dermatitis, eczema, and a variety of skin eruptions. Harvesting of the grindelia plant is usually carried out when the entire crop is in full bloom during the summer months. The herb can be used fresh and ground into an herbal poultice for topical problems. The dried herb is also used for preparing herbal infusions, tincture, and other remedies. The leaves and the flowering stems of the grindelia are the parts used in the preparation of the homeopathic remedy.

GUAVA - (PSIDIUM GUAVA)

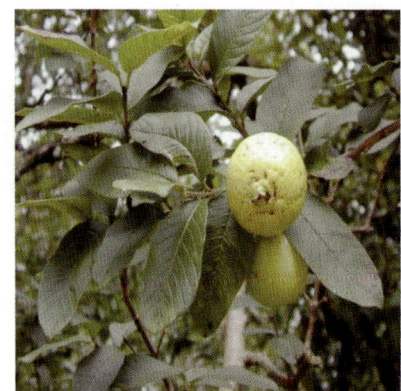

Guava is a shrub or small tree that sometimes grows as high as 30 feet, but usually no more than 10 to 15 feet.

The guava is highly adaptable to tropical and subtropical environments and can be grown outdoors as far North as the San Francisco Bay area in California, as most areas of Florida and Gulf Coast states. Protecting from temperatures below 30 degrees Fahrenheit is needed which can cause defoliation; harder freezes will kill the plant. In cool winter areas, guavas may partially defoliate, but should begin new growth flushes in spring and summer.

Guavas can be eaten fresh but are often used to flavor drinks, desserts, sauces, preserves, and many other food products.

GYMNEMA - (GYMNEMA SYLVESTRE)

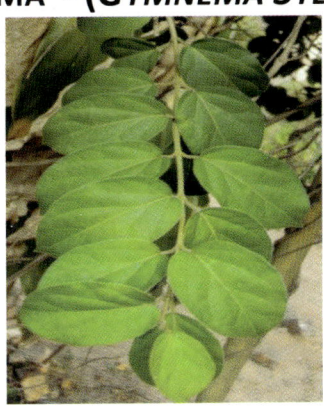

Gymnema sylvestre is also called gurmar, which is a Hindi name meaning "destroyer of sugar." It has been used for thousands of years as an herbal treatment for diabetes. It has the ability to block the absorption of glucose from the intestines and helps to reduce cravings for sugar. The reduction of sugar cravings also leads to the use of gymnema for herbal weight loss applications. Chewing the leaves, or even taking it in capsule form, can alter the taste of sugar when ingested and reduce the sweetness. Gymnema helps reduce the number of carbohydrates stored in fat stores and increases the amount burned for energy. This leads to a reduction in fat stores and increase in energy available. It has also been suggested that this herb may reduce the amount of triglycerides and LDLs, "bad cholesterol," in the bloodstream. This is an important step in combating cardiac problems, especially common in diabetics. It also has a slight diuretic effect and has been used to help with water retention. The leaves have been used to treat stomach ailments, constipation, and liver disease. Rheumatoid arthritis and gout have also been treated effectively using gymnema. The leaves have also demonstrated antibacterial and antiviral properties in liquid applications.

HAWTHORN - (CRATAEGUS MONOGYNA)

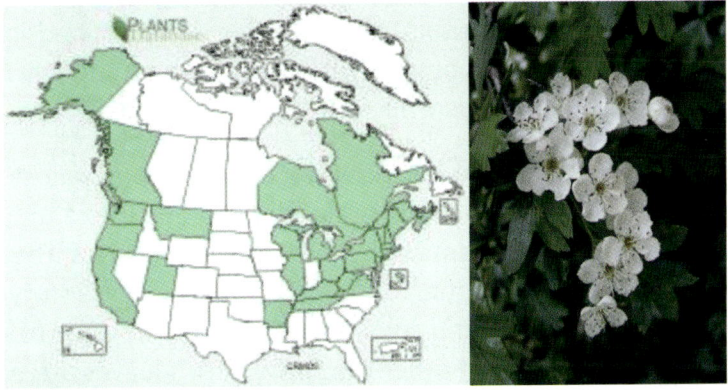

The hawthorn leaf and flower are used to make liquid extracts, usually with water and alcohol. Dry extracts can be put into capsules and tablets.

Hawthorn is considered safe for most adults when used for short periods. Side effects are rare and can include upset stomach, headache, and dizziness. Although drug interactions with hawthorn have not been thoroughly studied, there is evidence to suggest that hawthorn may interact with a number of different drugs, including certain heart medications.

Hawthorn fruit has been used for heart disease since the first century, also digestive and kidney problems. More recently, hawthorn leaf and flower have been used for heart failure, a weakness of the heart muscle that prevents the heart from pumping enough blood to the rest of the body that can lead to fatigue and limit physical activities. Hawthorn is also used for other heart conditions, including symptoms of coronary artery disease (such as angina).

Hawthorn contains the folowing minerals:

Calcium
Copper
Iron

Magnesium
Manganese
Potassium

Sodium

HEMIDESMUS – (HEMIDESMUS INDICUS)

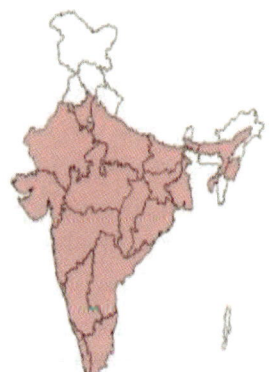
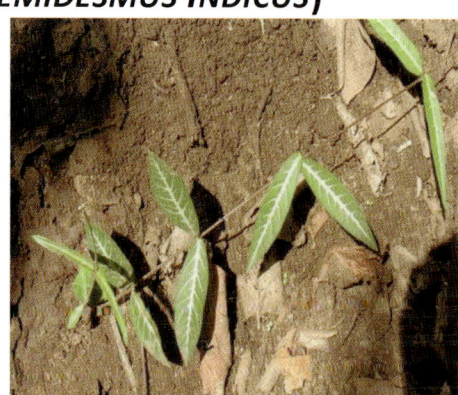

Hemidesmus is known in Ayurvedic medicine as Sugandi, and it has been valued for its medicinal properties for almost a 1000 years. In Ayurveda, it has been used medicinally to treat stomach problems, to cure rashes, and to calm the mind and induce deep meditation. It is also said to prepare the mind for the world of dreams. Sugandi root has an amazing, aromatic and sweet scent that reminds one of a combination of vanilla, almonds, and cinnamon. It tastes amazing made into a tea and has incredible effects on the dream state. The most noteworthy effects are the calming, clarifying, and tranquil feelings produced by drinking this tea. I generally take this tea an hour or so before bedtime. It produces an overall relaxing, calming sensation that envelopes me with euphoria and puts my mind at ease. It seems to help me to maintain mental clarity and focus while drifting off to sleep.

Ayurvedic medicine makes use of the hemidesmus in several different ways, most notably as a diuretic and a blood purifier. The herb, also known as false sarsaparilla, is also made into a tonic that is used to improve mental function, and it is employed in treatments to help ease skin infections, rheumatism, and urinary problems. Hemidesmus also is used in treatments for piles, insect bites, dysentery, gonorrhea and jaundice. Hemidesmus is given as an emetic, and sometimes it is given in place of ipecacuanha, from which syrup of ipecac, a common emetic, is made. At other times the herb's leaves are used medicinally for the treatment of whooping cough, bronchitis, and asthma. The leaves have a preventive effect in asthmatic patients, with a dose of three to six leaves proving effective in studies, with one leaf given per day. The studies noted some side effects, including vomiting and a loss of the sense of taste.

HOLY BASIL – (OCIMUM TENUIFLORUM)

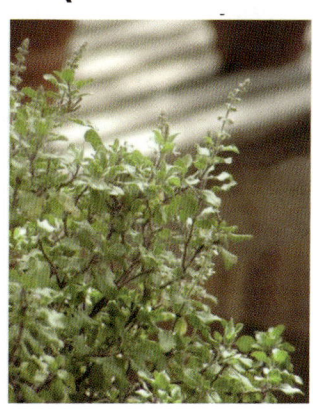

Holy basil is an aromatic plant in the family lamiaceae which is native throughout the old world tropics and widespread as a cultivated plant and an escaped weed. Tulsi is cultivated for religious and medicinal purposes and for its essential oil. It is widely known across South Asia as a medicinal plant and an herbal tea, commonly used in Ayurveda treatments. Scientific evidences are available on these various medicinal aspects:

- Adaptogenic
- Anti-carcinogenic
- Antidiabetic
- Anti-inflammatory
- Antimicrobial
- Cardio-protective
- Hepatoprotective
- Immunomodulatory
- Neuroprotective
- Radioprotective

Scientists at the Defense Research and Development Organization (DRDO) have developed a Holy basil herbal medicine for treating people exposed to radiations. According to scientists, Holy basil has antioxidant properties and can repair cells damaged by exposure to radiation. The medicines used for treating radiation-related ailments are very toxic in nature. These herbal medicines would change the way radiation treatment takes place as they would be quite safe.

HONEYSUCKLE - (LONICERA CAPRIFOLIUM)

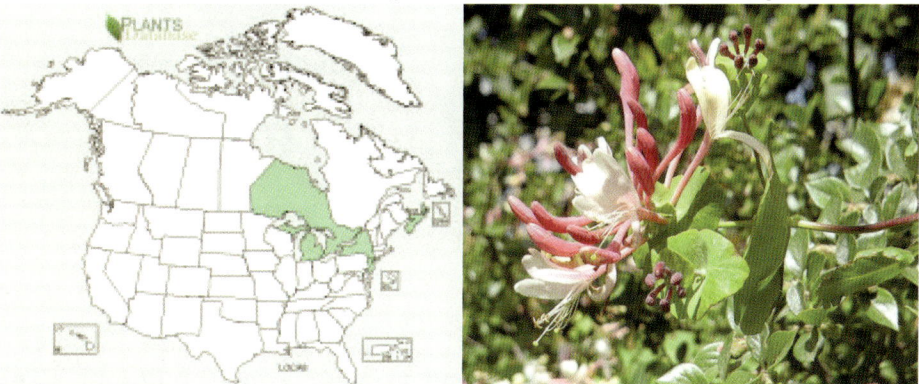

Honeysuckle is a fast-growing vine or shrub that can grow 15 to 20 feet high with a base between 2 to 10 feet wide. Honeysuckle is known for its colorful and fragrant blooms that flower in the spring and the fall. Honeysuckle wood can be used for gardening, craft projects, and even for herbal remedies.

Ground-up honeysuckle is used in Europe as an herbal remedy for asthma, urinary disorders, and labor pains. The variety of honeysuckle most commonly used for herbal remedies is jin yin, also known as

Chinese honeysuckle.

HOPS - (HUMULUS LUPULUS)

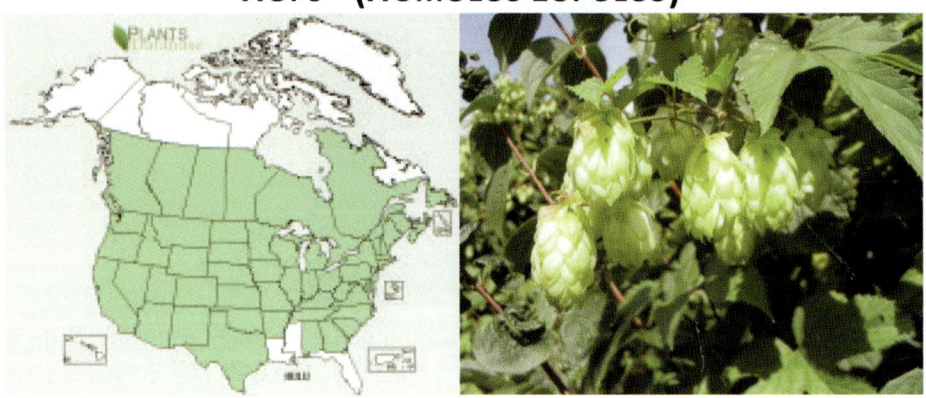

Hops are plants that grow throughout Europe and Asia. The female plant has flowers called strobilus that are used for medicinal purposes. They are harvested in early fall. Hops plants are usually tall and can grow as high as 22 feet.

As an infusion, drink one cup in the evening to aid sleep. As a tincture, take 20 drops in a glass of water 3 times daily for anxiety. Take 10 drops with water up to 5 times daily for digestion.

As a tablet, use for stress or as a sleep aid. As a capsule, take 500 milligrams 3 times daily before meals to help increase appetite. A sachet may be made and placed in your pillow to aid in sleep.

You should not use hops if you suffer from depression. As always, consult your health care provider before beginning use of any herb.

HOREHOUND - (MARRUBIUM VULGARE)

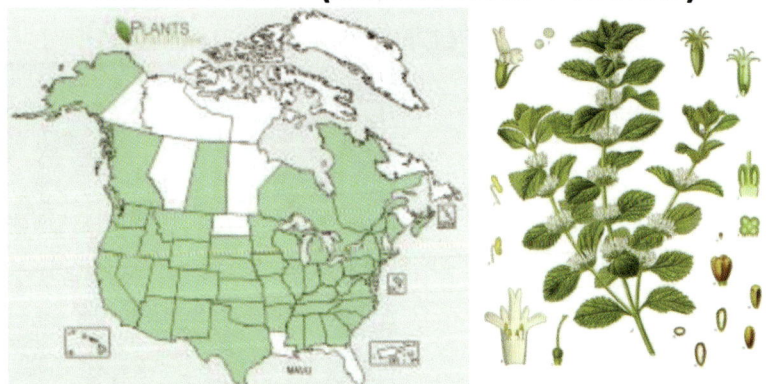

White horehound is a perennial herbaceous plant, found all over Europe and Britain. Like many other plants it flourishes in waste places and by roadsides. It is also cultivated in the corners of cottage gardens for making tea or candy for use in coughs and colds. Also brewed and made into horehound ale, an appetizing and healthful beverage, it has a curious, musky smell, which is diminished by drying and lost on keeping. Horehound flowers from June to September.

The Romans esteemed horehound for its medicinal properties in addition to its uses in coughs and colds. Horehound is a serviceable remedy against cankerworm in trees and it is stated that if it be put into new milk and set in a place pestered with flies, it will speedily kill them all.

HORSE CHESTNUT - (*AESCULUS HIPPOCASTANUM*)

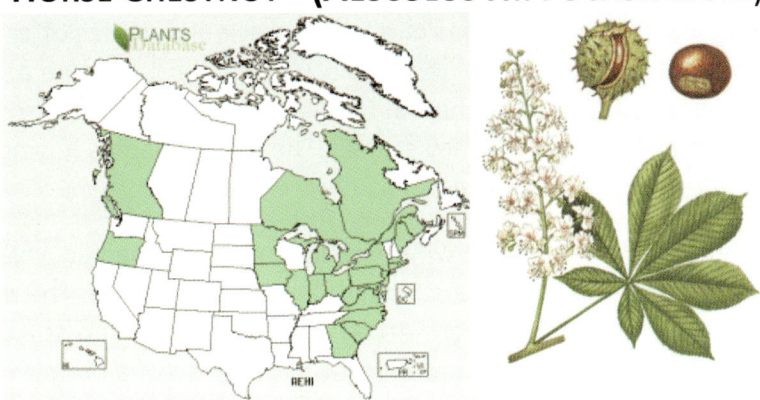

The horse chestnut tree is large with sticky buds and palm-like leaves. It has white flowers, with pink to yellow basal spots that appear in late spring while green-brown, spiny fruits follow, containing 1-3 shiny, and red-brown seeds.

Horse chestnut is a traditional remedy for leg vein health, toning, and protecting blood vessels. It is taken in small doses internally for the treatment of a wide range of venous diseases, including hardening of the arteries, varicose veins, leg ulcers, hemorrhoids, and frostbite.

Horse chestnut is a skin cleaner, anti-inflammatory herb that helps to tone the vein walls when slack or distended. The plant also reduces fluid retention by increasing the capillaries and allowing the re-absorption of excess fluid back into the circulatory system.

The seeds are decongestant, expectorant, and tonic. They have been used in the treatment of rheumatism, neuralgia, and hemorrhoids. A compound of the powdered roots is analgesic and has been used to treat chest pains. Extracts of the seeds are the source that promotes normal tone in the walls of the veins, thereby improving circulation through the veins and promoting the return of blood to the heart.

HORSEBALM AKA STONE ROOT - (*COLLINSONIA CANADENSIS*)

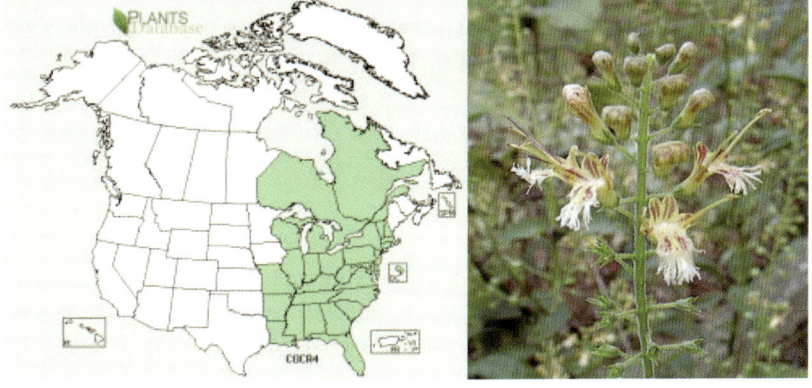

Stone root is a perennially growing herb that grows up to a maximum height of four feet. This herb has a solitary, straight stem that is square in form. The leaves of stone root are oval-shaped, jagged, and appear in opposite pairs on the stem and it ends in a cone-shaped, divided group of little, tubular, pale yellow flowers that appear during July/September. The blooms of this herb have a potent lemon-like aroma. This potent lemon aroma has helped the plant to earn another name, richweed. In effect, the lemon-like aroma is considered the most striking characteristic, native to America and in the mint family. The leaves as well as the rhizome (the underground stem) of stone root were once brewed to prepare therapeutic teas and rinses or ointments for treating wounds and cuts for numerous generations of the Native Americans as well as the pioneering while settlers from Europe in the rocky regions of Kentucky, Virginia, Tennessee, and the Carolinas. Like in the case of several other plants, the dissimilar names offer vital background. The common name stone root denotes either to the herb's knotty, rock-hard rhizome or to the mountaineers brewing the rhizome of the plant to prepare an herbal tea, which was used in the form of a diuretic in treating stone afflictions, such as bladder or kidney stones. The plant's names having "horse" and "ox" in them actually denote the large size of this species.

Both the Indians in North America as well as the white settlers from Europe had several uses with stone root to heal wounds. It was applied topically in the form of a wash or poultice. The rhizome of the herb was brewed to prepare an herbal tea, which when served hot not only worked as a diuretic in treating kidney and gallstones but was also used as a common tonic in the form of a purgative as well as a remedy for headaches.

HORSERADISH - (ARMORACIA RUSTICANA)

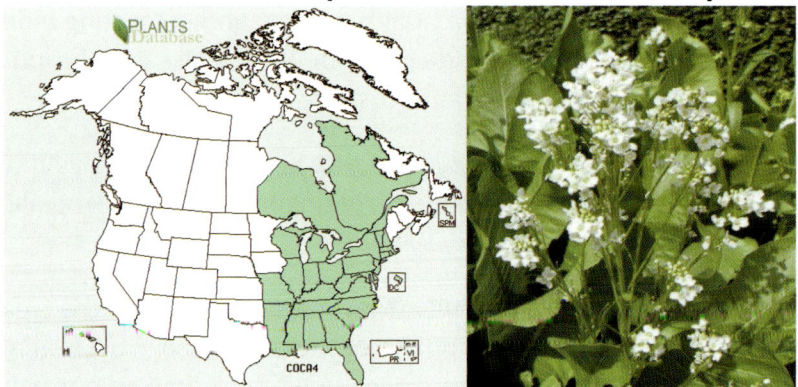

Horseradish is a perennial plant that grows up to two feet high. It has roots that are very deep and large leaves with white flowers. It is grown primarily in Asia and Europe. The root that is used for herbal medicine is harvested in the fall.

Horseradish must be eaten as a fresh root in order to have healing properties. The dried variety will not produce the same results. You may eat ½ to 1 teaspoon horseradish 3 times daily. Commonly used as a condiment with food, more is eaten in a prepared fashion.

As a poultice, wrap grated root in linen or cheesecloth and place on problem area until you feel a burning sensation. To make syrup, boil 1 teaspoon of root in ½ cup water for 2 hours in a covered pot. Strain and add sugar to taste.

You should not take horseradish internally unless supervised by a health professional. Too much horseradish can cause stomach and intestinal irritation. Do not use horseradish if you have an underactive thyroid. A horseradish poultice may cause blisters to form on the skin. Consult your health care provider before beginning use of this herb.

HORSETAIL AKA INDIAN ALMOND - (*EQUISETUM ARVENSE*)

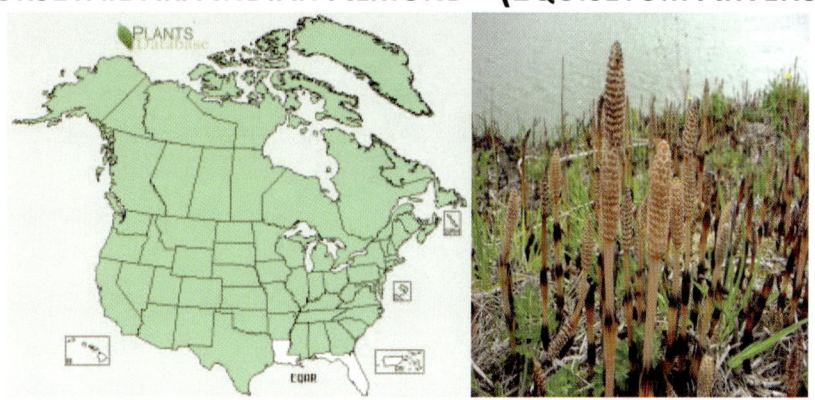

Horsetail is a sole survivor of a line of plants going way back. Several cultures have employed horsetail as a folk remedy for kidney, bladder troubles, arthritis, bleeding ulcers, and tuberculosis. The Chinese use it to cool fevers and as a remedy for eye inflammations such as cornea disorders, dysentery, flu, swellings, and hemorrhoids.

Because of its content of silica, this plant is recommended when it is necessary for the body to repair bony tissues that are in not well condition because of some trauma. Silica helps to fix calcium problems, so that the body can store more quantity of this mineral and it is able to form stronger bones or tendons. Equisetum hymale, a different variety of horsetail, can be used in a powdered form to rebuild tooth enamel. one teaspoon taken daily for 10 to 30 days, depending upon the severity of enamel loss, will rebuild tooth enamel. Strong tooth enamel is the first defense against tooth cavities. Once enamel is rebuilt, the frequency of using equisetum hymale should be reduced to 4 to 5 times a month for maintenance. Thios can also heal small cavities because of its mineral content. Horsetail is recommended for anemia. It has also been used to treat deep-seated lung damage such as tuberculosis.

Horsetail is a skin cleaner herb and has a diuretic action. It has an effect on the urinary tract where it can be used to sooth inflammation, hemorrhaging, ulcers, cystitis and treating infections. It is considered a specific remedy in cases of inflammation or benign enlargement of the prostate gland and is used to quicken the removal of kidney stones.

The plant contains the following minerals:

Aluminum	Iron	Potassium	Tin
Calcium	Magnesium	Selenium	Zinc
Chromium	Manganese	Silica	
Cobalt	Nitrogen	Sodium	

Ipecac - (Cephaelis Acuminata)

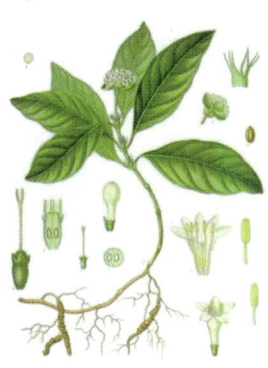

A Portuguese friar living in Brazil in the early 17th century first recorded the medicinal properties of ipecac, a traditional remedy used by Brazilian Indians. Its name is from the Portuguese for "sick-making plant," since in large doses it causes nausea, vomiting, and even cardiac failure. In conventional medicine, drugs derived from the root are used to loosen phlegm in the respiratory tract and to induce vomiting. Ipecac was used especially to relieve persistent nausea. Irritability is common in those who respond best to: ipecac and children suited to the remedy may scream and howl. When unwell, these people can be hard to please, asking for things and then changing their minds. Illness can prompt them to become depressed, impatient, and contemptuous of those around them. Physical symptoms generally linked with ipecac are persistent nausea, with or without vomiting and a tendency to hemorrhage. Despite any vomiting, the tongue is clean and unfurred. There is often oversensitivity to movement and a constant feeling of being hot on the inside and cold on the outside. These symptoms appear rapidly, are generally intermittent, and may include coughing fits and breathing difficulties. Ipecac is also used for headaches, migraines, and gynecological problems linked to the general tendency to bleed very easily.

The homeopathic remedy is made from the root, the most potent part of the plant. The root is dried and then ground into a coarse powder, which is diluted either in milk sugar to be used as a dry substance or in a water-and-alcohol base. Both preparations are weakened to a nontoxic level. Ipecac is an excellent remedy for nausea and vomiting. Physical symptoms helped include persistent nausea with a pale face and lips; cold or hot sweats and clamminess; nausea associated with migraines; nausea that is not relieved by vomiting; and vomiting that is worse when bending over. Stomach ailments accompanied by a weak pulse, lack of thirst, fainting, and constant saliva production are also helped by Ipecac. It is effective for breathing difficulties such as asthma, coughing that leads to choking, and a need to cough and vomit at the same time.

JABORANDI - (PILOCARPUS MICROPHYLLUS)

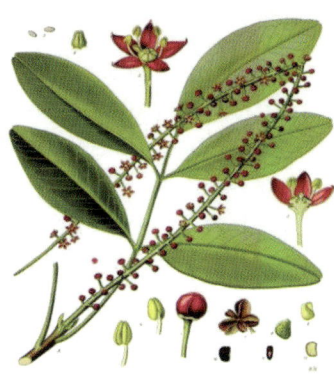

The herbal plant known as the jaborandi can reach heights of four to five feet tall. A perennial shrub grows in the Amazonian tropical forests. The jaborandi plant has distinct grayish-green colored, large sized leaves that are covered with many minute oil-secreting glands. The plant has a smooth textured and grayish colored bark; it bears small-sized reddish purple colored flowers when in bloom.

The harvesting of jaborandi leaves from the wild is just for the sake of getting this oil, which is used in herbal medicine as well as conventional medications. Various extracted substances from the oil are used in many kinds of useful medications; the oil is primary treatment in dealing with the dangerous blinding disease glaucom that affects thousands of people across the world.

An herbal jaborandi leaf tea has a long history of use in Brazilian traditional folk medicine. The indigenous peoples of the Amazon used the herbal tea in treating many different problems. The herbal tea can be consumed; when used in this manner; the jaborandi tea has a potent diuretic effect and induces perspiration in the body of the person. The herbal tea can also be used as a topical remedy and can help in preventing baldness if it is applied to the scalp; however, scientific studies have not substantiated this traditional belief in the herb. The herbal infusion prepared from the powdered down dried leaves of jaborandi has also been used as a stimulant and expectorant in other places. The infusion is often included in the herbal treatment regimens for a number of well-known diseases, such as rheumatism and pleurisy. The leaf extracts were at one time employed in the United States to stimulate urinary flow in patients with bladder dysfunction when bladder inactivity was induced by the shock of a surgical procedure. These days, this problem is treated using other techniques.

JEWELWEED - (IMPATIENS CAPENSIS)

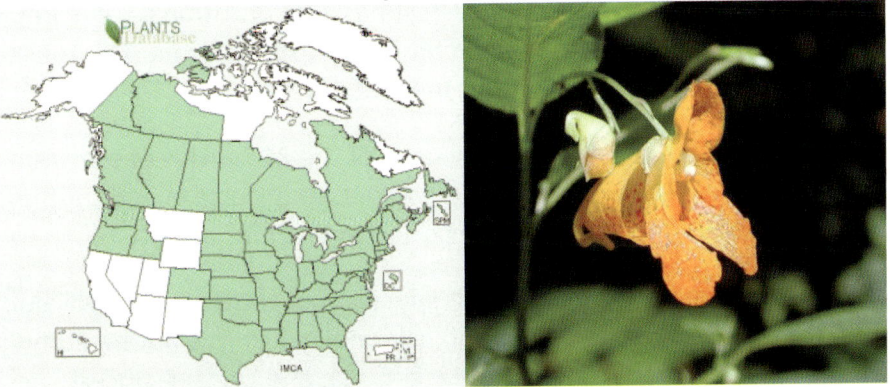

Jewelweed is best known for its skin-healing properties. Herbalists use the leaves and the juice from the stem of jewelweed as a treatment for poison ivy, oak, and other plant-induced rashes as well as many other types of dermatitis. Jewelweed works by counter-reacting with the chemicals in other plants that cause irritation. Poultices and salves from jewelweed are a folk remedy for bruises, burns, cuts, eczema, insect bites, sores, sprains, warts, and ringworm.

Jewelweed is a smooth annual, 3 to 5 feet in height with oval leaves. A bit trumpets-shaped, the flowers hang from the plant much as a jewel from a necklace, pale jewelweed has yellow flowers, and spotted touch-me-nots have orange flowers with dark red dots. The seeds will "pop" when touched; that is where the name touch-me-nots came from. The spotted jewelweed variety is most commonly used for treating poison ivy rashes, although the pale jewelweed may also have medicinal properties.

Jewelweed blooms May through October in the eastern part of North America from Southern Canada to the northern part of Florida. It is found most often in moist woods, usually near poison ivy or stinging nettle. It is commonly said that wherever you find poison ivy, you will find jewelweed; however, this is not true as jewelweed will not grow in dry places for long and does not thrive in direct sunlight. Poison ivy will grow in sun or shade. Jewelweed often grows on the edge of creek beds. There is plenty of jewelweed in the wild and it is not hard to find once you learn to identify it.

KAFFIR POTATO - (*PLECTRANTHUS ESCULENTUS*)

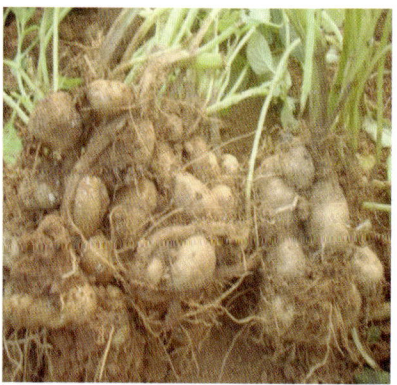

Livingstone potato is cultivated in Africa for its edible tubers, each of which may weigh up to 1.8 kilograms. The tubers persist underground even when the plant lacks leaves. They are dug up and usually boiled or roasted, and are often eaten as a substitute for sweet potato (ipomeas batatas) or potato (solanum tuberosum). Researchers in South Africa are continuing centuries of selection for its edible tubers to optimize the crop for local farmers.

Preliminary biochemical analysis of the species suggests it has high nutritional value being rich in carbohydrates, vitamin A, minerals, and is valuable in times of food shortage. This is especially true as the plant is well suited to local environmental conditions in areas where it has a long tradition of cultivation.

Plectranthus esculentus is one of the most frequently used of the 21 species of plectranthus employed in the treatment of disorders of the digestive system. It is also used in eastern and southern Africa as an antihelmintic to treat intestinal worms. It has cytotoxic and anti-tumor activity.

Further research is needed to determine whether this species is of wider medicinal value. The related species plectranthus barbatus contains the compound coleonol, which is a potent stimulant that has potential for the treatment of hypertension, glaucoma, asthma, and certain cancers.

KELP - (*FUCUS VESICULOSUS*)

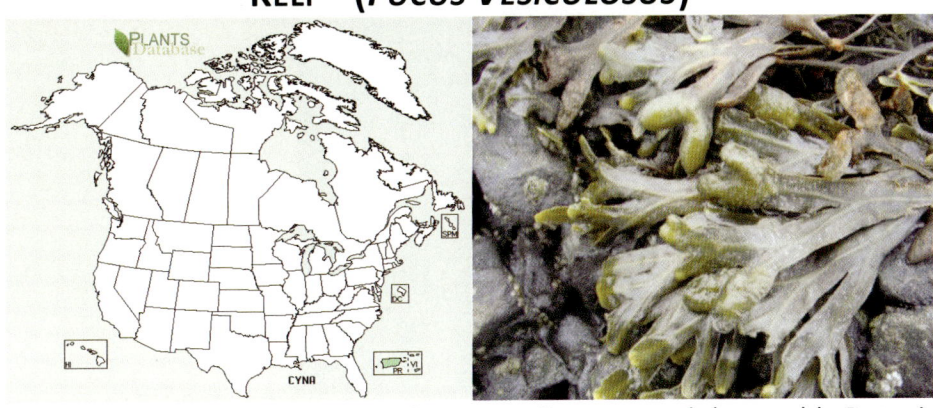

Kelp, commonly referred to as seaweed, grows along coastlines around the world. Botanically it is classified as algae. It is a rich source of natural vitamins and minerals, including essential trace minerals. Kelp is dependent upon the sea for its nourishment—an excellent source since the sea is the repository of all the minerals that have been washed from the land through the millennia. The plant can grow as much as two feet per day, and the entire plant is used as an herb. Kelp also makes a popular salt substitute. Because the plant's nutrients come in a natural form, they are easily assimilated by the body. Kelp is especially high in iodine, which must be present for proper thyroid function and metabolism.

Kelp contains the following minerals:

Aluminum	Cobalt	Rubidium
Antimony	Copper	Selenium
Arsenic	Iodine	Silver
Barium	Iron	Sodium
Beryllium	Lithium	Strontium
Bismuth	Magnesium	Sulphur
Boron	Manganese	Tin
Cadmium	Molybdenum	Vanadium
Cesium	Nickel	Zinc
Calcium	Phosphorus	
Chromium	Potassium	

Kelp is a source of the following vitamins:

Vitamin A	Vitamin D	Pantotene
Vitamin B_1, B_2, B_3, B_6	Vitamin E	Beta-carotene
Vitamin C	Choline	

Kelp amino acid content:

Alanine	Glutamic Acid	Proline
Arginine	Isoleucine	Serine
Aspartic Acid	Leucine	Threonine
Cystine	Lysine	Valine
Glycine	Methionine	

Khella - (Ammi Visnaga)

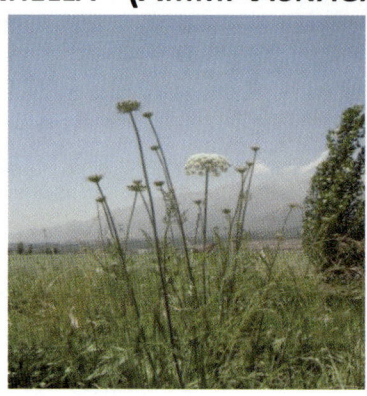

Khella is a bitter, aromatic plant that is native to the Mediterranean area of North Africa and the Middle East, and is cultivated in the United States, Mexico, Chile, and Argentina, thriving as a crop in well-drained soil in sun. The plant grows erect to a height of about five feet and bears wispy leaves and clusters of small white flowers and tiny fruits that are picked and dried for use in herbal medicines.

Khella's medicinal usage reaches back to antiquity. The herb appeared in the Egyptian time as a component in formulas to treat kidney stones, one of the very same uses that have echoed in traditional herbal therapy through the ages. The seeds contain a fatty oil, which includes khellin and research that was conducted in the 1950s led to its formulation in many commercial pharmaceuticals for dilating blood vessels.

Khella is reported to be very beneficial for good heart health. It has been used to assist the body's natural resources to relax the coronary arteries, reduce arterial plaque, and increase circulation to the heart without reducing blood pressure; and it is believed to support the body's natural ability to improve circulation in the heart muscle, giving a mild boost to the heart's pumping action. Khella also is believed to work with the body's own healing properties to improve a weak heart and relieve the pain of angina pectoris.

Further supporting coronary health, research has indicated that khella may act as a calcium channel blocker, which is thought to inhibit blood vessel constriction that could result in raised blood pressure. Moreover, the herb is thought to support the body's efforts to increase the ratio of HDL (high-density lipoprotein or "good" cholesterol) to LDL (low-density lipoprotein or "bad" cholesterol) in the blood, potentially helping to reduce plaque formation in the linings of arteries. This action is said toe diminish the risk of arteriosclerosis, stroke, and heart attack. In the management of kidney stones, khella is said to assist the body in its efforts to relax tubes and ducts to the bladder, which may allow the stones to pass while at the same time helping to relieve the pain caused by the trapped stone.

KUDZU - (*PUERARIA LOBATA*)

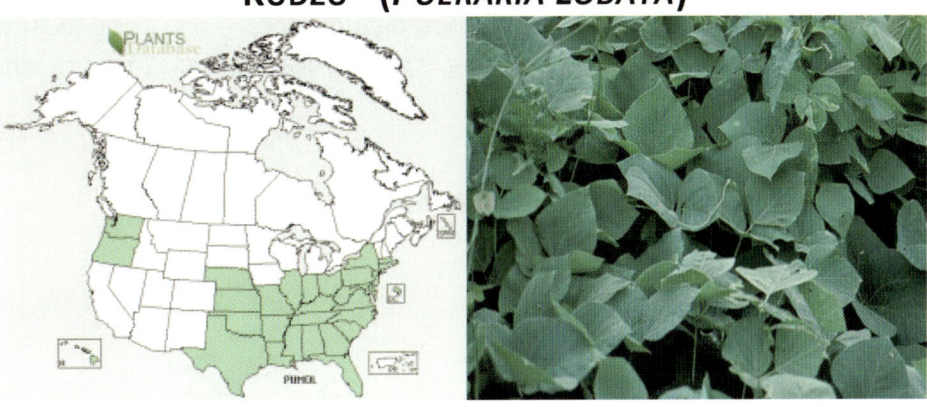

Kudzu is a vine. Under the right growing conditions, it spreads easily, covering virtually everything that does not move out of its path. Kudzu was introduced in North America in 1876 in the southeastern U.S. to prevent soil erosion. But kudzu spread quickly and overtook farms and buildings, leading some to call kudzu, "the vine that ate the South."

Kudzu's root, flower, and leaf are used to make medicine. It has been used in Chinese medicine since at least 200 B.C. As early as 600 A.D., it was used to treat alcoholism. Kudzu is used to treat alcoholism and to reduce symptoms of alcohol hangover including, headache, upset stomach, dizziness, and vomiting. Kudzu is also used for heart and circulatory problems, including high blood pressure, irregular heartbeat, and chest pain; for upper respiratory problems including sinus infections, the common cold, hay fever, flu, and swine flu; and for skin problems, including allergic skin rash, itchiness, and psoriasis.

Some people use kudzu for menopause, muscle pain, measles, dysentery, stomach pain, fever, diarrhea, thirst, neck stiffness, and to promote sweating. Other oral uses include treatment of polio, migraine, deafness, diabetes, and traumatic injuries.

Lavender – (*Lavandula Angustifolia*)

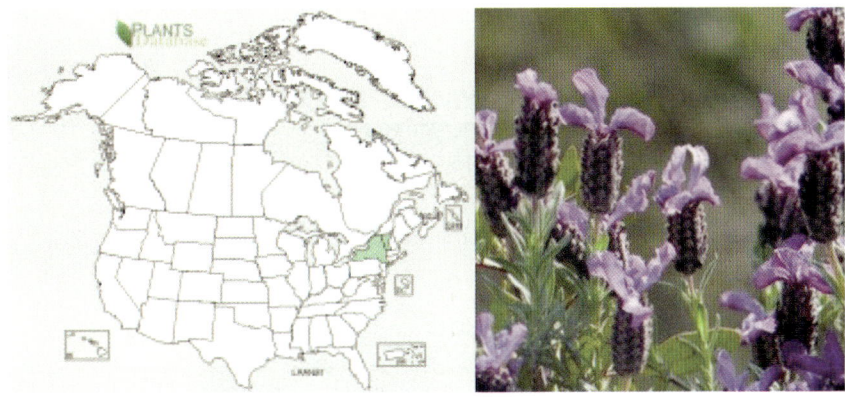

Lavender is indigenous to the mountain zones of the Mediterranean; lavender thrives in stony habitats that have access to lots of sunlight. Lavender can be found growing in the wild throughout southern Europe. Lavender is actually a shrub with heavy wood-like branches growing from the broad rootstock and green leaf-like shoots resembling rods protrude out from the branches. The narrow, grayish green leaves covered in a silver blanket-like substance taper down from the base. The leaves are oblong in shape and attach directly at the base in curled spiral-like patterns.

Hillman Health Food Store call 855-Amish-Dr (855-264-7437) www.emineral.info Vitamins and Minerals for Better Living

Lavender is frequently alluded to as a natural remedy for a large variety of ailments primarily used in connection with insomnia, anxiety, depression, and mood disturbances. This is due to studies showing lavender's effectiveness in producing calming, soothing, anticonvulsive effects in those who use it.

LEMON BALM - (MELISSA OFFICINALIS)

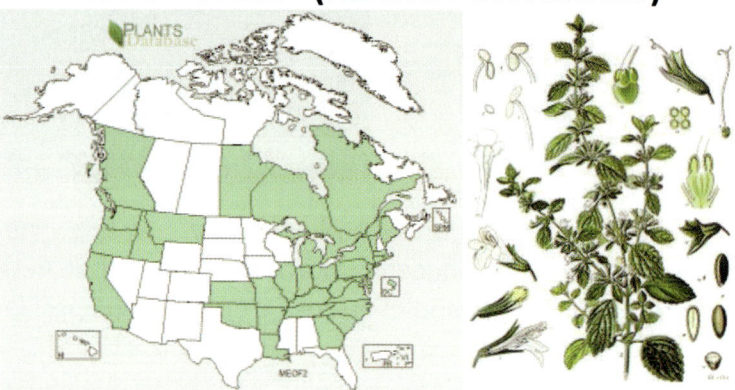

Lemon balm is a perennial herb from the mint family. The leaves, which have a mild lemon aroma, are used to make medicine. Lemon balm is used alone or as part of various multi-herb combination products. It is used for digestive problems including:

Bloating	Pain from including menstrual	Vomiting
Colic	cramps, headache, and toothaches	
Intestinal gas	Upset stomach	

Many people believe lemon balm has calming effects, so they take it for anxiety, sleep problems, and restlessness. It is also used for Alzheimer's disease, attention deficit-hyperactivity disorder, autoimmune disease involving the thyroid, swollen airways, rapid heartbeat due to nervousness, high blood pressure, sores, tumors, and insect bites. Some people apply lemon balm to their skin to treat cold sores. In foods and beverages, the oil extract is used for flavoring.

LEMONGRASS - (CYMBOPOGON CITRATUS)

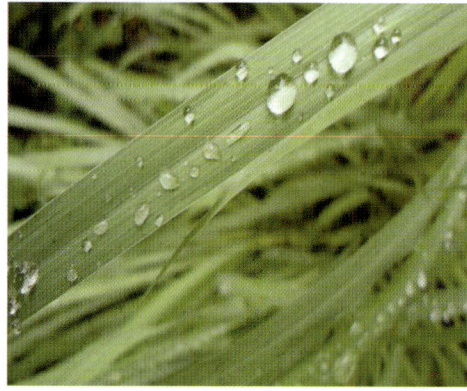

Lemon grass is an aromatic grass that grows naturally in India and Sri Lanka. It is now grown in tropical areas worldwide.

Lemon has a strong scent that most commonly is useful for food flavoring; however, it also works well for medicinal purposes.

Lemon grass is primarily used to treat digestive problems of cramps and gas. It is particularly helpful in treating upset stomach or intestines and can be used to help reduce fever. Lemon grass paste can be applied directly to the skin to treat ringworm and arthritis or applied to joints to reduce arthritic pain.

Do not take lemon grass essential oil internally!

Lesser Periwinkle - (Vinca Minor)

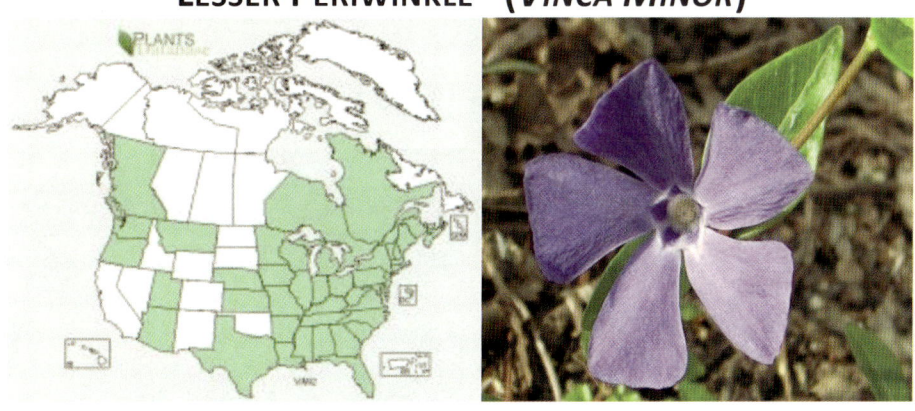

Periwinkle is an herb. The parts that grow above the ground are used to make medicine. Do not confuse periwinkle with Madagascar periwinkle (catharanthus roseus).

Despite serious safety concerns, periwinkle is used for brain health by increasing the blood flow to the brain, increasing mental productivity, preventing memory, concentration problems and feebleness, improving memory and thinking ability and preventing early aging of brain cells. Periwinkle is also used for treating diarrhea, vaginal discharge, throat ailments, tonsillitis, chest pain, high blood pressure, sore throat, intestinal pain and swelling (inflammation), toothache, and water retention. It is also used for promoting wound healing, improving the way the immune system defends the body and for "blood-purification."

Licorice - (Glycyrrhiza Glabra)

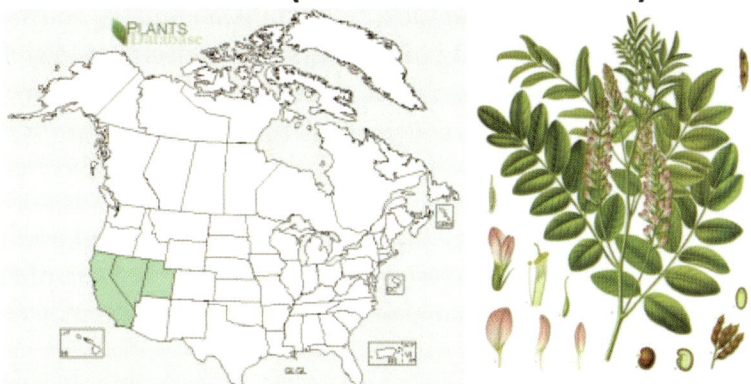

The use of licorice in cultural and traditional settings may differ from concepts accepted by current Western medicine. When considering the use of herbal supplements, consultation with a primary health care professional is advisable.

Licorice is also known as liquorice, American licorice, Spanish licorice, Russian licorice, sweet root, and glycyrrhiza glabra.

Licorice is a commonly used flavoring agent and food product, also available as an herbal supplement. The information contained refers to the use of licorice as an herbal supplement. When used as a food product the benefits and potential side effects of licorice may be less pronounced than when it is used as an herbal supplement.

Licorice has been used to loosen congestion that may occur with a cough or cold, to treat and prevent inflammation and/or ulceration of the stomach. Licorice has been used topically to suppress the production of oil on the scalp.

Lime Flowers – (*Tilia Cordata*)

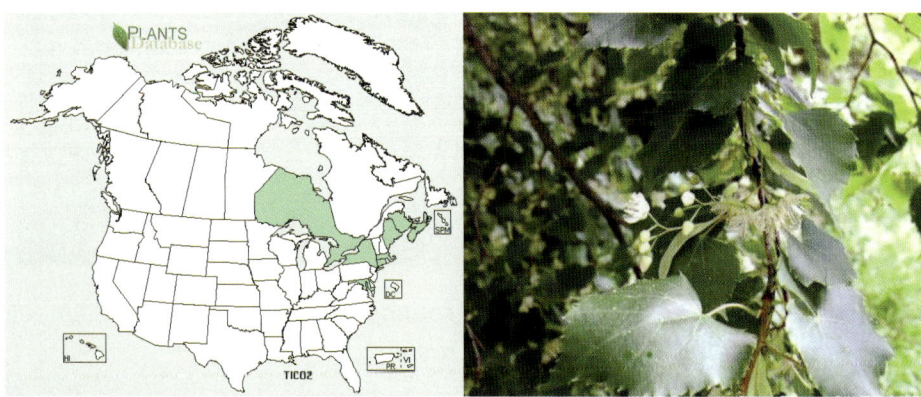

Linden is a tree belonging to different species of the genus tilia, also known as a lime or basswood tree. This herb has been used in European traditional medicine to cure an assortment of health conditions. An herbal tea prepared with dried linden flowers has been employed in the form of a diaphoretic (any medication that stimulates sweating) since the later part of the Middle Ages. In fact, the flowers of linden are prescribed for two opposing purposes—as a nervine (a sedative or medication for the nerves) and also in the form of a stimulant. Apart from these, linden flowers are regarded to be very effective in treating indigestion, headaches, diarrhea, and hysteria. There was a time when people believed that linden flowers were so useful in treating epilepsy that any individual enduring this medical condition could be cured just by sitting beneath a linden tree.

The flowers of linden are an excellent medication for treating tension and nervousness. At the same time, they also promote sleep (cure insomnia), alleviate restiveness and excitement in children, as well as facilitates in unwinding the tensed muscles. Blossoms of linden are also effective for treating medical condition related to tension, such as headaches, colic, menstrual pains and cramps.

The bioflavonoids present in linden flowers have soothing properties, which coupled with their favorable actions on the arteries make them an effective medication to lower high blood pressure as well as treat arteriosclerosis (a degenerating disease of the arteries). In addition, the flowers of linden also comfort/unwind the arteries of the heart, which make them helpful in treating palpitations and coronary heart ailments.

When taken in the form of a hot infusion, linden flowers promote sweating and improve blood circulation to the skin. The flowers of linden are also an effective medication to reduce fevers and especially in children, to clear catarrhal blocking. When ingested along with elderflowers, the blossoms of linden facilitate in treating colds, coughs as well as flu. When taken in the form of an infusion that is either cool or warm, linden flowers have a diuretic action and facilitate in getting rid of excessive fluid accumulation as well as toxic substances from the body by means of urination.

Uses of linden include:

- Alleviating colds and flu by lessening nasal blockage and reducing fever
- Anti-spasmodic remedy (lessening spasms of smooth muscles the length of the digestive tract)
- Colds
- Contagions
- Coughs
- Cure nervous palpitations
- Diaphoretic
- Diuretic (promoting urination)
- Headaches
- Headaches (especially migraine)
- Inflammation and hypertension (high blood pressure)
- Lower hypertension (high blood pressure), especially when emotional issues are concerned
- Tranquilizer (sedative)
- Tranquilizing attributes
- Treat fever
- Treating anxiety

Furthermore, the blooms of this plant are added to baths to alleviate hysteria and brewed in the form of tea to alleviate irregular heartbeat, indigestion, and vomiting related to anxiety. The leaves of linden are used to induce perspiration to reduce fevers. The wood of linden trees is employed to treat complaints of the liver and gallbladder as well as cellulitis. The log of linden trees is completely burned, pulverized into a powdered form, and consumed to cure intestinal complaints. In addition, the powder of the burnt wood of linden is also applied externally to heal infection, for instance, cellulitis (inflammation of cellular tissues), edema, or ulcers of the lower part of the leg.

It has been reported that very frequent use of the herbal tea prepared with blossoms of linden may harm the heart. While this only happens rarely and owing to drinking the beverage in excess, it is advisable that people having known cardiac disorder would be better off by keeping away from using linden flowers.

MALABAR NUT TREE, ADHATODA – (ADHATODA VASICA)

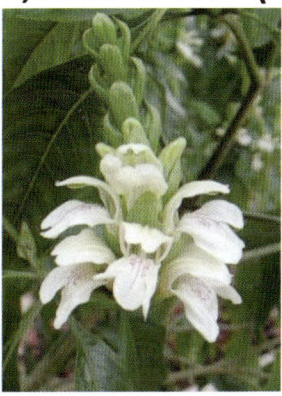

Plant parts that are used: The leaves, roots, flowers, and stem bark of this plant are used in medicinal applications.

The leaves, roots, and flowers have been used extensively in traditional Indian medicine for thousands of years to treat respiratory disorders such as asthma. Adhatoda vasica is thought to be useful in treating bronchitis, tube rculosis, and other lung and bronchiole disorders.

A decoction of the leaves may be used as an herbal treatment for cough and other symptoms of colds. The soothing action helps irritation in the throat and the expectorant will help loosen phlegm deposits in the airway which makes adhatoda a good remedy for sore throat. A poultice of the leaves may be applied to wounds for their antibacterial and anti-inflammatory properties. The poultice is also thought to be helpful in relieving rheumatic symptoms when applied to joints. It has been used to control both internal and external bleeding such as peptic ulcers, piles, and bleeding gums.

In Ayurvedic medicine, adhatoda vasica has been used for a multitude of disorders including:

Blood disorders	Jaundice	Mouth troubles
Fever	Leprosy	Sore-eye
Gonorrhea	Leucoderma	Tumors
Heart troubles	Loss of memory	Vomiting

This herb is known for its antispasmodic, expectorant, and blood-purifying qualities. A juice made from the leaves has been used as a treatment for diarrhea and dysentery, and in southern India the powdered leaves have been used to treat malaria. Additionally, it has been used as a folk medicine to speed delivery during childbirth.

Adhatoda vasica can be an ingredient in many herbal preparations and it may be listed under any of its names. It is important to follow the manufacturer's recommended dosing schedules if the herb is intended as an herbal medicine.

Marshmallow aka Mallow - (Althaea Officinalis)

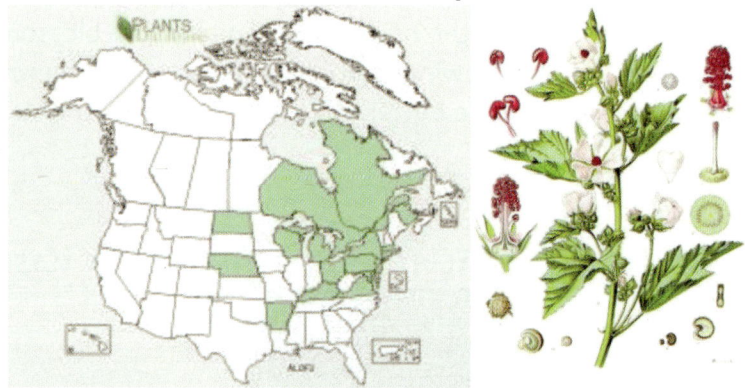

When most people hear marshmallow, they think of the white fluffy food treat commonly roasted at campfires. Marshmallow, however, is also a type of herb. An African plant with short roundish leaves and small pale flowers, it was originally used medicinally by the Egyptians. The French later adopted its usage; today it has a wide variety of medicinal uses.

Marshmallow is most commonly used to treat sore throats and dry coughs. Because of this, marshmallow has a soothing effect on inflamed membranes in the mouth and throat when ingested orally, specifically a sore throat. It also reduces dry coughing, preventing further irritation.

More recently, marshmallow has been used to treat certain digestive disorders including:

Crohn's disease	Indigestion	Ulcerative colitis
Heartburn	Stomach ulcers	

The mechanism by which it soothes sore throats applies to gastrointestinal mucosa as well and regular consumption of marshmallow can help with the pain of ulcerative colitis, Crohn's and prevent stomach ulcers from perforation. Marshmallow extract is sometimes added to creams and used to treat inflammatory skin conditions such as eczema and contact dermatitis. Additional uses are currently being investigated. There is evidence that marshmallow may also help with respiratory disorders such as asthma.

The leaf contains the following minerals:

- Aluminum
- Calcium
- Chromium
- Cobalt
- Iron
- Magnesium
- Manganese
- Nitrogen
- Potassium
- Selenium
- Silica
- Sodium
- Tin
- Zinc

MEADOWSWEET - (*FILIPENDULA ULMARIA*)

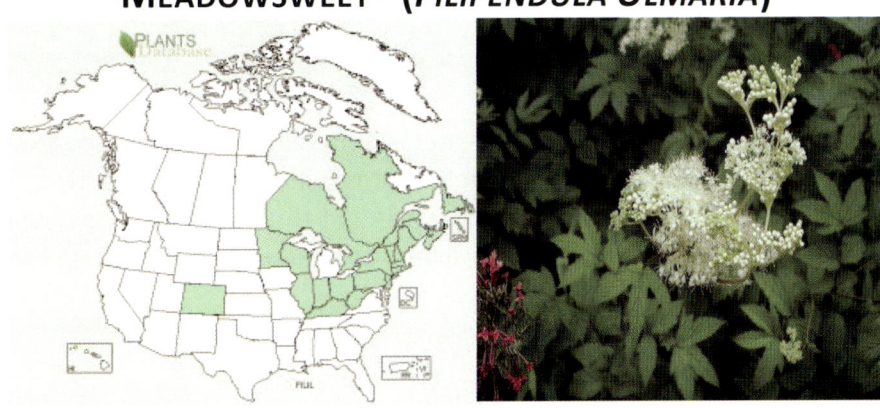

Meadowsweet is an herbaceous perennial shrub native to Europe, but also grows in North America. Meadowsweet's aromatic, ornamental wildflowers are creamy, yellow-white, and have an aroma reminiscent of oil of wintergreen. The dried herb consists of flower petals and some unopened buds that are used as the drug.

Queen Elizabeth adorned her apartments with meadowsweet. The flowers were used to flavor alcoholic beverages in England and Scandinavian countries. In the Middle Ages, meadowsweet was known as "meadwort" because it was used to flavor "mead," an alcoholic drink made by fermenting honey and fruit juices. In 1838, salicylic acid was isolated from the plant. In the 1890s, salicylic acid first was synthesized to make aspirin. The plant was used in folk medicine for cancer, tumors, rheumatism, skin diseases, diarrhea, and as a diuretic.

Meadowsweet is used as a digestive remedy for acid indigestion or peptic ulcers, supportive therapy for colds, respiratory problems, and as an analgesic for joint problems.

Meadowsweet has been used for centuries for cold therapy, gut disturbances, and joint problems. It also possesses bacterial actions and antitumor activity. Definitive clinical studies are needed to fully understand the many medicinal uses of meadowsweet.

MILK THISTLE - (*SILYBUM MARIANUM*)

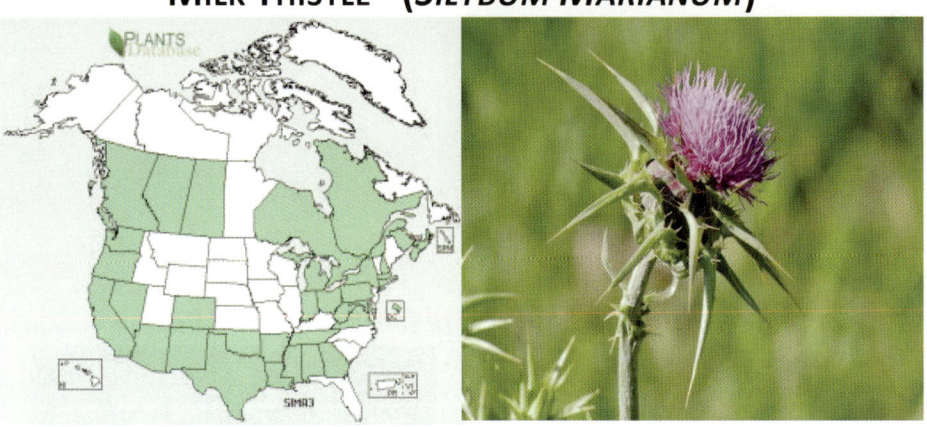

Milk thistle is unique in its ability to protect the liver and has no equivalent in the pharmaceutical drug world. In fact, in cases of poisoning with Amanita mushrooms, which destroy the liver, milk thistle is the only treatment option. It has been so dramatically effective that the treatment has never been disputed. Milk thistle was approved in 1986 as a treatment for liver disease and it is widely used to treat:

Alcoholic fatty liver	Cirrhosis	Viral hepatitis
Alcoholic hepatitis	Liver poisoning	

It has also been shown to protect the liver against medications such as acetaminophen, a non-aspirin pain reliever.

Milk thistle acts in a similar fashion to detoxify other synthetic chemicals that find their way into our bodies, from acetaminophen and alcohol to heavy metals and radiation.

MINTS - PEPPERMINT, SPEARMINT, APPLE MINT, AND PINEAPPLE MINT

Mint is one of the herbs that have it all. It grows like a weed, is perfectly safe for use, is an excellent remedy for reducing symptoms related to digestion and it tastes good going down! They do not serve after-dinner mints virtually everywhere you go for nothing. It is well known for its properties related to indigestion, stomach cramps, menstrual cramps, flatulence, upset stomach, nausea, vomiting, and colic in children. Make a tea out of fresh or dried leaves for a tasty and refreshing after-dinner stomach soother. For the younger crowd, it can also be heated with milk for the same effect (and they will like it).

Mint also can be used as an appetite stimulant. It reduces hunger for a short time, but when the effects wear off the hunger returns stronger than before. For those lucky enough to need to gain a few pounds, a tea might be tried 30 minutes before a meal for appetite stimulation.

Peppermint is much more effective as a medicinal herb than spearmint, which is mostly a culinary herb. However, use spearmint in place of peppermint in cases of digestive problems or colic in very small children as peppermint may be a bit too strong.

For a refreshing and cleansing facial wash, place a handful of bruised mint leaves (any kind) in a quart-sized pan of cool water. Let it sit for an hour or so, then chill in the refrigerator and use as desired. Mint combined with rosemary in vinegar is reported to help control dandruff (place the sprigs in a bottle that can be tightly sealed and let sit for at least a week out of direct sunlight).

New research indicates that mint oil used externally in a cold compress or rubbed directly into the skin can significantly reduce pain in cases of arthritis and chronic joint pain, with few if any side effects.

Peppermint - (*Mentha Piperita*)

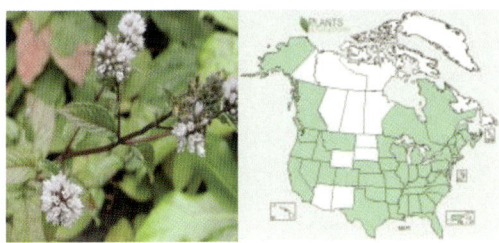

Spearmint - (*Mentha Apicata*)

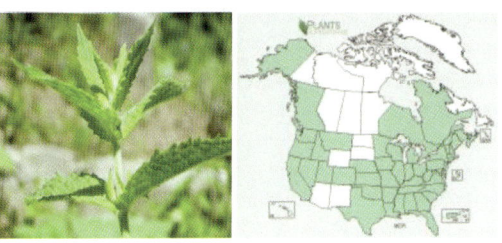

Apple Mint - (*Mentha Suaveolens*)

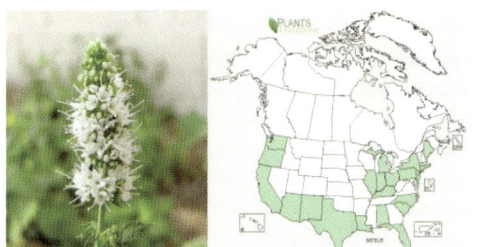

Mountain Mint - (*Pycnanthemum Virginianum*)

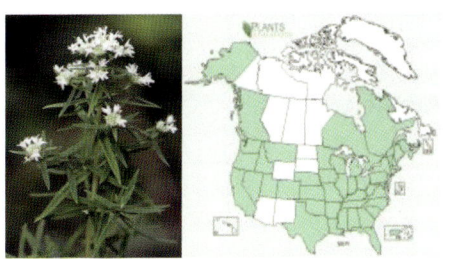

MISTLETOE – (*VISCUM ALBUM*)

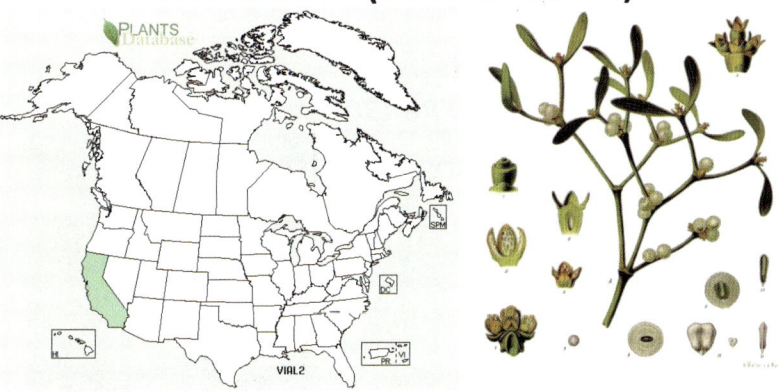

The English name is said to have come from the Anglo-Saxon misteltan, tan meaning "twig" and mistel from "mist" or from tan, "a twig" and mistl, meaning "different."

The major use of mistletoe, viscum album, is as a palliative cancer therapy. Historically it has been used to treat:

- Anxiety
- Arthritis
- Degenerative inflammation of the joints
- Epilepsy
- Exhaustion
- Hypertension
- Vertigo

Both European and American mistletoe contain toxic proteins which are similar in their chemical composition and produce similar effects, including:

- Bradycardia
- Hypotension
- Vasoconstriction

The German Commission E has approved mistletoe as a treatment for degenerative and inflamed joints and as a palliative therapy for malignant tumors.

Hillman Health Food Store call 855-Amish-Dr (855-264-7437) www.emineral.info Vitamins and Minerals for Better Living

MOTHERWORT – (LEONURUS CARDIACA)

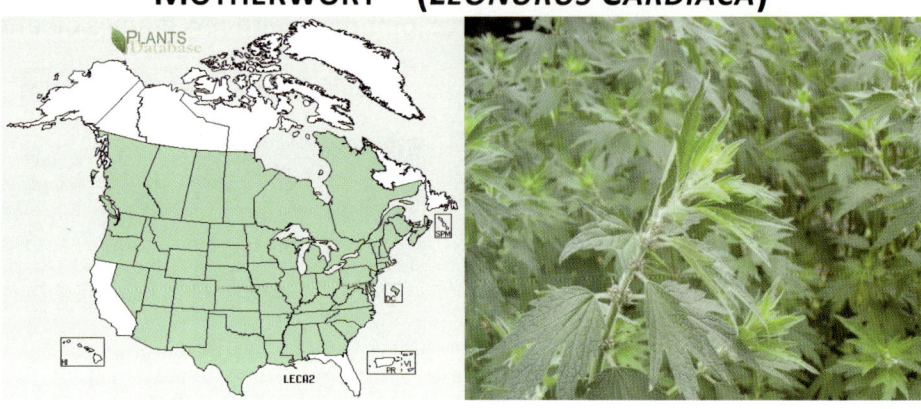

Motherwort is used for melancholy, restlessness, and disturbed sleep from emotional or physical ailments of the heart. It strengthens the heart.

The usages for motherwort are:

Antispasmodic
Congestive amenorrhea or dysmenorrhea
Diuretic
Emmenagogue

Female tonic
High blood pressure due to stress and nerve pain from herpes zoster and herpes simplex
Nervine

Nervous palpitations
Premenstrual nerve tension
Relieving premenstrual cramps with delayed menstruation

Contraindications: It is contraindicated in pregnancy due to the emmenagogue effect.

MULLEIN - (VERBASCUM THAPSUS)

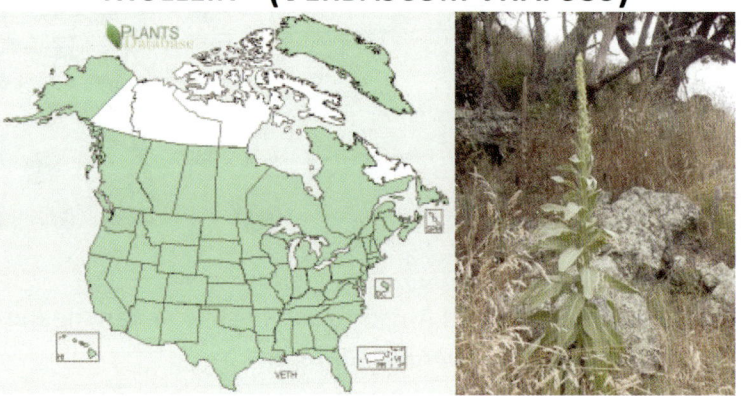

Mullein is an easily-grown plant found all over Europe and in temperate Asia in Himalayas and in North America. There are about 250 distinct species of mulleins. It can adapt to various environments, grows on roadsides, on waste ground, more likely on gravel, sand, or chalk. It can be found in natural meadows, forest openings, neglected pastures, road cuts, and industrial areas. It blossoms during July and August growing with its silver-gray leaves and its sturdy, towering height.

Fresh mullein leaves are used for making a homeopathic tincture. Mullein is commonly recognized by its tall flower spikes, which can be 10 feet tall. It has pretty flowers, but only a few blooms at a time.

Mullein is well known as a medicinal herb that has been used for centuries. The Greek physician, Dioscorides, mentioned the benefits of Mullein for "old coughs." Mullein tea is traditionally an effective treatment for coughs and lung disorders. Flowers and leaves from mullein are used for their strong mucilaginous (sticky and viscous) content against all forms of throat and lung irritation.

The leaf contains the following minerals:

Aluminum	Magnesium	Silica
Calcium	Manganese	Sodium
Chromium	Nitrogen	Tin
Cobalt	Potassium	Zinc
Iron	Selenium	

MYRRH – (COMMIPHORA MOLMOL)

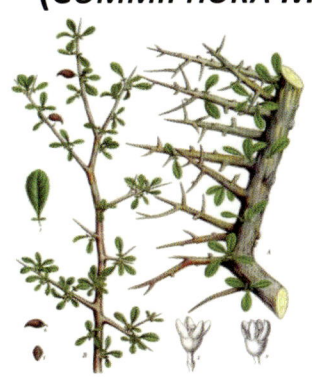

Alternative practitioners recommend the use of myrrh as an antiseptic. Myrrh forms an important ingredient of an ointment that is applied externally to cure hemorrhoids or swollen anus veins, and bed sores as well as wounds. The tincture prepared by steeping myrrh in alcohol is said to be an effective oral astringent (a substance that tightens affected tissues) and is generally used as a mouthwash or for curing a sore throat and other similar problems. Although internal use of myrrh is seldom recommended as the herb cannot be easily absorbed by the intestines, it is sometimes consumed to treat indigestion, ulcers, and also alleviate bronchial congestions. At times, myrrh is also used by physicians as an emmenagogue to invigorate menstrual flow in cases of delayed menstrual cycles or insufficient menstruation. There are many people who advocate the use of myrrh for therapeutic use in problems such as cancer, leprosy, and syphilis (a sexually-transmitted disease), but there is no scientific or whatsoever evidence in this regard.

MUSTARD AKA INDIAN MUSTARD - (BRASSICA JUNCEA)

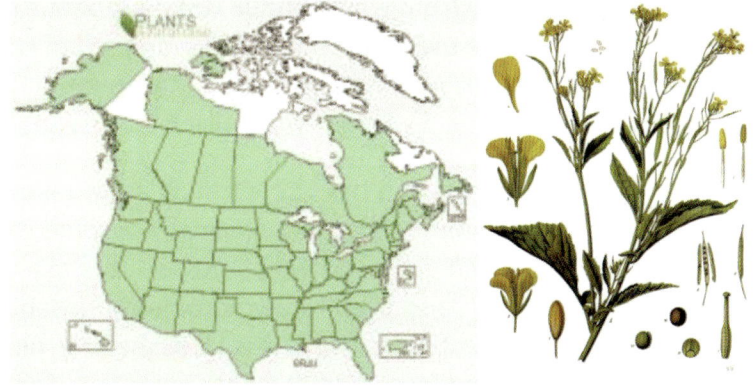

The mustard plant has been used since ancient times and is valued for its oil content. It is found growing wild in many parts of the world as it is widely cultivated, grown in just about every area of North America except the far northern parts, up to eight feet in height.

Common Herbs

There are many varieties of mustard. All have very pungent flavors. Some medicinal mustard compounds date back to at least 400 B.C. Other names for mustard are white mustard, yellow mustard, peppergrass, and hedge mustard. Mustard is the second most popular spice traded around the world. Pepper is the first.

Mustard helps to stimulate blood flow and is known to improve circulation. Believed to have strong aphrodisiac powers and has been included in many love potions. Because it is warming to the skin, it is often used to relieve sore joints and muscles when used as a mustard plaster.

As early as 1699, it was claimed that mustard seed could strengthen the memory, expel heaviness, and revive the spirits. Mustard seed was recommended in 1653 for toothaches, joint pain, skin problems, and stomach aches. Mustard plasters are used to clear up chest congestion, relieve arthritic and rheumatoid pain and soreness. Mustard seed is used to strengthen the digestive system as it can stimulate the flow of gastric juices so to aid with digestion and metabolizing fat in the body as well as encouraging a healthy appetite. While it calms the stomach, it can also act as a laxative. It has also been used to cure stubborn hiccups. Since mustard seed is a stimulant it will warm the circulatory system, this can result in dilated blood vessels, and a warmed system can help burn and metabolize fat in the body. As a warming herb, mustard seed will encourage perspiration that can lower fevers and cleanse the body of toxins, helping the body fight colds and flu.

Neem - (Azadirachta Indica)

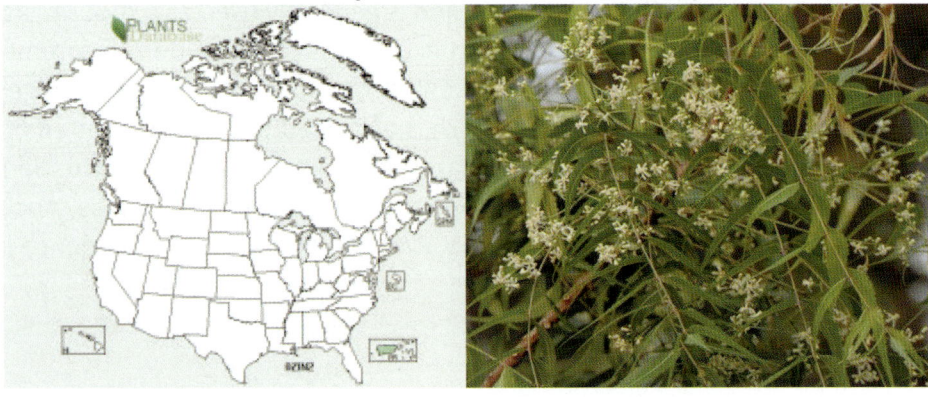

Neem has long been used in many countries, particularly India, to treat a wide range of health problems. Nearly every part of the tree is used medicinally from which about 700 therapeutic preparations have been listed. In addition, twigs from the neem tree are used as toothbrushes, and neem is applied topically as an insect repellent. Despite its broad usage, there is not enough scientific information to confirm the efficacy of neem for any health condition. Do not use Neem without supervision from a healthcare professional.

Other common names for neem include arishtha, bead tree, holy tree, margosa, Persian lilac, nim, and nimba. The bark, leaves, and seeds are more commonly used medicinally, but the root, flower, and fruit are also used. Neem leaf is used to treat stomach distress, liver ailments, intestinal worms, appetite loss, fever, gum disease, skin ulcers, and leprosy. It is also used for eye problems, nosebleeds, cardiovascular disease, and diabetes. Neem bark is used for treating conditions such as malaria, ulcers, skin disorders, and pain. Neem flower is used for decreasing bile and loosening phlegm. Twigs are used for cough, asthma, hemorrhoids, low sperm count, and urinary problems. Some use neem seeds for birth control.

There is not enough information from human studies to rate the effectiveness of neem for any health condition. According to the Natural Medicines Comprehensive Database, preliminary information suggests some benefit of neem for treating gum disease and for healing ulcers.

NUTS - (CYPERUS ROTUNDUS)

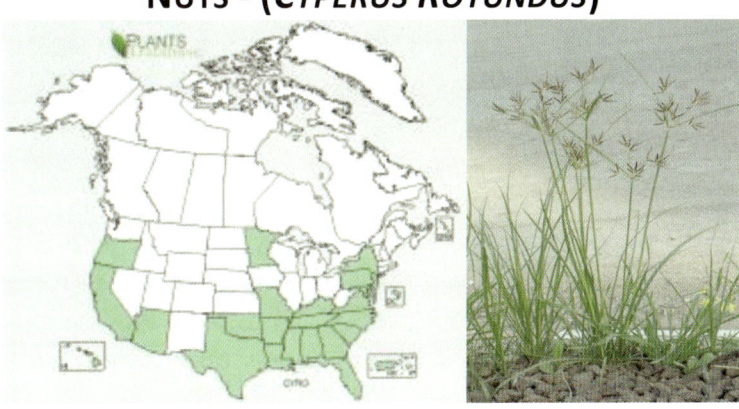

Nuts are also known by the names nutsedge and nut grass. Just munch a handful of nuts a day and you will be doing more than good to keep yourself healthy and stay fit.

Nuts are rich in energy, protein, packed with antioxidants, vitamins, minerals, and much discussed omega-3 fatty acids. Crunchy yet buttery, wonderfully delicious, nuts are wonderful gifts to humankind from God himself.

Nuts are nutritious and loaded with an excellent source of monounsaturated fatty acids, which help to lower LDL or "bad cholesterol" and increase HDL or "good cholesterol." Research studies suggest that a Mediterranean diet that is rich in monounsaturated fatty acids helps to prevent coronary artery disease and strokes by favoring healthy blood lipid profile.

They are rich source of the all important omega-3 essential fatty acids. Research studies have shown anti-inflammatory action helps to lower the risk of:

Blood pressure	Cancer of the breast, colon, and prostate	Coronary artery disease
Strokes		

Nuts are a storehouse of health benefits such as carotenes, resveratrol, and lutein. These compounds have been found to be protective against:

Alzheimer's disease	Degenerative nerve disease	Viral and or fungal infections
Cancers	Heart disease	

Studies suggests that resveratrol in peanuts reduces stroke risk by alteration of molecular mechanisms in the blood vessels, reducing their susceptibility to vascular damage.

Oats – (Avena Sativa)

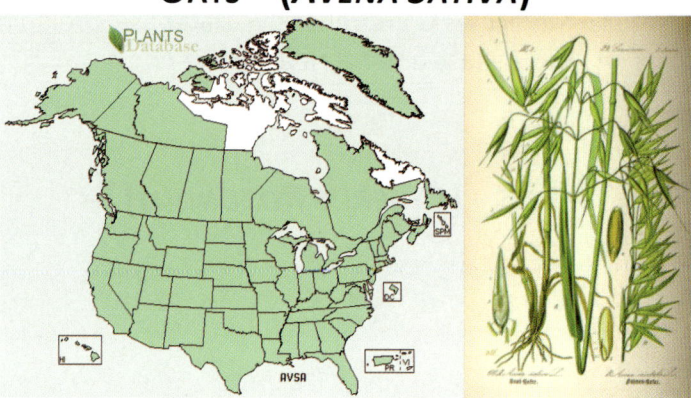

Little history of oat is known prior to the time of Christ. Oats did not become important to man as early as wheat or barley. Oats probably persisted as a weed-like plant in other cereals for centuries prior to being cultivated itself. Some authorities believe that our present cultivated oats developed as a mutation from wild oats. They think this may have taken place in Asia Minor or southeastern Europe not long before the birth of Christ.

Probably the oldest known oat grains were found in Egypt among remains of the 12th Dynasty, which was about 2000 B.C. These probably were weeds and not actually cultivated by the Egyptians. The oldest known cultivated oats were found in caves in Switzerland that are believed to belong to the Bronze Age.

The history of oats is somewhat clouded because there are so many different species and subspecies, which makes identification of old remains very difficult. The chief modern center of greatest variety of forms is in Asia Minor where most all subspecies are in contact with each other. Many feel that the area with the greatest diversity of types is most likely where a particular plant originated.

Oats were first brought to North America with other grains in 1602 and planted on the Elizabeth Islands off the coast of Massachusetts. As early as 1786, George Washington sowed 580 acres to oats. By the 1860s and 1870s, the westward shift of oat acreage in the United States had moved into the middle and upper Mississippi Valley, which is its major area of production today.

While most of us think of oats as a high fiber, low cholesterol breakfast cereal, herbalists have long made use of the grains and straw of avena sativa for their valuable medicinal properties. Oats are an annual grass that is high in calcium. Calcium-rich foods and herbs are the basis for remedies that relax the muscles and nervous system. Avena sativa should be thought of as the basis for every good nerve-relaxing formula.

Oatmeal or gruel is an ideal food for convalescents and can be flavored with raisins, lemon, butter, or maple syrup. It is easily digested and is a soothing food for those with fever and a good first food for those who have experienced intestinal illnesses or food poisoning. Oatmeal is an excellent alternative to eggs and sausages or bacon for those desiring a low fat, low cholesterol breakfast routine.

Oat straw tea is recommended by herbalists to soothe chest complaints, especially when mixed with a little lemon and honey. A strong brew can be added to the bath to benefit rheumatism, paralysis, liver ailments, gout, and kidney problems. Bladder and bowel conditions, intestinal colic, and bedwetting have all been helped by soaking in a bath of oat straw.

Oat straw makes a good wash for:

Chilblains	Frostbite	Wounds
Eye problems	Itching	
Flaky skin	Skin diseases	

Oat straw foot baths are recommended for tired or chronically cold feet. To make the tea, simmer the straw and grains in water for about an hour. For a bath, boil one to two pounds of the straw in three quarts of water for half an hour and add the brew to your tub.

OREGANO - (ORIGANUM VULGARE)

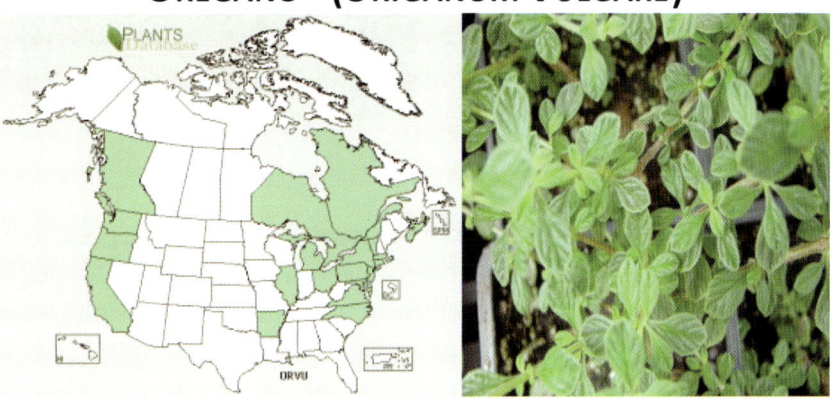

Oregano is usually thought of as a culinary herb and it has been used medicinally for thousands of years. Try a tea made with oregano for:

Bloating	Flatulence	Promoting menstruation
Bronchial problems	Headaches	Swollen glands
Coughs	Indigestion	Urinary problems

It has also been used in the past to relieve fevers, diarrhea, vomiting, and jaundice. Unsweetened tea can be used as a gargle or mouthwash. Alternatively, the leaves can be dried, pulverized, and made into capsule form for when it is inconvenient to make a tea.

Externally, oregano leaves can be pounded into a paste (add small amounts of hot water or tea to reach the desired consistency; oatmeal may also be added for consistency purposes). This paste can then be used for:

Aching muscles	Pain from rheumatism	Swelling
Itching	Sores	

The plant contains the following minerals:

Boron	Magnesium	Sodium
Calcium	Manganese	Zinc
Copper	Nitrogen	
Iron	Potassium	

OREGON GRAPE – (BERBERIS AQUIFOLIUM)

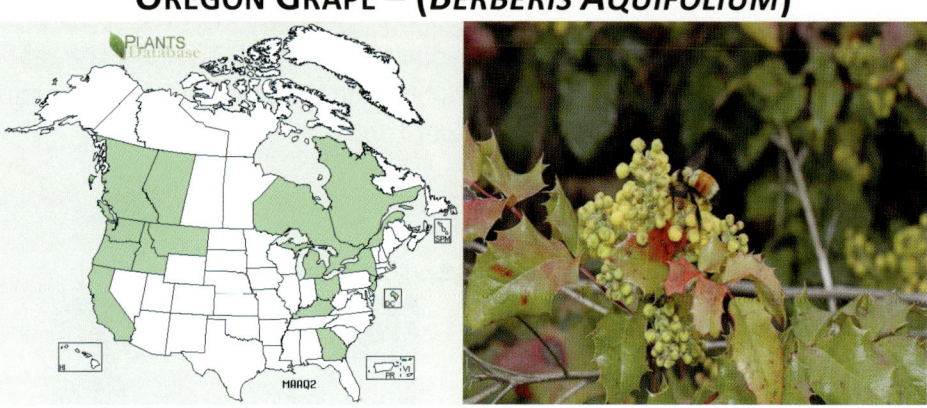

Traditional Role of Oregon grape:

The active constituents in Oregon grape are the alkaloids, berberine, berbamine, canadine, and hydrastine. Berberine can ease diarrhea caused by E. Coli by slowing the time food travels through the intestinal tract. It also inhibits bacteria from attaching to cells, specifically in the intestines, urinary tract, and throat, and boosts immune cell function. Topically, oregon grape has shown some promise for easing psoriasis problems like skin irritation, inflammation, and itching. The root of oregon grape is believed to stimulate digestive function.

Traditional Uses of Oregon grape:

Acne	Candidiasis	Herpes (topical)
Antibacterial and antifungal properties	Detoxification	Immune system
	Diarrhea	Intestinal parasites
Appetite stimulant	Digestive disorders	Liver and gallbladder
Arthritis	Eczema	Psoriasis
Boils	Fever	Urinary tract infections

Oregon grape is not recommended in large amounts or for long term use. It should not be used during pregnancy or lactation.

PANSY - (VIOLA TRICOLOR)

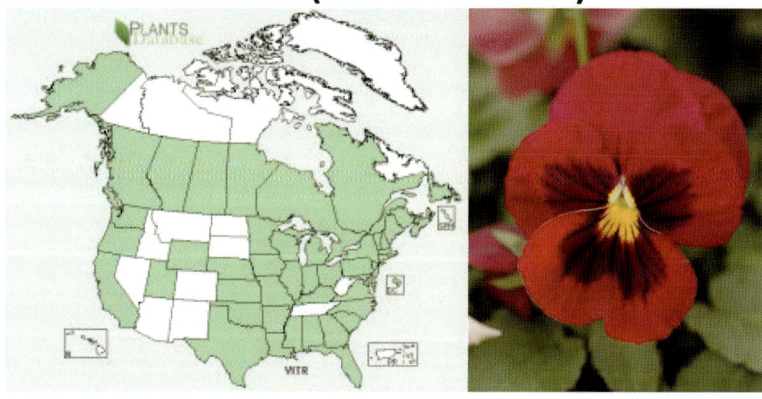

The pansy is an annual plant. The soft, angular, hollow stem, 4 to 12 inches high, bears alternate toothed leaves on the lower part of the plant and has a large, leaf like, and strongly divided. The flowers may be yellow, blue, violet, or two-colored with a flowering time from March to October.

It is widely cultivated as a garden ornamental, but also found wild in fields, meadows, heaths, moors, sunny banks, and along the edges of forests in North America, northern Asia, and Europe.

Although pansy is known as heart's ease, there is another herb known as heart's ease or lady's thumb. Lady's thumb is of the buckwheat family and has no similarity whatsoever to the pansy.

Used medicinally since ancient times, it was once used in love potions, hence the name of heart's ease.

An infusion is useful for:

Acne	Dry throat	Pleurisy
Arteriosclerosis	Epilepsy	Prevents colds
Asthma	Fevers	Psoriasis
Bedwetting	Gout	Retinal hemorrhages
Blemished skin	Heart palpitations	Rheumatic problems
Blood purifier	High blood pressure	Scaly skin diseases
Chest congestion	Hives	Skin eruptions
Convulsions	Hysteria	Sores
Cough	Itch	Tendency to bruise easily
Cradle cap in infants and children	Jaundice	Ulcers
Cramps in children	Lung inflammations	Urinary problems
Diaper rash	Mild sedative	Varicose veins
Diarrhea	Nervous complaints	

The dried and powdered plant can be applied to wounds or made into a salve with honey for external use.

PARSLEY - (PETROSELINUM CRISPUM)

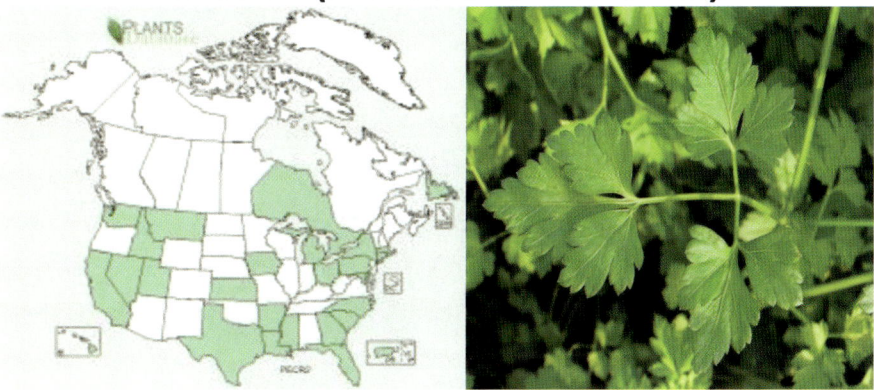

The leaf, seed, and root of parsley are used to make medicine for:

Asthma	Gastrointestinal disorders	Osteoarthritis
Colic	High blood pressure	Prostate conditions
Constipation	Indigestion	Spleen conditions
Cough	Intestinal gas	"Tired blood"
Diabetes	Jaundice	Urinary tract infection
Fluid retention	Kidney stones	

It is also used to start menstrual flow, to cause an abortion, as an aphrodisiac and as a breath freshener. Some people apply parsley directly to the skin for cracked or chapped skin, bruises, tumors, insect bites, lice, parasites, and to stimulate hair growth. In foods and beverages, parsley is widely used as a garnish, condiment, food, and flavoring. In manufacturing, parsley seed oil is used as a fragrance in soaps, cosmetics, and perfumes.

Parsley might help stimulate the appetite, improve digestion, increase urine production, reduce spasms, and increase menstrual flow.

PARTRIDGE BERRY - (MITCHELLA REPENS)

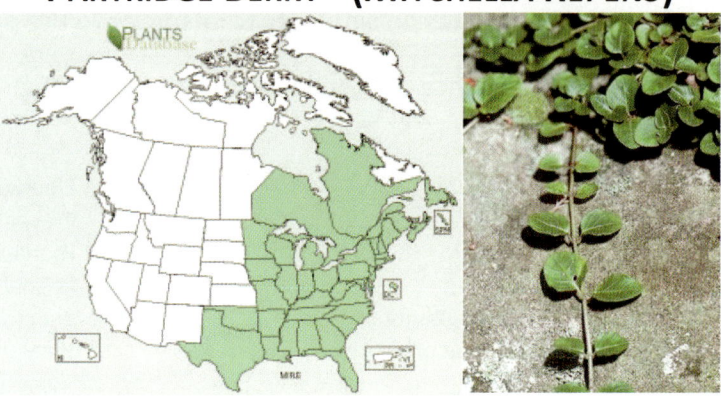

Partridge berry is a perennial evergreen found in the shady woods of the eastern U.S., with trailing roots, opposite leaves, white flowers, and red berries.

Partridge berry is one of the best known herbs for readying the uterus for childbirth. It was considered by some to increase the nervous tone of the uterus, taken during the final two months of pregnancy in preparation for childbirth and to facilitate labor. Partridge berry is also used as a preventative for threatened miscarriage. As a uterine relaxant, it is useful for both amenorrhea and painful periods. Naturopathic doctors have recommended it for prostatic enlargement with difficult urination in men who are mostly sedentary in habit.

CONSULT YOUR MIDWIFE BEFORE USAGE!

PASQUE FLOWER – (PULSATILLA VULGARIS)

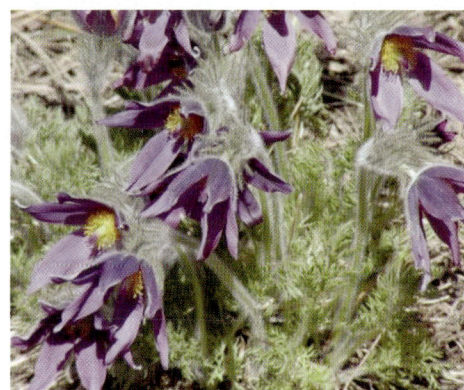

The pasque flower is native to northern and central Europe and western Asia. This very beautiful, perennial, early-flowering herb was given its common name ("pasque" is Old French for Easter) because it flowers near Easter, and it was once used to color Easter eggs. The Blackfeet Indians called the pasque flower "Napi" and used the leaves as a poultice as a counter-irritant for rheumatism. The fresh plant is the most active, but it is also highly irritating both externally and internally. The dried, powdered plant is sometimes used to promote the healing of wounds. Minute doses diluted in water have been used internally in homeopathic practice for:

Anxiety	Earache	Rheumatism
Asthma	Eye ailments	Skin eruptions
Bronchitis	Leukorrhea	Stress
Coughs	Obstructed menses	Tension

This pasque flower contains a poison that causes skin irritation and violent convulsions. It is used in homeopathic remedies. Grow only to enjoy its lovely purple bell-shaped flowers in early spring, and keep children away from the plantings.

Medicinal properties include:

Diaphoretic
Diuretic
Nervine

Rubefacient (causing redness of the skin)
Stimulant

PASSIONFLOWER - (*PASSIFLORA INCARNATA*)

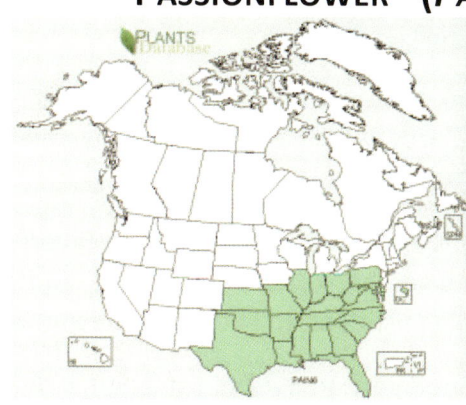 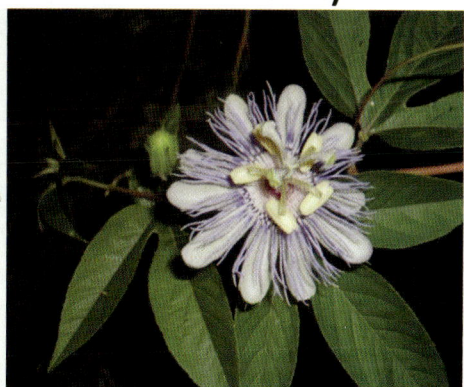

Passionflower is used in alternative medicine for:

Anxiety
Insomnia

Nervous disorders
Seizures

It is more commonly used in Europe than its native home, the United States, where it can be found growing profusely in fields and on fencerows. Passionflower has been approved by Germany's Commission E for the treatment of "nervous unrest."

Passionflower is said to be useful for back pain due to action on the nerves. The calming properties may also be helpful for attention deficit disorder and attention deficit hyperactivity disorder. However, since it has not been extensively studied it is not advisable to use on children without approval of their doctor.

Passionflower is not considered as strong in action as valerian or kava, but might be a good option for those who cannot stand the taste of the stronger herbs. It also has a reputation as an aphrodisiac.

Passionflower is both an edible and medicinal plant. As a tea, it is often blended with valerian, chamomile, lemon balm, skull cap, St. Johns wort, or other relaxing herbs. On its own in tea, it has a pleasant, very mild, but unusual taste, much like its fragrance that is hard to describe. The color of the infusion is a very pale green, lighter in color than most herbal teas. Some people say the scent is an aphrodisiac fragrance. The taste is not at all overwhelming so it could blend well with most any herb or iced tea.

The fruit contains calcium, iron, and nitrogen.

Pau d'Arco- (Tabebuia Avellanedae)

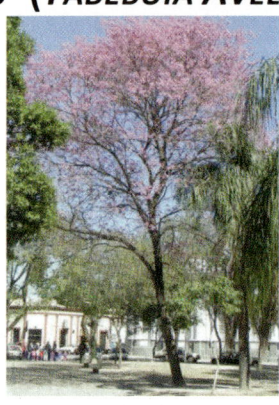

The pau d'arco tree is a beautiful tree with stunning pink trumpet or lily like flowers. It is native to South America. The inner bark is used as the source for pau d'arco, which was traditionally taken as a tea for ailments by many of the South American tribes for centuries.

Although the original and traditional use of this herb was exceptionally varied from fevers, pain relief colds and lung problems to more severe and often incurable diseases like cancer, arthritis, and syphilis, it has lately emerged predominantly as a means of combating cancer and to stimulate the immune system.

Although this herb was tested and passed by the U.S. Food and Drug Administration, it did cause diarrhea and nausea in some patients that were taking this herb in large quantities.

The bark contains the following minerals:

Aluminum	Magnesium	Silica
Calcium	Manganese	Sodium
Chromium	Nitrogen	Tin
Cobalt	Potassium	Zinc
Iron	Selenium	

Pineapple - (Ananas Comosus)

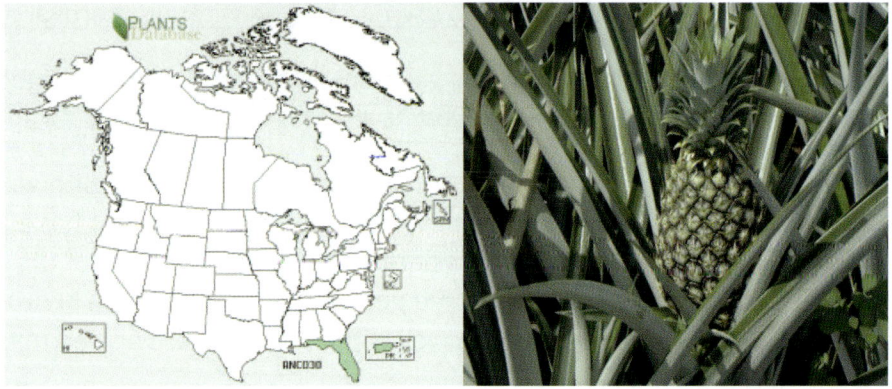

Pineapple plants grow to heights of 2 to 4 feet. The well-known fruit of the pineapple is actually a complex flower head that forms around the stem. The pineapple is the only cultivated fruit whose main stem runs completely through it. Each of the eyes on the surface is the dried base of a small flower. The top crown of leaves contains a bud, which when mature indicates the fruit is ready for cutting. Pineapples contain no seeds but are grown from their crowns.

Pineapples originated in South America and likely did not reach Hawaii until the 19th century. Europeans spread the plant throughout much of the world. Because of rising labor costs today, the bulk of pineapple production no longer occurs in Hawaii, but in regions of South America and the Philippines. The pineapple is cultivated for use in which juices, syrups, and candies are prepared.

The plant has a long history in traditional tropical medicine for the treatment of ailments ranging from constipation to jaundice. Pineapple has been used to:

Burn debridement	Prevent ulcers	Reduce soft tissue inflammation and irritation
Enhance fat excretion		

Pineapple extracts may produce:

Diarrhea	Skin rash	Uterine contractions
Nausea	Skin sensitization	Vomitting

Repeated exposure of pineapple cutters to bromelain can result in the obliteration of fingerprints and the hooked margins of the leaves can cause painful injury.

PLANTAIN - (PLANTAGO MAJOR)

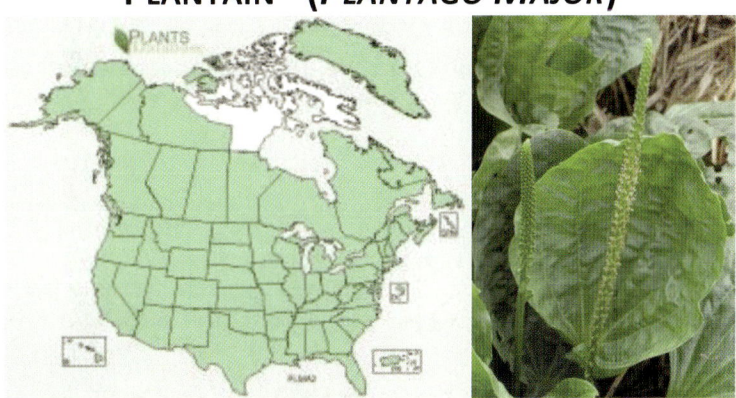

The plantain is very easy to cultivate. It succeeds in any soil and prefers a sunny location, and some varieties have been selected for their ornamental value. It is an important food plant for the caterpillars of many species of butterflies. Each tiny flower is brownish and bell-shaped with four stamens and purple anthers. Harvest the fresh young edible leaves in spring. Gather plantain after flower spike forms and dry for later herb use.

Young leaves are edible raw in salad or cooked as a potherb and very rich in B vitamins. The herb has a long history of use in alternative medicine dating back to ancient times. Being used as a medicine for everything in some cultures, one American Indian name for the plant translates to "life medicine." In addition, recent research indicates that this name may not be far from true due to its use as a powerful anti-toxin.

The leaves and the seed are used medicinally as:

Anti inflammatory	Astringent	Laxative
Antibacterial	Cardiac	Poultice
Antidote	Diuretic	
Antiseptic	Expectorant	

Medical evidence exists to confirm uses as an alternative medicine for:

Asthma	Bronchitis	Rheumatism
Bladder problems	Fever	
Blood sugar control	Hypertension	

The root is used in the treatment of a wide range of complaints including:

Asthma	Diarrhea	Hemorrhoids
Bronchitis	Dysentery	Irritable bowel syndrome
Catarrh	Gastritis	Peptic ulcers
Coughs	Hay fever	Sinusiti
Cystitis	Hemorrhage	

It also causes a natural aversion to tobacco and is currently being used in stop smoking preparations. Extracts of the plant have antibacterial activity, it is a safe and effective treatment to quickly stop bleeding and encourage the repair of damaged tissue. The heated leaves are used for the following:

A wet dressing for wounds	Promote healing without scars	Stings
Cuts	Skin inflammations	Swellings
Malignant ulcers		

A poultice of hot leaves is bound onto cuts and wounds to draw out thorns, splinters, and inflammation. The root is said to be used as anti-venom for the rattlesnake's bites. Plantain seeds contain up to 30% mucilage, which swells in the gut, acting as a bulk laxative and soothing irritated membranes. The seeds are used in the treatment of parasitic worms.

PLEURISY ROOT – (ASCLEPIAS TUBEROSE)

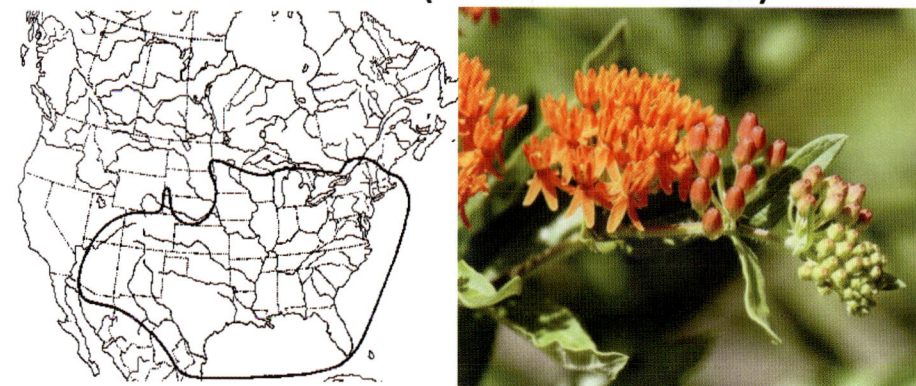

Commonly found from Canada southwards, it is known popularly as pleurisy root. It is also known from its medicinal uses against a wide range of respiratory and lung conditions specifically pleurisy, for which it was formerly official to the United States Pharmacopoeia.

Pleurisy root acts as an expectorant and relieves pain and congestion in the lungs, subduing inflammation, and exerting a general mild tonic effect, making it valuable in all chest complaints.

Pleurisy Root Side Effects: Large doses are emetic and purgative. The mature plant contains alkaloids that are toxic to livestock, and not recommended for women who are pregnant or breastfeeding, and children.

POKE ROOT – (PHYTOLACCA DECANDRA)

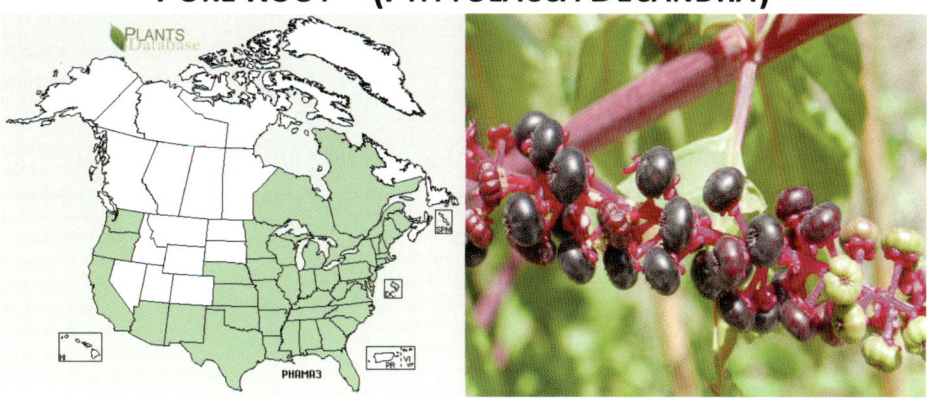

Phytolacca Americana is native to the eastern seaboard of the United States and Mexico. The plant is perennial and produces large tuberous roots weighing as much as 5 kilos. Any cleared land in the Southeastern United States is quickly colonized by this hardy perennial due to birds' fondness for its fruit and the veracity of the plants' growth habit.

Throughout its range, phytolacca is factored into domestic medicine. The Virginia tribes called it pokan which led to its English common name, pokeweed. The Pamunkey Tribe used the berries in a decoction to treat rheumatism. Initially the Colonials used the root of phytolacca to treat inflammatory conditions of the cow udder, specifically in the condition known as garge, hence its early common name: "garget plant." In time, this practice extended to women suffering from mastitis. As the colonial period progressed the root was used to treat all manner of inflammation, especially inflamed joints, applied topically and taken internally. The berry, macerated in alcohol, was a common domestic remedy for "rheumatism."

The uses of phytolacca decandra in early American medical circles include:

Anti-rheumatic	Discutient	Skin cancer
Cathartic	Emetic	Ulcers
Chronic rheumatism	Eruptive skin disease	Vulnerary
Chronic skin disease	Escharotic pathologies	
Discutient	Rheumatic conditions	

PRICKLY ASH – (ZANTHOXYLUM CLAVA-HERCULIS)

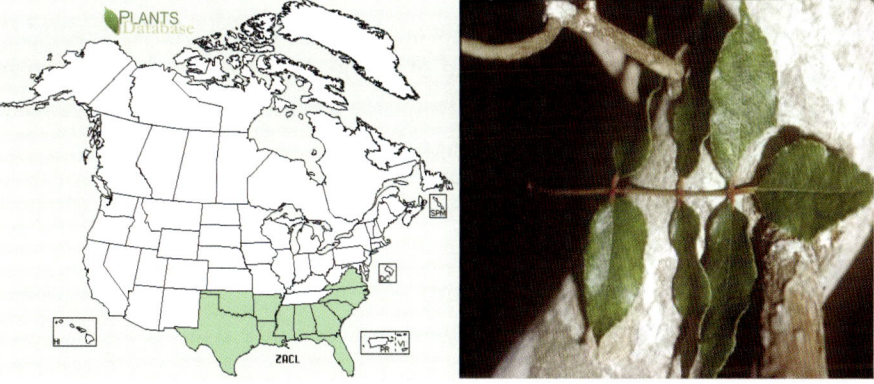

Prickly ash is indicated in relaxed, feeble conditions found with atonic digestive states where it improves digestion and circulation. It is specific for neuralgic pains.

The uses of prickly ash are:

Anti-inflammatory	Heartburn	Low Stomach Acidity
Antimicrobial	Immunomodulator	Restores vascular tone and
Diaphoretic	Indigestion	promotes capillary circulation

It is a good addition to formulas where a stimulating and tonifying alterative is needed for convalescence or the elderly. It is used for chronic rheumatic conditions, gastric irritation with gas and burping, loss of sensitivity in injured nerves and immune system support.

It is contraindicated in pregnancy due to the emmenagogue effect.

Psyllium - (Plantago Psyllium)

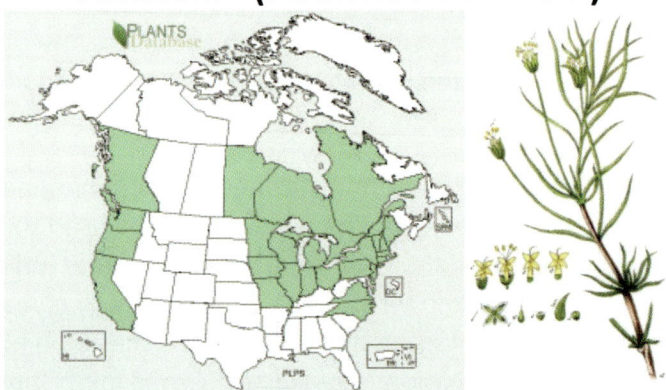

Psyllium is quickly becoming one of the top recommendations for low-carbohydrate diets. It is very difficult to get enough fiber in a diet when you eliminate the carbohydrates in cereals, whole grains, and fruits. Psyllium capsules are an easy way to take care of this problem. It fills you with fiber, reducing appetite without over stimulating the nervous system; a much healthier approach than formulas containing ephedra.

Psyllium is the husk of the seed of the plantain and is a top herb used in weight control and general intestinal health. It contains a spongy fiber that reduces appetite, improves digestion, cleanses the system, making it an excellent choice for healthy dieting. Psyllium can provide the missing fiber on low carbohydrate diets. Every 100 grams of psyllium provides 71 grams of soluble fiber; a similar amount of oat bran would contain only 5 grams of soluble fiber. Only recently have scientists learned that soluble fiber has unique effects on metabolism, providing a feeling of fullness that is helpful before meals. Just take one or two capsules with a glass of water or Yerba Mate tea, one half hour before meals. Psyllium is one of the simplest, healthiest, and most effective herbs for weight control.

Psyllium has also been used for irritable bowel syndrome (a stress-related disorder with alternating bouts of diarrhea and constipation). Because it will produce easy bowel movements with a loose stool, patients with anal fissures (cracks in the skin near the anus) and hemorrhoids use psyllium. Often recommended following anal or rectal surgery, during pregnancy and as a secondary treatment in certain types of diarrhea.

Psyllium soaks up a significant amount of water in the digestive tract, thereby making stools firmer and slower to pass. Psyllium also has the additional advantages over other sources of fiber of reducing flatulence and bloating. It may be recommended by a physician to help soften the stool and reduce pain associated with hemorrhoids.

PUMPKIN - (CUCURBITA PEPO)

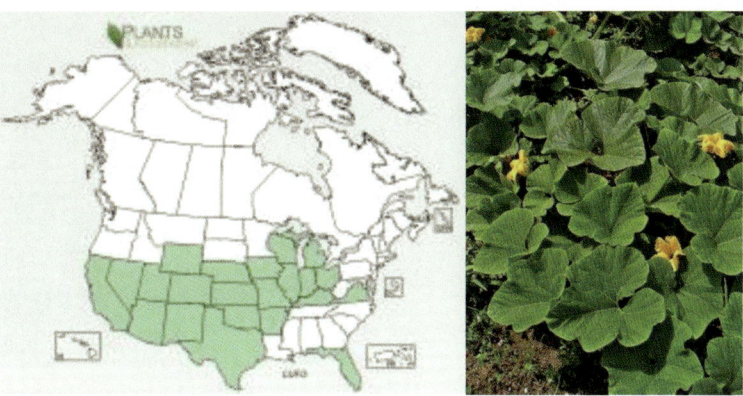

The plant is a vine, creeps on the surface in a similar fashion like that of other members of the family such as cucumber, squash, and cantaloupe. It is one of the most popular vegetables that are grown as a commercial field crop all over the world including in the USA.

Pumpkins vary greatly in shape, size, and colors. Great pumpkins generally weigh 4 to 6 pounds. With the largest capable of reaching weights over 25 pounds. Golden nugget pumpkins are flat, smaller in size, and have sweet creamy orange-colored flesh.

Pumpkin is incredibly rich in anti-oxidants and vitamins. The backyard vegetable is very low in calorie yet a good source of vitamin A, flavonoids, and antioxidants like lutein, xanthenes, and carotenes.

Although pumpkins in general feature orange or yellow color, some fruits are dark to pale green, orange-yellow, white, red, and gray. The rind is smooth and usually lightly ribbed. The color of pumpkins is due to yellow-orange pigments in their skin and pulp.

In structure, the pulp is golden-yellow to orange in color. The fruit has a hollow center with numerous, small, off-white colored seeds interspersed in the net like structure. Pumpkin seeds are a great source of protein, minerals, vitamins, and omega-3 fatty acids.

It is one of the vegetables which is very low in calories, providing just 26 calories per 100 grams, contains no saturated fats or cholesterol, is a rich source of dietary fiber, antioxidants, minerals and many anti-oxidant vitamins such as A, C, and E.

Research studies suggest natural foods rich in vitamin A help protect against lung and oral cavity cancers. It is also a rich source of minerals:

Calcium	Phosphorus
Copper	Potassium

PURSLANE - (PORTULACA OLERACEA)

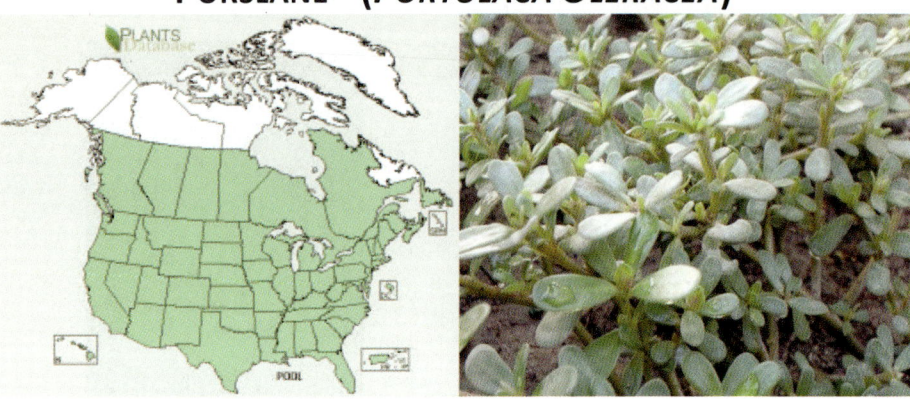

Purslane is a non-native weed plant, introduced to the United States from Europe in the 17th century. Purslane is easily identifiable and common throughout the U.S. Purslane forms spreading mats of stems and leaves that can grow 6 inches tall and cover an area from 2 to 3 ½ feet. It has round, reddish stems and one inch oval leaves.

You can find this plant growing wild along roadsides and in orchards, gardens, and crop fields. The plant has the ability to grow nearly any place it finds some amount of gravel, sand, or loam. Purslane readily withstands hot temperatures and dry conditions, because of the plant's ability to store water within its stems and leaves. On very hot and sunny days from May through September, you may observe purslane's flowers open from mid-morning through the afternoon. The blooms have five tiny yellow petals. Cultivated forms are eaten both raw and steamed, providing the best plant source for magnesium and omega-3-fatty acids. It is also rich in vitamin C, vitamin E, and potassium.

PYGEUM - (PRUNUS AFRICANA)

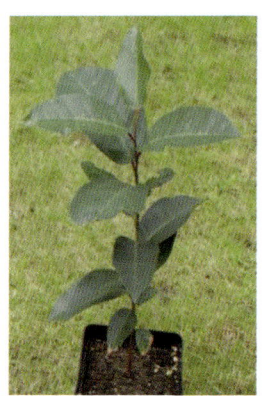

Pygeum is an evergreen tree native to African forest regions. It can grow to 150 feet in height. The thick leaves are oblong in shape with small, white flowers. Pygeum fruit is a red berry, resembling a cherry when ripe. The bark, the part of the plant used for medicinal purposes, is red, brown, or gray.

Its hard wood is valued in Africa and is often used to make wagons. African natives treat urinary problems using the powdered bark.

Pygeum has been used to improve benign prostate conditions and to improve sexual function. Usual dosage is 100 milligrams/day in 6 to 8 week cycles. Gastrointestinal irritation has been reported with the use of pygeum.

In human trials, a low incidence of toxicity has been demonstrated, with no side effects reported in 18 patients taking 200 milligrams/day of pygeum for 60 days. Gastrointestinal irritation ranging from nausea to severe stomach pain has been documented but with only a small percentage discontinuing therapy. In 263 patients, GI adverse effects occurred in five patients with only three patients having to stop treatment. It is recommended that pygeum be taken only under professional supervision.

This herb seems to be good for the following:

Anti-inflammatory
Helps reduce the size of prostate adenomas
Help to inhibit inflammation
Effective anti-edema agents

Increase the integrity of small veins and capillaries
Inhibiting the absorption and metabolism of cholesterol
Reduction in prostate size

QUEVRANCHO - (ASPIDOSPERMA QUEBRACHO-BLANCO)

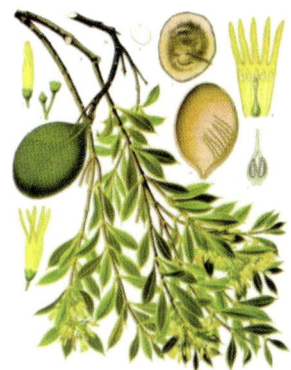

The bark of the quevrancho plant is used as medicine.

Be careful not to confuse quevrancho blanco (white quevrancho) with quevrancho Colorado (red quevrancho). Both are known as quevrancho, but they contain different chemicals. This information pertains to white quevrancho.

People take quevrancho for asthma and conditions of the lower respiratory tract to loosen chest congestion and as a respiratory tract stimulant.

Sometimes Quevrancho is used to treat:

Asthma
Cough
Fever
Fluid retention

High blood pressure
Increase sex drive
Lung disorders
Menstrual cramps

Pain
Spasms

Quevrancho is safe in food amounts, but there is not enough information to know if it is safe in medicinal amounts. It can cause some side effects including drooling, headache, sweating, dizziness, stupor, and sleepiness. In large doses, it can cause nausea and vomiting. Quevrancho is used as flavoring in foods and beverages.

RED CLOVER - (TRIFOLIUM PRATENSE)

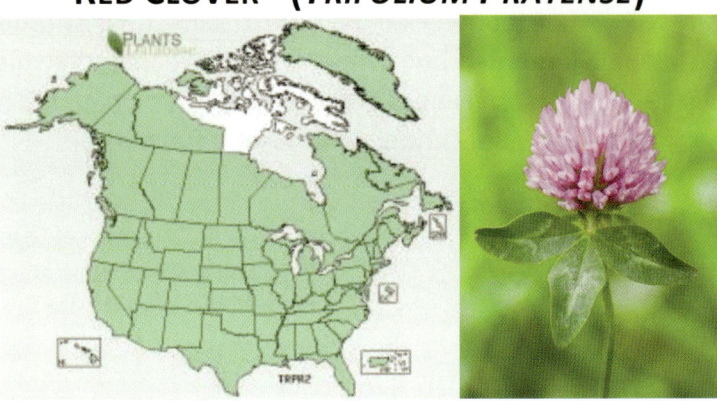

Red clover is native to Europe, Asia, and Africa and is naturalized in many other parts of the world. Herbalists use the flower heads, dried or fresh, to create herbal compounds. Use of the herb in the recommended dosages causes no known health hazards or side effects.

Red clover provides a rich source of plant-based estrogens and most extracts are standardized to contain specific amounts. A standard dose of the fresh or dried herb is 1 to 2 teaspoons of flower tops steeped in 8 ounces of water. Manufacturers provide standard dosage amounts for tinctures, capsules, powders, or extracts on the package label. Red clover may alleviate menopausal hot flashes, mood changes, night sweats, and vaginal dryness.

Research that is more independent is needed to confirm that red clover can reduce bone loss due to estrogen levels and movating the mineral boron. Researchers must also conduct more studies to determine how effective red clover is at reducing some cancer cells. Red clover contains vitamin A, B-complex, and vitamin C.

The red clover contains the following minerals:

Aluminum	Iron	Selenium
Boron	Magnesium	Silica
Calcium	Manganese	Sodium
Chromium	Nitrogen	Tin
Cobalt	Potassium	Zinc
Copper	Selenium	

REHMANNIA – (REHMANNIA GLUTINOSA)

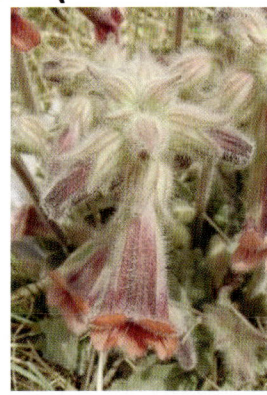

Rehmannia glutinosa is one of the 50 fundamental herbs used in traditional Chinese medicine. Rehmannia was known as dihuang (meaning earth yellow, or underground yellow) and disui (earth marrow) at the time the Shennong Bencao Jing was written (ca. 100 A.D.). Steamed roots of rehmannia glutinosa have been traditionally used in Oriental medicine for the treatment of auditory diseases such as tinnitus and hearing loss. Rehmannia rutinosa herb medical benefit and use as aphrodisiac, and rehmannia root powder has been used to enhance energy.

This plant is native to China, Japan, and Korea. Traditionally, the root has been used to replenish vitality, strengthen the liver, kidney, and heart, and for treatment of a variety of ailments like diabetes, anemia, and urinary tract problems. This herb is sometimes included in sexual enhancement products.

Rehmannia benefits:

- Ameliorates the progressive renal failure induced by 5/6 nephrectomy
- Certain hearing problems and for kidney disease
- Hypoglycemic effect of rehmannia glutinosa oligosaccharide in hyperglycemic and alloxan-induced diabetic rats and its mechanism
- Is involved in red blood cell regeneration
- Maintain healthy blood sugar levels
- May be involved in anti-tumor activity
- Passion Rx for sexual enhancement in a male and female
- Rehmannia glutinosa activates intracellular antioxidant enzyme systems in mouse auditory cells
- Rehmannia is used to enhance energy and sexuality, and it could also have benefits in terms of blood
- Sugar control

Rehmannia contains vitamins A, B, C, and amino acids.

REISHI - (GANODERMA LYCEUM)

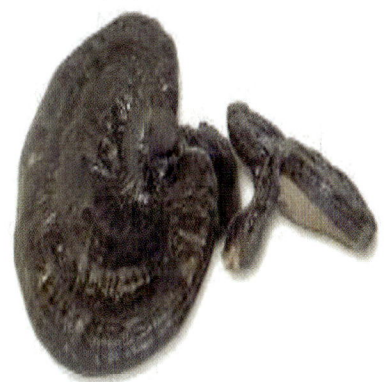

Reishi mushroom is a fungus that some people describe as "tough" and "woody" with a bitter taste. The fruiting body grows above ground and is used as medicine.

Reishi mushroom is used for:

Altitude sickness
Boosting the immune system
Cancer
Chronic fatigue syndrome
Heart disease and contributing conditions as high blood pressure and high cholesterol
Herpes pain
Kidney disease
Liver disease
Lung conditions including asthma, bronchitis
Poisoning
Preventing Fatigue
Reducing stress
Stomach ulcers
Trouble sleeping
Viral infections such as the fly and swine flu

In combination with other herbs, reishi mushroom has been used to treat prostate cancer.

Reishi mushroom is possibly safe for most people when used appropriately. It can cause some side effects including:

Bloody stools
Dryness of the mouth, throat, and nasal area
Itchiness
Nosebleeds
Stomach upset

Drinking reishi wine can cause a rash. Breathing in reishi spores can trigger allergies. Stay on the safe side and avoid use when pregnant. Reishi mushroom seems to be able to lower blood pressure. There is a concern that it might make low blood pressure worse and could interfere with treatment. If your blood pressure is too low, it is best to avoid reishi mushrooms.

Reishi contains vitamin B complex and vitamin D.

Reishi contains the following minerals:

Calcium
Copper
Iron
Phosphorus
Potassium
Selenium

RHODIOLA – (*RHODIOLA ROSEA*)

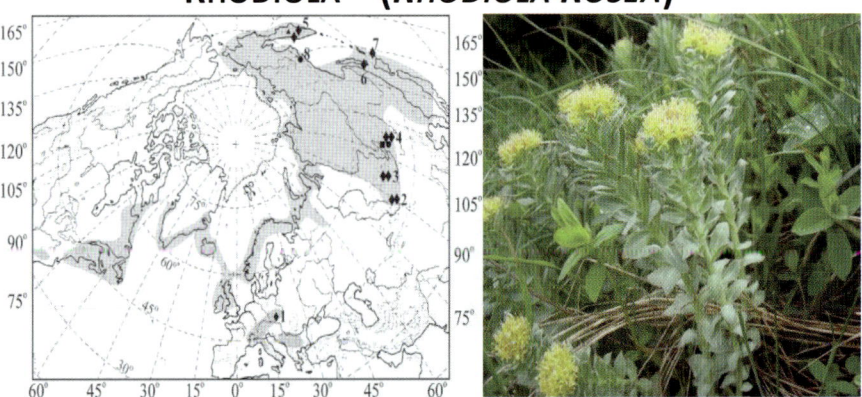

Rhodiola plant's roots are most valued for their purported medicinal properties. The roots contain numerous antioxidants, tannins, flavenoids, and rosavins, an active compound believed to produce antidepressant and anxiolytic (anti-anxiety) effects. A fixture of folk medicine traditions from Siberia to Scandinavia, rhodiola rosea was documented by the Romans as a headache remedy as early as the first century A.D. and thereafter as a general tonic, curing ailments ranging from fatigue to impotence to infection.

Nontoxic and non-addictive, antioxidant-rich rhodiola is considered to be an adaptogen. The term, coined in 1947 by Russian scientist N.V. Lazarev, refers to any plant that is safe for human consumption and does not cause side effects, treats a wide variety of illnesses and conditions, alleviates physical or mental stressors (including extremes of temperature, trauma, exposure to toxins, fatigue and sleep deprivation, infection, or psychological stress), and has a normalizing or "balancing" effect on the body. Like other adaptogens including ginseng, eleuthero, and ginger, rhodiola not only minimizes the harmful effects of stress and fatigue, it also restores the body to normal healthy function. Its most promising application, however, is in the treatment of depression and anxiety disorders. Rhodiola is thought to alleviate these conditions by targeting and inhibiting the enzymes responsible for decreasing the brain's levels of serotonin, norepinephrine, and dopamine.

Research including laboratory and animal studies suggest that rhodiola rosea, in addition to its antidepressant and anti-anxiety properties, may also inhibit the growth of cancer cells, prevent healthy cells from being damaged by toxins, correct enzyme imbalances in the body, and treat conditions such as Lyme disease. Human clinical trials suggest that rhodiola rosea has the potential to improve mental performance, decrease fatigue, and alleviate the symptoms of depression. In addition to these benefits, there is some indication that rhodiola may potentially play a role in treating erectile dysfunction and premature ejaculation as well as chronic fatigue. However, further studies are required in order to prove these claims.

While moderate use of rhodiola is considered safe, side effects such as irritability, insomnia, fatigue, and allergies may occur at higher doses or when consumed over a long period of time. Typically, those who take rhodiola do so at a low daily dose for a period of weeks or months, and later adopt a course of treatment that involves alternating intervals of consumption and abstinence—for example, three weeks of rhodiola followed by one week without. The logic behind this strategy is that it minimizes the chances of any harmful effects caused by long exposure to the chemical compounds in rhodiola.

RHUBARB - (RHEUM PALMATUM)

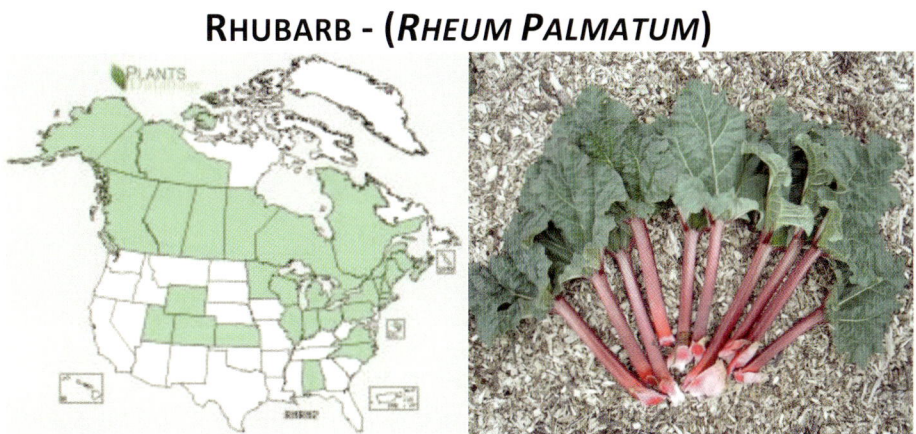

Rhubarb is a plant. The root and underground stem (rhizome) are used to make medicine.

Rhubarb is used primarily for digestive complaints including constipation, diarrhea, heartburn, stomach pain, gastrointestinal (GI) bleeding, and preparation GI diagnostic procedures. Some people use rhubarb so they have to strain less during bowel movements; this reduces pain from hemorrhoids or tears in the skin lining the anal canal. Rhubarb is sometimes applied to the skin to treat cold sores. In food, rhubarb stems are eaten in pie and other recipes. Rhubarb is also used as a flavoring agent.

ROSEMARY - (ROSMARINUS OFFICINALIS)

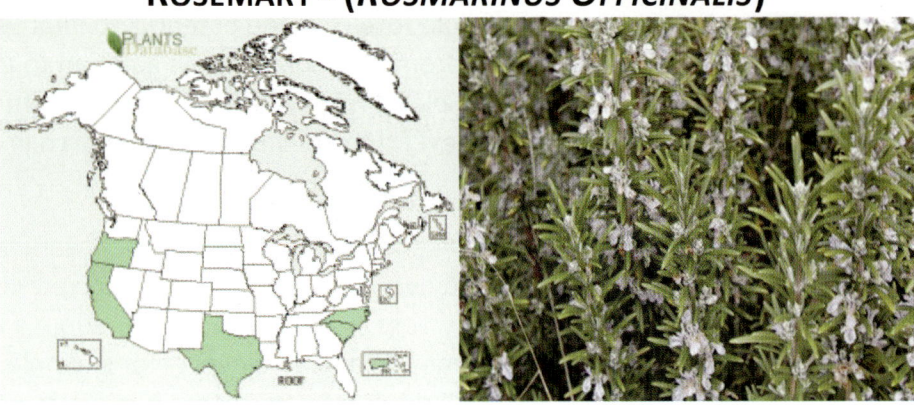

Rosemary is an herb. Oil is extracted from the leaf and used to make medicine.

Rosemary is used for:

Cough	Headache	Intestinal gas
Digestion problems	Heartburn	Liver/gallbladder complaints
Gout	High blood pressure	Loss of appetite

Some women use rosemary for increasing menstrual flow and causing abortion.

Rosemary is used topically for:

Circulation problems	Preventing and treating baldness	Skin conditions
Joint or muscle pain such as, sciatica and neuralgia	Toothache	

It is also used for wound healing in bath therapy and as an insect repellent.
In foods, rosemary is used as a spice. The leaf and oil are used in foods and the oil is used in beverages. In manufacturing, rosemary oil is used as a fragrant component in soaps and perfumes.

The plant contains the following minerals:

Boron	Magnesium	Sodium
Calcium	Manganese	Zinc
Copper	Nitrogen	
Iron	Potassium	

ROUGH PIGWEED - (AMARANTHUS HYBRIDUS)

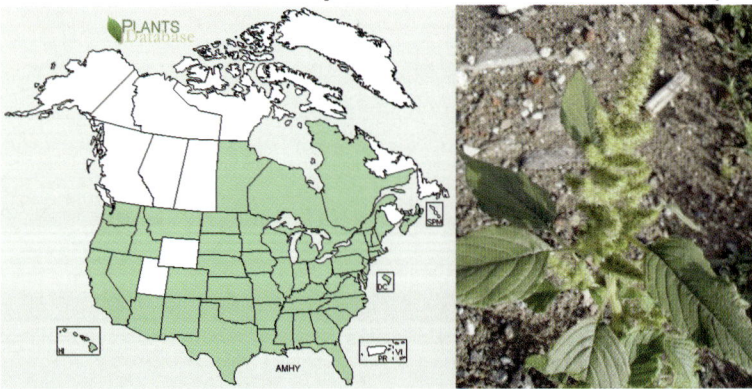

Rough pigweed can be used as a cereal substitute. The seed is usually ground into flour for use in porridge, bread, and baked goods. It is rather small but easy to harvest and very nutritious.

A tea made from the leaves of the rough pigweed and it is used for skin ailments. Pigweed is used to treat diarrhea, intestinal bleeding, and excessive menstration problems.

SAFFLOWER - (CARTHAMUS TINCTORIUS)

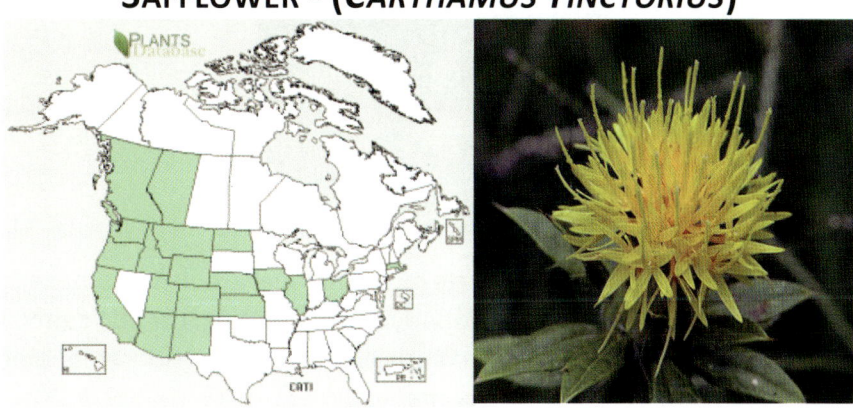

Safflower is a plant. The flower and oil from the seeds are used as medicine.

Safflower seed oil is used for preventing heart disease, including "hardening of the arteries", and stroke.

It is also used to treat:

Antiperspirant	Expectorant to help loosen phlegm	Pain
Breathing problems	Fever	Stimulant
Chest pain	Heart disease	Traumatic injuries
Clotting conditions	Inducing sweating	Tumors
Coughs	Laxative	

Women sometimes use safflower oil for absent or painful menstrual periods. Precaution: The use of safflower flower may cause a spontaneous abortion. In foods, safflower seed oil is used as cooking oil. In manufacturing, safflower flower is used to color cosmetics and dye fabrics. Safflower seed oil is used as a paint solvent. The linoleum acids in safflower seed oil might help lower cholesterol and reduce the risk of heart disease. Safflower contains chemicals that may thin the blood to prevent clots, widen blood vessels, lower blood pressure, and stimulate the heart. Safflower seed oil seems to be safe to take by mouth during pregnancy. However, do not take safflower flower, it can bring on menstrual periods, make the uterus contract, and cause miscarriage.

SAFFRON - (CROCUS SATIVUS)

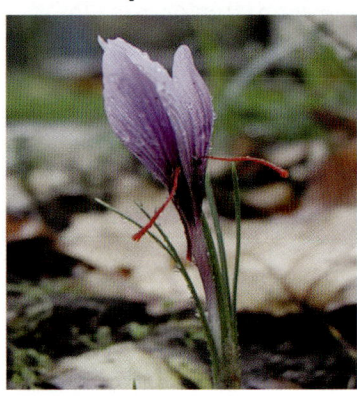

Saffron is a plant. The dried stigmas (thread-like parts of the flower) are used to make saffron spice. It can take 75,000 saffron blossoms to produce a single pound of saffron spice. Largely cultivated and harvested by hand, due to the amount of labor involved in harvesting, saffron is considered one of the world's most expensive spices. The stigmas are also used to make medicine.

Saffron is used for:

Alzheimer's disease	Fright	Shock
Asthma	Hardening of the arteries	Sleep problems (insomnia)
Cancer	Heartburn	Spitting up blood
Cough	Intestinal gas	Whooping cough
Depression	Loosening mucous	
Dry skin	Pain	

Women use saffron for menstrual cramps and premenstrual syndrome (PMS). Men use it to prevent early orgasm. Saffron is also used to increase interest in sex (as an aphrodisiac) and to induce sweating. Some people apply saffron directly to the scalp for baldness. In foods, saffron is used as a spice, yellow food coloring, and as a flavoring agent. In manufacturing, saffron extracts are used as fragrance in perfumes and as a dye for cloth. There is not enough information to know how saffron might work.

SAGE - (SALVIA OFFICINALIS)

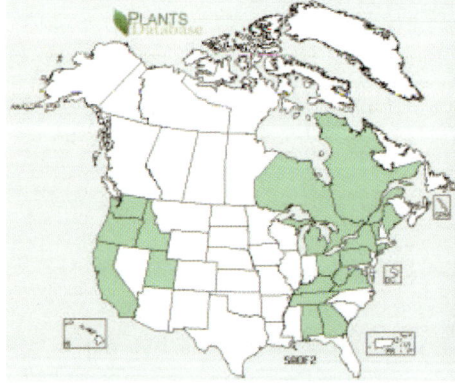
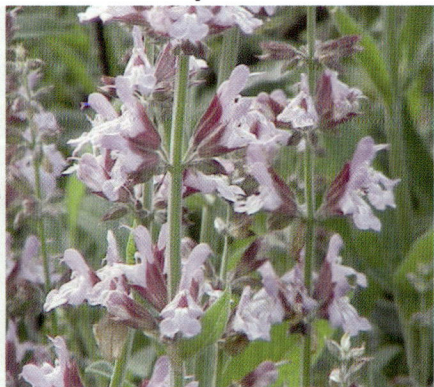

Sage is an herb. The leaf is used to make medicine. Sage is used for digestive problems including:

Alzheimer's disease	Gas	Reducing overproduction of perspiration and saliva
Bloating	Heartburn	
Depression	Loss of appetite	Stomach pain
Diarrhea	Memory loss	

Women use sage for painful menstrual periods and to correct excessive milk flow during nursing. Sage is applied directly to the skin for:

Cold sores	Sore mouth, throat or tongue
Gum disease	Swollen, painful nasal passages

Some people inhale sage to treat asthma.

In foods, sage is commonly used as a spice. In manufacturing, sage is used as a fragrance component in soaps and cosmetics. Sage might help chemical imbalances in the brain that causes Alzheimer's disease. Nevertheless, do not use sage in high doses or long-term. Some species of sage contain a chemical called thujone that can be poisonous if you get enough. This chemical can cause seizures and damage to the liver and nervous systems. The amount of thujone varies with the species of plant, time of harvest, growing conditions, and other factors.

The leaf contains the following minerals:

Aluminum	Iron	Silica
Boron	Magnesium	Sodium
Calcium	Manganese	Tin
Chromium	Nitrogen	Zinc
Cobalt	Potassium	
Copper	Silica	

Sarsaparilla – (Smilax Ornata)

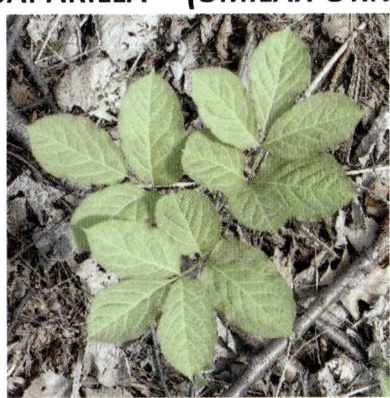

The Native Americans felt pretty strongly about sarsaparilla, believing it to be the supreme spring and blood tonic. The Chippewa, Meskwaki, Ojibwa, Potawatomi, and the Tete de Boule tribes all reported to the colonials that when an illness threatened to turn into consumption, sarsaparilla should be taken immediately. The belief was that any weakness could be turned into strength with the addition of some sarsaparilla. By the mid-1800s, its use had caught on among white physicians who, according to Gunn, prescribed it as a treatment "in constitutional diseases, such as scrofula, syphilis, skin diseases, and where an alternative and purifying medicine is needed." By the year 1868, the plant was esteemed highly enough that it was included in an official list of Canadian medicinal plants.

Sarsaparilla comes from the Spanish word "sarza," meaning bramble, and "parilla," meaning vine. It is thought that this plant was brought as a medicine to Spain from South America around 1573. One of its earliest uses was in the treatment of syphilis, but was advertised as a blood purifier; however, in recent studies it has not been shown to be effective as a treatment for syphilis, or as a blood purifier. Sarsaparilla root was also used by the indigenous peoples of Central and South America for treating sexual impotence, rheumatism, skin ailments, and as a general tonic for physical weakness. Tribes in Peru and Honduras have long since used sarsaparilla for headaches, joint pain, and the common cold. Shamans and medicine men in the Amazon use this root for leprosy and other skin problems, such as psoriasis and dermatitis. Today sarsaparilla is mainly used for the urinary system and is an important remedy for cystitis and renal colic from kidney stones. It is also used as a treatment for eczema with deep, bloody cracks on the hands, acne, dermatitis, and psoriasis. Rheumatic pain can be treated with sarsaparilla as well. Sarsaparilla is also used for sexual impotence. As a tonic, it is used for physical weakness, for enhancing the male reproductive system, and it aids in relieving low mood and debility associated with menopause. Sarsaparilla is also a cleansing remedy for skin and joint problems.

SAW PALMETTO - (SERENOA REPENS)

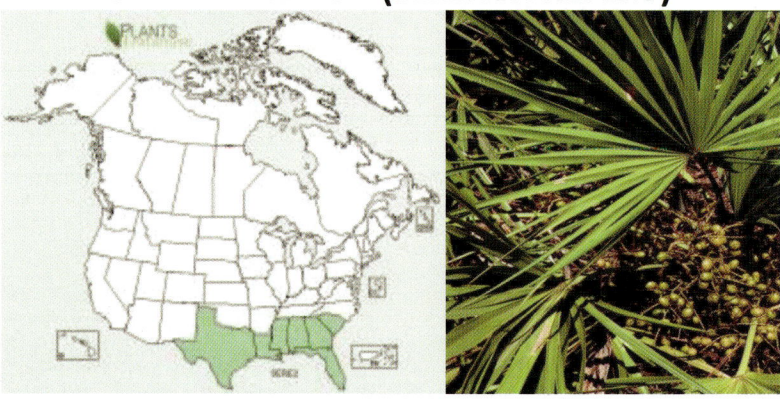

Saw palmetto is an extract derived from the deep purple berries of the saw palmetto fan palm, indigenous to the coastal regions of the southern United States and southern California.

Saw palmetto is used by natural health practitioners to treat a variety of ailments such as:

Aid digestion	Nutritive tonic	Stimulate the appetite
Balance the metabolism	Prostate health	Strengthen the thyroid gland
Coughs	Respiratory congestion	Testicular inflammation
Hair restoration	Sexual vigor	Urinary tract inflammation

Saw palmetto berry also tones the urethra and it may be used to uphold the healthy function of the thyroid gland and urinary system.

In the United States, its medicinal use is for its peculiar soothing power on the mucous membrane. It induces sleep, relieves the most troublesome coughs, promotes expectoration, and improves digestion. The great and diversified power of saw palmetto as a therapeutic agent seems strange that it should have so long escaped notice of the medical profession.

SAW PALMETTO – (SERENOA SERRULATA)

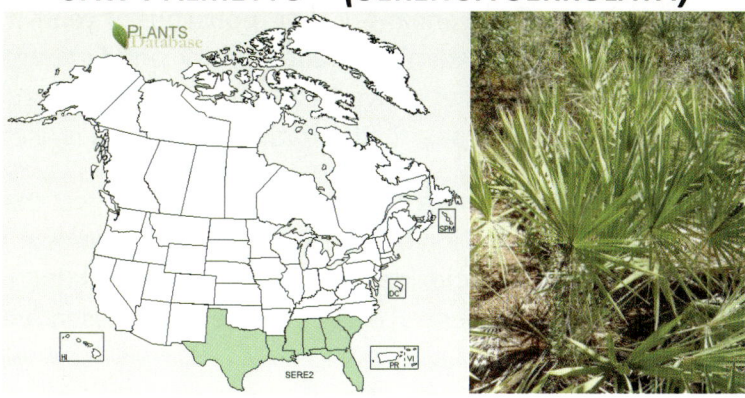

Saw palmetto is proven in many cases to be as effective in treating prostate disease as traditional medications without the harmful side effects and it is nature's answer to male reproductive problems. The American dwarf palm tree is native to the coastal regions of South Carolina to Florida in the Eastern United States, although it is currently being naturalized in other areas of the world.

Saw palmetto is named after the saw-like teeth that form its bony stems. This relatively large plant can reach heights of up to 10 feet in ideal climates. The saw palmetto bears fragrant ivory-colored flowers and yellowish berries resembling olives. When ripe, saw palmetto berries turn black, signaling harvesters they are ready to pick. The berries are then dried and ground into a powder from which liposterol, a fat-soluble steroid thought to contain the plant's medicinal properties, is removed.

Saw palmetto has long been used by Native Americans as a natural remedy for treating a variety of male conditions including impotence, inflammation, and infertility. By the late 19th Century, saw palmetto's beneficial effects on the genitourinary tract were generally recognized. In fact, up until the 1950s, saw palmetto was also widely used as a treatment for enlarged prostate, gonorrhea, cystitis, and conditions affecting the sensitive mucous membranes. Today, Germany's Commission still recognizes saw palmetto as the first-line treatment in 95 percent of benign prostatic hyperplasia cases.

SCHISANDRA - (SCHISANDRA CHINENSIS)

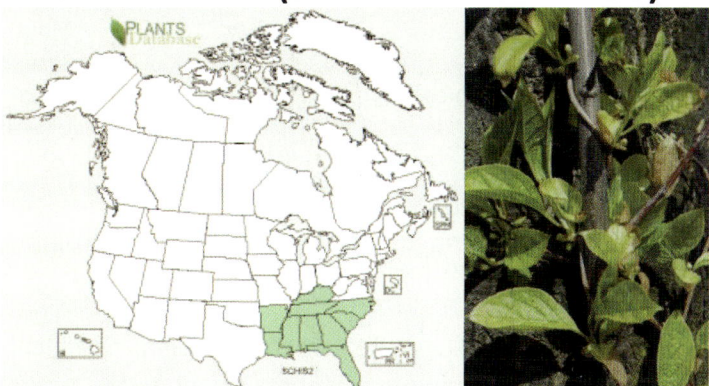

Schisandra berries and the beautiful vines upon which they grow are native to China, Russia, Korea, and some claim, to the eastern part of the United States. It is valued for its attractive flowers, foliage, and fruit, which are used in tasty and nutritious juices and as an important ingredient in herbal medicine. The plant is compact, adaptable to arbors and walls, and bears oval leaves, pink flowers, and spikes of red berries. The vine reaches a length of up to twenty-five feet and thrives in moist, well-drained soil in partial shade. The aromatic berries are dried and used medicinally.

Women in China rely on schisandra to preserve their beauty and maintain youth; both men and women are said to benefit from its qualities as a sexual enhancer. For thousands of years it has been cherished as an anti-aging tonic that is believed to increase stamina, mental clarity, and fight against fatigue and stress. Schisandra has a reputation as one of the most effective treatments for liver disorder. Because it helps the body to respond to stressful situations and act as a mild sedative, schisandra is used as an antidepressant.

Most research has been conducted in China where double blind studies suggest that schisandra has the ability to help those that suffer from inflammation of the liver. The berries appear to protect the liver by stimulating cells that produce much needed antioxidants. It has been implied that is stands next to medicines like ginseng as a stimulator for the central nervous system, increased brain efficiency, improved reflexes, and an accelerated rate of endurance.

The fruit contains the following minerals:

Aluminum	Iron	Silica
Calcium	Magnesium	Sodium
Chromium	Manganese	Silica
Cobalt	Nitrogen	Tin
Copper	Potassium	Zinc

SELF HEAL - (PRUNELLA VULGARIS)

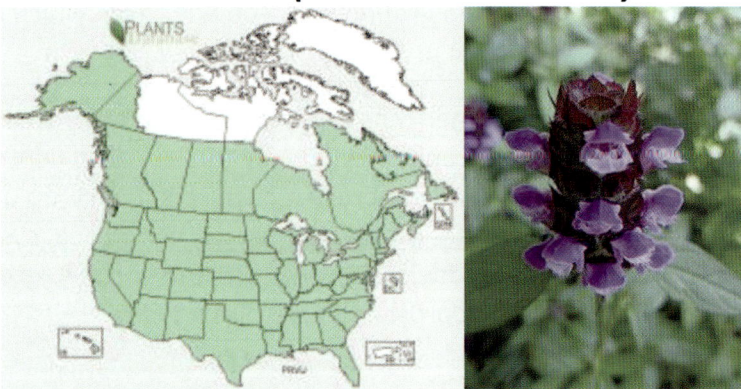

Self heal is an herb. The parts that grow above the ground are used to make medicine. Self-heal is used for:

Colic	Headaches	Mouth and throat ulcers
Crohn's disease	Inflammatory bowel disease	Sore throat
Diarrhea	Internal bleeding	Stomach upset
Dizziness	Irritation	Ulcerative colitis

It is also used to kill germs, loosen phlegm, tighten, and dry skin.
Self heal is applied directly to the skin for vaginal discharges and other disorders of women's reproductive systems as well as wounds and bruises.

Self-heal contains vitamins C, vitamin K, and B-complex. It also contains chemicals called tannins that might help reduce skin swelling and have a drying (astringent) effect on the tissues.

Self-heal seems to be safe for most people. Not enough is known about the use of self-heal during pregnancy and breast-feeding. Stay on the safe side and avoid use.

SESAME - (SESAMUM ORIENTALE)

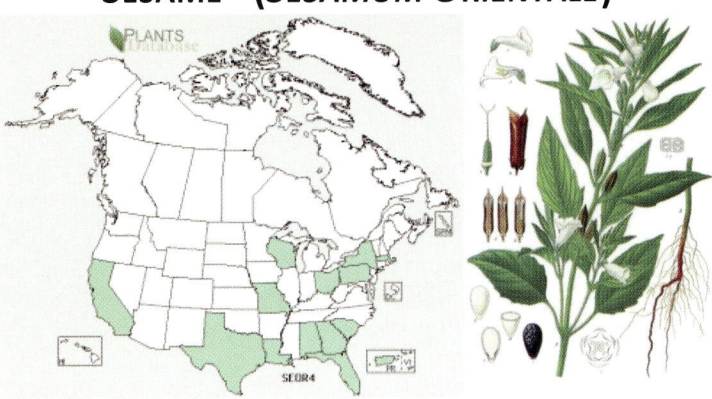

Sesame seeds are extracted from the sesame plant, which grows only in areas with 90 to 120 frost-free days per year. Sesame seeds grow inside pods of the plant containing 50 to 100 seeds and are extracted after drying the plant. The seeds can be stored at room temperature for about five years without loss of viability.

Sesame seeds are maybe most famous as a decoration on hamburger buns but have a wide range of uses in a great variety of different foods. They are rich in oil, proteins, B-vitamins, and vitamin E, therefore, a healthy basis or addition to any recipe.

Now, regions with the highest production of sesame seeds are Asia, Africa, and Latin America. Among the biggest consumers of sesame seeds are China, India, and the Middle East where sesame seeds are a basis of daily food consumption.

SHATAVARI – (ASPARAGUS RACEMOSUS)

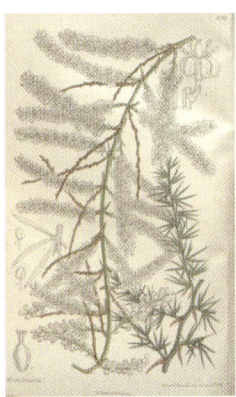

Shatavari is a galactagogue, aphrodisiac, anti-spasmodic, anti-allergic, nutritive, and demulcent. The baked leaves, along with ghee is externally applied over small abscess. The leaf juice together with milk is given internally to reduce the body heat and cure problems like leucorrhoea. The kizhangu or tuber of this plant is crushed and about 15 to 20 milliliters of juice is extracted which is mixed with equal amount of water and given internally for heartburn, burning sensation in abdomen, etc. For increasing the breast milk after delivery, the juice of the tuber is internally given with milk or ghee. The burning sensation produced in the sole of the foot can be cured by externally applying the juice of the tuber along with ramacham powder. The juice of the tuber along with sugar or honey is given for jaundice, hypertension, menorrhagia, leucorrhoea. The tuber is baked in milk and taken internally for diarrhea due to indigestion. One part of the juice of the tuber along with two parts of butter and nine parts of milk is prepared into a waxy consistency and mixed together with jaggery, honey, and piper longum and given internally to increase the sexual potency as well as to cure infertility, etc.

SHEPHERD'S PURSE – (CAPSELLA BURSA-PASTORIS)

People have been eating this plant for thousands of years and it is presently cultivated in a number of eastern countries. Shepherd's purse is one of the earliest wild greens in the spring. In the early spring, before the flower stalks appear, the leaves are good in salads or cooked as greens. When the plant flowers, the larger basal leaves tend to die off, leaving only the smaller leaves clasping the stem. They're still edible, but they get tougher, develop more flavor, and become labor-intensive to collect. Shepherd's purse is a member of the brassicaceae family and is one of the most common and widely-distributed flowering plants in the world. It has been used as a folk remedy to treat numerous conditions in humans, including diarrhea and bleeding, and to stimulate uterine contractions. Shepherd's purse is little used in herbalism, though it is a commonly used domestic remedy, being especially efficacious in the treatment of both internal and external bleeding, diarrhea, etc. A tea made from the whole plant is used for:

Antiscorbutic	Haemostatic	Vasoconstrictor
Astringent	Hypotensive	Vasodilator
Diuretic	Oxytocic	Vulnerary
Emmenagogue	Stimulant	

A tea made from the dried herb is considered to be a sovereign remedy against hemorrhages of all kinds: the stomach, the lungs, the uterus, and more especially the kidneys. The plant can be used fresh or dried. When dried it is harvested in the summer. The dried herb quickly loses its effectiveness and should not be stored for more than a year. The plant has been ranked 7th amongst 250 potential anti-fertility plants in China. It has proven uterine-contracting properties and is traditionally used during childbirth. The plant is a folk remedy for cancer; it contains fumaric acid which has markedly reduced growth and viability of Ehrlich tumors in mice. A homeopathic remedy is made from the fresh plant. It is used in the treatment of nose bleeds and urinary calculus. The German Commission E Monographs, a therapeutic guide to herbal medicine, approve capsella bursa-pastoris shepherd's purse for nose bleeds, premenstrual syndrome, wounds, and burns.

Shepherd's purse may cause low or high blood pressure. Caution is advised in patients taking drugs, herbs, or supplements that raise or lower blood pressure. Drowsiness or sedation may occur, so use caution if driving or operating heavy machinery. Use cautiously in patients taking diuretics, agents that affect the heart, or thyroid agents, as shepherd's purse may interfere with or enhance the effects of these types of agents. Use cautiously in patients with kidney stones. Avoid in pregnant women. Shepherd's purse has been used traditionally to stimulate menstrual flow, uterine contractions, and abortion. It may also improve uterine tone. Avoid in individuals with a known allergy or sensitivity to shepherd's purse, its constituents, or members of the brassicaceae family. Also, there is a lack of available evidence on the use of shepherd's purse in breastfeeding women.

SHIITAKE – (LENTINULA EDODES)

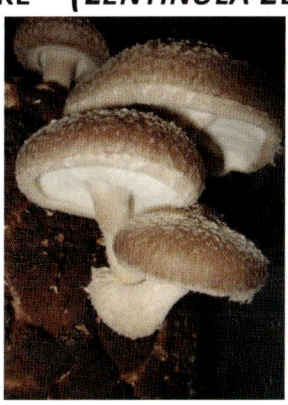

Shiitake, an edible mushroom indigenous to East Asia, is cultivated worldwide for its purported health benefits. The fresh and dried forms of the mushroom are commonly used in East Asian cooking. It is also valued as a medicinal mushroom. Shiitake is popular in many countries around the world and is commonly found in supermarkets and Asian grocery stores.

Studies of shiitake extracts may help:

- Anticaries
- Antimutagenic
- Antiproliferative
- Colorectal cancer
- Gastric cancer
- Hepatocellular carcinoma
- Hepatoprotective
- Immunostimulatory
- Pancreatic cancer
- Prostate cancer

SLIPPERY ELM - (ULMUS RUBRA)

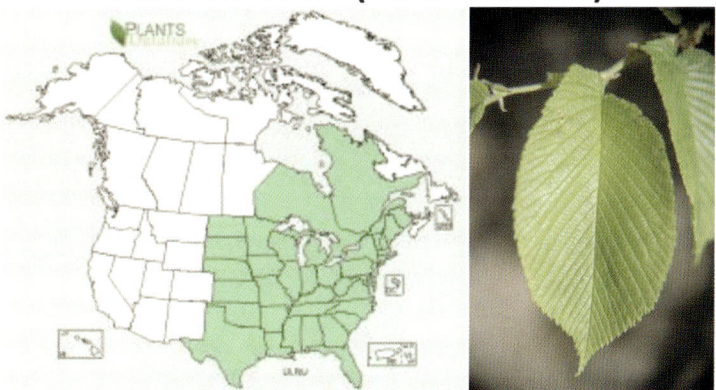

Slippery elm, an indigenous herb to North America, is also called moose elm, Indian elm, grey elm, or red elm. There are many claims to the health and healing properties of slippery elm, but as of 2009, the vast majority of these claims have not been evaluated or endorsed by the medical community. However, there does seem to be a general consensus among alternative practitioners and medical doctors alike that slippery elm is useful in resolving digestive upset.

Slippery elm comes from the inner bark of slippery elm trees. It has a long history of use as both a food substance and a medical agent. It contains a number of substances, the principal ingredient mucilage, a long chain of sugars that becomes slippery when mixed with water is responsible for slippery elm's success as a digestive aid. Some believe that George Washington, along with his army, ate slippery elm during a time of famine in Valley Forge. Other suggested historical uses include:

Alleviating coughs	Digestive upset	Inflammation
Cancer	Fever	Thinning of mucus

SOAPWORT - *(SAPONARIA)*

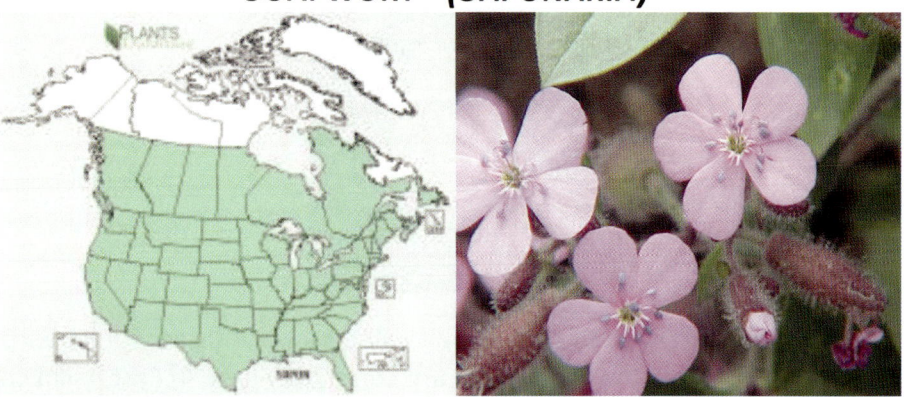

Soapwort is a perennial, European native herb that has become thoroughly naturalized in the United States. Found in moist ditches, along roadsides, waste places, near old home sites, in meadows, and as a planted ornamental, the root is harvested in the spring and can be dried for later herb use. Use the flowers and leaves fresh as body soap.

Soapwort root has been used as an alternative medicine since the time of Dioscorides, an herbalist in the days of the Roman Empire. It is medicinal as a diuretic, expectorant, purgative, and tonic. A decoction of the herb is applied externally to treat itchy skin. Soap can be obtained by boiling the whole plant (especially the root) in water. It is a gentle effective cleaner used on delicate fabrics that can be harmed by synthetic soaps. The best soap is obtained by infusing the plant in warm water. Soapwort is sometimes recommended as a hair shampoo though it can cause eye irritations.

Caution is advised. When taken in excess, this plant is POISONOUS; it destroys red blood cells and causes paralysis of the vasomotor center.

SPINY JUJUBE, ZIZYPHUS – *(ZIZYPHUS SPINOSA)*

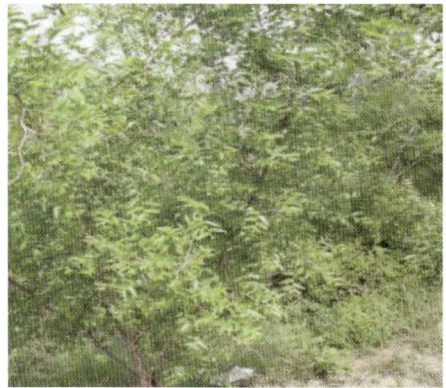

Jujube is known from Arabia to the Orient. The fruits are used as a tonic for the lungs and kidneys and as a good blood cleanser. The Chinese use jujube to tone the spleen and stomach, strengthen digestion, and calm the emotions. They are helpful for weakness, low energy, nervous exhaustion, and poor appetite. They can stabilize the emotions when feeling irritable, sad or crying for no reason. They are added like licorice to harmonize and sweeten other herbs in a formula. The whole jujube tree is medicinal. The leaves are said to kill parasites and worms in the intestinal tract, which cause diarrhea. The leaves are also used to treat children suffering from typhoid fever, inducing sweating to break the fever. The heartwood is a powerful blood tonic. The bark is said to be used as eyewash for inflamed eyes. The root helps promote hair growth and also is used for treating eruptive fevers of children in smallpox, measles, and chickenpox.

Other uses for jujube include:

- Asthma
- Circulatory problems including high blood pressure and anemia
- Digestive problems including lack of appetite and diarrhea
- Eye diseases
- Fatigue
- Fever
- Hysteria
- Improving muscular strength and weight
- Inflammation
- Preventing liver diseases and stress ulcers
- Sedative
- Skin conditions including dry and itchy skin, purpura, wounds, and ulcers

In manufacturing, jujube extracts are used in skin care products to reduce redness and swelling, wrinkles and dryness; and for relief from sunburn.

STEMONA – (STEMONA SESSILIFOLIA)

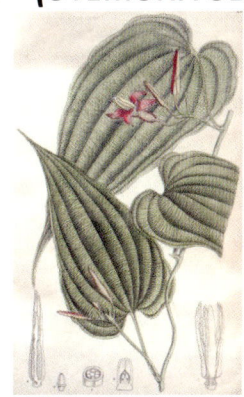

Stemona sessilifolia is used in Traditional Chinese Medicine mainly for the treatment of acute and chronic cough. Externally it is used for the treatment of fungal infections, lice infestation, and as an enema for pinworm infestation. In addition to its primary use for the treatment of cough, in Vietnam stemona japonica root is prescribed for Ascaris infestation and is used externally to treat scabies (mite infestation). It is primarily known for its use in traditional Chinese medicine and is considered one of the system's fifty fundamental herbs. Stemona root is primarily used in the lung organ of traditional Chinese medicine and therefore, most of its medicinal properties focus on the lungs and respiratory conditions. Stemona root is used to stop chronic and acute coughs, ventilate the lungs, and treat asthma.

ST. JOHN'S WORT - (HYPERICUM PERFORATUM)

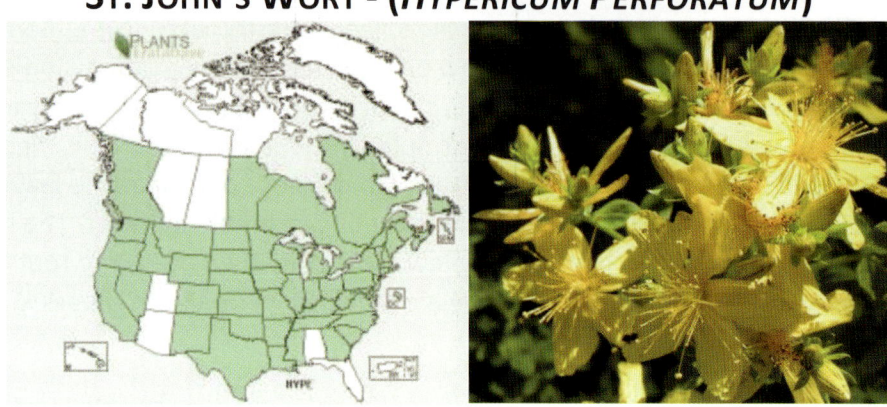

St. John's Wort has become popular again as an antidepressant being the number one treatment in Germany. In several studies of laboratory animals and humans, one or more of the chemicals in St. John's Wort appeared to delay or decrease re-absorption of the neurotransmitters, chemicals that carry messages from nerve cells to other cells. Ordinarily once the message has been delivered, neurotransmitters are re-absorbed and inactivated by the cells that released them. Chemicals in St. John's Wort may keep more of these antidepressant neurotransmitters available for the body to use. Multiple studies have shown that St. John's Wort may be effective in relieving mild to moderate depression, although maximum antidepressant effects may take several weeks to develop. St. John's Wort is an MAO inhibitor (monoamine oxidase inhibitors are a class of antidepressant drugs prescribed for the treatment of depression) and should not be used with alcohol and some other foods.

St. John's Wort has also been studied for the treatment of other emotional disorders such as anxiety, obsessive-compulsive disorder, menopausal mood swings, and premenstrual syndrome. In laboratory studies, it has shown some effectiveness for lessening the symptoms of nicotine withdrawal and for reducing the craving for alcohol in addicted animals. It is believed that chemicals in St. John's Wort may act like other chemicals that are associated with relieving emotional conditions.

SUNFLOWER - (HELIANTHUS ANNUUS)

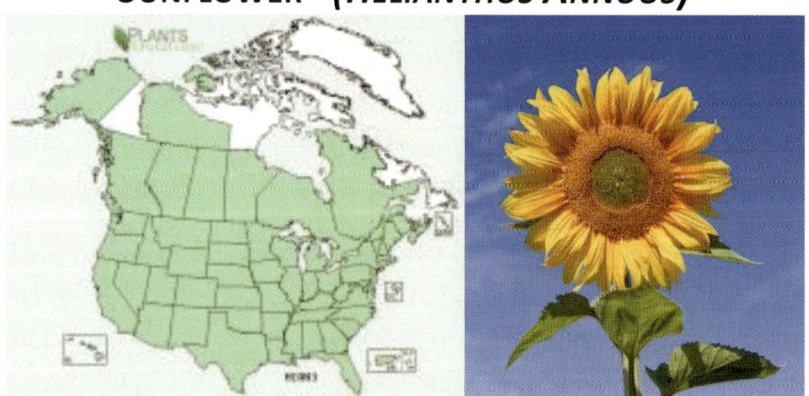

Looking for a health-promoting snack? A handful of sunflower seeds will take care of your hunger while also enhancing your health by supplying significant amounts of vitamin E, magnesium, and selenium.

Sunflower seeds are an excellent source of vitamin E, the body's primary fat-soluble antioxidant. Vitamin E travels throughout the body neutralizing free radicals that would otherwise damage fat-containing structures and molecules such as cell membranes, brain cells, and cholesterol. By protecting these cellular and molecular components, vitamin E has significant anti-inflammatory effects that result in the reduction of symptoms in asthma, osteoarthritis, and rheumatoid arthritis, conditions where free radicals and inflammation play a big role. Vitamin E has also been shown to reduce the risk of colon cancer, help decrease the severity and frequency of hot flashes in women going through menopause, and help reduce the development of diabetic complications.

Sunflower seeds are the gift of the beautiful sunflower that has rays of petals emanating from its bright yellow, seed-studded center. The flower produces grayish-green or black seeds encased in tear-dropped shaped gray or black shells that oftentimes feature black and white stripes. Since these seeds have very high oil content, they are one of the main sources of polyunsaturated oil.

SWEET FLAG - *(ACORUS CALAMUS)*

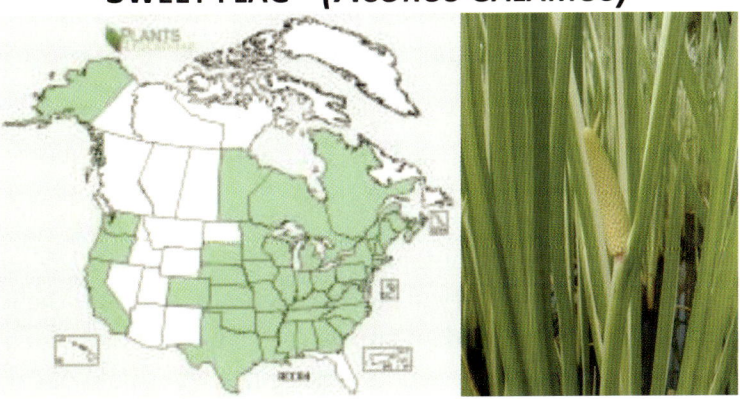

Sweet flag resembles the cattail or the iris, but it is actually related to the jack-in-the-pulpit and skunk cabbage. The entire plant has a spicy, lemon fragrance. Sweet flag also resembles the blue flag but it is not an iris.

It is particularly known for the beneficial effects on the stomach, especially heartburn; a few small pieces of the root being chewed and the juice swallowed will give prompt relief. The roots may be chewed several times a day for chronic conditions until the stomach is back in good healthy working order. It stimulates the appetite and helps to relieve acute or chronic colic. It is also used for:

Arthritis	Epilepsy	Neuralgia
Colds	Fevers	Shock
Coughs	Gastritis	Sinus headaches
Deafness	Hysteria	Sinusitis

For smokers, however, chewing the dried root tends to cause mild nausea, a property that makes sweet flag useful for breaking the smoking habit. A decoction of the rootstock makes a good bath additive for insomnia, malaria, cholera, typhus, flu, bronchitis, ague, diarrhea, dysentery, asthma, a general tonic, and tense nerves. It has also been used in baths for children with rickets. Externally, the tea is used for:

| Burns | Ulcers |
| Sores | Wounds |

SWEET VIOLET - (VIOLA ODORATA)

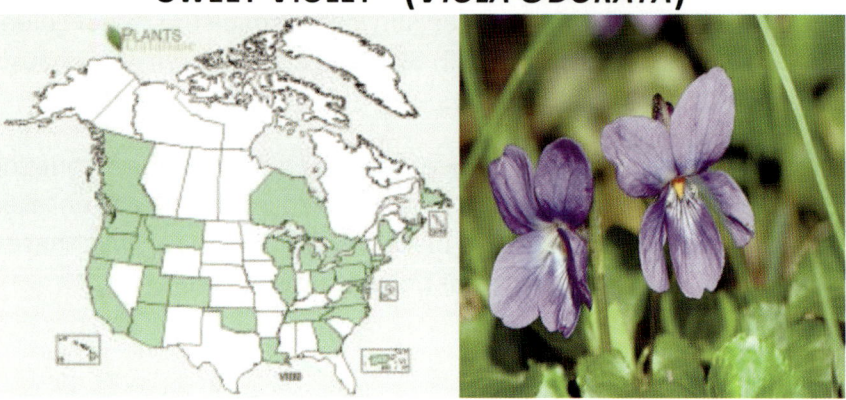

Native to Europe, sweet violet is commonly cultivated and grows wild in damp woods, shady places, meadows, thickets, hedges, along roadsides, and the edges of woods.

Medicinal uses are for:

Antiseptic	Laxative	Volatile oil
Expectorant	Mucilage	

It is rich in vitamins A and C. The flower also contains an aromatic compound called irone, a blue pigment. Garden violet is primarily an herb for respiratory problems. A tea made from the leaves is excellent as a soothing gargle for sore gums, canker sores and inflammations. For inflamed mucous tissue in the mouth, rinse with a tea made from the rootstock or the whole plant. It relieves pain of cancerous growths and works as a poultice to the back of the neck for headache. As a blood purifier it is good for treating:

Asthma	Pleurisy	Syphilis
Colds	Scrofula	Ulcers
Gout	Sores	

The flowers lower blood pressure and the flowers and seeds can be used as a mild laxative. A tonic of the rootstock makes a good expectorant and in large doses, the rootstock is emetic. A tea or syrup made from the plant, especially the rootstock and the flowers, is a soothing remedy for coughs and whooping cough. It is also a calming agent for insomnia and hysterical or nervous problems. Violet leaves are used in puddings, jellies, and salads. In addition, the candied form is used as a decorative garnish for desserts.

TEA TREE - (LEPTOSPERMUM SCOPARIUM)

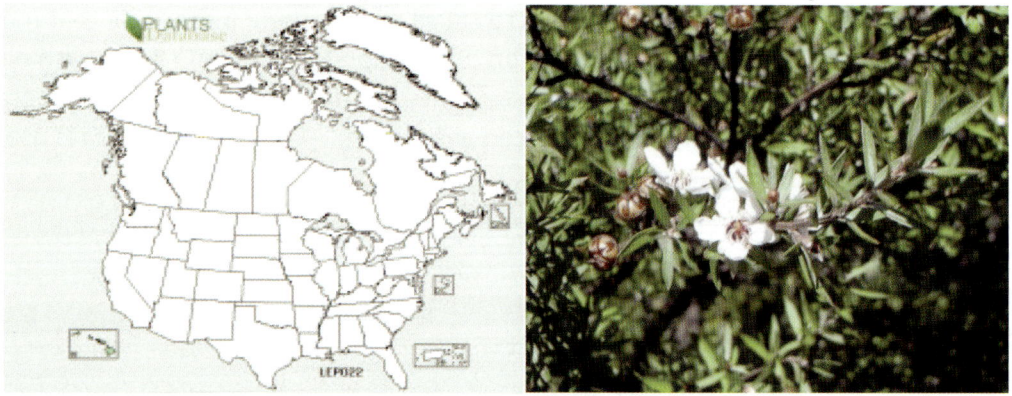

Tea tree oil is derived from the melaleuca tree that grows along streams and swampy flats in Australia and the north coast of New South Wales. The topical oil is obtained by the steam distillation of the tree's leaves and is known for having antiseptic properties that prevent and treat infections.

Tea tree oil helps treat a number of conditions such as:

Acne	Dandruff	Lice
Allergic skin reactions	Eye infections	Thrush
Athlete's foot	Fungal nail infections	Vaginal infections
Bad breath	Genital herpes	

It is applied topically and the chemicals in tea tree oil help fight infections by killing bacteria and fungus. Tea tree oil is applied topically to the skin. Side effects include skin rash, dryness, redness, blistering, itching, and irritation. Tea tree oil may interact with certain herbs and dietary supplements. Check with your health care provider before usage.

Tea tree oil should only be used in adults, 18 years or older. No proven effective dosage is known. Five to 10 percent tea tree oil is commonly used in gels and shampoos. For conditions such as fungal nail infections, 100 percent tea tree oil is used.

Tea tree oil should never be taken orally. Tea tree oil causes toxicity if consumed by mouth. Tea tree oil solution has been used in mouthwash; however, it should never be swallowed.

THYME - (*THYMUS VULGARIS*)

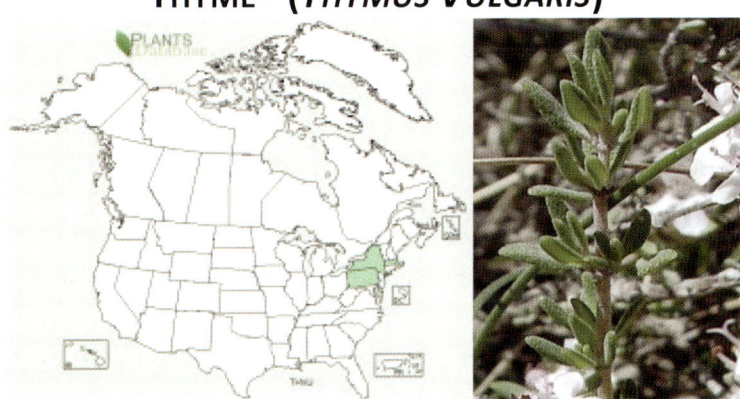

The origin of the name "thyme" has been traced to two possible sources. Thymus is a Greek name for "courage," but to the Greeks it also meant, "to fumigate." It has been used through the centuries as a remedy for many ailments from epilepsy to melancholy. Nowadays it is prescribed by herbalists for:

Bronchial problems	Gastrointestinal ailments	Lack of appetite
Diarrhea	Intestinal worms	Laryngitis

It has antiseptic properties and can be used as a(n):

Anti-fungal agent for athlete's foot	Anti-parasitic for lice, scabies, and crabs	Mouthwash
		Skin cleanser

The essential oil of thyme can cause adverse reactions if taken in its pure form, so use thyme-based medications sparingly. If taken in a tea, drink only once or twice per day, and if used on the skin, be aware that it may cause irritation.

Tienchi Ginseng – (Panax Notoginseng)

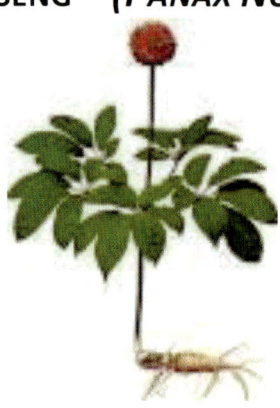

Notoginseng root is a frequently prescribed herb in Chinese medicine. Notoginseng grows naturally in China and Japan. The Chinese refer to it as "three-seven root" because the plant has three leaves on one side and four leaves on the other. The herb is a perennial with dark green leaves branching from a stem with a red cluster of berries in the middle. The root of the plant is used medicinally, and tea is sometimes made from the leaves. At the top of the root is a section called the "age root," which has notches that indicate the age of the particular root. Chinese herbalists consider roots older than three years to be the most effective medicinally. Notoginseng root has a very bitter flavor. Notoginseng root has been used in Chinese medicine for thousands of years. One of China's most famous herbalists said that the root was "more valuable than gold."

The herb is used as a general tonic, or a medicine to tone and strengthen the entire system. In particular, notoginseng is considered a blood and heart tonic. Research has pointed to notoginseng's benefits for the heart and circulatory system. Notoginseng also has been reported to have positive effects on the blood. It lowers cholesterol, and is believed to help dissolve clots. At the same time, it is reputed to stop bleeding both internally and externally. Notoginseng root is one of the main herbs prescribed in Chinese medicine for traumatic injuries. In fact, the root has been distributed to members of armed forces in Asian countries to be used in case of traumatic injury and bleeding.

Notoginseng is used to treat external and internal bleeding, including nosebleeds and bloody stools and urine. According to an American herbalist, notoginseng has been used in the United States for some years to control postpartum bleeding in women and heavy bleeding associated with menopause.

Precautions: Notoginseng root can be safely taken in large doses, but it should not be used during pregnancy, as it may contribute to miscarriage.

Tribulus – (Tribulus Terrestris)

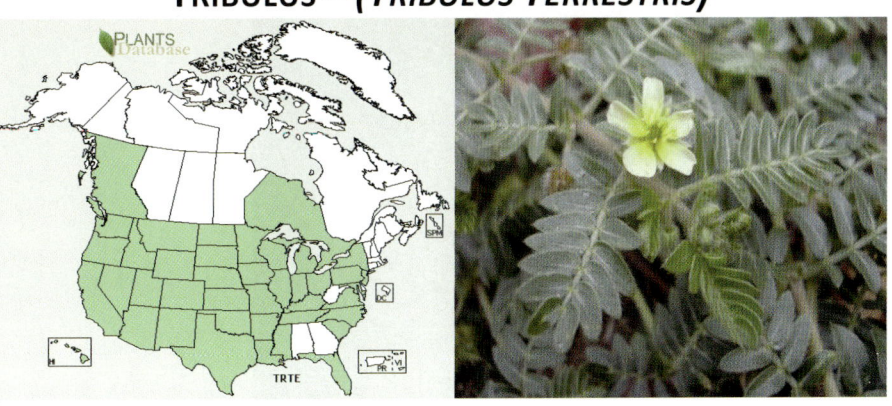

Tribulus terrestris has a long history of use for a variety of conditions. It has been suggested that it was used in ancient Greece and India as a physical rejuvenation tonic. In China, it is used as a component of therapy for conditions affecting the:

Cardiovascular system	Kidney
Immune systems	Liver

It has also been used in Eastern European folk medicine for increased muscle strength and sexual potency. Despite its history of use, there is limited human data available in order to evaluate its clinical effectiveness. It has been suggested that it was used in ancient Greece and India as a physical rejuvenation tonic.

While many men are embarrassed about it, about 50% of men from the ages of 40-70 suffer from a type of sexual dysfunction. Many of the problems can be aided by the use of tribulus terrestris. Almost all these erectile dysfunctions are linked with low testosterone levels. This particular sexual dysfunction is referred to as hypogonadism. A healthy male usually has a bloodstream testosterone level between 350 and 1,000 nanograms per deciliter. These levels decrease naturally as the male ages, but external factors can cause them to drop even lower, leading to multiple sexual problems. Males with low testosterone levels experience a lack of sexual appetite, inability to maintain an erection, and in some cases, inability to ejaculate. The modern society male can experience decreased testosterone levels due to several reasons. Sleep deprivation and stress is the main cause that impacts directly the sexual drive. For testosterone levels to be maintained at optimum levels the body needs 7 to 8 hours of sleep per night. Anything below this number can cause sexual disjunctions.

Besides sleep depravations, testosterone levels can decrease due to low fat diets and poor eating habits. The body needs dietary fat to produce testosterone. Also, alcohol has a similar effect as it has the ability to decrease these levels. Alcohol cripples the endocrine system causing the testicles to stop producing the male hormone.

Turmeric - (Curcuma Longa)

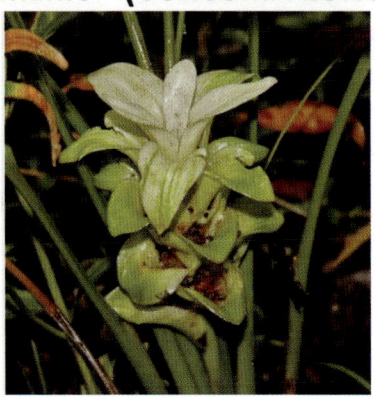

Turmeric produces a root used as a vibrant yellow culinary spice in curry dishes. Turmeric, native to India and parts of Asia, is a relative of cardamom and ginger. Today's herbalists and naturopaths consider turmeric to be one of nature's most potent anti-inflammatory and antioxidants. Turmeric may help treat a variety of conditions related to inflammation and antioxidant damage, including cataracts, arthritis, cancer, and heart disease. It is also used to treatment of:

Arthritis	Gallbladder problems	Scabies
Digestive disorders	Liver disorder	Strengthen the immune system
Dysentery	Promote wound healing	

Turmeric is a natural antioxidant, protecting the body from oxidative damage. Laboratory studies have found that turmeric inhibits the development of:

Breast cancer	Colon cancer
Cataracts	Lymphoma

In one study, smokers that took just 1 teaspoon of turmeric a day for 30 days had lower levels of cancer-causing agents. In another study, 500 milligrams each day significantly reduced participants' cholesterol levels in as little as 10 days. Some studies indicate that turmeric's ability to lower cholesterol may provide the same heart-protective benefits as its close relative ginger, including blood clot prevention and reduced blood pressure.

Turmeric helps detoxify the body and protects the liver from the damaging effects of alcohol, toxic chemicals, and some pharmaceutical drugs. Turmeric stimulates the production of bile, which is needed to digest fat. Turmeric also guards the stomach by killing salmonella bacteria and protozoa that can cause diarrhea.

The root contains the following mineral:
Boron

The rhizome contains the following minerals:

Calcium	Iron	Nitrogen	Zinc
Chromium	Manganese	Potassium	
Cobalt	Nickel	Sodium	

VALERIAN - (VALERIANA OFFICINALIS)

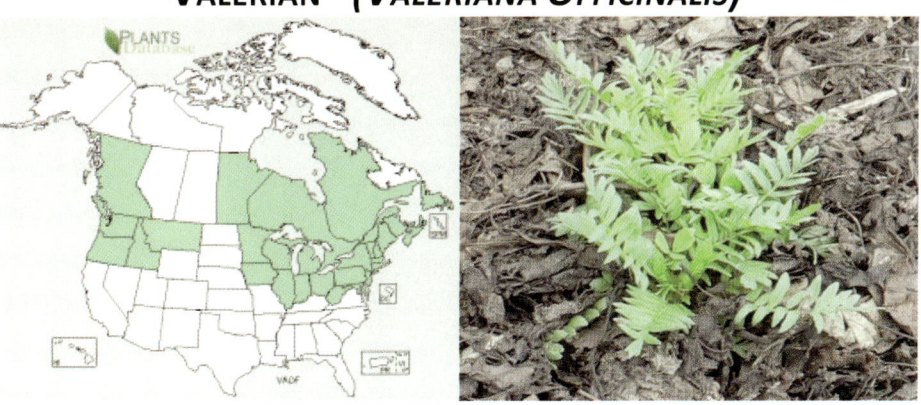

Valerian is well known for its sedative qualities and its ability to relax the central nervous system and the smooth muscle groups. It has been used as a sleeping aid for hundreds of years, especially when there is difficulty falling asleep due to nervousness. Over 120 chemical components are found in valerian. Although a very complex herb, it has not been found to have any negative side effects with moderate use.

It is calming without exerting too much of a sedative effect and is practically non-addictive. It is a valuable treatment for insomnia. At least two double-blind studies have demonstrated that valerian extract can significantly reduce the amount of time it takes people to fall asleep without changing the normal stages of sleep.

The root contains the following minerals:

Aluminum	Magnesium	Silica
Calcium	Manganese	Tin
Chromium	Potassium	Zinc
Cobalt	Selenium	
Iron	Sodium	

VERBENA - (SISAMBIGUATION)

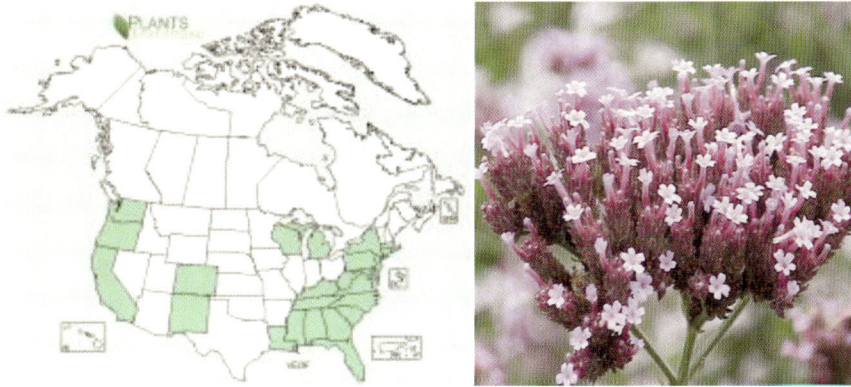

Verbena is said to be useful in fevers, ulcers, pleurisy. As a poultice, it is good for headache, earaches, and rheumatism. In this form, it colors the skin red, giving rise to the idea that it had the power of drawing blood outside. A decoction of two ounces to a quart, taken in the course of one day, is said to be a good medicine in easing pain of the bowels. It is often applied externally for piles. It is used in homoeopathy.

WHEATGRASS

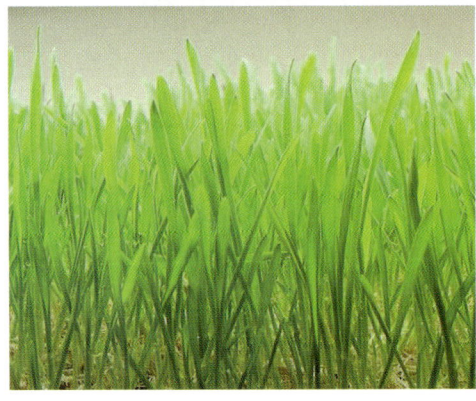

Wheatgrass is sold either as a juice or powder concentrate. Wheatgrass differs from wheat malt in that it is served freeze-dried or fresh, while wheat malt is convectively dried. Wheatgrass is also allowed to grow longer than malt is. It provides chlorophyll, amino acids, minerals, vitamins, and enzymes. Some consumers grow and juice wheatgrass in their homes. It is often available in juice bars, alone or in mixed fruit or vegetable drinks. It is also available in many health food stores as fresh produce, tablets, frozen juice, and powder. Wheatgrass contains no wheat gluten. Personal experience has shown when wheatgrass is grown with diluted ocean water it contains all 90 minerals found in ocean water. A press is used to extract the juice and further diluted with water to personal taste; it is a very sweet drink only when grown with diluted ocean water.

Nutrient comparison of 1 oz (28.35 g) of wheatgrass juice, broccoli, and spinach.			
Nutrient	Wheatgrass Juice	Broccoli	Spinach
Protein	860 mg	800 mg	810 mg
Beta-carotene	120 IU	177 IU	2658 IU
Vitamin E	880 mcg	220 mcg	580 mcg
Vitamin C	1 mg	25.3 mg	8 mg
Vitamin B_{12}	0.30 mcg	0 mcg	0 mcg
Phosphorus	21 mg	19 mg	14 mg
Magnesium	8 mg	6 mg	22 mg
Calcium	7.2 mg	13 mg	28 mg
Iron	0.66 mg	0.21 mg	0.77 mg
Potassium	42 mg	90 mg	158 mg

WHITE PEONY – (PAEONIA LACTIFLORA)

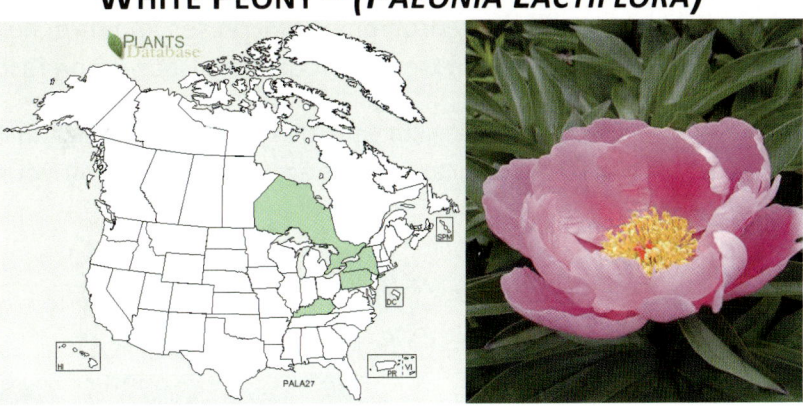

The root of Chinese peony has been used for over 1,500 years in Chinese medicine. It is known most widely as one of the herbs used to make "Four Things Soup," a woman's tonic, and it is also a remedy for gynecological problems and for cramps, pain, and giddiness. When the whole root is harvested it is called Chi Shao Yao. If the bark is removed during preparation, then it is called Bai Shao Yao.

The root is:

Analgesic	Antispasmodic	Expectorant
Anodyne	Astringent	Febrifuge
Antibacterial	Carminative	Hypotensive
Anti-inflammatory	Diuretic	Nervine
Antiseptic	Emmenagogue	Tonic

The most important ingredient medicinally in the root is paeoniflorin, which has been shown to have a strong antispasmodic effect on mammalian intestines. It also reduces blood pressure, reduces body temperature caused by fever, and protects against stress ulcers. It is taken internally in the treatment of:

High blood pressure	Liver disorders	Pre-menstrual tension
Injuries	Menstrual disorders	

It should only be used under the supervision of a qualified practitioner and should not be prescribed for pregnant women.

WILD ANGELICA - (ANGELICA SYLVESTRIS)

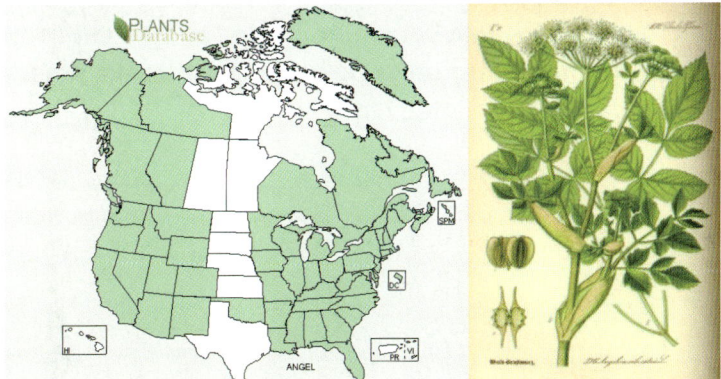

Wild angelica only lives for two years, growing up to 2 meters in height.

The plant is used successfully in treatments of intestinal and breathing conditions, helps with some stomach aches, dyspepsia, bowel gas, and urinary problems. It increases appetite, helps remove toxins from our body, and has shown to be very useful in treatment of skin diseases and rashes.

The plant contains fero-coumarins, which increase skin sensitivity to sunlight, and therefore could cause rashes. Some herbs could react with certain medication. It is advisable to consult your doctor before consumption of any herb.

WILD BERGAMOT - (MONARDA FISTULOSA)

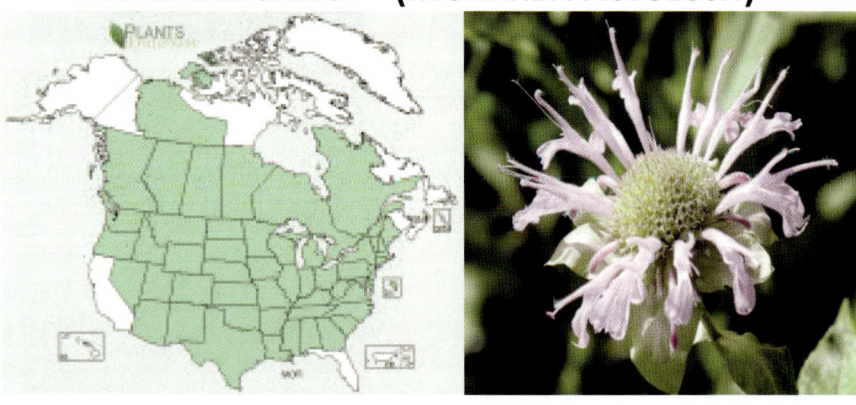

Wild bergamot is also known as bee balm, sweet leaf, horsemint, or oswego tea. Wild bergamot is an attractive, hardy, and easy-to-grow herb producing showy, long-lasting flowers, making it popular as an ornamental plant. Gardeners in the central and eastern United States and southern Canada who prefer to landscape with native plants are partial to wild bergamot, which is indigenous to the area. Wild bergamot tolerates drought and poor soil. Prone to mildew it needs plenty of air circulation and well-draining soil, thriving in full sun or partial shade. Butterflies, birds, and bees enjoy wild bergamot.

Wild bergamot is celebrated for its power to attract hummingbirds and butterflies. It is a mainstay of North American butterfly gardens. Its ability to draw bees has given rise to its alternate name, bee balm. Bees are important pollinators for a variety of plant species, while hummingbirds and butterflies are loved for their color and delicate beauty.

For the original inhabitants of its native range, wild bergamot was medicine. Members of the Chippewa tribe used the dried powdered leaves and flowers of this plant as a burn salve. A decoction brewed from its flowers and roots was used to expel parasites. The Ojibwa used a similar decoction to soothe stomach and intestinal pain. The Menominee drank wild bergamot leaf tea to cure catarrh, or inflammation of the mucus membranes; they also drank this tea for relieving headaches. Native Americans taught early European settlers to use wild bergamot as a remedy for:

Bronchial problems	Flatulence	Stomach aches
Cramps	Sinusitis	

WILD YAM - (DIOSCOREA VILLOSA)

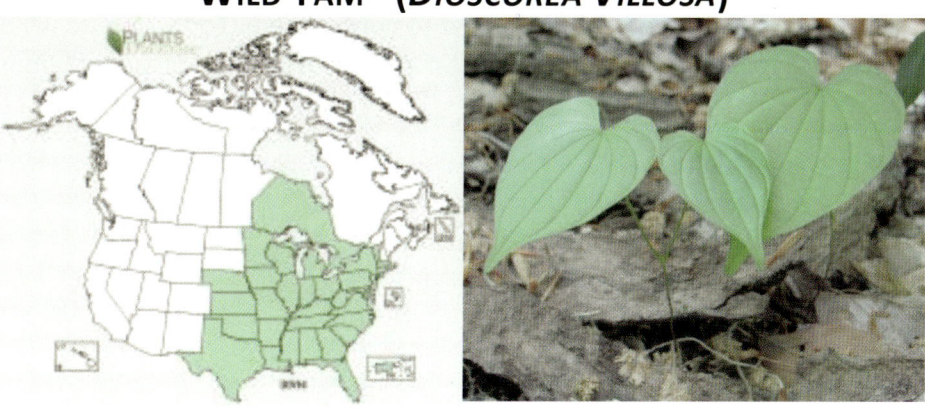

Wild yam is a perennial, tuberous, twining vine with pale-brown, knotty, woody, cylindrical tubers found in damp woodlands and thickets. This plant thrives in sunny conditions and rich soil. The tubers are crooked and bear horizontal branches with clusters of greenish-white or greenish-yellow flowers. The leaves, which are heart shaped, have a smooth top surface and downy under-surface. Native to North and Central America, it has become naturalized to many tropical, subtropical, and temperate areas throughout the world.

Traditionally this herb was used to treat colic and rheumatism, and may have been used by the Mayan and Aztec to treat pain. Wild yam's antispasmodic and anti-inflammatory actions make it useful for rheumatism and arthritis, cramps, and muscular pain.

It has also been used to treat digestive disorders including gallbladder inflammation, irritable bowel, and diverticulitis. The combination of its diuretic and anti-inflammatory effects makes it a good choice for urinary tract conditions.

Wild yam contains a compound, which is used in birth control pills and other steroid hormones. This supports the idea that wild yam may help regulate female sex hormones and is considered a good herb for many menopause symptoms. Also been shown to lower blood pressure and cholesterol, wild yam has also shown benefit to the spleen, kidneys, lungs, and stomach.

WILLOW BARK – (SALIX PURPUREA)

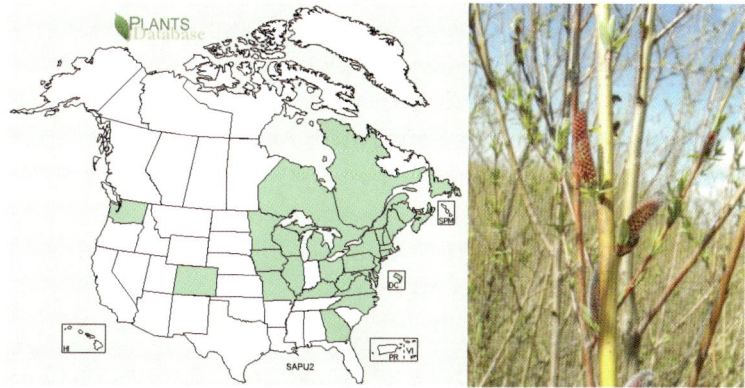

The white willow was introduced into the United States from Europe and can be found next to rivers and streams throughout the country. The bark is the part of the willow that is used, and is easily removed in the spring when the sap begins to flow. White willow bark contains salicin, which the body converts to salicylic acid and has the same effect on the body as aspirin without any of the side effects. In fact, white willow bark was the basis for the synthesis of aspirin. History of usage of white willow bark goes back as far as 500 B.C. when ancient Chinese healers began using it to control pain. Today, white willow bark is often used as a natural alternative to aspirin-one of the most common uses in dietary supplements is as an adjunct for weight loss.

For medicinal uses, the bark of willow is:

Anodyne
Anti-inflammatory
Antiperiodic
Astringent
Diuretic
Doaphoretic
Febrifuge
Hypnotic
Sedative
Tonic

Again, it is a very rich source of salicin, which is used in making aspirin.

It is taken internally in the treatment of:

Arthritis
Diarrhoea
Dysentery
Feverish illnesses
Gout
Headache
Inflammatory stages of auto-immune diseases
Neuralgia
Rheumatism

WINTERGREEN - (GAULTHERIA PROCUMBENS)

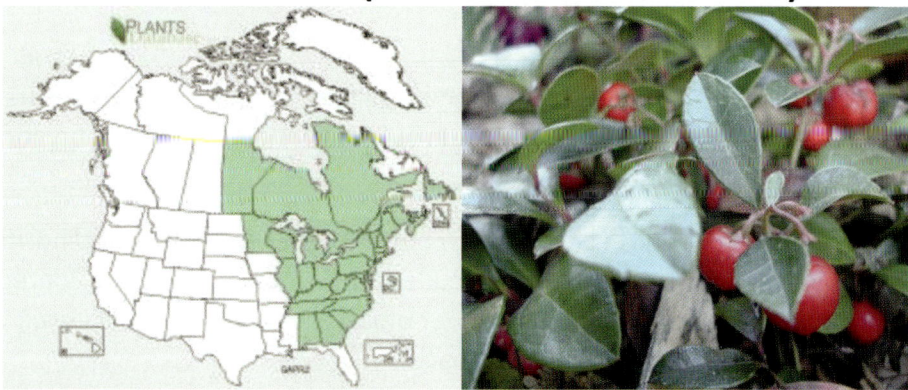

Wintergreen is a shrub-like plant that grows up to six inches in height and bears foliage round the year. When the plant is young it bears pale or yellowish green elliptical leaves that are delicately jagged or toothed. However, the mature leaves are rubbery and lustrous. The surface of the mature leaves is dark green in color, while below they are lighter. Wintergreen bears bell-shaped white flowers during the months of July and August and these are followed by red fruits.

Judging by the number of medications they used, the North American Indians appeared to be mostly suffering from painful disorders of the joints, muscles, or connective tissues and rheumatism. A tea prepared from the leaves of wintergreen herb was a widely used remedy for rheumatism. Interestingly, when the American nationalists boycotted the British tea during the American Revolution, they used the wintergreen tea as a substitute. Once acquainted with the properties of the tea, the American settlers also used it to cure headaches, muscle aches, and colds. Later, in the 1800s American pharmacologists ascertained that the oil extracted from the wintergreen leaves had properties of aspirin and this clarified the herb's effectiveness in alleviating pain. These days, it is suggested to use an external application of wintergreen oil to alleviate excruciating swellings from injury as well heal swollen joints and the muscles.

Earlier, wintergreen was also used to add essence to candies, cough drops, and toothpastes. Incidentally, the practice still continues as many such products available in the market suggest the usage of wintergreen extracts even today. However, over the years the herb has mostly been substituted by synthetic substances. Therefore, these days it is only animals like the deer and partridge that thrive on the original evergreen herb, serving as their staple food during the winter months.

WITCH HAZEL - (*HAMAMELIS VIRGINIANA*)

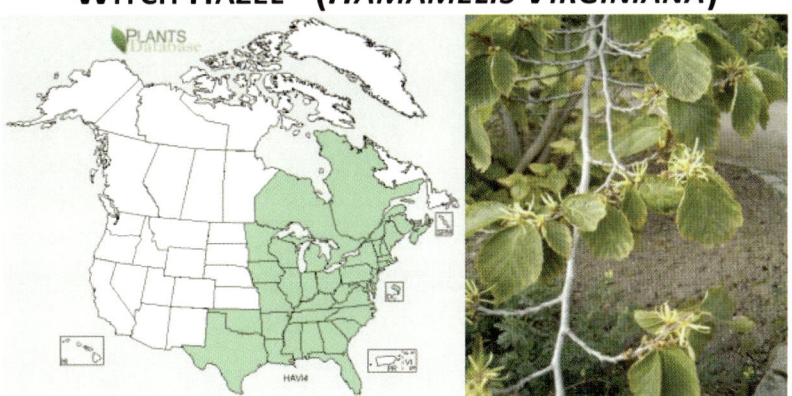

Witch hazel, a deciduous bush or small tree, is found throughout most of North America. It has broad, toothed oval leaves and golden yellow flowers. Brown fruit capsules appear after the flowers. The dried leaves, bark, and twigs are used medicinally.

Witch hazel is a widely-known plant with a lengthy history of use in the Americas. One source lists more than 30 traditional uses for it including the treatment of hemorrhoids, burns, cancers, tuberculosis, colds, and fever. Preparations have been used topically for symptomatic treatment of itching and other skin inflammations and in ophthalmic preparations for ocular irritations.

Traditionally, witch hazel was known to native North American people as a treatment for tumors and eye inflammations and used internally for hemorrhaging. Eighteenth century European settlers valued the plant for its astringency and it still is used today for this and other purposes.

These effects of astringency are thought to be because of the presence of a relatively high concentration of tannins in the leaf, bark, and extract as well as other unknown mechanisms of action. These properties make witch hazel potentially useful as a skin astringent to promote healing in hemorrhoid treatment, as well as skin inflammations such as eczema. The witch hazel involves tightening of skin proteins, which come together to form a protective covering that promotes skin healing. It is used to treat damaged veins by its ability to tighten distended veins and restore vessel tone. It is employed in varicose vein treatments and is valuable for bruises and sprains. It has also claimed to rapidly stop bleeding making it useful as an enema for inwardly bleeding piles. Witch hazel's action on skin lesions also protects against infection and skin lotions may contain witch hazel for this purpose.

Wolfberry - (Lycium Barbarum)

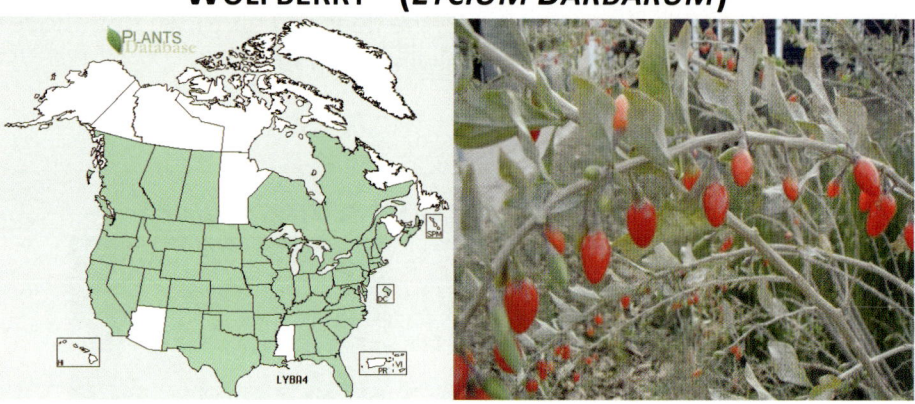

The Chinese wolfberry, also known as goji berry, contains more than 15% protein, 21 minerals, and 18 amino acids. This popular, nutrient-dense super food has been the subject of much interest for its high antioxidant content and other healthful attributes. Varieties of medicinal uses of wolfberry have been confirmed by scientific research. Consult a doctor before using it.

Wolfberry protects the retina from injury, of decreased blood supply, according to a study published in the January 2011, journal "PLoS One;" Lycium barbarum polysaccharides reduce neuronal damage, blood-retinal barrier disruption and oxidative stress in retinal ischemia/reperfusion injury. Li SY et al; Jan 2011. In the study, laboratory mice with ischemia that had consumed 1mg/kg body weight of wolfberry extract per day for one week showed retinal improvements such as decreased retinal cell death, decreased apoptosis, or cell death and decreased oxidative stress compared to a control group that did not receive wolfberry. The researchers concluded that the results of the experiment point to wolfberry's neuroprotective effects for vision, supporting the traditional Chinese medicinal use for wolfberry or goji berries.

Sciatica responds well to treatment with wolfberry. One of the fruit's main active constituents showed cell-toxic and tumor inhibiting effects on tissue cultures of a particular type of aggressive cervical cancer. The wolfberry extract inhibited tumor growth by inhibiting apoptosis of healthy cells and promoting apoptosis of cancer cells. Researchers concluded the potential of wolfberry is to be used as a dietary supplement for the prevention and treatment of cervical cancer; however, researchers noted that wolfberry was not effective on other cancer cell lines tested.

The wolfberry contains vitamins A, B-complex, C, and E. Additionally the Chinese wolfberry has protein and essential fatty acids including polyunsaturated fats and carbohydrates.

The minerals available in Chinese wolfberry include:

Calcium	Germanium	Copper	Iron
Magnesium	Phosphorus	Manganese	Zinc

WORMSEED - (CHENOPODIUM AMBROSIOIDES)

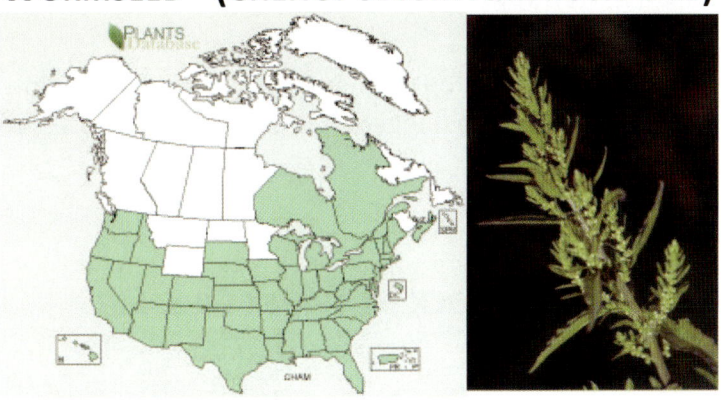

The oil of Chenopodium, derived from the seeds and other over ground parts of wormseed, is an excellent remedy for:

- Dwarf tapeworms
- Hookworms
- Intestinal amoeba
- Roundworms

It is not as effective against large tapeworms. Either the oil or an infusion of seeds with milk was used in treating worms in children. Now largely replaced by synthetics, wormseed is seldom used. Wormseed is also used as a mild cardiac stimulant and to promote secretions of skin and kidneys.

The herbal oil is highly toxic and may cause dermatitis, vertigo, or an allergic reaction. A dash of the leaves added as a culinary herb to Mexican bean dishes because it is believed to reduce gas.

WORMWOOD – (ARTEMISIA ABSINTHIUM)

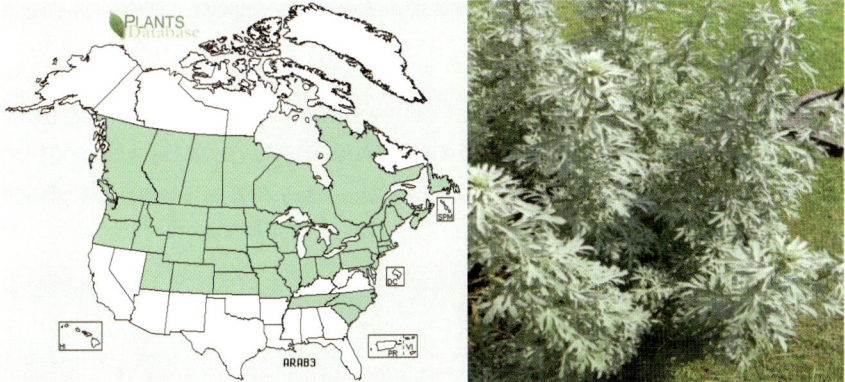

The medical use of the wormwood plant artemisia absinthium dates back to at least Roman times, while during the last century this tradition was seemingly on the decline due to fears of absinthism, a syndrome allegedly caused by the wormwood-flavored spirit absinthe and more specifically as a result of thujone, a monoterpene ketone often present in the essential oil of wormwood. Wormwood is native to temperate regions of Europe, Asia, and northern Africa. It can be found on waste places and uncultivated ground, on rocky slopes, roadsides, and at the edges of fields. Absinthe wormwood is considered to be a(n):

- Anthelmintic
- Antiseptic
- Antispasmodic
- Carminative
- Cholagogue
- Febrifuge
- Tonic and stomachic

It is often recommended in the treatment of indigestion and gastric pains. Wormwood tea can help alleviating labor pains. Oil made from the plant is used as a cardiac stimulant, improving blood circulation.

Combined with other herbs, wormwood can be an excellent remedy against heartburn and irritable bowel syndrome.

Safety: Pure wormwood oil is very poisonous, but with proper dosage and under the supervision of a health care professional, wormwood poses no danger. It is advisable to consult your doctor before consumption of any herb.

YELLOW DOCK – (RUMEX CRISPUS)

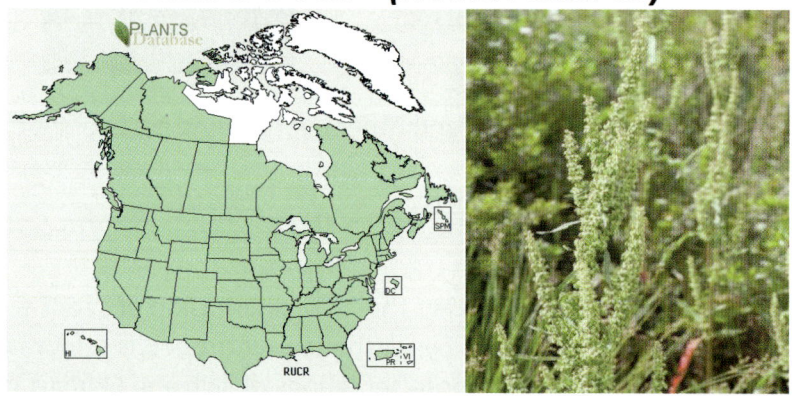

The Greek and Roman used yellow dock as far back as Herba Britannica of Pliny (AD 23). It was used as a pot herb by the English and Swedish settlers in North America in 1700-1900. The fresh leaves were boiled in lard or sweet cream for scrofulous ulcers, sore eyes, and glandular swellings. The roots and seeds were given in cases of dysentery. The Native American tribes used yellow dock as both a medicine and a dye. The bruised root was used as a poultice for abrasions and sores, itching of the skin, and eruptions. Dock plant is a common weed. You can find it growing all over the place, most often, as the name indicates, beside a dock.

During North America's colonial days, one plant that came as a real surprise to the Europeans, and an unpleasant surprise at that, was poison ivy. The old-time treatment for a bad case of poison ivy (and as these were people who went to the bathroom in the woods, they got some really serious cases) was yellow dock boiled with vinegar and applied to the sores. Dock leaves were likewise used to treat these conditions:

Itchy skin	Scrofulous	Sores
Glandular swellings	Sore eyes	

The Mennonites were quite familiar with this weed. They called it halwer gaul and considered it the best blood purifier on the planet. They used it to treat liver problems of all kinds along with the skin problems resulting from poor liver function, and still do to this day. It's interesting to note that Arab physicians recommend the same plant for hepatitis and poor digestion, and they are a long, long way from the Pennsylvania Dutch Country.

Good old Gerard recommended yellow dock as a key ingredient in a tonic which he claimed "cureth the dropsie, the yellow jaunders, all manner of itch, scabes, breaking out, and manginesse of the whole body… purifieth the blood from all corruption; prevaileth against the green sickness very greatly, and… maketh young wenches to look faire and cherrie like." I wonder if Gerard called all women wenches. I think not, but if you want your wench to look fine, or if you are a wench yourself and would like to look the same, this is the plant for you.

Various cultures around the world have used yellow dock for ailments ranging from cancer and tuberculosis to syphilis and leprosy to ringworm and hemorrhoids. In India, they even use the root juice for toothaches and the powdered roots for gingivitis and as a dentifrice. In what is perhaps a two-for-one deal, the Maori of New Zealand chew the leaf first and then apply it to wounds, which they claim can heal without visible scars. The overall universal conclusion is that this plant is one of the best. On a scientific level, researchers feel that herbal extracts may inhibit escherichia, salmonella, and staphylococcus. In other words, yellow dock contains several antimicrobial agents capable of killing off nasty little bacteria.

Medicinal uses of yellow dock include:

- A cleansing herb that is used as a laxative to treat constipation
- Arthritis
- Clear chronic skin problems
- Liver problems
- Remedy against internal parasites (tapeworm and roundworm)

Additionally, the whole plant is used for vascular disorders and internal bleeding. It is applied externally to ulcers, boils, and tumors.

YELLOWROOT - (*XANTHORHIZA SIMPLICISSIMA*)

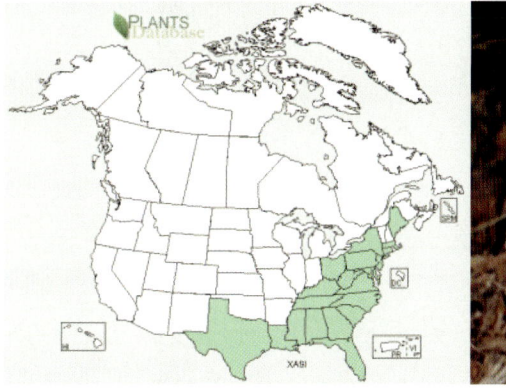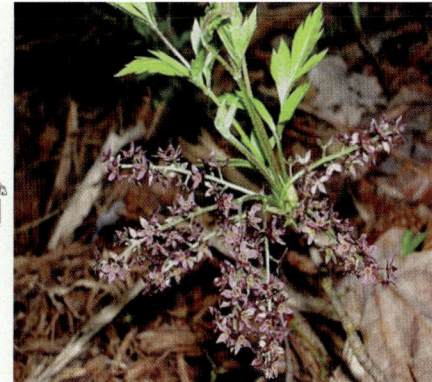

Yellowroot has been used to adulterate or as a substitute for goldenseal. Native Americans used it in a tea for stomach ulcers and ulcers of the mouth. It may have also been used as a tonic and externally on sores. It has been used in the southern U.S. as a folk remedy for diabetes and high blood pressure. The plant contains berberine that is:

- Anticonvulsant
- Anti-inflammatory
- Antimicrobial
- Astringent
- Haemostatic
- Immunostimulant
- Uterotonic

It also stimulates the secretion of bile and bilirubin, which may be helpful in cirrhosis of the liver. Warning: May be toxic in large doses.

Yohimbe - (Pausinystalia Yohimbe)

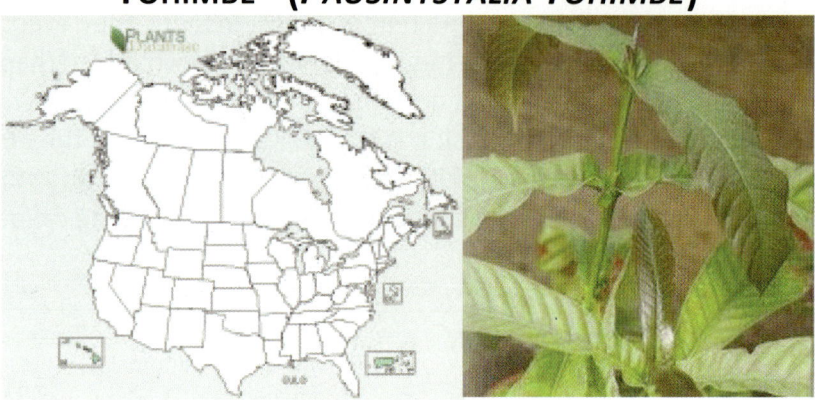

Yohimbe is a plant that is native to tropical West Africa and was frequently used by the Bantu people. Yohimbe bark has a long folk history of helping to increase libido or sexual energy and desire. Historically, yohimbe bark was used in western Africa for treatment of fevers, leprosy, and cough. It has also been used to dilate pupils and as a local anesthetic. It has a more recent history of use as a hallucinogen. Currently, Yohimbe is the only natural drug with enough credible evidence to be listed as a sensual stimulant and sexual booster.

CONDITIONS THAT CAN BE AFFECTED BY HERBS:

3 = 3 stars (best - for that indication)

2 = 2 stars (good - for that indication)

1 = 1 star (mediocre - for that indication)

AGING (SENESCENCE)
Ginkgo (3)
Echinacea (2)
Gotu Kola (2)
Ginseng (2)
Evening Primrose (2)
Milk Thistle (2)

ALLERGY
Garlic (2)
Ginkgo (2)
Stinging Nettle (2)
Horseradish (1)
Chamomile (1)
Feverfew (1)

ALTITUDE SICKNESS (SOROCHE)
Clove (2)
Horsebalm (2)
Garlic (2)
Reishi (2)
Ginkgo (1)

ALZHEIMER'S DISEASE (A/O SENILE DEMENTIA)
Horsebalm (3)
Rosemary (3)
Brazil Nut (2)
Ginkgo (2)
Dandelion (2)
Sage (2)

AMENORRHEA
Chasteberry (3)
Cohosh (Black & Blue) (2)
Celery (1)
Marshmallow (1)
Dill (1)
Assorted Herbs (1)

ANGINA
Angelica (2)
Garlic & Onion (2)
Kudzu (2)
Bilberry (2)
Ginger (2)
Willow (2)

ANKYLOSING SPONDYLITIS
Ginger (3)
Pineapple (3)
Corn (2)
Pigweed (2)
Vegetarianism (1)

ARTHRITIS
Ginger (3)
Red Pepper (3)
Stinging Nettle (3)
Pineapple (3)
Turmeric (3)
Celery Seed (2)

ASTHMA
Coffee, Tea, Etc. (3)
Ephedra (3)
Stinging Nettle (3)
Licorice (2)
Anise (2)
Ginkgo (1)

ATHLETE'S FOOT
Garlic (3)
Licorice (3)
Ginger (3)
Teatree (3)
Lemongrass (2)
Goldenseal (2)

Backache
Red Pepper (3)
Peppermint (3)
Willow (3)
Thyme (2)
Assorted Essentials Oils (1)

Bad breath
Cardamon (3)
Parsley (3)
Eucalyptus (3)
Coriander (2)
Peppermint (2)
Sage (2)

Baldness (Alopecia)
Saw Palmetto (3)
Rosemary (2)
Licorice (2)
Safflower (1)
Horsetail (1)
Sesame (1)

Bladder infections (Cystitis)
Blueberry (3)
Yogurt (3)
Parsley (2)
Bearberry (1)
Birch (1)
Couchgrass (1)

Body odor
Coriander (3)
Turnip Juice (1)
Baking Soda/Cornstarch (1)
Vegetables Containing Zinc (1)
Vinegar (1)

Breast enlargment (Micromastia)
Fenugreek (3)
Saw Palmetto (2)
Fennel (2)
Wild Yam (2)
Cumin (1)

Breast feeding problems (Dyslactea)
Fenugreek (3)
Garlic (3)
Anise (2)
Fennel (2)
Chasteberry (2)
Echinacea (2)

Bronchitis
Eucalyptus (2)
Mullein (2)
Garlic (2)
Stinging Nettle (2)
Marshmallow (1)

Bruises
Arnica (2)
Parsley (1)
St. John's Wort (1)
Comfrey (1)
Potato (1)
Witch Hazel (1)

Bunions
Calendula (2)
Red pepper (2)
Willow (2)
Pineapple (2)
Turmeric (2)
Ginger (1)

Burns - Amish Burn Ointment

There has been a lot of news recently about the extraordinary Amish burn remedy developed by John Keim. The Amish have successfully used it to treat third-degree burns, where skin grafting would ordinarily be required. This remedy, which uses a special burn salve together with burdock leaves, is not folklore. In fact, its success has been verified by doctors. However, this remedy for severe burns is not intended for self-treatment. Rather, third-degree burns should be treated only by trained practitioners. Nevertheless, anybody can use John Keim's burn ointment to treat minor burns. B&W's (Burn and Wound) ingredient label contains the following: Honey, lanolin, olive oil, wheat germ oil, aloe vera gel, marshmallow, wormwood, comfrey root, white oak bark, lobelia, vegetable glycerine, beeswax, and myrrh.

Bursitis and Tendinitis
Willow (3)
Ginger (2)
Echinacea (1)
Pineapple (1)
Licorice (1)
Turmeric (1)

Cancer Prevention
Cancer Prevention Herbal Salad (3)
Antioxidant Tea (2)

Canker Sores
Myrrh (2)
Tea (2)
Cankerroot (1)
Licorice (1)
Goldenseal (1)
Wild Geranium (1)

Cardiac Arrhythmia
Angelica (3)
Hawthorn (3)
Cinchona (3)
Khella (2)
Valerian (1)

Carpal tunnel syndrome
Willow (3)
Pineapple (2)
Turmeric (2)
Chamomile (2)
Red Pepper (2)
Cumin (1)

Cataracts
Bilberry (3)
Rosemary (3)
Catnip (3)
Carrot (2)
Brazil Nut (2)
Capers (1)

Chronic Fatigue Syndrome
Antiviral Herbs (2)
Purslane (1)
Ginseng (1)
Wheatgrass (1)
Spinach (1)

Colds and Flu
Echinacea (3)
Ginger (3)
Garlic (3)
Forsythia (2)
Elderberry (2)
Mullein (1)

Constipation
Flax (2)
Psyllium (2)
Fenugreek (1)
Rhubarb (1)
Aloe (Anthraquinones) (1)

Corns
Celandine (1)
Willow (1)
Fig (1)
Wintergreen (1)

Coughing
Elderberry (2)
Slippery Elm (2)
Ginger (2)
Licorice (2)
Stinging Nettle (1)
Mullein (1)

Cuts, scrapes, abscesses
Teatree (3)
Comfrey (2)
Horsebalm (2)
Calendula (2)
Goldenseal (2)
Gotu Kola (2)

Dandruff
Soybean (organic) (3)
Celandine (1)
Ginger/Sesame (1)
Comfrey (1)
Scarborough Shampoo (1)
Licorice (1)

Depression
Licorice (3)
St. John's Wort (3)
Ginger (2)
Purslane (2)
Rosemary (2)
Ginseng (1)

Diabetes
Fenugreek (3)
Onion (3)
Beans (2)
Peanut (2)
Garlic (2)
Bitter Gourd (2)

Diarrhea
Apple (1)
Blackberry (1)
Carrot (1)
Carob (1)
Bilberry (1)
Tea (1)

Diverticulitis
Flax (3)
Wheat (3)
Psyllium (3)
Slippery Elm (2)
Chamomile (1)
Wild Yam (1)

Dizziness (Vertigo)
Ginger (3)
Ginkgo (2)
Celery (1)
Assorted Herbs (1)
Pumpkin (1)

Dry mouth
Jaborandi (3)
Echinacea (1)
Multiflora Tose (1)
Yohimbe (1)
Evening Primrose (1)
Red Pepper (1)

Earache (Otalgia)
Goldenseal (?)
Forsythia /Gentian/ Garlic (2)
Echinacea (1)
Honeysuckle (1)
Ephedra (1)

Emphysema
Mullein (3)
Red Pepper (3)
Camu-Camu (2)
Licorice (2)
Peppermint (2)
Eucalyptus (2)

Endometriosis
Soybean (organic) (3)
Peanut (2)
Flax (2)
Evening Primrose (1)
Alfalfa (1)

Erection problems (Impotence)
Fava Bean (3)
Velvet Bean (3)
Ginkgo (3)
Yohimbe (3)
Cardamom (2)
Anise (2)

Fainting (Syncope)
Broomweed (2)
Country Mallow (2)
Eucalyptus (2)
Cardamom (2)
Coffee, Tea, Etc. (2)
Rosemary (2)

Fever
Willow (3)
Meadowsweet (2)
Elder (1)
Peppermint (1)
Ginger (1)
Red Pepper (1)

Flatulence (Gas)
Assorted Carminative Herbs (3)

Fungal infections (Mycoses)
Garlic (3)
Teatree (3)
Licorice (3)
Black Walnut (3)
Lemongrass (2)
Pau – D'arco (2)

Gallstones and kidney stones
Beggar - Lice (2)
Turmeric (2)
Celandine (2)
Peppermint (2)
Couchgrass (2)
Goldenrod (1)

Gential herpes and cold sores
Lemon Balm (3)
Mints (2)
St. John's Wort - (2)
Echinacea (2)
Red Pepper (2)
Garlic (1)

Gingivitis
Bloodroot (2)
Echinacea (2)
Purslane (2)
Chamomile (2)
Licorice (2)
Sage (2)

Glaucoma
Jaborandi (3)
Oregano (2)
Kaffir Potato (2)
Pansy (2)
Fruits/Veg/Vit.C (2)
Bilberry (1)

Gout (Podagrao)
Celery (3)
Chiso (2)
Turmeric (2)
Avocado (1)
Devil's Claw (1)
Cat's Claw (1)

Graves disease
Bugleweed (3)
Lemon Balm (3)
Self – Heal (3)
Verbena (2)
Kelp (2)
Broccoli (1)

Hangover
Cinchona (1)
Kudzu (1)
Folk Herbs (1)
Ginkgo (1)
Wintergreen (1)

Headache
Bay (3)
Willow (3)
Ginger (2)
Feverfew (3)
Evening Primrose (2)
Red Pepper (2)

Heartburn
Chamomile (2)
Peppermint (2)
Licorice (2)
Cardamom /Cinnamon (1)
Dill (1)
Fennel (1)

Heart disease
Pigweed (3)
Willow (3)
Angelica (2)
Hawthorn (2)
Grape (2)
Chicory (1)

Hemorrhoids
Comfrey (2)
Witch Hazel (2)
Psyllium (2)
Plantain (2)
Butcher's Broom (1)
Horse Chestnut (1)

High blood pressure
Celery (3)
Garlic (3)
Hawthorn (2)
Tomato (2)
Kudzu (2)
Saffron (1)

Conditions Affected by Herbs

High Cholesterol
Avocado (2)
Garlic (2)
Beans (2)
Celery (2)
Ginger (2)
Nuts (1)

Hives
Jewelweed (3)
Stinging Nettle (3)
Parsley (2)
Ginger (1)
Amaranth (1)

HIV Infection
Licorice (3)
St. John's Wort (3)
Oregano (3)
Echinacea (2)
Astragalus (2)
Burdock (2)

Hypothyroidism
Kelp (1)
Gentian (1)
Walnut (1)
Mustard (1)
Radish (1)
St. John's Wort (1)

Indigestion (Dyspepsia)
Chamomile (3)
Peppermint (3)
Ginger (2)
Angelica (2)
Red Pepper (1)
Coriander (1)

Infertility
Cauliflower (2)
Ginseng (2)
Spinach (2)
Ginger (2)
Guava (2)
Sunflower (2)

Inflammatory bowel disease (IBS)
Onion (1)
Tea (1)
Psyllium (1)
Valerian (1)

Inhibited sexual desire in women (Frigidity)
Chinese Angelica (2)
Quevrancho (2)
Damiana (2)
Ginseng (2)
Yohimbe (2)
Fenugreek (1)

Insect bites and stings (Bugbites)
Mountain Mint (3)
Citronella (2)
Garlic (2)
Basil (2)
Calendula (2)
Plantain (2)

Insomnia
Lemon Balm (3)
Valerian (3)
Lavender (2)
Passionflower (2)
Hops (1)
Chamomile (1)

Intermittent claudication
Garlic (3)
Ginkgo (3)
Ginger (2)
Purslane (2)
Hawthorn (2)

Intestinal parasites
Cinchona (3)
Ipecac (3)
Goldenseal (3)
Papaya (2)
Elecampane (2)
Cubeb (1)

Laryngitis
Cardamom (3)
Horehound (2)
Mullein (2)
Ginger (2)
Mallows (2)
Elecampane (1)

LICE
Neem (1)
Sweetflag (1)

LIVER PROBLEMS (HEPATOSIS)
Carrot (3)
Milk Thistle (3)
Schisandra (3)
Dandelion (3)
Indian Almond (3)
Licorice (2)

LYME'S DISEASE
Echinacea (3)
Cat's Claw (3)
Mountain Mint (3)
Garlic (3)
Licorice (2)

MACULAR DEGENERATION
Bilberry (3)
Ginkgo (2)
Greens (2)
Peanut (2)
Wolfberry (1)
Clove (1)

MENOPAUSE
Black Cohosh (2)
Licorice (2)
Alfalfa (1)
Chinese Angelica (1)
Chasteberry (1)
Red Clover (1)

MENSTRAL CRAMPS (DYSMENORRHEA)
Black Haw (3)
Chinese Angelica (3)
Raspberry (3)
Chasteberry (2)
Bilberry (2)
Red Clover (2)

MORNING SICKNESS
Ginger (3)
Peppermint (2)
Black Horehound (1)
Peach (1)
Cabbage (1)
Raspberry (1)

MOTION SICKNESS
Ginger (3)
Raspberry (1)

MULTIPLE SCLEROSIS
Stinging Nettle (3)
Blueberry (2)
Pineapple (2)
Black Current (2)
Evening Primrose (2)
Purslane (2)

NAUSEA
Ginger (3)
Peppermint (1)
Cinnamon (1)

OSTEOPOROSIS
Cabbage (3)
Pigweed (3)
Dandelion (3)
Soybean (2)
Avocado (2)
Parsley (1)

OVERWEIGHT (OBESITY)
Plantain (3)
Red Pepper (3)
Chickweed (2)
Pineapple (2)
Evening Primrose (2)
Walnut (2)

PAIN
Clove (3)
Willow (3)
Red pepper (3)
Ginger (2)
Evening Primrose (2)
Mountain Mint (2)

Parkinson's disease
Fava Bean (3)
Velvet Bean (3)
Evening Primrose (2)
Passionflower (1)
Ginkgo (1),
St. John's Wort (1)

PNEUMONIA
Astragalus (2)
Dandelion (2)
Garlic (2)
Baikal Skullcap (2)
Echinacea (2)
Honeysuckle (2)

POISON IVY, POISON OAK, AND POISON SUMAC
Jewelweed (3)
Plantain (2)
Aloe (2)
Soapwort (2)

PREGNANCY AND DELIVERY
Partridge Berry (3)
Raspberry (3)
Black Haw (2)
Blue Cohosh (2)
Spinach (2)

Premenstrual syndrome (PMS)
Chasteberry (3)
Chinese Angelica (3)
Evening Primrose (3)
Stinging Nettle (2)
Burdock (1)
Raspberry (1)

PROSTATE ENLARGEMENT (BPH) (PROSTATITIS)
Pumpkin (3)
Licorice (3)
Saw Palmetto (3)
Stinging Nettle (2)
Pygeum (2)
Evening Primrose (2)

PSORIASIS
Red Pepper (3)
Bishop's Weed (3)
Avocado (2)
Licorice (2)
Brazil Nut (2)
Purslane (2)

RAYNAUD'S DISEASE
Garlic (3)
Evening Primrose (3)
Ginkgo (3)
Mustard (2)
Borage (2)
Red Pepper (2)

SCABIES
Evening Primrose (3)
Onion (3)
Neem (3)
American Pennyroyal (2)
Teatree Oil (2)
Mountain Mint (2)

SCIATICA
Willow (3)
Stinging Nettle (3)
Wintergreen (3)
Mustard (2)
Country Mallow (2)

SHINGLES
Lemon Balm (3)
Red Pepper (3)
Chinese Angelica (2)
Licorice (2)
Baikal Skullcap (2)
Passionflower (2)

SINUSITIS
Garlic (3)
Goldenseal (3)
Eucalyptus / Peppermint (2)
Oregano (2)
Echinacea (2)
Horseradish (1)

SKIN PROBLEMS (DERMATOSES)
Aloe (3)
Evening Primrose (3)
Avocado (2)
Chamomile (2)
Calendula (2)
Witch Hazel (2)

SMOKING
Licorice (3)
Red Clover (3)

SORES
Calendula (3)
Dragon's Blood (3)
Comfrey (3)
Ginkgo (2)
Teatree (2)
Gotu Kola (1)

SORE THROAT
Eucalyptus (3)
Honeysuckle (3)
Slippery Elm (3)
Licorice (3)
Marsh Mallow (2)
Burnet - Saxifrage (2)

STIES
Echinacea (3)
Potato (3)
Goldenseal (3)
Thyme (3)
Garlic (1)
Chamomile (1)

STROKE
Garlic (3)
Pigweed (3)
Ginkgo (3)
Willow (3)
Carrot (2)
Evening Primrose (1)

SUNBURN
Tea (3)
Black Nightshade (2)
Eggplant (2)
Aloe (2)
Calendula (2)
Plantain (2)

SWELLING
Ginger (3)
Turmeric (2)
Pineapple (2)
Arnica (1)
Aloe (1)
Cat's Claw (1)

TINNITUS
Ginkgo (3)
Sesame (2)
Black Cohosh (1)
Lesser Periwinkle (1)
Goldenseal (1)
Spinach (1)

TONSILLITIS
Echinacea (3)
Honeysuckle (2)
Citrus (Vitamin C) (2)
Garlic (2)
Sage (2)
Elderberry (1)

TOOTHACHE
Clove (3)
Red Pepper (2)
Willow (2)
Ginger (2)
Toothache Tree (2)
Sesame (1)

TOOTH DECAY (CARIES)
Tea (3)
Bloodroot (2)
Wild Bergamot (2)
Bay (2)
Licorice (2)
Chaparral (1)

TUBERCULOSIS
Echinacea (3)
Garlic (3)
Licorice (3)
Forsythia (3)
Honeysuckle (3)
Eucalyptus (2)

ULCERS
Licorice (3)
Ginger (3)
Yellowroot (3)
Cabbage (2)
Banana (2)
Garlic (2)

VAGINITIS
Teatree (3)
Garlic (3)
Cardamom (2)
Apple Cider Vinegar (1)
Goldenseal (2)
Lavender (1)

Varicose veins
Horse Chestnut (3)　　Witch Hazel (3)　　Butcher's Broom (2)
Violet (3)　　Ginkgo (2)　　Goto Kola (1)

Viral infections
Echinacea (3)　　Licorice (2)　　Dragon's Blood (2)
Goldenseal (2)　　Garlic (2)　　Lemon balm (2)

Warts
Birch (3)　　Pineapple (2)　　Celandine (2)
Castor (2)　　Bloodroot (2)　　Banana (1)

Worms
Pumpkin (3)　　Wormseed (3)　　Garlic (2)
Ginger (3)　　Papaya (2)　　Clove (1)

Wrinkles
Horse Chestnut (3)　　Sage (2)　　Cucumber (2)
Cocoa (2)　　Carrot (2)　　Rosemary (2)

Yeast infections
Echinacea (3)　　Cranberry (2)　　Goldenseal (2)
Garlic (3)　　Pau-D'Arco (2)　　Purslane (2)

Melatonin

Melatonin is a natural hormone created by the pineal gland, located deep within the brain. Its main purpose is to regulate the human body clock and help bring about sleep.

Levels of melatonin fluctuate over time; lower melatonin levels are found during the day, while the highest melatonin levels are present in the body during the night. Melatonin is associated with the sleep cycle in humans. Several double-blind, controlled studies have shown that melatonin reduces the time people need to go to sleep and improves the quality of a person's sleep. It can also reduce the effects of jet lag and help people recover their energy levels.

Melatonin may also work on a variety of other conditions. Some studies have shown that melatonin supplements can reduce the number of cluster headaches and tension headaches in people with sleep disorders. Test-tube studies suggest that melatonin can reduce the production of breast cancer cells and increase survival rates in people with lung cancer and brain cancer. In addition, it may effectively treat fibromyalgia and a pediatric disorder called Angelman's syndrome (a neuro-genetic disorder characterized by intellectual and developmental disability, sleep disturbance, seizures, jerky movements [especially hand-flapping], frequent laughter or smiling, and usually a happy demeanor). Melatonin is able to reset the biological clocks and be taken to restore daytime and night time cycles.

How much melatonin should I take? Normally, the body secretes melatonin for several hours per day in healthy people. For people who have a melatonin deficiency or trouble sleeping, most practitioners recommend between 1 and 3 milligrams of a melatonin supplement each night, taken one to two hours before bedtime. People with cancer often take large amounts of melatonin—up to 20 milligrams per night. Melatonin should not be taken during the day, and should only be taken under the care of a licensed health care provider.

What forms of melatonin are available? Melatonin is available in some foods, but only in trace amounts. Synthesized melatonin supplements are available at some health food stores. However, in many countries, melatonin supplements can only be obtained through a doctor's prescription.

What can happen if I take too much melatonin? Are there any interactions I should be aware of? What precautions should I take? Melatonin supplements have been associated with a wide range of side effects, ranging from drowsiness and confusion, to decreased sperm counts and sperm quality, to headaches and abdominal cramps. As a result, melatonin should not be taken by the following people: women who are pregnant or breastfeeding, people diagnosed with depression or schizophrenia, people diagnosed with autoimmune diseases (such as lupus), people with neurological disorders, and people with fibromyalgia. Diabetics should take melatonin supplements only under the care and supervision of a licensed health care provider.

Melatonin may also interact with certain medications, particularly chemotherapy drugs and medications used to treat breast cancer. As such, melatonin uptake should be monitored closely by any patients taking these or other medications. As always, make sure to speak with a licensed health care provider before taking melatonin or any other dietary supplement or herbal remedy.

Methoxyisoflavone

Methoxyisoflavone is a chemical substance that belongs to the flavonoid family. Flavonoids are water-soluble plant pigments, some of which are believed to possess anti-inflammatory and antiviral properties; others help strengthen the immune system and promote the growth of connective tissues.

Methoxyisoflavone is believed to help increase athletic performance. Animal studies have shown that methoxyisoflavone has anabolic properties (i.e., it helps to build muscle and bone), without any of the side effects reported with androgenic hormones. Other studies have shown that a daily dose of methoxyisoflavone can reduce body fat. However, the results of these studies have yet to be carried out in a controlled, double-blind setting.

How much methoxyisoflavone should I take? Because methoxyisoflavone is not an essential nutrient, suggested daily allowances have yet to be established. There have been studies that have examined methoxyisoflavone in athletes that have used daily doses of 800 milligrams.

What forms of methoxyisoflavone are available? Substances similar to methoxyisoflavone have been found in soybeans and other plant foods. However, methoxyisoflavone does not appear to occur naturally. It is available as a dietary supplement, usually in tablet or capsule form.

What can happen if I take too much methoxyisoflavone? Are there any interactions I should be aware of? What precautions should I take? Because of the relatively low number of studies on methoxyisoflavone, side effects connected with the supplement have yet to be investigated thoroughly. However, other substances that have anabolic effects may cause unwanted side effects, ranging from acne and hair loss to reduced levels of HDL cholesterol in the blood. As such, methoxyisoflavone should only be taken under the supervision of a licensed health care provider. As of this writing, there are no well-known drug interactions linked with methoxyisoflavone. As always, make sure to speak with a licensed health care provider before taking methoxyisoflavone or any other herbal remedy or dietary supplement.

Milk

Cow's Milk

I think you will find a book, "The Devils in the Milk," by Keith Woodford, very interesting as this relates to all dairy products coming from cow's milk. Approximately 500 New Zealand dairy farmers are converting their herds to eliminate production of the A1 Beta-Casein within the milk as well as many U.S. organic farmers. The alternative casein is A2 beta-casein, and the associated milk is known as A2 milk. A2 milk can be considered the original milk before a mutation affected some antecedents of modern European breeds. There are now more than 100 relevant papers in peer reviewed journals. Healthy cows are called A-2 cows. A1 cows (Beta-casomorphin – 7) is implicated in many illnesses:

- Autism
- Coeliac disease
- Crohn's disease
- Delayed development in genetically susceptible babies fed infant formula
- Hardening of the arteries
- Heart disease
- Lactose intolerance
- Milk intolerance
- Mucus production
- Schizophrenia
- Some auto-immune diseases
- Type 1 diabetes

And the list goes on. Also, I do not recommend drinking pasteurized milk of any kind because the pasteurization process, which entails heating the milk to a temperature of 145 degrees to 150 degrees F. and keeping it there for at least half an hour, completely changes the structure of the milk proteins into something far less than healthy. Pasteurized cow's milk may be the number one allergic food in the United States. It has been associated with a number of symptoms and illnesses including:

Arthritis	Diarrhea	Osteoporosis
Bloating	Gas	Recurrent ear infections and colic in
Cancer	Infertility	infants and children
Cramps	Leukemia	Rheumatoid arthritis

The healthy alternative to pasteurized milk is raw milk (organic if possible), which is an outstanding source of nutrients including beneficial bacteria such as lactobacillus acidolphilus, vitamins and enzymes, and it is, in my estimation, one of the finest sources of calcium available. Raw milk (A2) is generally not associated with any of the above health problems, and even people who have been allergic to pasteurized milk for many years can typically tolerate and even thrive on raw milk. Yet, there are those people who still have trouble drinking raw milk. That piece, it turns out, may very well be related to the type of cow your milk comes from. A1 Vs. A2 Cows - Dairy cows must be genetically tested and the test can be done thru the A1A2 Gene Testing Company. For more information on wholesome milk, please contact the Weston A. Price Foundation.

Other forms of milk substitution are as follows:

Almond milk	Goat Milk	Rice Milk
Coconut Milk	Hemp Milk	Soy Milk

ALMOND MILK

Almond milk is a beverage made from ground almonds, often used as a substitute for milk.
Unlike animal milk, almond milk contains neither cholesterol nor lactose. As it does not contain any animal products, it is suitable for vegans and vegetarians who abstain from dairy products. Commercial almond milk products often come in plain, vanilla, or chocolate flavors and are sometimes enriched with vitamins. Almond milk can also be made at home by combining ground almonds with water in a blender. Vanilla flavoring and sweeteners are often added. It's a healthy alternative to cow's milk and contains more vitamins and minerals than soy and
rice milks. Many people who've tried almond milk prefer the flavor of almond milk to that of soy and rice milk. Almond milk is one of the most nutritious milk substitutes available. It doesn't contain saturated fats or cholesterol, but it does contain omega-3 fatty acids, so it's very good for your heart. Almond milk is high in protein; the typical eight-ounce serving of almond milk
contains about one gram of protein. One serving of almond milk also contains about one gram of dietary fiber. Almond milk is very low in calories; it contains only about 40 calories per serving, and it's low in carbs at only two grams per serving. Almond milk contains about three grams of fat per eight-ounce serving, making its fat content equivalent to that of rice milk.
Almonds are rich in vitamins and minerals, so almond milk doesn't need to be fortified. Almonds contain:

Calcium	Manganese	Vitamin E
Fiber	Phosphorous	Zinc
Iron	Potassium	
Magnesium	Selenium	

The flavonoids in almond milk help prevent cancer and slow the signs of aging. The high levels of antioxidant vitamin E found in almond milk make it very effective in the prevention of cancer.

Coconut Milk

Coconut milk is extracted by grating mature coconuts and squeezing them by using cheesecloth or both bare hands. It is used in several food recipes like sauces, delicious curries, and desserts. Apart from making foods tastier and creamier, coconut milk is also a healthy addition to various food preparations. Coconut milk contains a large proportion of lauric acid, a saturated fat that raises blood cholesterol levels by increasing the amount of high-density lipoprotein cholesterol that is also found in significant amounts in breast milk and sebaceous gland secretions. This may create a more favorable blood cholesterol profile, though it is unclear if coconut oil may promote atherosclerosis through other pathways. Because much of the saturated fat of coconut oil is in the form of lauric acid, coconut oil may be a better alternative to partially hydrogenated vegetable oil when solid fats are required. In addition, virgin coconut oil is composed mainly of medium-chain triglycerides, which may not carry the same risks as other saturated fats. Early studies on the health effects of coconut oil used partially hydrogenated coconut oil, which creates trans fats, and not virgin coconut oil, which has a different health risk profile.

Coconut milk has a long-standing cultural association with health in the Ayurveda tradition. This natural drink is usually recommended for maintaining electrolyte balance and can also be used in case of dehydration. Some recent studies have suggested that coconut milk has hyperlipidemic balancing qualities, antimicrobial properties in the gastrointestinal tract or by topical application, and it has been used as a home remedy for healing mouth ulcers. In a study with rats, two coconut based preparations (a crude warm water extract of coconut milk and coconut water dispersion) were studied for their protective effects on drug-induced gastric ulceration. Both substances offered protection against ulceration, with coconut milk producing a 54% reduction vs. 39% for coconut water. In addition, the saturated fat in coconut milk is mostly lauric acid, which was found to have positive effects on the cardiovascular system.

While it is important to note that there is conflicting evidence on the claimed health effects of consuming significant amounts of coconut milk, coconut is rich in medium-chain fatty acids (MCFAs), which the body processes differently than other saturated fats. MCFAs promote weight maintenance without raising cholesterol levels.

Goat Milk

Goat milk is an alternative to cow's milk. Goat milk and goat cheese have been made and consumed for generation upon generations. There is no fear of the A1 in goat milk as the A1 gene is only cow related problema. Goats produce about 2% of the world's total annual milk supply. Some goats are bred specifically for milk. If the strong-smelling buck is not separated from the does, his scent will affect the milk. Doe milk naturally has small, well-emulsified fat globules, which means the cream remains suspended in the milk, instead of rising to the top, as in raw cow's milk; therefore, it does not need to be homogenized. Indeed, if the milk is to be used to make cheese, homogenization is not recommended, as it changes the structure of the milk, impacting the culture's ability to coagulate the milk and the final quality and yield of cheese. Dairy goats in their prime (generally around the third or fourth lactation cycle) average 6 to 8 lb (2.7 to 3.6 kg) of milk production daily (roughly 3 to 4 US quarts (2.7 to 3.6 liters)) during a ten-month lactation, producing more just after freshening and gradually dropping in production toward the end of their lactation. The milk generally averages 3.5% butterfat.

Hemp Milk

Hemp milk, or hemp seed milk, is a drink made from hemp seeds that are soaked and ground into water, yielding a creamy nutty beverage. Hemp seeds contain no THC (delta-9-tetrahydrocannabinol), the psychoactive substance found in marijuana but instead contain a three-to-one ratio of omega-6 and omega-3 essential fatty acids and other nutrients including:

Beta-carotene	Magnesium	Vitamin B_1
Calcium	Phosphorus	Vitamin B_2
Fiber	Phytosterols	Vitamin B_3
Iron	Potassium	Vitamin C

Hemp milk also contains 10 essential amino acids, making it a good vegan source of protein as hemp protein does not contain phytates, enzyme inhibitors found in some soy protein that can interfere with the absorption of essential minerals. Hemp protein may also be more digestible than soy protein because unlike soy, it doesn't contain oligosaccharides, complex sugars that can cause flatulence if not properly broken down during digestion. As far as allergies are concerned, hemp seeds do not pose the threat that tree nuts do and that anyone allergic to soy or dairy should be able to safely consume hemp milk.

Soy Milk

Soy milk (also called soya milk, soymilk, soybean milk, or soy bean juice and sometimes referred to as soy drink/beverage) is a beverage made from soybeans. A traditional staple of Asian cuisine, it is a stable emulsion of oil, water, and protein. It is produced by soaking dry soybeans and grinding them with water. Soy milk contains about the same proportion of protein as cow's milk: around 3.5%; also 2% fat, 2.9% carbohydrate, and 0.5% ash. Soy milk can be made at home with traditional kitchen tools or with a soy milk machine. Soy milk has about the same amount of protein as cow's milk, though the amino acid profile differs. Natural soy milk contains little digestible calcium as it is bound to the bean's pulp, which is insoluble in humans. To counter this, many manufacturers enrich their products with calcium carbonate available to human digestion.

Unlike cow's milk, it has little saturated fat and no cholesterol. Soy products contain sucrose as the basic disaccharide, which breaks down into glucose and fructose. Since soy doesn't contain galactose, a product of lactose breakdown, soy-based infant formulas can safely replace breast milk in children with galactosemia. Like lactose-free cow's milk, soy milk contains no lactose, which makes it a good alternative for lactose-intolerant people. For patients without conditions that limit which sugars they can consume, there is no evidence to support any sugar-related health benefit or detriment to consuming soy milk instead of cow's milk.

The American Academy of Pediatrics considers soy milk a suitable alternative for children who cannot tolerate human or cow's milk, or whose parents opt for a vegan diet. They find no medical benefit to using soy milk instead of human or cow's milk. Soy milk, like cow's milk, varies in fat content, but the most commonly sold varieties have less fat than whole milk, similar fat content to 2% milk, and more fat than skim/nonfat milk. Though it has been suggested that soy consumption is associated with a reduction in low-density lipoprotein ("bad cholesterol") and triglycerides, a 2006 study of a decade of soy protein consumption found no association between soy intake and health benefits such as cardiovascular health or cancer rates, and no benefit for women undergoing menopause. Soy was able to replace animal protein, foods high in saturated fats, and other sources of dietary fiber, vitamins and minerals. However, much of the mineral content in soy milk is unassimilable because of high content of phytic acid in soy milk. If soy milk is made into tempeh, the phytic acid content is cut in half.

Rice Milk

Rice milk is a kind of grain milk processed from rice. It is mostly made from brown rice and commonly unsweetened. The sweetness in most rice milk varieties is generated by a natural enzymatic process, cleaving the carbohydrates into sugars, especially glucose, similar to the Japanese amazake. Some rice milk kinds may nevertheless be sweetened with sugarcane syrup or other sugars. Compared to cow's milk, rice milk contains more carbohydrates, but does not contain significant amounts of calcium or protein, and no cholesterol or lactose. Commercial brands of rice milk, however, are often fortified with vitamins and minerals, including:

Calcium
Iron
Vitamin B_3
Vitamin B_{12}

Rice milk is often consumed by people who are lactose intolerant, allergic to soy, or have PKU. It is also used as a dairy substitute by vegans. Rice milk doesn't contain as much calcium or protein as cow's milk. Since rice milk doesn't contain a lot of protein, those who use rice milk as a milk substitute must plan to include more protein in their diet through other means. Most commercial brands of rice milk, however, are fortified with calcium. This is why a serving of fortified rice milk provides the same amount of calcium as a serving of cow's milk. Rice milk is also often fortified with:

Iron
Vitamin A
Vitamin B_{12}
Vitamin B_3
Vitamin D

Naringin

Naringin is a type of flavonoid, a water-soluble pigment, found in grapefruits. By itself, naringin has little nutritional value, other than being responsible for giving grapefruit its bitter flavor, and possibly enhancing one's sense of taste. As a dietary supplement, however, naringin has a wide range of benefits.

Naringin appears to interfere with the activity of several enzymes that are responsible for the breakdown of certain nutrients in the intestines, along with many types of drugs, resulting in higher levels of those substances in the blood. As such, naringin is used to improve the effectiveness and increase the half-life of several supplements and related substances, such as caffeine.

How much naringin should I take? Most studies have shown that a dose of 25 milligrams of naringin is enough to increase the bioavailability and half-life of certain nutrients and/or drugs consumed with it.

What forms of naringin are available? The main source of naringin is pure grapefruit juice. However, many types of grapefruit juice are either blended with other juices, or use grapefruits that have low naringin levels, to help remove bitterness and improve taste. Naringin supplements are also available, and are sold in pill, liquid, and capsule form.

What can happen if I take too much naringin? Are there any interactions I should be aware of? What precautions should I take? Because naringin can change the metabolism of certain drugs so that they remain in the bloodstream longer, taking naringin supplements can result in higher-than-expected levels of those drugs in the blood, which may cause a variety of unwanted side effects. As a result, patients should not take any drugs with naringin or grapefruit juice without first speaking with a licensed health care provider. In addition, the effects of taking naringin and/or drinking grapefruit juice are related; the more naringin that is ingested, the greater its interaction with certain drugs and other nutrients.

Among the drugs known to be affected by naringin are calcium channel blockers; estrogen supplements; sedatives; high blood pressure medications; and cholesterol-lowering medications. As always, make sure to consult with a licensed health care provider before taking naringin or any other herbal remedy or dietary supplement.

OCTACOSANOL

Octacosanol is a solid, insoluble waxy substance that belongs to the fatty alcohol family. It is isolated from the wax usually found on the green blades of wheat and can also be found in wheat germ oil. It is the primary component of a sugar cane extract called policosanol.

While the exact action of octacosanol is unknown, research conducted in the 1970s suggested that it could improve endurance, increase reaction time, and help athletes train longer. Other studies have shown that it could improve grip strength and visual sharpness. Unreliable research suggests that octacosanol may lower blood cholesterol levels and may benefit patients with Parkinson's disease, but more research needs to be performed in these areas.

How much octacosanol should I take? Most practitioners recommend between 1 and 8 milligrams of octacosanol daily, taken with food. Doses of 20 milligrams or more should not be exceeded. When taken as part of policosanol, slightly higher doses may be consumed.

What forms of octacosanol are available? Octacosanol is most often available as a tablet or capsule. It is occasionally blended with other fatty alcohols as part of a larger supplement.

What can happen if I take too much octacosanol? Are there any interactions I should be aware of? What precautions should I take? Octacosanol should not be taken by children or women who are pregnant or nursing. Some studies have shown that patients with Parkinson's disease who take octacosanol supplements may experience dizziness and increased nervousness. Octacosonal may also interact with the drug levadopa; patients taking this medication should consult with a licensed health care provider before taking octacosanol. No other drug interactions are known to exist as of this writing.

Oryzanol

Oryzanol (also referred to as gamma oryzanol) is a naturally occurring mixture of various plant chemicals, includes sterols and esters. It is found in a variety of plant foods such as rice bran, corn, and barley, but the body does not easily absorb it.

Some research suggests that oryzanol stimulates the release of natural pain-relieving substances called endorphins. Other studies suggest that oryzanol can increase testosterone levels and increase the growth of muscle tissue in athletes. Some bodybuilders and weightlifters use oryzanol to increase athletic performance and reduce tiredness; however, there is no final evidence that oryzanol helps to improve strength or increase endurance. There is also evidence that oryzanol may reduce cholesterol levels in the blood.

How much oryzanol should I take? Because oryzanol is not an essential nutrient, suggested daily allowance levels have yet to be established. The bulk of research into oryzanol has used supplements ranging from 300 mg to 600 mg per day.

What forms of oryzanol are available? Oryzanol occurs naturally in some plant foods, including rice bran, corn and barley, and some plant oils. Oryzanol is also available as a dietary supplement, usually as a capsule or liquid.

What can happen if I take too much oryzanol? Are there any interactions I should be aware of? What precautions should I take? Research suggests that high amounts of oryzanol (>600 milligrams per day) for long-drawn-out periods of time (6 months) may cause a variety of unpleasant side effects, including dry mouth, irritability, and light-headedness. If such side effects occur, patients should consult with a health care provider about lowering dosage or stopping use of oryzanol. As of this writing, there are no known drug interactions linked with oryzanol. As always, make sure to speak with a licensed health care provider before taking oryzanol or any other dietary supplement or herbal remedy.

Oligosaccharides

Oligosaccharides are short chains of sugar molecules. There are several kinds of oligosaccharides, each made from different types of sugars.

Fructo-oligosaccharides and inulin oligosaccharides consist of short chains of fructose molecules, while galacto-oligosaccharides consist of short chains of galactose molecules. All three types of oligosaccharides occur naturally, but they can be only partially digested by humans. The undigested portions remain in the body and serve as food for probiotics and other "friendly" intestinal bacteria.

Research has established a positive relationship between oligosaccharides and friendly bacteria; intake of oligosaccharides can increase the amount of friendly bacteria in the gut, while at the same time reducing the number of harmful bacteria. Oligosaccharide supplements may also increase creation of several fatty acids, increase the intake of magnesium and calcium, and lower blood sugar levels in people with diabetes. In addition, oligosaccharides may reduce cholesterol and triglyceride levels in the blood. These results are best seen in people with high triglyceride/cholesterol levels, or people with diabetes.

How many oligosaccharides should I take? Scientists estimate that the average American ingests between 800 and 1,000 milligrams of oligosaccharides per day. To promote growth of friendly intestinal bacteria, some practitioners recommend higher doses—between 2,000 to 3,000 milligrams per day, eaten with meals. Some studies have used much higher amounts—8 to 20 grams per day.

What forms of oligosaccharides are available? Oligosaccharides are found in a variety of fruits and vegetables. Inulin oligosaccharides and fructo-oligosaccharides are present in artichokes, leeks, onions, asparagus, and chicory. Galacto-oligosaccharides are found in soybeans and can be synthesized from lactose. All three types of oligosaccharides are also available as supplements, either in capsule, tablet, or powder form.

What can happen if I take too many oligosaccharides? Are there any interactions I should be aware of? What precautions should I take? Oligosaccharide supplements are usually well tolerated by individuals, although they may cause flatulence and bloating in some people. High levels (.40 grams per day) may cause diarrhea. In addition, some people may be allergic to fructo-oligosaccharides; in these cases, supplementation should be avoided. As of this writing, there are no well-known drug interactions with oligosaccharides. As always, make sure to speak with a licensed health care provider before taking oligosaccharides or any other dietary supplement or herbal remedy.

OLIVE LEAF EXTRACT

Also known as, oleuropein, olive leaf extract comes from the leaves of the olive tree. There are about 800 million olive trees in existence, the vast majority of which are located in and about the Mediterranean region. Olive leaf extract is usually removed from the leaves of the mission and manzanillo varieties of olive tree.

Olive leaf extract has been shown to display antibiotic, antibacterial, antiviral, and antifungal properties. When ingested, olive leaf extract is changed by the body into elonolic acid, which helps strengthen the immune system. It has been prescribed to treat a number of infectious conditions, including chlamydia, strep throat, herpes, and yeast infections. Other practitioners have used it to treat chronic fatigue syndrome and fibromyalgia.

How much olive leaf extract should I take? The typical suggested dose of olive leaf extract is between 500 milligrams and 1,000 milligrams daily, usually for preventive purposes. For specific conditions, some practitioners may recommend between 2 and 6 grams per day.

What forms of olive leaf extract are available? Olive leaf extract is available as a capsule or liquid extract.

What can happen if I take too much olive leaf extract? Are there any interactions I should be aware of? What precautions should I take? As of this writing, there are no known side effects associated with olive leaf extract. Because olive leaf extract can reduce the effect of certain antibiotics, it should not be used while a person is also taking antibiotics. As always, make sure to speak with a licensed health care provider before taking olive leaf extracts or any other dietary supplements or herbal remedies.

Phosphatidylserine

Phosphatidylserine is a type of phospholipid, a fat-soluble substance necessary for the growth of cell membranes. Normally, the body makes phosphatidylserine from other components of phospholipids. It is found in high concentrations in the brain and elsewhere in the body.

Most research relating to phosphatidylserine has examined its role in mental function and the treatment of Alzheimer's disease. Placebo-controlled studies have suggested that phosphatidylserine may have a moderate effect in improving mental function in Alzheimer's, with the effects lasting up to three months after the end of the study. However, phosphatidylserine is not a cure for Alzheimer's disease; at best, it appears to slow mental deterioration. (Coconut Oil has shown promise improving early onset Alzheimer's)

Phosphatidylserine also appears to affect the levels of certain neurotransmitters that are related to mood. For this reason, it may be of benefit in the treatment of depression.

How much phosphatidylserine should I take? Because phosphatidylserine is manufactured naturally by the body, shortages caused by diet usually do not exist. Most studies of phosphatidylserine have used 300 milligrams or 600 milligrams per day, usually derived from genetically modified organism (GMO) soy.

What forms of phosphatidylserine are available? The body forms phosphatidylserine naturally. Dietary forms are rather uncommon. Very small amounts of phosphatidylserine are found in lecithin. Most clinical studies have used phosphatidylserine derived from bovine animals, specifically, bovine brain tissue. As a dietary supplement, phosphatidylserine is usually derived from soy. It is available in capsule, tablet, and liquid forms.

What can happen if I take too much phosphatidylserine? Are there any interactions I should be aware of? What precautions should I take? Because of concerns about mad cow disease, bovine-based forms of phosphatidylserine are not available in the United States. As of this writing, no major side effects have been reported in people taking phosphatidylserine, nor are there any known drug interactions. As always, make sure to speak with a licensed health care provider before taking phosphatidylserine or any other dietary supplement or herbal remedy.

Phytic Acid

Phytic acid is a naturally forming element found in plant fiber. It is known by several other names, including phytate, vitamin B_8, and IP-6. While somewhat little human research with phytic acid has been conducted, it is believed to possess some of the properties of well-known antioxidants, in addition to other as-yet-unknown benefits.

Many animal studies have shown that phytic acid can protect against some types of cancer, including cancers of the breast and colon. Injections of phytic acid have also showed the ability to reduce the size of cancerous tumors in mice. Phytic acid may also have a positive effect on controlling blood sugar, and may reduce the frequency of kidney stones. As of this writing, however, nearly all research on phytic acid has involved the use of animals. As a result, it is not known how well humans can absorb or use phytic acid, if at all.

How much phytic acid should I take? Because most of the research on phytic acid has been conducted on animals, scientists have been unable to decide an optimal amount of phytic acid intake. The typical diet provides between 1 and 1.5 grams of phytic acid per day, much of it coming from grains and legumes.

What forms of phytic acid are available? Phytic acid is available in a wide range of plant foods, including wheat bran, whole grain, and legumes. Nuts and seeds also contain phytic acid, but in smaller amounts compared to bran and grains.

Side Note: Phytic acid not only grabs on to or chelates important minerals, but it also inhibits enzymes that we need to digest our food, including pepsin, needed for the breakdown of proteins in the stomach, and amylase, needed for the breakdown of starch into sugar. Trypsin, needed for protein digestion in the small intestine, is also inhibited by phytates. High-phytate diets result in mineral deficiencies. In populations where cereal grains provide a major source of calories, rickets and osteoporosis are common. Soaking grains and flour in an acid medium at very warm temperatures, as in the sourdough process, also activates phytase and reduces or even eliminates phytic acid.

What can happen if I take too much phytic acid? Are there any interactions I should be aware of? What precautions should I take? In animal studies, phytic acid intake has been connected with reduced absorption of certain minerals, especially iron. As a result, people who are anemic or have a shortage of iron should talk with a health care provider about increasing iron supplementation before taking phytic acid supplements. As of this writing, there are no known drug interactions with phytic acid. As always, make sure to speak with a licensed health care provider before taking phytic acid or any other dietary supplement or herbal remedy.

POLICOSANOL

Policosanol is a popular dietary supplement that consists of a mixture of alcohols and beeswax. Many of the alcohols are derived from sugar cane, and include policosanol, hexacosanol, triocontanol, and quite a few others.

As a dietary supplement, policosanol has been used to lower levels of low-density lipoprotein (LDL) cholesterol in the blood. Studies have shown that policosanol supplementation can reduce both total cholesterol and LDL levels, while raising HDL cholesterol levels, with positive results lasting up to two years. These results have been seen in various patient populations, ranging from postmenopausal women to patients with Type 2 diabetes.

Clinical studies have shown that policosanol may benefit patients suffering from other conditions, as well. It appears to reduce the formation of blood clots, and shows a synergistic effect when used with aspirin for this purpose. Policosanol may also reduce inflammation and protect the body from certain types of viruses.

How much policosanol should I take? The suggested dose of policosanol is 10 milligrams once per day, usually taken during the evening, with meals. Animal studies using much higher doses for extended amounts of time have shown no unpleasant side effects or signs of toxicity.

What forms of policosanol are available? Policosanol is available in supplement form as a tablet, capsule, or pill. Policosanol is often sold as part of a larger dietary supplement that includes coenzyme Q_{10} and various antioxidants.

What can happen if I take too much policosanol? Are there any interactions I should be aware of? What precautions should I take? Some minor side effects have been associated with long-term policosanol use, including dizziness, upset stomach, and headaches. Because policosanol acts as a blood thinner, patients using blood-thinning medications such as warfarin or coumadin, or non-steroidal anti-inflammatory drugs such as naproxen or ibuprofen, without first consulting with a licensed health care provider, should not take it. In addition, because policosanol is made in part from beeswax, some patients who are allergic to bee stings or bee products may have an allergic reaction to policosanol.

As of this writing, there are no known drug interactions with policosanol. As always, make sure to speak with a licensed health care provider before taking policosanol or any other dietary supplement or herbal remedy.

Propolis

Propolis is the name given to the resinous material that is collected by bees from the leaf buds and barks of trees, such as poplars and conifers. The bees use the propolis and combine it with beeswax to help build their hives. It contains a variety of vitamins, minerals, proteins, and amino acids. Because of this, some people use propolis as a dietary supplement.

Propolis has been shown to have both antibiotic and antimicrobial properties. Test-tube studies have shown that propolis is successful against certain bacteria and yeasts associated with dental cavities, periodontal disease, and gingivitis, and that it may help mouth wounds heal faster. Other studies have shown that propolis extracts can treat giardiasis, a common intestinal parasite found in children. Topical application of propolis may reduce inflammation of the skin and treat conditions such as genital herpes and rheumatoid arthritis.

How much propolis should I take? Because propolis is not considered an essential nutrient, shortage levels and suggested daily allowance levels have yet to be decided. However, many supplement manufacturers recommend a dosage of 500 milligrams of propolis taken orally, once or twice daily. For topical applications, patients should follow the instructions on the product label.

What forms of propolis are available? Commercially prepared propolis is available in a liquid extract, as well as in capsules and tablets. Topical creams and sprays containing propolis are also available.

What can happen if I take too much propolis? Are there any interactions I should be aware of? What precautions should I take? Proplis is usually thought of as non-toxic, although it may cause allergic reactions such as skin rashes. People who are allergic to bee stings, bee pollen, royal jelly, honey, or conifer and poplar trees should not use propolis unless being tested by an allergy specialist first. In addition, because the effects of propolis have not been determined in women who are pregnant or breastfeeding, it should be avoided by women during these times. As of this writing, there are no well-known drug interactions with propolis. As always, make sure to speak with a licensed health care provider before taking propolis or any other herbal remedy or dietary supplement.

Psyllium – (Psyllium Seed)

Psyllium (also known as psyllium seed) is a soluble fiber. It comes from a shrub like herb called the plantain (no relation to the plant that produces edible plantains). Its ingredients include alkaloids, amino acids, oils, protein, tannins, flavonoids, and a variety of sugars and carbohydrates.

Psyllium seeds are oval-shaped, odorless, practically tasteless, and are coated with mucilage. Unlike wheat bran and other fibers, psyllium does not cause excessive gas and bloating.

Used as a dietary fiber, psyllium makes stools softer, which helps relieve constipation, irritable bowel syndrome, hemorrhoids, and other intestinal disorders. It is considered a good intestinal cleanser in that it speeds waste matter through the digestive system, shortening the amount of time toxic substances stay in the body and thereby reducing the risk of colon cancer and other diseases.

Soluble fibers such as psyllium can also help prevent the intestine from absorbing cholesterol. Studies have found that adding psyllium to one's diet can reduce the amount of cholesterol in the blood; when taken in combination with certain medications, it can reduce blood cholesterol levels even further.

How much psyllium should I take? There is no recommended daily allowance, but many herbalists and health professionals recommend taking between one to two teaspoons of psyllium one or two times a day. The best times to take it are early in the morning and just before going to bed.

What are some good sources of psyllium? Psyllium seed or husks are the two dietary sources of psyllium fiber.

What can happen if we do not get enough psyllium? There are no studies that have documented the effects of psyllium deficiency.

Do not take psyllium at the same time (or within an hour of the time) you take other medications: it can interfere with the way drugs are absorbed and make some medications less effective. Always take psyllium with a full eight-ounce glass of water, and make sure to drink at least six to eight glasses of water a day.

Another fiber supplement, guar works the same way psyllium does. If you are already taking guar, do not take psyllium (and vice-versa). Do not give psyllium to a child. For more information on psyllium, please speak with your health care provider.

QUERCETIN

Quercetin is a flavanoid, a substance found in fruits, flowers, and vegetables. Among other things, flavonoids give objects their color. Most flavonoids have been found to work as both antioxidants and anti-inflammatory, which are useful in treating or preventing a variety of health problems.

Quercetin is useful in reducing allergic reactions and may be helpful in treating canker sores, hives, asthma, and other inflammatory responses. Other conditions for which quercetin may be helpful includes diabetes, dysentery, gout, cataracts, and atopic dermatitis.

Recent research has focused on quercetin's ability to fight certain forms of cancer. In one study, it helped prevent the formation of skin cancer. In another, it was helpful against the formation of tumors in patients with ovarian cancer and hepatoma.

How much quercetin should I take? Most health practitioners recommend 100-250 milligrams of quercetin daily as a general supplement. For other conditions, the dosage can be increased:

*For lowered histamine levels and allergy symptoms: 250-600 milligrams.

*For treatment of gout: 200-400 milligrams of quercetin taken with bromelain between meals.

*For treatment of chronic hives: 200-400 milligrams of quercetin taken approximately 20 minutes before each meal.

What are some good sources of quercetin? Quercetin can be found in fruits and vegetables (mainly citrus fruits), apples, onions (especially the outer skin), parsley, green tea, and red wine. Flavonoid rich extracts, such as those from grape seed, bilberry, and ginkgo biloba, are also good sources of quercetin.

What can happen if we do not get enough quercetin? No side effects have been reported on the subject of quercetin shortage.

What can happen if I take too much? Are there any side effects I should be aware of? No side effects have been connected with quercetin. No problems with excess amounts of quercetin have been recorded. For more information on quercetin, please speak with your health care provider.

RESVERATROL

Resveratrol is a polyphenolic compound found in grapes, red wine, purple grape juice, peanuts, and some berries. When taken orally, resveratrol appears to be well-absorbed by humans, but its bioavailability is relatively low because it is rapidly metabolized and eliminated. Resveratrol is produced naturally by several plants when under attack by pathogens such as bacteria or fungi. The first mention of resveratrol was in a Japanese article in 1939 by Michio Takaoka, who isolated it from the poisonous, but medicinal, Veratrum album, variety grandiflorum. The name presumably comes from the fact that it is a resorcinol derivative coming from a Veratrum species.

The effects of resveratrol are currently a topic of numerous animal and human studies. In mouse and rat experiments, anticancer, anti-inflammatory, blood sugar-lowering and other beneficial cardiovascular effects of resveratrol have been reported. Resveratrol is found in the skin of red grapes and in other fruits, and it is sold as a nutritional supplement derived primarily from Japanese knotweed.

Resveratrol is thhought to have profound effects on the following concerns:

- Antidiabetic effects
- Anti-inflammatory effects
- Cancer prevention
- Cardioprotective effects
- Effect on testosterone levels
- Neuroprotective effects
- Opioid tolerance reduction

The secret to anti-aging lies with trans-resveratrol, the active form of resveratrol polyphenols found in the skins, seeds and stems of red wine grapes. Trans-resveratrol remains active only when sheltered from the sun, light and oxygen. In this pure, ultra beneficial form, trans-resveratrol has been proven in studies to activate longevity genes and enhance cellular productivity. Make sure that the label has no *cis*-resveratrol on the label as you will not be able to use any of the *cis* type.

How much resveratrol should I take? While a recommended daily allowance has not been decided, researchers believe a minimum of 500 milligrams of resveratrol should be taken to help reduce the risk of cancer. A glass of red wine contains approximately 640 micrograms of resveratrol; a handful of peanuts supplies nearly 75 micrograms.

What are some good sources of resveratrol? What forms are available? Grapes and peanuts are the two main food sources of resveratrol. Resveratrol is concentrated in grape skin. Since the manufacturing process of red wine includes extended contact with grape skins, red wine contains far higher amounts of resveratrol than white wine. Resveratrol supplements are also available; they are usually found in combination with grape extracts or other antioxidants.

What can happen if I do not get enough resveratrol? What can happen if I take too much? Are there any side effects I should be aware of? Since resveratrol is not classified as an essential nutrient, no exact deficiency or toxicity levels have been established. At the time of this writing, there are no known adverse reactions or drug interactions associated with resveratrol.

SOLUBLE FIBER

Fiber is divided into two general categories water soluble and water insoluble. This section will discuss soluble fiber. Soluble fibers are those that dissolve in water or swell when placed in water. They are found in various types of plants and gums, along with some cereals, jams, and jellies.

One of the main properties of soluble fiber is its ability to lower cholesterol. Dozens of studies have shown that soluble fiber lowers cholesterol, but the level of reduction can vary depending on the type of fiber. Soluble fiber can also lower blood sugar levels in people by slowing the intake of glucose from the small intestine. This lessens the body's need for insulin and may be of help to people with diabetes. Another function of soluble fiber is to help promote weight loss. Because fiber creates a feeling that one's stomach is full, it is believed to help decrease appetite, leading to weight loss. However, an exact link between soluble fiber intake and weight loss has yet to be established.

How much soluble fiber should I take? High amounts of soluble fiber can help decrease blood cholesterol. The amount of fiber to be taken depends on the food from which it is derived. For oat bran, for example, some practitioners may suggest between 80 and 100 grams per day, which translates into about three-quarters of a cup of uncooked oats. For beans, approximately 1.5 cups (150 grams) will provide enough fiber to help lower cholesterol levels.

What forms of soluble fiber are available? Soluble fiber is plentiful in foods such as oats, barley, beans, whole fruits, and psyllium. Soluble fiber is also available as a supplement in powder, pill, and capsule form.

What can happen if I take too much soluble fiber? Are there any interactions I should be aware of? What precautions should I take? Some people may be allergic to foods that are high in fiber; these foods should be avoided. In addition, some foods such as beans contain sugars that are not easily digested, which can lead to flatulence and bloating. Fiber may also reduce the intake of some minerals, such as calcium and magnesium. People who do not get enough calcium in their diet should consult with a licensed health care provider before taking large amounts of fiber. In addition, people with scleroderma should speak with a health care provider before taking fiber supplements or engaging in a high-fiber diet. Generally, however, high-fiber diets are more likely to improve a person's health, rather than cause any health problems.

Certain medications, such as Lovastatin, Verapamil, and Propoxyphene may interact with fiber supplements. As always, make sure to speak with a licensed health care provider before taking soluble fiber or any other herbal remedy or dietary supplement.

Spirulina

Spirulina is a type of blue-green algae, of which there are several species. The most popular are spirulina maxima (which is cultivated in Mexico) and spirulina platensis (which is cultivated in California). It grows best in warm climates and areas with warm, alkaline water.

Spirulina is a rich source of nutrients, especially protein. Sixty-two percent of its composition consists of nonessential amino acids; it is also rich in vitamins, beta-carotene, zinc, manganese, copper, iron, selenium, and essential fatty acids such as GLA. Because of its high nutrient content, and because the cellular walls of spirulina are made up of complex proteins and sugars instead of cellulose, it is easily digested by the body and is considered a vital food source for vegetarians. Many weightlifters also use spirulina as a protein source.

Spirulina is currently being studied to determine its effects on a number of clinical conditions. One recent study suggested that calcium spirulina, a part of spirulina, could protect the body against human immunodeficiency virus (HIV). Animal studies have showed that another component of spirulina, C-phycocyanin, can reduce inflammation in the colon. Other clinical trials suggest that spirulina can slow the growth of some forms of cancers and can reduce the risk of oral cancer in people who chew tobacco.

How much spirulina should I take? A standard dosage of spirulina is 4-6 tablets (500milligrams) per day. However, patients should always consult with a health care provider before taking spirulina supplements.

What are some good sources of spirulina? What forms are available? Spirulina is an algae. Although it can be found growing in warm climates, most spirulina consumed in the U.S. is cultivated in a laboratory. It is readily available in pill or powder form at most health food stores.

What can happen if I do not get enough spirulina? What can happen if I take too much? Are there any side effects I should be aware of? To date, there are no known side effects or interactions reported with spirulina. However, women who are pregnant or breast-feeding should speak with a health care provider before taking spirulina supplements.

Sulforaphane

Sulforaphane is a compound that was discovered by accident by a group of scientists in the United States in the mid-1990s. At the time, scientists were researching the anticancer compounds in broccoli, when they discovered that broccoli sprouts contain between 30 and 50 times the concentration of protective compounds compared to mature broccoli plants. One of those compounds was sulforaphane. Sulforaphane is considered an antioxidant, and also helps promote the production of detoxifying enzymes, which are believed to reduce the risk of cancer. Animal studies have shown that sulforaphane extracts can reduce the frequency, size, and amount of cancerous tumors in rats, but these results have yet to be copied in humans. Some studies suggest that an increased intake of broccoli and broccoli sprouts that contain sulforaphane may dramatically reduce one's risk of cancer.

How much sulforaphane should I take? Although recommended daily intake levels have not been established, some providers recommend between 200 and 400 micrograms of sulforaphane daily.

What forms of sulforaphane are available? Broccoli and broccoli sprouts.

Sulforaphane extracts are also available in some nutritional stores.

What can happen if I take too much sulforaphane? Are there any interactions I should be aware of? What precautions should I take? Because sulforaphane is not an essential nutrient, deficiency and toxicity levels have not been established. However, many practitioners recommend between 200 and 400 micrograms of sulforaphane daily. As of this writing, no side effects or drug interactions with sulforaphane have been reported; however, people taking prescription drugs should consult with a licensed health care provider before taking sulforaphane supplements. As always, make sure to consult with a licensed health care practitioner before taking sulforaphane or any other dietary supplement or herbal remedy.

Velver Antler (Deer – Elk)

The production of elk and deer velvet antler as a dietary supplement or medicinal substance constitutes a major industry in Asia, and the history of velvet antler use in Asian countries dates back more than 2,000 years.

The first documented evidence of velvet antler's use as a health tonic was found on a Chinese silk scroll dated at 168 B.C. In Russia, documented use dates to the late 1400's, when antlers were referred to as "horns of gold." Medicinal use of antler became so common that deer farming was introduced to Russia in the 1840s.

Unlike the horns of cattle or sheep, which grow throughout the life of the animal, the antlers of deer and elk are grown new every spring and then cast off. For thousands of years, traditional Asian herbalists have harvested antler growth in the early stage, before it hardens into bone. Antler velvet, as this naturally-regenerated, early-stage growth is known, has been prized in traditional Chinese herbalism, as well as in countries including Korea, Russia, and Japan. Used predominantly as a vitalizing tonic, its traditional uses have also included reducing the negative effects of stress, improving mental function, and improving circulation.

Velvet antler contains key compounds including:

All the essential amino acids	Glucosamine sulfate	Potassium
Calcium	Iron	Selenium
Chondroitin sulfate	Magnesium	Sodium
Cobalt	Manganese	Sulfur
Copper	Phosphorus	Zinc

DEFINITIONS OF HUMAN CONDITIONS

Abortifacient - Causing abortion.

Abscesses - A localized collection of pus in the tissues of the body often accompanied by swelling and inflammation and frequently caused by bacteria.

Absorbent - Material capable of absorbing moisture.

Acrochordons - Also known as a cutaneous skin tag, a small benign tumor that forms primarily in areas where the skin forms creases, such as the neck, armpit, and groin. They may also occur on the face, usually on the eyelids. Acrochorda are harmless and typically painless, and do not grow or change over time.

Ague gue - A fever (such as from malaria) that is marked by paroxysms of chills, fever, and sweating recurring at regular intervals.

Alexiteric - A preservative against infectious diseases or a preservative against the effects of poison, or the effects of venom.

Alopecia - Loss of hair from the head or body and can mean baldness. Compulsive pulling of hair can also produce hair loss.

Amebic dysentery - Amoebic dysentery is a type of dysentery caused primarily by the amoeba entamoeba histolytica. Amoebic dysentery is transmitted through contaminated food and water. Amoebae spread by forming infective cysts which can be found in stools, and spread if whoever touches them does not sanitize their hands. Amoebic dysentery is most common in developing countries although it is occasionally seen in industrialized countries, and not just in travellers. Although it is commonly associated with tropical climates, the first documented case was in St. Petersburg, Russia.

Amygdalitis - An acute inflammation of the amygdala, the emotional center of the brain, usually triggered by being told "no" or being asked to stop playing some game. This is a common psychiatric diagnosis in those who work with children, or adults, who loose physical or emotional control regularly.

Anesthetic - A substance that causes lack of feeling or awareness; a person who is anesthetic barely has feelings.

Anodyne - A source of soothing comfort.

Antihelmintic - Drugs that expel parasitic worms (helminths) from the body, by either stunning or killing them.

Antiscorbutic - Relating to, resembling, or affected by scurvy.

Anticholinergic - Anticholinergics are a class of medications that inhibit parasympathetic nerve impulses by selectively blocking the binding of the neurotransmitter acetylcholine to its receptor in nerve cells. The nerve fibers of the parasympathetic system are responsible for the involuntary movements of smooth muscles present in the gastrointestinal tract, urinary tract, lungs, etc.

Antihepatotoxin - Liver-healing properties.

Antirheumatic - Relieving or preventing rheumatism.

Antiscorbutic - Having the effect of preventing or curing scurvy.

Antitussive - Capable of relieving or suppressing coughing.

Antivinous - Treating alcohol addiction.

Aperitive - Having a stimulating effect on the appetite.

Aphrodisiac - An aphrodisiac is a substance that increases sexual desire. Throughout history, many foods, drinks, and behaviors have had a reputation for making sex more attainable and/or pleasurable.

Aphthae - Canker sores.

Apoplexy - A medical term, which can be used to describe "bleeding" in a stroke (described as a cerebrovascular accident).

Apostemes - An abscess; a swelling filled with purulent matter.

Ascites - Ascites is excess fluid in the space between the tissues lining the abdomen and abdominal organs (the peritoneal cavity). A person with ascites usually has severe liver disease.

Astringent - A substance chemical compound that tends to shrink or constrict body tissues, usually locally after topical medicinal application. The word "astringent" derives from Latin adstringere, meaning "to bind fast."

Atherosclerosis - (also known as arteriosclerotic vascular disease or ASVD) is a condition in which an artery wall thickens as a result of the accumulation of fatty materials such as cholesterol.

Atheroma - In pathology, a "tumor full gruel-like matter" is an accumulation and swelling in artery walls made up of debris, and contain cholesterol and fatty acids, calcium, and a variable amount of fibrous connective tissue. Atheroma occurs in atherosclerosis.

Atitiperiodic - Preventing the regular recurrence of symptoms.

Atropine - Atropine is a naturally-occurring tropane alkaloid extracted from deadly nightshade (atropa belladonna), jimson weed (datura stramonium), mandrake (mandragora officinarum) and other plants of the family solanaceae. It is a secondary metabolite of these plants and serves as a drug with a wide variety of effects.

Barrenness - Not producing offspring, incapable of producing offspring.

Belpharitis - Blepharitis is an ocular condition characterized by chronic inflammation of the eyelid, the severity and time course of which can vary.

Benzoin - Benzoin is a balsamic resin. Normally the trees do not produce it or any substance analogous to it, but the infliction of a wound sufficiently severe to injure the cambium results in the formation of numerous oleoresin ducts in which the secretion is produced, it is, therefore, a pathological product. The trunk of the tree is hacked with an axe, and after a time the liquid benzoin either accumulates beneath the bark or exudes from the incisions. When it has sufficiently hardened it is collected and exported, either in the form of loose pieces (tears) or in masses packed in oblong boxes or in tins; several varieties are known, but Siam and Sumatra benzoins are the most important.

Biliousness - A term pertaining to bad digestion, stomach pains, constipation, and excessive flatulence (passing gas). The quantity or quality of the bile was thought to be at fault for the condition. Hence, the name "biliousness." ("Bilious" derives from the French "bilieux," which in turn came from "bilis," the Latin term for "bile.") Biliousness was generally laid to high living.

Boils - A boil is a localized infection in the skin that begins as a reddened, tender area. Over time, the area becomes firm, hard, and more tender. Eventually, the center of the boil softens and becomes filled with infection-fighting white blood cells from the bloodstream to eradicate the infection. This collection of white blood cells, bacteria, and proteins is known as pus. Finally, the pus "forms a head," which can be surgically opened or spontaneously drain out through the surface of the skin. Pus enclosed within tissue is referred to as an abscess. A boil is also referred to as a skin abscess.

Bronchitis - Bronchitis is inflammation of the mucous membranes of the bronchi, the airways that carry airflow from the trachea into the lungs. Bronchitis can be divided into two categories, acute and chronic, each of which has distinct etiologies, pathologies, and therapies.

Cachexia - Wasting syndrome is loss of weight, muscle atrophy, fatigue, weakness, and significant loss of appetite in someone who is not actively trying to lose weight. The formal definition of cachexia is the loss of body mass that cannot be reversed nutritionally: Even if the affected patient eats more food.

Cacoethes - An uncontrollable urge or desire, especially for something harmful like smoking.

Cancer - A broad group of various diseases, all involving unregulated cell growth. In cancer, cells divide and grow uncontrollably, forming malignant tumors, and invade nearby parts of the body. The cancer may also spread to more distant parts of the body through the lymphatic system or bloodstream. Not all tumors are cancerous. Benign tumors do not grow uncontrollably, do not invade neighboring tissues, and do not spread throughout the body. There are over 200 different known cancers that afflict humans.

Carbuncles - A carbuncle is an abscess larger than a boil, usually with one or more openings draining pus onto the skin. It is usually caused by bacterial infection, most commonly Staphylococcus infection. The infection is contagious and may spread to other areas of the body or other people. Because the condition is contagious, family members may develop carbuncles at the same time.

Cardiotonic - Relating to or having a favorable effect upon the action of the heart.

Carminative - A carminative, also known as carminativum (plural carminativa), is a herb or preparation that either prevents formation of gas in the gastrointestinal tract or facilitates the expulsion of said gas, thereby combatting flatulence. Carminatives have been shown to decrease lower esophageal pressure.

Cataplasm - Cataplasm is a poultice.

Cathartic - In medicine, a cathartic is a substance that accelerates defecation. This is in contrast to a laxative, which is a substance which eases defecation, usually by softening feces. It is possible for a substance to be both a laxative and a cathartic. However, agents such as psyllium seed husks increase the bulk of the feces.

Chancre - The primary sore of syphilis, occurring at the site of entry of the infection.

Chilblains - Chilblains are acral ulcers (that is, ulcers affecting the extremities) that occur when a predisposed individual is exposed to cold and humidity. The cold exposure damages capillary beds in the skin, which in turn can cause redness, itching, blisters, and inflammation.

Chorea - Chorea is an abnormal involuntary movement disorder, one of a group of neurological disorders called dyskinesias. The term "chorea" is derived from the Greek word "χορεία" which equals the words dance, as the quick movements of the feet or hands are comparable to dancing.

Cicatrizant - A cicatrizant is the term used to describe a product that promotes healing through the formation of scar tissue. Sandalwood is a natural cicatrizant. It derives its name from the word "cicatrix," which is another word for "scar."

Cinchona - Cinchona are medicinal plants, known as sources for quinine and other compounds.

Colic - Colic (also known as infantile colic) is a condition in which an otherwise healthy baby cries or displays symptoms of distress (cramping, moaning, etc.) frequently and for extended periods, without any discernible reason. The condition typically appears within the first month of life and often disappears rather suddenly, before the baby is three to four months old, but can last up to 12 months of life. One study concludes that babies who are not breastfed are almost twice as likely to have colic. Folklore suggests that chocolate, brassica, onions, and cow's milk are among the foods that a lactating mother may need to avoid. The crying often increases during a specific period of the day, particularly the early evening. Symptoms may worsen soon after feeding, especially in babies that do not belch easily.

Collagen - Collagen is the main structural protein found in the connective tissues of the body (skin, bones, cartilage, tendons, and ligaments). Hydrolyzed collagen protein (gelatin) is a modified form that has been broken down into smaller pieces, making it easier to digest and absorb. Collagen and gelatin are inexpensive ingredients used to support joint health, nourish bones and the tendons and ligaments surrounding them, and aid in recovery from exercise and injury.

Collyrium - In eye care, collyrium is an word for a lotion or liquid wash used as a cleanser for the eyes, particularly in diseases of the eye. The same name was also given to unguents used for the same purpose, such as unguent of tutty. Lastly, the name was given, though improperly, to some liquid medicines used against venereal diseases. Pre-modern medicine distinguished two kinds of collyriums: the one liquid, the other dry. Liquid collyriums were composed of ophthalmic powders, or waters, such as rose-water, plantain-water, that of fennel, eyebright, etc, in which was dissolved tutty, white vitriol, or some other proper powder. Dry collyriums were pastilles of Rhasis, sugar-candy, iris, tutty prepared and blown into the eye with a little pipe.

Condyloma - Condyloma refers to an infection of the genitals.

Condylomata - Genital warts is a highly contagious sexually-transmitted disease caused by some sub-types of human papillomavirus. It is spread through direct skin-to-skin contact during sex with an person. Warts are the most easily recognized symptom of genital papillomavirus infection.

Conjunctivitis - Conjunctivitis (also called pink eye). This is inflammation of the conjunctiva (the outermost layer of the eye and the inner surface of the eyelids). It is most commonly due to an infection (usually viral, but sometimes bacterial) or an allergic reaction.

Consumption - A progressive wasting away of the body especially from pulmonary tuberculosis.

Contagion - The communication of disease by direct or indirect contact.

Convulsions - A convulsion is a medical condition where body muscles contract and relax rapidly and repeatedly, resulting in an uncontrolled shaking of the body. Because a convulsion is often a symptom of an epileptic seizure, the term convulsion is sometimes used as a synonym for seizure. However, not all epileptic seizures lead to convulsions, and not all convulsions are caused by epileptic seizures. Convulsions are also consistent with an electric shock. For non-epileptic convulsions, see non-epileptic seizures. The word "fit" is sometimes used to mean a convulsion or epileptic seizure.

Cordial - From Middle French cordial ("stimulating the heart").

Corns - Corns and calluses (hyperkeratosis) are painful areas of thickened skin that appear between the toes, on the soles of the feet.

Cyanogenetic - Capable of producing cyanide; amygdalin is a cyanogenetic glucoside.

Cystitis - Cystitis is a urinary bladder inflammation that can result from any one of a number of distinct syndromes. It is most commonly caused by a bacterial infection in which case it is referred to as a urinary tract infection.

Decoction - Decoction is a method of extraction, by boiling, of dissolved chemicals, or herbal or plant material, which may include stems, roots, bark, and rhizomes.

Delirium - Delirium is most often caused by physical or mental illness and is usually temporary and reversible.

Demulcent - Serving to soothe or soften. n. A soothing, usually mucilaginous or oily substance, such as glycerin or lanolin.

Deobstruent - Removing obstructions; having power to clear or open the natural ducts of the fluids and secretions of the body.

Depilatory creams - A cosmetic preparation used to remove the hair from the skin on the human body.

Depurative - Depurative herbs help cleanse waste products and toxins from our body, and are a staple of herbal medicine. Depurative herbs work by supporting the natural cleansing functions of the kidneys, large intestines, and increase tissue blood flow and lymph drainage. They also seem to function as general, nonspecific "blood purifiers and cleansers." By lessening the toxic load of the body many root causes of disease can be addressed.

Diaphoretic - Pertaining to, characterized by, or promoting sweating.

Dioestrus - A period of sexual inactivity between recurrent periods of oestrus.

Discutient - An agent that dissolves or causes something, such as a tumor, to disappear.

Diuretic - A diuretic provides a means of forced diuresis which elevates the rate of urination.

Dropsy - A term for the swelling of soft tissues due to the accumulation of excess water.

Dyschezia - Dyschezia refers to excessive straining with stools, specifically referring to a very common problem of newborns.

Dysuria - Dysuria refers to painful urination.

Ecbolic - A drug that tends to increase uterine contractions and that is used especially to facilitate delivery of a new born.

Egilops - An abscess in the inner canthus of the eye; fistula lachrymalis.

Emetic - Inducing to vomit; exciting the stomach to discharge its contents by the oesophagus and mouth.

Emmenagogue - A medicine that promotes the menstrual discharge.

Emollient - Softening; making supple; relaxing the solids. Barley is emollient.

Epistaxis - To bleed from the nose.

Epitheliomas - Epitheliomas can be benign growths or malignant carcinomas. They are classified according to the specific type of epithelial cells that are affected. The most common epitheliomas are basal cell carcinoma and squamous cell carcinoma (skin cancers).

Ergot - A stub, like a piece of soft horn, about the size of a chestnut.

Ergotism - A logical inference; a conclusion.

Erysipelas - A disease called St. Anthony's fire; a diffused inflammation with fever of two or three days, generally with coma or delirium; an eruption of a fiery acrid humor, on some part of the body, but chiefly on the face. One species of erysipelas is called shingles, or eruption with small vesicles.

Excrescences - An outgrowth, especially of this skin, such as occurs in any abnormal fleshy excrescence or tuberosity. Carnosity comes from the word carnose which means a build up of flesh.

Excoriations - An injury to a surface of the body caused by trauma, such as scratching, abrasion, or a chemical or thermal burn.

Expectorant - Having the quality of promoting discharges from the lungs.

Fauces - The isthmus of the fauces or the oropharyngeal isthmus is a part of the oropharynx directly behind the mouth cavity, bounded superiorly by the soft palate, laterally by the palatoglossal arches, and inferiorly by the tongue.

Febrifuge - Any medicine that mitigates or removes fever.

Fluxes - Dysentery (formerly known as flux or the bloody flux) is an inflammatory disorder of the intestine, especially of the colon, that results in severe diarrhea containing mucus and/or blood in the feces with fever, abdominal pain, and rectal tenesmus. If left untreated, dysentery can be fatal.

Fungoids - Mycosis fungoides was first described in 1806 by French dermatologist Jean-Louis-Marc Alibert. The name mycosis fungoides is somewhat misleading—it loosely means "mushroom-like fungal disease." The disease, however, is not a fungal infection but rather a type of non-Hodgkin's lymphoma. It was so named because Alibert described the skin tumors of a severe case as having a mushroom-like appearance.

Furuncles - A boil, also called a furuncle, is a deep folliculitis, infection of the hair follicle. It is most commonly caused by infection by the bacterium staphylococcus aureus, resulting in a painful swollen area on the skin caused by an accumulation of pus and dead tissue.

Gangrene - A mortification of living flesh, or of some part of a living animal body. It is particularly applied to the first state of mortification, before the life of the part is completely extinct. When the part is completely dead, it is called sphacelus.

Goiter - A large tumor that forms gradually on the human throat between the trachea and the skin.

Gonorrhea - A morbid discharge in venereal complaints.

Gravel - Small stones or fragments of stone or very small pebbles, larger than the particles of sand, but often intermixed with them. In medicine, small calculous concretions in the kidneys and bladder.

Gruel - A kind of light food made by boiling meal in water. It is usually made of the meal of oats or maiz.

Gynecopathy - Any disease unique to women.

Hemorrhoids - A discharge of blood from the vessels of the anus. The term is also applied to tumors formed by a morbid dilatation of the hemorrhoidal veins. When they do not discharge blood, they are called blind piles, when they occasionally emit blood, bleeding, or open piles.

Heinoptysis – Also known as hemoptysis which is the expectoration (coughing up) of blood or of blood-stained sputum from the bronchi, larynx, trachea, or lungs (e.g., in tuberculosis or other respiratory infections or cardiovascular pathologies).

Hemicranias - Hemicrania continua is a persistent unilateral. It is usually unremitting, but rare cases of remission have been documented. Hemicrania continua is considered a primary headache disorder, meaning that it is not caused by another condition.

Hepatitis - Hepatitis (plural hepatitides) is a medical condition defined by the inflammation of the liver and characterized by the presence of inflammatory cells in the tissue of the organ. The name is from the Greek hepar, the root being hepat, meaning liver, and suffix -itis, meaning "inflammation." The condition can be self-limiting (healing on its own) or can progress to fibrosis (scarring) and cirrhosis.

Idiocy - A defect of understanding; properly, a natural defect.

Impetigo - Impetigo is a highly contagious bacterial skin infection most common among pre-school children. People who play close contact sports such as rugby, American football, and wrestling are also susceptible, regardless of age. Impetigo is not as common in adults. The name derives from the Latin "impetere" (assail). It is also known as school sores.

Impostumes - Middle English "emposteme," ultimately from Greek "apostema," from "aphistanai" to remove, from "apo- + histanai" to cause to stand.

Indolent - Habitually idle or indisposed to labor; lazy; listless; sluggish; indulging in ease; applied to persons.

Indurations - The process of or condition produced by growing hard; specifically, sclerosis especially when associated with inflammation.

Insecticidal - Destroying or controlling insects.

Insipid - Tasteless; destitute of taste; wanting the qualities which affect the organs of taste; vapid; as insipid liquor.

Insolation - The act of exposing to the rays of the sun for drying or maturing, as fruits, drugs, etc., or for rendering acid, as vinegar, or for promoting some chemical action of one substance on another.

Jaundice - A disease which is characterized by a suffusion of bile over the coats of the eye and the whole surface of the body, by which they are tinged with a yellow color.

Labor - Exertion of muscular strength, or bodily exertion (child birth) which occasions weariness; particularly, the exertion of the limbs in occupations by which subsistence is obtained, as in agriculture and manufactures, in distinction from exertions of strength in play or amusements, which are denominated exercise, rather than labor. Toilsome work; pains; travail; any bodily exertion which is attended with fatigue. After the labors of the day, the farmer retires, and rest is sweet. Moderate labor contributes to health.

Lactagogue - An agent that promotes the secretion of breast milk.

Laxative - Having the power or quality of loosening or opening the bowels, and relieving from constipation.

Leucoderma - Partial or total loss or absence of pigmentation that is marked especially by white patches of skin.

Leucorrhea - Leukorrhea is a medical term that denotes a thick, whitish or yellowish vaginal discharge. There are many causes of leukorrhea, the usual one being estrogen imbalance. The amount of discharge may increase due to vaginal infection.

Leprosy - A foul cutaneous disease, appearing in dry, white, thin, scurfy scabs, attended with violent itching. It sometimes covers the whole body, rarely the face. One species of it is called elephantiasis.

Masticatory - Chewing; adapted to perform the office of chewing food. A substance to be chewed to increase the saliva.

Mastitis - Mastitis is the inflammation of breast tissue.

Medulla - Medulla refers to the middle of something and derives from the Latin word for marrow.

Melancholy - A gloomy state of mind, often a gloomy state that is of some continuance, or habitual; depression of spirits induced by grief; dejection of spirits. This was formerly supposed to proceed from a redundance of black bile. Melancholy, when extreme and of long continuance, is a disease, sometimes accompanied with partial insanity. Cullen defines it, partial insanity without dyspepsy.

Melanosis - Melanosis is a form of hyperpigmentation associated with increased melanin.

Meningitis - Meningitis is inflammation of the protective membranes covering the brain and spinal cord.

Menopause - Menopause is a term used to describe the permanent cessation of the primary functions of the human ovaries.

Mucilage - In chemistry, one of the proximate elements of vegetables. The same substance is a gum when solid, and a mucilage when in solution. Both the ingredients improve one another; for the mucilage adds to the lubricity of the oil, and the oil preserves the mucilage from inspissation. Mucilage is obtained from vegetable or animal substances.

Mucilaginous - Pertaining to or secreting mucilage; as the mucilaginous glands. Slimy; ropy; moist, soft and lubricous; partaking of the nature of mucilage; as a mucilaginous gum.

Mydriatic - Mydriasis is a dilation of the pupil, usually defined as when having a non-physiological cause, but sometimes defined as potentially being a physiological pupillary response.

Narcissus - In botany, the daffodil, a genus of plants of several species. They are of the bulbous rooted tribe, perennial in root, but with annual leaves and flower stalks.

Narcotic - A medicine which stupefies the senses and renders insensible to pain; hence, a medicine which induces sleep; a soporific; and opiate.

Nervine - That has the quality of relieving in disorders of the nerves. A medicine that affords relief from disorders of the nerves.

Neuralgia - Neuralgia is pain in one or more nerves that occurs without stimulation of pain receptor cells.

Neurasthenia - Neurasthenia is a term that was first used at least as early as 1829 to label a mechanical weakness of the actual nerves.

Niter - In Hebrew, the verb under which this word appears signifies to spring, leap, shake, and to strip or break. A salt, called also salt-peter, and in the modern nomenclature of chemistry, nitrate of potash. It exists in large quantities in the earth, and is continually formed in inhabited places, on walls sheltered from rain, and in all situations where animal matters are decomposed, under stables and barns. It is of great use in the arts; is the principal ingredient in gunpowder, and is useful in medicines, in preserving meat, butter. It is a white substance and has an acrid, bitter taste.

Orchitis - Orchitis is swelling (inflammation) of one or both of the testicles.

Orgiastic - Tending to arouse or excite unrestrained emotion: orgiastic rhythms.

Oxyuriasis - Symptoms of pinworm infections which are caused by a small, white intestinal worm enterobius vermicularis. Pinworms are about the length of a staple and live in the intestines of humans; they do not live in any other species. While an infected person sleeps, female pinworms leave the intestines through the anus and deposit large numbers of eggs on the surrounding skin.

Parasiticide - An agent or preparation that destroys parasites.

Parotitis - Parotitis is an inflammation of one or both parotid glands, the major salivary glands located on either side of the face.

Pediculicide - Pediculicides are substances used to treat lice.

Peroxidases - Enzymes that use peroxide to break down bacteria and other harmful material.

Pertussis - Pertussis, also known as whooping cough, is a highly contagious bacterial disease.

Phlegmasia - Phlegmasia alba dolens (also known as milk leg or white leg) is part of a spectrum of diseases related to deep vein thrombosis.

Photophobia - A symptom of abnormal intolerance to visual perception of light.

Piscicide - A piscicide is a chemical substance which is poisonous to fish.

Phthisis - A consumption occasioned by ulcerated lungs.

Poultice - A cataplasm; a soft composition of meal, bran, or the like substance, to be applied to sores, inflamed parts of the body.

Prebiotic - Prebiotics are sources of non-digestible, soluble fiber that serve as food for the probiotics or "good" bugs in the large intestine, keeping them healthy. Examples of prebiotics are arabinogalactan, fructooligosaccharides (FOS), inulin, mannanoligosaccharides (MOS), pectin and psyllium.

Probiotic - Probiotics are live microorganisms (bacteria and yeast) fed to promote healthy digestive and immune function. When these "good" bugs break down food ingredients that the body normally can't, they produce energy and vitamins for the body, food for cells in the cecum and colon, and byproducts that keep the "bad" bugs from growing. Research suggests probiotics are useful in repopulating the intestine with "good" bugs after antibiotic use and may benefit people with diarrhea.

Procuring - Getting; gaining; obtaining. Causing to come or to be done. That causes to come; bringing on.

Puerperium - The state of a woman during childbirth or immediately thereafter.

Purgative - Having the power of cleansing; usually, having the power of evacuating the bowels; cathartic.

Putrid - In a state of dissolution or disorganization, as animal and vegetable bodies; corrupt; rotten; as putrid flesh. Indicating a state of dissolution; tending to disorganize the substances composing the body; malignant; as a putrid fever.

Pyelitis - Acute inflammation of the pelvis of the kidney, caused by bacterial infection.

Refrigerant - Cooling; allaying heat. Among physicians, a medicine which abates heat and refreshes the patient.

Rheumatism - A painful disease affecting muscles and joints of the human body, chiefly the larger joints, as the hips, knees, shoulders.

Rubefacient - In medicine, a substance or external application which excites redness of the skin.

Scabies – Scabies, known colloquially as the seven-year itch, is a contagious skin infection that occurs among humans and other animals. It has been classified by the World Health Orginazation (WHO) as a water-related disease. It is caused by a tiny and usually not directly visible parasite.

Scalds - Scald burns are more common in children, especially "spill scalds" from hot drinks and bath water scalds.

Schizophrenia - A mental disorder characterized by a breakdown of thought processes and by poor emotional responsiveness. It most commonly manifests itself as auditory hallucinations, paranoid or bizarre delusions, or disorganized speech and thinking, and it is accompanied by significant social or occupational dysfunction.

Sciatica - Rheumatism in the hip.

Scirrhi - A hard dense cancerous growth usually arising from connective tissue.

Scrofula - A disease, called vulgarly the king's evil, characterized by hard, scirrhous, and often indolent tumors in the glands of the neck, under the chin, in the arm-pits.

Scirrhus - A large, hard, and painless swelling. Apparently refers in this case to a carcinoma of the stomach. The closely related word scirrhous was used to refer to a growth, often a carcinoma, that was hard and strong due to dense fibrous tissue.

Sclerosis - A thickening or hardening of a body part, as of an artery, especially from excessive formation of fibrous interstitial tissue.

Sedative - In medicine, moderating muscular action or animal energy.

Sialogogue - A medicing that promotes the salivary discharge.

Spasms - In medicine a spasm is a sudden, involuntary contraction of a muscle, a group of muscles, or a hollow organ such as a heart, or a similarly sudden contraction of an orifice. It most commonly refers to a muscle cramp which is often accompanied by a sudden burst of pain, but is usually harmless and ceases after a few minutes. There is a variety of other causes of involuntary muscle contractions, which may be more serious, depending on the cause. The word "spasm" may also refer to a temporary burst of energy, activity, emotion, eustress, stress, or anxiety unrelated to, or as a consequence of, involuntary muscle activity.

Splenomegaly - Plenomegaly is an enlargement of the spleen. The spleen usually lies in the left upper quadrant of the human abdomen. It is one of the four cardinal signs of hypersplenism, some reduction in the number of circulating blood cells affecting granulocytes, erythrocytes or platelets in any combination; a compensatory proliferative response in the bone marrow; and the potential for correction of these abnormalities by splenectomy. Splenomegaly is usually associated with increased workload (such as in hemolytic anemias), which suggests that it is a response to hyperfunction. It is therefore not surprising that splenomegaly is associated with any disease process that involves abnormal red blood cells being destroyed in the spleen. Other common causes include congestion due to portal hypertension and infiltration by leukemias and lymphomas. Thus, the finding of an enlarged spleen; along with caput medusa; is an important sign of portal hypertension.

Staphylococcus - A genus of gram-positive bacteria. Under the microscope, they appear round (cocci), and form in grape-like clusters. The staphylococcus genus includes at least 40 species. Of these, nine have two subspecies and one has three subspecies. Most are harmless and reside normally on the skin and mucous membranes of humans and other organisms. Found worldwide, they are a small component of soil microbial flora.

Streptococcus - Treptococcus is a genus of spherical Gram-positive bacteria belonging to the phylum firmicutes and the lactic acid bacteria group. Cellular division occurs along a single axis in these bacteria, and thus they grow in chains or pairs, hence the name — from Greek streptos, meaning easily bent or twisted, like a chain (twisted chain). Contrast this with staphylococci, which divide along multiple axes and generate grape-like clusters of cells. Most streptococci are oxidase- and catalase-negative, and many are facultative anaerobes. In 1984, many organisms formerly considered Streptococcus were separated out into the genera Enterococcus and Lactococcus.

Stomachic - Pertaining to the stomach; as stomachic vessels. Strengthening to the stomach; exciting the action of the stomach.

Strangury - Literally, a discharge of urine by drops; a difficulty of discharging urine, attended with pain.

Styptic - That stops bleeding; having the quality of restraining hemorrhage.

Sudorific - A medicine that produces sweat or sensible perspiration.

Sunstroke - Heat illness or heat-related illness is a spectrum of disorders due to environmental heat exposure. It includes minor conditions such as heat cramps, heat syncope, and heat exhaustion as well as the more severe condition known as heat stroke. Heat stroke is defined as a body temperature of greater than 40.6° C (105.1° F) due to environmental heat exposure with lack of thermoregulation. This is distinct from a fever, where there is a physiological increase in the temperature set point of the body.

Suppurative - A medicine that promotes the discharge of pus.

Tenesmus - A painful, ineffectual, and repeated effort, or a continual and urgent desire to go to stool.

Tertian - A disease or fever whose paroxysms return every other day; an intermittent occurring after intervals of about forty-eight hours.

Ulcers - A break in skin or mucous membrane with loss of surface tissue, disintegration and necrosis of epithelial tissue, and often pus.

Venery - The pleasures of the bed. Contentment, without the pleasure of lawful venery, is continence; of unlawful, chastity.

Vermifuge - A medicine or substance that destroys or expels worms from animal bodies; an anthelmintic.

Vervain - (also known as verbena) is an herb used for many reasons in people. Characterized as a "nervine," an herb with specific actions on the nervous system, several compounds have been isolated from the plant and shown to have actions on nerve cells.

Voluptuousness - Luxuriousness; addictedness to pleasure or sensual gratification. Where no voluptuousness, yet all delight.

Vulnerary - Useful in healing wounds; adapted to the cure of external injuries; as vulnerary plants or potions. Any plant, drug, or composition that is useful in the cure of wounds. Certain unguents, balsams and the like are used as vulneraries.

E= Edible
M= Medicial
T= Toxic

Sourcing the Elements

PLANTS CONTAINING ALUMINUM

Species	Part	Ordered by quantity
Cucumber - Cucumis Sativus - E	Fruit	21,000 ppm
Coneflower, Echinacea - Echinacea ssp - M	Root	12,900 ppm
Red Cedar - Juniperus Virginiana Amphicarpaea Bracteata - E - M - T	Shoot	8,800 ppm
Red Pignut Hickory - Carya Glabra - E	Shoot	7,700 ppm
Buckbush - Symphoricarpos Orbiculatus - M	Stem	4,400 ppm
Shortleaf Pine - Pinus Echinata - M	Shoot	4,200 ppm
Butter Bean, Lima Bean - Phaseolus Lunatus - E	Seed	3,000 ppm
Black Gum, Black Tupelo - Nyssa Sylvatica - E - M	Leaf	2,730 ppm
Gotu Kola, Pennywort - Centella Asiatica - E - M	Leaf	2,060 ppm
Chickweed, Common Chickweed - Stellaria Media - E	Plant	1,960 ppm
Dwarf Sumac, Winged Sumac - Rhus Copallina - E - M	Leaf	1,920 ppm
European Pennyroyal - Mentha Pulegium - E - M - T	Plant	1,850 ppm
American Styrax, Sweetgum - Liquidambar Styraciflua - E - M	Stem	1,800 ppm
Tomato - Lycopersicon Esculentum - E - M - T	Fruit	1,700 ppm
Black Cherry, Wild Cherry - Prunus Serotina - E - M - T	Leaf	1,440 ppm
Buchu, Honey Buchu, Mountain Buchu - Agathosma Bbetulina - M	Leaf	1,360 ppm
Sassafras - Sassafras Albidum - E - M - T	Leaf	1,360 ppm
Box-Holly, Butcher's broom - Ruscus Aculeatus - E - M	Root	1,310 ppm
American Styrax, Sweetgum - Liquidambar Styraciflua - E - M	Leaf	1,230 ppm
Flannelleaf, Flannelplant, Great mullein, Mullein, Velvet Verbascum Thapsus - M	Leaf	1,090 ppm
White Oak - Quercus Alba - M	Stem	1,064 ppm
Carrot - Daucus Carota - E	Root	1,050 ppm
Black bean, Dwarf bean, Field bean, Flageolet bean, French bean, Garden bean, Green bean, Haricot, Haricot bean, Haricot vert, Kidney bean, Navy bean, Pop bean, Popping bean, Snap bean, String bean, Wax bean - Phaseolus Vulgaris - E	Fruit	1,050 ppm
Peach - Prunus Persica - E - M - T	Fruit	1,050 ppm
European Grape, Grape, Grapevine, Vigne Vinifere, Wine Grape - Vitis Vinifera - E - M	Stem	1,030 ppm
Smooth Sumac - Rhus Glabra - E - M	Stem	1,005 ppm
Devil's claw, Grapple Harpagophytum Procumbens - M	Root	939 ppm
Common thyme, Garden thyme, Thyme - Thymus Vulgaris - E - M	Leaf	920 ppm
Post Oak - Quercus Stellata - E - M	Stem	840 ppm
Asparagus bean, Pea bean, Yardlong bean - Vigna Unguiculata subsp. Sesquipedalis - E	Seed	840 ppm
Blue Cohosh - Caulophyllum Thalictroides M	Root	762 ppm
Sarsaparilla - Smilax spp - E - M	Root	745 ppm
Sassafras - Sassafras Albidum - E - M - T	Stem	740 ppm
Bearberry, Uva ursi - Arctostaphylos Uva-Ursi - M	Leaf	719 ppm
Crampbark, European Cranberry Bush, Guelder Rose, Snowballbush - Viburnum Opulus subsp. var. Opulus - E - M - T	Bark	702 ppm
Asparagus - Asparagus Officinalis - E	Shoot	700 ppm
Tea - Camellia Sinensis - E - E	Leaf	690 ppm
Marshmallow, White Mallow - Althaea Officinalis - E	Root	680 ppm
Ginger - Zingiber Officinale - E	Rhizome	663 ppm
Black Gum, Black Tupelo - Nyssa Sylvatica - E - M	Stem	660 ppm
Northern Red Oak - Quercus Rubra - E - M	Stem	660 ppm
Dandelion - Taraxacum Officinale - E - M	Root	656 ppm
Bladderwrack, Kelp - Fucus Vesiculosus - E - M	Plant	631 ppm
Dulse - Rhodymenia Palmata - E	Plant	615 ppm

Species	Part	Quantity
Dwarf Sumac, Winged Sumac - Rhus Copallina - E - M	Stem	610 ppm
Damiana - Turnera Diffusa - M	Leaf	605 ppm
Black Cherry, Wild Cherry - Prunus Serotina - E - M - T	Stem	540 ppm
Lemongrass, West Indian Lemongrass - Cymbopogon Citratus - E - M	Plant	515 ppm
Barberry - Berberis Vulgaris - M	Root	489 ppm
Black Oak - Quercus Velutina - E - M	Stem	434 ppm
Chinese Angelica, Dong Gui, Dong quai - Angelica Sinensis - M	Root	422 ppm
Common Valerian, Garden-Heliotrope, Valerian - Valeriana Officinalis - M	Root	422 ppm
Beet, Beetroot, Garden Beet, Sugar Beet - Beta Vulgaris - E	Root	420 ppm
Coca - Erythroxylum Coca var. Coca - E - M	Leaf	420 ppm
Willow Oak - Quercus Phellos - E - M	Stem	420 ppm
Raspberry, Red raspberry - Rubus Idaeus - E - M	Leaf	392 ppm
Parsley - Petroselinum Crispum - E	Plant	390 ppm
Curly Dock, Lengua De Vaca, Sour Dock, Yellow Dock - Rumex Crispus - M - T - E - M - T	Root	390 ppm
Onion, Shallot - Allium Cepa - Shallot Bulb - E	Bulb	385 ppm
American Persimmon - Diospyros Virginiana - E - M	Stem	378 ppm
Field Horsetail, Horsetail - Equisetum Arvense - M	Plant	378 ppm
Irish moss - Chondrus Crispus - E	Plant	355 ppm
Alholva, Bockshornklee, Fenugreek, Greek Clover, Greek Trigonella Foenum-Graecum - E - M	Seed	350 ppm
European Nettle, Stinging Nettle - Urtica Dioica - E - M	Leaf	345 ppm
Couchgrass, Doggrass, Quackgrass, Twitchgrass, Wheatgrass - Elytrigia Repens - E - M	Plant	331 ppm
Grape Citrus Paradisi - E	Fruit	330 ppm
Goldenseal - Hydrastis Canadensis - M	Root	325 ppm
Gentian, Yellow Gentian - Gentiana Lutea - M	Root	291 ppm
Chaparral, Creosote Bush - Larrea Tridentata M	Plant	290 ppm
American Ginseng, Ginseng - Panax Quinquefolius - M	Plant	285 ppm
European Mistletoe - Viscum Album - M - T	Leaf	283 ppm
Corn - Zea Mays - E	Seed	275 ppm
Spinach - Spinacia Oleracea - E	Leaf	270 ppm
Lady's Thistle, Milk Thistle - Silybum Marianum - M	Plant	267 ppm
Mad-Dog Skullcap, Scullcap - Scutellaria lateriflora - M - M	Plant	258 ppm

PLANTS CONTAINING ANTIMONY

Species	Part	Quantity
Cashew - Anacardium Occidentale - E	Seed	Trace
Pecan - Carya Illinoensis - E	Seed	Trace
Northern Red Oak - Quercus Rubra - E - M	Seed	Trace
Brazilnut, Brazilnut-Tree, Creamnut, Paranut - Bertholletia Eexcelsa - E	Seed	Trace
Shagbark Hickory - Carya Ovata - E	Seed	Trace
Coconut, Coconut Palm - Cocos Nucifera - E	Seed	Trace
Cobnut, English Filbert, European Filbert, European Hazel, Hazel - Corylus Avellana - E	Seed	Trace
Black Walnut - Juglans Nigra - E	Seed	Trace
Almond - Prunus Dulcis - E - M - T	Seed	Trace
Butternut - Juglans Cinerea - E	Seed	Trace
Pistachio - Pistacia Vera - E	Seed	Trace
Asparagus bean, Pea bean, Yardlong bean - Vigna Unguiculata subsp. Sesquipedalis - E	Seed	Trace

PLANTS CONTAINING ARSENIC

Species	Part	Quantity
Dyer's Woad - Isatis Tinctoria - M	Root	132 ppm
Bladderwrack, Kelp - Fucus Vesiculosus - E - M	Plant	68 ppm
Dulse - Rhodymenia Palmata - E	Plant	33 ppm
Irish moss - Chondrus Crispus - E	Plant	10 ppm
Bai-Wei, Pai-Wei - Cynanchum Atratum - E - M	Root	4.85 ppm
Grape Citrus Paradisi - E	Fruit	4.4 ppm
Chinese Spikenard - Nardostachys Chinensis - M	Rhizome	2.11 ppm
Mongoloid Dandelion - Taraxacum Mongolicum - E - M	Plant	1.95 ppm

ARSENIC CONTINUED

Species	Part	Quantity
Asian Plantain - Plantago Asiatica - E - M	Plant	1.71 ppm
Citron - Citrus Medica - E	Fruit	1.64 ppm
Broadbean, Faba Bean, Habas - Vicia Faba - E	Fruit	1.4 ppm
Hardy Orchid, Hyacinth Bletilla, Hyacinth Orchid, Shiran - Bletilla Striata - M	Tuber	1.35 ppm
Climbing Fern - Lygodium Japonicum - Pollen or Spore - M	Pollen Or Spore	1.17 ppm
Chinese Anemone - Pulsatilla Chinensis - M	Root	1.14 ppm
Calamus, Flagroot, Myrtle Flag, Sweet Calamus, Sweetflag, Sweet Acorus Calamus - M	Rhizome	1.13 ppm
Madder - Rubia Cordifolia - M	Root	1.1 ppm
Japanese Gentian - Gentiana Scabra - E	Root	1.06 ppm
Carrot - Daucus Carota - E	Root	1 ppm
Jussiaeae Herba, Pond Dragon - Jussiaea Repens - M	Plant	1 ppm

Species	Part	Quantity
Red Cedar - Juniperus Virginiana Amphicarpaea Bracteata - E - M - T	Shoot	880 ppm
Black Gum, Black Tupelo - Nyssa Sylvatica - E - M	Stem	880 ppm
Black Cherry, Wild Cherry - Prunus Serotina - E - M - T	Stem	810 ppm
Dwarf Sumac, Winged Sumac - Rhus Copallina - E - M	Leaf	672 ppm
Northern Red Oak - Quercus Rubra - E - M	Stem	660 ppm
Black Oak - Quercus Velutina - E - M	Stem	620 ppm
American Styrax, Sweetgum - Liquidambar Styraciflua - E - M	Leaf	574 ppm
Post Oak - Quercus Stellata - E - M	Stem	420 ppm
Sassafras - Sassafras Albidum - E - M - T	Stem	370 ppm
Smooth Sumac - Rhus Glabra - E - M	Stem	335 ppm
Willow Oak - Quercus Phellos - E - M	Stem	210 ppm
Sassafras - Sassafras Albidum - E - M - T	Leaf	204 ppm
Carrot - Daucus Carota - E	Root	150 ppm
Lettuce - Lactuca Sativa - E	Leaf	145 ppm
Cassia, Cassia Bark, Cassia Lignea, China Junk Cassia, Chinazimt, Chinese Cassia - Cinnamomum Aromaticum	Bark	140 ppm
Soybean - Glycine Max - E	Seed	90 ppm
Chinese Polystichum - Polystichum Polyblepharum - T	Plant	90 ppm
Alehoof - Glechoma Hederacea - M	Plant	89 ppm
Cabbage, Red Cabbage, White Cabbage - Brassica Oleracea var. Capitata - E	Leaf	87 ppm
Japanese Cinnamon - Cinnamomum Sieboldii - E - M - T	Root Bark	80 ppm
Dandelion - Taraxacum Officinale - E - M	Leaf	80 ppm
Asparagus - Asparagus Officinalis - E	Shoot	70 ppm
Beet, Beetroot, Garden Beet, Sugar Beet - Beta Vulgaris - E	Root	70 ppm
Cucumber - Cucumis Sativus - E	Fruit	70 ppm
Ceylon Cinnamon, Cinnamon - Cinnamomum Verum - E - M - T	Bark	60 ppm
Tomato - Lycopersicon Esculentum - E - M - T	Fruit	60 ppm
Potato - Solanum Tuberosum - E	Tuber	60 ppm
Asparagus bean, Pea bean, Yardlong bean - Vigna Unguiculata subsp. Sesquipedalis - E	Seed	60 ppm

PLANTS CONTAINING BARIUM

Species	Part	Quantity
Buckbush - Symphoricarpos Orbiculatus - M	Stem	2,640 ppm
Brazilnut, Brazilnut-Tree, Creamnut, Paranut - Bertholletia Eexcelsa - E	Seed	2,600 ppm
Red Pignut Hickory - Carya Glabra - E	Shoot	2,200 ppm
Shagbark Hickory - Carya Ovata - E	Shoot	1,800 ppm
American Styrax, Sweetgum - Liquidambar Styraciflua - E - M	Stem	1,200 ppm
White Oak - Quercus Alba - M	Stem	1,140 ppm
American Persimmon - Diospyros Virginiana - E - M	Stem	1,080 ppm
Black Cherry, Wild Cherry - Prunus Serotina - E - M - T	Leaf	960 ppm
Dwarf Sumac, Winged Sumac - Rhus Copallina - E - M	Stem	915 ppm
American Persimmon - Diospyros Virginiana - E - M	Leaf	910 ppm
Black Gum, Black Tupelo - Nyssa Sylvatica - E - M	Leaf	910 ppm

Species	Part	Quantity
Japanese Cinnamon - Cinnamomum Sieboldii - E - M - T	Bark	55 ppm
Mugwort - Artemisia Vulgaris - M	Plant	50 ppm
Java Cinnamon, Padang Cassia - Cinnamomum Burmannii - E - M - T	Bark	50 ppm
Butterbur - Petasites Japonicus - T	Plant	50 ppm
Coca - Erythroxylum Coca var. Coca - E - M	Leaf	48 ppm
Ramie - Boehmeria Nivea - M	Plant	46 ppm
Black bean, Dwarf bean, Field bean, Flageolet bean, French bean, Garden bean, Green bean, Haricot, Haricot bean, Haricot vert, Kidney bean, Navy bean, Pop bean, Popping bean, Snap bean, String bean, Wax bean - Phaseolus Vulgaris - E	Fruit	45 ppm
Qian Hu - Peucedanum Decursivum - M	Plant	41 ppm
Parsley - Petroselinum Crispum - E	Plant	40 ppm
Giant Knotweed, Hu-Zhang, Japanese Knotweed, Mexican Bamboo - Polygonum Cuspidatum - E - M - T	Plant	32 ppm
Butter Bean, Lima Bean - Phaseolus Lunatus - E	Seed	30 ppm
Peach - Prunus Persica - E - M - T	Fruit	30 ppm
Clove, Clovetree - Syzygium Aromaticum - E	Flower	30 ppm
Onion, Shallot - Allium Cepa - Shallot Bulb - E	Bulb	28 ppm
Plum - Prunus Domestica - E - M	Fruit	25.5 ppm
Endive, Escarole - Cichorium Endivia - M	Leaf	24 ppm
Grape Citrus Paradisi - E	Fruit	22 ppm
Chinese Cabbage - Brassica Pekinensis - E	Leaf	21 ppm
Shortleaf Pine - Pinus Echinata - M	Shoot	21 ppm
Allspice, Clover-Pepper, Jamaica-Pepper, Pimenta, Pimento - Pimenta Dioica - E	Plant	20 ppm
Orange - Citrus Sinensis - E	Fruit	16.5 ppm
European Grape, Grape, Grapevine, Vigne Vinifere, Wine Grape - Vitis Vinifera - E - M	Fruit	15.4 ppm
Pecan - Carya Illinoensis - E	Seed	14 ppm
Corn - Zea Mays - E	Seed	14 ppm
Pear - Pyrus Communis - E	Fruit	11 ppm
Black Walnut - Juglans Nigra - E	Seed	8.7 ppm
Apple - Malus Domestica - E	Fruit	8.6 ppm
Bell Pepper, Cherry Pepper, Cone Pepper, Green Pepper, Paprika, Sweet Pepper - Capsicum Annuum - E	Fruit	8 ppm
Cantaloupe, Melon, Muskmelon, Netted Melon, Nutmeg Melon, Persian Melon - Cucumis Melo subsp. ssp Melo var. Ccantalupensis - Friut - E	Fruit	7.7 ppm
Black bean, Dwarf bean, Field bean, Flageolet bean, French bean, Garden bean, Green bean, Haricot, Haricot bean, Haricot vert, Kidney bean, Navy bean, Pop bean, Popping bean, Snap bean, String bean, Wax bean - Phaseolus Vulgaris - E	Seed	7.3 ppm
Aubergine, Egg Solanum Melongena - E	Fruit	5.6 ppm
Almond - Prunus Dulcis - E - M - T	Seed	2.6 ppm
Butternut - Juglans Cinerea - E	Seed	1.6 ppm
Cobnut, English Filbert, European Filbert, European Hazel, Hazel - Corylus Avellana - E	Seed	1.1 ppm

PLANTS CONTAINING BORON

Species	Part	Quantity
Corn Salad, Lamb's Lettuce - Valerianella Locusta - E	Plant	350 ppm
Plum - Prunus Domestica - E - M	Fruit	255 ppm
Quince - Cydonia Oblonga - E	Fruit	160 ppm
Strawberry - Fragaria spp. - E	Fruit	160 ppm
Peach - Prunus Persica - E - M - T	Fruit	150 ppm
Cabbage, Red Cabbage, White Cabbage - Brassica Oleracea var. Capitata - E	Leaf	145 ppm
Black Gum, Black Tupelo - Nyssa Sylvatica - E - M	Leaf	136 ppm
Dandelion - Taraxacum Officinale - E - M	Leaf	125 ppm
Apple - Malus Domestica - E	Fruit	110 ppm
Sugar-Apple, Sweetsop - Annona Squamosa - E	Leaf	107 ppm
Asparagus - Asparagus Officinalis - E	Shoot	104 ppm
Celery - Apium Graveolens - E	Root	103 ppm
Fig - Ficus Carica - E	Fruit	100 ppm

BORON CONTINUED

Tomato - Lycopersicon Esculentum - E - M - T	Fruit	96 ppm
American Ginseng, Ginseng - Panax Quinquefolius - M	Plant	96 ppm
Opium Poppy, Poppyseed Poppy - Papaver Somniferum - E	Seed	95 ppm
Lettuce - Lactuca Sativa - E	Leaf	87 ppm
Cauli Brassica Oleracea var. Botrytis - E	Leaf	85 ppm
American Styrax, Sweetgum - Liquidambar Styraciflua - E - M	Leaf	84 ppm
Red Mangrove - Rhizophora Mangle - M	Leaf	83 ppm
Pear - Pyrus Communis - E	Fruit	82 ppm
Beet, Beetroot, Garden Beet, Sugar Beet - Beta Vulgaris - E	Root	80 ppm
Sour Cherry - Prunus Cerasus - E - M - T	Fruit	80 ppm
Red Currant, White Currant - Ribes Rubrum - E	Fruit	80 ppm
Red Pignut Hickory - Carya Glabra - E	Shoot	77 ppm
Cauli Brassica Oleracea var. Botrytis - E	Flower	76 ppm
Apricot - Prunus Armeniaca - E - M - T	Fruit	70 ppm
Dwarf Sumac, Winged Sumac - Rhus Copallina - E - M	Leaf	67 ppm
Northern Red Oak - Quercus Rubra - E - M	Stem	66 ppm
Radish - Raphanus Sativus - E	Root	64 ppm
Black Currant - Ribes Nigrum - E	Fruit	64 ppm
Shagbark Hickory - Carya Ovata - E	Shoot	63 ppm
Celery - Apium Graveolens - E	Seed	61 ppm
American Styrax, Sweetgum - Liquidambar Styraciflua - E - M	Stem	60 ppm
Asparagus bean, Pea bean, Yardlong bean - Vigna Unguiculata subsp. Sesquipedalis - E	Seed	60 ppm
Brussel-Sprout - Brassica Oleracea var. Gemmifera - E	Leaf	57 ppm
Coca - Erythroxylum Coca var. Coca - E - M	Leaf	57 ppm
Parsley - Petroselinum Crispum - E	Plant	54 ppm
Black Cherry, Wild Cherry - Prunus Serotina - E - M - T	Stem	54 ppm
Rutabaga, Swede, Swedish Turnip - Brassica Napus var. Napobrassica - E	Leaf	52 ppm
Dill, Garden Dill - Anethum Graveolens - E	Seed	50 ppm
Cumin - Cuminum Cyminum - E - M	Fruit	50 ppm
American Persimmon - Diospyros Virginiana - E - M	Leaf	50 ppm
European Grape, Grape, Grapevine, Vigne Vinifere, Wine Grape - Vitis Vinifera - E - M	Fruit	50 ppm
Marjoram, Sweet Marjoram - Origanum Majorana - E	Plant	48 ppm
Oregano, Pot Marjoram - Origanum Onites	Plant	48 ppm
Black Cherry, Wild Cherry - Prunus Serotina - E - M - T	Leaf	48 ppm
Sassafras - Sassafras Albidum - E - M - T	Leaf	48 ppm
Common thyme, Garden thyme, Thyme - Thymus Vulgaris - E - M	Plant	48 ppm
Cucumber - Cucumis Sativus - E	Fruit	46 ppm
Onion, Shallot - Allium Cepa - Shallot Bulb - E	Bulb	45 ppm
Alfalfa, Lucerne - Medicago Sativa subsp. Sativa - E	Plant	45 ppm
Black bean, Dwarf bean, Field bean, Flageolet bean, French bean, Garden bean, Green bean, Haricot, Haricot bean, Haricot vert, Kidney bean, Navy bean, Pop bean, Popping bean, Snap bean, String bean, Wax bean - Phaseolus Vulgaris - E	Fruit	45 ppm
Red Cedar - Juniperus Virginiana Amphicarpaea Bracteata- E - M - T	Shoot	44 ppm
Black bean, Dwarf bean, Field bean, Flageolet bean, French bean, Garden bean, Green bean, Haricot, Haricot bean, Haricot vert, Kidney bean, Navy bean, Pop bean, Popping bean, Snap bean, String bean, Wax bean - Phaseolus Vulgaris - E	Seed	43 ppm
Evening-Primrose - Oenothera Biennis - E - M	Seed	41 ppm
Common Turkish Oregano, European Oregano, Oregano, Pot Marjoram, Wild Marjoram, Wild Oregano - Origanum Vulgare - E	Plant	41 ppm
Sage - Salvia Officinalis - E - M	Leaf	41 ppm
Spinach - Spinacia Oleracea - E	Leaf	40 ppm
Clove, Clovetree - Syzygium Aromaticum - E	Flower	40 ppm
Rosemary - Rosmarinus Officinalis - E - M	Plant	39 ppm
American Persimmon - Diospyros Virginiana - E - M	Stem	38 ppm

Almond - Prunus Dulcis - E - M - T	Seed	38 ppm
White Oak - Quercus Alba - M	Stem	38 ppm
Summer Savory - Satureja Hortensis - E	Plant	37 ppm
Savory, Winter Savory - *Satureja Montana*	Plant	37 ppm
Carrot - Daucus Carota - E	Root	36 ppm
Fennel - Foeniculum Vulgare - M	Leaf	36 ppm
Rhubarb - Rheum Rhabarbarum - E	Pt	36 ppm
European Nettle, Stinging Nettle - Urtica Dioica - E - M	Leaf	36 ppm
Dill, Garden Dill - Anethum Graveolens - E	Plant	35 ppm
Smooth Sumac - Rhus Glabra - E - M	Stem	34 ppm
Grape Citrus Paradisi - E	Fruit	33 ppm
White Tephrosia - Tephrosia Candida - M - T	Plant	32 ppm
Black Gum, Black Tupelo - Nyssa Sylvatica - E - M	Stem	31 ppm
Basil, Cuban Basil, Sweet Basil - Ocimum Basilicum - E	Plant	31 ppm
Black Oak - Quercus Velutina - E - M	Stem	31 ppm
Rutabaga, Swede, Swedish Turnip - Brassica Napus var. Napobrassica - E	Root	30 ppm
Butter Bean, Lima Bean - Phaseolus Lunatus - E	Seed	30 ppm
Dwarf Sumac, Winged Sumac - Rhus Copallina - E - M	Stem	30 ppm
Chinese Parsley, Cilantro, Coriander - Coriandrum Sativum E	Seed	29 ppm
Orange - Citrus Sinensis - E	Fruit	27.5 ppm
Horseradish - Armoracia Rusticana - E	Root	27 ppm
Sassafras - Sassafras Albidum - E - M - T	Stem	26 ppm
Buckbush - Symphoricarpos Orbiculatus - M	Stem	26 ppm
Alfalfa, Lucerne - Medicago Sativa subsp. Sativa - E	Leaf	25 ppm
Parsnip - Pastinaca Sativa - E	Root	25 ppm
Allspice, Clover-Pepper, Jamaica-Pepper, Pimenta, Pimento - Pimenta Dioica - E	Fruit	25 ppm
Post Oak - Quercus Stellata - E - M	Stem	25 ppm
Rutabaga, Swede, Swedish Turnip - Brassica Napus var. Napobrassica - E	Stem	24 ppm
Endive, Escarole - Cichorium Endivia - M	Leaf	24 ppm
Rowan Berry - Sorbus Aucubaria - E - M - T	Fruit	24 ppm
Bread Artocarpus Altilis - E	Fruit	23 ppm
Pea - Pisum Sativum - E	Seed	23 ppm
Cowgrass, Peavine Clover, Purple Clover, Red Clover - Trifolium Pratense - E - M	Leaf	23 ppm
Dog Rose, Dogbrier, Rose - Rosa Canina - E - M	Fruit	22 ppm
Cauli Brassica Oleracea var. Botrytis - E	Stem	21 ppm
Brussel-Sprout - Brassica Oleracea var. Gemmifera - E	Stem	21 ppm
Chinese Cabbage - Brassica Pekinensis - E	Leaf	21 ppm
Cobnut, English Filbert, European Filbert, European Hazel, Hazel - Corylus Avellana - E	Seed	21 ppm
Shortleaf Pine - Pinus Echinata - M	Shoot	21 ppm
Willow Oak - Quercus Phellos - E - M	Stem	21 ppm
Blackberry - *Rubus Fruticosus*	Fruit	21 ppm
Rapini, Seven-Top Turnip, Turnip - Brassica Rapa - E	Root	20 ppm
Chicory, Succory, Witloof - Cichorium Intybus - E - M	Root	20 ppm
Sweet Potato - Ipomoea Batatas - E	Root	20 ppm
Anise, Sweet Cumin - Pimpinella Anisum - E - M	Fruit	20 ppm
Groundnut, Peanut - Arachis Hypogaea - E - M	Seed	18 ppm
Bell Pepper, Cherry Pepper, Cone Pepper, Green Pepper, Paprika, Sweet Pepper - Capsicum Annuum - E	Fruit	18 ppm
Soybean - Glycine Max - E	Seed	18 ppm
Black Pepper, Pepper, White Pepper - Piper Nigrum - E - M	Fruit	18 ppm
Northern Red Oak - Quercus Rubra - E - M	Seed	18 ppm
Banana, Plantain - Musa x Paradisiaca - E	Fruit	17.7 ppm
Mango - Mangifera Indica - E - M	Fruit	17.5 ppm
Cayenne, Chili, Hot Pepper, Red Chili, Spur Pepper, Tabasco - Capsicum Frutescens - E	Fruit	17 ppm
Cantaloupe, Melon, Muskmelon, Netted Melon, Nutmeg Melon, Persian Melon - Cucumis Melo subsp. ssp Melo var.Ccantalupensis - Friut - E	Fruit	16.5 ppm
Bay, Bay Laurel, Bayleaf, Grecian Laurel, Laurel, Sweet Bay *Laurus Nobilis*	Leaf	16 ppm
Cowgrass, Peavine Clover, Purple Clover, Red Clover - Trifolium Pratense - E - M	Stem	16 ppm
Wheat - Triticum Aestivum - E - M	Seed	16 ppm

BORON CONTINUED

Species	Part	Quantity
Papaya - Carica Papaya - E - M	Fruit	15 ppm
Ceylon Cinnamon, Cinnamon - Cinnamomum Verum - E - M - T	Bark	15 ppm
Genipap, Jagua - Genipa Americana - E - M	Seed	15 ppm
Gooseberry - Ribes Uva-Crispa - E	Fruit	15 ppm
Corn - Zea Mays - E	Seed	15 ppm
Mandarin, Tangerine - Citrus Reticulata - E	Fruit	14 ppm
Cardamom - Elettaria Cardamomum - E - M	Seed	14 ppm
Genipap, Jagua - Genipa Americana - E - M	Fruit	14 ppm
Alfalfa, Lucerne - Medicago Sativa subsp. Sativa - E	Stem	14 ppm
Mace, Nutmeg - Myristica Fragrans - E	Seed	13 ppm
Avocado - Persea Americana - E - M - T	Fruit	13 ppm
Raspberry, Red raspberry - Rubus Idaeus - E - M	Fruit	13 ppm
Sesame - Sesamum Indicum - E - M	Seed	13 ppm
Blueberry - Vaccinium Corymbosum - E	Fruit	13 ppm
English Walnut - Juglans Rregia - E	Seed	12 ppm
Cloudberry - Rubus Chamaemorus - E - M	Fruit	12 ppm
Emblic, Myrobalan - Phyllanthus Emblica - E	Fruit	11 ppm
Pistachio - Pistacia Vera - E	Seed	11 ppm
Cowberry, Lingen, Lingonberry - Vaccinium Vitis-Idaea var. Minus - E - M	Fruit	11 ppm
Bilberry, Dwarf Bilberry, Whortleberry - Vaccinium Myrtillus - E - M	Fruit	10 ppm
Shagbark Hickory - Carya Ovata - E	Seed	8.5 ppm
Buckwheat - Fagopyrum Esculentum - E	Seed	8.5 ppm
Aubergine, Egg Solanum Melongena - E	Fruit	13.8-16.6 ppm
Potato - Solanum Tuberosum - E	Tuber	8 ppm
American Cranberry, Cranberry, Large Cranberry - Vaccinium Macrocarpon - E	Fruit	8 ppm
Elephant-Foot Yam - Amorphophallus Campanulatus - E - M - T	Root	8 ppm
Pecan - Carya Illinoensis - E	Seed	8 ppm
Russian Olive - Elaeagnus Umbellatus - E - M	Fruit	7.7 ppm
Cassava, Tapioca, Yuca - Manihot Esculenta - E	Root	7.6 ppm
Oats - Avena Sativa - E - M	Seed	2-15 ppm
Taro - Colocasia Esculenta - E	Root	7.5 ppm
Greater Yam, Winged Yam - Dioscorea Alata - E	Root	7 ppm
Butternut - Juglans Cinerea - E	Seed	7 ppm
Date Palm - Phoenix Dactylifera - E	Fruit	7 ppm
Malanga, Tannia, Yautia - Xanthosoma Sagittifolium - E	Root	7 ppm
Corn Salad, Lamb's Lettuce - Valerianella Locusta - E	Plant	7 ppm
Garlic - Allium Sativum Bulb - E	Bulb	6.5 ppm
Indian Saffron, Turmeric - Curcuma Longa - E	Root	12-12.2 ppm
Barley, Barleygrass - Hordeum Vulgare - E - M	Seed	6 ppm
Coconut, Coconut Palm - Cocos Nucifera - E	Seed	6 ppm
Artichoke - Cynara Cardunculus - E	Flower	6 ppm
Black Walnut - Juglans Nigra - E	Seed	5.2 ppm
Carambola, Star Averrhoa Carambola - E	Fruit	5 ppm
Watermelon - Citrullus Lanatus - E	Fruit	4.7 ppm
Swamp Taro - Cyrtosperma Chamissonis - E	Root	0.6-8 ppm
Olive - Olea Europaea - E	Fruit	4 ppm
Ginger - Zingiber Officinale - E	Rhizome	4 ppm
Taro - Colocasia Esculenta - E	Leaf	4 ppm
Giant Taro - Alocasia Macrorrhiza - E	Root	4 ppm
Cashew - Anacardium Occidentale - E	Seed	3.6 ppm
Soursop - Annona Muricata - E	Fruit	3.3 ppm
Jerusalem Artichoke - Helianthus Tuberosus E	Root	3.2 ppm
Brazilnut, Brazilnut-Tree, Creamnut, Paranut - Bertholletia Eexcelsa - E	Seed	3 ppm
Ambarella - Spondias Dulcis - E	Fruit	3 ppm
Imbu, Umbu - Spondias Tuberosa - E	Fruit	2.7 ppm
Pumpkin - Cucurbita Pepo - E	Fruit	1.9 ppm
Pineapple - Ananas Comosus - E	Fruit	1.45 ppm
Black Cutch, Catechu - Acacia Catechu - M	Plant	1 ppm

PLANTS CONTAINING BROMINE

Species	Part	Quantity
Bladderwrack, Kelp - Fucus Vesiculosus - E - M	Plant	150 ppm

Bell Pepper, Cherry Pepper, Cone Pepper, Green Pepper, Paprika, Sweet Pepper - Capsicum Annuum - E	Fruit	111 ppm
European Nettle, Stinging Nettle - Urtica Dioica - E - M	Leaf	110 ppm
Brazilnut, Brazilnut-Tree, Creamnut, Paranut - Bertholletia Eexcelsa - E	Seed	87 ppm
Giant Knotweed, Hu-Zhang, Japanese Knotweed, Mexican Bamboo - Polygonum Cuspidatum - E - M - T	Plant	80 ppm
Dandelion - Taraxacum Officinale - E - M	Leaf	80 ppm
Butterbur - Petasites Japonicus - T	Plant	40 ppm
Mugwort - Artemisia Vulgaris - M	Plant	38 ppm
Cabbage, Red Cabbage, White Cabbage - Brassica Oleracea var. Capitata - E	Leaf	37 ppm
Potato - Solanum Tuberosum - E	Tuber	30 ppm
Banana, Plantain - Musa x Paradisiaca - E	Fruit	27 ppm
Qian Hu - Peucedanum Decursivum - M	Plant	23 ppm
Parsley - Petroselinum Crispum - E	Plant	21 ppm
Java Cinnamon, Padang Cassia - Cinnamomum Burmannii - E - M - T	Bark	20 ppm
Black bean, Dwarf bean, Field bean, Flageolet bean, French bean, Garden bean, Green bean, Haricot, Haricot bean, Haricot vert, Kidney bean, Navy bean, Pop bean, Popping bean, Snap bean, String bean, Wax bean - Phaseolus Vulgaris - E	Fruit	20 ppm
Almond - Prunus Dulcis - E - M - T	Seed	20 ppm
Rhubarb - Rheum Rhabarbarum - E	Pt	20 ppm
Horseradish - Armoracia Rusticana - E	Root	19 ppm
Alehoof - Glechoma Hederacea - M	Plant	19 ppm
Beet, Beetroot, Garden Beet, Sugar Beet - Beta Vulgaris - E	Root	16 ppm
Pistachio - Pistacia Vera - E	Seed	16 ppm
Onion, Shallot - Allium Cepa - Shallot Bulb - E	Bulb	15 ppm
Ramie - Boehmeria Nivea - M	Plant	14 ppm
Pea - Pisum Sativum - E	Seed	12 ppm
Cassia, Cassia Bark, Cassia Lignea, China Junk Cassia, Chinazimt, Chinese Cassia - Cinnamomum Aromaticuminnamon - E - M - T	Bark	10 ppm
Ceylon Cinnamon, Cinnamon - Cinnamomum Verum - E - M - T	Bark	10 ppm
Chinese Polystichum - Polystichum Polyblepharum - T	Plant	10 ppm
Carrot - Daucus Carota - E	Root	9 ppm
Dill, Garden Dill - Anethum Graveolens - E	Plant	6 ppm
Japanese Cinnamon - Cinnamomum Sieboldii - E - M - T	Root Bark	5 ppm
Dog Rose, Dogbrier, Rose - Rosa Canina - E - M	Fruit	5 ppm
Coconut, Coconut Palm - Cocos Nucifera - E	Seed	4 ppm
Rowan Berry - Sorbus Aucubaria - E - M - T	Fruit	4 ppm
Spinach - Spinacia Oleracea - E	Leaf	4 ppm
Black Walnut - Juglans Nigra - E	Seed	2.5 ppm
Shagbark Hickory - Carya Ovata - E	Seed	1.8 ppm
Cobnut, English Filbert, European Filbert, European Hazel, Hazel - Corylus Avellana - E	Seed	1.8 ppm
Northern Red Oak - Quercus Rubra - E - M	Seed	1.6 ppm
Pecan - Carya Illinoensis - E	Seed	1.5 ppm
Butternut - Juglans Cinerea - E	Seed	1.5 ppm
Cashew - Anacardium Occidentale - E	Seed	1.2 ppm
Mandarin, Tangerine - Citrus Reticulata - E	Fruit	1 ppm
Celery - Apium Graveolens - E	Root	Trace
Rutabaga, Swede, Swedish Turnip - Brassica Napus var. Napobrassica - E	Root	Trace
Cauli Brassica Oleracea var. Botrytis - E	Flower	Trace
Rapini, Seven-Top Turnip, Turnip - Brassica Rapa - E	Root	Trace
Japanese Cinnamon - Cinnamomum Sieboldii - E - M - T	Bark	Trace
Grape Citrus Paradisi - E	Fruit	Trace
Orange - Citrus Sinensis - E	Fruit	Trace
Strawberry - Fragaria spp. - E	Fruit	Trace
Lettuce - Lactuca Sativa - E	Leaf	Trace
Apple - Malus Domestica - E	Fruit	Trace
Parsnip - Pastinaca Sativa - E	Root	Trace
Plum - Prunus Domestica - E - M	Fruit	Trace

BROMINE CONTINUED

Species	Part	Quantity
Peach - Prunus Persica - E - M - T	Fruit	Trace
Pear - Pyrus Communis - E	Fruit	Trace
Radish - Raphanus Sativus - E	Root	Trace
Black Currant - Ribes Nigrum - E	Fruit	Trace
Red Currant, White Currant - Ribes Rubrum - E	Fruit	Trace
Gooseberry - Ribes Uva-Crispa - E	Fruit	Trace
Cloudberry - Rubus Chamaemorus - E - M	Fruit	Trace
Bilberry, Dwarf Bilberry, Whortleberry - Vaccinium Myrtillus - E - M	Fruit	Trace
Cowberry, Lingen, Lingonberry - Vaccinium Vitis-Idaea var. Minus - E - M	Fruit	Trace
European Grape, Grape, Grapevine, Vigne Vinifere, Wine Grape - Vitis Vinifera - E - M	Fruit	Trace

PLANTS CONTAINING CALCIUM

Species	Part	Quantity
Tomato - Lycopersicon Esculentum - E - M - T	Leaf	60,800 ppm
Brigham Tea, Mormon Tea - Ephedra Nevadensis - M	Plant	58,100 ppm
Luffa, Smooth Loofah, Vegetable Sponge - Luffa Aegyptiaca - E	Leaf	55,000 ppm
Huaca-Mullo - Mimulus Glabratus - M	Shoot	54,300 ppm
Cauli Brassica Oleracea var. Botrytis - E	Leaf	54,247 ppm
Chinese Boxthorn, Chinese Matrimony Vine, Chinese Wolfberry - Lycium Chinense - E - M	Root Bark	53,900 ppm
Pigweed - Amaranthus sp. - E - M	Leaf	53,333 ppm
Chaff Achyranthes Bidentata - M	Root	52,200 ppm
Angel Of Death, Bolek Hena, Curia - Justicia Pectoralis - M	Leaf	44,200 ppm
American Styrax, Sweetgum - Liquidambar Styraciflua - E - M	Stem	42,000 ppm
Common Valerian, Garden-Heliotrope, Valerian - Valeriana Officinalis - E - M	Root	42,000 ppm
Red Pignut Hickory - Carya Glabra - E	Shoot	40,700 ppm
Common Garden Peony, Peony, White Peony - Paeonia Lactiflora - M	Root	40,600 ppm
Ramie - Boehmeria Nivea - M	Plant	39,000 ppm
Buchu, Honey Buchu, Mountain Buchu - Agathosma Betulina	Leaf	38,800 ppm
Buchu, Honey Buchu, Mountain Buchu - Agathosma Betulina - M		
Buffalo Gourd - Cucurbita Foetidissima - E - M - T	Leaf	0-77,600 ppm
Chinese Ash - Fraxinus Rhynchophylla - M - E	Bark	38,600 ppm
Madder - Rubia Cordifolia - M	Root	37,800 ppm
White Oak - Quercus Alba - M	Bark	37,000 ppm
Mimosa - Albizia Julibrissin - E - M	Bark	35,500 ppm
Lambsquarter - Chenopodium Album - E - M - T	Leaf	33,800 ppm
Shagbark Hickory - Carya Ovata - E	Shoot	33,300 ppm
European Nettle, Stinging Nettle - Urtica Dioica - E - M	Leaf	33,000 ppm
Black Cherry, Wild Cherry - Prunus Serotina - E - M - T	Leaf	32,640 ppm
Pau D'Arco - Tabebuia Heptaphylla - M	Bark	32,600 ppm
Chai-Hu - Bupleurum - M	Root	32,100 ppm
Post Oak - Quercus Stellata - E - M	Stem	31,920 ppm
Red Cedar - Juniperus Virginiana Amphicarpaea Bracteata - E - M - T	Shoot	31,680 ppm
Fig - Ficus Carica - E	Leaf	31,600 ppm
Groundnut, Peanut - Arachis Hypogaea - E - M	Plant	31,500 ppm
Broadbean, Faba Bean, Habas - Vicia Faba - E	Seed	31,160 ppm
Calendula, Pot-Marigold - Calendula Officinalis - E - M	Leaf	30,400 ppm
Bladderwrack, Kelp - Fucus Vesiculosus - E - M	Plant	30,400 ppm
Gum Ghatti - Anogeissus Latifolia - E - M - M	Leaf	30,300 ppm
Qian Hu - Peucedanum Decursivum - M	Plant	30,000 ppm
Mango - Mangifera Indica - E - M	Leaf	29,300 ppm
Sickle Senna - Cassia Tora - Sprout - Seedling - M	Sprout Seedling	28,100 ppm
Black Cutch, Catechu - Acacia Catechu - M	Leaf	27,400 ppm
White Mulberry - Morus Alba - E - M	Leaf	27,400 ppm
White Oak - Quercus Alba - M	Stem	27,360 ppm
Black Gram - Vigna Mungo - E	Fruit	27,100 ppm
Paper Mulberry - Broussonetia Papyrifera - E - M	Fruit	26,900 ppm
Castorbean - Ricinus Communis - T	Leaf	26,700 ppm

Spiny Pigweed - Amaranthus Spinosus - E - M	Leaf	4,760-53,335 ppm
Neem - Azadirachta Indica - M	Leaf	26,500 ppm
Chinaberry - Melia Azedarach - T	Leaf	25,500 ppm
Dwarf Sumac, Winged Sumac - Rhus Copallina - E - M	Leaf	24,960 ppm
Smooth Sumac - Rhus Glabra - E - M	Stem	24,790 ppm
Field Horsetail, Horsetail - Equisetum Arvense - M	Plant	24,000 ppm
Berro, Watercress - Nasturtium Officinale - E	Herb	24,000 ppm
Papaya - Carica Papaya - E - M	Leaf	23,800 ppm
Sensitive Mimosa Pudica - M	Leaf	23,800 ppm
Northern Red Oak - Quercus Rubra - E - M	Stem	23,760 ppm
Mat Bean, Moth Bean - Vigna Aconitifolia - E	Plant	23,700 ppm
Cheeseweed - Malva Parviflora - E - M	Plant	23,650 ppm
Marjoram, Sweet Marjoram - Origanum Majorana - E	Plant	23,625 ppm
Crampbark, European Cranberry bush, Guelder Rose, Snowballbush - Viburnum Opulus - E - M - T	Bark	23,540 ppm
Broomweed, Tea Sida Rhombifolia - M	Leaf	23,535 ppm
Chinese Licorice - Glycyrrhiza Uralensis - M	Root	23,500 ppm
Summer Savory - Satureja Hortensis - E	Plant	23,429 ppm
Evening-Primrose - Oenothera Biennis - E - M	Plant	23,400 ppm
Mat Bean, Moth Bean - Vigna Aconitifolia - E	Leaf	23,400 ppm
Alehoof - Glechoma Hederacea - M	Plant	23,000 ppm
Indian Tamarind, Kilytree, Tamarind - Tamarindus Indica - M	Leaf	23,000 ppm
Black Oak - Quercus Velutina - E - M	Stem	22,940 ppm
Cowgrass, Peavine Clover, Purple Clover, Red Clover - Trifolium Pratense - E - M	Shoot	22,900 ppm
Buckbush - Symphoricarpos Orbiculatus - M	Stem	22,880 ppm
Black Gum, Black Tupelo - Nyssa Sylvatica - E - M	Leaf	22,750 ppm
Umbrella Thorn - Acacia Tortilis - M	Leaf	22,700 ppm
Common thyme, Garden thyme, Thyme - Thymus Vulgaris - E - M	Plant	22,534 ppm
Bok-Choy, Celery Cabbage, Celery Mustard, Chinese Cabbage, Chinese Mustard, Chinese White Cabbage, Pak-Choi - Brassica Chinensis - E	Leaf	22,440 ppm
Basil, Cuban Basil, Sweet Basil - Ocimum Basilicum - E	Leaf	22,112 ppm
Loquat - Eriobotrya Japonica - E	Leaf	21,900 ppm
Da-Zao, Jujube, Ta-Tsao - Zizyphus Jujuba - E - M	Shoot	21,600 ppm
Groundnut, Peanut - Arachis Hypogaea - E - M	Leaf	21,500 ppm
Dill, Garden Dill - Anethum Graveolens - E	Plant	21,453 ppm
Dwarf Sumac, Winged Sumac - Rhus Copallina - E - M	Stem	21,350 ppm
Sugar-Apple, Sweetsop - Annona Squamosa - E	Leaf	21,200 ppm
Chaya - Cnidoscolus Chayamansa - E	Leaf	21,050 ppm
Epazote, Worm Chenopodium Ambrosioides - E - M - T	Leaf	21,000 ppm
Dandelion - Taraxacum Officinale - E - M	Plant	21,000 ppm
Purslane, Verdolaga - Portulaca Oleracea - E	Herb	20,800 ppm
Mesquite - Prosopis Juliflora - M	Leaf	20,800 ppm
Celery - Apium Graveolens - E	Seed	20,776 ppm
Black bean, Dwarf bean, Field bean, Flageolet bean, French bean, Garden bean, Green bean, Haricot, Haricot bean, Haricot vert, Kidney bean, Navy bean, Pop bean, Popping bean, Snap bean, String bean, Wax bean - Phaseolus Vulgaris - E	Leaf	20,758 ppm
Amboini Coleus, Country Borage, Cuban Oregano, French Thyme, Indian Borage, Mexican Mint, Soup Mint, Spanish Thyme - Plectranthus amboinicus - E	Leaf	2,320-41,430 ppm
Florida Eryngium - Eryngium Floridanum - M	Shoot	20,600 ppm
Coffee - Coffea Arabica - E - M	Leaf	20,406 ppm
Garden Cress - Lepidium Sativum - E	Leaf	20,340 ppm
Mat Bean, Moth Bean - Vigna Aconitifolia - E	Fruit	20,100 ppm
Da-Zao, Jujube, Ta-Tsao - Zizyphus Jujuba - E - M	Leaf	19,700 ppm
Cerraja, Sow Thistle - Sonchus Oleraceus - E - M	Leaf	19,265 ppm
Burn Mouth Vine - Rhynchosia Minima - M - T	Shoot	19,200 ppm

CALCIUM CONTINUED

Plant	Part	ppm	Plant	Part	ppm
Collards, Cow Cabbage, Spring-Heading Cabbage, Tall Kale, Tree Kale - Brassica Oleracea - E	Leaf	19,180 ppm	Black Mustard - Brassica Nigra - E	Leaf	17,867 ppm
			American Persimmon - Diospyros Virginiana - E - M	Stem	17,820 ppm
Lettuce - Lactuca Sativa - E	Leaf	19,140 ppm	Malanga, Tannia, Yautia - Xanthosoma Sagittifolium - E	Leaf	17,800 ppm
Radish - Raphanus Sativus - E	Leaf	19,130 ppm			
Barberry - Berberis Vulgaris - M	Root	19,100 ppm	European Grape, Grape, Grapevine, Vigne Vinifere, Wine Grape - Vitis Vinifera - E - M	Stem	17,700 ppm
Chocolate Vine - Akebia Quinata - M	Stem	19,000 ppm			
Black Locust - Robinia Pseudoacacia - T	Seed	19,000 ppm	Sassafras - Sassafras Albidum - E - M - T	Leaf	17,680 ppm
Bourbon Vanilla, Vanilla - Vanilla Planifolia - E	Fruit	19,000 ppm	Dill, Garden Dill - Anethum Graveolens - E	Fruit	17,671 ppm
Chicory, Succory, Witloof - Cichorium Intybus - E - M	Leaf	18,900 ppm	Shepherd's Purse - Capsella Bursa-Pastoris - E - M	Plant	17,627 ppm
American Styrax, Sweetgum - Liquidambar Styraciflua - E - M	Leaf	18,860 ppm	Taro - Colocasia Esculenta - E	Leaf	17,400 ppm
Irish moss - Chondrus Crispus - E	Plant	18,820 ppm	Indian Sorrel, Jamaica Sorrel, Kharkadi, Red Sorrel, Sorrel - Hibiscus Sabdariffa - E	Flower	17,400 ppm
Common Turkish Oregano, European Oregano, Oregano, Pot Marjoram, Wild Marjoram, Wild Oregano - Origanum Vulgare - E	Plant	18,794 ppm	Black Gram - Vigna Mungo - E	Plant	17,400 ppm
			Beet, Beetroot, Garden Beet, Sugar Beet - Beta Vulgaris - E	Leaf	17,368 ppm
Butterbur - Petasites Japonicus - T	Pt	18,725 ppm	Alfalfa, Lucerne - Medicago Sativa subsp. Sativa - E	Plant	17,200 ppm
Bitter Melon, Sorosi - Momordica Charantia - E	Leaf	18,701 ppm	SafCarthamus Tinctorius - M	Plant	17,000 ppm
Aubergine, Egg Solanum Melongena - E	Leaf	18,676 ppm	Java Cinnamon, Padang Cassia - Cinnamomum Burmannii - E - M - T	Bark	17,000 ppm
Shan Dou Gen - Sophora Subprostrata - M - T	Root	18,600 ppm			
Rhubarb - Rheum Rhabarbarum - E	Pt	18,462 ppm	Gennoshiouko, Oriental Geranium - Geranium Thunbergii - E - M	Plant	16,900 ppm
Jew's Mallow, Mulukiya, Nalta Jute - Corchorus Olitorius - E - M	Leaf	18,365 ppm	Mongoloid Dandelion - Taraxacum Mongolicum - E - M	Plant	16,900 ppm
Black Cherry, Wild Cherry - Prunus Serotina - E - M - T	Stem	18,360 ppm	European Pennyroyal - Mentha pulegium - E - M- T	Plant	16,870 ppm
Rice Paper Tree, Tong-Cao, Tung-Tsao - Tetrapanax Papyrifera M	Pith	18,300 ppm	Parsley - Petroselinum Crispum - E	Plant	16,850 ppm
Damiana - Turnera Diffusa - M	Leaf	18,100 ppm	Chinese Cabbage - Brassica Pekinensis - E	Leaf	16,800 ppm
Evening-Primrose - Oenothera Biennis - E - M	Seed	18,000 ppm	Ladyslipper Cypripedium Pubescens - M	Root	16,800 ppm
Black bean, Dwarf bean, Field bean, Flageolet bean, French bean, Garden bean, Green bean, Haricot, Haricot bean, Haricot vert, Kidney bean, Navy bean, Pop bean, Popping bean, Snap bean, String bean, Wax bean - Phaseolus Vulgaris - E	Fruit	18,000 ppm	Moutan, Tree Peony - Paeonia Moutan - M	Root Bark	16,700 ppm
			Moutan, Moutan Peony, Tree Peony - *Paeonia Suffruticosa*	Root Bark	16,700 ppm
			Common thyme, Garden thyme, Thyme - Thymus Vulgaris - E - M	Leaf	16,700 ppm
			White Mulberry - Morus Alba - E - M	Root Bark	16,500 ppm
Asian Plantain - Plantago Asiatica - E - M	Plant	18,000 ppm	Purple Tephrosia, Wild Indigo - Tephrosia Purpurea - M - T	Leaf	16,500 ppm
Sage - Salvia Officinalis - E - M	Leaf	17,957 ppm			
			Ajwan - Trachyspermum Ammi - E - M	Fruit	16,469 ppm
Sweet Potato - Ipomoea Batatas - E	Leaf	17,900 ppm			

Name	Part	ppm
Texas Colubrina - *Colubrina Texensis*	Shoot	0-32,900 ppm
Chaparral, Creosote Bush - Larrea Tridentata - M	Plant	16,400 ppm
Dyer's Woad - Isatis Tinctoria - M	Root	16,300 ppm
Applemint - Mentha x Rotundifolia - E - M - T	Leaf	16,300 ppm
Opium Poppy, Poppyseed Poppy - Papaver Somniferum - E	Seed	16,214 ppm
Peppermint - Mentha x Piperita subsp. Nothosubsp. Piperita - E - M - T	Leaf	16,200 ppm
Chinese Anemone - Pulsatilla Chinensis - M	Root	16,200 ppm
Rosemary - Rosmarinus Officinalis - E - M	Plant	16,150 ppm
Antler Herb, Clubmoss - Lycopodium Clavatum - M - T	Plant	16,020 ppm
Fortune's Fern - Drynaria Fortunei - M	Rhizome	16,000 ppm
Gotu Kola, Pennywort - Centella Asiatica - E - M	Leaf	15,888 ppm
Vinespinach - Basella Alba - E - M	Leaf	15,800 ppm
Wild Pineapple - Bromelia Pinguin - E - M	Shoot	15,800 ppm
Betel Pepper - Piper Betel - E - M	Leaf	15,750 ppm
Giant Taro - Alocasia Macrorrhiza - E	Leaf	15,700 ppm
Spinach - Spinacia Oleracea - E	Plant	15,700 ppm
Cumin - Cuminum Cyminum - E - M	Fruit	15,511 ppm
Horsetail, Scouring Rush - Equisetum Hyemale - M	Plant	15,500 ppm
Ching-Feng-Teng - Sinomenium Acutum - E - M	Rhizome	15,400 ppm
Kapok, Silk-Cotton Tree - Ceiba Pentandra - M - E	Shoot	15,400 ppm
Chinese Cornbind, Chinese Knotweed, Fleeceflower, Fo Ti, He Shou Wu - Polygonum Multiflorum - E - M - T	Rhizome	15,300 ppm
Elephant-Foot Yam - Amorphophallus Campanulatus - E - M- T	Shoot	15,200 ppm
Capillary Wormwood - Artemisia Capillaris - M	Plant	15,200 ppm
Black Locust - Robinia Pseudoacacia - T	Leaf	15,000 ppm
Cascara Buckthorn, Cascara Sagrada - Frangula Purshiana - M	Bark	14,800 ppm
Indian Sorrel, Jamaica Sorrel, Kharkadi, Red Sorrel, Sorrel Hibiscus Sabdariffa - E	Leaf	14,792 ppm
Willow Oak - Quercus Phellos - E - M	Stem	14,700 ppm
Coca - Erythroxylum Novogranatense var. Truxillense - E - M	Leaf	14,600 ppm
Black Gum, Black Tupelo - Nyssa Sylvatica - E - M	Stem	14,520 ppm
Chervil - Anthriscus Cerefolium - E	Leaf	14,509 ppm
Heal-All, Self-Heal - Prunella Vulgaris - E - M	Flower	14,500 ppm
Chinese Parsley, Cilantro, Coriander - Coriandrum Sativum E	Seed	14,469 ppm
Cordoncillo, Hierba Santa, Hoja Santa - Piper Auritum - E - M	Leaf	14,440 ppm
Jussiaeae Herba, Pond Dragon - Jussiaea Repens - M	Plant	14,400 ppm
Rhubarb - Rheum Rhabarbarum - E	Leaf	14,400 ppm
Black Nightshade - Solanum Nigrum - E	Leaf	14,400 ppm
Oats - Avena Sativa - E - M	Plant	14,300 ppm
Chinese Boxthorn, Chinese Matrimony Vine, Chinese Wolfberry - Lycium Chinense - E - M	Leaf	14,231 ppm
Amur Cork Tree, Huang Bai, Huang Po, Po Mu - Phellodendron Amurense - M	Bark	14,100 ppm
Pea - Pisum Sativum - E	Plant	14,100 ppm
White Willow - Salix Alba - M	Bark	14,100 ppm
Perilla - Perilla Frutescens - E - M - T	Leaf	14,071 ppm
Japanese Cinnamon - Cinnamomum Sieboldii - E - M - T	Bark	14,000 ppm
Butterbur - Petasites Japonicus - T	Plant	14,000 ppm
Fennel - Foeniculum Vulgare - M	Fruit	13,941 ppm
Cassia, Cassia Bark, Cassia Lignea, China Junk Cassia, Chinazimt, Chinese Cassia - Cinnamomum Aromaticuminnamon- E - M - T	Bark	13,569 ppm
Cornmint, Field Mint, Japanese Mint - Mentha Arvensis var. Piperascens - E - M- T	Plant	13,500 ppm
Red Mangrove - Rhizophora Mangle - M	Leaf	13,500 ppm
Chinese Parsley, Cilantro, Coriander - Coriandrum Sativum E	Leaf	13,441 ppm
Small-Flowered Melilot - Melilotus Indica - E - M - T	Plant	13,400 ppm
Water Lotus - Nelumbo Nucifera - E - M	Seed	13,333 ppm
Flannelleaf, Flannelplant, Great mullein, Mullein, Velvet Verbascum Thapsus - M	Leaf	13,300 ppm

CALCIUM CONTINUED

Gum Arabic, Gum Arabic Tree, Kher, Senegal Gum, Sudan Gum Arabic - Acacia Senegal - M	Leaf	13,200 ppm
Cowgrass, Peavine Clover, Purple Clover, Red Clover - Trifolium Pratense - E - M	Flower	13,100 ppm
Coca - Erythroxylum Novogranatense var. Novogranatense - E - M	Leaf	13,000 ppm
Soybean - Glycine Max - E	Plant	13,000 ppm
Dandelion - Taraxacum Officinale - E - M	Leaf	13,000 ppm
Asian Wild Ginger - Asiasarum Heterotropoides - M	Root	12,900 ppm
Siebold's Wild Ginger - Asiasarum Sieboldii - M	Root	12,900 ppm
Alholva, Bockshornklee, Fenugreek, Greek Clover, Greek Trigonella Foenum-Graecum - E - M	Leaf	12,900 ppm
Perilla - Perilla Frutescens - E - M - T	Plant	12,670 ppm
Swamp Cabbage, Water Spinach - Ipomoea Aquatica - E	Leaf	12,665 ppm
Sesame - Sesamum Indicum - E - M	Seed	12,638 ppm
Wu Chia Pi - Acanthopanax Gracilistylis - M	Root Bark	12,600 ppm
American Persimmon - Diospyros Virginiana - E - M	Leaf	12,500 ppm
Chinese Rhubarb - Rheum Palmatum - E	Rhizome	12,400 ppm
Tarragon - Artemisia Dracunculus - M	Plant	12,340 ppm
Raspberry, Red raspberry - Rubus Idaeus - E - M	Leaf	12,100 ppm
Chickweed, Common Chickweed - Stellaria Media - E	Plant	12,100 ppm
Giant Knotweed, Hu-Zhang, Japanese Knotweed, Mexican Bamboo - Polygonum Cuspidatum - E - M - T	Plant	12,000 ppm
Celery - Apium Graveolens - E	Pt	11,918 ppm
Olive - Olea Europaea - E	Leaf	11,800 ppm
Spearmint - Mentha Spicata - E - M- T	Plant	11,760 ppm
Shortleaf Pine - Pinus Echinata - M	Shoot	11,760 ppm
Sickle Senna - Cassia Tora - Sprout - Seedling - M	Seed	11,700 ppm
Chih-Mu, Zhi-Mu - Anemarrhena Asphodeloides - M	Rhizome	11,600 ppm
Bai-Zhu, Pai-Chu - Atractylodes Ovata - M	Rhizome	11,600 ppm
Wou Chou Yu - Euodia Rutaecarpa - E	Fruit	11,600 ppm
Banana, Plantain - Musa x Paradisiaca - E	Sprout Seedling	11,600 ppm
Chinese Spikenard - Nardostachys Chinensis - M	Rhizome	11,600 ppm
Ma-Huang - Ephedra spp. - M	Plant	11,500 ppm
Eyebright - Euphrasia Officinalis - M	Plant	11,500 ppm
Asparagus Pea, Goa Bean, Winged Bean - Psophocarpus Tetragonolobus - E	Leaf	11,383 ppm
Cang Zhu - Atractylodes Lancea - M	Rhizome	11,300 ppm
Comfrey - Symphytum Officinale - E - M - T	Root	11,300 ppm
Blessed Thistle - Cnicus Benedictus - M	Plant	11,200 ppm
Bayberry, Candle-Berry, Southern Bayberry, Wax Myrtle - Myrica Cerifera - E - M	Bark	11,200 ppm
Hsi Chien, Saint Paul'Swort - Siegesbeckia Orientalis - M	Plant	11,100 ppm
Mugwort - Artemisia Vulgaris - M	Plant	11,000 ppm
Barley, Barleygrass - Hordeum Vulgare - E - M	Stem	11,000 ppm
Bearberry, Uva Uursi - Arctostaphylos Uva-Ursi - M	Leaf	10,900 ppm
Ching-Chieh, Jing-Jie - Schizonepeta Tenuifolia - E - M	Plant	10,900 ppm
American Ginseng, Ginseng - Panax Quinquefolius - M	Plant	10,800 ppm
High Mallow - Malva Sylvestris - E - M	Leaf	10,715 ppm
Swamp Taro - Cyrtosperma Chamissonis - E	Root	10,630 ppm
Black Caraway, Black Cumin, Fennel-Flower, Nutmeg-Flower, Roman Coriander - Nigella Sativa - E - M	Seed	10,600 ppm
Fennel - Foeniculum Vulgare - M	Leaf	10,556 ppm
Guinea Grass - Panicum Maximum - M	Leaf	7,100-20,900 ppm
Barley, Barleygrass - Hordeum Vulgare - E - M	Plant	10,400 ppm
Wheat - Triticum Aestivum - E - M	Plant	10,400 ppm
Chives - Allium Schoenoprasum - E	Leaf	10,375 ppm
Sassafras - Sassafras Albidum - E - M - T	Stem	10,360 ppm
Baikal Skullcap, Chinese Skullcap, Huang Qin - Scutellaria Baicalensis - M	Root	10,300 ppm
Du Zhong, Gutta-Percha Tree, Tu Chung - Eucommia Ulmoides - M	Bark	10,200 ppm
Radish - Raphanus Sativus - E	Fruit	10,130 ppm
Endive, Escarole - Cichorium Endivia - M	Leaf	10,080 ppm

Name	Part	ppm
Cucumber - Cucumis Sativus - E	Fruit	10,000 ppm
Cassava, Tapioca, Yuca - Manihot Esculenta - E	Leaf	10,000 ppm
Morinda - Morinda spp. - M	Root	10,000 ppm
Ban-Xia, Pan-Hsia - Pinellia Ternata - E - M - T	Tuber	10,000 ppm
Curly Dock, Lengua De Vaca, Sour Dock, Yellow Dock - Rumex Crispus - M - T	Leaf	10,000 ppm
Bai-Wei, Pai-Wei - Cynanchum Atratum - E - M	Root	9,900 ppm
Red Elm, Slippery Elm - Ulmus Rubra - M	Bark	9,770 ppm
Sheng Ma - Cimicifuga Dahurica - M	Rhizome	9,750 ppm
Narrowleaf Sophora - Sophora Angustifolia - M - T- M - T	Root	9,710 ppm
Garland Chrysanthemum - Chrysanthemum Coronarium - Bud - E	Leaf	9,690 ppm
New Zealand Spinach - Tetragonia Tetragonioides - E	Leaf	9,665 ppm
Jerusalem Artichoke - Helianthus Tuberosus E	Tuber	9,600 ppm
Calico Bush, Mountain Laurel, Spoonwood - *Kalmia Latifolia*	Leaf	9,600 ppm
Clove, Clovetree - Syzygium Aromaticum - E	Flower	9,540 ppm
Pothomorphe sp. -- Santiago	Leaf	9,440 ppm
ElytriCouchgrass, Doggrass, Quackgrass, Twitchgrass, Wheatgrass - Elytrigia Repens - E - M	Plant	9,280 ppm
Snakegourd - Trichosanthes Anguina - E - M	Fruit	9,260 ppm
Japanese Cinnamon - Cinnamomum Sieboldii - E - M - T	Root Bark	9,000 ppm
Chayote - Sechium Edule - E - M	Shoot	8,920 ppm
Cockscomb - Celosia Cristata - M	Flower	8,910 ppm
European Mistletoe - Viscum Album - M - T	Leaf	8,910 ppm
Pigeonpea - Cajanus Vajan - E	Plant	8,900 ppm
Peach - Prunus Persica - E - M - T	Fruit	8,850 ppm
Ben Nut, Benzolive Tree, Drumstick Tree, Horseradish Tree, Moringa, West Indian Ben - Moringa Oleifera - E	Leaf	4,400-17,600 ppm
Commom Licorice, Licorice, Licorice-Root, Smooth Licorice - Glycyrrhiza Glabra - M	Root	8,780 ppm
Dog Rose, Dogbrier, Rose - Rosa Canina - E - M	Fruit	8,750 ppm
Milfoil, Yarrow - Achillea Millefolium - M	Plant	8,670 ppm
Amphicarpaea Bracteata- E - M	Shoot	0-17,300 ppm
Mugwort - Artemisia Vulgaris - M	Shoot	8,600 ppm
Butter Bean, Lima Bean - Phaseolus Lunatus - E	Seed	8,600 ppm
Asparagus Pea, Goa Bean, Winged Bean - Psophocarpus Tetragonolobus - E	Seed	8,586 ppm
Radish - Raphanus Sativus - E	Root	8,570 ppm
Burdock, Gobo, Great Burdock - Arctium lappa - E - M - T	Root	8,510 ppm
Common Juniper, Juniper - Juniperus Communis - E - M - T	Fruit	8,490 ppm
Chinese Kudzu - Pueraria Pseudohirsuta - E - M	Root	8,300 ppm
Kuan Chung, Shield Fernle - Blechnum Orientale - E - M - T	Rhizome	8,280 ppm
Banana Yucca, Blue Yucca, Spanish Bayonet, Yucca - Yucca Baccata - E - M - T	Root	8,260 ppm
Elephant Apple, Manzana De Elefante, Wood-Apple - Limonia acidissima - Wood - Apple - E - M	Seed	15,800-16,460 ppm
Marshmallow, White Mallow - Althaea Officinalis - M	Root	8,160 ppm
Caraway, Carum - Carum Carvi - E	Fruit	8,160 ppm
Gentian, Yellow Gentian - Gentiana Lutea - M	Root	8,140 ppm
Okra - Abelmoschus Esculentus - Friut - E - M	Fruit	8,100 ppm
Pumpkin - Cucurbita Pepo - E	Flower	8,041 ppm
Hsin-I, Xin-Yi - Magnolia Denudata - E - M	Flower	8,040 ppm
Hsin-I, Xin-Yi - Magnolia Fargesii - E - M	Flower	8,040 ppm
Magnolia kobus DC. -- Hsin-I, Xin-Yi	Flower	8,040 ppm
Allspice, Clover-Pepper, Jamaica-Pepper, Pimenta, Pimento - Pimenta Dioica - E	Fruit	8,000 ppm
Pepper Elder, Yerba De La Plata - Peperomia Pelucida - Leaf	Leaf	1,240-15,900 ppm
Umbrella Thorn - Acacia Tortilis - M	Fruit	7,900 ppm
Anise, Sweet Cumin - Pimpinella Anisum - E - M	Fruit	7,843 ppm
Puncture-Vine - Tribulus Terrestris - Leaf	Leaf	33,500-15,550 ppm
Coneflower, Echinacea - Echinacea ssp - M	Root	7,760 ppm

CALCIUM CONTINUED

Curly Kale, Kale, Kitchen Kale, Scotch Kale - Brassica Oleracea var. Sabellica l. var. Acephala - E	Leaf	7,725 ppm
SafCarthamus Tinctorius - M	Flower	7,700 ppm
Cherokee Rose - Rosa Laevigata - E - M	Fruit	7,620 ppm
Commelina benghalensis L. -- Benghal dayflower	Leaf	2,100-15,215 ppm
Garland Chrysanthemum - Chrysanthemum Coronarium - Bud - E	Bud	7,525 ppm
Cabbage, Red Cabbage, White Cabbage - Brassica Oleracea var. Capitata - E	Leaf	7,500 ppm
Banana, Plantain - Musa x Paradisiaca - E	Leaf	7,500 ppm
Japanese Gentian - Gentiana Scabra - E	Root	7,490 ppm
Chinese Raspberry - Rubus Cchingii - E - M	Fruit	7,490 ppm
Coffee Senna - Senna Occidentalis - E - T	Seed	7,450 ppm
Henbane - Hyoscyamus Niger - E - M	Seed	7,420 ppm
Japanese Honeysuckle - Lonicera Japonica - M	Flower	7,390 ppm
Box-Holly, Butcher's broom - Ruscus aculeatus - E - M	Root	7,250 ppm
Flax, Lin Linum Usitatissimum - E	Hay	7,200 ppm
Susumba, Wild Egg Solanum Torvum - Friut - E	Fruit	7,125 ppm
Calamus, Flagroot, Myrtle Flag, Sweet Calamus, Sweetflag, Sweet Acorus Calamus - M	Rhizome	7,040 ppm
Indian Tobacco, Lobelia - Lobelia Inflata - M - T	Leaf	7,020 ppm
Calamansi, Calamondin - Citrus Mitis - Friut - E	Fruit	1,400-14,000 ppm
Japanese Ginseng - Panax Japonicus - M	Rhizome	7,000 ppm
Chinese Polystichum - Polystichum Polyblepharum - T	Plant	6,900 ppm
Indian Snakeroot, Serpentine Wood - Rauvolfia Serpentina - Seed	Seed	6,900 ppm
Citron - Citrus Medica - E	Fruit	6,840 ppm
Pito - Erythrina Berteroana - E	Shoot	6,835 ppm
Garden Camomile, Perennial Camomile, Roman Camomile - Chamaemelum Nobile M	Flower	6,720 ppm
Sicklepod - Senna Obtusifolia - E - T	Seed	6,590 ppm
Devil's Tongue, Elephant Yam, Konjac, Leopard Palm, Snake Palm, Umbrella Arum - Amorphophallus Konjac - E - M - T	Leaf	6,538 ppm
Noble Dendrobium - Dendrobium Nobile - M	Stem	6,530 ppm
Genet, Spanish Broom, Weaver's Broom - Spartium Junceum - Stem	Stem	6,500 ppm
Hydrangea, Smooth Hydrangea - Hydrangea Arborescens - E - M	Root	6,460 ppm
Lady's Thistle, Milk Thistle - Silybum Marianum - M	Plant	6,460 ppm
Mugwort - Artemisia Vulgaris - M	Leaf	6,455 ppm
White Mulberry - Morus Alba - E - M	Fruit	6,400 ppm
Chinese Magnolia, Hou Pu, Magnolia- Magnolia Officinalis - E - M	Bark	6,350 ppm
Dulse - Rhodymenia Palmata - E	Plant	6,320 ppm
Pokeweed - Phytolacca Americana - E - M- T	Shoot	6,307 ppm
Manioc Hibiscus - Abelmoschus Manihot - E - M	Leaf	6,241 ppm
Hops - Humulus Lupulus - E - M - T	Fruit	6,222 ppm
Blackberry Lily, Shenan - Belamcanda Chinensis - M	Rhizome	6,170 ppm
Asparagus bean, Pea bean, Yardlong bean - Vigna Unguiculata subsp. Sesquipedalis - E	Shoot	6,164 ppm
Catnip Nepeta Cataria - M	Plant	6,160 ppm
Dandelion - Taraxacum Officinale - E - M	Root	6,140 ppm
Lantana, Wild Sage - Lantana Camara - M	Shoot	6,100 ppm
Devil's claw, Grapple Harpagophytum procumbens - M	Root	6,060 ppm
Rutabaga, Swede, Swedish Turnip - Brassica Napus var. Napobrassica - E	Root	6,040 ppm
Ceylon Cinnamon, Cinnamon - Cinnamomum Verum - E - M - T	Bark	6,000 ppm
Indian Sorrel, Jamaica Sorrel, Kharkadi, Red Sorrel, Sorrel - Hibiscus Sabdariffa - E	Seed	6,000 ppm
Black Cohosh, Black Snake Cimicifuga Racemosa - E - M	Root	5,970 ppm
White Mustard - Sinapis Alba - E - M - T	Seed	5,850 ppm
Calabash Gourd, White-Flowered Gourd - Lagenaria Siceraria - E	Fruit	5,830 ppm
Feverfew - Chrysanthemum Parthenium - M	Plant	5,810 ppm
Tamarillo, Tree Tomato - Cyphomandra Betacea - Fruit	Fruit	5,780 ppm
Elephant-Foot Yam - Amorphophallus Campanulatus - E - M- T	Root	5,720 ppm

Plant	Part	ppm
Carrot - Daucus Carota - E	Root	5,710 ppm
Aubergine, Egg Solanum Melongena - E	Fruit	5,706 ppm
Orange - Citrus Sinensis - E	Fruit	5,615 ppm
Umbrella Thorn - Acacia Tortilis - M	Seed	5,600 ppm
Peganum harmala L. -- Harmel, Syrian Rue	Plant	5,600 ppm
English Hawthorn, Hawthorn, Whitethorn, Woodland Hawthorn - Crataegus Laevigata - M	Fruit	5,570 ppm
Mustard Greens - Brassica Juncea - E	Leaf	5,565 ppm
Horseradish - Armoracia Rusticana - E	Root	5,512 ppm
Cassie, Huisache, Opopanax, Popinac, Sweet Acacia - Acacia Farnesiana - M	Seed	5,500 ppm
Elephant Garlic, Kurrat - Allium Ampeloprasum - E	Leaf	5,472 ppm
Indian Sorrel, Jamaica Sorrel, Stevia, Sweet Leaf of Paraguay - Stevia Rebaudiana - E	Leaf	5,440 ppm
Onion, Shallot - Allium Cepa - Shallot Bulb - E	Leaf	5,385 ppm
Pyrethrum - Chrysanthemum Cinerariifolium - M	Shoot	5,300 ppm
Artichoke - Cynara Cardunculus - E	Flower	5,286 ppm
Jack Bean - Canavalia Ensiformis - E	Fruit	5,263 ppm
Balloon Flower, Chieh-Keng, Jie-Geng - Platycodon Grandiflorum - E - M - T	Root	5,240 ppm
Breadroot, Indian Bread-Root, Indian Turnip, Prairie Apple, Prairie Potato, Prairie Turnip - Psoralea Esculenta - E - M - T	Root	5,100 ppm
Terminalia catappa L. -- Indian Almond, Malabar Almond, Tropical Almond	Seed	5,100 ppm
Bastard Cardamom, Chin Kousha, Malabar Cardamom, Tavoy Cardamom - Amomum Xanthioides - E	Seed	5,090 ppm
Beebread, Beeplant, Borage, Talewort - Borago Officinalis - E - M - T	Leaf	5,005 ppm
Cassie, Huisache, Opopanax, Popinac, Sweet Acacia - Acacia Farnesiana - M	Leaf	5,003 ppm
Perejil - Peperomia Pereskiifolia - Leaf	Leaf	1,500-10,000 ppm
Ambarella - Spondias Dulcis - E	Seed	5,000 ppm
Black Pepper, Pepper, White Pepper - Piper Nigrum - E - M	Fruit	4,989 ppm
Garlic - Allium Sativum Bulb - E	Bulb	4,947 ppm
Giant Reed - Arundo Donax - Plant	Plant	4,900 ppm
Waxgourd - Benincasa Hispida - Fruit	Fruit	4,870 ppm
Oats - Avena Sativa - E - M	Seed	4,800 ppm
Desert Date, Soapberry Tree - Balanites Aegyptiacus - Seed	Shoot	4,800 ppm
European Grape, Grape, Grapevine, Vigne Vinifere, Wine Grape - Vitis Vinifera - E - M	Fruit	4,774 ppm
Black Currant - Ribes Nigrum - E	Fruit	4,720 ppm
Cape Jasmine, Gardenia, Jasmin, Shan-Chih-Tzu, Shan-Zhi-Zi, Zhi Zi - Gardenia Jasminoides - M	Fruit	4,710 ppm
Aloe, Bitter Aloes - Aloe Vera - E - M	Leaf	4,600 ppm
Mad-Dog Skullcap, Scullcap - Scutellaria lateriflora - M	Plant	4,550 ppm
Soybean - Glycine Max - E	Seed	4,440 ppm
Hardy Orchid, Hyacinth Bletilla, Hyacinth Orchid, Shiran - Bletilla Striata - M	Tuber	4,400 ppm
Chinese Ephedra, Ma Huang - Ephedra Sinica - M	Plant	4,390 ppm
Lian-Jiao, Lien-Chiao - Forsythia Suspensa - M	Fruit	4,380 ppm
Bitter Melon, Sorosi - Momordica Charantia - E	Fruit	4,333 ppm
Garden Sorrel - Rumex Acetosa - E - M - T	Leaf	4,300 ppm
Ambarella - Spondias Dulcis - E	Fruit	4,275 ppm
Grape Citrus Paradisi - E	Fruit	4,270 ppm
Garlic - Allium Sativum Bulb - E	Leaf	4,265 ppm
Pea - Pisum Sativum - E	Fruit	4,253 ppm
Bitter Orange, Petitgrain - Citrus Aurantium - E	Fruit	4,230 ppm
Fig - Ficus Carica - E	Fruit	4,228 ppm
Beet, Beetroot, Garden Beet, Sugar Beet - Beta Vulgaris - E	Root	4,200 ppm
Cardamom - Elettaria Cardamomum - E - M	Seed	4,177 ppm
Chinese Ginseng, Ginseng, Korean Ginseng, Oriental Ginseng - Panax Ginseng - M	Root	4,140 ppm
Bonavist Bean, Hyacinth Bean, Lablab Bean - Lablab Purpureus - E - M - T	Seed	4,122 ppm
Gooseberry - Ribes Uva-Crispa - E	Fruit	4,122 ppm
Asparagus bean, Pea bean, Yardlong bean - Vigna Unguiculata subsp. Sesquipedalis - E	Fruit	4,115 ppm
Barley, Barleygrass - Hordeum Vulgare - E - M	Seed	4,100 ppm

Hillman Health Food Store call 855-Amish-Dr (855-264-7437) www.emineral.info Vitamins and Minerals for Better Living

CALCIUM CONTINUED

Wheat - Triticum Aestivum - E - M	Seed	4,100 ppm	
Bolsa Mullaca, Winter Cherry - Physalis Angulata - E	Fruit	810-8,100 ppm	
Cauli Brassica Oleracea var. Botrytis - E	Flower	4,040 ppm	
Luffa, Smooth Loofah, Vegetable Sponge - Luffa Aegyptiaca - E	Fruit	4,000 ppm	
Malanga, Tannia, Yautia - Xanthosoma Sagittifolium - E	Root	4,000 ppm	
Flax, Lin Linum Usitatissimum - E	Seed	3,969 ppm	
Blue Cohosh - Caulophyllum Thalictroides - M	Root	3,890 ppm	
Qiang Huo - Notopterygium Incisum - M	Rhizome	3,850 ppm	
Asparagus - Asparagus Officinalis - E	Shoot	3,840 ppm	
Tu Huo - Angelica Laxiflora - M	Root	3,800 ppm	
Desert Date, Soapberry Tree - Balanites Aegyptiacus - Seed	Fruit	3,800 ppm	
Elephant Garlic, Kurrat - Allium Ampeloprasum - E	Root	3,796 ppm	
Taro - Colocasia Esculenta - E	Root	3,780 ppm	
Hawthorn - Crataegus Cuneata - M	Fruit	3,770 ppm	
Yellow Mombin, Yellow Plum - Spondias Pinnata - E	Fruit	3,710 ppm	
Water Lotus - Nelumbo Nucifera - E - M	Rhizome	3,704 ppm	
Genipap, Jagua - Genipa Americana - E - M	Fruit	3,700 ppm	
Rapini, Seven-Top Turnip, Turnip - Brassica Rapa - E	Root	3,690 ppm	
Lemongrass, West indian lemongrass - Cymbopogon Citratus - E - M	Plant	3,680 ppm	
Radish - Raphanus Sativus - E	Seed	3,670 ppm	
Coltsfoot - Tussilago Farfara - M - T	Flower	3,670 ppm	
Celery - Apium Graveolens - E	Root	3,635 ppm	
Corn Salad, Lamb's Lettuce - Valerianella Locusta - E	Plant	6,410-7,139 ppm	
Parsnip - Pastinaca Sativa - E	Root	3,525 ppm	
Soybean - Glycine Max - E	Sprout Seedling	3,504 ppm	
Perilla - Perilla Frutescens - E - M - T	Seed	3,500 ppm	
Mat Bean, Moth Bean - Vigna Aconitifolia - E	Seed	3,500 ppm	
Ginger - Zingiber Officinale - E	Rhizome	3,458 ppm	
Mai-Men-Dong, Mai-Men-Tung - Ophiopogon Japonicus - M	Tuber	3,450 ppm	
Mud Plantain, Tse-Hsieh, Water Plantain, Ze-Xie - Alisma Plantago-Aquatica - M	Rhizome	3,430 ppm	
Broadbean, Faba Bean, Habas - Vicia Faba - E	Fruit	3,425 ppm	
Chinese Senega - Polygala Tenuifolia - M	Root	3,420 ppm	
Chinese Goldthread, Huang-Lian, Huang-Lien - Coptis Chinensis - M	Rhizome	3,410 ppm	
Huang-Lia, Huang-Lian, Huang-Lien, Japanese Goldthread - Coptis Japonica - M	Rhizome	3,410 ppm	
Generic Goldthread - Coptis spp. - M	Rhizome	3,410 ppm	
Neem - Azadirachta Indica - M	Fruit	3,400 ppm	
Watermelon - Citrullus Lanatus - E	Fruit	3,400 ppm	
Strawberry Guava - Psidium Cattleianum - E	Fruit	3,400 ppm	
Chinese Cornbind, Chinese Knotweed, Fleeceflower, Fo Ti, He Shou Wu - Polygonum Multiflorum - E - M - T	Root	3,370 ppm	
Chayote - Sechium Edule - E - M	Leaf	3,345 ppm	
Psyllium - Plantago Psyllium - E - M	Seed	3,340 ppm	
Rice - Oryza Sativa - E	Plant	3,300 ppm	
Black bean, Dwarf bean, Field bean, Flageolet bean, French bean, Garden bean, Green bean, Haricot, Haricot bean, Haricot vert, Kidney bean, Navy bean, Pop bean, Popping bean, Snap bean, String bean, Wax bean - Phaseolus Vulgaris - E	Seed	3,295 ppm	
Garden Cress - Lepidium Sativum - E	Seed	3,290 ppm	
Elephant Apple, Manzana De Elefante, Wood-Apple - Limonia acidissima - Wood - Apple - E - M	Fruit	1,300-6,540 ppm	
Chinese Dogwood - Cornus Officinalis - E - M	Fruit	3,250 ppm	
Pawpaw - Asimina Triloba - Friut - E	Fruit	3,248 ppm	
Lemon - Citrus Limon - E	Fruit	3,227 ppm	
Nutsedge - Cyperus Rotundus - E - M	Rhizome	3,180 ppm	
Brussel-Sprout - Brassica Oleracea var. Gemmifera - E	Leaf	3,177 ppm	
Summer Squash - Cucurbita spp. - E	Fruit	3,165 ppm	
Achocha - Cyclanthera Pedata - Friut - E - M	Fruit	3,160 ppm	

Species	Part	Quantity
Stillingia sylvatica GARDEN EX L. -- Queen's-Delight, Queen's-Root, Stillingia, Yawroot	Plant	3,100 ppm
Cus-Cus, Cuscus Grass, Vetiver - Vetiveria Zizanioides - E	Leaf	3,100 ppm
Jack Bean - Canavalia Ensiformis - E	Seed	3,090 ppm
Black Walnut - Juglans Nigra - E	Hull Husk	3,090 ppm
Lime - Citrus Aurantiifolia - E	Fruit	3,084 ppm
Cantaloupe, Melon, Muskmelon, Netted Melon, Nutmeg Melon, Persian Melon - Cucumis Melo subsp. ssp Melo var.Ccantalupensis - Friut - E	Fruit	3,080 ppm
Erythrina fusca LOUR. -- Coral Bean, Gallito	Leaf	3,080 ppm
Mandarin, Tangerine - Citrus Reticulata - E	Fruit	3,077 ppm
Indian Fig, Nopal, Nopalito, Prickly Pear - Opuntia Ficus-Indica - E - M	Fruit	3,065 ppm
Wild Yam - Dioscorea sp. - E	Root	3,060 ppm
Climbing Fern - Lygodium Japonicum - Pollen or Spore - M	Pollen Or Spore	3,060 ppm
Psyllium - Plantago Psyllium - E - M	Hull Husk	3,059 ppm
Equatorial Ivory Palm - Phytelephas Aequatorialis - E	Flower	1,780-6,095 ppm
Japanese Privet, Ligustri Fructus - Ligustrum Japonicum - M	Fruit	3,040 ppm
Chinese Privet, Glossy Privet, Ligustri Fructus, Privet, White Waxtree - Ligustrum Lucidum - M	Fruit	3,040 ppm
Butter Bean, Lima Bean - Phaseolus Lunatus - E	Sprout Seedling	3,028 ppm
Onion, Shallot - Allium Cepa - Shallot Bulb - E	Bulb	3,008 ppm
Lambsquarter - Chenopodium Album - E - M - T	Seed	3,000 ppm
Sarsaparilla - Smilax spp - E - M	Root	2,980 ppm
Goldenseal - Hydrastis Canadensis - M	Root	2,970 ppm
Almond - Prunus Dulcis - E - M - T	Seed	2,962 ppm
Bactris gasipaes HBK. -- Peach palm, Pejibaye	Fruit	89-5,820 ppm
Khat - Catha Edulis - E	Leaf	2,900 ppm
Strawberry - Fragaria spp. - E	Fruit	2,900 ppm
Indian Saffron, Turmeric - Curcuma Longa - E	Rhizome	2,898 ppm
Hsin-Pa-Pi, Kisasage - Catalpa Ovata - E - M	Fruit	2,890 ppm
Cassava, Tapioca, Yuca - Manihot Esculenta - E	Root	2,890 ppm
Red Currant, White Currant - Ribes Rubrum - E	Fruit	2,875 ppm
Butter Bean, Lima Bean - Phaseolus Lunatus - E	Leaf	2,857 ppm
Bonavist Bean, Hyacinth Bean, Lablab Bean - Lablab Purpureus - E - M - T	Fruit	2,841 ppm
Indian Tamarind, Kilytree, Tamarind - Tamarindus Indica - M	Fruit	2,829 ppm
Chinese Angelica, Dong Gui, Dong Quai - Angelica Sinensis - M	Root	2,820 ppm
Muntingia calabura L. -- Cereso, Jamaica cherry, Yumansa	Fruit	640-5,615 ppm
Honey Locust - Gleditsia Triacanthos - M	Seed	2,800 ppm
Olive - Olea Europaea - E	Fruit	2,798 ppm
Papaya - Carica Papaya - E - M	Fruit	2,792 ppm
Dan-Shen, Red Sage, Tan-Shen - Salvia Miltiorrhiza - E - M	Root	2,780 ppm
Udo - Aralia Cordata - E - M	Leaf	2,765 ppm
Chayote - Sechium Edule - E - M	Fruit	2,715 ppm
Hsuan-Shen, Yuan-Shen - Scrophularia Buergeriana - M	Root	2,670 ppm
Kohlrabi - Brassica Oleracea var. Gongylodes - E	Stem	2,665 ppm
Coral Beadplant, Crab's Eye, Indian Licorice, Jequerity, Jequirity Bean, Licorice Vine, Love Bean, Lucky Bean, Minnie-Minnies, Prayer Beads, Precatory Bean, Red Beadvine, Rosary Pea, Weatherplant, Weathervine - Abrus Precatorius - Leaf	Leaf	2,660 ppm
Emblic, Myrobalan - Phyllanthus Emblica - E	Fruit	2,660 ppm
Indian Tamarind, Kilytree, Tamarind - Tamarindus Indica - M	Flower	2,650 ppm
Japanese Pagoda Tree - Sophora Japonica - M - T	Seed	2,649 ppm

PLANTS CONTAINING CESIUM

Species	Part	Quantity
Brazilnut, Brazilnut-Tree, Creamnut, Paranut - Bertholletia Eexcelsa - E	Seed	1.3 ppm
Pecan - Carya Illinoensis - E	Seed	Trace

CESIUM CONTINUED

Species	Part	Quantity
Asparagus bean, Pea bean, Yardlong bean - Vigna Unguiculata subsp. Sesquipedalis - E	Seed	Trace
Cashew - Anacardium Occidentale - E	Seed	Trace
Shagbark Hickory - Carya Ovata - E	Seed	Trace
Coconut, Coconut Palm - Cocos Nucifera - E	Seed	Trace
Black Walnut - Juglans Nigra - E	Seed	Trace
Pistachio - Pistacia Vera - E	Seed	Trace
Almond - Prunus Dulcis - E - M - T	Seed	Trace
Butternut - Juglans Cinerea - E	Seed	Trace
Cobnut, English Filbert, European Filbert, European Hazel, Hazel - Corylus Avellana - E	Seed	Trace

PLANTS CONTAINING CHLORINE

Species	Part	Quantity
Dandelion - Taraxacum Officinale - E - M	Leaf	22,000 ppm
Chickweed, Common Chickweed - Stellaria Media - E	Plant	12,936 ppm
Ramie - Boehmeria Nivea - M	Plant	12,000 ppm
Mugwort - Artemisia Vulgaris - M	Plant	11,000 ppm
Butterbur - Petasites Japonicus - T	Plant	11,000 ppm
Purslane, Verdolaga - Portulaca Oleracea - E	Herb	7,300 ppm
Spinach - Spinacia Oleracea - E	Plant	6,835 ppm
Alehoof - Glechoma Hederacea - M	Plant	1,100 ppm
Giant Knotweed, Hu-Zhang, Japanese Knotweed, Mexican Bamboo - Polygonum Cuspidatum - E - M - T	Plant	6,000 ppm
Oats - Avena Sativa - E - M	Plant	5,700 ppm
Black Pepper, Pepper, White Pepper - Piper Nigrum - E - M	Fruit	5,100 ppm
Chinese Polystichum - Polystichum Polyblepharum - T	Plant	4,700 ppm
Qian Hu - Peucedanum Decursivum - M	Plant	4,000 ppm
Snakegourd - Trichosanthes Anguina - E - M	Fruit	3,890 ppm
Wheat - Triticum Aestivum - E - M	Plant	3,400 ppm
Broadbean, Faba Bean, Habas - Vicia Faba - E	Fruit	2,945 ppm
Guinea Grass - Panicum Maximum - M	Leaf	0-5,600 ppm
European Nettle, Stinging Nettle - Urtica Dioica - E - M	Leaf	2,700 ppm
Oats - Avena Sativa - E - M	Seed	1,900 ppm
Wheat - Triticum Aestivum - E - M	Seed	1,800 ppm
Alholva, Bockshornklee, Fenugreek, Greek Clover, Greek Trigonella Foenum-Graecum - E - M	Leaf	1,650 ppm
Banana, Plantain - Musa x Paradisiaca - E	Fruit	1,250 ppm
Coconut, Coconut Palm - Cocos Nucifera - E	Seed	1,007 ppm
Indian Tamarind, Kilytree, Tamarind - Tamarindus Indica - M	Leaf	940 ppm
Red Currant, White Currant - Ribes Rubrum - E	Fruit	910 ppm
Chaparral, Creosote Bush - Larrea Tridentata - M	Plant	900 ppm
Gooseberry - Ribes Uva-Crispa - E	Fruit	882 ppm
Sweet Potato - Ipomoea Batatas - E	Root	850 ppm
Lentil - Lens Culinaris - E	Seed	636 ppm
Pea - Pisum Sativum - E	Seed	590 ppm
Aubergine, Egg Solanum Melongena - E	Fruit	520 ppm
Tomato - Lycopersicon Esculentum - E M T	Fruit	510 ppm
Alholva, Bockshornklee, Fenugreek, Greek Clover, Greek Trigonella Foenum-Graecum - E - M	Seed	500 ppm
Pineapple - Ananas Comosus - E	Fruit	460 ppm
Salsify - Tragopogon Porrifolius - E	Root	460 ppm
Pistachio - Pistacia Vera - E	Seed	408 ppm
Cotton - Gossypium spp. - - T	Seed	400 ppm
Lettuce - Lactuca Sativa - E	Leaf	395 ppm
Corn - Zea Mays - E	Fruit	330 ppm
Dog Rose, Dogbrier, Rose - Rosa Canina - E - M	Fruit	313 ppm
Date Palm - Phoenix Dactylifera - E	Fruit	310 ppm
Japanese Cinnamon - Cinnamomum Sieboldii - E - M - T	Root Bark	300 ppm
Ceylon Cinnamon, Cinnamon - Cinnamomum Verum - E - M - T	Bark	300 ppm
Green Gram, Mungbean - Vigna Radiata - E	Seed	278 ppm
Brazilnut, Brazilnut-Tree, Creamnut, Paranut - Bertholletia Eexcelsa - E	Seed	246 ppm
Aceituna Dulce, Jambolan, Java Plum - Syzygium Cumini - E	Fruit	80-490 ppm
English Walnut - Juglans Rregia - E	Seed	230 ppm

Species	Part	Quantity
Mango - Mangifera Indica - E - M	Fruit	205 ppm
Java Cinnamon, Padang Cassia - Cinnamomum Burmannii - E - M - T	Bark	200 ppm
Japanese Cinnamon - Cinnamomum Sieboldii - E - M - T	Bark	200 ppm
Soybean - Glycine Max - E	Seed	200 ppm
Cashew - Anacardium Occidentale - E	Seed	184 ppm
Buckwheat - Fagopyrum Esculentum - E	Seed	138 ppm
Pomarrosa, Rose Apple - Syzygium Jambos - E	Fruit	40-258 ppm
Mat Bean, Moth Bean - Vigna Aconitifolia - E	Seed	101 ppm
Black Gram - Vigna Mungo - E	Seed	101 ppm
Asparagus bean, Pea bean, Yardlong bean - Vigna Unguiculata subsp. Sesquipedalis - E	Seed	100 ppm
Butternut - Juglans Cinerea - E	Seed	78 ppm
Flax, Lin Linum Usitatissimum - E	Seed	78 ppm
Shagbark Hickory - Carya Ovata - E	Seed	71 ppm
Cassia, Cassia Bark, Cassia Lignea, China Junk Cassia, Chinazimt, Chinese Cassia - Cinnamomum Aromaticuminnamon- E - M - T	Bark	70 ppm
Black Walnut - Juglans Nigra - E	Seed	54 ppm
Northern Red Oak - Quercus Rubra - E - M	Seed	49 ppm
Pecan - Carya Illinoensis - E	Seed	46 ppm
Cobnut, English Filbert, European Filbert, European Hazel, Hazel - Corylus Avellana - E	Seed	41 ppm
Guavas - Psidium Guajava - E	Fruit	40 ppm
Orange - Citrus Sinensis - E	Fruit	32 ppm
Almond - Prunus Dulcis - E - M - T	Seed	28 ppm
Mandarin, Tangerine - Citrus Reticulata - E	Fruit	24 ppm
Pomegranate - Punica Granatum - E	Fruit	20 ppm
Potato - Solanum Tuberosum - E	Tuber	16 ppm
Grape Citrus Paradisi - E	Plant	6 ppm

PLANTS CONTAINING CHROMIUM

Species	Part	Quantity
Indian Sorrel, Jamaica Sorrel, Kharkadi, Red Sorrel, Sorrel - Hibiscus Sabdariffa - E	Flower	54 ppm
Dandelion - Taraxacum Officinale - E - M	Leaf	50 ppm
Oats - Avena Sativa - E - M	Plant	39 ppm
Indian Sorrel, Jamaica Sorrel, Stevia, Sweet Leaf of Paraguay - Stevia Rebaudiana - E	Leaf	39 ppm
Lemongrass, West indian lemongrass - Cymbopogon Citratus - E - M	Plant	37 ppm
ElytriCouchgrass, Doggrass, Quackgrass, Twitchgrass, Wheatgrass - Elytrigia Repens - E - M	Plant	37 ppm
Peach - Prunus Persica - E - M - T	Bark	35 ppm
Common Juniper, Juniper - Juniperus Communis - E - M - T	Fruit	32 ppm
Cowgrass, Peavine Clover, Purple Clover, Red Clover - Trifolium Pratense - E - M	Flower	32 ppm
SafCarthamus Tinctorius - M	Flower	31 ppm
Barley, Barleygrass - Hordeum Vulgare - E - M	Stem	31 ppm
Ajwan - Trachyspermum Ammi - E - M	Fruit	31 ppm
Damiana - Turnera Diffusa - M	Leaf	31 ppm
Cardamom - Elettaria Cardamomum - E - M	Fruit	29.5 ppm
Buchu, Honey Buchu, Mountain Buchu - Agathosma Betulina Buchu, Honey Buchu, Mountain Buchu - Agathosma Betulina - M	Leaf	29 ppm
Chinese Parsley, Cilantro, Coriander - Coriandrum Sativum E	Seed	28.8 ppm
Catnip - Nepeta Cataria - M	Plant	27 ppm
Dulse - Rhodymenia Palmata - E	Plant	27 ppm
Wild Yam - Dioscorea sp. - E	Root	26 ppm
Milfoil, Yarrow - Achillea Millefolium - M	Plant	25 ppm
Hydrangea, Smooth Hydrangea - Hydrangea Arborescens - E - M	Root	25 ppm
Box-Holly, Butcher's broom - Ruscus aculeatus - E - M	Root	25 ppm
Butterbur - Petasites Japonicus - T	Plant	23 ppm
Mugwort - Artemisia Vulgaris - M	Plant	22 ppm
Field Horsetail, Horsetail - Equisetum Arvense - M	Plant	22 ppm
Lady's Thistle, Milk Thistle - Silybum Marianum - M	Plant	22 ppm

CHROMIUM CONTINUED

Plant	Part	ppm
Crampbark, European Cranberry bush, Guelder Rose, Snowballbush - Viburnum Opulus - E - M - T	Bark	21 ppm
Burdock, Gobo, Great burdock - Arctium Lappa - M	Root	20 ppm
Lettuce - Lactuca Sativa - E	Leaf	20 ppm
Chinese Polystichum - Polystichum Polyblepharum - T	Plant	20 ppm
Common thyme, Garden thyme, Thyme - Thymus Vulgaris - E - M	Leaf	20 ppm
Ginger - Zingiber Officinale - E	Rhizome	20 ppm
Coneflower, Echinacea - Echinacea ssp - M	Root	19 ppm
European Mistletoe - Viscum Album - M - T	Leaf	19 ppm
White Mustard - Sinapis Alba - E - M - T	Seed	18.6 ppm
Black Cohosh, Black Snake Cimicifuga Racemosa - E - M	Root	18 ppm
Chinese Magnolia Vine, Five-Flavor-Fruit, Magnolia Vine, Schizandra, Wu Wei Zi, Wu Wei Zu - Schisandra Chinensis - M	Fruit	18 ppm
Common Valerian, Garden-Heliotrope, Valerian - Valeriana Officinalis - E - M	Root	18 ppm
Feverfew - Chrysanthemum Parthenium - M	Plant	17 ppm
English Hawthorn, Hawthorn, Whitethorn, Woodland Hawthorn - Crataegus Laevigata - M	Fruit	17 ppm
Pumpkin - Cucurbita Pepo - E	Seed	17 ppm
Commom Licorice, Licorice, Licorice-Root, Smooth Licorice - Glycyrrhiza Glabra - M	Root	17 ppm
European Pennyroyal - Mentha pulegium - E - M - T	Plant	17 ppm
Sarsaparilla - Smilax spp - E - M	Root	17 ppm
Mace, Nutmeg - Myristica Fragrans - E	Seed	16.4 ppm
Ramie - Boehmeria Nivea - M	Plant	16 ppm
Blessed Thistle - Cnicus Benedictus - M	Plant	16 ppm
Qian Hu - Peucedanum Decursivum - M	Plant	16 ppm
Caraway, Carum - Carum Carvi - E	Fruit	15.5 ppm
Garlic - Allium Sativum Bulb - E	Bulb	15 ppm
Marshmallow, White Mallow - Althaea Officinalis - M	Root	15 ppm
Bayberry, Candle-Berry, Southern Bayberry, Wax Myrtle - Myrica Cerifera - E - M	Bark	15 ppm
Ceylon Cinnamon, Cinnamon - Cinnamomum Verum - E - M - T	Leaf	14.4 ppm
Giant Knotweed, Hu-Zhang, Japanese Knotweed, Mexican Bamboo - Polygonum Cuspidatum - E - M - T	Plant	14 ppm
Flannelleaf, Flannelplant, Great mullein, Mullein, Velvet Verbascum Thapsus - M	Leaf	14 ppm
Opium Poppy, Poppyseed Poppy - Papaver Somniferum - E	Seed	13.4 ppm
Mace, Nutmeg - Myristica Fragrans - E	Aril	13.2 ppm
Gentian, Yellow Gentian - Gentiana Lutea - M	Root	13 ppm
Raspberry, Red raspberry - Rubus Idaeus - E - M	Leaf	13 ppm
Corn - Zea Mays - E	Silk Stigma Style	13 ppm
Bearberry, Uva Uursi - Arctostaphylos Uva-Ursi - M	Leaf	12 ppm
Barberry - Berberis Vulgaris - M	Root	12 ppm
Blue Cohosh - Caulophyllum Thalictroides - M	Root	12 ppm
Irish moss - Chondrus Crispus - E	Plant	12 ppm
Devil's claw, Grapple Harpagophytum procumbens - M	Root	12 ppm
Chinese Ginseng, Ginseng, Korean Ginseng, Oriental Ginseng - Panax Ginseng - M	Root	11 ppm
Chickweed, Common Chickweed - Stellaria Media - E	Plant	11 ppm
Smooth Sumac - Rhus Glabra - E - M	Stem	10.05 ppm
Gotu Kola, Pennywort - Centella Asiatica - E - M	Leaf	10 ppm
Ceylon Cinnamon, Cinnamon - Cinnamomum Verum - E - M - T	Bark	10 ppm
Ladyslipper - Cypripedium Pubescens - M	Root	10 ppm
Red Elm, Slippery Elm - Ulmus Rubra - M	Bark	10 ppm
Chinese Angelica, Dong Gui, Dong Quai - Angelica Sinensis - M	Root	9 ppm
Goldenseal - Hydrastis Canadensis - M	Root	9 ppm
Black Walnut - Juglans Nigra - E	Hull Husk	9 ppm

Alfalfa, Lucerne - Medicago Sativa subsp. Sativa - E	Plant	9 ppm
Pau D'Arco - Tabebuia Heptaphylla - M	Bark	9 ppm
Dandelion - Taraxacum Officinale - E - M	Root	9 ppm
European Grape, Grape, Grapevine, Vigne Vinifere, Wine Grape - Vitis Vinifera - E - M	Stem	9 ppm
Cabbage, Red Cabbage, White Cabbage - Brassica Oleracea var. Capitata - E	Leaf	8.7 ppm
Cumin - Cuminum Cyminum - E - M	Fruit	8.4 ppm
American Styrax, Sweetgum - Liquidambar Styraciflua - E - M	Leaf	8.2 ppm
Chaparral, Creosote Bush - Larrea Tridentata - M	Bark	8 ppm
Psyllium - Plantago Psyllium - E - M	Seed	8 ppm
Comfrey - Symphytum Officinale - E - M - T	Root	8 ppm
Eyebright - Euphrasia Officinalis - M	Plant	7 ppm
Bladderwrack, Kelp - Fucus Vesiculosus - E - M	Plant	7 ppm
Hops - Humulus Lupulus - E - M - T	Fruit	7 ppm
Mad-Dog Skullcap, Scullcap - Scutellaria lateriflora - M	Plant	7 ppm
Black Gum, Black Tupelo - Nyssa Sylvatica - E - M	Leaf	6.37 ppm
Buckbush - Symphoricarpos Orbiculatus - M	Stem	6.16 ppm
Garden Camomile, Perennial Camomile, Roman Camomile - Chamaemelum Nobile M	Flower	6 ppm
Indian Saffron, Turmeric - Curcuma Longa - E	Rhizome	6 ppm
Cascara Buckthorn, Cascara Sagrada - Frangula Purshiana - M	Bark	6 ppm
Red Pignut Hickory - Carya Glabra - E	Shoot	5.5 ppm
White Oak - Quercus Alba - M	Stem	5.32 ppm
Fennel - Foeniculum Vulgare - M	Fruit	5 ppm
Indian Tobacco, Lobelia - Lobelia Inflata - M - T	Leaf	5 ppm
Butter Bean, Lima Bean - Phaseolus Lunatus - E	Seed	5 ppm
Allspice, Clover-Pepper, Jamaica-Pepper, Pimenta, Pimento - Pimenta Dioica - E	Plant	5 ppm
Clove, Clovetree - Syzygium Aromaticum - E	Flower	5 ppm
Black bean, Dwarf bean, Field bean, Flageolet bean, French bean, Garden bean, Green bean, Haricot, Haricot bean, Haricot vert, Kidney bean, Navy bean, Pop bean, Popping bean, Snap bean, String bean, Wax bean - Phaseolus Vulgaris - E	Seed	4.9 ppm
Onion, Shallot - Allium Cepa - Shallot Bulb - E	Seed	4.8 ppm
Black Gum, Black Tupelo - Nyssa Sylvatica - E - M	Stem	4.4 ppm
Onion, Shallot - Allium Cepa - Shallot Bulb - E	Bulb	4 ppm
Alehoof - Glechoma Hederacea - M	Plant	4 ppm
Alholva, Bockshornklee, Fenugreek, Greek Clover, Greek Trigonella Foenum-Graecum - E - M	Seed	4 ppm
Coca - Erythroxylum Coca var. Coca - E - M	Leaf	3.8 ppm
American Styrax, Sweetgum - Liquidambar Styraciflua - E - M	Stem	3.6 ppm
Asparagus bean, Pea bean, Yardlong bean - Vigna Unguiculata subsp. Sesquipedalis - E	Seed	3.6 ppm
Cayenne, Chili, Hot Pepper, Red Chili, Spur Pepper, Tabasco - Capsicum Frutescens - E	Fruit	3.5 ppm
Black Pepper, Pepper, White Pepper - Piper Nigrum - E - M	Fruit	3.5 ppm
Northern Red Oak - Quercus Rubra - E - M	Stem	3.3 ppm
Japanese Cinnamon - Cinnamomum Sieboldii - E - M - T	Root Bark	3 ppm
Tomato - Lycopersicon Esculentum - E - M - T	Fruit	3 ppm
White Oak - Quercus Alba - M	Bark	3 ppm
Sage - Salvia Officinalis - E - M	Leaf	3 ppm
Black Cherry, Wild Cherry - Prunus Serotina - E - M - T	Leaf	2.88 ppm
Sarson - Brassica Rapa - E	Seed	2.8 ppm
Shagbark Hickory - Carya Ovata - E	Shoot	2.7 ppm
American Persimmon - Diospyros Virginiana - E - M	Stem	2.7 ppm
Red Cedar - Juniperus Virginiana Amphicarpaea Bracteata - E - M - T	Shoot	2.64 ppm
Sassafras - Sassafras Albidum - E - M - T	Stem	2.59 ppm
Peach - Prunus Persica - E - M - T	Fruit	2.25 ppm
Sassafras - Sassafras Albidum - E - M - T	Leaf	2.04 ppm

CHROMIUM CONTINUED

Species	Part	Quantity
Dwarf Sumac, Winged Sumac - Rhus Copallina - E - M	Leaf	1.92 ppm
Black Oak - Quercus Velutina - E - M	Stem	1.73 ppm
Almond - Prunus Dulcis - E - M - T	Seed	1.7 ppm
Post Oak - Quercus Stellata - E - M	Stem	1.68 ppm
Corn - Zea Mays - E	Seed	1.65 ppm
Shagbark Hickory - Carya Ovata - E	Seed	1.6 ppm
Carrot - Daucus Carota - E	Root	1.5 ppm
Black bean, Dwarf bean, Field bean, Flageolet bean, French bean, Garden bean, Green bean, Haricot, Haricot bean, Haricot vert, Kidney bean, Navy bean, Pop bean, Popping bean, Snap bean, String bean, Wax bean - Phaseolus Vulgaris - E	Fruit	1.5 ppm
Butternut - Juglans Cinerea - E	Seed	1.4 ppm
Sesame - Sesamum Indicum - E - M	Seed	1.4 ppm
Potato - Solanum Tuberosum - E	Tuber	1.4 ppm
Shortleaf Pine - Pinus Echinata - M	Shoot	1.26 ppm
Dwarf Sumac, Winged Sumac - Rhus Copallina - E - M	Stem	1.22 ppm
Plum - Prunus Domestica - E - M	Fruit	1.19 ppm
Cassia, Cassia Bark, Cassia Lignea, China Junk Cassia, Chinazimt, Chinese Cassia - Cinnamomum Aromaticuminnamon- E - M - T	Bark	1 ppm
American Persimmon - Diospyros Virginiana - E - M	Leaf	1 ppm
Black Walnut - Juglans Nigra - E	Seed	1 ppm
European Nettle, Stinging Nettle - Urtica Dioica - E - M	Leaf	1 ppm

PLANTS CONTAINING COBALT

Species	Part	Quantity
Black Gum, Black Tupelo - Nyssa Sylvatica - E - M	Leaf	910 ppm
Goldenseal - Hydrastis Canadensis - M	Root	153 ppm
Sarsaparilla - Smilax spp - E - M	Root	152 ppm
Chinese Angelica, Dong Gui, Dong Quai - Angelica Sinensis - M	Root	151 ppm
Pau D'Arco - Tabebuia Heptaphylla - M	Bark	151 ppm
Dulse - Rhodymenia Palmata - E	Plant	150 ppm
Coneflower, Echinacea - Echinacea ssp - M	Root	148 ppm
Wild Yam - Dioscorea sp. - E	Root	147 ppm
Eyebright - Euphrasia Officinalis - M	Plant	147 ppm
Devil's claw, Grapple - Harpagophytum procumbens - M	Root	145 ppm
Chinese Cornbind, Chinese Knotweed, Fleeceflower, Fo Ti, He Shou Wu - Polygonum Multiflorum - E - M - T	Root	145 ppm
Pumpkin - Cucurbita Pepo - E	Seed	143 ppm
Comfrey - Symphytum Officinale - E - M - T	Root	129 ppm
Damiana - Turnera Diffusa - M	Leaf	129 ppm
Box-Holly, Butcher's broom - Ruscus aculeatus - E - M	Root	128 ppm
Flannelleaf, Flannelplant, Great mullein, Mullein, Velvet - Verbascum Thapsus - M	Leaf	128 ppm
Devil's Tongue, Elephant Yam, Konjac, Leopard Palm, Snake Palm, Umbrella Arum - Amorphophallus Konjac - E - M - T	Root	125 ppm
Common Juniper, Juniper - Juniperus Communis - E - M - T	Fruit	123 ppm
Chickweed, Common Chickweed - Stellaria Media - E	Plant	121 ppm
Burdock, Gobo, Great Burdock - Arctium lappa - E - M - T	Root	120 ppm
Catnip - Nepeta Cataria - M	Plant	118 ppm
Cascara Buckthorn, Cascara Sagrada - Frangula Purshiana - M	Bark	116 ppm
Alfalfa, Lucerne - Medicago Sativa subsp. Sativa - E	Plant	115 ppm
Crampbark, European Cranberry bush, Guelder Rose, Snowballbush - Viburnum Opulus - E - M - T	Bark	115 ppm
Common thyme, Garden thyme, Thyme - Thymus Vulgaris - E - M	Leaf	113 ppm
Chinese Magnolia Vine, Five-Flavor-Fruit, Magnolia Vine, Schizandra, Wu Wei Zi, Wu Wei Zu - Schisandra Chinensis - M	Fruit	104 ppm
Commom Licorice, Licorice, Licorice-Root, Smooth Licorice - Glycyrrhiza Glabra - M	Root	101 ppm

Plant	Part	ppm
Garlic - Allium Sativum Bulb - E	Bulb	100 ppm
American Persimmon - Diospyros Virginiana - E - M	Leaf	100 ppm
White Willow - Salix Alba - M	Bark	98 ppm
Chaparral, Creosote Bush - Larrea Tridentata - M	Bark	93 ppm
Peppermint - Mentha x Piperita subsp. Nothosubsp. Piperita - E - M - T	Leaf	93 ppm
European Mistletoe - Viscum Album - M - T	Leaf	92 ppm
Buchu, Honey Buchu, Mountain Buchu - Agathosma Betulina Buchu, Honey Buchu, Mountain Buchu - Agathosma Betulina - M	Leaf	87 ppm
Dandelion - Taraxacum Officinale - E - M	Root	80 ppm
Gotu Kola, Pennywort - Centella Asiatica - E - M	Leaf	73 ppm
Irish moss - Chondrus Crispus - E	Plant	70 ppm
Black Gum, Black Tupelo - Nyssa Sylvatica - E - M	Stem	66 ppm
Corn - Zea Mays - E	Silk Stigma Style	64 ppm
Garden Camomile, Perennial Camomile, Roman Camomile - Chamaemelum Nobile M	Flower	58 ppm
American Persimmon - Diospyros Virginiana - E - M	Stem	54 ppm
Field Horsetail, Horsetail - Equisetum Arvense - M	Plant	53 ppm
Barley, Barleygrass - Hordeum Vulgare - E - M	Stem	49 ppm
Lemongrass, West indian lemongrass - Cymbopogon Citratus - E - M	Plant	48 ppm
Common Valerian, Garden-Heliotrope, Valerian - Valeriana Officinalis - E - M	Root	48 ppm
Barberry - Berberis Vulgaris - M	Root	42 ppm
Ginger - Zingiber Officinale - E	Rhizome	42 ppm
Lady's Thistle, Milk Thistle - Silybum Marianum - M	Plant	41 ppm
Chinese Ephedra, Ma Huang - Ephedra Sinica - M	Plant	40 ppm
Black Cohosh, Black Snake - Cimicifuga Racemosa - E - M	Root	38 ppm
Blessed Thistle - Cnicus Benedictus - M	Plant	38 ppm
Indian Sorrel, Jamaica Sorrel, Kharkadi, Red Sorrel, Sorrel - Hibiscus Sabdariffa - E	Flower	38 ppm
Hydrangea, Smooth Hydrangea - Hydrangea Arborescens - E - M	Root	38 ppm
Blue Cohosh - Caulophyllum Thalictroides - M	Root	36 ppm
Black Walnut - Juglans Nigra - E	Fruit	36 ppm
Bayberry, Candle-Berry, Southern Bayberry, Wax Myrtle - Myrica Cerifera - E - M	Bark	35 ppm
Curly Dock, Lengua De Vaca, Sour Dock, Yellow Dock - Rumex Crispus - M - T	Root	35 ppm
Raspberry, Red raspberry - Rubus Idaeus - E - M	Leaf	34 ppm
Marshmallow, White Mallow - Althaea Officinalis - M	Root	33 ppm
European Grape, Grape, Grapevine, Vigne Vinifere, Wine Grape - Vitis Vinifera - E - M	Stem	33 ppm
Milfoil, Yarrow - Achillea Millefolium - M	Plant	31 ppm
Fennel - Foeniculum Vulgare - M	Fruit	31 ppm
Chinese Ginseng, Ginseng, Korean Ginseng, Oriental Ginseng - Panax Ginseng - M	Root	31 ppm
SafCarthamus Tinctorius - M	Flower	26 ppm
Psyllium - Plantago Psyllium - E - M	Seed	25 ppm
Indian Sorrel, Jamaica Sorrel, Stevia, Sweet Leaf of Paraguay - Stevia Rebaudiana - E	Leaf	25 ppm
Hops - Humulus Lupulus - E - M - T	Fruit	24 ppm
Indian Tobacco, Lobelia - Lobelia Inflata - M - T	Leaf	22 ppm
English Hawthorn, Hawthorn, Whitethorn, Woodland Hawthorn - Crataegus Laevigata - M	Fruit	20 ppm
Peach - Prunus Persica - E - M - T	Bark	20 ppm
ElytriCouchgrass, Doggrass, Quackgrass, Twitchgrass, Wheatgrass - Elytrigia Repens - E - M	Plant	18 ppm
Cowgrass, Peavine Clover, Purple Clover, Red Clover - Trifolium Pratense - E - M	Flower	18 ppm
Alholva, Bockshornklee, Fenugreek, Greek Clover, Greek - Trigonella Foenum-Graecum - E - M	Seed	18 ppm
Red Elm, Slippery Elm - Ulmus Rubra - M	Bark	18 ppm

COBALT CONTINUED

Species	Part	Quantity
Bearberry, Uva Uursi - Arctostaphylos Uva-Ursi - M	Leaf	17 ppm
Red Pignut Hickory - Carya Glabra - E	Shoot	16.5 ppm
Bladderwrack, Kelp - Fucus Vesiculosus - E - M	Plant	16 ppm
Gentian, Yellow Gentian - Gentiana Lutea - M	Root	14 ppm
European Pennyroyal - Mentha pulegium - E - M- T	Plant	14 ppm
Shagbark Hickory - Carya Ovata - E	Shoot	13.5 ppm
Banana Yucca, Blue Yucca, Spanish Bayonet, Yucca - Yucca Baccata - E - M - T	Root	12 ppm
Mad-Dog Skullcap, Scullcap - Scutellaria lateriflora - M	Plant	11 ppm
Black bean, Dwarf bean, Field bean, Flageolet bean, French bean, Garden bean, Green bean, Haricot, Haricot bean, Haricot vert, Kidney bean, Navy bean, Pop bean, Popping bean, Snap bean, String bean, Wax bean - Phaseolus Vulgaris - E	Fruit	10.5 ppm
White Oak - Quercus Alba - M	Bark	9.2 ppm
Ladyslipper - Cypripedium Pubescens - M	Root	9 ppm
Black Cherry, Wild Cherry - Prunus Serotina - E - M - T	Stem	5.4 ppm
White Oak - Quercus Alba - M	Stem	5.32 ppm
Red Mangrove - Rhizophora Mangle - M	Leaf	5 ppm
American Styrax, Sweetgum - Liquidambar Styraciflua - E - M	Stem	3.6 ppm
Northern Red Oak - Quercus Rubra - E - M	Stem	3.3 ppm
Cabbage, Red Cabbage, White Cabbage - Brassica Oleracea var. Capitata - E	Leaf	2.9 ppm
Onion, Shallot - Allium Cepa - Shallot Bulb - E	Seed	2.5 ppm
Buckbush - Symphoricarpos Orbiculatus - M	Stem	2.4 ppm
Black Oak - Quercus Velutina - E - M	Stem	2.29 ppm
Cumin - Cuminum Cyminum - E - M	Fruit	2.2 ppm
Strawberry - Fragaria spp. - E	Fruit	2 ppm
Brazilnut, Brazilnut-Tree, Creamnut, Paranut - Bertholletia Eexcelsa - E	Seed	1.9 ppm
Tomato - Lycopersicon Esculentum - E - M - T	Fruit	1.4 ppm
Red Cedar - Juniperus Virginiana Amphicarpaea Bracteata- E - M - T	Shoot	1.32 ppm
Shortleaf Pine - Pinus Echinata - M	Shoot	1.26 ppm
Spinach - Spinacia Oleracea - E	Plant	1.2 ppm
Asparagus bean, Pea bean, Yardlong bean - Vigna Unguiculata subsp. Sesquipedalis - E	Seed	1.2 ppm
Ceylon Cinnamon, Cinnamon - Cinnamomum Verum - E - M - T	Leaf	1.1 ppm
White Mustard - Sinapis Alba - E - M - T	Seed	1.1 ppm
Black bean, Dwarf bean, Field bean, Flageolet bean, French bean, Garden bean, Green bean, Haricot, Haricot bean, Haricot vert, Kidney bean, Navy bean, Pop bean, Popping bean, Snap bean, String bean, Wax bean - Phaseolus Vulgaris - E	Seed	1.05 ppm
Caraway, Carum - Carum Carvi - E	Fruit	1 ppm
Indian Saffron, Turmeric - Curcuma Longa - E	Rhizome	1 ppm
Butter Bean, Lima Bean - Phaseolus Lunatus - E	Seed	1 ppm

PLANTS CONTAINING COPPER

Species	Part	Quantity
Black Cherry, Wild Cherry - Prunus Serotina - E - M - T	Stem	378 ppm
American Styrax, Sweetgum - Liquidambar Styraciflua - E - M	Stem	360 ppm
Black Gum, Black Tupelo - Nyssa Sylvatica - E - M	Leaf	182 ppm
American Styrax, Sweetgum - Liquidambar Styraciflua - E - M	Leaf	164 ppm
Buckbush - Symphoricarpos Orbiculatus - M	Stem	132 ppm
American Persimmon - Diospyros Virginiana - E - M	Stem	108 ppm
Sassafras - Sassafras Albidum - E - M - T	Leaf	102 ppm
Tomato - Lycopersicon Esculentum - E - M - T	Fruit	100 ppm
Cabbage, Red Cabbage, White Cabbage - Brassica Oleracea var. Capitata - E	Leaf	87 ppm
Cobnut, English Filbert, European Filbert, European Hazel, Hazel - Corylus Avellana - E	Seed	82 ppm
Sassafras - Sassafras Albidum - E - M - T	Stem	56 ppm
Sesame - Sesamum Indicum - E - M	Plant	56 ppm
Red Pignut Hickory - Carya Glabra - E	Shoot	55 ppm

Cauli Brassica Oleracea var. Botrytis - E	Leaf	52 ppm
Shagbark Hickory - Carya Ovata - E	Shoot	45 ppm
Black bean, Dwarf bean, Field bean, Flageolet bean, French bean, Garden bean, Green bean, Haricot, Haricot bean, Haricot vert, Kidney bean, Navy bean, Pop bean, Popping bean, Snap bean, String bean, Wax bean - Phaseolus Vulgaris - E	Fruit	45 ppm
Collards, Cow Cabbage, Spring-Heading Cabbage, Tall Kale, Tree Kale - Brassica Oleracea - E	Leaf	43 ppm
Cucumber - Cucumis Sativus - E	Fruit	42 ppm
Post Oak - Quercus Stellata - E - M	Stem	42 ppm
Cashew - Anacardium Occidentale - E	Seed	37 ppm
Dog Rose, Dogbrier, Rose - Rosa Canina - E - M	Fruit	36 ppm
Red Mangrove - Rhizophora Mangle - M	Leaf	35 ppm
Plum - Prunus Domestica - E - M	Fruit	34 ppm
Coconut, Coconut Palm - Cocos Nucifera - E	Seed	33 ppm
Pistachio - Pistacia Vera - E	Seed	33 ppm
Asparagus Pea, Goa Bean, Winged Bean - Psophocarpus Tetragonolobus - E	Seed	33 ppm
Sicklepod - Senna Obtusifolia - E - T	Seed	32 ppm
Black Gum, Black Tupelo - Nyssa Sylvatica - E - M	Stem	31 ppm
Black Oak - Quercus Velutina - E - M	Stem	31 ppm
Pumpkin - Cucurbita Maxima - E	Leaf	30 ppm
Jerusalem Artichoke - Helianthus Tuberosus E	Plant	30 ppm
Bitter Melon, Sorosi - Momordica Charantia - E	Fruit	30 ppm
Peach - Prunus Persica - E - M - T	Fruit	30 ppm
Dwarf Sumac, Winged Sumac - Rhus Copallina - E - M	Stem	30 ppm
Garden Sorrel - Rumex Acetosa - E - M - T	Leaf	30 ppm
Burdock, Gobo, Great Burdock - Arctium lappa - E - M - T	Root	29 ppm
Lettuce - Lactuca Sativa - E	Leaf	29 ppm
Black Cherry, Wild Cherry - Prunus Serotina - E - M - T	Leaf	29 ppm
Willow Oak - Quercus Phellos - E - M	Stem	29 ppm
SafCarthamus Tinctorius - M	Flower	26 ppm
Dokudami, Fishwort, Yu Xing Cao - Houttuynia Cordata - E - M	Plant	26 ppm
Henbane - Hyoscyamus Niger - E - M	Seed	26 ppm
Oats - Avena Sativa - E - M	Seed	25.7 ppm
Mace, Nutmeg - Myristica Fragrans - E	Aril	25 ppm
Yambean - Pachyrhizus Erosus - E	Tuber	25 ppm
Asparagus - Asparagus Officinalis - E	Shoot	24 ppm
Chinese Quince, Mu-Kua - Chaenomeles Lagenaria - E	Fruit	24 ppm
Artichoke - Cynara Cardunculus - E	Flower	24 ppm
Fennel - Foeniculum Vulgare - M	Fruit	24 ppm
Spinach - Spinacia Oleracea - E	Plant	24 ppm
Cacao - Theobroma Ccacao - E	Seed	24 ppm
Gennoshiouko, Oriental Geranium - Geranium Thunbergii - E - M	Plant	23 ppm
Opium Poppy, Poppyseed Poppy - Papaver Somniferum - E	Seed	23 ppm
Ching-Chieh, Jing-Jie - Schizonepeta Tenuifolia - E - M	Plant	23 ppm
Green Gram, Mungbean - Vigna Radiata - E	Sprout Seedling	23 ppm
Manioc Hibiscus - Abelmoschus Manihot - E - M	Leaf	21.5 ppm
Mace, Nutmeg - Myristica Fragrans - E	Seed	21 ppm
Indian Tamarind, Kilytree, Tamarind - Tamarindus Indica - M	Leaf	21 ppm
Mugwort - Artemisia Vulgaris - M	Plant	20 ppm
Curly Kale, Kale, Kitchen Kale, Scotch Kale - Brassica Oleracea var. Sabellica l. var. Acephala - E	Leaf	20 ppm
Tea - Camellia Sinensis - E	Leaf	20 ppm
Bell Pepper, Cherry Pepper, Cone Pepper, Green Pepper, Paprika, Sweet Pepper - Capsicum Annuum - E	Fruit	20 ppm
Barley, Barleygrass - Hordeum Vulgare - E - M	Seed	20 ppm
Cornmint, Field Mint, Japanese Mint - Mentha Arvensis var. Piperascens - E - M- T	Plant	20 ppm
Black Pepper, Pepper, White Pepper - Piper Nigrum - E - M	Fruit	20 ppm
Smooth Sumac - Rhus Glabra - E - M	Stem	20 ppm

COPPER CONTINUED

Name	Part	ppm
Aubergine, Egg Solanum Melongena - E	Fruit	20 ppm
Snakegourd - Trichosanthes Anguina - E - M	Fruit	20 ppm
Coltsfoot - Tussilago Farfara - M - T	Flower	20 ppm
Corn - Zea Mays - E	Fruit	20 ppm
Pigweed - Amaranthus sp. - E - M	Leaf	19 ppm
Lian-Jiao, Lien-Chiao - Forsythia Suspensa - M	Fruit	19 ppm
Girasol, Sun Helianthus Annuus - E	Seed	19 ppm
Swamp Cabbage, Water Spinach - Ipomoea Aquatica - E	Leaf	19 ppm
Black Walnut - Juglans Nigra - E	Seed	19 ppm
Purslane, Verdolaga - Portulaca Oleracea - E	Herb	19 ppm
Dwarf Sumac, Winged Sumac - Rhus Copallina - E - M	Leaf	19 ppm
Mongoloid Dandelion - Taraxacum Mongolicum - E - M	Plant	19 ppm
Onion, Shallot - Allium Cepa - Shallot Bulb - E	Seed	18.2 ppm
Bai-Zhu, Pai-Chu - Atractylodes Ovata - M	Rhizome	18 ppm
Brazilnut, Brazilnut-Tree, Creamnut, Paranut - Bertholletia Eexcelsa - E	Seed	18 ppm
Chinese Parsley, Cilantro, Coriander - Coriandrum Sativum E	Leaf	18 ppm
Carrot - Daucus Carota - E	Root	18 ppm
Japanese Gentian - Gentiana Scabra - E	Root	18 ppm
Soybean - Glycine Max - E	Seed	18 ppm
Baikal Skullcap, Chinese Skullcap, Huang Qin - Scutellaria Baicalensis - M	Root	18 ppm
Cowgrass, Peavine Clover, Purple Clover, Red Clover - Trifolium Pratense - E - M	Hay	18 ppm
Red Cedar - Juniperus Virginiana Amphicarpaea Bracteata- E - M - T	Shoot	17.6 ppm
Jack Na Bush - Eupatorium Odoratum - M	Leaf	0-35 ppm
Dill, Garden Dill - Anethum Graveolens - E	Plant	17 ppm
Beet, Beetroot, Garden Beet, Sugar Beet - Beta Vulgaris - E	Root	17 ppm
Chinese Goldthread, Huang-Lian, Huang-Lien - Coptis Chinensis - M	Rhizome	17 ppm
Huang-Lia, Huang-Lian, Huang-Lien, Japanese Goldthread - Coptis Japonica - M	Rhizome	17 ppm
Generic Goldthread - Coptis spp. - M	Rhizome	17 ppm
Indian Saffron, Turmeric - Curcuma Longa - E	Rhizome	17 ppm
Strawberry - Fragaria spp. - E	Fruit	17 ppm
Chinese Boxthorn, Chinese Matrimony Vine, Chinese Wolfberry - Lycium Chinense - E - M	Root Bark	17 ppm
Water Lotus - Nelumbo Nucifera - E - M	Seed	17 ppm
Chinese Ginseng, Ginseng, Korean Ginseng, Oriental Ginseng - Panax Ginseng - M	Root	17 ppm
Perilla - Perilla Frutescens - E - M - T	Plant	17 ppm
Endive, Escarole - Cichorium Endivia - M	Leaf	16.8 ppm
Wheat - Triticum Aestivum - E - M	Seed	16.7 ppm
Mango - Mangifera Indica - E - M	Fruit	16.6 ppm
Chai-Hu - Bupleurum - M	Root	16 ppm
Cumin - Cuminum Cyminum - E - M	Fruit	16 ppm
Wou Chou Yu - Euodia Rutaecarpa - E	Fruit	16 ppm
Bonavist Bean, Hyacinth Bean, Lablab Bean - Lablab Purpureus - E - M - T	Seed	16 ppm
Hsin-I, Xin-Yi - Magnolia Denudata - E - M	Flower	16 ppm
Hsin-I, Xin-Yi - Magnolia Fargesii - E - M	Flower	16 ppm
Magnolia kobus DC. -- Hsin-I, Xin-Yi	Flower	16 ppm
Butterbur - Petasites Japonicus - T	Plant	16 ppm
Tomatillo - Physalis Ixocarpa - E	Fruit	16 ppm
Apricot - Prunus Armeniaca - E - M - T	Seed	16 ppm
Ching-Feng-Teng - Sinomenium Acutum - E - M	Rhizome	16 ppm
Ginger - Zingiber Officinale - E	Rhizome	16 ppm
Cardamom - Elettaria Cardamomum - E - M	Fruit	15.4 ppm
White Oak - Quercus Alba - M	Stem	15.2 ppm
Mud Plantain, Tse-Hsieh, Water Plantain, Ze-Xie - Alisma Plantago-Aquatica - M	Rhizome	15 ppm
Betel Nut, Pin-Lang - Areca Catechu Amphicarpaea Bracteata- E - M	Seed	15 ppm
Pecan - Carya Illinoensis - E	Seed	15 ppm
Pumpkin - Cucurbita Pepo - E	Seed	15 ppm
Chinese Parasol - Firmiana Simplex - E - M	Seed	15 ppm
Bei Sha Shen - Glehnia Littoralis - E - M	Root	15 ppm

Jussiaeae Herba, Pond Dragon - Jussiaea Repens - M	Plant	15 ppm
Chinese Boxthorn, Chinese Matrimony Vine, Chinese Wolfberry - Lycium Chinense - E - M	Fruit	15 ppm
Butter Bean, Lima Bean - Phaseolus Lunatus - E	Seed	15 ppm
Black bean, Dwarf bean, Field bean, Flageolet bean, French bean, Garden bean, Green bean, Haricot, Haricot bean, Haricot vert, Kidney bean, Navy bean, Pop bean, Popping bean, Snap bean, String bean, Wax bean - Phaseolus Vulgaris - E	Seed	15 ppm
Madder - Rubia Cordifolia - M	Root	15 ppm
Coffee Senna - Senna Occidentalis - E - T	Seed	15 ppm
European Nettle, Stinging Nettle - Urtica Dioica - E - M	Leaf	15 ppm
Wu Chia Pi - Acanthopanax Gracilistylis - M	Root Bark	14 ppm
Celery - Apium Graveolens - E	Seed	14 ppm
Chinese Birthwort - Aristolochia Debilis - E - M - T	Fruit	14 ppm
Desert Wormwood - Artemisia Herba-Alba - M	Plant	14 ppm
Asian Wild Ginger - Asiasarum Heterotropoides - M	Root	14 ppm
Siebold's Wild Ginger - Asiasarum Sieboldii - M	Root	14 ppm
Mustard Greens - Brassica Juncea - E	Leaf	14 ppm
Cayenne, Chili, Hot Pepper, Red Chili, Spur Pepper, Tabasco - Capsicum Frutescens - E	Fruit	14 ppm
Chinese Licorice - Glycyrrhiza Uralensis - M	Root	14 ppm
Basil, Cuban Basil, Sweet Basil - Ocimum Basilicum - E	Leaf	14 ppm
Emblic, Myrobalan - Phyllanthus Emblica - E	Fruit	14 ppm
Asian Plantain - Plantago Asiatica E M	Plant	14 ppm
Potato - Solanum Tuberosum - E	Tuber	14 ppm
Malanga, Tannia, Yautia - Xanthosoma Sagittifolium - E	Root	14 ppm
Caraway, Carum - Carum Carvi - E	Fruit	13.8 ppm
Northern Red Oak - Quercus Rubra - E - M	Stem	13.2 ppm
Ramie - Boehmeria Nivea - M	Plant	13 ppm
Chinese Parsley, Cilantro, Coriander - Coriandrum Sativum E	Fruit	13 ppm
Coca - Erythroxylum Coca var. Coca - E - M	Leaf	13 ppm
Cape Jasmine, Gardenia, Jasmin, Shan-Chih-Tzu, Shan-Zhi-Zi, Zhi Zi - Gardenia Jasminoides - M	Fruit	13 ppm
Japanese Honeysuckle - Lonicera Japonica - M	Flower	13 ppm
Climbing Fern - Lygodium Japonicum - Pollen or Spore - M	Pollen Or Spore	13 ppm
Evening-Primrose - Oenothera Biennis - E - M	Seed	13 ppm
American Ginseng, Ginseng - Panax Quinquefolius - M	Plant	13 ppm
Chinese Kudzu - Pueraria Pseudohirsuta - E - M	Root	13 ppm
Rangoon Creeper - Quisqualis Indica - E - T	Fruit	13 ppm
Adzuki Bean - Vigna Angularis - E	Seed	13 ppm
Green Gram, Mungbean - Vigna Radiata - E	Seed	13 ppm
Aconite, Fu-Tsu - Aconitum Carmichaelii - E - M	Tuber	12 ppm
Cang Zhu - Atractylodes Lancea - M	Rhizome	12 ppm
Hardy Orchid, Hyacinth Bletilla, Hyacinth Orchid, Shiran - Bletilla Striata - M	Tuber	12 ppm
Paper Mulberry - Broussonetia Papyrifera - E - M	Fruit	12 ppm
Pigeonpea - Cajanus Vajan - E	Seed	12 ppm
Summer Squash - Cucurbita spp. - E	Fruit	12 ppm
Bai-Wei, Pai-Wei - Cynanchum Atratum - E - M	Root	12 ppm
Bei-Mu, Fritillary - Fritillaria Thunbergii - Blub - E - M	Bulb	12 ppm
Lentil - Lens Culinaris - E	Sprout Seedling	12 ppm
Japanese Privet, Ligustri Fructus - Ligustrum Japonicum - M	Fruit	12 ppm
Chinese Privet, Glossy Privet, Ligustri Fructus, Privet, White Waxtree - Ligustrum Lucidum - M	Fruit	12 ppm
White Lupine - Lupinus Albus - M - T	Seed	12 ppm
Parsnip - Pastinaca Sativa - E	Root	12 ppm
Parsley - Petroselinum Crispum - E	Plant	12 ppm
Chinese Raspberry - Rubus Cchingii - E - M	Fruit	12 ppm
Dandelion - Taraxacum Officinale - E - M	Leaf	12 ppm

COPPER CONTINUED

Name	Part	ppm
Grapevine, Vigne Vinifere, Wine Grape - Vitis Vinifera - E - M		11.6 ppm
Guanique - Chamissoa Altissima - M	Leaf	2-23 ppm
Black Mustard - Brassica Nigra - E	Leaf	11.2 ppm
White Tephrosia - Tephrosia Candida - M - T	Plant	11.2 ppm
Pear - Pyrus Communis - E	Fruit	11.1 ppm
Chaff Achyranthes Bidentata - M	Root	11 ppm
Onion, Shallot - Allium Cepa - Shallot Bulb - E	Bulb	11 ppm
Celery - Apium Graveolens - E	Root	11 ppm
Groundnut, Peanut - Arachis Hypogaea - E - M	Seed	11 ppm
Alehoof - Glechoma Hederacea - M	Plant	11 ppm
Marjoram, Sweet Marjoram - Origanum Majorana - E	Plant	11 ppm
Avocado - Persea Americana - E - M - T	Fruit	11 ppm
Cape Gooseberry, Ground Cherry - Physalis Peruviana - E	Fruit	11 ppm
Almond - Prunus Dulcis - E - M - T	Seed	11 ppm
Chinese Magnolia Vine, Five-Flavor-Fruit, Magnolia Vine, Schizandra, Wu Wei Zi, Wu Wei Zu - Schisandra Chinensis - M	Fruit	11 ppm
Alholva, Bockshornklee, Fenugreek, Greek Clover, Greek Trigonella Foenum-Graecum - E - M	Seed	11 ppm
Ceylon Cinnamon, Cinnamon - Cinnamomum Verum - E - M - T	Leaf	10.9 ppm
Greater Yam, Winged Yam - Dioscorea Alata - E	Root	10.7 ppm
Amphicarpaea Bracteata - E - M	Shoot	0-20 ppm
Bai Zhi - Angelica Dahurica - M	Root	10 ppm
Sickle Senna - Cassia Tora - Sprout - Seedling - M	Seed	10 ppm
Chickpea, Garbanzo - Cicer Arietinum - E	Seed	10 ppm
Cassia, Cassia Bark, Cassia Lignea, China Junk Cassia, Chinazimt, Chinese Cassia - Cinnamomum Aromaticuminnamon - E - M - T	Bark	10 ppm
Bitter Orange, Petitgrain - Citrus Aurantium - E	Fruit	10 ppm
Nutsedge - Cyperus Rotundus - E - M	Rhizome	10 ppm
Fortune's Fern - Drynaria Fortunei - M	Rhizome	10 ppm
Dyer's Woad - Isatis Tinctoria - M	Root	10 ppm
Chinese Spikenard - Nardostachys Chinensis - M	Rhizome	10 ppm
Qian Hu - Peucedanum Decursivum - M	Plant	10 ppm
Allspice, Clover-Pepper, Jamaica-Pepper, Pimenta, Pimento - Pimenta Dioica - E	Bud	10 ppm
Pea - Pisum Sativum - E	Seed	10 ppm
Balloon Flower, Chieh-Keng, Jie-Geng - Platycodon Grandiflorum - E - M - T	Root	10 ppm
Giant Knotweed, Hu-Zhang, Japanese Knotweed, Mexican Bamboo - Polygonum Cuspidatum - E - M - T	Plant	10 ppm
Chinese Polystichum - Polystichum Polyblepharum - T	Plant	10 ppm
Peach - Prunus Persica - E - M - T	Seed	10 ppm
Chinese Rhubarb - Rheum Palmatum - E	Rhizome	10 ppm
Chayote - Sechium Edule - E - M	Leaf	10 ppm
Hsi Chien, Saint Paul'Swort - Siegesbeckia Orientalis - M	Plant	10 ppm
Jojoba - Simmondsia Chinensis Seed	Seed	10 ppm
Narrowleaf Sophora - Sophora Angustifolia - M - T- M - T	Root	10 ppm
Asparagus bean, Pea bean, Yardlong bean - Vigna Unguiculata subsp. Sesquipedalis - E	Seed	10 ppm
Garlic - Allium Sativum Bulb - E	Bulb	9.7 ppm
Ajwan - Trachyspermum Ammi - E - M	Fruit	9.1 ppm
Okra - Abelmoschus Esculentus - Friut - F - M	Fruit	9 ppm
Chih-Mu, Zhi-Mu - Anemarrhena Asphodeloides - M	Rhizome	9 ppm
Tu Huo - Angelica Laxiflora - M	Root	9 ppm
Horseradish - Armoracia Rusticana - E	Root	9 ppm
Cockscomb - Celosia Cristata - M	Flower	9 ppm
Japanese Cinnamon - Cinnamomum Sieboldii - E - M - T	Root Bark	9 ppm
Ceylon Cinnamon, Cinnamon - Cinnamomum Verum - E - M - T	Bark	9 ppm
Citron - Citrus Medica - E	Fruit	9 ppm
Jih-Chiung - Cnidium Officinale - M	Rhizome	9 ppm
Noble Dendrobium - Dendrobium Nobile - M	Stem	9 ppm

Name	Part	ppm
Oriental Pipewort - Eriocaulon spp. - M	Leaf	9 ppm
Lentil - Lens Culinaris - E	Seed	9 ppm
Dan Zhu Ye - Lophatherum Gracile - M	Plant	9 ppm
Common Turkish Oregano, European Oregano, Oregano, Pot Marjoram, Wild Marjoram, Wild Oregano - Origanum Vulgare - E	Plant	9 ppm
Peganum harmala L. -- Harmel, Syrian Rue	Plant	9 ppm
Anise, Sweet Cumin - Pimpinella Anisum - E - M	Seed	9 ppm
Chinese Senega - Polygala Tenuifolia - M	Root	9 ppm
Guavas - Psidium Guajava - E	Fruit	9 ppm
Chinese Anemone - Pulsatilla Chinensis - M	Root	9 ppm
Cherokee Rose - Rosa Laevigata - E - M	Fruit	9 ppm
Summer Savory - Satureja Hortensis - E	Leaf	9 ppm
Savory, Winter Savory - Satureja Montana	Leaf	9 ppm
Clove, Clovetree - Syzygium Aromaticum - E	Flower	9 ppm
Common thyme, Garden thyme, Thyme - Thymus Vulgaris - E - M	Plant	9 ppm
Mat Bean, Moth Bean - Vigna Aconitifolia - E	Seed	9 ppm
Pineapple - Ananas Comosus - E	Fruit	8.8 ppm
Butternut - Juglans Cinerea - E	Seed	8.4 ppm
Bastard Cardamom, Chin Kousha, Malabar Cardamom, Tavoy Cardamom - Amomum Xanthioides - E	Seed	8 ppm
Elephant-Foot Yam - Amorphophallus Campanulatus - E - M- T	Root	8 ppm
Dill, Garden Dill - Anethum Graveolens - E	Fruit	8 ppm
Capillary Wormwood - Artemisia Capillaris - M	Plant	8 ppm
Kuan Chung, Shield Fernle - Blechnum Orientale - E - M - T	Rhizome	8 ppm
Cauli Brassica Oleracea var. Botrytis - E	Flower	8 ppm
Jack Bean - Canavalia Ensiformis - E	Seed	8 ppm
Sheng Ma - Cimicifuga Dahurica - M	Rhizome	8 ppm
Broomrape, Cistanchis Herba, Jou Tsung Jung - Cistanche Salsa - M	Plant	8 ppm
Taro - Colocasia Esculenta - E	Root	8 ppm
Hawthorn - Crataegus Cuneata - M	Fruit	8 ppm
Air Potato, Potato Yam - Dioscorea Bulbifera - E	Rhizome	8 ppm
Barley, Barleygrass - Hordeum Vulgare - E - M	Sprout Seedling	8 ppm
Rush - Juncus Effusus E - M - T	Pith	8 ppm
Antler Herb, Clubmoss - Lycopodium Clavatum - M - T	Plant	8 ppm
Chinese Magnolia, Hou Pu, Magnolia- Magnolia Officinalis - E - M	Bark	8 ppm
Heal-All, Self-Heal - Prunella Vulgaris - E - M	Flower	8 ppm
Radish - Raphanus Sativus - E	Root	8 ppm
Dan-Shen, Red Sage, Tan-Shen - Salvia Miltiorrhiza - E - M	Root	8 ppm
Sage - Salvia Officinalis - E - M	Leaf	8 ppm
White Mustard - Sinapis Alba - E - M - T	Seed	8 ppm
Rice Paper Tree, Tong-Cao, Tung-Tsao - Tetrapanax Papyrifera M	Pith	8 ppm
Black Gram - Vigna Mungo - E	Seed	8 ppm
Shagbark Hickory - Carya Ovata - E	Seed	7.8 ppm
Grape Citrus Paradisi - E	Fruit	7.7 ppm
Cantaloupe, Melon, Muskmelon, Netted Melon, Nutmeg Melon, Persian Melon - Cucumis Melo subsp. ssp Melo var.Ccantalupensis - Friut - E	Fruit	7.7 ppm
Bread Artocarpus Altilis - E	Fruit	7.5 ppm
Carambola, Star Averrhoa Carambola - E	Fruit	1-15 ppm
American Persimmon - Diospyros Virginiana - E - M	Leaf	7.5 ppm
Chocolate Vine - Akebia Quinata - M	Stem	7 ppm
Celery - Apium Graveolens - E	Pt	7 ppm
Chinese Jack-In-The-Pulpit - Arisaema Consanguineum - E - M - T	Rhizome	7 ppm
Tarragon - Artemisia Dracunculus - M	Plant	7 ppm
Jack Artocarpus Heterophyllus - E	Fruit	7 ppm
American Chestnut - Castanea Dentata - E - M	Seed	7 ppm
Japanese Cinnamon - Cinnamomum Sieboldii - E - M - T	Bark	7 ppm
Loquat - Eriobotrya Japonica - E	Leaf	7 ppm
Sweet Potato - Ipomoea Batatas - E	Root	7 ppm
Morinda - Morinda spp. - M	Root	7 ppm

COPPER CONTINUED

Name	Part	ppm
Paradisiaca - E		7 ppm
Qiang Huo - Notopterygium Incisum - M	Rhizome	7 ppm
Northern Red Oak - Quercus Rubra - E - M	Seed	7 ppm
Black Currant - Ribes Nigrum - E	Fruit	7 ppm
Red Currant, White Currant - Ribes Rubrum - E	Fruit	7 ppm
Aceituna Dulce, Jambolan, Java Plum - Syzygium Cumini - E	Fruit	2.3-14 ppm
Da-Zao, Jujube, Ta-Tsao - Zizyphus Jujuba - E - M	Fruit	7 ppm
Corn Salad, Lamb's Lettuce - Valerianella Locusta - E	Plant	13-13.2 ppm
Russian Olive - Elaeagnus Umbellatus - E - M	Fruit	2-13 ppm
Bilberry, Dwarf Bilberry, Whortleberry - Vaccinium Myrtillus - E - M	Fruit	6.3 ppm
Mimosa - Albizia Julibrissin - E - M	Bark	6 ppm
Blackberry Lily, Shenan - Belamcanda Chinensis - M	Rhizome	6 ppm
Sarson - Brassica Rapa - E	Seed	6 ppm
Chinese Chestnut - Castanea Mollisima - M	Seed	6 ppm
Lime - Citrus Aurantiifolia - E	Fruit	6 ppm
Chinese Dogwood - Cornus Officinalis - E - M	Fruit	6 ppm
Chinese Ash - Fraxinus Rhynchophylla - M - E	Bark	6 ppm
Ginkgo, Maidenhair Tree - Ginkgo Biloba - Tree - E - M - T	Seed	6 ppm
White Mulberry - Morus Alba - E - M	Root Bark	6 ppm
Curry Murraya spp. - E - M	Fruit	6 ppm
Common Garden Peony, Peony, White Peony - Paeonia Lactiflora - M	Root	6 ppm
Moutan, Tree Peony - Paeonia Moutan - M	Root Bark	6 ppm
Moutan, Moutan Peony, Tree Peony - Paeonia Suffruticosa	Root Bark	6 ppm
Japanese Ginseng - Panax Japonicus - M	Rhizome	6 ppm
Amur Cork Tree, Huang Bai, Huang Po, Po Mu - Phellodendron Amurense - M	Bark	6 ppm
Pinyon Pine - Pinus Edulis	Seed	10-12 ppm
Radish - Raphanus Sativus - E	Seed	6 ppm
Gooseberry - Ribes Uva-Crispa - E	Fruit	6 ppm
Rosemary - Rosmarinus Officinalis - E - M	Plant	6 ppm
Hsuan-Shen, Yuan-Shen - Scrophularia Buergeriana - M	Root	6 ppm
Valerianella radicata	Plant	11.1-11.3 ppm
Cloudberry - Rubus Chamaemorus - E - M	Fruit	5.6 ppm
Orange - Citrus Sinensis - E	Fruit	5.5 ppm
Italian Stone Pine, Pignolia - Pinus Pinea - M	Seed	10-11 ppm
Rhubarb - Rheum Rhabarbarum - E	Pt	5.2 ppm
Cowberry, Lingen, Lingonberry - Vaccinium Vitis-Idaea var. Minus - E - M	Fruit	5.2 ppm
Chinese Angelica, Dong Gui, Dong Quai - Angelica Sinensis - M	Root	5 ppm
Asparagus lucidus LINDL. -- Lucid Asparagus	Root	5 ppm
Brussel-Sprout - Brassica Oleracea var. Gemmifera - E	Leaf	5 ppm
Papaya - Carica Papaya - E - M	Fruit	5 ppm
European Chestnut - Castanea Sativa - E - M	Seed	5 ppm
Lambsquarter - Chenopodium Album - E - M - T	Seed	5 ppm
Java Cinnamon, Padang Cassia - Cinnamomum Burmannii - E - M - T	Bark	5 ppm
Adlay, Adlay Millet, Job's-Tears, Yi-Yi-Ren - Coix Lacryma-Jobi - E - M	Seed	5 ppm
Du Zhong, Gutta-Percha Tree, Tu Chung - Eucommia Ulmoides - M	Bark	5 ppm
Chinese Cornbind, Chinese Knotweed, Fleeceflower, Fo Ti, He Shou Wu - Polygonum Multiflorum - E - M - T	Rhizome	5 ppm
Shan Dou Gen - Sophora Subprostrata - M - T	Root	5 ppm
Mandarin, Tangerine - Citrus Reticulata - E	Fruit	4.8 ppm
American Cranberry, Cranberry, Large Cranberry - Vaccinium Macrocarpon - E	Fruit	4.7 ppm
Chervil - Anthriscus Cerefolium - E	Leaf	4.4 ppm
Swamp Taro - Cyrtosperma Chamissonis - E	Root	4.4 ppm
Calamus, Flagroot, Myrtle Flag, Sweet Calamus, Sweetflag, Sweet Acorus Calamus - M	Rhizome	4 ppm
Oats - Avena Sativa - E - M	Plant	4 ppm
Rutabaga, Swede, Swedish Turnip - Brassica Napus var. Napobrassica - E	Root	4 ppm
Rapini, Seven-Top Turnip, Turnip - Brassica Rapa - E	Root	4 ppm
Watermelon - Citrullus Lanatus - E	Fruit	4 ppm

Species	Part	Quantity
Horsetail, Scouring Rush - Equisetum Hyemale - M	Plant	4 ppm
Tian Ma - Gastrodia Elata - Rhizome	Rhizome	4 ppm
Bay, Bay Laurel, Bayleaf, Grecian Laurel, Laurel, Sweet Bay - Laurus Nobilis	Leaf	4 ppm
Apple - Malus Domestica - E	Fruit	4 ppm
Mai-Men-Dong, Mai-Men-Tung - Ophiopogon Japonicus - M	Tuber	4 ppm
Date Palm - Phoenix Dactylifera - E	Fruit	4 ppm
Ban-Xia, Pan-Hsia - Pinellia Ternata - E - M - T	Tuber	4 ppm
Chinese Foxglove - Rehmannia Glutinosa - M	Root	4 ppm
Rowan Berry - Sorbus Aucubaria - E - M - T	Fruit	4 ppm
Wheat - Triticum Aestivum - E - M	Plant	4 ppm
Blueberry - Vaccinium Corymbosum - E	Fruit	4 ppm
Cassava, Tapioca, Yuca - Manihot Esculenta - E	Root	3.8 ppm
Fig - Ficus Carica - E	Fruit	3.6 ppm
Indian Fig, Nopal, Nopalito, Prickly Pear - Opuntia Ficus-Indica - E - M	Seed	3.4 ppm
Chinese Cabbage - Brassica Pekinensis - E	Leaf	3.15 ppm
Saffron - Crocus Sativus - Style	Silk Stigma Style	3 ppm
English Walnut - Juglans Rregia - E	Seed	3 ppm
Macadamia - Macadamia spp. - E	Seed	3 ppm
Alholva, Bockshornklee, Fenugreek, Greek Clover, Greek Trigonella Foenum-Graecum - E - M	Leaf	3 ppm
Coca - Erythroxylum Novogranatense var. Truxillense - E - M	Leaf	2.9 ppm
Coca - Erythroxylum Novogranatense var. Novogranatense - E - M	Leaf	2.7 ppm
Rye - Secale Cereale - E	Seed	4-5 ppm
Giant Taro - Alocasia Macrorrhiza - E	Root	2.4 ppm
Shortleaf Pine - Pinus Echinata - M	Shoot	2.1 ppm
Ma-Huang - Ephedra spp. - M	Plant	2 ppm
Spearmint - Mentha Spicata - E - M - T	Plant	2 ppm
Ben Nut, Benzolive Tree, Drumstick Tree, Horseradish Tree, Moringa, West Indian Ben - Moringa Oleifera - E	Leaf	1-4 ppm
Date Palm - Phoenix Dactylifera - E	Seed	2 ppm
Pomegranate - Punica Granatum - E	Fruit	2 ppm
Broadbean, Faba Bean, Habas - Vicia Faba - E	Fruit	1.7 ppm
Soursop - Annona Muricata - E	Fruit	1.6 ppm
Taro - Colocasia Esculenta - E	Leaf	1.5 ppm
Huang Qi, Huang-Chi - Astragalus Membranaceus - M	Root	1 ppm
Genipap, Jagua - Genipa Americana - E - M	Fruit	1 ppm
Salsify - Tragopogon Porrifolius - E	Root	1 ppm

PLANTS CONTAINING FLUORINE

Species	Part	Quantity
Lettuce - Lactuca Sativa - E	Leaf	8 ppm
Parsley - Petroselinum Crispum - E	Plant	7.8 ppm
European Nettle, Stinging Nettle - Urtica Dioica - E - M	Leaf	7.8 ppm
Spinach - Spinacia Oleracea - E	Leaf	5.7 ppm
Dill, Garden Dill - Anethum Graveolens - E	Plant	5.3 ppm
Allspice, Clover-Pepper, Jamaica-Pepper, Pimenta, Pimento - Pimenta Dioica - E	Plant	5 ppm
Bitter Melon, Sorosi - Momordica Charantia - E	Fruit	4.8 ppm
Rhubarb - Rheum Rhabarbarum - E	Pt	4 ppm
Pistachio - Pistacia Vera - E	Seed	3.8 ppm
Black Currant - Ribes Nigrum - E	Fruit	2.8 ppm
Coconut, Coconut Palm - Cocos Nucifera - E	Seed	2.7 ppm
Cauli Brassica Oleracea var. Botrytis - E	Flower	2.5 ppm
Cabbage, Red Cabbage, White Cabbage - Brassica Oleracea var. Capitata - E	Leaf	2.5 ppm
Apple - Malus Domestica - E	Fruit	2.1 ppm
Ben Nut, Benzolive Tree, Drumstick Tree, Horseradish Tree, Moringa, West Indian Ben - Moringa Oleifera - E	Leaf	0-4 ppm
Black bean, Dwarf bean, Field bean, Flageolet bean, French bean, Garden bean, Green bean, Haricot, Haricot bean, Haricot vert, Kidney bean, Navy bean, Pop bean, Popping bean, Snap bean, String bean, Wax bean - Phaseolus Vulgaris - E	Fruit	2 ppm

FLUORINE CONTINUED

Species	Part	Quantity
Ginger - Zingiber Officinale - E	Rhizome	2 ppm
Cloudberry - Rubus Chamaemorus - E - M	Fruit	1.9 ppm
Carrot - Daucus Carota - E	Root	1.8 ppm
Red Currant, White Currant - Ribes Rubrum - E	Fruit	1.8 ppm
Brazilnut, Brazilnut-Tree, Creamnut, Paranut - Bertholletia Eexcelsa - E	Seed	1.7 ppm
Tomato - Lycopersicon Esculentum - E - M - T	Fruit	1.7 ppm
Pecan - Carya Illinoensis - E	Seed	1.6 ppm
Black Walnut - Juglans Nigra - E	Seed	1.6 ppm
Dog Rose, Dogbrier, Rose - Rosa Canina - E - M	Fruit	1.5 ppm
Rowan Berry - Sorbus Aucubaria - E - M - T	Fruit	1.5 ppm
Cashew - Anacardium Occidentale - E	Seed	1.4 ppm
Shagbark Hickory - Carya Ovata - E	Seed	1.3 ppm
Almond - Prunus Dulcis - E - M - T	Seed	1.3 ppm
Northern Red Oak - Quercus Rubra - E - M	Seed	1.3 ppm
Cobnut, English Filbert, European Filbert, European Hazel, Hazel - Corylus Avellana - E	Seed	1.2 ppm
Butternut - Juglans Cinerea - E	Seed	1.1 ppm
Bell Pepper, Cherry Pepper, Cone Pepper, Green Pepper, Paprika, Sweet Pepper - Capsicum Annuum - E	Fruit	1 ppm
Pea - Pisum Sativum - E	Seed	1 ppm
American Styrax, Sweetgum - Liquidambar Styraciflua - E - M	Stem	6 ppm
Shortleaf Pine - Pinus Echinata - M	Shoot	6 ppm
White Oak - Quercus Alba - M	Stem	6 ppm
Willow Oak - Quercus Phellos - E - M	Stem	6 ppm
Smooth Sumac - Rhus Glabra - E - M	Stem	6 ppm
Buckbush - Symphoricarpos Orbiculatus - M	Stem	6 ppm
Red Pignut Hickory - Carya Glabra - E	Shoot	5 ppm
Shagbark Hickory - Carya Ovata - E	Shoot	5 ppm
Northern Red Oak - Quercus Rubra - E - M	Stem	5 ppm
Post Oak - Quercus Stellata - E - M	Stem	5 ppm
Black Oak - Quercus Velutina - E - M	Stem	5 ppm
Japanese Cinnamon - Cinnamomum Sieboldii - E - M - T	Root Bark	4 ppm
Ceylon Cinnamon, Cinnamon - Cinnamomum Verum - E - M - T	Bark	3 ppm
Garden Sorrel - Rumex Acetosa - E - M - T	Leaf	2 ppm
Swamp Cabbage, Water Spinach - Ipomoea Aquatica - E	Leaf	1.5 ppm
Calabash Gourd, White Flowered Gourd - Lagenaria Siceraria - E	Fruit	1.12 ppm
Pineapple - Ananas Comosus - E	Fruit	1 ppm
Cassia, Cassia Bark, Cassia Lignea, China Junk Cassia, Chinazimt, Chinese Cassia - Cinnamomum Aromaticuminnamon- E - M - T	Bark	1 ppm

PLANTS CONTAINING GERMANIUM

Species	Part	Quantity
Ginger - Zingiber Officinale - E	Rhizome	169 ppm
Garlic Allium Sativum Bulb E	Bulb	Trace
American Ginseng, Ginseng - Panax Quinquefolius - M	Plant	Trace

PLANTS CONTAINING IODINE

Species	Part	Quantity
Bladderwrack, Kelp - Fucus Vesiculosus - E - M	Plant	5,400 ppm
Pistachio - Pistacia Vera - E	Seed	51 ppm
Soybean - Glycine Max - E	Seed	16 ppm
Red Cedar - Juniperus Virginiana Amphicarpaea Bracteata- E - M - T	Shoot	10 ppm

PLANTS CONTAINING IRON

Species	Part	Quantity
Dandelion - Taraxacum Officinale - E - M	Leaf	5,000 ppm
Coneflower, Echinacea - Echinacea ssp - M	Root	4,800 ppm
Buckbush - Symphoricarpos Orbiculatus - M	Stem	4,400 ppm
Mugwort - Artemisia Vulgaris - M	Plant	3,900 ppm
Ramie - Boehmeria Nivea - M	Plant	3,500 ppm
Tomatillo - Physalis Ixocarpa - E	Fruit	2,974 ppm

Devil's claw, Grapple Harpagophytum procumbens - M	Root	2,900 ppm
Asian Wild Ginger - Asiasarum Heterotropoides - M	Root	2,800 ppm
Siebold's Wild Ginger - Asiasarum Sieboldii - M	Root	2,800 ppm
Chickweed, Common Chickweed - Stellaria Media - E	Plant	2,530 ppm
Flannelleaf, Flannelplant, Great mullein, Mullein, Velvet Verbascum Thapsus - M	Leaf	2,360 ppm
European Pennyroyal - Mentha pulegium - E - M- T	Plant	2,310 ppm
SafCarthamus Tinctorius - M	Flower	2,200 ppm
Butterbur - Petasites Japonicus - T	Plant	2,100 ppm
Corn Salad, Lamb's Lettuce - Valerianella Locusta - E	Plant	3,519-4,143 ppm
Chinese Polystichum - Polystichum Polyblepharum - T	Plant	1,900 ppm
Cowgrass, Peavine Clover, Purple Clover, Red Clover - Trifolium Pratense - E - M	Shoot	1,850 ppm
Black Gum, Black Tupelo - Nyssa Sylvatica - E - M	Leaf	1,820 ppm
Bai Zhi - Angelica Dahurica - M	Root	1,800 ppm
Ching-Chieh, Jing-Jie - Schizonepeta Tenuifolia - E - M	Plant	1,700 ppm
Blue Cohosh - Caulophyllum Thalictroides - M	Root	1,640 ppm
Box-Holly, Butcher's broom - Ruscus aculeatus - E - M	Root	1,640 ppm
American Persimmon - Diospyros Virginiana - E - M	Stem	1,620 ppm
Pigweed - Amaranthus sp. - E - M	Leaf	1,527 ppm
Common thyme, Garden thyme, Thyme - Thymus Vulgaris - E - M	Plant	1,508 ppm
Tea - Camellia Sinensis - E	Leaf	1,500 ppm
Cassava, Tapioca, Yuca - Manihot Esculenta - E	Leaf	1,500 ppm
Burdock, Gobo, Great Burdock - Arctium lappa - E - M - T	Root	1,470 ppm
Black Cherry, Wild Cherry - Prunus Serotina - E - M - T	Leaf	1,440 ppm
Barberry - Berberis Vulgaris - M	Root	1,410 ppm
Chih-Mu, Zhi-Mu - Anemarrhena Asphodeloides - M	Rhizome	1,400 ppm
Qian Hu - Peucedanum Decursivum - M	Plant	1,400 ppm
Catnip - Nepeta Cataria - M	Plant	1,380 ppm
Bai-Wei, Pai-Wei - Cynanchum Atratum - E - M	Root	1,350 ppm
Red Cedar - Juniperus Virginiana Amphicarpaea Bracteata- E - M - T	Shoot	1,320 ppm
Giant Knotweed, Hu-Zhang, Japanese Knotweed, Mexican Bamboo - Polygonum Cuspidatum - E - M - T	Plant	1,300 ppm
Coffee Senna - Senna Occidentalis - E - T	Seed	1,300 ppm
Field Horsetail, Horsetail - Equisetum Arvense - M	Plant	1,230 ppm
Chinese Spikenard - Nardostachys Chinensis - M	Rhizome	1,210 ppm
Chai-Hu - Bupleurum - M	Root	1,200 ppm
Luffa, Smooth Loofah, Vegetable Sponge - Luffa Aegyptiaca - E	Leaf	1,162 ppm
Marshmallow, White Mallow - Althaea Officinalis - M	Root	1,150 ppm
Aubergine, Egg Solanum Melongena - E	Leaf	1,140 ppm
Climbing Fern - Lygodium Japonicum - Pollen or Spore - M	Pollen Or Spore	1,090 ppm
Lady's Thistle, Milk Thistle - Silybum Marianum - M	Plant	1,060 ppm
Bearberry, Uva Uursi - Arctostaphylos Uva-Ursi - M	Leaf	1,050 ppm
Black bean, Dwarf bean, Field bean, Flageolet bean, French bean, Garden bean, Green bean, Haricot, Haricot bean, Haricot vert, Kidney bean, Navy bean, Pop bean, Popping bean, Snap bean, String bean, Wax bean - Phaseolus Vulgaris - E	Fruit	1,050 ppm
Chinese Anemone - Pulsatilla Chinensis - M	Root	1,050 ppm
Coffee - Coffea Arabica - E - M	Leaf	1,032 ppm
Sassafras - Sassafras Albidum - E - M - T	Leaf	1,020 ppm
Raspberry, Red raspberry - Rubus Idaeus - E - M	Leaf	1,010 ppm
Butter Bean, Lima Bean - Phaseolus Lunatus - E	Seed	1,000 ppm
Oats - Avena Sativa - E - M	Plant	990 ppm
Spiny Pigweed - Amaranthus Spinosus - E - M	Leaf	22-1,965 ppm
Marjoram, Sweet Marjoram - Origanum Majorana - E	Plant	975 ppm
Dandelion - Taraxacum Officinale - E - M	Root	960 ppm
Chinese Foxglove - Rehmannia Glutinosa - M	Root	920 ppm
Spearmint - Mentha Spicata - E - M- T	Plant	918 ppm

IRON CONTINUED

Name	Part	ppm
Bastard Cardamom, Chin Kousha, Malabar Cardamom, Tavoy Cardamom - Amomum Xanthioides - E	Seed	910 ppm
Japanese Gentian - Gentiana Scabra - E	Root	910 ppm
Mongoloid Dandelion - Taraxacum Mongolicum - E - M	Plant	910 ppm
Sarsaparilla - Smilax spp - E - M	Root	905 ppm
European Grape, Grape, Grapevine, Vigne Vinifere, Wine Grape - Vitis Vinifera - E - M	Stem	900 ppm
Asian Plantain - Plantago Asiatica - E - M	Plant	890 ppm
Chinese Angelica, Dong Gui, Dong Quai - Angelica Sinensis - M	Root	880 ppm
Commom Licorice, Licorice, Licorice-Root, Smooth Licorice - Glycyrrhiza Glabra - M	Root	880 ppm
Damiana - Turnera Diffusa - M	Leaf	880 ppm
Crampbark, European Cranberry bush, Guelder Rose, Snowballbush - Viburnum Opulus - E - M - T	Bark	880 ppm
Irish moss - Chondrus Crispus - E	Plant	874 ppm
Buchu, Honey Buchu, Mountain Buchu - Agathosma Betulina Buchu, Honey Buchu, Mountain Buchu - Agathosma Betulina - M	Leaf	867 ppm
Narrowleaf Sophora - Sophora Angustifolia - M - T - M - T	Root	860 ppm
Rush - Juncus Effusus E - M - T	Pith	840 ppm
Butter Bean, Lima Bean - Phaseolus Lunatus - E	Leaf	821 ppm
Desert Wormwood - Artemisia Herba-Alba - M	Plant	820 ppm
Bei Sha Shen - Glehnia Littoralis - E - M	Root	820 ppm
Black Cherry, Wild Cherry - Prunus Serotina - E - M - T	Stem	810 ppm
Comfrey - Symphytum Officinale - E - M - T	Root	810 ppm
Tomato - Lycopersicon Esculentum - E - M - T	Fruit	800 ppm
Dulse - Rhodymenia Palmata - E	Plant	792 ppm
Bai-Zhu, Pai-Chu - Atractylodes Ovata - M	Rhizome	780 ppm
Wheat - Triticum Aestivum - E - M	Plant	770 ppm
Curly Dock, Lengua De Vaca, Sour Dock, Yellow Dock - Rumex Crispus - M - T	Root	760 ppm
Dill, Garden Dill - Anethum Graveolens - E	Plant	755 ppm
Cumin - Cuminum Cyminum - E - M	Fruit	748 ppm
Sassafras - Sassafras Albidum - E - M - T	Stem	740 ppm
Madder - Rubia Cordifolia - M	Root	720 ppm
Spirulina - Spirulina Pratensis - E	Plant	713 ppm
Jussiaeae Herba, Pond Dragon - Jussiaea Repens - M	Plant	700 ppm
Black bean, Dwarf bean, Field bean, Flageolet bean, French bean, Garden bean, Green bean, Haricot, Haricot bean, Haricot vert, Kidney bean, Navy bean, Pop bean, Popping bean, Snap bean, String bean, Wax bean - Phaseolus Vulgaris - E	Leaf	697 ppm
Guanique - Chamissoa Altissima - M	Leaf	137-1,370 ppm
Sheng Ma - Cimicifuga Dahurica - M	Rhizome	680 ppm
Chinese Boxthorn, Chinese Matrimony Vine, Chinese Wolfberry - Lycium Chinense - E - M	Root Bark	670 ppm
Huaca-Mullo - Mimulus Glabratus - M	Shoot	660 ppm
Black Nightshade - Solanum Nigrum - E	Leaf	660 ppm
Antler Herb, Clubmoss - Lycopodium Clavatum - M - T	Plant	650 ppm
Heal-All, Self-Heal - Prunella Vulgaris - E - M	Flower	640 ppm
Shortleaf Pine - Pinus Echinata - M	Shoot	630 ppm
Goldenseal - Hydrastis Canadensis - M	Root	610 ppm
Chinese Jack-In-The-Pulpit - Arisaema Consanguineum - E - M - T	Rhizome	600 ppm
Chaya - Cnidoscolus Chayamansa - E	Leaf	600 ppm
Ma-Huang - Ephedra spp. - M	Plant	600 ppm
Peppermint - Mentha x Piperita subsp. Nothosubsp. Piperita - E - M - T	Leaf	600 ppm
Common Turkish Oregano, European Oregano, Oregano, Pot Marjoram, Wild Marjoram, Wild Oregano - Origanum Vulgare - E	Plant	598 ppm
Chaparral, Creosote Bush - Larrea Tridentata - M	Plant	580 ppm
Celery - Apium Graveolens - E	Seed	571 ppm

Name	Part	ppm
Paper Mulberry - Broussonetia Papyrifera - E - M	Fruit	560 ppm
Bitter Melon, Sorosi - Momordica Charantia - E	Fruit	560 ppm
Alholva, Bockshornklee, Fenugreek, Greek Clover, Greek Trigonella Foenum-Graecum - E - M	Seed	560 ppm
Flax, Lin Linum Usitatissimum - E	Seed	549 ppm
Lemongrass, West indian lemongrass - Cymbopogon Citratus - E - M	Plant	543 ppm
Swamp Cabbage, Water Spinach - Ipomoea Aquatica - E	Leaf	540 ppm
Indian Sorrel, Jamaica Sorrel, Kharkadi, Red Sorrel, Sorrel - Hibiscus Sabdariffa - E	Flower	536 ppm
Chinese Parsley, Cilantro, Coriander - Coriandrum Sativum E	Leaf	528 ppm
Chinese Boxthorn, Chinese Matrimony Vine, Chinese Wolfberry - Lycium Chinense - E - M	Leaf	519 ppm
Corn - Zea Mays - E	Silk Stigma Style	504 ppm
Japanese Cinnamon - Cinnamomum Sieboldii - E - M - T	Root Bark	500 ppm
American Persimmon - Diospyros Virginiana - E - M	Leaf	500 ppm
Alehoof - Glechoma Hederacea - M	Plant	500 ppm
Dokudami, Fishwort, Yu Xing Cao - Houttuynia Cordata - E - M	Plant	500 ppm
Angel Of Death, Bolek Hena, Curia - Justicia Pectoralis - M	Leaf	495 ppm
Coca - Erythroxylum Coca var. Coca - E - M	Leaf	490 ppm
Jew's Mallow, Mulukiya, Nalta Jute - Corchorus Olitorius - E - M	Leaf	485 ppm
Common Valerian, Garden-Heliotrope, Valerian - Valeriana Officinalis - E - M	Root	480 ppm
Perilla - Perilla Frutescens - E - M - T	Leaf	479 ppm
Basil, Cuban Basil, Sweet Basil - Ocimum Basilicum - E	Leaf	478 ppm
Beebread, Beeplant, Borage, Talewort - Borago Officinalis - E - M - T	Leaf	472 ppm
Bayberry, Candle-Berry, Southern Bayberry, Wax Myrtle - Myrica Cerifera - E - M	Bark	470 ppm
Indian Saffron, Turmeric - Curcuma Longa - E	Rhizome	467 ppm
Purslane, Verdolaga - Portulaca Oleracea - E	Herb	467 ppm
Huang Qi, Huang-Chi - Astragalus Membranaceus - M	Root	460 ppm
Perilla - Perilla Frutescens - E - M - T	Plant	460 ppm
European Mistletoe - Viscum Album - M - T	Leaf	460 ppm
Black Walnut - Juglans Nigra - E	Fruit	455 ppm
Cerraja, Sow Thistle - Sonchus Oleraceus - E - M	Leaf	455 ppm
Lian-Jiao, Lien-Chiao - Forsythia Suspensa - M	Fruit	440 ppm
High Mallow - Malva Sylvestris - E - M	Leaf	440 ppm
Black Gum, Black Tupelo - Nyssa Sylvatica - E - M	Stem	440 ppm
Onion, Shallot - Allium Cepa - Shallot Bulb - E	Leaf	436 ppm
Nutsedge - Cyperus Rotundus - E - M	Rhizome	430 ppm
Red Pignut Hickory - Carya Glabra - E	Shoot	429 ppm
Cassia, Cassia Bark, Cassia Lignea, China Junk Cassia, Chinazimt, Chinese Cassia - Cinnamomum Aromaticuminnamon- E - M - T	Bark	421 ppm
Ceylon Cinnamon, Cinnamon - Cinnamomum Verum - E - M - T	Bark	421 ppm
Garland Chrysanthemum - Chrysanthemum Coronarium - Bud - E	Bud	420 ppm
Cucumber - Cucumis Sativus - E	Fruit	420 ppm
Post Oak - Quercus Stellata - E - M	Stem	420 ppm
European Nettle, Stinging Nettle - Urtica Dioica - E - M	Leaf	418 ppm
Summer Savory - Satureja Hortensis - E	Plant	416 ppm
Anise, Sweet Cumin - Pimpinella Anisum - E - M	Fruit	409 ppm
Shepherd's Purse - Capsella Bursa-Pastoris - E - M	Plant	407 ppm
American Ginseng, Ginseng - Panax Quinquefolius - M	Plant	407 ppm
Black Pepper, Pepper, White Pepper - Piper Nigrum - E - M	Fruit	407 ppm
Florida Eryngium - Eryngium Floridanum - M	Shoot	400 ppm
Gennoshiouko, Oriental Geranium - Geranium Thunbergii - E - M	Plant	400 ppm
Cornmint, Field Mint, Japanese Mint - Mentha Arvensis var. Piperascens - E - M- T	Plant	400 ppm
Pea - Pisum Sativum - E	Plant	400 ppm

IRON CONTINUED

Plant	Part	ppm
Rosemary - Rosmarinus Officinalis - E - M	Plant	400 ppm
Yellow Mombin, Yellow Plum - Spondias Pinnata - E	Fruit	400 ppm
Beet, Beetroot, Garden Beet, Sugar Beet - Beta Vulgaris - E	Leaf	392 ppm
Evening-Primrose - Oenothera Biennis - E - M	Seed	390 ppm
Garland Chrysanthemum - Chrysanthemum Coronarium - Bud - E	Leaf	385 ppm
Spinach - Spinacia Oleracea - E	Plant	384 ppm
Black Cohosh, Black Snake - Cimicifuga Racemosa - E - M	Root	380 ppm
White Oak - Quercus Alba - M	Stem	380 ppm
Indian Gooseberry, Otaheite Gooseberry - Phyllanthus Acidus - E	Fruit	372 ppm
Gentian, Yellow Gentian - Gentiana Lutea - M	Root	370 ppm
White Mustard - Sinapis Alba - E - M - T	Seed	370 ppm
Coltsfoot - Tussilago Farfara - M - T	Flower	370 ppm
Sweet Potato - Ipomoea Batatas - E	Leaf	365 ppm
Malanga, Tannia, Yautia - Xanthosoma Sagittifolium - E	Leaf	365 ppm
Endive, Escarole - Cichorium Endivia - M	Leaf	360 ppm
Japanese Ginseng - Panax Japonicus - M	Rhizome	360 ppm
Bitter Melon, Sorosi - Momordica Charantia - E	Leaf	357 ppm
Radish - Raphanus Sativus - E	Leaf	357 ppm
Calamus, Flagroot, Myrtle Flag, Sweet Calamus, Sweetflag, Sweet Acorus Calamus - M	Rhizome	350 ppm
Tarragon - Artemisia Dracunculus - M	Plant	350 ppm
Japanese Honeysuckle - Lonicera Japonica - M	Flower	350 ppm
Chinese Magnolia Vine, Five-Flavor-Fruit, Magnolia Vine, Schizandra, Wu Wei Zi, Wu Wei Zu - Schisandra Chinensis - M	Fruit	350 ppm
Amboini Coleus, Country Borage, Cuban Oregano, French Thyme, Indian Borage, Mexican Mint, Soup Mint, Spanish Thyme - Plectranthus amboinicus - E	Leaf	39-695 ppm
Celery - Apium Graveolens - E	Pt	347 ppm
Chervil - Anthriscus Cerefolium - E	Leaf	345 ppm
Northern Red Oak - Quercus Rubra - E - M	Stem	343 ppm
Mai-Men-Dong, Mai-Men-Tung - Ophiopogon Japonicus - M	Tuber	340 ppm
Indian Sorrel, Jamaica Sorrel, Kharkadi, Red Sorrel, Sorrel - Hibiscus Sabdariffa - E	Leaf	333 ppm
Alfalfa, Lucerne - Medicago Sativa subsp. Sativa - E	Plant	333 ppm
Chinese Goldthread, Huang-Lian, Huang-Lien - Coptis Chinensis - M	Rhizome	320 ppm
Huang-Lia, Huang-Lian, Huang-Lien, Japanese Goldthread - Coptis Japonica - M	Rhizome	320 ppm
Generic Goldthread - Coptis spp. - M	Rhizome	320 ppm
Hsin-I, Xin-Yi - Magnolia Denudata - E - M	Flower	320 ppm
Morinda - Morinda spp. - M	Root	320 ppm
Wild Yam - Dioscorea sp. - E	Root	315 ppm
Cordoncillo, Hierba Santa, Hoja Santa - Piper Auritum - E - M	Leaf	315 ppm
Susumba, Wild Egg Solanum Torvum - Friut - E	Fruit	315 ppm
ElytriCouchgrass, Doggrass, Quackgrass, Twitchgrass, Wheatgrass - Elytrigia Repens - E - M	Plant	311 ppm
Aconite, Fu-Tsu - Aconitum Carmichaelii - E - M	Tuber	310 ppm
Eyebright - Euphrasia Officinalis - M	Plant	310 ppm
Indian Tobacco, Lobelia - Lobelia Inflata - M - T	Leaf	310 ppm
Pawpaw - Asimina Triloba - Friut - E	Fruit	308 ppm
Sage - Salvia Officinalis - E - M	Leaf	305 ppm
Aloe, Bitter Aloes - Aloe Vera - E - M	Leaf	300 ppm
Oats - Avena Sativa - E - M	Seed	300 ppm
Carrot - Daucus Carota - E	Root	300 ppm
Du Zhong, Gutta-Percha Tree, Tu Chung - Eucommia Ulmoides - M	Bark	300 ppm
Ajwan - Trachyspermum Ammi - E - M	Fruit	299 ppm
Radish - Raphanus Sativus - E	Fruit	295 ppm
Willow Oak - Quercus Phellos - E - M	Stem	294 ppm
Cang Zhu - Atractylodes Lancea - M	Rhizome	290 ppm
Gotu Kola, Pennywort - Centella Asiatica - E - M	Leaf	290 ppm
White Mulberry - Morus Alba - E - M	Root Bark	290 ppm
Chinese Senega - Polygala Tenuifolia - M	Root	290 ppm

Plant	Part	ppm
Bell Pepper, Cherry Pepper, Cone Pepper, Green Pepper, Paprika, Sweet Pepper - Capsicum Annuum - E	Fruit	286 ppm
Caraway, Carum - Carum Carvi - E	Fruit	286 ppm
Garden Cress - Lepidium Sativum - E	Leaf	286 ppm
Manioc Hibiscus - Abelmoschus Manihot - E - M	Leaf	284 ppm
Chinese Licorice - Glycyrrhiza Uralensis - M	Root	280 ppm
Qiang Huo - Notopterygium Incisum - M	Rhizome	280 ppm
Cherimoya - Annona Cherimola - E	Seed	270 ppm
Fennel - Foeniculum Vulgare - M	Plant	270 ppm
Guinea Grass - Panicum Maximum - M	Leaf	0-525 ppm
Berro, Watercress - Nasturtium Officinale - E	Herb	262 ppm
Chayote - Sechium Edule - E - M	Leaf	262 ppm
Bitter Orange, Petitgrain - Citrus Aurantium - E	Fruit	260 ppm
Asparagus Pea, Goa Bean, Winged Bean - Psophocarpus Tetragonolobus - E	Leaf	259 ppm
Elephant Garlic, Kurrat - Allium Ampeloprasum - E	Leaf	255 ppm
Broomweed, Tea Sida - Sida Rhombifolia - M	Leaf	253 ppm
Wu Chia Pi - Acanthopanax Gracilistylis - M	Root Bark	250 ppm
Lambsquarter - Chenopodium Album - E - M - T	Leaf	250 ppm
Parsley - Petroselinum Crispum - E	Plant	250 ppm
Rhubarb - Rheum Rhabarbarum - E	Leaf	250 ppm
Mad-Dog Skullcap, Scullcap - Scutellaria lateriflora - M	Plant	250 ppm
Bilberry, Dwarf Bilberry, Whortleberry - Vaccinium Myrtillus - E - M	Leaf	250 ppm
Cowberry, Lingen, Lingonberry - Vaccinium Vitis-Idaea var. Minus - E - M	Leaf	250 ppm
White Mulberry - Morus Alba - E - M	Fruit	247 ppm
Chicory, Succory, Witloof - Cichorium Intybus - E - M	Leaf	246 ppm
Two-Flowered Sandspur - Cenchrus Biflorus - E	Seed	245 ppm
Mango - Mangifera Indica - E - M	Fruit	243 ppm
Asparagus - Asparagus Officinalis - E	Shoot	240 ppm
Blessed Thistle - Cnicus Benedictus - M	Plant	240 ppm
Jih-Chiung - Cnidium Officinale - M	Rhizome	240 ppm
Fennel - Foeniculum Vulgare - M	Fruit	240 ppm
Dan Zhu Ye - Lophatherum Gracile - M	Plant	240 ppm
Betel Pepper - Piper Betel - E - M	Leaf	240 ppm
Black Oak - Quercus Velutina - E - M	Stem	236 ppm
Onion, Shallot - Allium Cepa - Shallot Bulb - E	Seed	235 ppm
Dill, Garden Dill - Anethum Graveolens - E	Fruit	230 ppm
Tu Huo - Angelica Laxiflora - M	Root	230 ppm
Cascara Buckthorn, Cascara Sagrada - Frangula Purshiana - M	Bark	230 ppm
Dan-Shen, Red Sage, Tan-Shen - Salvia Miltiorrhiza - E - M	Root	230 ppm
Butter Bean, Lima Bean - Phaseolus Lunatus - E	Sprout Seedling	228 ppm
Chinese Parsley, Cilantro, Coriander - Coriandrum Sativum E	Fruit	227 ppm
Baikal Skullcap, Chinese Skullcap, Huang Qin - Scutellaria Baicalensis - M	Root	220 ppm
Hawthorn - Crataegus Cuneata - M	Fruit	210 ppm
Achocha - Cyclanthera Pedata - Friut - E - M	Fruit	210 ppm
Chinese Ephedra, Ma Huang - Ephedra Sinica - M	Plant	210 ppm
Soybean - Glycine Max - E	Plant	210 ppm
Amur Cork Tree, Huang Bai, Huang Po, Po Mu - Phellodendron Amurense - M	Bark	210 ppm
White Willow - Salix Alba - M	Bark	210 ppm
Black Mustard - Brassica Nigra - E	Leaf	209 ppm
Pea - Pisum Sativum - E	Fruit	206 ppm
Pepper Elder, Yerba De La Plata - Peperomia Pelucida - Leaf	Leaf	30-410 ppm
Pokeweed - Phytolacca Americana - E - M- T	Shoot	202 ppm
Chives - Allium Schoenoprasum - E	Leaf	200 ppm
Capillary Wormwood - Artemisia Capillaris - M	Plant	200 ppm
Taro - Colocasia Esculenta - E	Leaf	200 ppm
Loquat - Eriobotrya Japonica - E	Leaf	200 ppm
Macadamia - Macadamia spp. - E	Seed	200 ppm
Cowage, Velvetbean - Mucuna Pruriens - E	Seed	200 ppm
Psyllium - Plantago Psyllium - E - M	Seed	200 ppm

Hillman Health Food Store call 855-Amish-Dr (855-264-7437) www.emineral.info Vitamins and Minerals for Better Living

IRON CONTINUED

Plant	Part	ppm
Balloon Flower, Chieh-Keng, Jie-Geng - Platycodon Grandiflorum - E - M - T	Root	200 ppm
Snakegourd - Trichosanthes Anguina - E - M	Fruit	200 ppm
Cassie, Huisache, Opopanax, Popinac, Sweet Acacia - Acacia Farnesiana - M	Leaf	199 ppm
Cashew - Anacardium Occidentale - E	Seed	195 ppm
Groundnut, Peanut - Arachis Hypogaea - E - M	Leaf	195 ppm
Cheeseweed - Malva Parviflora - E - M	Plant	195 ppm
Chinese Birthwort - Aristolochia Debilis - E - M - T	Fruit	190 ppm
Perejil - Peperomia Pereskiifolia - Leaf	Leaf	57-380 ppm
Hsi Chien, Saint Paul'Swort - Siegesbeckia Orientalis - M	Plant	190 ppm
Radish - Raphanus Sativus - E	Root	189 ppm
Asparagus bean, Pea bean, Yardlong bean - Vigna Unguiculata subsp. Sesquipedalis - E	Shoot	188 ppm
Khat - Catha Edulis - E	Leaf	185 ppm
Psyllium - Plantago Psyllium - E - M	Hull Husk	183 ppm
Chaff Achyranthes Bidentata - M	Root	180 ppm
Amphicarpaea Bracteata - E - M	Shoot	0-360 ppm
Cockscomb - Celosia Cristata - M	Flower	180 ppm
Soybean - Glycine Max - E	Seed	180 ppm
Henbane - Hyoscyamus Niger - E - M	Seed	180 ppm
Chinese Ginseng, Ginseng, Korean Ginseng, Oriental Ginseng - Panax Ginseng - M	Root	180 ppm
Chinese Rhubarb - Rheum Palmatum - E	Rhizome	180 ppm
Hydrangea, Smooth Hydrangea - Hydrangea Arborescens - E - M	Root	179 ppm
Lettuce - Lactuca Sativa - E	Leaf	176 ppm
Vinespinach - Basella Alba - E - M	Leaf	175 ppm
Jack Bean - Canavalia Ensiformis - E	Fruit	175 ppm
Mustard Greens - Brassica Juncea - E	Leaf	174 ppm
Akee, Seso Vegetal - Blighia Sapida - M	Seed	173 ppm
Pumpkin - Cucurbita Pepo - E	Seed	172 ppm
Bok-Choy, Celery Cabbage, Celery Mustard, Chinese Cabbage, Chinese Mustard, Chinese White Cabbage, Pak-Choi - Brassica Chinensis - E	Leaf	171 ppm
Garden Camomile, Perennial Camomile, Roman Camomile - Chamaemelum Nobile M	Flower	170 ppm
Da-Zao, Jujube, Ta-Tsao - Zizyphus Jujuba - E - M	Fruit	170 ppm
Sesame - Sesamum Indicum - E - M	Seed	169 ppm
Jerusalem Artichoke - Helianthus Tuberosus E	Tuber	168 ppm
Beet, Beetroot, Garden Beet, Sugar Beet - Beta Vulgaris - E	Root	165 ppm
Emblic, Myrobalan - Phyllanthus Emblica - E	Fruit	163 ppm
Ginger - Zingiber Officinale - E	Rhizome	162 ppm
Genipap, Jagua - Genipa Americana - E - M	Fruit	160 ppm
Barley, Barleygrass - Hordeum Vulgare - E - M	Stem	160 ppm
Garden Sorrel - Rumex Acetosa - E - M - T	Leaf	160 ppm
Asparagus Pea, Goa Bean, Winged Bean - Psophocarpus Tetragonolobus - E	Seed	158 ppm
Elephant Apple, Manzana De Elefante, Wood-Apple - Limonia acidissima - Wood - Apple - E - M	Seed	300-312 ppm
Chinese Cornbind, Chinese Knotweed, Fleeceflower, Fo Ti, He Shou Wu - Polygonum Multiflorum - E - M - T	Root	156 ppm
Rhubarb - Rheum Rhabarbarum - E	Pt	154 ppm
European Grape, Grape, Grapevine, Vigne Vinifere, Wine Grape - Vitis Vinifera - E - M	Fruit	154 ppm
Cardamom - Elettaria Cardamomum - E - M	Seed	153 ppm
Red Mangrove - Rhizophora Mangle - M	Leaf	152 ppm
Cabbage, Red Cabbage, White Cabbage - Brassica Oleracea var. Capitata - E	Leaf	151 ppm
Date Palm - Phoenix Dactylifera - E	Fruit	151 ppm
Okra - Abelmoschus Esculentus - Friut - E - M	Fruit	150 ppm
Chocolate Vine - Akebia Quinata - M	Stem	150 ppm
Blackberry Lily, Shenan - Belamcanda Chinensis - M	Rhizome	150 ppm
Calamansi, Calamondin - Citrus Mitis - Friut - E	Fruit	30-300 ppm

Bladderwrack, Kelp - Fucus Vesiculosus - E - M	Plant	150 ppm
Dyer's Woad - Isatis Tinctoria - M	Root	150 ppm
Common Juniper, Juniper - Juniperus Communis - E - M - T	Fruit	150 ppm
Chinese Cornbind, Chinese Knotweed, Fleeceflower, Fo Ti, He Shou Wu - Polygonum Multiflorum - E - M - T	Rhizome	150 ppm
Ching-Feng-Teng - Sinomenium Acutum - E - M	Rhizome	150 ppm
Clove, Clovetree - Syzygium Aromaticum - E	Flower	150 ppm
Greater Galangal, Languas, Siamese Ginger - Alpinia Galanga - M	Rhizome	149 ppm
Betel Nut, Pin-Lang - Areca Catechu Amphicarpaea Bracteata- E - M	Shoot	147 ppm
Black bean, Dwarf bean, Field bean, Flageolet bean, French bean, Garden bean, Green bean, Haricot, Haricot bean, Haricot vert, Kidney bean, Navy bean, Pop bean, Popping bean, Snap bean, String bean, Wax bean - Phaseolus Vulgaris - E	Seed	147 ppm
Pumpkin - Cucurbita Maxima - E	Leaf	145 ppm
Pumpkin - Cucurbita Pepo - E	Flower	144 ppm
Watermelon - Citrullus Lanatus - E	Fruit	143 ppm
Opium Poppy, Poppyseed Poppy - Papaver Somniferum - E	Seed	143 ppm
Granadilla - Passiflora Quadrangularis - E	Fruit	143 ppm
Mat Bean, Moth Bean - Vigna Aconitifolia - E	Seed	143 ppm
Hsin-Pa-Pi, Kisasage - Catalpa Ovata - E - M	Fruit	140 ppm
Horsetail, Scouring Rush - Equisetum Hyemale - M	Plant	140 ppm
Pito - Erythrina Berteroana - E	Shoot	140 ppm
Chinese Boxthorn, Chinese Matrimony Vine, Chinese Wolfberry - Lycium Chinense - E - M	Fruit	140 ppm
Ben Nut, Benzolive Tree, Drumstick Tree, Horseradish Tree, Moringa, West Indian Ben - Moringa Oleifera - E	Leaf	70-280 ppm
Mace, Nutmeg - Myristica Fragrans - E	Aril	140 ppm
Black Caraway, Black Cumin, Fennel-Flower, Nutmeg-Flower, Roman Coriander - Nigella Sativa - E - M	Seed	140 ppm
Hsuan-Shen, Yuan-Shen - Scrophularia Buergeriana - M	Root	140 ppm
Hemp, Indian Hemp, Marihuana, Marijuana - Cannabis Sativa - M	Seed	139 ppm
Pistachio - Pistacia Vera - E	Seed	137 ppm
Aubergine, Egg Solanum Melongena - E	Fruit	137 ppm
Brussel-Sprout - Brassica Oleracea var. Gemmifera - E	Leaf	136 ppm
Bambarra Groundnut, Groundbean - Vigna Subterranea - E	Seed	136 ppm
Onion, Shallot - Allium Cepa - Shallot Bulb - E	Bulb	135 ppm
Cayenne, Chili, Hot Pepper, Red Chili, Spur Pepper, Tabasco - Capsicum Frutescens - E	Fruit	135 ppm
Perilla - Perilla Frutescens - E - M - T	Seed	135 ppm
Granadilla - Passiflora Quadrangularis - E	Seed	134 ppm
New Zealand Spinach - Tetragonia Tetragonioides - E	Leaf	133 ppm
Buckwheat - Fagopyrum Esculentum - E	Seed	132 ppm
Green Gram, Mungbean - Vigna Radiata - E	Sprout Seedling	132 ppm
Akee, Seso Vegetal - Blighia Sapida - M	Aril	130 ppm
Cape Jasmine, Gardenia, Jasmin, Shan-Chih-Tzu, Shan-Zhi-Zi, Zhi Zi - Gardenia Jasminoides - M	Fruit	130 ppm
Shan Dou Gen - Sophora Subprostrata - M - T	Root	130 ppm
Garlic - Allium Sativum Bulb - E	Bulb	129 ppm
Mata Raton - Gliricidia Sepium - M	Flower	129 ppm
Potato - Solanum Tuberosum - E	Tuber	128 ppm
Yellow Mombin, Yellow Plum - Spondias Mombin - E	Fruit	127 ppm
Waxgourd - Benincasa Hispida - Fruit	Fruit	125 ppm
Barbados Gooseberry, Grosela Americana - Pereskia Aculeata - E - M	Fruit	0-250 ppm
Ramie - Boehmeria Nivea - M	Leaf	123 ppm
Apple - Malus Domestica - E	Fruit	123 ppm
Cauli Brassica Oleracea var. Botrytis - E	Flower	122 ppm

IRON CONTINUED

Plant	Part	ppm
Chinese Ash - Fraxinus Rhynchophylla - M - E	Bark	120 ppm
Japanese Privet, Ligustri Fructus - Ligustrum Japonicum - M	Fruit	120 ppm
Chinese Privet, Glossy Privet, Ligustri Fructus, Privet, White Waxtree - Ligustrum Lucidum - M	Fruit	120 ppm
Chinese Magnolia, Hou Pu, Magnolia- Magnolia Officinalis - E - M	Bark	120 ppm
Moutan, Moutan Peony, Tree Peony - Paeonia Suffruticosa - M	Root Bark	120 ppm
Radish - Raphanus Sativus - E	Seed	120 ppm
Wheat - Triticum Aestivum - E - M	Seed	120 ppm
Mugwort - Artemisia Vulgaris - M	Leaf	118 ppm
Ladyslipper - Cypripedium Pubescens - M	Root	117 ppm
Peach - Prunus Persica - E - M - T	Bark	117 ppm
Lentil - Lens Culinaris - E	Sprout Seedling	116 ppm
Devil's Tongue, Elephant Yam, Konjac, Leopard Palm, Snake Palm, Umbrella Arum - Amorphophallus Konjac - E - M - T	Leaf	115 ppm
Cape Gooseberry, Ground Cherry - Physalis Peruviana - E	Fruit	115 ppm
Cassava, Tapioca, Yuca - Manihot Esculenta - E	Root	114 ppm
Elephant-Foot Yam - Amorphophallus Campanulatus - E - M- T	Root	112 ppm
Parsnip - Pastinaca Sativa - E	Root	112 ppm
Mud Plantain, Tse-Hsieh, Water Plantain, Ze-Xie - Alisma Plantago Aquatica M	Rhizome	110 ppm
Curly Kale, Kale, Kitchen Kale, Scotch Kale - Brassica Oleracea var. Sabellica l. var. Acephala - E	Leaf	110 ppm
Chinese Quince, Mu-Kua - Chaenomeles Lagenaria - E	Fruit	110 ppm
Chinese Raspberry - Rubus Cchingii - E - M	Fruit	110 ppm
Cauli Brassica Oleracea var. Botrytis - E	Leaf	109 ppm
Indian Tamarind, Kilytree, Tamarind - Tamarindus Indica - M	Fruit	109 ppm
Black Currant - Ribes Nigrum - E	Fruit	108 ppm
Horseradish - Armoracia Rusticana - E	Root	106 ppm
Lentil - Lens Culinaris - E	Seed	106 ppm
Scarlet Runner Bean - Phaseolus Coccineus - E	Seed	103 ppm
Collards, Cow Cabbage, Spring-Heading Cabbage, Tall Kale, Tree Kale - Brassica Oleracea - E	Leaf	102 ppm
SafCarthamus Tinctorius - M	Seed	102 ppm
Black Gram - Vigna Mungo - E	Seed	102 ppm
Artichoke - Cynara Cardunculus - E	Flower	101 ppm
Mimosa - Albizia Julibrissin - E - M	Bark	100 ppm
Hardy Orchid, Hyacinth Bletilla, Hyacinth Orchid, Shiran - Bletilla Striata - M	Tuber	100 ppm
Java Cinnamon, Padang Cassia - Cinnamomum Burmannii - E - M - T	Bark	100 ppm
Strawberry - Fragaria spp. - E	Fruit	100 ppm
Genipap, Jagua - Genipa Americana - E - M	Seed	100 ppm
Barley, Barleygrass - Hordeum Vulgare - E - M	Seed	100 ppm
Indian Mulberry, Noni - Morinda Citrifolia - M	Leaf	100 ppm
Indian Fig, Nopal, Nopalito, Prickly Pear - Opuntia Ficus-Indica - E - M	Seed	100 ppm
Broadbean, Faba Bean, Habas - Vicia Faba - E	Seed	100 ppm
Cobnut, English Filbert, European Filbert, European Hazel, Hazel - Corylus Avellana - E	Seed	99 ppm
Peach - Prunus Persica - E - M - T	Fruit	99 ppm
Jack Bean - Canavalia Ensiformis - E	Seed	97 ppm
Jicaro - Crescentia Alata - M	Seed	97 ppm
Coca - Erythroxylum Novogranatense var. Novogranatense E M	Leaf	97 ppm
Ban-Xla, Pan-Hsla - Pinellia Ternata - E - M - T	Tuber	95 ppm
Terminalia catappa L. -- Indian Almond, Malabar Almond, Tropical Almond	Seed	95 ppm
Kapok, Silk-Cotton Tree - Ceiba Pentandra - M - E	Shoot	95 ppm
Bonavist Bean, Hyacinth Bean, Lablab Bean - Lablab Purpureus - E - M - T	Fruit	94.9 ppm
Asparagus bean, Pea bean, Yardlong bean - Vigna Unguiculata subsp. Sesquipedalis - E	Seed	94 ppm
Brazilnut, Brazilnut-Tree, Creamnut, Paranut - Bertholletia Eexcelsa - E	Seed	93 ppm
Sarson - Brassica Rapa - E	Seed	93 ppm

Plant	Part	ppm
Ben Nut, Benzolive Tree, Drumstick Tree, Horseradish Tree, Moringa, West Indian Ben - Moringa Oleifera - E	Shoot	40-185 ppm
Soybean - Glycine Max - E	Fruit	91 ppm
Chinese Dogwood - Cornus Officinalis - E - M	Fruit	90 ppm
Noble Dendrobium - Dendrobium Nobile - M	Stem	90 ppm
Maracuya, Passion Passiflora Edulis - E	Seed	0-180 ppm
Pea - Pisum Sativum - E	Seed	90 ppm
Rice Paper Tree, Tong-Cao, Tung-Tsao - Tetrapanax Papyrifera M	Pith	90 ppm
Grape Citrus Paradisi - E	Fruit	88 ppm
Indian Tamarind, Kilytree, Tamarind - Tamarindus Indica - M	Leaf	88 ppm
Black bean, Dwarf bean, Field bean, Flageolet bean, French bean, Garden bean, Green bean, Haricot, Haricot bean, Haricot vert, Kidney bean, Navy bean, Pop bean, Popping bean, Snap bean, String bean, Wax bean - Phaseolus Vulgaris - E	Sprout Seedling	87 ppm
Wou Chou Yu - Euodia Rutaecarpa - E	Fruit	86 ppm
Rice - Oryza Sativa - E	Seed	85 ppm
Allspice, Clover-Pepper, Jamaica-Pepper, Pimenta, Pimento - Pimenta Dioica - E	Fruit	85 ppm
Plum - Prunus Domestica - E - M	Fruit	85 ppm
Anu, Mashua - Tropaeolum Tuberosum - E	Root	85 ppm
Green Gram, Mungbean - Vigna Radiata - E	Seed	84 ppm
Carambola, Star Averrhoa Carambola - E	Fruit	1-165 ppm
Chinese Hibiscus, Shoe- Hibiscus Rosa-Sinensis - E	Flower	17-165 ppm
Strawberry Guava - Psidium Cattleianum - E	Fruit	82 ppm
Coca - Erythroxylum Novogranatense var. Truxillense - E - M	Leaf	81 ppm
Northern Red Oak - Quercus Rubra - E - M	Seed	81 ppm
Elephant Garlic, Kurrat - Allium Ampeloprasum - E	Root	80 ppm
Luffa, Smooth Loofah, Vegetable Sponge - Luffa Aegyptiaca - E	Fruit	80 ppm
Peach - Prunus Persica - E - M - T	Seed	80 ppm
Mandarin, Tangerine - Citrus Reticulata - E	Fruit	79 ppm
Apricot - Prunus Armeniaca - E - M - T	Fruit	79 ppm
American Elder, American Elderberry, Elderberry, Sweet Elder - Sambucus Canadensis - E	Plant	79 ppm
Garlic - Allium Sativum Bulb - E	Flower	78 ppm
Sour Cherry - Prunus Cerasus - E - M - T	Fruit	78 ppm
White Tephrosia - Tephrosia Candida - M - T	Plant	78 ppm
Cashew - Anacardium Occidentale - E	Fruit	77 ppm
Garlic - Allium Sativum Bulb - E	Shoot	76 ppm
Butternut - Juglans Cinerea - E	Seed	76 ppm
Wild Pineapple - Bromelia Pinguin - E - M	Shoot	75 ppm
Watermelon - Citrullus Lanatus - E	Seed	75 ppm
Pineapple - Ananas Comosus - E	Fruit	73 ppm
Pecan - Carya Illinoensis - E	Seed	73 ppm
Summer Squash - Cucurbita spp. - E	Fruit	73 ppm
Soybean - Glycine Max - E	Sprout Seedling	73 ppm
Black Walnut - Juglans Nigra - E	Seed	73 ppm
Olive - Olea Europaea - E	Fruit	73 ppm
Banana Yucca, Blue Yucca, Spanish Bayonet, Yucca - Yucca Baccata - E - M - T	Root	73 ppm
Chickpea, Garbanzo - Cicer Arietinum - E	Seed	72 ppm
Lemon - Citrus Limon - E	Fruit	72 ppm
Girasol, Sun Helianthus Annuus - E	Seed	71 ppm
Water Lotus - Nelumbo Nucifera - E - M	Seed	71 ppm
Avocado - Persea Americana - E - M - T	Fruit	71 ppm
Betel Nut, Pin-Lang - Areca Catechu Amphicarpaea Bracteata- E - M	Seed	70 ppm
Kuan Chung, Shield Fernle - Blechnum Orientale - E - M - T	Rhizome	70 ppm
American Persimmon - Diospyros Virginiana - E - M	Fruit	70 ppm
Oriental Pipewort - Eriocaulon spp. - M	Leaf	70 ppm
Chinese Parasol - Firmiana Simplex - E - M	Seed	70 ppm
Water Lotus - Nelumbo Nucifera - E - M	Rhizome	70 ppm
Indian Tamarind, Kilytree, Tamarind - Tamarindus Indica - M	Flower	70 ppm
Asparagus bean, Pea bean, Yardlong bean - Vigna Unguiculata subsp. Sesquipedalis - E	Fruit	69 ppm

IRON CONTINUED

Species	Part	Quantity
Adlay, Adlay Millet, Job's-Tears, Yi-Yi-Ren - Coix Lacryma-Jobi - E - M	Seed	68 ppm
Chinese Kudzu - Pueraria Pseudohirsuta - E - M	Root	68 ppm
Red Currant, White Currant - Ribes Rubrum - E	Fruit	68 ppm
Lime - Citrus Aurantiifolia - E	Fruit	67 ppm
Loquat - Eriobotrya Japonica - E	Fruit	67 ppm
Salsify - Tragopogon Porrifolius - E	Root	67 ppm
Sugar-Apple, Sweetsop - Annona Squamosa - E	Fruit	66 ppm
Cardamom - Elettaria Cardamomum - E - M	Fruit	66 ppm
Andean Lupine, Chocho, Tarhui - Lupinus Mutabilis - E - T	Fruit	66 ppm
Northern Red Oak - Quercus Rubra - E - M	Seed	Trace
Shagbark Hickory - Carya Ovata - E	Seed	Trace
Coconut, Coconut Palm - Cocos Nucifera - E	Seed	Trace
Butternut - Juglans Cinerea - E	Seed	Trace
Black Walnut - Juglans Nigra - E	Seed	Trace
Almond - Prunus Dulcis - E - M - T	Seed	Trace
Cashew - Anacardium Occidentale - E	Seed	Trace
Pecan - Carya Illinoensis - E	Seed	Trace
Cobnut, English Filbert, European Filbert, European Hazel, Hazel - Corylus Avellana - E	Seed	Trace
Pistachio - Pistacia Vera - E	Seed	Trace

PLANTS CONTAINING LANTHANUM

Species	Part	Quantity
Red Pignut Hickory - Carya Glabra - E	Shoot	220 ppm
Shagbark Hickory - Carya Ovata - E	Shoot	90 ppm
Dwarf Sumac, Winged Sumac - Rhus Copallina - E - M	Leaf	29 ppm
White Oak - Quercus Alba - M	Stem	23.6 ppm
Cabbage, Red Cabbage, White Cabbage - Brassica Oleracea var. Capitata - E	Leaf	20.3 ppm
Lettuce - Lactuca Sativa - E	Leaf	20.3 ppm
Northern Red Oak - Quercus Rubra - E - M	Stem	19.8 ppm
Black Cherry, Wild Cherry - Prunus Serotina - E - M - T	Leaf	19 ppm
American Styrax, Sweetgum - Liquidambar Styraciflua - E - M	Stem	18 ppm
American Persimmon - Diospyros Virginiana - E - M	Stem	16.2 ppm
Black Cherry, Wild Cherry - Prunus Serotina - E - M - T	Stem	16 ppm
American Persimmon - Diospyros Virginiana - E - M	Leaf	15 ppm
Black Oak - Quercus Velutina - E - M	Stem	14.9 ppm
Plum - Prunus Domestica - E - M	Fruit	12 ppm
Dwarf Sumac, Winged Sumac - Rhus Copallina - E - M	Stem	9.2 ppm
American Styrax, Sweetgum - Liquidambar Styraciflua - E - M	Leaf	8.2 ppm
Brazilnut, Brazilnut-Tree, Creamnut, Paranut - Bertholletia Eexcelsa - E	Seed	Trace

PLANTS CONTAINING LITHIUM

Species	Part	Quantity
Guanique - Chamissoa Altissima - M	Leaf	13-132 ppm
Shagbark Hickory - Carya Ovata - E	Shoot	11.7 ppm
Red Pignut Hickory - Carya Glabra - E	Shoot	6.6 ppm
Black Oak - Quercus Velutina - E - M	Stem	5.2 ppm
White Oak - Quercus Alba - M	Stem	4.94 ppm
Common thyme, Garden thyme, Thyme - Thymus Vulgaris - E - M	Plant	4 ppm
Northern Red Oak - Quercus Rubra - E - M	Stem	3.96 ppm
Black bean, Dwarf bean, Field bean, Flageolet bean, French bean, Garden bean, Green bean, Haricot, Haricot bean, Haricot vert, Kidney bean, Navy bean, Pop bean, Popping bean, Snap bean, String bean, Wax bean - Phaseolus Vulgaris - E	Fruit	2.7 ppm
Lettuce - Lactuca Sativa - E	Leaf	2.6 ppm
Black bean, Dwarf bean, Field bean, Flageolet bean, French bean, Garden bean, Green bean, Haricot, Haricot bean, Haricot vert, Kidney bean, Navy bean, Pop bean, Popping bean, Snap bean, String bean, Wax bean - Phaseolus Vulgaris - E	Seed	2.45 ppm
Grape Citrus Paradisi - E	Fruit	2.31 ppm
Orange - Citrus Sinensis - E	Fruit	1.54 ppm

Species	Part	Quantity
Cabbage, Red Cabbage, White Cabbage - Brassica Oleracea var. Capitata - E	Leaf	1.4 ppm
Buckbush - Symphoricarpos Orbiculatus - M	Stem	1.06 ppm
Endive, Escarole - Cichorium Endivia - M	Leaf	Trace
Chinese Cabbage - Brassica Pekinensis - E	Leaf	Trace
Parsley - Petroselinum Crispum - E	Plant	Trace
Tomato - Lycopersicon Esculentum - E - M - T	Fruit	Trace
Plum - Prunus Domestica - E - M	Fruit	Trace
Asparagus - Asparagus Officinalis - E	Shoot	Trace
Beet, Beetroot, Garden Beet, Sugar Beet - Beta Vulgaris - E	Root	Trace
Carrot - Daucus Carota - E	Root	Trace
Peach - Prunus Persica - E - M - T	Fruit	Trace
Cucumber - Cucumis Sativus - E	Fruit	Trace
Cantaloupe, Melon, Muskmelon, Netted Melon, Nutmeg Melon, Persian Melon - Cucumis Melo subsp. ssp Melo var.Ccantalupensis - Friut - E	Fruit	Trace
Shortleaf Pine - Pinus Echinata - M	Shoot	Trace
Bell Pepper, Cherry Pepper, Cone Pepper, Green Pepper, Paprika, Sweet Pepper - Capsicum Annuum - E	Fruit	Trace
Red Cedar - Juniperus Virginiana Amphicarpaea Bracteata- E - M - T	Shoot	Trace
Onion, Shallot - Allium Cepa - Shallot Bulb - E	Bulb	Trace
Aubergine, Egg Solanum Melongena - E	Fruit	Trace
European Grape, Grape, Grapevine, Vigne Vinifere,Wine Grape - Vitis Vinifera - E - M	Fruit	Trace
Potato - Solanum Tuberosum - E	Tuber	Trace
Corn - Zea Mays - E	Seed	Trace
Pear - Pyrus Communis - E	Fruit	Trace
Apple - Malus Domestica - E	Fruit	Trace
Cayenne, Chili, Hot Pepper, Red Chili, Spur Pepper, Tabasco - Capsicum Frutescens - E	Fruit	Trace
Flax, Lin Linum Usitatissimum - E	Seed	Trace

Plants Containing

LUTETIUM

Species	Part	Quantity
Black Walnut - Juglans Nigra - E	Seed	Trace
Cashew - Anacardium Occidentale - E	Seed	Trace
Brazilnut, Brazilnut-Tree, Creamnut, Paranut - Bertholletia Eexcelsa - E	Seed	Trace
Pecan - Carya Illinoensis - E	Seed	Trace
Shagbark Hickory - Carya Ovata - E	Seed	Trace
Coconut, Coconut Palm - Cocos Nucifera - E	Seed	Trace
Pistachio - Pistacia Vera - E	Seed	Trace
Almond - Prunus Dulcis - E - M - T	Seed	Trace
Northern Red Oak - Quercus Rubra - E - M	Seed	Trace
Butternut - Juglans Cinerea - E	Seed	Trace
Cobnut, English Filbert, European Filbert, European Hazel, Hazel - Corylus Avellana - E	Seed	Trace

PLANTS CONTAINING MAGNESIUM

Species	Part	Quantity
Red Pignut Hickory - Carya Glabra - E	Shoot	24,200 ppm
Shagbark Hickory - Carya Ovata - E	Shoot	21,600 ppm
Irish moss - Chondrus Crispus - E	Plant	19,600 ppm
Purslane, Verdolaga - Portulaca Oleracea - E	Herb	18,700 ppm
Black bean, Dwarf bean, Field bean, Flageolet bean, French bean, Garden bean, Green bean, Haricot, Haricot bean, Haricot vert, Kidney bean, Navy bean, Pop bean, Popping bean, Snap bean, String bean, Wax bean - Phaseolus Vulgaris - E	Fruit	18,000 ppm
Opium Poppy, Poppyseed Poppy - Papaver Somniferum - E	Seed	15,600 ppm
Oats - Avena Sativa - E - M	Plant	14,800 ppm
Spinach - Spinacia Oleracea - E	Plant	11,000 ppm
Purple Tephrosia, Wild Indigo - Tephrosia Purpurea - M - T	Leaf	10,300 ppm
Snakegourd - Trichosanthes Anguina - E - M	Fruit	9,815 ppm

MAGNESIUM CONTINUED

Commom Licorice, Licorice, Licorice-Root, Smooth Licorice - Glycyrrhiza Glabra - M	Root	9,650 ppm
Black Cherry, Wild Cherry - Prunus Serotina - E - M - T	Leaf	9,600 ppm
Dwarf Sumac, Winged Sumac - Rhus Copallina - E - M	Leaf	9,600 ppm
Black Gum, Black Tupelo - Nyssa Sylvatica - E - M	Leaf	9,100 ppm
Red Cedar - Juniperus Virginiana Amphicarpaea Bracteata- E - M - T	Shoot	8,800 ppm
Red Mangrove - Rhizophora Mangle - M	Leaf	8,800 ppm
Buckbush - Symphoricarpos Orbiculatus - M	Stem	8,800 ppm
Groundnut, Peanut - Arachis Hypogaea - E - M	Plant	8,700 ppm
Lettuce - Lactuca Sativa - E	Leaf	8,700 ppm
Bladderwrack, Kelp - Fucus Vesiculosus - E - M	Plant	8,670 ppm
European Nettle, Stinging Nettle - Urtica Dioica - E - M	Leaf	8,600 ppm
Northern Red Oak - Quercus Rubra - E - M	Stem	8,580 ppm
American Styrax, Sweetgum - Liquidambar Styraciflua - E - M	Stem	8,400 ppm
Cowgrass, Peavine Clover, Purple Clover, Red Clover - Trifolium Pratense - E - M	Hay	8,100 ppm
ElytriCouchgrass, Doggrass, Quackgrass, Twitchgrass, Wheatgrass - Elytrigia Repens - E - M	Plant	7,570 ppm
Chinese Parsley, Cilantro, Coriander - Coriandrum Sativum E	Leaf	7,488 ppm
Beebread, Beeplant, Borage, Talewort - Borago Officinalis - E - M - T	Leaf	7,436 ppm
Baikal Skullcap, Chinese Skullcap, Huang Qin - Scutellaria Baicalensis - M	Root	7,220 ppm
Neem - Azadirachta Indica - M	Leaf	7,100 ppm
Flax, Lin Linum Usitatissimum - E	Seed	7,002 ppm
Asparagus - Asparagus Officinalis - E	Shoot	7,000 ppm
Cucumber - Cucumis Sativus - E	Fruit	7,000 ppm
Butter Bean, Lima Bean - Phaseolus Lunatus - E	Seed	7,000 ppm
Wheat - Triticum Aestivum - E - M	Plant	7,000 ppm
Coca - Erythroxylum Novogranatense var. Novogranatense - E - M	Leaf	6,900 ppm
Chives - Allium Schoenoprasum - E	Leaf	6,875 ppm
Black Oak - Quercus Velutina - E - M	Stem	6,820 ppm
Sassafras - Sassafras Albidum - E - M - T	Leaf	6,800 ppm
Coca - Erythroxylum Novogranatense var. Truxillense - E - M	Leaf	6,700 ppm
Pigweed - Amaranthus sp. - E - M	Leaf	6,616 ppm
Peppermint - Mentha x Piperita subsp. Nothosubsp. Piperita - E - M - T	Leaf	6,610 ppm
New Zealand Spinach - Tetragonia Tetragonioides - E	Leaf	6,500 ppm
Dill, Garden Dill - Anethum Graveolens - E	Plant	6,470 ppm
Cockscomb - Celosia Cristata - M	Flower	6,080 ppm
Okra - Abelmoschus Esculentus - Friut - E - M	Fruit	6,000 ppm
Tomato - Lycopersicon Esculentum - E - M - T	Fruit	6,000 ppm
Dulse - Rhodymenia Palmata - E	Plant	5,930 ppm
Post Oak - Quercus Stellata - E - M	Stem	5,880 ppm
Bok-Choy, Celery Cabbage, Celery Mustard, Chinese Cabbage, Chinese Mustard, Chinese White Cabbage, Pak-Choi - Brassica Chinensis - E	Leaf	5,844 ppm
Pumpkin - Cucurbita Pepo - E	Seed	5,748 ppm
American Styrax, Sweetgum - Liquidambar Styraciflua - E - M	Leaf	5,740 ppm
Chaff Achyranthes Bidentata - M	Root	5,730 ppm
Coca - Erythroxylum Coca var. Coca - E - M	Leaf	5,700 ppm
White Willow - Salix Alba - M	Bark	5,600 ppm
Parsley - Petroselinum Crispum - E	Plant	5,577 ppm
Bonavist Bean, Hyacinth Bean, Lablab Bean - Lablab Purpureus - E - M - T	Seed	5,505 ppm
European Pennyroyal - Mentha pulegium - E - M- T	Plant	5,500 ppm
Devil's claw, Grapple Harpagophytum procumbens - M	Root	5,440 ppm
American Persimmon - Diospyros Virginiana - E - M	Stem	5,400 ppm
Black Cherry, Wild Cherry - Prunus Serotina - E - M - T	Stem	5,400 ppm
Burdock, Gobo, Great Burdock - Arctium lappa - E - M - T	Root	5,370 ppm
Asian Plantain - Plantago Asiatica - E - M	Plant	5,320 ppm
White Oak - Quercus Alba - M	Stem	5,320 ppm
Evening-Primrose - Oenothera Biennis - E - M	Seed	5,300 ppm

Plant	Part	ppm
Chickweed, Common Chickweed - Stellaria Media - E	Plant	5,290 ppm
Henbane - Hyoscyamus Niger - E - M	Seed	5,250 ppm
Jew's Mallow, Mulukiya, Nalta Jute - Corchorus Olitorius - E - M	Leaf	5,200 ppm
Marshmallow, White Mallow - Althaea Officinalis - M	Root	5,180 ppm
Girasol, Sun Helianthus Annuus - E	Seed	5,176 ppm
Pawpaw - Asimina Triloba - Friut - E	Fruit	5,128 ppm
Chinese Licorice - Glycyrrhiza Uralensis - M	Root	5,070 ppm
Fennel - Foeniculum Vulgare - M	Fruit	5,012 ppm
American Persimmon - Diospyros Virginiana - E - M	Leaf	5,000 ppm
Mat Bean, Moth Bean - Vigna Aconitifolia - E	Seed	4,962 ppm
Pumpkin - Cucurbita Pepo - E	Flower	4,950 ppm
Wou Chou Yu - Euodia Rutaecarpa - E	Fruit	4,950 ppm
Celery - Apium Graveolens - E	Seed	4,903 ppm
Waxgourd - Benincasa Hispida - Fruit	Fruit	4,870 ppm
Manioc Hibiscus - Abelmoschus Manihot - E - M	Leaf	4,862 ppm
Ma-Huang - Ephedra spp. - M	Plant	4,780 ppm
Sassafras - Sassafras Albidum - E - M - T	Stem	4,760 ppm
Smooth Sumac - Rhus Glabra - E - M	Stem	4,690 ppm
Garden Sorrel - Rumex Acetosa - E - M - T	Leaf	4,600 ppm
Heal-All, Self-Heal - Prunella Vulgaris - E - M	Flower	4,560 ppm
Chinese Parasol - Firmiana Simplex - E - M	Seed	4,480 ppm
Dyer's Woad - Isatis Tinctoria - M	Root	4,410 ppm
Alfalfa, Lucerne - Medicago Sativa subsp. Sativa - E	Plant	4,400 ppm
Black Gum, Black Tupelo - Nyssa Sylvatica - E - M	Stem	4,400 ppm
Field Horsetail, Horsetail - Equisetum Arvense - M	Plant	4,370 ppm
Common thyme, Garden thyme, Thyme - Thymus Vulgaris - E - M	Leaf	4,360 ppm
European Grape, Grape, Grapevine, Vigne Vinifere, Wine Grape - Vitis Vinifera - E - M	Stem	4,360 ppm
Basil, Cuban Basil, Sweet Basil - Ocimum Basilicum - E	Leaf	4,340 ppm
Tomato - Lycopersicon Esculentum - E - M - T	Leaf	4,300 ppm
Artichoke - Cynara Cardunculus - E	Flower	4,275 ppm
Dwarf Sumac, Winged Sumac - Rhus Copallina - E - M	Stem	4,270 ppm
Potato - Solanum Tuberosum - E	Tuber	4,250 ppm
Peach - Prunus Persica - E - M - T	Bark	4,220 ppm
Asparagus bean, Pea bean, Yardlong bean - Vigna Unguiculata subsp. Sesquipedalis - E	Shoot	4,207 ppm
Beet, Beetroot, Garden Beet, Sugar Beet - Beta Vulgaris - E	Root	4,200 ppm
Berro, Watercress - Nasturtium Officinale - E	Herb	4,200 ppm
Eyebright - Euphrasia Officinalis - M	Plant	4,160 ppm
Asparagus bean, Pea bean, Yardlong bean - Vigna Unguiculata subsp. Sesquipedalis - E	Fruit	4,160 ppm
Fortune's Fern - Drynaria Fortunei - M	Rhizome	4,140 ppm
Sesame - Sesamum Indicum - E - M	Seed	4,082 ppm
Mongoloid Dandelion - Taraxacum Mongolicum - E - M	Plant	4,050 ppm
Paper Mulberry - Broussonetia Papyrifera - E - M	Fruit	4,030 ppm
Lady's Thistle, Milk Thistle - Silybum Marianum - M	Plant	4,030 ppm
Chinese Parsley, Cilantro, Coriander - Coriandrum Sativum E	Fruit	4,016 ppm
Neem - Azadirachta Indica - M	Fruit	4,000 ppm
Radish - Raphanus Sativus - E	Seed	3,960 ppm
Asparagus bean, Pea bean, Yardlong bean - Vigna Unguiculata subsp. Sesquipedalis - E	Seed	3,952 ppm
Evening-Primrose - Oenothera Biennis - E - M	Herb	3,900 ppm
Marjoram, Sweet Marjoram - Origanum Majorana - E	Plant	3,900 ppm
Mustard Greens - Brassica Juncea - E	Leaf	3,837 ppm
Perilla - Perilla Frutescens - E - M - T	Plant	3,830 ppm
Swamp Cabbage, Water Spinach - Ipomoea Aquatica - E	Leaf	3,810 ppm
Peach - Prunus Persica - E - M - T	Seed	3,810 ppm
Bitter Melon, Sorosi - Momordica Charantia - E	Fruit	3,800 ppm
Chayote - Sechium Edule - E - M	Leaf	3,785 ppm

Hillman Health Food Store call 855-Amish-Dr (855-264-7437) www.emineral.info Vitamins and Minerals for Better Living

MAGNESIUM CONTINUED

Name	Part	ppm
Narrowleaf Sophora - Sophora Angustifolia - M - T- M - T	Root	3,720 ppm
Pea - Pisum Sativum - E	Plant	3,700 ppm
Chinese Kudzu - Pueraria Pseudohirsuta - E - M	Root	3,690 ppm
Summer Squash - Cucurbita spp. - E	Fruit	3,640 ppm
Jussiaeae Herba, Pond Dragon - Jussiaea Repens - M	Plant	3,590 ppm
Radish - Raphanus Sativus - E	Root	3,570 ppm
Bastard Cardamom, Chin Kousha, Malabar Cardamom, Tavoy Cardamom - Amomum Xanthioides - E	Seed	3,540 ppm
Wheat - Triticum Aestivum - E - M	Seed	3,500 ppm
Indian Sorrel, Jamaica Sorrel, Stevia, Sweet Leaf of Paraguay - Stevia Rebaudiana - E	Leaf	3,490 ppm
Cowgrass, Peavine Clover, Purple Clover, Red Clover - Trifolium Pratense - E - M	Flower	3,490 ppm
Tarragon - Artemisia Dracunculus - M	Plant	3,470 ppm
Ben Nut, Benzolive Tree, Drumstick Tree, Horseradish Tree, Moringa, West Indian Ben - Moringa Oleifera - E	Shoot	1,470-6,890 ppm
Dokudami, Fishwort, Yu Xing Cao - Houttuynia Cordata - E - M	Plant	3,430 ppm
Black bean, Dwarf bean, Field bean, Flageolet bean, French bean, Garden bean, Green bean, Haricot, Haricot bean, Haricot vert, Kidney bean, Navy bean, Pop bean, Popping bean, Snap bean, String bean, Wax bean - Phaseolus Vulgaris - E	Seed	3,430 ppm
Plum - Prunus Domestica - E - M	Fruit	3,400 ppm
Chai-Hu - Bupleurum - M	Root	3,390 ppm
Ching-Chieh, Jing-Jie - Schizonepeta Tenuifolia - E - M	Plant	3,390 ppm
Brazilnut, Brazilnut-Tree, Creamnut, Paranut - Bertholletia Eexcelsa - E	Seed	3,370 ppm
Lemongrass, West indian lemongrass - Cymbopogon Citratus - E - M	Plant	3,310 ppm
Cantaloupe, Melon, Muskmelon, Netted Melon, Nutmeg Melon, Persian Melon - Cucumis Melo subsp. ssp Melo var.Ccantalupensis - Friut - E	Fruit	3,300 ppm
White Mustard - Sinapis Alba - E - M - T	Seed	3,282 ppm
Dan-Shen, Red Sage, Tan-Shen - Salvia Miltiorrhiza - E - M	Root	3,230 ppm
Flannelleaf, Flannelplant, Great mullein, Mullein, Velvet Verbascum Thapsus - M	Leaf	3,230 ppm
Sicklepod - Senna Obtusifolia - E - T	Seed	3,220 ppm
Gotu Kola, Pennywort - Centella Asiatica - E - M	Leaf	3,200 ppm
Curly Dock, Lengua De Vaca, Sour Dock, Yellow Dock - Rumex Crispus - M - T	Root	3,200 ppm
Chinese Anemone - Pulsatilla Chinensis - M	Root	3,190 ppm
Raspberry, Red raspberry - Rubus Idaeus - E - M	Leaf	3,190 ppm
Sickle Senna - Cassia Tora - Sprout - Seedling - M	Seed	3,180 ppm
Common Valerian, Garden-Heliotrope, Valerian - Valeriana Officinalis - E - M	Root	3,180 ppm
Malanga, Tannia, Yautia - Xanthosoma Sagittifolium - E	Leaf	3,170 ppm
Soybean - Glycine Max - E	Seed	3,160 ppm
Cobnut, English Filbert, European Filbert, European Hazel, Hazel - Corylus Avellana - E	Seed	3,156 ppm
Chinese Cabbage - Brassica Pekinensis - E	Leaf	3,150 ppm
Taro - Colocasia Esculenta - E	Leaf	3,140 ppm
Almond - Prunus Dulcis - E - M - T	Seed	3,126 ppm
Elephant-Foot Yam - Amorphophallus Campanulatus - E - M - T	Root	3,120 ppm
Crampbark, European Cranberry bush, Guelder Rose, Snowballbush - Viburnum Opulus - E - M - T	Bark	3,110 ppm
European Mistletoe - Viscum Album - M - T	Leaf	3,110 ppm
Flax, Lin Linum Usitatissimum - E	Hay	3,100 ppm
Cauli Brassica Oleracea var. Botrytis - E	Leaf	3,072 ppm
Clove, Clovetree - Syzygium Aromaticum - E	Flower	3,020 ppm
Common Turkish Oregano, European Oregano, Oregano, Pot Marjoram, Wild Marjoram, Wild Oregano - Origanum Vulgare - E	Plant	3,016 ppm
Common thyme, Garden thyme, Thyme - Thymus Vulgaris - E - M	Plant	2,992 ppm
Japanese Honeysuckle - Lonicera Japonica - M	Flower	2,990 ppm

Name	Part	ppm
Qiang Huo - Notopterygium Incisum - M	Rhizome	2,980 ppm
Goldenseal - Hydrastis Canadensis - M	Root	2,940 ppm
Willow Oak - Quercus Phellos - E - M	Stem	2,940 ppm
Garden Camomile, Perennial Camomile, Roman Camomile - Chamaemelum Nobile M	Flower	2,920 ppm
Lambsquarter - Chenopodium Album - E - M - T	Seed	2,920 ppm
Oats - Avena Sativa - E - M	Seed	2,900 ppm
Genipap, Jagua - Genipa Americana - E - M	Fruit	2,900 ppm
Dill, Garden Dill - Anethum Graveolens - E	Fruit	2,893 ppm
Coffee Senna - Senna Occidentalis - E - T	Seed	2,880 ppm
Caraway, Carum - Carum Carvi - E	Fruit	2,863 ppm
Wu Chia Pi - Acanthopanax Gracilistylis - M	Root Bark	2,840 ppm
Cornmint, Field Mint, Japanese Mint - Mentha Arvensis var. Piperascens - E - M- T	Plant	2,830 ppm
Cherokee Rose - Rosa Laevigata - E - M	Fruit	2,830 ppm
Sage - Salvia Officinalis - E - M	Leaf	2,830 ppm
Luffa, Smooth Loofah, Vegetable Sponge - Luffa Aegyptiaca - E	Fruit	2,800 ppm
Collards, Cow Cabbage, Spring-Heading Cabbage, Tall Kale, Tree Kale - Brassica Oleracea - E	Leaf	2,786 ppm
Alholva, Bockshornklee, Fenugreek, Greek Clover, Greek Trigonella Foenum-Graecum - E - M	Seed	2,780 ppm
Chinese Magnolia Vine, Five-Flavor-Fruit, Magnolia Vine, Schizandra, Wu Wei Zi, Wu Wei Zu - Schisandra Chinensis - M	Fruit	2,760 ppm
Pumpkin - Cucurbita Maxima - E	Leaf	2,752 ppm
Gentian, Yellow Gentian - Gentiana Lutea - M	Root	2,740 ppm
Chinese Raspberry - Rubus Cchingii - E - M	Fruit	2,740 ppm
Mugwort - Artemisia Vulgaris - M	Shoot	2,700 ppm
Ginger - Zingiber Officinale - E	Rhizome	2,690 ppm
Butternut - Juglans Cinerea - E	Seed	2,676 ppm
Hsi Chien, Saint Paul'Swort - Siegesbeckia Orientalis - M	Plant	2,660 ppm
Chicory, Succory, Witloof - Cichorium Intybus - E - M	Leaf	2,652 ppm
Chinese Angelica, Dong Gui, Dong Quai - Angelica Sinensis - M	Root	2,650 ppm
Celery - Apium Graveolens - E	Leaf	2,650 ppm
Water Lotus - Nelumbo Nucifera - E - M	Seed	2,650 ppm
Asparagus Pea, Goa Bean, Winged Bean - Psophocarpus Tetragonolobus - E	Seed	2,623 ppm
Rutabaga, Swede, Swedish Turnip - Brassica Napus var. Napobrassica - E	Root	2,610 ppm
Chinese Boxthorn, Chinese Matrimony Vine, Chinese Wolfberry - Lycium Chinense - E - M	Root Bark	2,610 ppm
Asian Wild Ginger - Asiasarum Heterotropoides - M	Root	2,600 ppm
Siebold's Wild Ginger - Asiasarum Sieboldii - M	Root	2,600 ppm
Pea - Pisum Sativum - E	Fruit	2,591 ppm
Chinese Spikenard - Nardostachys Chinensis - M	Rhizome	2,590 ppm
Kuan Chung, Shield Fernle - Blechnum Orientale - E - M - T	Rhizome	2,580 ppm
Chinese Rhubarb - Rheum Palmatum - E	Rhizome	2,560 ppm
Green Gram, Mungbean - Vigna Radiata - E	Sprout Seedling	2,560 ppm
Spirulina - Spirulina Pratensis - E	Plant	2,550 ppm
Butterbur - Petasites Japonicus - T	Pt	2,545 ppm
Dandelion - Taraxacum Officinale - E - M	Leaf	2,500 ppm
Dan Zhu Ye - Lophatherum Gracile - M	Plant	2,490 ppm
Rosemary - Rosmarinus Officinalis - E - M	Plant	2,483 ppm
Loquat - Eriobotrya Japonica - E	Leaf	2,480 ppm
Black Mustard - Brassica Nigra - E	Leaf	2,471 ppm
Calabash Gourd, White-Flowered Gourd - Lagenaria Siceraria - E	Fruit	2,465 ppm
White Mulberry - Morus Alba - E - M	Root Bark	2,450 ppm
Chinese Goldthread, Huang-Lian, Huang-Lien - Coptis Chinensis - M	Rhizome	2,420 ppm
Huang-Lia, Huang-Lian, Huang-Lien, Japanese Goldthread - Coptis Japonica - M	Rhizome	2,420 ppm
Generic Goldthread - Coptis spp. - M	Rhizome	2,420 ppm
Soursop - Annona Muricata - E	Fruit	2,400 ppm

MAGNESIUM CONTINUED

Plant	Part	ppm
Feverfew - Chrysanthemum Parthenium - M	Plant	2,400 ppm
Endive, Escarole - Cichorium Endivia - M	Leaf	2,400 ppm
Japanese Ginseng - Panax Japonicus - M	Rhizome	2,400 ppm
Hops - Humulus Lupulus - E - M - T	Fruit	2,380 ppm
Bell Pepper, Cherry Pepper, Cone Pepper, Green Pepper, Paprika, Sweet Pepper - Capsicum Annuum - E	Fruit	2,340 ppm
Antler Herb, Clubmoss - Lycopodium Clavatum - M - T	Plant	2,340 ppm
Chinese Cornbind, Chinese Knotweed, Fleeceflower, Fo Ti, He Shou Wu - Polygonum Multiflorum - E - M - T	Root	2,340 ppm
Box-Holly, Butcher's broom - Ruscus aculeatus - E - M	Root	2,340 ppm
Black Pepper, Pepper, White Pepper - Piper Nigrum - E - M	Fruit	2,319 ppm
European Grape, Grape, Grapevine, Vigne Vinifere, Wine Grape - Vitis Vinifera - E - M	Fruit	2,310 ppm
Barley, Barleygrass - Hordeum Vulgare - E - M	Seed	2,300 ppm
Garland Chrysanthemum - Chrysanthemum Coronarium - Bud - E	Bud	2,285 ppm
Climbing Fern - Lygodium Japonicum - Pollen or Spore - M	Pollen Or Spore	2,270 ppm
Cashew - Anacardium Occidentale - E	Seed	1,886 ppm
SafCarthamus Tinctorius - M	Flower	2,260 ppm
Broadbean, Faba Bean, Habas - Vicia Faba - E	Fruit	2,260 ppm
Black bean, Dwarf bean, Field bean, Flageolet bean, French bean, Garden bean, Green bean, Haricot, Haricot bean, Haricot vert, Kidney bean, Navy bean, Pop bean, Popping bean, Snap bean, String bean, Wax bean - Phaseolus Vulgaris - E	Sprout Seedling	2,258 ppm
Cauli Brassica Oleracea var. Botrytis - E	Flower	2,250 ppm
Barley, Barleygrass - Hordeum Vulgare - E - M	Stem	2,250 ppm
Guinea Grass - Panicum Maximum - M	Leaf	0-4,500 ppm
Indian Sorrel, Jamaica Sorrel, Kharkadi, Red Sorrel, Sorrel - Hibiscus Sabdariffa - E	Flower	2,240 ppm
Cabbage, Red Cabbage, White Cabbage - Brassica Oleracea var. Capitata - E	Leaf	2,228 ppm
Buchu, Honey Buchu, Mountain Buchu - Agathosma Betulina Buchu, Honey Buchu, Mountain Buchu - Agathosma Betulina - M	Leaf	2,210 ppm
Bai-Wei, Pai-Wei - Cynanchum Atratum - E - M	Root	2,210 ppm
Cayenne, Chili, Hot Pepper, Red Chili, Spur Pepper, Tabasco - Capsicum Frutescens - E	Fruit	2,203 ppm
Green Gram, Mungbean - Vigna Radiata - E	Seed	2,203 ppm
Tea - Camellia Sinensis - E	Leaf	2,200 ppm
White Lupine - Lupinus Albus - M - T	Seed	2,200 ppm
Rice - Oryza Sativa - E	Plant	2,200 ppm
American Ginseng, Ginseng - Panax Quinquefolius - M	Plant	2,200 ppm
Curly Kale, Kale, Kitchen Kale, Scotch Kale - Brassica Oleracea var. Sabellica l. var. Acephala - E	Leaf	2,190 ppm
Jack Bean - Canavalia Ensiformis - E	Seed	2,190 ppm
Cape Jasmine, Gardenia, Jasmin, Shan-Chih-Tzu, Shan-Zhi-Zi, Zhi Zi - Gardenia Jasminoides - M	Fruit	2,170 ppm
Tomatillo - Physalis Ixocarpa - E	Fruit	2,150 ppm
Hsin-I, Xin-Yi - Magnolia Denudata - E - M	Flower	2,120 ppm
Hsin-I, Xin-Yi - Magnolia Fargesii - E - M	Flower	2,120 ppm
Rice Paper Tree, Tong-Cao, Tung-Tsao - Tetrapanax Papyrifera M	Pith	2,120 ppm
Groundnut, Peanut - Arachis Hypogaea - E - M	Seed	2,110 ppm
Kohlrabi - Brassica Oleracea var. Gongylodes - E	Stem	2,110 ppm
Chinese Ephedra, Ma Huang - Ephedra Sinica - M	Plant	2,110 ppm
Cassava, Tapioca, Yuca - Manihot Esculenta - E	Root	2,100 ppm
Parsnip - Pastinaca Sativa - E	Root	2,100 ppm
Shortleaf Pine - Pinus Echinata - M	Shoot	2,100 ppm
Malanga, Tannia, Yautia - Xanthosoma Sagittifolium - E	Root	2,100 ppm
Acerola - Malpighia Glabra - E - M	Fruit	2,095 ppm
Dog Rose, Dogbrier, Rose - Rosa Canina - E - M	Fruit	2,090 ppm
Du Zhong, Gutta-Percha Tree, Tu Chung - Eucommia Ulmoides - M	Bark	2,080 ppm

Name	Part	PPM
Black Gram - Vigna Mungo - E	Seed	2,076 ppm
Chinese Ash - Fraxinus Rhynchophylla - M - E	Bark	2,070 ppm
Catnip - Nepeta Cataria - M	Plant	2,070 ppm
Desert Wormwood - Artemisia Herba-Alba - M	Plant	2,060 ppm
Hsuan-Shen, Yuan-Shen - Scrophularia Buergeriana - M	Root	2,060 ppm
Amphicarpaea Bracteata - E - M	Shoot	0-4,100 ppm
Damiana - Turnera Diffusa - M	Leaf	2,040 ppm
Mace, Nutmeg - Myristica Fragrans - E	Seed	2,030 ppm
Rapini, Seven-Top Turnip, Turnip - Brassica Rapa - E	Root	2,000 ppm
Chayote - Sechium Edule - E - M	Fruit	2,000 ppm
Broadbean, Faba Bean, Habas - Vicia Faba - E	Seed	2,000 ppm
Carrot - Daucus Carota - E	Root	1,980 ppm
Rhubarb - Rheum Rhabarbarum - E	Pt	1,975 ppm
Hsin-Pa-Pi, Kisasage - Catalpa Ovata - E - M	Fruit	1,960 ppm
Tu Huo - Angelica Laxiflora - M	Root	1,950 ppm
Chinese Ginseng, Ginseng, Korean Ginseng, Oriental Ginseng - Panax Ginseng - M	Root	1,950 ppm
Milfoil, Yarrow - Achillea Millefolium - M	Plant	1,920 ppm
Ben Nut, Benzolive Tree, Drumstick Tree, Horseradish Tree, Moringa, West Indian Ben - Moringa Oleifera - E	Fruit	450-3,815 ppm
Corn Salad, Lamb's Lettuce - Valerianella Locusta - E	Plant	3,773-3,798 ppm
Hardy Orchid, Hyacinth Bletilla, Hyacinth Orchid, Shiran - Bletilla Striata - M	Tuber	1,890 ppm
Chinese Birthwort - Aristolochia Debilis - E - M - T	Fruit	1,880 ppm
Shan Dou Gen - Sophora Subprostrata - M - T	Root	1,880 ppm
Anise, Sweet Cumin - Pimpinella Anisum - E - M	Fruit	1,878 ppm
Cloudberry - Rubus Chamaemorus - E - M	Fruit	1,875 ppm
Madder - Rubia Cordifolia - M	Root	1,870 ppm
Huang Qi, Huang-Chi - Astragalus Membranaceus - M	Root	1,860 ppm
Coneflower, Echinacea - Echinacea ssp - M	Root	1,860 ppm
Cape Gooseberry, Ground Cherry - Physalis Peruviana - E	Fruit	1,810 ppm
Jerusalem Artichoke - Helianthus Tuberosus E	Tuber	1,800 ppm
Black Walnut - Juglans Nigra - E	Seed	1,794 ppm
Corn - Zea Mays - E	Silk Stigma Style	1,790 ppm
Scarlet Runner Bean - Phaseolus Coccineus - E	Seed	1,780 ppm
Kiwi - Actinidia Chinensis - E	Fruit	1,770 ppm
Blessed Thistle - Cnicus Benedictus - M	Plant	1,770 ppm
Giant Taro - Alocasia Macrorrhiza - E	Root	1,750 ppm
Apricot - Prunus Armeniaca - E - M - T	Seed	1,750 ppm
Mud Plantain, Tse-Hsieh, Water Plantain, Ze-Xie - Alisma Plantago-Aquatica - M	Rhizome	1,740 ppm
Black Cohosh, Black Snake - Cimicifuga Racemosa - E - M	Root	1,740 ppm
Avocado - Persea Americana - E - M - T	Fruit	1,740 ppm
Bitter Orange, Petitgrain - Citrus Aurantium - E	Fruit	1,730 ppm
Chaparral, Creosote Bush - Larrea Tridentata - M	Plant	1,720 ppm
Black Currant - Ribes Nigrum - E	Fruit	1,720 ppm
Pea - Pisum Sativum - E	Seed	1,700 ppm
Comfrey - Symphytum Officinale - E - M - T	Root	1,700 ppm
Horseradish - Armoracia Rusticana - E	Root	1,690 ppm
Cassia, Cassia Bark, Cassia Lignea, China Junk Cassia, Chinazimt, Chinese Cassia - Cinnamomum Aromaticuminnamon - E - M - T	Bark	1,680 ppm
Barley, Barleygrass - Hordeum Vulgare - E - M	Sprout Seedling	1,670 ppm
Sarsaparilla - Smilax spp - E - M	Root	1,670 ppm
Gennoshiouko, Oriental Geranium - Geranium Thunbergii - E - M	Plant	1,660 ppm
Bei Sha Shen - Glehnia Littoralis - E - M	Root	1,650 ppm
Pistachio - Pistacia Vera - E	Seed	1,644 ppm
Brussel-Sprout - Brassica Oleracea var. Gemmifera - E	Leaf	1,642 ppm
Celery - Apium Graveolens - E	Root	1,635 ppm
Wild Yam - Dioscorea sp. - E	Root	1,630 ppm
Mace, Nutmeg - Myristica Fragrans - E	Aril	1,630 ppm
Hydrangea, Smooth Hydrangea - Hydrangea Arborescens - E - M	Root	1,620 ppm
Indian Tobacco, Lobelia - Lobelia Inflata - M - T	Leaf	1,620 ppm

MAGNESIUM CONTINUED

Plant	Part	PPM
Jack Na Bush - Eupatorium Odoratum - M	Leaf	0-3,200 ppm
Corn - Zea Mays - E	Seed	1,600 ppm
Cascara Buckthorn, Cascara Sagrada - Frangula Purshiana - M	Bark	1,590 ppm
Dandelion - Taraxacum Officinale - E - M	Root	1,570 ppm
Aubergine, Egg Solanum Melongena - E	Fruit	1,563 ppm
Strawberry - Fragaria spp. - E	Fruit	1,545 ppm
Chinese Chestnut - Castanea Mollisima - M	Seed	1,531 ppm
Balloon Flower, Chieh-Keng, Jie-Geng - Platycodon Grandiflorum - E - M - T	Root	1,510 ppm
Watermelon - Citrullus Lanatus - E	Fruit	1,500 ppm
Nutsedge - Cyperus Rotundus - E - M	Rhizome	1,500 ppm
Genipap, Jagua - Genipa Americana - E - M	Seed	1,500 ppm
Adlay, Adlay Millet, Job's-Tears, Yi-Yi-Ren - Coix Lacryma-Jobi - E - M	Seed	1,490 ppm
Allspice, Clover-Pepper, Jamaica-Pepper, Pimenta, Pimento - Pimenta Dioica - E	Fruit	1,480 ppm
Yambean - Pachyrhizus Erosus - E	Tuber	1,475 ppm
Adzuki Bean - Vigna Angularis - E	Seed	1,467 ppm
Banana, Plantain - Musa x Paradisiaca - E	Fruit	1,465 ppm
Lantana, Wild Sage - Lantana Camara - M	Fruit	1,460 ppm
Sheng Ma - Cimicifuga Dahurica - M	Rhizome	1,450 ppm
Barberry - Berberis Vulgaris - M	Root	1,430 ppm
Pumpkin - Cucurbita Pepo - E	Fruit	1,429 ppm
Indian Fig, Nopal, Nopalito, Prickly Pear - Opuntia Ficus-Indica - E - M	Bud	1,420 ppm
Mandarin, Tangerine - Citrus Reticulata - E	Fruit	1,416 ppm
Jojoba - Simmondsia Chinensis Seed	Seed	1,410 ppm
American Chestnut - Castanea Dentata - E - M	Seed	1,406 ppm
Chervil - Anthriscus Cerefolium - E	Leaf	1,400 ppm
Breadroot, Indian Bread-Root, Indian Turnip, Prairie Apple, Prairie Potato, Prairie Turnip - Psoralea Esculenta - E - M - T	Root	1,400 ppm
Jack Artocarpus Heterophyllus - E	Fruit	1,380 ppm
Grape Citrus Paradisi - E	Fruit	1,360 ppm
Taro - Colocasia Esculenta - E	Root	1,350 ppm
Chickpea, Garbanzo - Cicer Arietinum - E	Seed	1,348 ppm
Indian Tamarind, Kilytree, Tamarind - Tamarindus Indica - M	Fruit	1,341 ppm
Tamarindus Indica - Indian Tamarind, Kilytree, Tamaring - M	Seed	2,180-2,650 ppm
Lentil - Lens Culinaris - E	Sprout Seedling	1,323 ppm
English Walnut - Juglans Rregia - E	Seed	1,310 ppm
Blue Cohosh - Caulophyllum Thalictroides - M	Root	1,300 ppm
Lentil - Lens Culinaris - E	Seed	1,280 ppm
Onion, Shallot - Allium Cepa - Shallot Bulb - E	Bulb	1,230 ppm
Swamp Taro - Cyrtosperma Chamissonis - E	Root	1,215 ppm
Water Lotus - Nelumbo Nucifera - E - M	Rhizome	1,215 ppm
Garlic - Allium Sativum Bulb - E	Bulb	1,210 ppm
Bearberry, Uva Uursi - Arctostaphylos Uva-Ursi - M	Leaf	1,210 ppm
Chih-Mu, Zhi-Mu - Anemarrhena Asphodeloides - M	Rhizome	1,200 ppm
Morinda - Morinda spp. - M	Root	1,200 ppm
Ambarella - Spondias Dulcis - E	Seed	1,200 ppm
Macadamia - Macadamia spp. - E	Seed	1,190 ppm
Chinese Foxglove - Rehmannia Glutinosa - M	Root	1,190 ppm
Rowan Berry - Sorbus Aucubaria - E - M - T	Fruit	1,190 ppm
Moutan, Tree Peony - Paeonia Moutan - M	Root Bark	1,180 ppm
Moutan, Moutan Peony, Tree Peony - Paeonia Suffruticosa	Root Bark	1,180 ppm
Lian-Jiao, Lien-Chiao - Forsythia Suspensa - M	Fruit	1,160 ppm
Japanese Gentian - Gentiana Scabra - E	Root	1,150 ppm
Mad-Dog Skullcap, Scullcap - Scutellaria lateriflora - M	Plant	1,130 ppm
Curry Murraya spp. - E - M	Fruit	1,118 ppm
Pear - Pyrus Communis - E	Fruit	1,110 ppm
Calamus, Flagroot, Myrtle Flag, Sweet Calamus, Sweetflag, Sweet Acorus Calamus - M	Rhizome	1,100 ppm
Chicory, Succory, Witloof - Cichorium Intybus - E - M	Root	1,100 ppm
Mimosa - Albizia Julibrissin - E - M	Bark	1,090 ppm
Ladyslipper - Cypripedium Pubescens - M	Root	1,090 ppm
Coltsfoot - Tussilago Farfara - M - T	Flower	1,080 ppm

Name	Part	ppm
Pineapple - Ananas Comosus - E	Fruit	1,075 ppm
Orange - Citrus Sinensis - E	Fruit	1,075 ppm
Aceituna Dulce, Jambolan, Java Plum - Syzygium Cumini - E	Fruit	350-2,145 ppm
Chinese Boxthorn, Chinese Matrimony Vine, Chinese Wolfberry - Lycium Chinense - E - M	Fruit	1,060 ppm
Papaya - Carica Papaya - E - M	Fruit	1,058 ppm
Cherimoya - Annona Cherimola - E	Seed	1,045 ppm
Rangoon Creeper - Quisqualis Indica - E - T	Fruit	1,040 ppm
Japanese Privet, Ligustri Fructus - Ligustrum Japonicum - M	Fruit	1,020 ppm
Chinese Privet, Glossy Privet, Ligustri Fructus, Privet, White Waxtree - Ligustrum Lucidum - M	Fruit	1,020 ppm
Horsetail, Scouring Rush - Equisetum Hyemale - M	Plant	1,010 ppm
Cherimoya - Annona Cherimola - E	Fruit	1,000 ppm
Capillary Wormwood - Artemisia Capillaris - M	Plant	1,000 ppm
Salsify - Tragopogon Porrifolius - E	Root	1,000 ppm
Chinese Quince, Mu-Kua - Chaenomeles Lagenaria - E	Fruit	990 ppm
Common Garden Peony, Peony, White Peony - Paeonia Lactiflora - M	Root	990 ppm
Pecan - Carya Illinoensis - E	Seed	980 ppm
Bread Artocarpus Altilis - E	Fruit	975 ppm
Blackberry Lily, Shenan - Belamcanda Chinensis - M	Rhizome	970 ppm
Bai-Zhu, Pai-Chu - Atractylodes Ovata - M	Rhizome	960 ppm
Chinese Senega - Polygala Tenuifolia - M	Root	960 ppm
Citron - Citrus Medica - E	Fruit	950 ppm
English Hawthorn, Hawthorn, Whitethorn, Woodland Hawthorn - Crataegus Laevigata - M	Fruit	940 ppm
Gooseberry - Ribes Uva-Crispa - E	Fruit	938 ppm
Red Currant, White Currant - Ribes Rubrum - E	Fruit	935 ppm
Aloe, Bitter Aloes - Aloe Vera - E - M	Leaf	930 ppm
Common Juniper, Juniper - Juniperus Communis - E - M - T	Fruit	930 ppm
Rush - Juncus Effusus E - M - T	Pith	920 ppm
Shagbark Hickory - Carya Ovata - E	Seed	900 ppm
Chinese Cornbind, Chinese Knotweed, Fleeceflower, Fo Ti, He Shou Wu - Polygonum Multiflorum - E - M - T	Rhizome	890 ppm
Strawberry Guava - Psidium Cattleianum - E	Fruit	880 ppm
Mango - Mangifera Indica - E - M	Fruit	875 ppm
Fig - Ficus Carica - E	Fruit	872 ppm
Rye - Secale Cereale - E	Seed	1,185-1,740 ppm
Jih-Chiung - Cnidium Officinale - M	Rhizome	850 ppm
Peach - Prunus Persica - E - M - T	Fruit	850 ppm
Kudsu, Kudzu - Pueraria Montana subsp. var. Lobata - E - M	Shoot	850 ppm
Chocolate Vine - Akebia Quinata - M	Stem	840 ppm
Chinese Dogwood - Cornus Officinalis - E - M	Fruit	830 ppm
Greater Yam, Winged Yam - Dioscorea Alata - E	Root	827 ppm
Broomrape, Cistanchis Herba, Jou Tsung Jung - Cistanche Salsa - M	Plant	810 ppm
Pau D'Arco - Tabebuia Heptaphylla - M	Bark	810 ppm
Mountain Yam - Dioscorea Pentaphylla - E	Root	792 ppm
Cang Zhu - Atractylodes Lancea - M	Rhizome	790 ppm
Indian Fig, Nopal, Nopalito, Prickly Pear - Opuntia Ficus-Indica - E - M	Seed	790 ppm
Date Palm - Phoenix Dactylifera - E	Fruit	790 ppm
Sugar-Apple, Sweetsop - Annona Squamosa - E	Fruit	785 ppm
Coconut, Coconut Palm - Cocos Nucifera - E	Seed	770 ppm
Hawthorn - Crataegus Cuneata - M	Fruit	760 ppm
Equatorial Ivory Palm - Phytelephas Aequatorialis - E	Flower	440-1,505 ppm
Guavas - Psidium Guajava - E	Fruit	735 ppm
Sweet Potato - Ipomoea Batatas - E	Root	710 ppm
Ban-Xia, Pan-Hsia - Pinellia Ternata - E - M - T	Tuber	710 ppm
Indian Tamarind, Kilytree, Tamarind - Tamarindus Indica - M	Leaf	710 ppm
European Chestnut - Castanea Sativa - E - M	Seed	704 ppm
Bilberry, Dwarf Bilberry, Whortleberry - Vaccinium Myrtillus - E - M	Fruit	700 ppm
Chinese Magnolia, Hou Pu, Magnolia- Magnolia Officinalis - E - M	Bark	690 ppm

MAGNESIUM CONTINUED

Species	Part	Quantity
American Cranberry, Cranberry, Large Cranberry - Vaccinium Macrocarpon - E	Fruit	690 ppm
Oriental Pipewort - Eriocaulon spp. - M	Leaf	670 ppm
Amur Cork Tree, Huang Bai, Huang Po, Po Mu - Phellodendron Amurense - M	Bark	650 ppm
Sour Cherry - Prunus Cerasus - E - M - T	Fruit	648 ppm
Custard Apple - Annona Reticulata - E	Fruit	630 ppm
Sweet Potato - Ipomoea Batatas - E	Leaf	620 ppm
Da-Zao, Jujube, Ta-Tsao - Zizyphus Jujuba - E - M	Fruit	620 ppm
Apricot - Prunus Armeniaca - E - M - T	Fruit	615 ppm
Ginkgo, Maidenhair Tree - Ginkgo Biloba - Tree - E - M - T	Seed	602 ppm
Carambola, Star Averrhoa Carambola - E	Fruit	80-1,200 ppm
Cowberry, Lingen, Lingonberry - Vaccinium Vitis-Idaea var. Minus - E - M	Fruit	600 ppm
Tian Ma - Gastrodia Elata - Rhizome	Rhizome	590 ppm
Emblic, Myrobalan - Phyllanthus Emblica - E	Fruit	584 ppm
Red Elm, Slippery Elm - Ulmus Rubra - M	Bark	580 ppm
Noble Dendrobium - Dendrobium Nobile - M	Stem	520 ppm
Psyllium - Plantago Psyllium - E - M	Seed	510 ppm
Banana Yucca, Blue Yucca, Spanish Bayonet, Yucca - Yucca Baccata - E - M - T	Root	510 ppm
Russian Olive - Elaeagnus Umbellatus - E - M	Fruit	170-1,010 ppm
Equatorial Ivory Palm - Phytelephas Aequatorialis - E	Mesocarp	320-1,005 ppm
Betel Nut, Pin-Lang - Areca Catechu Amphicarpaea Bracteata- E - M	Seed	500 ppm
Squaw Perideridia Gairdneri - E - M	Root	500 ppm
Northern Red Oak - Quercus Rubra - E - M	Seed	500 ppm
Aconite, Fu-Tsu - Aconitum Carmichaelii - E - M	Tuber	490 ppm
Bayberry, Candle-Berry, Southern Bayberry, Wax Myrtle - Myrica Cerifera - E - M	Bark	490 ppm
Apple - Malus Domestica - E	Fruit	478 ppm
Black Walnut - Juglans Nigra - E	Fruit	440 ppm
Mai-Men-Dong, Mai-Men-Tung - Ophiopogon Japonicus - M	Tuber	410 ppm
Air Potato, Potato Yam - Dioscorea Bulbifera - E	Rhizome	370 ppm
Bei-Mu, Fritillary - Fritillaria Thunbergii - Blub - E - M	Bulb	370 ppm
Ching-Feng-Teng - Sinomenium Acutum - E - M	Rhizome	360 ppm
Guanique - Chamissoa Altissima - M	Leaf	70-715 ppm
Asparagus Pea, Goa Bean, Winged Bean - Psophocarpus Tetragonolobus - E	Leaf	346 ppm
Blueberry - Vaccinium Corymbosum - E	Fruit	332 ppm
Ambarella - Spondias Dulcis - E	Fruit	240 ppm
White Oak - Quercus Alba - M	Bark	160 ppm
Pomarrosa, Rose Apple - Syzygium Jambos - E	Fruit	40-260 ppm
Pomegranate - Punica Granatum - E	Fruit	120 ppm
Chinese Jack-In-The-Pulpit - Arisaema Consanguineum - E - M - T	Rhizome	100 ppm
Imbu, Umbu - Spondias Tuberosa - E	Fruit	90 ppm
Bai Zhi - Angelica Dahurica - M	Root	3.67 ppm

PLANTS CONTAINING MANGANESE

Species	Part	Quantity
White Oak - Quercus Alba - M	Stem	3,800 ppm
Red Pignut Hickory - Carya Glabra - E	Shoot	3,300 ppm
Northern Red Oak - Quercus Rubra - E - M	Stem	3,300 ppm
Black Gum, Black Tupelo - Nyssa Sylvatica - E - M	Leaf	2,730 ppm
Shagbark Hickory - Carya Ovata - E	Shoot	2,700 ppm
Red Cedar - Juniperus Virginiana Amphicarpaea Bracteata- E - M - T	Shoot	2,640 ppm
Buckbush - Symphoricarpos Orbiculatus - M	Stem	2,640 ppm
Bilberry, Dwarf Bilberry, Whortleberry - Vaccinium Myrtillus - E - M	Leaf	2,500 ppm
Cowberry, Lingen, Lingonberry - Vaccinium Vitis-Idaea var. Minus - E - M	Leaf	2,500 ppm
American Styrax, Sweetgum - Liquidambar Styraciflua - E - M	Stem	2,460 ppm

Black Oak - Quercus Velutina - E - M	Stem	1,984 ppm
Post Oak - Quercus Stellata - E - M	Stem	1,680 ppm
American Persimmon - Diospyros Virginiana - E - M	Leaf	1,500 ppm
Black Gum, Black Tupelo - Nyssa Sylvatica - E - M	Stem	1,320 ppm
Shortleaf Pine - Pinus Echinata - M	Shoot	1,260 ppm
Tea - Camellia Sinensis - E	Leaf	1,200 ppm
Clove, Clovetree - Syzygium Aromaticum - E	Flower	1,200 ppm
American Persimmon - Diospyros Virginiana - E - M	Stem	1,080 ppm
Sassafras - Sassafras Albidum - E - M - T	Leaf	1,020 ppm
European Grape, Grape, Grapevine, Vigne Vinifere, Wine Grape - Vitis Vinifera - E - M	Stem	986 ppm
Dwarf Sumac, Winged Sumac - Rhus Copallina - E - M	Stem	915 ppm
Jussiaeae Herba, Pond Dragon - Jussiaea Repens - M	Plant	799 ppm
Fennel - Foeniculum Vulgare - M	Fruit	721 ppm
Sassafras - Sassafras Albidum - E - M - T	Stem	680 ppm
Buchu, Honey Buchu, Mountain Buchu - Agathosma Betulina Buchu, Honey Buchu, Mountain Buchu - Agathosma Betulina - M	Leaf	675 ppm
Cassia, Cassia Bark, Cassia Lignea, China Junk Cassia, Chinazimt, Chinese Cassia - Cinnamomum Aromaticuminnamon- E - M - T	Bark	600 ppm
Bastard Cardamom, Chin Kousha, Malabar Cardamom, Tavoy Cardamom - Amomum Xanthioides - E	Seed	565 ppm
Morinda - Morinda spp. - M	Root	520 ppm
Spinach - Spinacia Oleracea - E	Plant	485 ppm
Dwarf Sumac, Winged Sumac - Rhus Copallina - E - M	Leaf	480 ppm
Mud Plantain, Tse-Hsieh, Water Plantain, Ze-Xie - Alisma Plantago-Aquatica - M	Rhizome	479 ppm
Cowgrass, Peavine Clover, Purple Clover, Red Clover - Trifolium Pratense - E - M	Hay	464 ppm
Dan Zhu Ye - Lophatherum Gracile - M	Plant	445 ppm
Dill, Garden Dill - Anethum Graveolens - E	Plant	435 ppm
Lantana, Wild Sage - Lantana Camara - M	Shoot	412 ppm
Chinese Goldthread, Huang-Lian, Huang-Lien - Coptis Chinensis - M	Rhizome	398 ppm
Huang-Lia, Huang-Lian, Huang-Lien, Japanese Goldthread - Coptis Japonica - M	Rhizome	398 ppm
Generic Goldthread - Coptis spp. - M	Rhizome	398 ppm
Parsley - Petroselinum Crispum - E	Plant	375 ppm
Catnip - Nepeta Cataria - M	Plant	374 ppm
Bilberry, Dwarf Bilberry, Whortleberry - Vaccinium Myrtillus - E - M	Fruit	370 ppm
Japanese Cinnamon - Cinnamomum Sieboldii - E - M - T	Bark	360 ppm
Ginger - Zingiber Officinale - E	Rhizome	350 ppm
Bai-Wei, Pai-Wei - Cynanchum Atratum - E - M	Root	341 ppm
Giant Knotweed, Hu-Zhang, Japanese Knotweed, Mexican Bamboo - Polygonum Cuspidatum - E - M - T	Plant	330 ppm
Chocolate Vine - Akebia Quinata - M	Stem	310 ppm
Calamus, Flagroot, Myrtle Flag, Sweet Calamus, Sweetflag, Sweet Acorus Calamus - M	Rhizome	309 ppm
Red Mangrove - Rhizophora Mangle - M	Leaf	300 ppm
Chinese Raspberry - Rubus Cchingii - E - M	Fruit	287 ppm
Saffron - Crocus Sativus - Style	Silk Stigma Style	284 ppm
Cardamom - Elettaria Cardamomum - E - M	Fruit	280 ppm
Gotu Kola, Pennywort - Centella Asiatica - E - M	Leaf	277 ppm
Sugar-Apple, Sweetsop - Annona Squamosa - E	Leaf	253 ppm
White Oak - Quercus Alba - M	Bark	253 ppm
Cowberry, Lingen, Lingonberry - Vaccinium Vitis-Idaea var. Minus - E - M	Fruit	250 ppm
Asian Wild Ginger - Asiasarum Heterotropoides - M	Root	248 ppm
Siebold's Wild Ginger - Asiasarum Sieboldii - M	Root	248 ppm
Lettuce - Lactuca Sativa - E	Leaf	240 ppm
Blue Cohosh - Caulophyllum Thalictroides - M	Root	237 ppm
Hsi Chien, Saint Paul'Swort - Siegesbeckia Orientalis - M	Plant	231 ppm

MANGANESE CONTINUED

Plant	Part	ppm
Jerusalem Artichoke - Helianthus Tuberosus E	Tuber	228 ppm
Loquat - Eriobotrya Japonica - E	Leaf	224 ppm
Japanese Cinnamon - Cinnamomum Sieboldii - E - M - T	Root Bark	220 ppm
Pineapple - Ananas Comosus - E	Fruit	209 ppm
Ladyslipper - Cypripedium Pubescens - M	Root	209 ppm
Oats - Avena Sativa - E - M	Seed	204 ppm
American Cranberry, Cranberry, Large Cranberry - Vaccinium Macrocarpon - E	Fruit	200 ppm
Climbing Fern - Lygodium Japonicum - Pollen or Spore - M	Pollen Or Spore	191 ppm
ElytriCouchgrass, Doggrass, Quackgrass, Twitchgrass, Wheatgrass - Elytrigia Repens - E - M	Plant	188 ppm
Hydrangea, Smooth Hydrangea - Hydrangea Arborescens - E - M	Root	187 ppm
Dyer's Woad - Isatis Tinctoria - M	Root	181 ppm
Chinese Ginseng, Ginseng, Korean Ginseng, Oriental Ginseng - Panax Ginseng - M	Root	180 ppm
Perilla - Perilla Frutescens - E - M - T	Plant	180 ppm
Mongoloid Dandelion - Taraxacum Mongolicum - E - M	Plant	178 ppm
European Nettle, Stinging Nettle - Urtica Dioica - E - M	Leaf	172 ppm
Rush - Juncus Effusus E - M - T	Pith	171 ppm
Mugwort - Artemisia Vulgaris - M	Plant	170 ppm
Java Cinnamon, Padang Cassia - Cinnamomum Burmannii - E - M - T	Bark	170 ppm
Oats - Avena Sativa - E - M	Plant	168 ppm
Evening-Primrose - Oenothera Biennis - E - M	Seed	168 ppm
Henbane - Hyoscyamus Niger - E - M	Seed	166 ppm
Bearberry, Uva Uursi - Arctostaphylos Uva-Ursi - M	Leaf	165 ppm
European Mistletoe - Viscum Album - M - T	Leaf	159 ppm
American Ginseng, Ginseng - Panax Quinquefolius - M	Plant	156 ppm
Chickweed, Common Chickweed - Stellaria Media - E	Plant	153 ppm
Indian Sorrel, Jamaica Sorrel, Kharkadi, Red Sorrel, Sorrel - Hibiscus Sabdariffa - E	Flower	151 ppm
Black bean, Dwarf bean, Field bean, Flageolet bean, French bean, Garden bean, Green bean, Haricot, Haricot bean, Haricot vert, Kidney bean, Navy bean, Pop bean, Popping bean, Snap bean, String bean, Wax bean - Phaseolus Vulgaris - E	Fruit	150 ppm
Lady's Thistle, Milk Thistle - Silybum Marianum - M	Plant	147 ppm
Indian Sorrel, Jamaica Sorrel, Stevia, Sweet Leaf of Paraguay - Stevia Rebaudiana - E	Leaf	147 ppm
Raspberry, Red raspberry - Rubus Idaeus - E - M	Leaf	146 ppm
Curly Dock, Lengua De Vaca, Sour Dock, Yellow Dock - Rumex Crispus - M - T	Root	145 ppm
Chinese Spikenard - Nardostachys Chinensis - M	Rhizome	141 ppm
Ramie - Boehmeria Nivea - M	Plant	140 ppm
Ceylon Cinnamon, Cinnamon - Cinnamomum Verum - E - M - T	Bark	140 ppm
Bai-Zhu, Pai-Chu - Atractylodes Ovata - M	Rhizome	139 ppm
Du Zhong, Gutta-Percha Tree, Tu Chung - Eucommia Ulmoides - M	Bark	135 ppm
Smooth Sumac - Rhus Glabra - E - M	Stem	134 ppm
Dandelion - Taraxacum Officinale - E - M	Plant	130 ppm
Eyebright - Euphrasia Officinalis - M	Plant	126 ppm
Strawberry - Fragaria spp. - E	Fruit	125 ppm
Water Lotus - Nelumbo Nucifera - E - M	Seed	125 ppm
Cloudberry - Rubus Chamaemorus - E - M	Fruit	125 ppm
Lian-Jiao, Lien-Chiao - Forsythia Suspensa - M	Fruit	120 ppm
Barley, Barleygrass - Hordeum Vulgare - E - M	Seed	120 ppm
Dokudami, Fishwort, Yu Xing Cao - Houttuynia Cordata - E - M	Plant	120 ppm
Chinese Magnolia, Hou Pu, Magnolia- Magnolia Officinalis - E - M	Bark	120 ppm
Flannelleaf, Flannelplant, Great mullein, Mullein, Velvet Verbascum Thapsus - M	Leaf	120 ppm
Chinese Anemone - Pulsatilla Chinensis - M	Root	119 ppm
Chai-Hu - Bupleurum - M	Root	114 ppm
Pawpaw - Asimina Triloba - Friut - E	Fruit	111 ppm

Name	Part	ppm
Bai Zhi - Angelica Dahurica - M	Root	110 ppm
Cockscomb - Celosia Cristata - M	Flower	109 ppm
Wheat - Triticum Aestivum - E - M	Plant	105 ppm
Lemongrass, West indian lemongrass - Cymbopogon Citratus - E - M	Plant	104 ppm
Ceylon Cinnamon, Cinnamon - Cinnamomum Verum - E - M - T	Leaf	101.6 ppm
Coneflower, Echinacea - Echinacea ssp - M	Root	101 ppm
Corn Salad, Lamb's Lettuce - Valerianella Locusta - E	Plant	179-201 ppm
Okra - Abelmoschus Esculentus - Friut - E - M	Fruit	100 ppm
Cherimoya - Annona Cherimola - E	Seed	100 ppm
Asparagus - Asparagus Officinalis - E	Shoot	100 ppm
Cobnut, English Filbert, European Filbert, European Hazel, Hazel - Corylus Avellana - E	Seed	100 ppm
Alehoof - Glechoma Hederacea - M	Plant	100 ppm
Tomato - Lycopersicon Esculentum - E - M - T	Fruit	100 ppm
Antler Herb, Clubmoss - Lycopodium Clavatum - M - T	Plant	100 ppm
Butterbur - Petasites Japonicus - T	Plant	100 ppm
Butter Bean, Lima Bean - Phaseolus Lunatus - E	Seed	100 ppm
Cucumber - Cucumis Sativus - E	Fruit	98 ppm
Japanese Gentian - Gentiana Scabra - E	Root	98 ppm
Oriental Pipewort - Eriocaulon spp. - M	Leaf	96 ppm
Heal-All, Self-Heal - Prunella Vulgaris - E - M	Flower	96 ppm
Chinese Magnolia Vine, Five-Flavor-Fruit, Magnolia Vine, Schizandra, Wu Wei Zi, Wu Wei Zu - Schisandra Chinensis - M	Fruit	96 ppm
Madder - Rubia Cordifolia - M	Root	94 ppm
Chinese Boxthorn, Chinese Matrimony Vine, Chinese Wolfberry - Lycium Chinense - E - M	Root Bark	91 ppm
Beet, Beetroot, Garden Beet, Sugar Beet - Beta Vulgaris - E	Root	90 ppm
Chinese Ash - Fraxinus Rhynchophylla - M - E	Bark	89 ppm
Wheat - Triticum Aestivum - E - M	Seed	86 ppm
Goldenseal - Hydrastis Canadensis - M	Root	85 ppm
Pea - Pisum Sativum - E	Plant	85 ppm
Tu Huo - Angelica Laxiflora - M	Root	83 ppm
European Pennyroyal - Mentha pulegium - E - M- T	Plant	83 ppm
Bay, Bay Laurel, Bayleaf, Grecian Laurel, Laurel, Sweet Bay - Laurus Nobilis	Leaf	82 ppm
Paper Mulberry - Broussonetia Papyrifera - E - M	Fruit	81 ppm
Feverfew - Chrysanthemum Parthenium - M	Plant	81 ppm
Hops - Humulus Lupulus - E - M - T	Fruit	81 ppm
Tarragon - Artemisia Dracunculus - M	Plant	80 ppm
Cauli Brassica Oleracea var. Botrytis - E	Leaf	80 ppm
Indian Tobacco, Lobelia - Lobelia Inflata - M - T	Leaf	80 ppm
Common thyme, Garden thyme, Thyme - Thymus Vulgaris - E - M	Leaf	79 ppm
Indian Saffron, Turmeric - Curcuma Longa - E	Rhizome	78 ppm
Devil's claw, Grapple Harpagophytum procumbens - M	Root	77 ppm
Celery - Apium Graveolens - E	Seed	76 ppm
Bladderwrack, Kelp - Fucus Vesiculosus - E - M	Plant	76 ppm
Rowan Berry - Sorbus Aucubaria - E - M - T	Fruit	75 ppm
Wu Chia Pi - Acanthopanax Gracilistylis - M	Root Bark	74 ppm
Sheng Ma - Cimicifuga Dahurica - M	Rhizome	74 ppm
Asian Plantain - Plantago Asiatica - E - M	Plant	74 ppm
Endive, Escarole - Cichorium Endivia - M	Leaf	72 ppm
Butternut - Juglans Cinerea - E	Seed	72 ppm
Chinese Angelica, Dong Gui, Dong Quai - Angelica Sinensis - M	Root	71 ppm
Coca - Erythroxylum Coca var. Coca - E - M	Leaf	71 ppm
Bei Sha Shen - Glehnia Littoralis - E - M	Root	70 ppm
Japanese Honeysuckle - Lonicera Japonica - M	Flower	70 ppm
Allspice, Clover-Pepper, Jamaica-Pepper, Pimenta, Pimento - Pimenta Dioica - E	Bud	70 ppm
Box-Holly, Butcher's broom - Ruscus aculeatus - E - M	Root	70 ppm
Field Horsetail, Horsetail - Equisetum Arvense - M	Plant	69 ppm
Qian Hu - Peucedanum Decursivum - M	Plant	69 ppm
Opium Poppy, Poppyseed Poppy - Papaver Somniferum - E	Seed	68 ppm

MANGANESE CONTINUED

Ching-Chieh, Jing-Jie - Schizonepeta Tenuifolia - E - M	Plant	68 ppm
Dandelion - Taraxacum Officinale - E - M	Root	68 ppm
Betel Nut, Pin-Lang - Areca Catechu Amphicarpaea Bracteata- E - M	Seed	67 ppm
Comfrey - Symphytum Officinale - E - M - T	Root	67 ppm
Chaff Achyranthes Bidentata - M	Root	66 ppm
White Willow - Salix Alba - M	Bark	66 ppm
Chinese Parsley, Cilantro, Coriander - Coriandrum Sativum E	Leaf	64 ppm
Wild Yam - Dioscorea sp. - E	Root	64 ppm
Bayberry, Candle-Berry, Southern Bayberry, Wax Myrtle - Myrica Cerifera - E - M	Bark	64 ppm
Wou Chou Yu - Euodia Rutaecarpa - E	Fruit	63 ppm
Common Juniper, Juniper - Juniperus Communis - E - M - T	Fruit	63 ppm
Corn - Zea Mays - E	Seed	63 ppm
Carrot - Daucus Carota - E	Root	62 ppm
Chinese Polystichum - Polystichum Polyblepharum - T	Plant	62 ppm
Peppermint - Mentha x Piperita subsp. Nothosubsp. Piperita - E - M - T	Leaf	61 ppm
Summer Savory - Satureja Hortensis - E	Leaf	61 ppm
Savory, Winter Savory - Satureja Montana	Plant	61 ppm
Amphicarpaea Bracteata- E - M	Shoot	0-120 ppm
Burdock, Gobo, Great Burdock - Arctium lappa - E - M - T	Root	60 ppm
Barberry - Berberis Vulgaris - M	Root	60 ppm
Collards, Cow Cabbage, Spring-Heading Cabbage, Tall Kale, Tree Kale - Brassica Oleracea - E	Leaf	60 ppm
Soybean - Glycine Max - E	Seed	60 ppm
Barley, Barleygrass - Hordeum Vulgare - E - M	Stem	60 ppm
Garden Sorrel - Rumex Acetosa - E - M - T	Leaf	60 ppm
Cherokee Rose - Rosa Laevigata - E - M	Fruit	59 ppm
Cowgrass, Peavine Clover, Purple Clover, Red Clover - Trifolium Pratense - E - M	Flower	59 ppm
Shagbark Hickory - Carya Ovata - E	Seed	58 ppm
Sarsaparilla - Smilax spp - E - M	Root	57 ppm
Black Pepper, Pepper, White Pepper - Piper Nigrum - E - M	Fruit	56 ppm
Common Valerian, Garden-Heliotrope, Valerian - Valeriana Officinalis - E - M	Root	56 ppm
Coca - Erythroxylum Novogranatense var. Novogranatense - E - M	Leaf	55 ppm
Emblic, Myrobalan - Phyllanthus Emblica - E	Fruit	55 ppm
Chinese Ephedra, Ma Huang - Ephedra Sinica - M	Plant	54 ppm
Marjoram, Sweet Marjoram - Origanum Majorana - E	Plant	54 ppm
Peach - Prunus Persica - E - M - T	Bark	54 ppm
Damiana - Turnera Diffusa - M	Leaf	54 ppm
European Grape, Grape, Grapevine, Vigne Vinifere, Wine Grape - Vitis Vinifera - E - M	Fruit	54 ppm
Black Mustard - Brassica Nigra - E	Leaf	53 ppm
SafCarthamus Tinctorius - M	Flower	53 ppm
Noble Dendrobium - Dendrobium Nobile - M	Stem	53 ppm
Garden Camomile, Perennial Camomile, Roman Camomile - Chamaemelum Nobile M	Flower	52 ppm
Chaparral, Creosote Bush - Larrea Tridentata - M	Plant	52 ppm
Milfoil, Yarrow - Achillea Millefolium - M	Plant	50 ppm
Curly Kale, Kale, Kitchen Kale, Scotch Kale - Brassica Oleracea var. Sabellica l. var. Acephala - E	Leaf	50 ppm
Gennoshiouko, Oriental Geranium - Geranium Thunbergii - E - M	Plant	49 ppm
Crampbark, European Cranberry bush, Guelder Rose, Snowballbush - Viburnum Opulus - E - M - T	Bark	49 ppm
Cauli Brassica Oleracea var. Botrytis - E	Flower	48 ppm
Commom Licorice, Licorice, Licorice-Root, Smooth Licorice - Glycyrrhiza Glabra - M	Root	47 ppm
Common Turkish Oregano, European Oregano, Oregano, Pot Marjoram, Wild Marjoram, Wild Oregano - Origanum Vulgare - E	Plant	47 ppm
Mad-Dog Skullcap, Scullcap - Scutellaria lateriflora - M	Plant	47 ppm
Ban-Xia, Pan-Hsia - Pinellia Ternata - E - M - T	Tuber	46 ppm

Name	Part	ppm
Chinese Rhubarb - Rheum Palmatum - E	Rhizome	46 ppm
Cabbage, Red Cabbage, White Cabbage - Brassica Oleracea var. Capitata - E	Leaf	45 ppm
Taro - Colocasia Esculenta - E	Leaf	45 ppm
Date Palm - Phoenix Dactylifera - E	Fruit	45 ppm
Marshmallow, White Mallow - Althaea Officinalis - M	Root	44 ppm
American Chestnut - Castanea Dentata - E - M	Seed	44 ppm
Cornmint, Field Mint, Japanese Mint - Mentha Arvensis var. Piperascens - E - M- T	Plant	44 ppm
Asparagus Pea, Goa Bean, Winged Bean - Psophocarpus Tetragonolobus - E	Seed	44 ppm
Japanese Ginseng - Panax Japonicus - M	Rhizome	43 ppm
Rice Paper Tree, Tong-Cao, Tung-Tsao - Tetrapanax Papyrifera M	Pith	43 ppm
Hsin-I, Xin-Yi - Magnolia Denudata - E - M	Flower	42 ppm
Hsin-I, Xin-Yi - Magnolia Fargesii - E - M	Flower	42 ppm
Magnolia kobus DC. -- Hsin-I, Xin-Yi	Flower	42 ppm
Coffee Senna - Senna Occidentalis - E - T	Seed	42 ppm
Narrowleaf Sophora - Sophora Angustifolia - M - T- M - T	Root	42 ppm
White Mustard - Sinapis Alba - E - M - T	Seed	41 ppm
Chih-Mu, Zhi-Mu - Anemarrhena Asphodeloides - M	Rhizome	40 ppm
Pumpkin - Cucurbita Pepo - E	Seed	40 ppm
Radish - Raphanus Sativus - E	Seed	40 ppm
Dog Rose, Dogbrier, Rose - Rosa Canina - E - M	Fruit	40 ppm
Aubergine, Egg Solanum Melongena - E	Fruit	40 ppm
Cang Zhu - Atractylodes Lancea - M	Rhizome	39 ppm
Bell Pepper, Cherry Pepper, Cone Pepper, Green Pepper, Paprika, Sweet Pepper - Capsicum Annuum - E	Fruit	39 ppm
Fortune's Fern - Drynaria Fortunei - M	Rhizome	39 ppm
Bonavist Bean, Hyacinth Bean, Lablab Bean - Lablab Purpureus - E - M - T	Seed	39 ppm
Qiang Huo - Notopterygium Incisum - M	Rhizome	39 ppm
Onion, Shallot - Allium Cepa - Shallot Bulb - E	Bulb	38 ppm
Irish moss - Chondrus Crispus - E	Plant	38 ppm
White Tephrosia - Tephrosia Candida - M - T	Plant	38 ppm
Capillary Wormwood - Artemisia Capillaris - M	Plant	37 ppm
Ma-Huang - Ephedra spp. - M	Plant	37 ppm
White Mulberry - Morus Alba - E - M	Root Bark	37 ppm
Dulse - Rhodymenia Palmata - E	Plant	37 ppm
Chinese Chestnut - Castanea Mollisima - M	Seed	36 ppm
Coca - Erythroxylum Novogranatense var. Truxillense - E - M	Leaf	36 ppm
Jack Na Bush - Eupatorium Odoratum - M	Leaf	0-70 ppm
Rhubarb - Rheum Rhabarbarum - E	Pt	35 ppm
Caraway, Carum - Carum Carvi - E	Fruit	34 ppm
Moutan, Tree Peony - Paeonia Moutan - M	Root Bark	34 ppm
Moutan, Moutan Peony, Tree Peony - Paeonia Suffruticosa	Root Bark	34 ppm
Corn - Zea Mays - E	Silk Stigma Style	34 ppm
Ajwan - Trachyspermum Ammi - E - M	Fruit	33.1 ppm
Mimosa - Albizia Julibrissin - E - M	Bark	33 ppm
Celery - Apium Graveolens - E	Pt	33 ppm
Chinese Birthwort - Aristolochia Debilis - E - M - T	Fruit	33 ppm
Cumin - Cuminum Cyminum - E - M	Fruit	33 ppm
Parsnip - Pastinaca Sativa - E	Root	33 ppm
Rangoon Creeper - Quisqualis Indica - E - T	Fruit	33 ppm
Basil, Cuban Basil, Sweet Basil - Ocimum Basilicum - E	Leaf	32 ppm
Almond - Prunus Dulcis - E - M - T	Seed	32 ppm
Sage - Salvia Officinalis - E - M	Leaf	31 ppm
Groundnut, Peanut - Arachis Hypogaea - E - M	Seed	30 ppm
Pecan - Carya Illinoensis - E	Seed	30 ppm
Jih-Chiung - Cnidium Officinale - M	Rhizome	30 ppm
Black Walnut - Juglans Nigra - E	Seed	30 ppm
Balloon Flower, Chieh-Keng, Jie-Geng - Platycodon Grandiflorum - E - M - T	Root	30 ppm

MANGANESE CONTINUED

Name	Part	ppm
Huang Qi, Huang-Chi - Astragalus Membranaceus - M	Root	29 ppm
Apple - Malus Domestica - E	Fruit	29 ppm
Mace, Nutmeg - Myristica Fragrans - E	Seed	29 ppm
Baikal Skullcap, Chinese Skullcap, Huang Qin - Scutellaria Baicalensis - M	Root	29 ppm
Kuan Chung, Shield Fernle - Blechnum Orientale - E - M - T	Rhizome	28 ppm
Nutsedge - Cyperus Rotundus - E - M	Rhizome	28 ppm
Summer Squash - Cucurbita spp. - E	Fruit	27 ppm
Mai-Men-Dong, Mai-Men-Tung - Ophiopogon Japonicus - M	Tuber	27 ppm
Black Currant - Ribes Nigrum - E	Fruit	27 ppm
Pau D'Arco - Tabebuia Heptaphylla - M	Bark	27 ppm
Chickpea, Garbanzo - Cicer Arietinum - E	Seed	26 ppm
Adlay, Adlay Millet, Job's-Tears, Yi-Yi-Ren - Coix Lacryma-Jobi - E - M	Seed	26 ppm
Tian Ma - Gastrodia Elata - Rhizome	Rhizome	26 ppm
Chinese Licorice - Glycyrrhiza Uralensis - M	Root	26 ppm
Barley, Barleygrass - Hordeum Vulgare - E - M	Sprout Seedling	26 ppm
Japanese Privet, Ligustri Fructus - Ligustrum Japonicum - M	Fruit	26 ppm
Chinese Privet, Glossy Privet, Ligustri Fructus, Privet, White Waxtree - Ligustrum Lucidum - M	Fruit	26 ppm
Chinese Cornbind, Chinese Knotweed, Fleeceflower, Fo Ti, He Shou Wu - Polygonum Multiflorum - E - M - T	Rhizome	26 ppm
Plum - Prunus Domestica - E - M	Fruit	25.5 ppm
Alfalfa, Lucerne - Medicago Sativa subsp. Sativa - E	Plant	25.3 ppm
Coltsfoot - Tussilago Farfara - M - T	Flower	25 ppm
Green Gram, Mungbean - Vigna Radiata - E	Sprout Seedling	25 ppm
Brussel-Sprout - Brassica Oleracea var. Gemmifera - E	Leaf	24 ppm
Sickle Senna - Cassia Tora - Sprout - Seedling - M	Seed	24 ppm
Black Walnut - Juglans Nigra - E	Fruit	24 ppm
Black bean, Dwarf bean, Field bean, Flageolet bean, French bean, Garden bean, Green bean, Haricot, Haricot bean, Haricot vert, Kidney bean, Navy bean, Pop bean, Popping bean, Snap bean, String bean, Wax bean - Phaseolus Vulgaris - E	Seed	24 ppm
Chinese Senega - Polygala Tenuifolia - M	Root	24 ppm
Chinese Foxglove - Rehmannia Glutinosa - M	Root	24 ppm
Celery - Apium Graveolens - E	Root	23 ppm
Chinese Parasol - Firmiana Simplex - E - M	Seed	23 ppm
Gentian, Yellow Gentian - Gentiana Lutea - M	Root	23 ppm
Anise, Sweet Cumin - Pimpinella Anisum - E - M	Fruit	23 ppm
Dan-Shen, Red Sage, Tan-Shen - Salvia Miltiorrhiza - E - M	Root	23 ppm
Peach - Prunus Persica - E - M - T	Fruit	22.5 ppm
Potato - Solanum Tuberosum - E	Tuber	22 ppm
Giant Taro - Alocasia Macrorrhiza - E	Root	21 ppm
Chervil - Anthriscus Cerefolium - E	Leaf	21 ppm
Pigeonpea - Cajanus Vajan - E	Seed	21 ppm
Lambsquarter - Chenopodium Album - E - M - T	Seed	21 ppm
Blessed Thistle - Cnicus Benedictus - M	Plant	21 ppm
Coconut, Coconut Palm - Cocos Nucifera - E	Seed	21 ppm
Girasol, Sun Helianthus Annuus - E	Seed	21 ppm
Chinese Boxthorn, Chinese Matrimony Vine, Chinese Wolfberry - Lycium Chinense - E - M	Fruit	21 ppm
Pea - Pisum Sativum - E	Seed	21 ppm
Chinese Cornbind, Chinese Knotweed, Fleeceflower, Fo Ti, He Shou Wu - Polygonum Multiflorum - E - M - T	Root	21 ppm
Ching-Feng-Teng - Sinomenium Acutum - E - M	Rhizome	21 ppm
Alholva, Bockshornklee, Fenugreek, Greek Clover, Greek Trigonella Foenum-Graecum - E - M	Seed	21 ppm
Sarson - Brassica Rapa - E	Seed	20 ppm
Cayenne, Chili, Hot Pepper, Red Chili, Spur Pepper, Tabasco - Capsicum Frutescens - E	Fruit	20 ppm

Broomrape, Cistanchis Herba, Jou Tsung Jung - Cistanche Salsa - M	Plant	20 ppm
Common Garden Peony, Peony, White Peony - Paeonia Lactiflora - M	Root	20 ppm
Amur Cork Tree, Huang Bai, Huang Po, Po Mu - Phellodendron Amurense - M	Bark	20 ppm
Radish - Raphanus Sativus - E	Root	20 ppm
Blueberry - Vaccinium Corymbosum - E	Fruit	20 ppm
Mat Bean, Moth Bean - Vigna Aconitifolia - E	Seed	20 ppm
Adzuki Bean - Vigna Angularis - E	Seed	20 ppm
Onion, Shallot - Allium Cepa - Shallot Bulb - E	Seed	19.4 ppm
Horseradish - Armoracia Rusticana - E	Root	19 ppm
Chinese Parsley, Cilantro, Coriander - Coriandrum Sativum E	Fruit	19 ppm
Cape Jasmine, Gardenia, Jasmin, Shan-Chih-Tzu, Shan-Zhi-Zi, Zhi Zi - Gardenia Jasminoides - M	Fruit	19 ppm
Rosemary - Rosmarinus Officinalis - E - M	Plant	19 ppm
Red Elm, Slippery Elm - Ulmus Rubra - M	Bark	19 ppm
Aconite, Fu-Tsu - Aconitum Carmichaelii - E - M	Tuber	18 ppm
Dill, Garden Dill - Anethum Graveolens - E	Fruit	18 ppm
Lentil - Lens Culinaris - E	Sprout Seedling	18 ppm
Banana, Plantain - Musa x Paradisiaca - E	Fruit	18 ppm
Raspberry, Red raspberry - Rubus Idaeus - E - M	Fruit	18 ppm
Hsuan-Shen, Yuan-Shen - Scrophularia Buergeriana - M	Root	18 ppm
Rutabaga, Swede, Swedish Turnip - Brassica Napus var. Napobrassica - E	Root	17 ppm
Artichoke - Cynara Cardunculus - E	Flower	17 ppm
Russian Olive - Elaeagnus Umbellatus - E - M	Fruit	6-34 ppm
Peach - Prunus Persica - E - M - T	Seed	17 ppm
Asparagus bean, Pea bean, Yardlong bean - Vigna Unguiculata subsp. Sesquipedalis - E	Seed	17 ppm
Date Palm - Phoenix Dactylifera - E	Seed	16 ppm
Psyllium - Plantago Psyllium - E - M	Seed	16 ppm
Gooseberry - Ribes Uva-Crispa - E	Fruit	16 ppm
Garlic - Allium Sativum Bulb - E	Bulb	15.3 ppm
Chinese Quince, Mu-Kua - Chaenomeles Lagenaria - E	Fruit	15 ppm
Sweet Potato - Ipomoea Batatas - E	Root	15 ppm
Red Currant, White Currant - Ribes Rubrum - E	Fruit	15 ppm
Rye - Secale Cereale - E	Seed	25-30 ppm
Valerianella radicata	Plant	27.1-28.6 ppm
Elephant-Foot Yam - Amorphophallus Campanulatus - E - M- T	Root	14 ppm
Hsin-Pa-Pi, Kisasage - Catalpa Ovata - E - M	Fruit	14 ppm
Black Cohosh, Black Snake - Cimicifuga Racemosa - E - M	Root	14 ppm
English Hawthorn, Hawthorn, Whitethorn, Woodland Hawthorn - Crataegus Laevigata - M	Fruit	14 ppm
Cascara Buckthorn, Cascara Sagrada - Frangula Purshiana - M	Bark	14 ppm
Mace, Nutmeg - Myristica Fragrans - E	Aril	14 ppm
Sicklepod - Senna Obtusifolia - E - T	Seed	14 ppm
Sesame - Sesamum Indicum - E - M	Seed	14 ppm
Shan Dou Gen - Sophora Subprostrata - M - T	Root	14 ppm
Blackberry Lily, Shenan - Belamcanda Chinensis - M	Rhizome	13 ppm
European Chestnut - Castanea Sativa - E - M	Seed	13 ppm
Mango - Mangifera Indica - E - M	Fruit	12.2 ppm
Green Gram, Mungbean - Vigna Radiata - E	Seed	12.2 ppm
Hawthorn - Crataegus Cuneata - M	Fruit	12 ppm
Swamp Taro - Cyrtosperma Chamissonis - E	Root	12 ppm
Horsetail, Scouring Rush - Equisetum Hyemale - M	Plant	12 ppm
Bei-Mu, Fritillary - Fritillaria Thunbergii - Blub - E - M	Bulb	12 ppm
Guavas - Psidium Guajava - E	Fruit	12 ppm
Salsify - Tragopogon Porrifolius - E	Root	12 ppm
Malanga, Tannia, Yautia - Xanthosoma Sagittifolium - E	Root	11.3 ppm
Jack Bean - Canavalia Ensiformis - E	Seed	11 ppm
Chinese Dogwood - Cornus Officinalis - E - M	Fruit	11 ppm
Apricot - Prunus Armeniaca - E - M - T	Seed	11 ppm
Chinese Cabbage - Brassica Pekinensis - E	Leaf	10.5 ppm

MANGANESE CONTINUED

Species	Part	Quantity
Asparagus lucidus LINDL. -- Lucid Asparagus	Root	10 ppm
Hardy Orchid, Hyacinth Bletilla, Hyacinth Orchid, Shiran - Bletilla Striata - M	Tuber	10 ppm
Bitter Melon, Sorosi - Momordica Charantia - E	Fruit	10 ppm
Avocado - Persea Americana - E - M - T	Fruit	10 ppm
Da-Zao, Jujube, Ta-Tsao - Zizyphus Jujuba - E - M	Fruit	10 ppm
Citron - Citrus Medica - E	Fruit	9 ppm
Cashew - Anacardium Occidentale - E	Seed	8.4 ppm
Flax, Lin Linum Usitatissimum - E	Hay	8.1 ppm
Brazilnut, Brazilnut-Tree, Creamnut, Paranut - Bertholletia Eexcelsa - E	Seed	8 ppm
Bitter Orange, Petitgrain - Citrus Aurantium - E	Fruit	8 ppm
Orange - Citrus Sinensis - E	Fruit	8 ppm
Sour Cherry - Prunus Cerasus - E - M - T	Fruit	8 ppm
Cantaloupe, Melon, Muskmelon, Netted Melon, Nutmeg Melon, Persian Melon - Cucumis Melo subsp. ssp Melo var.Ccantalupensis - Friut - E	Fruit	7.7 ppm
Taro - Colocasia Esculenta - E	Root	7.6 ppm
Jack Artocarpus Heterophyllus - E	Fruit	7 ppm
Rapini, Seven-Top Turnip, Turnip - Brassica Rapa - E	Root	7 ppm
Fig - Ficus Carica - E	Fruit	7 ppm
Aloe, Bitter Aloes - Aloe Vera - E - M	Leaf	6 ppm
Genipap, Jagua - Genipa Americana - E - M	Seed	6 ppm
Banana Yucca, Blue Yucca, Spanish Bayonet, Yucca - Yucca Baccata - E - M - T	Root	6 ppm
Pear - Pyrus Communis - E	Fruit	5.55 ppm
Carambola, Star Averrhoa Carambola - E	Fruit	1-11 ppm
Cherimoya - Annona Cherimola - E	Fruit	5 ppm
Grape Citrus Paradisi - E	Fruit	5 ppm
Chinese Kudzu - Pueraria Pseudohirsuta - E - M	Root	5 ppm
Mandarin, Tangerine - Citrus Reticulata - E	Fruit	4.6 ppm
Chinese Jack-In-The-Pulpit - Arisaema Consanguineum - E - M - T	Rhizome	4 ppm
Watermelon - Citrullus Lanatus - E	Fruit	4 ppm
Air Potato, Potato Yam - Dioscorea Bulbifera - E	Rhizome	4 ppm
Northern Red Oak - Quercus Rubra - E - M	Seed	3.9 ppm
Bread Artocarpus Altilis - E	Fruit	3.5 ppm
Pistachio - Pistacia Vera - E	Seed	3.4 ppm
Scarlet Runner Bean - Phaseolus Coccineus - E	Seed	3.2 ppm
Ginkgo, Maidenhair Tree - Ginkgo Biloba - Tree - E - M - T	Seed	3 ppm
Soursop - Annona Muricata - E	Fruit	2.7 ppm
Cassava, Tapioca, Yuca - Manihot Esculenta - E	Root	2.5 ppm
Curry Murraya spp. - E - M	Fruit	1.8 ppm
Ambarella - Spondias Dulcis - E	Fruit	1.2 ppm
Papaya - Carica Papaya - E - M	Fruit	1.1 ppm
Genipap, Jagua - Genipa Americana - E - M	Fruit	1 ppm

PLANTS CONTAINING MOLYBDENUM

Species	Part	Quantity
Red Pignut Hickory - Carya Glabra - E	Shoot	33 ppm
Black bean, Dwarf bean, Field bean, Flageolet bean, French bean, Garden bean, Green bean, Haricot, Haricot bean, Haricot vert, Kidney bean, Navy bean, Pop bean, Popping bean, Snap bean, String bean, Wax bean - Phaseolus Vulgaris - E	Fruit	20 ppm
Shagbark Hickory - Carya Ovata - E	Shoot	18 ppm
Bell Pepper, Cherry Pepper, Cone Pepper, Green Pepper, Paprika, Sweet Pepper - Capsicum Annuum - E	Fruit	15 ppm
Butter Bean, Lima Bean - Phaseolus Lunatus - E	Seed	15 ppm
American Ginseng, Ginseng - Panax Quinquefolius - M	Plant	14 ppm
Parsley - Petroselinum Crispum - E	Plant	14 ppm
Black bean, Dwarf bean, Field bean, Flageolet bean, French bean, Garden bean, Green bean, Haricot, Haricot bean, Haricot vert, Kidney bean, Navy bean, Pop bean, Popping bean, Snap bean, String bean, Wax bean - Phaseolus Vulgaris - E	Seed	14 ppm
White Oak - Quercus Alba - M	Stem	9.12 ppm
Cabbage, Red Cabbage, White Cabbage - Brassica Oleracea var. Capitata - E	Leaf	8.7 ppm

Asparagus bean, Pea bean, Yardlong bean - Vigna Unguiculata subsp. Sesquipedalis - E	Seed	8 ppm
Corn - Zea Mays - E	Seed	6.3 ppm
Black Oak - Quercus Velutina - E - M	Stem	6.2 ppm
Tomato - Lycopersicon Esculentum - E - M - T	Fruit	6 ppm
Buckwheat - Fagopyrum Esculentum - E	Seed	5.5 ppm
Smooth Sumac - Rhus Glabra - E - M	Stem	4.69 ppm
Northern Red Oak - Quercus Rubra - E - M	Stem	4.62 ppm
Soybean - Glycine Max - E	Seed	4 ppm
Cauli Brassica Oleracea var. Botrytis - E	Leaf	3.76 ppm
Pea - Pisum Sativum - E	Seed	3 ppm
Cucumber - Cucumis Sativus - E	Fruit	2.8 ppm
Red Cedar - Juniperus Virginiana Amphicarpaea Bracteata- E - M - T	Shoot	2.64 ppm
Onion, Shallot - Allium Cepa - Shallot Bulb - E	Bulb	2.3 ppm
Potato - Solanum Tuberosum - E	Tuber	2.1 ppm
Lettuce - Lactuca Sativa - E	Leaf	2 ppm
Black Cherry, Wild Cherry - Prunus Serotina - E - M - T	Leaf	1.9 ppm
Asparagus - Asparagus Officinalis - E	Shoot	1.8 ppm
Cauli Brassica Oleracea var. Botrytis - E	Stem	1.76 ppm
Plum - Prunus Domestica - E - M	Fruit	1.7 ppm
Endive, Escarole - Cichorium Endivia - M	Leaf	1.68 ppm
Chinese Cabbage - Brassica Pekinensis - E	Leaf	1.47 ppm
Black Gum, Black Tupelo - Nyssa Sylvatica - E - M	Leaf	1.4 ppm
White Tephrosia - Tephrosia Candida - M - T	Plant	1.25 ppm
Corn Salad, Lamb's Lettuce - Valerianella Locusta - E	Plant	2.35-2.41 ppm
American Persimmon - Diospyros Virginiana - E - M	Stem	1.08 ppm
Peach - Prunus Persica - E - M - T	Fruit	1.05 ppm
Rapini, Seven-Top Turnip, Turnip - Brassica Rapa - E	Root	1 ppm
Valerianella radicata	Plant	1.59-1.82 ppm
Brussel-Sprout - Brassica Oleracea var. Gemmifera - E	Leaf	Trace
Spinach - Spinacia Oleracea - E	Plant	Trace
Grape Citrus Paradisi - E	Fruit	Trace
Cantaloupe, Melon, Muskmelon, Netted Melon, Nutmeg Melon, Persian Melon - Cucumis Melo subsp. ssp Melo var.Ccantalupensis - Friut - E	Fruit	Trace
Sassafras - Sassafras Albidum - E - M - T	Stem	Trace
Carrot - Daucus Carota - E	Root	Trace
American Cranberry, Cranberry, Large Cranberry - Vaccinium Macrocarpon - E	Fruit	Trace
Lambsquarter - Chenopodium Album - E - M - T	Plant	Trace
Rutabaga, Swede, Swedish Turnip - Brassica Napus var. Napobrassica - E	Leaf	Trace
Cobnut, English Filbert, European Filbert, European Hazel, Hazel - Corylus Avellana - E	Seed	Trace
Northern Red Oak - Quercus Rubra - E - M	Seed	Trace
Black Currant - Ribes Nigrum - E	Fruit	Trace
Red Currant, White Currant - Ribes Rubrum - E	Fruit	Trace
Cloudberry - Rubus Chamaemorus - E - M	Fruit	Trace
Aubergine, Egg Solanum Melongena - E	Fruit	Trace
European Grape, Grape, Grapevine, Vigne Vinifere, Wine Grape - Vitis Vinifera - E - M	Fruit	Trace
Parsnip - Pastinaca Sativa - E	Root	Trace
Dwarf Sumac, Winged Sumac - Rhus Copallina - E - M	Stem	Trace
Sassafras - Sassafras Albidum - E - M - T	Leaf	Trace
Black Gum, Black Tupelo - Nyssa Sylvatica - E - M	Stem	Trace
Apple - Malus Domestica - E	Fruit	Trace
Butternut - Juglans Cinerea - E	Seed	Trace
Black Walnut - Juglans Nigra - E	Seed	Trace
Orange - Citrus Sinensis - E	Fruit	Trace
Brussel-Sprout - Brassica Oleracea var. Gemmifera - E	Stem	Trace
Rutabaga, Swede, Swedish Turnip - Brassica Napus var. Napobrassica - E	Stem	Trace
Almond - Prunus Dulcis - E - M - T	Seed	Trace
Pear - Pyrus Communis - E	Fruit	Trace
Black Cherry, Wild Cherry - Prunus Serotina - E - M - T	Stem	Trace

MOLYBDENUM CONTINUED

Species	Part	Quantity
Cowgrass, Peavine Clover, Purple Clover, Red Clover - Trifolium Pratense - E - M	Stem	Trace
Cashew - Anacardium Occidentale - E	Seed	Trace
Cauli Brassica Oleracea var. Botrytis - E	Flower	Trace
Shagbark Hickory - Carya Ovata - E	Seed	Trace
Rhubarb - Rheum Rhabarbarum - E	Pt	Trace
Coconut, Coconut Palm - Cocos Nucifera - E	Seed	Trace
Alfalfa, Lucerne - Medicago Sativa subsp. Sativa - E	Leaf	Trace
Dill, Garden Dill - Anethum Graveolens - E	Plant	Trace
Celery - Apium Graveolens - E	Root	Trace
Horseradish - Armoracia Rusticana - E	Root	Trace
Mugwort - Artemisia Vulgaris - M	Plant	Trace
Beet, Beetroot, Garden Beet, Sugar Beet - Beta Vulgaris - E	Root	Trace
Ramie - Boehmeria Nivea - M	Plant	Trace
Rutabaga, Swede, Swedish Turnip - Brassica Napus var. Napobrassica - E	Root	Trace
Pecan - Carya Illinoensis - E	Plant	Trace
Mandarin, Tangerine - Citrus Reticulata - E	Fruit	Trace
Strawberry - Fragaria spp. - E	Fruit	Trace
Alehoof - Glechoma Hederacea - M	Plant	Trace
Flax, Lin Linum Usitatissimum - E	Seed	Trace
Banana, Plantain - Musa x Paradisiaca - E	Fruit	Trace
Butterbur - Petasites Japonicus - T	Plant	Trace
Qian Hu - Peucedanum Decursivum - M	Plant	Trace
Giant Knotweed, Hu-Zhang, Japanese Knotweed, Mexican Bamboo - Polygonum Cuspidatum - E - M - T	Plant	Trace
Chinese Polystichum - Polystichum Polyblepharum - T	Plant	Trace
Radish - Raphanus Sativus - E	Root	Trace
Gooseberry - Ribes Uva-Crispa - E	Fruit	Trace
Dog Rose, Dogbrier, Rose - Rosa Canina - E - M	Fruit	Trace
Rowan Berry - Sorbus Aucubaria - E - M - T	Fruit	Trace
Dandelion - Taraxacum Officinale - E - M	Plant	Trace
European Nettle, Stinging Nettle - Urtica Dioica - E - M	Leaf	Trace
Bilberry, Dwarf Bilberry, Whortleberry - Vaccinium Myrtillus - E - M	Fruit	Trace
Cowberry, Lingen, Lingonberry - Vaccinium Vitis-Idaea var. Minus - E - M	Fruit	Trace

PLANTS CONTAINING NITROGEN

Species	Part	Quantity
Cucumber - Cucumis Sativus - E	Fruit	80,000 ppm
Purple Tephrosia, Wild Indigo - Tephrosia Purpurea - M - T	Leaf	72,500 ppm
Cauli Brassica Oleracea var. Botrytis - E	Leaf	71,800 ppm
Cassie, Huisache, Opopanax, Popinac, Sweet Acacia - Acacia Farnesiana - M	Leaf	68,800 ppm
European Nettle, Stinging Nettle - Urtica Dioica - E - M	Leaf	55,555 ppm
Dill, Garden Dill - Anethum Graveolens - E	Plant	55,300 ppm
Lettuce - Lactuca Sativa - E	Leaf	54,000 ppm
Common Indigo - Indigofera Tinctoria - Leaf	Leaf	51,100 ppm
Pea - Pisum Sativum - E	Seed	50,000 ppm
Cauli Brassica Oleracea var. Botrytis - E	Flower	47,500 ppm
Spinach - Spinacia Oleracea - E	Leaf	45,700 ppm
Black bean, Dwarf bean, Field bean, Flageolet bean, French bean, Garden bean, Green bean, Haricot, Haricot bean, Haricot vert, Kidney bean, Navy bean, Pop bean, Popping bean, Snap bean, String bean, Wax bean - Phaseolus Vulgaris - E	Fruit	41,000 ppm
Parsley - Petroselinum Crispum - E	Leaf	40,700 ppm
Groundnut, Peanut - Arachis Hypogaea - E - M	Seed	40,000 ppm
Tobacco - Nicotiana Tabacum - Leaf	Leaf	40,000 ppm
Radish - Raphanus Sativus - E	Root	38,570 ppm
Horseradish - Armoracia Rusticana - E	Root	38,461 ppm
Cabbage, Red Cabbage, White Cabbage - Brassica Oleracea var. Capitata - E	Leaf	37,500 ppm
Sugar-Apple, Sweetsop - Annona Squamosa - E	Leaf	36,000 ppm
Beet, Beetroot, Garden Beet, Sugar Beet - Beta Vulgaris - E	Root	35,830 ppm

Wild Pineapple - Bromelia Pinguin - E - M	Shoot	35,800 ppm
Bitter Melon, Sorosi - Momordica Charantia - E	Fruit	33,800 ppm
Small-Flowered Melilot - Melilotus Indica - E - M - T	Plant	33,600 ppm
Parsnip - Pastinaca Sativa - E	Root	33,160 ppm
Indian Sorrel, Jamaica Sorrel, Kharkadi, Red Sorrel, Sorrel - Hibiscus Sabdariffa - E	Seed	32,900 ppm
Sicklepod - Senna Obtusifolia - E - T	Seed	31,300 ppm
Mate, Paraguay Tea, South American Holly - Ilex Paraguariensis - M	Leaf	30,000 ppm
Cobnut, English Filbert, European Filbert, European Hazel, Hazel - Corylus Avellana - E	Seed	28,000 ppm
Loquat - Eriobotrya Japonica - E	Seed	26,000 ppm
Tomato - Lycopersicon Esculentum - E - M - T	Leaf	26,000 ppm
Achiote, Annato, Annatto, Annoto, Arnato, Bija, Lipstick Pod, Lipsticktree - Bixa Orellana - E	Seed	25,200 ppm
Rutabaga, Swede, Swedish Turnip - Brassica Napus var. Napobrassica - E	Root	25,000 ppm
Indian Kino, Malabar Kinol - Pterocarpus Marsupium - Leaf	Leaf	25,000 ppm
Ginger - Zingiber Officinale - E	Rhizome	24,440 ppm
Saffron - Crocus Sativus - Style	Silk Stigma Style	24,300 ppm
White Tephrosia - Tephrosia Candida - M - T	Plant	23,600 ppm
Bell Pepper, Cherry Pepper, Cone Pepper, Green Pepper, Paprika, Sweet Pepper - Capsicum Annuum - E	Fruit	23,330 ppm
Tomato - Lycopersicon Esculentum - E - M - T	Fruit	23,330 ppm
Coffee - Coffea Arabica - E - M	Seed	23,000 ppm
Cacao - Theobroma Ccacao - E	Seed	22,800 ppm
Rhubarb - Rheum Rhabarbarum - E	Pt	22,000 ppm
Carrot - Daucus Carota - E	Root	20,000 ppm
American Ginseng, Ginseng - Panax Quinquefolius - M	Plant	20,000 ppm
Red Currant, White Currant - Ribes Rubrum - E	Fruit	20,000 ppm
Celery - Apium Graveolens - E	Root	19,090 ppm
Cloudberry - Rubus Chamaemorus - E - M	Fruit	18,125 ppm
Rapini, Seven-Top Turnip, Turnip - Brassica Rapa - E	Root	18,000 ppm
Ambarella - Spondias Dulcis - E	Fruit	17,900 ppm
Onion, Shallot - Allium Cepa - Shallot Bulb - E	Bulb	17,690 ppm
Potato - Solanum Tuberosum - E	Tuber	17,000 ppm
Grape Citrus Paradisi - E	Fruit	16,360 ppm
Indian Snakeroot, Serpentine Wood - Rauvolfia Serpentina - Seed	Seed	16,000 ppm
Banana, Plantain - Musa x Paradisiaca - E	Fruit	15,000 ppm
Gooseberry - Ribes Uva-Crispa - E	Fruit	15,000 ppm
Genipap, Jagua - Genipa Americana - E - M	Fruit	13,900 ppm
Orange - Citrus Sinensis - E	Fruit	13,845 ppm
Amphicarpaea Bracteata- E - M	Shoot	0-26,500 ppm
Mandarin, Tangerine - Citrus Reticulata - E	Fruit	13,075 ppm
Peach - Prunus Persica - E - M - T	Fruit	13,075 ppm
Black Currant - Ribes Nigrum - E	Fruit	12,775 ppm
Rowan Berry - Sorbus Aucubaria - E - M - T	Fruit	11,900 ppm
Genipap, Jagua - Genipa Americana - E - M	Seed	11,100 ppm
Aubergine, Egg Solanum Melongena - E	Fruit	10,250 ppm
Gru-Gru Nut, Mbocaya - Acrocomia Totai - E	Seed	0-20,200 ppm
Strawberry - Fragaria spp. - E	Fruit	10,000 ppm
Plum - Prunus Domestica - E - M	Fruit	10,000 ppm
Cheeseweed - Malva Parviflora - E - M	Plant	9,400 ppm
Dog Rose, Dogbrier, Rose - Rosa Canina - E - M	Fruit	9,000 ppm
Lantana, Wild Sage - Lantana Camara - M	Shoot	8,800 ppm
White Melilot - Melilotus alba Medic - E - M - T	Plant	8,300 ppm
European Grape, Grape, Grapevine, Vigne Vinifere, Wine Grape - Vitis Vinifera - E - M	Fruit	7,220 ppm
Carambola, Star Averrhoa Carambola - E	Fruit	10,200-12,800 ppm
Ambarella - Spondias Dulcis - E	Seed	6,200 ppm
Emblic, Myrobalan - Phyllanthus Emblica - E	Fruit	5,445 ppm
American Cranberry, Cranberry, Large Cranberry - Vaccinium Macrocarpon - E	Fruit	5,000 ppm
Tamarillo, Tree Tomato - Cyphomandra Betacea - Fruit	Fruit	4,450 ppm
Palta De Monte, Wild Avocado, Wild Pear - Persea Schiedeana - E	Fruit	1,910-8,680 ppm

NITROGEN CONTINUED

Species	Part	Quantity
Almond - Prunus Dulcis - E - M - T	Seed	4,315 ppm
Cheeses, Common Mallow - Malva Neglecta - E - M	Plant	4,200 ppm
Apple - Malus Domestica - E	Fruit	4,000 ppm
Gru-Gru Nut, Mbocaya - Acrocomia Totai - E	Fruit	0-6,700 ppm
High Mallow - Malva Sylvestris - E - M	Leaf	3,300 ppm
Chinese Hibiscus, Shoe- Hibiscus Rosa-Sinensis - E	Flower	640-6,275 ppm
Pear - Pyrus Communis - E	Fruit	3,000 ppm
Soursop - Annona Muricata - E	Fruit	2,700 ppm
Cherimoya - Annona Cherimola - E	Fruit	2,270 ppm
Pineapple - Ananas Comosus - E	Fruit	1,150 ppm
Coconut, Coconut Palm - Cocos Nucifera - E	Hull Husk	1,100 ppm
Imbu, Umbu - Spondias Tuberosa - E	Fruit	1,100 ppm
Maracuya, Passion Passiflora Edulis - E	Plant	960-1,920 ppm
Black bean, Dwarf bean, Field bean, Flageolet bean, French bean, Garden bean, Green bean, Haricot, Haricot bean, Haricot vert, Kidney bean, Navy bean, Pop bean, Popping bean, Snap bean, String bean, Wax bean - Phaseolus Vulgaris - E	Fruit	13,500 ppm
Marula - Sclerocarya Caffra - Seed	Seed	12,985 ppm
Pumpkin - Cucurbita Pepo - E	Seed	12,982 ppm
Cucumber - Cucumis Sativus - E	Fruit	12,600 ppm
Swamp Cabbage, Water Spinach - Ipomoea Aquatica - E	Leaf	12,360 ppm
Berro, Watercress - Nasturtium Officinale - E	Herb	12,000 ppm
Hemp, Indian Hemp, Marihuana, Marijuana - Cannabis Sativa - M	Seed	11,227 ppm
Butter Bean, Lima Bean - Phaseolus Lunatus - E	Sprout Seedling	10,611 ppm
Radish - Raphanus Sativus - E	Fruit	10,526 ppm
Asparagus - Asparagus Officinalis - E	Shoot	10,244 ppm
Oats - Avena Sativa - E - M	Seed	10,200 ppm
Pumpkin - Cucurbita Pepo - E	Flower	10,100 ppm
Pigweed - Amaranthus sp. - E - M	Leaf	10,082 ppm
Jicaro - Crescentia Alata - M	Seed	10,020 ppm
Groundnut, Peanut - Arachis Hypogaea - E - M	Plant	10,000 ppm

PLANTS CONTAINING PHOSPHORUS

Species	Part	Quantity
Beet, Beetroot, Garden Beet, Sugar Beet - Beta Vulgaris - E	Root	45,580 ppm
Malanga, Tannia, Yautia - Xanthosoma Sagittifolium - E	Leaf	38,416 ppm
Lambsquarter - Chenopodium Album - E - M - T	Leaf	36,833 ppm
Bitter Melon, Sorosi - Momordica Charantia - E	Leaf	33,467 ppm
Tomatillo - Physalis Ixocarpa - E	Fruit	30,250 ppm
Flax, Lin Linum Usitatissimum - E	Seed	20,335 ppm
Luffa, Smooth Loofah, Vegetable Sponge - Luffa Aegyptiaca - E	Seed	18,300 ppm
Garden Cress - Lepidium Sativum - E	Seed	17,500 ppm
Field Horsetail, Horsetail - Equisetum Arvense - M	Plant	14,762 ppm
Watermelon - Citrullus Lanatus - E	Seed	14,600 ppm
Luffa, Smooth Loofah, Vegetable Sponge - Luffa Aegyptiaca - E	Leaf	14,141 ppm
Sesame - Sesamum Indicum - E - M	Leaf	14,000 ppm
Lettuce - Lactuca Sativa - E	Leaf	13,920 ppm
Terminalia catappa L. -- Indian Almond, Malabar Almond, Tropical Almond	Seed	9,835 ppm
Coca - Erythroxylum Coca var. Coca - E - M	Leaf	9,740 ppm
ElytriCouchgrass, Doggrass, Quackgrass, Twitchgrass, Wheatgrass - Elytrigia Repens - E - M	Plant	9,510 ppm
White Mustard - Sinapis Alba - E - M - T	Seed	9,330 ppm
Opium Poppy, Poppyseed Poppy - Papaver Somniferum - E	Seed	9,277 ppm
Barley, Barleygrass - Hordeum Vulgare - E - M	Seed	9,200 ppm
Cauli Brassica Oleracea var. Botrytis - E	Leaf	9,090 ppm
Butter Bean, Lima Bean - Phaseolus Lunatus - E	Seed	9,000 ppm
Sesame - Sesamum Indicum - E - M	Seed	8,898 ppm
Oats - Avena Sativa - E - M	Plant	8,800 ppm
Date Palm - Phoenix Dactylifera - E	Fruit	8,795 ppm

Plant	Part	ppm
Almond - Prunus Dulcis - E - M - T	Seed	8,735 ppm
Tomato - Lycopersicon Esculentum - E - M - T	Fruit	8,400 ppm
Bitter Melon, Sorosi - Momordica Charantia - E	Fruit	8,333 ppm
Elephant-Foot Yam - Amorphophallus Campanulatus - E - M- T	Shoot	8,100 ppm
Soybean - Glycine Max - E	Seed	8,040 ppm
Bok-Choy, Celery Cabbage, Celery Mustard, Chinese Cabbage, Chinese Mustard, Chinese White Cabbage, Pak-Choi - Brassica Chinensis - E	Leaf	7,907 ppm
Okra - Abelmoschus Esculentus - Friut - E - M	Seed	7,900 ppm
Celery - Apium Graveolens - E	Root	7,900 ppm
Purslane, Verdolaga - Portulaca Oleracea - E	Herb	7,740 ppm
Peppermint - Mentha x Piperita subsp. Nothosubsp. Piperita - E - M - T	Leaf	7,720 ppm
Dill, Garden Dill - Anethum Graveolens - E	Plant	7,625 ppm
Beebread, Beeplant, Borage, Talewort - Borago Officinalis - E - M - T	Leaf	7,579 ppm
Curly Dock, Lengua De Vaca, Sour Dock, Yellow Dock - Rumex Crispus - M - T	Root	7,570 ppm
Chinese Cabbage - Brassica Pekinensis - E	Leaf	7,560 ppm
Vinespinach - Basella Alba - E - M	Leaf	7,535 ppm
Girasol, Sun Helianthus Annuus - E	Seed	7,449 ppm
Elephant Apple, Manzana De Elefante, Wood-Apple - Limonia acidissima - Wood - Apple - E - M	Seed	14,300-14,895 ppm
Cauli Brassica Oleracea var. Botrytis - E	Flower	7,375 ppm
Parsnip - Pastinaca Sativa - E	Root	7,365 ppm
Soybean - Glycine Max - E	Fruit	7,305 ppm
Umbrella Thorn - Acacia Tortilis - M	Seed	7,300 ppm
Shepherd's Purse - Capsella Bursa-Pastoris - E - M	Plant	7,288 ppm
Evening-Primrose - Oenothera Biennis - E - M	Seed	7,257 ppm
Rutabaga, Swede, Swedish Turnip - Brassica Napus var. Napobrassica - E	Root	7,250 ppm
Wheat - Triticum Aestivum - E - M	Plant	7,200 ppm
Garden Cress - Lepidium Sativum - E	Leaf	7,170 ppm
Water Lotus - Nelumbo Nucifera - E - M	Seed	7,130 ppm
Andean Lupine, Chocho, Tarhui - Lupinus Mutabilis - E - T	Seed	7,100 ppm
Lady's Thistle, Milk Thistle - Silybum Marianum - M	Plant	7,060 ppm
Barley, Barleygrass - Hordeum Vulgare - E - M	Plant	6,900 ppm
Celery - Apium Graveolens - E	Pt	6,849 ppm
Wheat - Triticum Aestivum - E - M	Seed	6,800 ppm
European Nettle, Stinging Nettle - Urtica Dioica - E - M	Leaf	6,800 ppm
Buchu, Honey Buchu, Mountain Buchu - Agathosma Betulina Buchu, Honey Buchu, Mountain Buchu - Agathosma Betulina - M	Leaf	6,780 ppm
Jew's Mallow, Mulukiya, Nalta Jute - Corchorus Olitorius - E - M	Leaf	6,755 ppm
Bolsa Mullaca, Winter Cherry - Physalis Angulata - E	Fruit	1,350-13,500 ppm
Green Gram, Mungbean - Vigna Radiata - E	Sprout Seedling	6,560 ppm
Cabbage, Red Cabbage, White Cabbage - Brassica Oleracea var. Capitata - E	Leaf	6,500 ppm
Brazilnut, Brazilnut-Tree, Creamnut, Paranut - Bertholletia Eexcelsa - E	Seed	6,208 ppm
Indian Sorrel, Jamaica Sorrel, Kharkadi, Red Sorrel, Sorrel - Hibiscus Sabdariffa - E	Leaf	6,458 ppm
Chinese Parsley, Cilantro, Coriander - Coriandrum Sativum E	Leaf	6,452 ppm
Chives - Allium Schoenoprasum - E	Leaf	6,437 ppm
Parsley - Petroselinum Crispum - E	Plant	6,425 ppm
Luffa, Smooth Loofah, Vegetable Sponge - Luffa Aegyptiaca - E	Fruit	6,400 ppm
Pea - Pisum Sativum - E	Plant	6,400 ppm
Asparagus bean, Pea bean, Yardlong bean - Vigna Unguiculata subsp. Sesquipedalis - E	Seed	6,375 ppm
Chayote - Sechium Edule - E - M	Shoot	6,350 ppm
Kapok, Silk-Cotton Tree - Ceiba Pentandra - M	Seed	9,700-12,690 ppm
Papaya - Carica Papaya - E - M	Leaf	6,311 ppm
Indian Saffron, Turmeric - Curcuma Longa - E	Rhizome	6,307 ppm
Caraway, Carum - Carum Carvi - E	Fruit	6,302 ppm
Okra - Abelmoschus Esculentus - Friut - E - M	Fruit	6,300 ppm

PHOSPHORUS CONTINUED

Cashew - Anacardium Occidentale - E	Seed	6,255 ppm
Pea - Pisum Sativum - E	Seed	6,250 ppm
Artichoke - Cynara Cardunculus - E	Flower	6,240 ppm
Spinach - Spinacia Oleracea - E	Plant	6,232 ppm
Kapok, Silk-Cotton Tree - Ceiba Pentandra - M - E	Shoot	6,200 ppm
Lentil - Lens Culinaris - E	Sprout Seedling	6,165 ppm
Sweet Potato - Ipomoea Batatas - E	Leaf	6,090 ppm
Bambarra Groundnut, Groundbean - Vigna Subterranea - E	Seed	6,042 ppm
Gru-Gru Nut, Mbocaya - Acrocomia Totai - E	Fruit	0-12,000 ppm
Indian Sorrel, Jamaica Sorrel, Kharkadi, Red Sorrel, Sorrel - Hibiscus Sabdariffa - E	Seed	6,000 ppm
Cus-Cus, Cuscus Grass, Vetiver - Vetiveria Zizanioides - E	Fruit	6,000 ppm
Fennel - Foeniculum Vulgare - M	Fruit	5,960 ppm
Barley, Barleygrass - Hordeum Vulgare - E - M	Stem	5,950 ppm
Beet, Beetroot, Garden Beet, Sugar Beet - Beta Vulgaris - E	Leaf	5,946 ppm
Black Walnut - Juglans Nigra - E	Seed	5,882 ppm
Black bean, Dwarf bean, Field bean, Flageolet bean, French bean, Garden bean, Green bean, Haricot, Haricot bean, Haricot vert, Kidney bean, Navy bean, Pop bean, Popping bean, Snap bean, String bean, Wax bean - Phaseolus Vulgaris - E	Seed	5,880 ppm
Andean Lupine, Chocho, Tarhui - Lupinus Mutabilis - E - T	Fruit	5,875 ppm
Radish - Raphanus Sativus - E	Root	5,850 ppm
Aubergine, Egg Solanum Melongena - E	Fruit	5,836 ppm
Taro - Colocasia Esculenta - E	Leaf	5,800 ppm
Endive, Escarole - Cichorium Endivia - M	Leaf	5,760 ppm
Sickle Senna - Cassia Tora - Sprout - Seedling - M	Sprout Seedling	5,700 ppm
Flannelleaf, Flannelplant, Great mullein, Mullein, Velvet - Verbascum Thapsus - M	Leaf	5,700 ppm
Black bean, Dwarf bean, Field bean, Flageolet bean, French bean, Garden bean, Green bean, Haricot, Haricot bean, Haricot vert, Kidney bean, Navy bean, Pop bean, Popping bean, Snap bean, String bean, Wax bean - Phaseolus Vulgaris - E	Leaf	5,682 ppm
Cumin - Cuminum Cyminum - E - M	Fruit	5,673 ppm
Achocha - Cyclanthera Pedata - Friut - E - M	Fruit	5,615 ppm
Rice - Oryza Sativa - E	Seed	5,588 ppm
Cacao - Theobroma Ccacao - E	Seed	5,571 ppm
Summer Squash - Cucurbita spp. - E	Fruit	5,540 ppm
Onion, Shallot - Allium Cepa - Shallot Bulb - E	Leaf	5,513 ppm
Tomato - Lycopersicon Esculentum - E - M - T	Leaf	5,500 ppm
Cerraja, Sow Thistle - Sonchus Oleraceus - E - M	Leaf	5,440 ppm
Mat Bean, Moth Bean - Vigna Aconitifolia - E	Seed	5,418 ppm
Soybean - Glycine Max - E	Plant	5,410 ppm
Mat Bean, Moth Bean - Vigna Aconitifolia - E	Plant	5,400 ppm
Perilla - Perilla Frutescens - E - M - T	Seed	5,339 ppm
Ginger - Zingiber Officinale - E	Rhizome	5,323 ppm
Udo - Aralia Cordata - E - M	Leaf	5,320 ppm
Pistachio - Pistacia Vera - E	Seed	5,280 ppm
Lentil - Lens Culinaris - E	Seed	5,275 ppm
Pea - Pisum Sativum - E	Fruit	5,240 ppm
Pumpkin - Cucurbita Pepo - E	Fruit	5,238 ppm
Pokeweed - Phytolacca Americana - E - M - T	Shoot	5,238 ppm
Garland Chrysanthemum - Chrysanthemum Coronarium - Bud - E	Leaf	5,230 ppm
Garlic - Allium Sativum Bulb - E	Bulb	5,220 ppm
Perilla - Perilla Frutescens - E - M - T	Leaf	5,214 ppm
Taro - Colocasia Esculenta - E	Root	5,204 ppm
Jerusalem Artichoke - Helianthus Tuberosus E	Tuber	5,200 ppm
Huaca-Mullo - Mimulus Glabratus - M	Shoot	5,200 ppm
American Ginseng, Ginseng - Panax Quinquefolius - M	Plant	5,200 ppm
Purple Tephrosia, Wild Indigo - Tephrosia Purpurea - M - T	Leaf	5,200 ppm
Dog Rose, Dogbrier, Rose - Rosa Canina - E - M	Fruit	5,180 ppm
Basil, Cuban Basil, Sweet Basil - Ocimum Basilicum - E	Leaf	5,168 ppm

Name	Part	ppm
Ambarella - Spondias Dulcis - E	Fruit	5,115 ppm
Kohlrabi - Brassica Oleracea var. Gongylodes - E	Stem	5,110 ppm
Fennel - Foeniculum Vulgare - M	Plant	5,100 ppm
English Walnut - Juglans Rregia - E	Seed	5,100 ppm
Carrot - Daucus Carota - E	Root	5,090 ppm
Broadbean, Faba Bean, Habas - Vicia Faba - E	Fruit	5,070 ppm
Pito - Erythrina Berteroana - E	Shoot	5,060 ppm
Asparagus Pea, Goa Bean, Winged Bean - Psophocarpus Tetragonolobus - E	Seed	5,058 ppm
Feverfew - Chrysanthemum Parthenium - M	Plant	5,010 ppm
Horseradish - Armoracia Rusticana - E	Root	5,000 ppm
Rapini, Seven-Top Turnip, Turnip - Brassica Rapa - E	Root	5,000 ppm
Wild Pineapple - Bromelia Pinguin - E - M	Shoot	5,000 ppm
Adlay, Adlay Millet, Job's-Tears, Yi-Yi-Ren - Coix Lacryma-Jobi - E - M	Seed	5,000 ppm
Brigham Tea, Mormon Tea - Ephedra Nevadensis - M	Plant	5,000 ppm
High Mallow - Malva Sylvestris - E - M	Leaf	5,000 ppm
Broadbean, Faba Bean, Habas - Vicia Faba - E	Seed	5,000 ppm
Brussel-Sprout - Brassica Oleracea var. Gemmifera - E	Leaf	4,927 ppm
White Lupine - Lupinus Albus - M - T	Seed	4,900 ppm
Soybean - Glycine Max - E	Sprout Seedling	4,891 ppm
Cheeseweed - Malva Parviflora - E - M	Plant	4,891 ppm
Pigeonpea - Cajanus Vajan - E	Fruit	4,888 ppm
Waxgourd - Benincasa Hispida - Fruit	Fruit	4,870 ppm
Anise, Sweet Cumin - Pimpinella Anisum - E - M	Fruit	4,862 ppm
Asparagus bean, Pea bean, Yardlong bean - Vigna Unguiculata subsp. Sesquipedalis - E	Fruit	4,856 ppm
Chervil - Anthriscus Cerefolium - E	Leaf	4,850 ppm
Butternut - Juglans Cinerea - E	Seed	4,834 ppm
Bonavist Bean, Hyacinth Bean, Lablab Bean - Lablab Purpureus - E - M - T	Seed	4,800 ppm
Susumba, Wild Egg Solanum Torvum - Friut - E	Fruit	4,795 ppm
Water Lotus - Nelumbo Nucifera - E - M	Rhizome	4,785 ppm
Ajwan - Trachyspermum Ammi - E - M	Fruit	4,784 ppm
Hops - Humulus Lupulus - E - M - T	Fruit	4,760 ppm
Spearmint - Mentha Spicata - E - M- T	Plant	4,706 ppm
Cowage, Velvetbean - Mucuna Pruriens - E	Seed	4,700 ppm
Malanga, Tannia, Yautia - Xanthosoma Sagittifolium - E	Root	4,700 ppm
Chinese Parsley, Cilantro, Coriander - Coriandrum Sativum E	Fruit	4,687 ppm
New Zealand Spinach - Tetragonia Tetragonioides - E	Leaf	4,665 ppm
Cobnut, English Filbert, European Filbert, European Hazel, Hazel - Corylus Avellana - E	Seed	4,622 ppm
Black Cherry, Wild Cherry - Prunus Serotina - E - M - T	Leaf	4,608 ppm
Castorbean - Ricinus Communis - T	Leaf	4,600 ppm
Dandelion - Taraxacum Officinale - E - M	Leaf	4,583 ppm
Black Mustard - Brassica Nigra - E	Leaf	4,563 ppm
Elephant Garlic, Kurrat - Allium Ampeloprasum - E	Leaf	4,528 ppm
Cassie, Huisache, Opopanax, Popinac, Sweet Acacia - Acacia Farnesiana - M	Leaf	4,519 ppm
Pigeonpea - Cajanus Vajan - E	Seed	4,500 ppm
White Mulberry - Morus Alba - E - M	Leaf	4,500 ppm
Cowgrass, Peavine Clover, Purple Clover, Red Clover - Trifolium Pratense - E - M	Shoot	4,500 ppm
Green Gram, Mungbean - Vigna Radiata - E	Seed	4,500 ppm
Chickweed, Common Chickweed - Stellaria Media - E	Plant	4,480 ppm
Adzuki Bean - Vigna Angularis - E	Seed	4,402 ppm
African Yam Bean, Yam Pea - Sphenostylis Stenocarpa - Seed	Seed	4,393 ppm
Burdock, Gobo, Great Burdock - Arctium lappa - E - M - T	Root	4,370 ppm
Indian Sorrel, Jamaica Sorrel, Kharkadi, Red Sorrel, Sorrel - Hibiscus Sabdariffa - E	Flower	4,348 ppm
Black Gram - Vigna Mungo - E	Seed	4,321 ppm
Garland Chrysanthemum - Chrysanthemum Coronarium - Bud - E	Bud	4,300 ppm

PHOSPHORUS CONTINUED

Name	Part	ppm
Alholva, Bockshornklee, Fenugreek, Greek Clover, Greek Trigonella Foenum-Graecum - E - M	Seed	4,285 ppm
Chicory, Succory, Witloof - Cichorium Intybus - E - M	Leaf	4,284 ppm
Chickpea, Garbanzo - Cicer Arietinum - E	Seed	4,275 ppm
Chinese Magnolia Vine, Five-Flavor-Fruit, Magnolia Vine, Schizandra, Wu Wei Zi, Wu Wei Zu - Schisandra Chinensis - M	Fruit	4,260 ppm
Groundnut, Peanut - Arachis Hypogaea - E - M	Seed	4,248 ppm
Buckbush - Symphoricarpos Orbiculatus - M	Stem	4,224 ppm
Cape Gooseberry, Ground Cherry - Physalis Peruviana - E	Fruit	4,215 ppm
Potato - Solanum Tuberosum - E	Tuber	4,200 ppm
Lambsquarter - Chenopodium Album - E - M - T	Seed	4,160 ppm
Tea - Camellia Sinensis - E	Leaf	4,150 ppm
Chinese Boxthorn, Chinese Matrimony Vine, Chinese Wolfberry - Lycium Chinense - E - M	Leaf	4,135 ppm
Chaya - Cnidoscolus Chayamansa - E	Leaf	4,100 ppm
White Willow - Salix Alba - M	Bark	4,100 ppm
Plum - Prunus Domestica - E - M	Fruit	4,080 ppm
Corn - Zea Mays - E	Seed	4,066 ppm
Scarlet Runner Bean - Phaseolus Coccineus - E	Seed	4,046 ppm
Onion, Shallot - Allium Cepa - Shallot Bulb - E	Bulb	4,038 ppm
Desert Date, Soapberry Tree - Balanites Aegyptiacus - Seed	Fruit	4,000 ppm
Black Nightshade - Solanum Nigrum - E	Leaf	4,000 ppm
Black bean, Dwarf bean, Field bean, Flageolet bean, French bean, Garden bean, Green bean, Haricot, Haricot bean, Haricot vert, Kidney bean, Navy bean, Pop bean, Popping bean, Snap bean, String bean, Wax bean - Phaseolus Vulgaris - E	Sprout Seedling	3,978 ppm
Garlic - Allium Sativum Bulb - E	Flower	3,966 ppm
Jack Bean - Canavalia Ensiformis - E	Seed	3,898 ppm
Bell Pepper, Cherry Pepper, Cone Pepper, Green Pepper, Paprika, Sweet Pepper - Capsicum Annuum - E	Fruit	3,885 ppm
Dulse - Rhodymenia Palmata - E	Plant	3,860 ppm
Groundnut, Peanut - Arachis Hypogaea - E - M	Leaf	3,814 ppm
Mango - Mangifera Indica - E - M	Leaf	3,800 ppm
Cayenne, Chili, Hot Pepper, Red Chili, Spur Pepper, Tabasco - Capsicum Frutescens - E	Fruit	3,794 ppm
Marjoram, Sweet Marjoram - Origanum Majorana - E	Plant	3,725 ppm
Dill, Garden Dill - Anethum Graveolens - E	Fruit	3,723 ppm
Chayote - Sechium Edule - E - M	Fruit	3,715 ppm
Evening-Primrose - Oenothera Biennis - E - M	Plant	3,700 ppm
Snakegourd - Trichosanthes Anguina - E - M	Fruit	3,700 ppm
Elephant Garlic, Kurrat - Allium Ampeloprasum - E	Root	3,650 ppm
Dandelion - Taraxacum Officinale - E - M	Root	3,620 ppm
Curly Kale, Kale, Kitchen Kale, Scotch Kale - Brassica Oleracea var. Sabellica l. var. Acephala - E	Leaf	3,600 ppm
Epazote, Worm Chenopodium Ambrosioides - E - M - T	Leaf	3,585 ppm
SafCarthamus Tinctorius - M	Seed	3,526 ppm
Jack Bean - Canavalia Ensiformis - E	Fruit	3,509 ppm
Calamansi, Calamondin - Citrus Mitis - Friut - E	Fruit	700-7,000 ppm
Alehoof - Glechoma Hederacea - M	Plant	3,500 ppm
Small-Flowered Melilot - Melilotus Indica - E - M - T	Plant	3,500 ppm
Black Currant - Ribes Nigrum - E	Fruit	3,500 ppm
Achlote, Annato, Annatto, Annoto, Arnato, Bija, Lipstick Pod, Lipsticktree - Bixa Orellana - E	Seed	3,490 ppm
Rice - Oryza Sativa - E	Plant	3,478 ppm
Rhubarb - Rheum Rhabarbarum - E	Leaf	3,472 ppm
Ramie - Boehmeria Nivea - M	Leaf	3,460 ppm
Dwarf Sumac, Winged Sumac - Rhus Copallina - E - M	Leaf	3,456 ppm
Bonavist Bean, Hyacinth Bean, Lablab Bean - Lablab Purpureus - E - M - T	Fruit	3,409 ppm
Umbrella Thorn - Acacia Tortilis - M	Fruit	3,400 ppm
Soursop - Annona Muricata - E	Fruit	3,400 ppm
Gum Ghatti - Anogeissus Latifolia - E - M - M	Leaf	3,400 ppm

SafCarthamus Tinctorius - M	Plant	3,400 ppm
Tamarillo, Tree Tomato - Cyphomandra Betacea - Fruit	Fruit	3,400 ppm
Tarragon - Artemisia Dracunculus - M	Plant	3,391 ppm
Garlic - Allium Sativum Bulb - E	Leaf	3,382 ppm
Chinese Angelica, Dong Gui, Dong Quai - Angelica Sinensis - M	Root	3,340 ppm
Pecan - Carya Illinoensis - E	Seed	3,340 ppm
Red Currant, White Currant - Ribes Rubrum - E	Fruit	3,310 ppm
Ginkgo, Maidenhair Tree - Ginkgo Biloba - Tree - E - M - T	Seed	3,268 ppm
Water Lotus - Nelumbo Nucifera - E - M	Fruit	3,267 ppm
Sassafras - Sassafras Albidum - E - M - T	Stem	3,264 ppm
Salsify - Tragopogon Porrifolius - E	Root	3,262 ppm
Yellow Mombin, Yellow Plum - Spondias Mombin - E	Fruit	3,250 ppm
Garden Camomile, Perennial Camomile, Roman Camomile - Chamaemelum Nobile M	Flower	3,220 ppm
Cowgrass, Peavine Clover, Purple Clover, Red Clover - Trifolium Pratense - E - M	Flower	3,220 ppm
Florida Eryngium - Eryngium Floridanum - M	Shoot	3,215 ppm
Buckwheat - Fagopyrum Esculentum - E	Seed	3,200 ppm
Honey Locust - Gleditsia Triacanthos - M	Seed	3,200 ppm
White Mulberry - Morus Alba - E - M	Fruit	3,200 ppm
Maracuya, Passion Passiflora Edulis - E	Seed	0-6,400 ppm
Black Locust - Robinia Pseudoacacia - T	Leaf	3,200 ppm
Strawberry - Fragaria spp. - E	Fruit	3,191 ppm
Spirulina - Spirulina Pratensis - E	Plant	3,190 ppm
Chufle - Calathea Macrosepala - Flower	Flower	490-6,365 ppm
Pomegranate - Punica Granatum - E	Fruit	3,182 ppm
Indian Sorrel, Jamaica Sorrel, Stevia, Sweet Leaf of Paraguay - Stevia Rebaudiana - E	Leaf	3,180 ppm
Asparagus Pea, Goa Bean, Winged Bean - Psophocarpus Tetragonolobus - E	Leaf	3,175 ppm
Red Cedar - Juniperus Virginiana Amphicarpaea Bracteata- E - M - T	Shoot	3,168 ppm
Mugwort - Artemisia Vulgaris - M	Leaf	3,150 ppm
Peach - Prunus Persica - E - M - T	Bark	3,150 ppm
Giant Taro - Alocasia Macrorrhiza - E	Root	3,125 ppm
Cashew - Anacardium Occidentale - E	Fruit	3,125 ppm
Mexican Pinyon - Pinus Cembroides - M	Seed	5,150-6,235 ppm
Gum Arabic, Gum Arabic Tree, Kher, Senegal Gum, Sudan Gum Arabic - Acacia Senegal - M	Seed	3,100 ppm
Alfalfa, Lucerne - Medicago Sativa subsp. Sativa - E	Plant	3,100 ppm
Qian Hu - Peucedanum Decursivum - M	Plant	3,100 ppm
Kiwi - Actinidia Chinensis - E	Fruit	3,060 ppm
Chicory, Succory, Witloof - Cichorium Intybus - E - M	Root	3,050 ppm
Granadilla, Sweet Granadilla - Passiflora Ligularis - E	Fruit	300-6,095 ppm
Granadilla - Passiflora Quadrangularis - E	Fruit	3,035 ppm
Avocado - Persea Americana - E - M - T	Cr	3,030 ppm
Large-Fruited Provision Tree - Pachira Macrocarpa - E	Seed	3,025 ppm
Elephant-Foot Yam - Amorphophallus Campanulatus - E - M- T	Root	3,020 ppm
Genipap, Jagua - Genipa Americana - E - M	Fruit	3,000 ppm
Apricot - Prunus Armeniaca - E - M - T	Seed	3,000 ppm
Anu, Mashua - Tropaeolum Tuberosum - E	Root	3,000 ppm
Two-Flowered Sandspur - Cenchrus Biflorus - E	Seed	2,990 ppm
Apricot - Prunus Armeniaca - E - M - T	Fruit	2,982 ppm
American Styrax, Sweetgum - Liquidambar Styraciflua - E - M	Leaf	2,952 ppm
Milfoil, Yarrow - Achillea Millefolium - M	Plant	2,950 ppm
Broomweed, Tea Sida Rhombifolia - M	Leaf	2,930 ppm
Cordoncillo, Hierba Santa, Hoja Santa - Piper Auritum - E - M	Leaf	2,920 ppm
Calabash Gourd, White-Flowered Gourd - Lagenaria Siceraria - E	Fruit	2,915 ppm
Watermelon - Citrullus Lanatus - E	Fruit	2,900 ppm
American Styrax, Sweetgum - Liquidambar Styraciflua - E - M	Stem	2,880 ppm
Nicaraguan Cacao, Pataste - Theobroma Bicolor - E	Seed	5,490-5,695 ppm

PHOSPHORUS CONTINUED

Name	Part	ppm
Gotu Kola, Pennywort - Centella Asiatica - E - M	Leaf	2,804 ppm
Cassava, Tapioca, Yuca - Manihot Esculenta - E	Leaf	2,800 ppm
Guinea Grass - Panicum Maximum - M	Leaf	0-5,600 ppm
Giant Knotweed, Hu-Zhang, Japanese Knotweed, Mexican Bamboo - Polygonum Cuspidatum - E - M - T	Plant	2,800 ppm
Aubergine, Egg Solanum Melongena - E	Leaf	2,794 ppm
Melloco, Ulluco - Ullucus Tuberosus - E	Root	2,775 ppm
Scarlet Runner Bean - Phaseolus Coccineus - E	Fruit	2,770 ppm
Fig - Ficus Carica - E	Fruit	2,764 ppm
Betel Pepper - Piper Betel - E - M	Leaf	2,740 ppm
Japanese Pagoda Tree - Sophora Japonica - M - T	Seed	2,723 ppm
Italian Stone Pine, Pignolia - Pinus Pinea - M	Seed	5,080-5,445 ppm
Cassie, Huisache, Opopanax, Popinac, Sweet Acacia - Acacia Farnesiana - M	Seed	2,700 ppm
Blessed Thistle - Cnicus Benedictus - M	Plant	2,700 ppm
Gentian, Yellow Gentian - Gentiana Lutea - M	Root	2,700 ppm
Bread Artocarpus Altilis - E	Seed	1,750-5,385 ppm
Devil's Tongue, Elephant Yam, Konjac, Leopard Palm, Snake Palm, Umbrella Arum - Amorphophallus Konjac - E - M - T	Leaf	2,692 ppm
Jack Artocarpus Heterophyllus - E	Seed	2,685 ppm
Loquat - Eriobotrya Japonica - E	Fruit	2,667 ppm
Gooseberry - Ribes Uva-Crispa - E	Fruit	2,665 ppm
Mata Raton - Gliricidia Sepium - M	Flower	2,645 ppm
Red Pignut Hickory - Carya Glabra - E	Shoot	2,640 ppm
Cantaloupe, Melon, Muskmelon, Netted Melon, Nutmeg Melon, Persian Melon - Cucumis Melo subsp. ssp Melo var.Ccantalupensis - Friut - E	Fruit	2,640 ppm
Collards, Cow Cabbage, Spring-Heading Cabbage, Tall Kale, Tree Kale - Brassica Oleracea - E	Leaf	2,622 ppm
Radish - Raphanus Sativus - E	Leaf	2,609 ppm
Squaw Perideridia Gairdneri - E - M	Root	2,600 ppm
Genet, Spanish Broom, Weaver's Broom - Spartium Junceum - Stem	Stem	2,600 ppm
American Persimmon - Diospyros Virginiana - E - M	Stem	2,592 ppm
Black Cherry, Wild Cherry - Prunus Serotina - E - M - T	Stem	2,592 ppm
Marshmallow, White Mallow - Althaea Officinalis - M	Root	2,560 ppm
Grape Citrus Paradisi - E	Fruit	2,545 ppm
European Pennyroyal - Mentha pulegium - E - M- T	Plant	2,520 ppm
Common thyme, Garden thyme, Thyme - Thymus Vulgaris - E - M	Plant	2,502 ppm
Cloudberry - Rubus Chamaemorus - E - M	Fruit	2,500 ppm
Mat Bean, Moth Bean - Vigna Aconitifolia - E	Fruit	2,500 ppm
Balloon Flower, Chieh-Keng, Jie-Geng - Platycodon Grandiflorum - E - M - T	Root	2,493 ppm
Bladderwrack, Kelp - Fucus Vesiculosus - E - M	Plant	2,490 ppm
Akee, Seso Vegetal - Blighia Sapida - M	Seed	2,455 ppm
Indian Gooseberry, Otaheite Gooseberry - Phyllanthus Acidus - E	Fruit	2,442 ppm
Kudsu, Kudzu - Pueraria Montana subsp. var. Lobata - E - M	Shoot	2,440 ppm
White Oak - Quercus Alba - M	Stem	2,432 ppm
Smooth Sumac - Rhus Glabra - E - M	Stem	2,412 ppm
Catnip - Nepeta Cataria - M	Plant	2,410 ppm
Common Turkish Oregano, European Oregano, Oregano, Pot Marjoram, Wild Marjoram, Wild Oregano - Origanum Vulgare - E	Plant	2,402 ppm
Neem - Azadirachta Indica - M	Fruit	2,400 ppm
Ramie - Boehmeria Nivea - M	Shoot	2,400 ppm
Pigeonpea - Cajanus Vajan - E	Plant	2,400 ppm
Pyrethrum - Chrysanthemum Cinerariifolium - M	Shoot	2,400 ppm
Coconut, Coconut Palm - Cocos Nucifera - E	Seed	2,400 ppm
Banana, Plantain - Musa x Paradisiaca - E	Leaf	2,400 ppm
Mace, Nutmeg - Myristica Fragrans - E	Seed	2,400 ppm
Burn Mouth Vine - Rhynchosia Minima - M- T	Shoot	2,400 ppm
Stillingia sylvatica GARDEN EX L. -- Queen's-Delight, Queen's-Root, Stillingia, Yawroot	Plant	2,400 ppm

Species	Part	Quantity
European Mistletoe - Viscum Album - M - T	Leaf	2,400 ppm
SafCarthamus Tinctorius - M	Flower	2,370 ppm
Indian Tamarind, Kilytree, Tamarind - Tamarindus Indica - M	Seed	2,370 ppm
Raspberry, Red raspberry - Rubus Idaeus - E - M	Leaf	2,340 ppm
Angel Of Death, Bolek Hena, Curia - Justicia Pectoralis - M	Leaf	2,335 ppm
Garlic - Allium Sativum Bulb - E	Shoot	2,332 ppm
Strawberry Guava - Psidium Cattleianum - E	Fruit	2,305 ppm
Sour Cherry - Prunus Cerasus - E - M - T	Fruit	2,302 ppm
Spiny Pigweed - Amaranthus Spinosus - E - M	Leaf	500-4,600 ppm
Akee, Seso Vegetal - Blighia Sapida - M	Aril	2,300 ppm
Chinaberry - Melia Azedarach - T	Leaf	2,300 ppm
Da-Zao, Jujube, Ta-Tsao - Zizyphus Jujuba - E - M	Shoot	2,300 ppm
Indian Tamarind, Kilytree, Tamarind - Tamarindus Indica - M	Leaf	2,281 ppm
Pawpaw - Asimina Triloba - Friut - E	Fruit	2,265 ppm
Elephant Garlic, Kurrat - Allium Ampeloprasum - E	Flower	2,249 ppm
Cassava, Tapioca, Yuca - Manihot Esculenta - E	Root	2,225 ppm
Erythrina fusca LOUR. -- Coral Bean, Gallito	Leaf	2,220 ppm
Mata Raton - Gliricidia Sepium - M	Leaf	2,220 ppm
Mesquite - Prosopis Juliflora - M	Leaf	2,200 ppm
Indian Tamarind, Kilytree, Tamarind - Tamarindus Indica - M	Flower	2,200 ppm
Greater Yam, Winged Yam - Dioscorea Alata - E	Root	2,190 ppm
Black Gum, Black Tupelo - Nyssa Sylvatica - E - M	Leaf	2,184 ppm

PLANTS CONTAINING POTASSIUM

Species	Part	Quantity
Lettuce - Lactuca Sativa - E	Leaf	121,800 ppm
Endive, Escarole - Cichorium Endivia - M	Leaf	96,000 ppm
Black Gram - Vigna Mungo - E	Seed	89,790 ppm
Lambsquarter - Chenopodium Album - E - M - T	Leaf	87,100 ppm
Radish - Raphanus Sativus - E	Root	85,700 ppm
Chinese Cabbage - Brassica Pekinensis - E	Leaf	81,900 ppm
Purslane, Verdolaga - Portulaca Oleracea - E	Herb	81,200 ppm
Oats - Avena Sativa - E - M	Plant	78,900 ppm
Garland Chrysanthemum - Chrysanthemum Coronarium - Bud - E	Bud	76,745 ppm
Dill, Garden Dill - Anethum Graveolens - E	Plant	76,450 ppm
Dandelion - Taraxacum Officinale - E - M	Root	75,000 ppm
Pigweed - Amaranthus sp. - E - M	Leaf	73,503 ppm
Cucumber - Cucumis Sativus - E	Fruit	72,500 ppm
Bok-Choy, Celery Cabbage, Celery Mustard, Chinese Cabbage, Chinese Mustard, Chinese White Cabbage, Pak-Choi - Brassica Chinensis - E	Leaf	69,143 ppm
Spinach - Spinacia Oleracea - E	Plant	69,077 ppm
Beebread, Beeplant, Borage, Talewort - Borago Officinalis - E - M - T	Leaf	67,210 ppm
Rhubarb - Rheum Rhabarbarum - E	Pt	66,400 ppm
Berro, Watercress - Nasturtium Officinale - E	Herb	66,000 ppm
Udo - Aralia Cordata - E - M	Leaf	65,950 ppm
Beet, Beetroot, Garden Beet, Sugar Beet - Beta Vulgaris - E	Leaf	61,798 ppm
Tomato - Lycopersicon Esculentum - E - M - T	Fruit	58,800 ppm
Black bean, Dwarf bean, Field bean, Flageolet bean, French bean, Garden bean, Green bean, Haricot, Haricot bean, Haricot vert, Kidney bean, Navy bean, Pop bean, Popping bean, Snap bean, String bean, Wax bean - Phaseolus Vulgaris - E	Fruit	58,500 ppm
Celery - Apium Graveolens - E	Pt	57,800 ppm
Garden Cress - Lepidium Sativum - E	Leaf	57,170 ppm
Celery - Apium Graveolens - E	Root	56,360 ppm
Asparagus - Asparagus Officinalis - E	Shoot	55,200 ppm
Dokudami, Fishwort, Yu Xing Cao - Houttuynia Cordata - E - M	Plant	54,300 ppm
Parsley - Petroselinum Crispum - E	Plant	53,833 ppm
Taro - Colocasia Esculenta - E	Leaf	51,774 ppm
Chervil - Anthriscus Cerefolium - E	Leaf	51,200 ppm

POTASSIUM CONTINUED

Beet, Beetroot, Garden Beet, Sugar Beet - Beta Vulgaris - E	Root	50,000 ppm
Chinese Boxthorn, Chinese Matrimony Vine, Chinese Wolfberry - Lycium Chinense - E - M	Leaf	49,808 ppm
Swamp Cabbage, Water Spinach - Ipomoea Aquatica - E	Leaf	49,200 ppm
Cauli Brassica Oleracea var. Botrytis - E	Flower	49,080 ppm
Chinese Parsley, Cilantro, Coriander - Coriandrum Sativum E	Leaf	48,177 ppm
Tomato - Lycopersicon Esculentum - E - M - T	Leaf	47,000 ppm
Perilla - Perilla Frutescens - E - M - T	Leaf	46,429 ppm
Carrot - Daucus Carota - E	Root	46,360 ppm
Alehoof - Glechoma Hederacea - M	Plant	46,000 ppm
Jew's Mallow, Mulukiya, Nalta Jute - Corchorus Olitorius - E - M	Leaf	45,500 ppm
Bitter Melon, Sorosi - Momordica Charantia - E	Fruit	45,000 ppm
Asparagus bean, Pea bean, Yardlong bean - Vigna Unguiculata subsp. Sesquipedalis - E	Shoot	44,520 ppm
Plum - Prunus Domestica - E - M	Fruit	44,200 ppm
Cantaloupe, Melon, Muskmelon, Netted Melon, Nutmeg Melon, Persian Melon - Cucumis Melo subsp. ssp Melo var.Ccantalupensis - Friut - E	Fruit	44,000 ppm
Barley, Barleygrass - Hordeum Vulgare - E - M	Plant	44,000 ppm
Rutabaga, Swede, Swedish Turnip - Brassica Napus var. Napobrassica - E	Root	43,850 ppm
Wheat - Triticum Aestivum - E - M	Plant	43,500 ppm
Radish - Raphanus Sativus - E	Leaf	43,478 ppm
Basil, Cuban Basil, Sweet Basil - Ocimum Basilicum - E	Leaf	42,900 ppm
Cabbage, Red Cabbage, White Cabbage - Brassica Oleracea var. Capitata - E	Leaf	42,500 ppm
Sweet Potato - Ipomoea Batatas - E	Leaf	42,256 ppm
Butterbur - Petasites Japonicus - T	Plant	42,000 ppm
Chayote - Sechium Edule - E - M	Shoot	41,890 ppm
Indian Saffron, Turmeric - Curcuma Longa - E	Rhizome	41,271 ppm
Mugwort - Artemisia Vulgaris - M	Plant	41,000 ppm
Pumpkin - Cucurbita Pepo - E	Fruit	40,476 ppm
Parsnip - Pastinaca Sativa - E	Root	40,000 ppm
Garden Sorrel - Rumex Acetosa - E - M - T	Leaf	40,000 ppm
Fennel - Foeniculum Vulgare - M	Plant	39,700 ppm
Jerusalem Artichoke - Helianthus Tuberosus E	Tuber	39,700 ppm
Garland Chrysanthemum - Chrysanthemum Coronarium - Bud - E	Leaf	39,385 ppm
Malanga, Tannia, Yautia - Xanthosoma Sagittifolium - E	Root	39,100 ppm
Butter Bean, Lima Bean - Phaseolus Lunatus - E	Seed	39,000 ppm
Kohlrabi - Brassica Oleracea var. Gongylodes - E	Stem	38,890 ppm
Gotu Kola, Pennywort - Centella Asiatica - E - M	Leaf	38,693 ppm
Cherimoya - Annona Cherimola - E	Seed	38,000 ppm
Cauli Brassica Oleracea var. Botrytis - E	Leaf	37,270 ppm
European Nettle, Stinging Nettle - Urtica Dioica - E - M	Leaf	37,220 ppm
Chicory, Succory, Witloof - Cichorium Intybus - E - M	Leaf	37,128 ppm
Tomatillo - Physalis Ixocarpa - E	Fruit	36,250 ppm
Kudsu, Kudzu - Pueraria Montana subsp. var. Lobata - E - M	Shoot	36,050 ppm
Soursop - Annona Muricata - E	Fruit	36,000 ppm
Scarlet Runner Bean - Phaseolus Coccineus - E	Seed	35,807 ppm
Pumpkin - Cucurbita Pepo - E	Flower	35,670 ppm
Cornmint, Field Mint, Japanese Mint - Mentha Arvensis var. Piperascens - E - M- T	Plant	35,100 ppm
Evening-Primrose - Oenothera Biennis - E - M	Herb	35,100 ppm
Bell Pepper, Cherry Pepper, Cone Pepper, Green Pepper, Paprika, Sweet Pepper - Capsicum Annuum - E	Fruit	35,000 ppm
Water Lotus - Nelumbo Nucifera - E - M	Rhizome	34,925 ppm
Cayenne, Chili, Hot Pepper, Red Chili, Spur Pepper, Tabasco - Capsicum Frutescens - E	Fruit	34,272 ppm
American Ginseng, Ginseng - Panax Quinquefolius - M	Plant	33,800 ppm
Purple Tephrosia, Wild Indigo - Tephrosia Purpurea - M - T	Leaf	33,800 ppm

Name	Part	ppm
Calabash Gourd, White-Flowered Gourd - Lagenaria Siceraria - E	Fruit	33,635 ppm
American Styrax, Sweetgum - Liquidambar Styraciflua - E - M	Stem	33,600 ppm
Shepherd's Purse - Capsella Bursa-Pastoris - E - M	Plant	33,390 ppm
Bitter Melon, Sorosi - Momordica Charantia - E	Leaf	33,117 ppm
Tarragon - Artemisia Dracunculus - M	Plant	32,719 ppm
Okra - Abelmoschus Esculentus - Friut - E - M	Fruit	32,500 ppm
Aubergine, Egg Solanum Melongena - E	Fruit	32,000 ppm
Chives - Allium Schoenoprasum - E	Leaf	31,250 ppm
Horseradish - Armoracia Rusticana - E	Root	31,150 ppm
Summer Squash - Cucurbita spp. - E	Fruit	30,855 ppm
Curly Kale, Kale, Kitchen Kale, Scotch Kale - Brassica Oleracea var. Sabellica l. var. Acephala - E	Leaf	30,000 ppm
Rapini, Seven-Top Turnip, Turnip - Brassica Rapa - E	Root	30,000 ppm
Potato - Solanum Tuberosum - E	Tuber	30,000 ppm
Elephant Garlic, Kurrat - Allium Ampeloprasum - E	Leaf	29,811 ppm
Artichoke - Cynara Cardunculus - E	Flower	29,780 ppm
Dwarf Sumac, Winged Sumac - Rhus Copallina - E - M	Leaf	29,760 ppm
Qian Hu - Peucedanum Decursivum - M	Plant	29,600 ppm
Brussel-Sprout - Brassica Oleracea var. Gemmifera - E	Leaf	29,343 ppm
Papaya - Carica Papaya - E - M	Leaf	28,978 ppm
Waxgourd - Benincasa Hispida - Fruit	Fruit	28,450 ppm
Black Mustard - Brassica Nigra - E	Leaf	28,215 ppm
Bastard Cardamom, Chin Kousha, Malabar Cardamom, Tavoy Cardamom - Amomum Xanthioides - E	Seed	28,100 ppm
Elephant-Foot Yam - Amorphophallus Campanulatus - E - M- T	Root	28,020 ppm
Luffa, Smooth Loofah, Vegetable Sponge - Luffa Aegyptiaca - E	Fruit	27,800 ppm
Loquat - Eriobotrya Japonica - E	Fruit	27,632 ppm
Soybean - Glycine Max - E	Seed	27,600 ppm
Dandelion - Taraxacum Officinale - E - M	Leaf	27,569 ppm
Avocado - Persea Americana - E - M - T	Fruit	27,470 ppm
Black Cherry, Wild Cherry - Prunus Serotina - E - M - T	Leaf	26,880 ppm
Cowgrass, Peavine Clover, Purple Clover, Red Clover - Trifolium Pratense - E - M	Shoot	26,700 ppm
Bai Zhi - Angelica Dahurica - M	Root	26,600 ppm
Perilla - Perilla Frutescens - E - M - T	Plant	26,100 ppm
Blessed Thistle - Cnicus Benedictus - M	Plant	26,000 ppm
Giant Reed - Arundo Donax - Plant	Plant	25,500 ppm
Black Gum, Black Tupelo - Nyssa Sylvatica - E - M	Leaf	25,480 ppm
Papaya - Carica Papaya - E - M	Fruit	25,469 ppm
Mountain Yam - Dioscorea Pentaphylla - E	Root	25,350 ppm
Pea - Pisum Sativum - E	Plant	25,200 ppm
Ginger - Zingiber Officinale - E	Rhizome	25,079 ppm
Barley, Barleygrass - Hordeum Vulgare - E - M	Stem	25,000 ppm
Sage - Salvia Officinalis - E - M	Leaf	24,700 ppm
European Grape, Grape, Grapevine, Vigne Vinifere, Wine Grape - Vitis Vinifera - E - M	Fruit	24,640 ppm
Corn Salad, Lamb's Lettuce - Valerianella Locusta - E	Plant	4,573-48,864 ppm
Acerola - Malpighia Glabra - E - M	Fruit	24,345 ppm
Cassava, Tapioca, Yuca - Manihot Esculenta - E	Root	24,260 ppm
Collards, Cow Cabbage, Spring-Heading Cabbage, Tall Kale, Tree Kale - Brassica Oleracea - E	Leaf	24,257 ppm
Garlic - Allium Sativum Bulb - E	Leaf	23,971 ppm
Catnip - Nepeta Cataria - M	Plant	23,500 ppm
Lemongrass, West indian lemongrass - Cymbopogon Citratus - E - M	Plant	23,000 ppm
Genipap, Jagua - Genipa Americana - E - M	Fruit	22,900 ppm
Custard Apple - Annona Reticulata - E	Fruit	22,810 ppm
Mongoloid Dandelion - Taraxacum Mongolicum - E - M	Plant	22,800 ppm
Pea - Pisum Sativum - E	Fruit	22,737 ppm
Dulse - Rhodymenia Palmata - E	Plant	22,700 ppm
Peppermint - Mentha x Piperita subsp. Nothosubsp. Piperita - E - M - T	Leaf	22,600 ppm
Apricot - Prunus Armeniaca - E - M - T	Fruit	22,565 ppm
Feverfew - Chrysanthemum Parthenium - M	Plant	22,500 ppm

POTASSIUM CONTINUED

Strawberry - Fragaria spp. - E	Leaf	22,500 ppm
SafCarthamus Tinctorius - M	Flower	22,400 ppm
Dan Zhu Ye - Lophatherum Gracile - M	Plant	22,400 ppm
Equatorial Ivory Palm - Phytelephas Aequatorialis - E	Mesocarp	2,510-44,590 ppm
Asparagus bean, Pea bean, Yardlong bean - Vigna Unguiculata subsp. Sesquipedalis - E	Fruit	22,212 ppm
Onion, Shallot - Allium Cepa - Shallot Bulb - E	Bulb	22,164 ppm
Peach - Prunus Persica - E - M - T	Fruit	22,072 ppm
Capillary Wormwood - Artemisia Capillaris - M	Plant	22,000 ppm
Mugwort - Artemisia Vulgaris - M	Shoot	22,000 ppm
Giant Knotweed, Hu-Zhang, Japanese Knotweed, Mexican Bamboo - Polygonum Cuspidatum - E - M - T	Plant	22,000 ppm
Mad-Dog Skullcap, Scullcap - Scutellaria lateriflora - M	Plant	21,800 ppm
Taro - Colocasia Esculenta - E	Root	21,760 ppm
Sassafras - Sassafras Albidum - E - M - T	Leaf	21,760 ppm
New Zealand Spinach - Tetragonia Tetragonioides - E	Leaf	21,665 ppm
Guavas - Psidium Guajava - E	Fruit	21,658 ppm
Coca - Erythroxylum Coca var. Coca - E - M	Leaf	21,600 ppm
Chinese Rhubarb - Rheum Palmatum - E	Rhizome	21,600 ppm
Chinese Birthwort - Aristolochia Debilis - E - M - T	Fruit	21,500 ppm
Chayote - Sechium Edule - E - M	Fruit	21,430 ppm
Red Currant, White Currant - Ribes Rubrum - E	Fruit	21,250 ppm
Black Currant - Ribes Nigrum - E	Fruit	21,110 ppm
Bladderwrack, Kelp - Fucus Vesiculosus - E - M	Plant	21,100 ppm
Black bean, Dwarf bean, Field bean, Flageolet bean, French bean, Garden bean, Green bean, Haricot, Haricot bean, Haricot vert, Kidney bean, Navy bean, Pop bean, Popping bean, Snap bean, String bean, Wax bean - Phaseolus Vulgaris - E	Seed	21,070 ppm
Dog Rose, Dogbrier, Rose - Rosa Canina - E - M	Fruit	21,000 ppm
Cumin - Cuminum Cyminum - E - M	Fruit	20,916 ppm
Gooseberry - Ribes Uva-Crispa - E	Fruit	20,830 ppm
Bonavist Bean, Hyacinth Bean, Lablab Bean - Lablab Purpureus - E - M - T	Seed	20,775 ppm
Dwarf Sumac, Winged Sumac - Rhus Copallina - E - M	Stem	20,740 ppm
Ambarella - Spondias Dulcis - E	Fruit	20,700 ppm
Cockscomb - Celosia Cristata - M	Flower	20,600 ppm
Radish - Raphanus Sativus - E	Fruit	20,495 ppm
Hsi Chien, Saint Paul'Swort - Siegesbeckia Orientalis - M	Plant	20,400 ppm
Hops - Humulus Lupulus - E - M - T	Fruit	20,350 ppm
Tu Huo - Angelica Laxiflora - M	Root	20,300 ppm
Alfalfa, Lucerne - Medicago Sativa subsp. Sativa - E	Plant	20,300 ppm
Black bean, Dwarf bean, Field bean, Flageolet bean, French bean, Garden bean, Green bean, Haricot, Haricot bean, Haricot vert, Kidney bean, Navy bean, Pop bean, Popping bean, Snap bean, String bean, Wax bean - Phaseolus Vulgaris - E	Sprout Seedling	20,108 ppm
Japanese Honeysuckle - Lonicera Japonica - M	Flower	20,100 ppm
European Grape, Grape, Grapevine, Vigne Vinifere, Wine Grape - Vitis Vinifera - E - M	Stem	20,100 ppm
Chaff Achyranthes Bidentata - M	Root	20,000 ppm
Chinese Polystichum - Polystichum Polyblepharum - T	Plant	20,000 ppm
Cowgrass, Peavine Clover, Purple Clover, Red Clover - Trifolium Pratense - E - M	Flower	20,000 ppm
Rangoon Creeper - Quisqualis Indica - E - T	Fruit	19,900 ppm
Kiwi - Actinidia Chinensis - E	Fruit	19,600 ppm
Asian Plantain - Plantago Asiatica - E - M	Plant	19,600 ppm
Ben Nut, Benzolive Tree, Drumstick Tree, Horseradish Tree, Moringa, West Indian Ben - Moringa Oleifera - E	Fruit	4,610-39,065 ppm
Chinese Dogwood - Cornus Officinalis - E - M	Fruit	19,500 ppm
Fennel - Foeniculum Vulgare - M	Fruit	19,400 ppm
Peach - Prunus Persica - E - M - T	Bark	19,400 ppm
Buckbush - Symphoricarpos Orbiculatus - M	Stem	19,360 ppm

Sour Cherry - Prunus Cerasus - E - M - T	Fruit	19,277 ppm
Chai-Hu - Bupleurum - M	Root	19,200 ppm
Jussiaeae Herba, Pond Dragon - Jussiaea Repens - M	Plant	19,200 ppm
Pomegranate - Punica Granatum - E	Fruit	18,950 ppm
Asparagus Pea, Goa Bean, Winged Bean - Psophocarpus Tetragonolobus - E	Seed	18,873 ppm
American Styrax, Sweetgum - Liquidambar Styraciflua - E - M	Leaf	18,860 ppm
Cape Gooseberry, Ground Cherry - Physalis Peruviana - E	Fruit	18,710 ppm
Red Pignut Hickory - Carya Glabra - E	Shoot	18,700 ppm
Common Turkish Oregano, European Oregano, Oregano, Pot Marjoram, Wild Marjoram, Wild Oregano - Origanum Vulgare - E	Plant	18,647 ppm
Sheng Ma - Cimicifuga Dahurica - M	Rhizome	18,600 ppm
Chickweed, Common Chickweed - Stellaria Media - E	Plant	18,400 ppm
Perejil - Peperomia Pereskiifolia - Leaf	Leaf	5,480-36,535 ppm
Asian Wild Ginger - Asiasarum Heterotropoides - M	Root	18,200 ppm
Siebold's Wild Ginger - Asiasarum Sieboldii - M	Root	18,200 ppm
Coltsfoot - Tussilago Farfara - M - T	Flower	18,200 ppm
Pigeonpea - Cajanus Vajan - E	Seed	18,103 ppm
Green Gram, Mungbean - Vigna Radiata - E	Sprout Seedling	18,092 ppm
Watermelon - Citrullus Lanatus - E	Fruit	18,000 ppm
Field Horsetail, Horsetail - Equisetum Arvense - M	Plant	18,000 ppm
Antler Herb, Clubmoss - Lycopodium Clavatum - M - T	Plant	18,000 ppm
Milfoil, Yarrow - Achillea Millefolium - M	Plant	17,800 ppm
Indian Sorrel, Jamaica Sorrel, Stevia, Sweet Leaf of Paraguay - Stevia Rebaudiana - E	Leaf	17,800 ppm
Pepper Elder, Yerba De La Plata - Peperomia Pelucida - Leaf	Leaf	2,770-35,510 ppm
Spiny Pigweed - Amaranthus Spinosus - E - M	Leaf	3,370-35,276 ppm
Tea - Camellia Sinensis - E	Plant	17,600 ppm
Groundnut, Peanut - Arachis Hypogaea - E - M	Plant	17,500 ppm
Pigeonpea - Cajanus Vajan - E	Fruit	17,472 ppm
Flax, Lin Linum Usitatissimum - E	Hay	17,400 ppm
Chinese Magnolia Vine, Five-Flavor-Fruit, Magnolia Vine, Schizandra, Wu Wei Zi, Wu Wei Zu - Schisandra Chinensis - M	Fruit	17,400 ppm
Marjoram, Sweet Marjoram - Origanum Majorana - E	Plant	17,225 ppm
Broomrape, Cistanchis Herba, Jou Tsung Jung - Cistanche Salsa - M	Plant	17,100 ppm
Applemint - Mentha x Rotundifolia - E - M - T	Leaf	17,100 ppm
Salsify - Tragopogon Porrifolius - E	Root	16,964 ppm
Fortune's Fern - Drynaria Fortunei - M	Rhizome	16,900 ppm
Chinese Angelica, Dong Gui, Dong Quai - Angelica Sinensis - M	Root	16,800 ppm
Burdock, Gobo, Great Burdock - Arctium lappa - E - M - T	Root	16,800 ppm
Japanese Privet, Ligustri Fructus - Ligustrum Japonicum - M	Fruit	16,800 ppm
Chinese Privet, Glossy Privet, Ligustri Fructus, Privet, White Waxtree - Ligustrum Lucidum - M	Fruit	16,800 ppm
Bread Artocarpus Altilis - E	Fruit	16,700 ppm
Chinese Boxthorn, Chinese Matrimony Vine, Chinese Wolfberry - Lycium Chinense - E - M	Fruit	16,700 ppm
Imbu, Umbu - Spondias Tuberosa - E	Fruit	16,700 ppm
Water Lotus - Nelumbo Nucifera - E - M	Seed	16,652 ppm
Jack Bean - Canavalia Ensiformis - E	Seed	16,600 ppm
Grape Citrus Paradisi - E	Fruit	16,360 ppm
Dyer's Woad - Isatis Tinctoria - M	Root	16,300 ppm
American Persimmon - Diospyros Virginiana - E - M	Stem	16,200 ppm
Clove, Clovetree - Syzygium Aromaticum - E	Flower	16,200 ppm
Banana, Plantain - Musa x Paradisiaca - E	Fruit	16,150 ppm
Yambean - Pachyrhizus Erosus - E	Tuber	16,130 ppm
Calamus, Flagroot, Myrtle Flag, Sweet Calamus, Sweetflag, Sweet Acorus Calamus - M	Rhizome	16,000 ppm
American Persimmon - Diospyros Virginiana - E - M	Leaf	16,000 ppm
Anise, Sweet Cumin - Pimpinella Anisum - E - M	Fruit	15,923 ppm

POTASSIUM CONTINUED

Comfrey - Symphytum Officinale - E - M - T	Root	15,900 ppm
Indian Gooseberry, Otaheite Gooseberry - Phyllanthus Acidus - E	Fruit	15,895 ppm
Strawberry Guava - Psidium Cattleianum - E	Fruit	15,880 ppm
Pea - Pisum Sativum - E	Seed	15,830 ppm
Sweet Potato - Ipomoea Batatas - E	Root	15,740 ppm
Pawpaw - Asimina Triloba - Friut - E	Fruit	15,726 ppm
Caraway, Carum - Carum Carvi - E	Fruit	15,665 ppm
Curry Murraya spp. - E - M	Fruit	15,612 ppm
Cassia, Cassia Bark, Cassia Lignea, China Junk Cassia, Chinazimt, Chinese Cassia - Cinnamomum Aromaticuminnamon- E - M - T	Bark	15,500 ppm
Citron - Citrus Medica - E	Fruit	15,500 ppm
Loquat - Eriobotrya Japonica - E	Leaf	15,500 ppm
Indian Tamarind, Kilytree, Tamarind - Tamarindus Indica - M	Fruit	15,415 ppm
Celery - Apium Graveolens - E	Seed	15,330 ppm
European Pennyroyal - Mentha pulegium - E - M- T	Plant	15,310 ppm
Wu Chia Pi - Acanthopanax Gracilistylis - M	Root Bark	15,300 ppm
Cape Jasmine, Gardenia, Jasmin, Shan-Chih-Tzu, Shan-Zhi-Zi, Zhi Zi - Gardenia Jasminoides - M	Fruit	15,300 ppm
Jack Artocarpus Heterophyllus - E	Fruit	15,125 ppm
Black Cherry, Wild Cherry - Prunus Serotina - E - M - T	Stem	15,120 ppm
Soybean - Glycine Max - E	Sprout Seedling	15,081 ppm
Black Pepper, Pepper, White Pepper - Piper Nigrum - E - M	Fruit	15,077 ppm
Greater Yam, Winged Yam - Dioscorea Alata - E	Root	15,040 ppm
Ajwan - Trachyspermum Ammi - E - M	Fruit	15,011 ppm
Flax, Lin Linum Usitatissimum - E	Seed	15,009 ppm
Horsetail, Scouring Rush - Equisetum Hyemale - M	Plant	14,900 ppm
Gennoshiouko, Oriental Geranium - Geranium Thunbergii - E - M	Plant	14,900 ppm
Black Walnut - Juglans Nigra - E	Hull Husk	14,900 ppm
Chinese Parsley, Cilantro, Coriander - Coriandrum Sativum E	Fruit	14,781 ppm
Smooth Sumac - Rhus Glabra - E - M	Stem	14,740 ppm
Lemon - Citrus Limon - E	Fruit	14,700 ppm
Wou Chou Yu - Euodia Rutaecarpa - E	Fruit	14,600 ppm
Guinea Grass - Panicum Maximum - M	Leaf	5,900-29,200 ppm
Chicory, Succory, Witloof - Cichorium Intybus - E - M	Root	14,500 ppm
Chinese Parasol - Firmiana Simplex - E - M	Seed	14,500 ppm
Hsuan-Shen, Yuan-Shen - Scrophularia Buergeriana - M	Root	14,500 ppm
Adzuki Bean - Vigna Angularis - E	Seed	14,487 ppm
Shagbark Hickory - Carya Ovata - E	Shoot	14,400 ppm
American Elder, American Elderberry, Elderberry, Sweet Elder - Sambucus Canadensis - E	Fruit	14,356 ppm
Mat Bean, Moth Bean - Vigna Aconitifolia - E	Seed	14,230 ppm
Chinese Anemone - Pulsatilla Chinensis - M	Root	14,200 ppm
Puncture-Vine - Tribulus Terrestris - Leaf	Leaf	0-28,400 ppm
Green Gram, Mungbean - Vigna Radiata - E	Seed	14,170 ppm
Dill, Garden Dill - Anethum Graveolens - E	Fruit	14,122 ppm
Red Cedar - Juniperus Virginiana Amphicarpaea Bracteata- E - M - T	Shoot	14,080 ppm
Emblic, Myrobalan - Phyllanthus Emblica - E	Fruit	13,960 ppm
Bei Sha Shen - Glehnia Littoralis - E - M	Root	13,900 ppm
Bitter Orange, Petitgrain - Citrus Aurantium - E	Fruit	13,800 ppm
Orange - Citrus Sinensis - E	Fruit	13,772 ppm
Chaparral, Creosote Bush - Larrea Tridentata - M	Plant	13,700 ppm
Garlic - Allium Sativum Bulb - E	Bulb	13,669 ppm
Raspberry, Red raspberry - Rubus Idaeus - E - M	Leaf	13,400 ppm
Irish moss - Chondrus Crispus - E	Plant	13,310 ppm
Ma-Huang - Ephedra spp. - M	Plant	13,300 ppm
Sugar-Apple, Sweetsop - Annona Squamosa - E	Fruit	13,290 ppm
Chinese Quince, Mu-Kua - Chaenomeles Lagenaria - E	Fruit	13,200 ppm
Garden Camomile, Perennial Camomile, Roman Camomile - Chamaemelum Nobile M	Flower	13,200 ppm
Bai-Wei, Pai-Wei - Cynanchum Atratum - E - M	Root	13,200 ppm
Chinese Ephedra, Ma Huang - Ephedra Sinica - M	Plant	13,200 ppm
Flannelleaf, Flannelplant, Great mullein, Mullein, Velvet Verbascum Thapsus - M	Leaf	13,200 ppm

Name	Part	ppm
Broadbean, Faba Bean, Habas - Vicia Faba - E	Seed	13,160 ppm
Mandarin, Tangerine - Citrus Reticulata - E	Fruit	13,127 ppm
Rowan Berry - Sorbus Aucubaria - E - M - T	Fruit	13,075 ppm
Hsin-Pa-Pi, Kisasage - Catalpa Ovata - E - M	Fruit	13,000 ppm
Eyebright - Euphrasia Officinalis - M	Plant	13,000 ppm
Cherokee Rose - Rosa Laevigata - E - M	Fruit	13,000 ppm
Tian Ma - Gastrodia Elata - Rhizome	Rhizome	12,900 ppm
Squaw Perideridia Gairdneri - E - M	Root	12,900 ppm
Cardamom - Elettaria Cardamomum - E - M	Seed	12,857 ppm
Water Chestnut - Eleocharis Dulcis - Tuber	Tuber	4,810-25,450 ppm
Sickle Senna - Cassia Tora - Sprout - Seedling - M	Seed	12,700 ppm
Indian Tamarind, Kilytree, Tamarind - Tamarindus Indica - M	Flower	12,700 ppm
Buffalo Gourd - Cucurbita Foetidissima - E - M - T	Leaf	0-25,300 ppm
Asparagus bean, Pea bean, Yardlong bean - Vigna Unguiculata subsp. Sesquipedalis - E	Seed	12,635 ppm
Indian Tobacco, Lobelia - Lobelia Inflata - M - T	Leaf	12,600 ppm
Rice - Oryza Sativa - E	Plant	12,600 ppm
Madder - Rubia Cordifolia - M	Root	12,600 ppm
Sassafras - Sassafras Albidum - E - M - T	Stem	12,580 ppm
Chinese Raspberry - Rubus Cchingii - E - M	Fruit	12,500 ppm
Desert Wormwood - Artemisia Herba-Alba - M	Plant	12,400 ppm
Garlic - Allium Sativum Bulb - E	Shoot	12,242 ppm
Curly Dock, Lengua De Vaca, Sour Dock, Yellow Dock - Rumex Crispus - M - T	Root	12,200 ppm
European Mistletoe - Viscum Album - M - T	Leaf	12,200 ppm
Corn - Zea Mays - E	Silk Stigma Style	12,200 ppm
Quince - Cydonia Oblonga - E	Fruit	12,160 ppm
Apple - Malus Domestica - E	Fruit	12,140 ppm
Marshmallow, White Mallow - Althaea Officinalis - M	Root	12,100 ppm
Da-Zao, Jujube, Ta-Tsao - Zizyphus Jujuba - E - M	Fruit	12,035 ppm
Indian Tamarind, Kilytree, Tamarind - Tamarindus Indica - M	Leaf	11,974 ppm
Hawthorn - Crataegus Cuneata - M	Fruit	11,900 ppm
Butterbur - Petasites Japonicus - T	Pt	11,900 ppm
Heal-All, Self-Heal - Prunella Vulgaris - E - M	Flower	11,900 ppm
Radish - Raphanus Sativus - E	Seed	11,900 ppm
Cloudberry - Rubus Chamaemorus - E - M	Fruit	11,875 ppm
Carambola, Star Averrhoa Carambola - E	Fruit	1,400-23,500 ppm
Buchu, Honey Buchu, Mountain Buchu - Agathosma Betulina Buchu, Honey Buchu, Mountain Buchu - Agathosma Betulina - M	Leaf	11,700 ppm
Bai-Zhu, Pai-Chu - Atractylodes Ovata - M	Rhizome	11,700 ppm
Buchu - Barosma Betulina	Leaf	11,700 ppm
Dan-Shen, Red Sage, Tan-Shen - Salvia Miltiorrhiza - E - M	Root	11,700 ppm
Fig - Ficus Carica - E	Fruit	11,662 ppm
Sage - Salvia Officinalis - E - M	Plant	11,630 ppm
Summer Savory - Satureja Hortensis - E	Plant	11,549 ppm
Lentil - Lens Culinaris - E	Sprout Seedling	11,495 ppm
Pistachio - Pistacia Vera - E	Seed	11,493 ppm
Coconut, Coconut Palm - Cocos Nucifera - E	Seed	11,491 ppm
Corn - Zea Mays - E	Seed	11,450 ppm
Commom Licorice, Licorice, Licorice-Root, Smooth Licorice - Glycyrrhiza Glabra - M	Plant	11,400 ppm
Sensitive Mimosa Pudica - M	Leaf	11,400 ppm
Ginkgo, Maidenhair Tree - Ginkgo Biloba - Tree - E - M - T	Seed	11,394 ppm
White Lupine - Lupinus Albus - M - T	Seed	11,300 ppm
Rosemary - Rosmarinus Officinalis - E - M	Plant	11,284 ppm
Pear - Pyrus Communis - E	Fruit	11,250 ppm
Mud Plantain, Tse-Hsieh, Water Plantain, Ze-Xie - Alisma Plantago Aquatica - M	Rhizome	11,200 ppm
Chinese Kudzu - Pueraria Pseudohirsuta - E - M	Root	11,200 ppm
Purple Jobo, Purple Plum - Spondias Purpurea - E	Fruit	11,155 ppm
English Hawthorn, Hawthorn, Whitethorn, Woodland Hawthorn - Crataegus Laevigata - M	Fruit	11,000 ppm
Japanese Ginseng - Panax Japonicus - M	Rhizome	11,000 ppm
Gru-Gru Nut, Mbocaya - Acrocomia Totai - E	Fruit	0-21,800 ppm

POTASSIUM CONTINUED

Name	Part	ppm
Chinese Spikenard - Nardostachys Chinensis - M	Rhizome	10,800 ppm
Chinese Cornbind, Chinese Knotweed, Fleeceflower, Fo Ti, He Shou Wu - Polygonum Multiflorum - E - M - T	Root	10,800 ppm
Chinese Ginseng, Ginseng, Korean Ginseng, Oriental Ginseng - Panax Ginseng - M	Root	10,700 ppm
Japanese Pagoda Tree - Sophora Japonica - M - T	Seed	10,660 ppm
Soybean - Glycine Max - E	Plant	10,600 ppm
Mai-Men-Dong, Mai-Men-Tung - Ophiopogon Japonicus - M	Tuber	10,600 ppm
Ching-Chieh, Jing-Jie - Schizonepeta Tenuifolia - E - M	Plant	10,600 ppm
Lentil - Lens Culinaris - E	Seed	10,440 ppm
Cobnut, English Filbert, European Filbert, European Hazel, Hazel - Corylus Avellana - E	Seed	10,433 ppm
Black Cohosh, Black Snake - Cimicifuga Racemosa - E - M	Root	10,300 ppm
Common Valerian, Garden-Heliotrope, Valerian - Valeriana Officinalis - E - M	Root	10,300 ppm
Chickpea, Garbanzo - Cicer Arietinum - E	Seed	10,220 ppm
Qiang Huo - Notopterygium Incisum - M	Rhizome	10,200 ppm
Alholva, Bockshornklee, Fenugreek, Greek Clover, Greek Trigonella Foenum-Graecum - E - M	Seed	10,200 ppm
White Mulberry - Morus Alba - E - M	Fruit	10,133 ppm
Chih-Mu, Zhi-Mu - Anemarrhena Asphodeloides - M	Rhizome	10,100 ppm
Nutsedge - Cyperus Rotundus - E - M	Rhizome	10,100 ppm
Huang Qi, Huang-Chi - Astragalus Membranaceus - M	Root	10,000 ppm
Pineapple - Ananas Comosus - E	Fruit	9,932 ppm
Devil's claw, Grapple - Harpagophytum procumbens - M	Root	9,910 ppm
Cherimoya - Annona Cherimola - E	Fruit	9,900 ppm
Barley, Barleygrass - Hordeum Vulgare - E - M	Seed	9,900 ppm
White Willow - Salix Alba - M	Bark	9,830 ppm
ElytriCouchgrass, Doggrass, Quackgrass, Twitchgrass, Wheatgrass - Elytrigia Repens - E - M	Plant	9,780 ppm
Hsin-I, Xin-Yi - Magnolia Denudata - E - M	Flower	9,780 ppm
Hsin-I, Xin-Yi - Magnolia Fargesii - E - M	Flower	9,780 ppm
Chinese Foxglove - Rehmannia Glutinosa - M	Root	9,730 ppm
Common thyme, Garden thyme, Thyme - Thymus Vulgaris - E - M	Leaf	9,680 ppm
Common Juniper, Juniper - Juniperus Communis - E - M - T	Fruit	9,570 ppm
Lian-Jiao, Lien-Chiao - Forsythia Suspensa - M	Fruit	9,560 ppm
Coffee Senna - Senna Occidentalis - E - T	Seed	9,560 ppm
Lime - Citrus Aurantiifolia - E	Fruit	9,533 ppm
Sarsaparilla - Smilax spp - E - M	Root	9,530 ppm
Mango - Mangifera Indica - E - M	Fruit	9,475 ppm
Genipap, Jagua - Genipa Americana - E - M	Seed	9,400 ppm
Indian Sorrel, Jamaica Sorrel, Kharkadi, Red Sorrel, Sorrel - Hibiscus Sabdariffa - E	Flower	9,400 ppm
Ladyslipper - Cypripedium Pubescens - M	Root	9,340 ppm
Box-Holly, Butcher's broom - Ruscus aculeatus - E - M	Root	9,340 ppm
Common thyme, Garden thyme, Thyme - Thymus Vulgaris - E - M	Plant	9,302 ppm
Black Gum, Black Tupelo - Nyssa Sylvatica - E - M	Stem	9,240 ppm
Northern Red Oak - Quercus Rubra - E - M	Stem	9,240 ppm
Post Oak - Quercus Stellata - E - M	Stem	9,240 ppm
Sicklepod - Senna Obtusifolia - E - T	Seed	9,200 ppm
White Mustard - Sinapis Alba - E - M - T	Seed	9,130 ppm
Chinese Cornbind, Chinese Knotweed, Fleeceflower, Fo Ti, He Shou Wu - Polygonum Multiflorum - E - M - T	Rhizome	9,120 ppm
Baikal Skullcap, Chinese Skullcap, Huang Qin - Scutellaria Baicalensis - M	Root	9,120 ppm
Giant Taro - Alocasia Macrorrhiza - E	Root	9,000 ppm
Lantana, Wild Sage - Lantana Camara - M	Shoot	9,000 ppm
Japanese Gentian - Gentiana Scabra - E	Root	8,980 ppm
Blackberry Lily, Shenan - Belamcanda Chinensis - M	Rhizome	8,940 ppm
Oats - Avena Sativa - E - M	Seed	8,900 ppm
Date Palm - Phoenix Dactylifera - E	Fruit	8,780 ppm
Gentian, Yellow Gentian - Gentiana Lutea - M	Root	8,770 ppm

Jih-Chiung - Cnidium Officinale - M	Rhizome	8,750 ppm
American Persimmon - Diospyros Virginiana - E - M	Fruit	8,710 ppm
Equatorial Ivory Palm - Phytelephas Aequatorialis - E	Flower	5,070-17,365 ppm
Pumpkin - Cucurbita Pepo - E	Seed	8,670 ppm
European Chestnut - Castanea Sativa - E - M	Seed	8,646 ppm
Almond - Prunus Dulcis - E - M - T	Seed	8,560 ppm
Northern Red Oak - Quercus Rubra - E - M	Seed	8,485 ppm
Bilberry, Dwarf Bilberry, Whortleberry - Vaccinium Myrtillus - E - M	Fruit	8,460 ppm
Shortleaf Pine - Pinus Echinata - M	Shoot	8,400 ppm
Lady's Thistle, Milk Thistle - Silybum Marianum - M	Plant	8,330 ppm
Chinese Chestnut - Castanea Mollisima - M	Seed	8,224 ppm
Okra - Abelmoschus Esculentus - Friut - E - M	Seed	8,200 ppm
Opium Poppy, Poppyseed Poppy - Papaver Somniferum - E	Seed	8,179 ppm
Terminalia catappa L. -- Indian Almond, Malabar Almond, Tropical Almond	Seed	8,165 ppm
Chinese Boxthorn, Chinese Matrimony Vine, Chinese Wolfberry - Lycium Chinense - E - M	Root Bark	8,110 ppm
Psyllium - Plantago Psyllium - E - M	Seed	8,110 ppm
Coneflower, Echinacea - Echinacea ssp - M	Root	8,090 ppm
Black Oak - Quercus Velutina - E - M	Stem	8,060 ppm
Wheat - Triticum Aestivum - E - M	Seed	7,900 ppm
Ben Nut, Benzolive Tree, Drumstick Tree, Horseradish Tree, Moringa, West Indian Ben - Moringa Oleifera - E	Shoot	3,370-15,790 ppm
Common Garden Peony, Peony, White Peony - Paeonia Lactiflora - M	Root	7,860 ppm
Coca - Erythroxylum Novogranatense var. Novogranatense - E - M	Leaf	7,800 ppm
Apricot - Prunus Armeniaca - E - M - T	Seed	7,783 ppm
Damiana - Turnera Diffusa - M	Leaf	7,760 ppm
Groundnut, Peanut - Arachis Hypogaea - E - M	Seed	7,681 ppm
Sesame - Sesamum Indicum - E - M	Seed	7,664 ppm
Rush - Juncus Effusus E - M - T	Pith	7,620 ppm
Asparagus Pea, Goa Bean, Winged Bean - Psophocarpus Tetragonolobus - E	Leaf	7,602 ppm
Evening-Primrose - Oenothera Biennis - E - M	Seed	7,577 ppm
American Chestnut - Castanea Dentata - E - M	Seed	7,541 ppm
Butternut - Juglans Cinerea - E	Seed	7,493 ppm
Hardy Orchid, Hyacinth Bletilla, Hyacinth Orchid, Shiran - Bletilla Striata - M	Tuber	7,380 ppm
Climbing Fern - Lygodium Japonicum - Pollen or Spore - M	Pollen Or Spore	7,380 ppm
Crampbark, European Cranberry bush, Guelder Rose, Snowballbush - Viburnum Opulus - E - M - T	Bark	7,360 ppm
Paper Mulberry - Broussonetia Papyrifera - E - M	Fruit	7,340 ppm
White Oak - Quercus Alba - M	Stem	7,296 ppm
Girasol, Sun Helianthus Annuus - E	Seed	7,280 ppm
Blue Cohosh - Caulophyllum Thalictroides - M	Root	7,250 ppm
Noble Dendrobium - Dendrobium Nobile - M	Stem	7,200 ppm
Amphicarpaea Bracteata- E - M	Shoot	0-14,200 ppm
Peach - Prunus Persica - E - M - T	Seed	7,010 ppm
Japanese Cinnamon - Cinnamomum Sieboldii - E - M - T	Root Bark	7,000 ppm
Large-Fruited Provision Tree - Pachira Macrocarpa - E	Seed	7,000 ppm
Maracuya, Passion Passiflora Edulis - E	Fruit	3,480-13,975 ppm
English Walnut - Juglans Rregia - E	Seed	6,870 ppm
Chinese Goldthread, Huang-Lian, Huang-Lien - Coptis Chinensis - M	Rhizome	6,840 ppm
Huang-Lia, Huang-Lian, Huang-Lien, Japanese Goldthread - Coptis Japonica - M	Rhizome	6,840 ppm
Generic Goldthread - Coptis spp. - M	Rhizome	6,840 ppm
Cashew - Anacardium Occidentale - E	Seed	6,815 ppm
Gru-Gru Nut, Mbocaya - Acrocomia Totai - E	Seed	0-13,600 ppm
American Cranberry, Cranberry, Large Cranberry - Vaccinium Macrocarpon - E	Fruit	6,777 ppm
Betel Nut, Pin-Lang - Areca Catechu Amphicarpaea Bracteata- E - M	Seed	6,700 ppm

Hillman Health Food Store call 855-Amish-Dr (855-264-7437) www.emineral.info Vitamins and Minerals for Better Living

POTASSIUM CONTINUED

Moutan, Tree Peony - Paeonia Moutan - M	Root Bark	6,700 ppm
Moutan, Moutan Peony, Tree Peony - Paeonia Suffruticosa	Root Bark	6,700 ppm
Balloon Flower, Chieh-Keng, Jie-Geng - Platycodon Grandiflorum - E - M - T	Root	6,660 ppm
Indian Fig, Nopal, Nopalito, Prickly Pear - Opuntia Ficus-Indica - E - M	Fruit	6,615 ppm
Jojoba - Simmondsia Chinensis Seed	Seed	6,610 ppm
Red Mangrove - Rhizophora Mangle - M	Leaf	6,500 ppm
Brazilnut, Brazilnut-Tree, Creamnut, Paranut - Bertholletia Eexcelsa - E	Seed	6,208 ppm
Snakegourd - Trichosanthes Anguina - E - M	Fruit	6,300 ppm
Pecan - Carya Illinoensis - E	Seed	6,242 ppm
Cang Zhu - Atractylodes Lancea - M	Rhizome	6,210 ppm
Cowberry, Lingen, Lingonberry - Vaccinium Vitis-Idaea var. Minus - E - M	Fruit	6,200 ppm
Goldenseal - Hydrastis Canadensis - M	Root	6,180 ppm
Du Zhong, Gutta-Percha Tree, Tu Chung - Eucommia Ulmoides - M	Bark	6,170 ppm
Kuan Chung, Shield Fernle - Blechnum Orientale - E - M - T	Rhizome	6,150 ppm
Barley, Barleygrass - Hordeum Vulgare - E - M	Sprout Seedling	6,130 ppm
Chinese Ash - Fraxinus Rhynchophylla - M - E	Bark	6,080 ppm
Oriental Pipewort - Eriocaulon spp. - M	Leaf	6,050 ppm
Java Cinnamon, Padang Cassia - Cinnamomum Burmannii - E - M - T	Bark	6,000 ppm
Japanese Cinnamon - Cinnamomum Sieboldii - E - M - T	Bark	6,000 ppm
Ceylon Cinnamon, Cinnamon - Cinnamomum Verum - E - M - T	Bark	6,000 ppm
Bei-Mu, Fritillary - Fritillaria Thunbergii - Blub - E - M	Tuber	5,980 ppm
Willow Oak - Quercus Phellos - E - M	Stem	5,880 ppm
Blueberry - Vaccinium Corymbosum - E	Fruit	5,859 ppm
Black Caraway, Black Cumin, Fennel-Flower, Nutmeg-Flower, Roman Coriander - Nigella Sativa - E - M	Seed	5,820 ppm
Hydrangea, Smooth Hydrangea - Hydrangea Arborescens - E - M	Root	5,810 ppm
Ambarella - Spondias Dulcis - E	Seed	5,800 ppm
Rye - Secale Cereale - E	Leaf	0-11,500 ppm
Henbane - Hyoscyamus Niger - E - M	Seed	5,680 ppm
Morinda - Morinda spp. - M	Root	5,660 ppm
Ching-Feng-Teng - Sinomenium Acutum - E - M	Rhizome	5,560 ppm
Wild Yam - Dioscorea sp. - E	Root	5,420 ppm
Shagbark Hickory - Carya Ovata - E	Seed	5,361 ppm
White Mulberry - Morus Alba - E - M	Root Bark	5,270 ppm
Mace, Nutmeg - Myristica Fragrans - E	Seed	5,210 ppm
Black Walnut - Juglans Nigra - E	Seed	5,154 ppm
Narrowleaf Sophora - Sophora Angustifolia - M - T- M - T	Root	4,740 ppm
Mace, Nutmeg - Myristica Fragrans - E	Aril	4,630 ppm
Buckwheat - Fagopyrum Esculentum - E	Seed	4,480 ppm
Barberry - Berberis Vulgaris - M	Root	4,370 ppm
Amur Cork Tree, Huang Bai, Huang Po, Po Mu - Phellodendron Amurense - M	Bark	4,370 ppm
Cascara Buckthorn, Cascara Sagrada - Frangula Purshiana - M	Bark	3,980 ppm
Bearberry, Uva Uursi - Arctostaphylos Uva-Ursi - M	Leaf	3,830 ppm
Macadamia - Macadamia spp. - E	Seed	3,785 ppm
Chrysophyllum cainito RADLK. -- Caimito, Star Apple	Fruit	1,400-7,565 ppm
Air Potato, Potato Yam - Dioscorea Bulbifera - E	Rhizome	3,570 ppm
Aceituna Dulce, Jambolan, Java Plum - Syzygium Cumini - E	Fruit	550-6,705 ppm
Italian Stone Pine, Pignolia - Pinus Pinea - M	Seed	5,990-6,420 ppm
Chinese Licorice - Glycyrrhiza Uralensis - M	Root	3,140 ppm
Rice Paper Tree, Tong-Cao, Tung-Tsao - Tetrapanax Papyrifera M	Pith	3,040 ppm
Chinese Senega - Polygala Tenuifolia - M	Root	2,900 ppm
Breadroot, Indian Bread-Root, Indian Turnip, Prairie Apple, Prairie Potato, Prairie Turnip - Psoralea Esculenta - E - M - T	Root	2,800 ppm

Species	Part	Quantity
Red Elm, Slippery Elm - Ulmus Rubra - M	Bark	2,710 ppm
Broadbean, Faba Bean, Habas - Vicia Faba - E	Fruit	2,670 ppm
Coca Erythroxylum Novogranatense var. Truxillense - E - M	Leaf	2,600 ppm
Indian Fig, Nopal, Nopalito, Prickly Pear - Opuntia Ficus-Indica - E - M	Bud	2,600 ppm
Swamp Taro - Cyrtosperma Chamissonis - E	Root	2,575 ppm
Chinese Magnolia, Hou Pu, Magnolia- Magnolia Officinalis - E - M	Bark	2,560 ppm
Rye - Secale Cereale - E	Seed	2,500-5,090 ppm
Olive - Olea Europaea - E	Fruit	2,523 ppm
Date Palm - Phoenix Dactylifera - E	Seed	2,440 ppm
Rice - Oryza Sativa - E	Seed	2,431 ppm
Chocolate Vine - Akebia Quinata - M	Stem	2,410 ppm
Adlay, Adlay Millet, Job's-Tears, Yi-Yi-Ren - Coix Lacryma-Jobi - E - M	Seed	2,360 ppm
Mimosa - Albizia Julibrissin - E - M	Bark	1,990 ppm
Bayberry, Candle-Berry, Southern Bayberry, Wax Myrtle - Myrica Cerifera - E - M	Bark	1,960 ppm
Ban-Xia, Pan-Hsia - Pinellia Ternata - E - M - T	Tuber	1,940 ppm
White Oak - Quercus Alba - M	Bark	1,900 ppm
Pau D'Arco - Tabebuia Heptaphylla - M	Bark	1,850 ppm
Devil's Tongue, Elephant Yam, Konjac, Leopard Palm, Snake Palm, Umbrella Arum - Amorphophallus Konjac - E - M - T	Root	1,740 ppm
Indian Fig, Nopal, Nopalito, Prickly Pear - Opuntia Ficus-Indica - E - M	Seed	1,720 ppm
Mamey - Mammea Americana - Fruit	Fruit	470-3,405 ppm
Guanique - Chamissoa Altissima - M	Leaf	328-3,280 ppm
Pomarrosa, Rose Apple - Syzygium Jambos - E	Fruit	500-3,225 ppm
Spirulina - Spirulina Pratensis - E	Plant	1,600 ppm
Ramie - Boehmeria Nivea - M	Plant	1,300 ppm
Aloe, Bitter Aloes - Aloe Vera - E - M	Leaf	850 ppm
Shan Dou Gen - Sophora Subprostrata - M - T	Root	820 ppm
Russian Olive - Elaeagnus Umbellatus - E - M	Fruit	2,010-1,125 ppm
Chinese Jack-In-The-Pulpit - Arisaema Consanguineum - E - M - T	Rhizome	180 ppm
Aconite, Fu-Tsu - Aconitum Carmichaelii - E - M	Tuber	170 ppm
Banana Yucca, Blue Yucca, Spanish Bayonet, Yucca - Yucca Baccata - E - M - T	Root	160 ppm
Gum Arabic, Gum Arabic Tree, Kher, Senegal Gum, Sudan Gum Arabic - Acacia Senegal - M	Plant	
Yellow Mombin, Yellow Plum - Spondias Mombin - E	Fruit	
Yellow Mombin, Yellow Plum - Spondias Pinnata - E	Fruit	

PLANTS CONTAINING RUBIDIUM

Species	Part	Quantity
Shagbark Hickory - Carya Ovata - E	Shoot	192 ppm
Spinach - Spinacia Oleracea - E	Leaf	90 ppm
Parsley - Petroselinum Crispum - E	Leaf	65 ppm
Bilberry, Dwarf Bilberry, Whortleberry - Vaccinium Myrtillus - E - M	Fruit	60 ppm
Rhubarb - Rheum Rhabarbarum - E	Pt	58 ppm
Dandelion - Taraxacum Officinale - E - M	Plant	50 ppm
White Oak - Quercus Alba - M	Stem	40 ppm
Asparagus bean, Pea bean, Yardlong bean - Vigna Unguiculata subsp. Sesquipedalis - E	Seed	39 ppm
Cloudberry - Rubus Chamaemorus - E - M	Fruit	38 ppm
Cashew - Anacardium Occidentale - E	Seed	35 ppm
Giant Knotweed, Hu-Zhang, Japanese Knotweed, Mexican Bamboo - Polygonum Cuspidatum - E - M - T	Plant	33 ppm
Rowan Berry - Sorbus Aucubaria - E - M - T	Fruit	33 ppm
Beet, Beetroot, Garden Beet, Sugar Beet - Beta Vulgaris - E	Root	32 ppm
Cassia, Cassia Bark, Cassia Lignea, China Junk Cassia, Chinazimt, Chinese Cassia - Cinnamomum Aromaticuminnamon- E - M - T	Bark	30 ppm
Dill, Garden Dill - Anethum Graveolens - E	Plant	28 ppm
Black Currant - Ribes Nigrum - E	Fruit	28 ppm

RUBIDIUM CONTINUED

Cabbage, Red Cabbage, White Cabbage - Brassica Oleracea var. Capitata - E	Leaf	27.5 ppm
Butterbur - Petasites Japonicus - T	Plant	26 ppm
Northern Red Oak - Quercus Rubra - E - M	Stem	26 ppm
Dog Rose, Dogbrier, Rose - Rosa Canina - E - M	Fruit	25 ppm
Cauli Brassica Oleracea var. Botrytis - E	Leaf	23 ppm
Red Currant, White Currant - Ribes Rubrum - E	Fruit	23 ppm
Potato - Solanum Tuberosum - E	Tuber	23 ppm
Pecan - Carya Illinoensis - E	Seed	22 ppm
Grape Citrus Paradisi - E	Fruit	22 ppm
Tomato - Lycopersicon Esculentum - E - M - T	Fruit	22 ppm
Cowberry, Lingen, Lingonberry - Vaccinium Vitis-Idaea var. Minus - E - M	Fruit	22 ppm
Black Oak - Quercus Velutina - E - M	Stem	21 ppm
Java Cinnamon, Padang Cassia - Cinnamomum Burmannii - E - M - T	Bark	20 ppm
Ceylon Cinnamon, Cinnamon - Cinnamomum Verum - E - M - T	Bark	20 ppm
Banana, Plantain - Musa x Paradisiaca - E	Fruit	20 ppm
Pear - Pyrus Communis - E	Fruit	20 ppm
Mugwort - Artemisia Vulgaris - M	Plant	19 ppm
Cucumber - Cucumis Sativus - E	Fruit	19 ppm
Qian Hu - Peucedanum Decursivum - M	Plant	18 ppm
European Nettle, Stinging Nettle - Urtica Dioica - E - M	Leaf	17.8 ppm
Red Pignut Hickory - Carya Glabra - E	Shoot	17 ppm
Coconut, Coconut Palm - Cocos Nucifera - E	Seed	16 ppm
Radish - Raphanus Sativus - E	Root	15.7 ppm
Plum - Prunus Domestica - E - M	Fruit	15 ppm
Ramie - Boehmeria Nivea - M	Plant	14 ppm
Groundnut, Peanut - Arachis Hypogaea - E - M	Seed	13 ppm
Chinese Polystichum - Polystichum Polyblepharum - T	Plant	13 ppm
Almond - Prunus Dulcis - E - M - T	Seed	13 ppm
Carrot - Daucus Carota - E	Root	12.7 ppm
Cauli Brassica Oleracea var. Botrytis - E	Flower	11 ppm
Cobnut, English Filbert, European Filbert, European Hazel, Hazel - Corylus Avellana - E	Seed	11 ppm
Alehoof - Glechoma Hederacea - M	Plant	11 ppm
Rutabaga, Swede, Swedish Turnip - Brassica Napus var. Napobrassica - E	Root	10 ppm
Rapini, Seven-Top Turnip, Turnip - Brassica Rapa - E	Root	10 ppm
Bell Pepper, Cherry Pepper, Cone Pepper, Green Pepper, Paprika, Sweet Pepper - Capsicum Annuum - E	Fruit	10 ppm
Apple - Malus Domestica - E	Fruit	10 ppm
Parsnip - Pastinaca Sativa - E	Root	10 ppm
Pistachio - Pistacia Vera - E	Seed	10 ppm
Pea - Pisum Sativum - E	Seed	10 ppm
Black Walnut - Juglans Nigra - E	Seed	9.3 ppm
Celery - Apium Graveolens - E	Root	9 ppm
Japanese Cinnamon - Cinnamomum Sieboldii - E - M - T	Root Bark	9 ppm
Orange - Citrus Sinensis - E	Fruit	7.7 ppm
Black bean, Dwarf bean, Field bean, Flageolet bean, French bean, Garden bean, Green bean, Haricot, Haricot bean, Haricot vert, Kidney bean, Navy bean, Pop bean, Popping bean, Snap bean, String bean, Wax bean - Phaseolus Vulgaris - E	Fruit	7 ppm
Onion, Shallot - Allium Cepa - Shallot Bulb - E	Bulb	6.6 ppm
Strawberry - Fragaria spp. - E	Fruit	6.5 ppm
European Grape, Grape, Grapevine, Vigne Vinifere, Wine Grape - Vitis Vinifera - E - M	Fruit	5.5 ppm
Northern Red Oak - Quercus Rubra - E - M	Seed	5 ppm
Horseradish - Armoracia Rusticana - E	Root	4.6 ppm
Shagbark Hickory - Carya Ovata - E	Seed	4 ppm
American Cranberry, Cranberry, Large Cranberry - Vaccinium Macrocarpon - E	Fruit	3.5 ppm
Japanese Cinnamon - Cinnamomum Sieboldii - E - M - T	Bark	3 ppm
Butternut - Juglans Cinerea - E	Seed	2.5 ppm
Mandarin, Tangerine - Citrus Reticulata - E	Fruit	2.4 ppm

PLANTS CONTAINING SCANDIUM

Species	Part	Quantity
Dwarf Sumac, Winged Sumac - Rhus Copallina - E - M	Plant	Trace
Black Gum, Black Tupelo - Nyssa Sylvatica - E - M	Leaf	Trace
Sassafras - Sassafras Albidum - E - M - T	Leaf	Trace
Brazilnut, Brazilnut-Tree, Creamnut, Paranut - Bertholletia Eexcelsa - E	Seed	Trace
Asparagus bean, Pea bean, Yardlong bean - Vigna Unguiculata subsp. Sesquipedalis - E	Seed	Trace
Pecan - Carya Illinoensis - E	Seed	Trace
Shagbark Hickory - Carya Ovata - E	Seed	Trace
Cobnut, English Filbert, European Filbert, European Hazel, Hazel - Corylus Avellana - E	Seed	Trace
Black Walnut - Juglans Nigra - E	Seed	Trace
Pistachio - Pistacia Vera - E	Seed	Trace
Butternut - Juglans Cinerea - E	Seed	Trace
Almond - Prunus Dulcis - E - M - T	Seed	Trace
Northern Red Oak - Quercus Rubra - E - M	Seed	Trace
Cashew - Anacardium Occidentale - E	Seed	Trace
Coconut, Coconut Palm - Cocos Nucifera - E	Seed	Trace

PLANTS CONTAINING SELENIUM

Species	Part	Quantity
Brazilnut, Brazilnut-Tree, Creamnut, Paranut - Bertholletia Eexcelsa - E	Seed	497 ppm
Catnip - Nepeta Cataria - M	Plant	123 ppm
Lady's Thistle, Milk Thistle - Silybum Marianum - M	Plant	171 ppm
Indian Sorrel, Jamaica Sorrel, Kharkadi, Red Sorrel, Sorrel - Hibiscus Sabdariffa - E	Flower	143 ppm
ElytriCouchgrass, Doggrass, Quackgrass, Twitchgrass, Wheatgrass - Elytrigia Repens - E - M	Plant	102 ppm
Chinese Cornbind, Chinese Knotweed, Fleeceflower, Fo Ti, He Shou Wu - Polygonum Multiflorum - E - M - T	Root	74 ppm
Buchu, Honey Buchu, Mountain Buchu - Agathosma Betulina Buchu, Honey Buchu, Mountain Buchu - Agathosma Betulina - M	Leaf	70 ppm
Lemongrass, West indian lemongrass - Cymbopogon Citratus - E - M	Plant	62 ppm
European Pennyroyal - Mentha pulegium - E - M- T	Plant	25 ppm
Ladyslipper - Cypripedium Pubescens - M	Root	49 ppm
Common Valerian, Garden-Heliotrope, Valerian - Valeriana Officinalis - E - M	Root	44 ppm
Blue Cohosh - Caulophyllum Thalictroides - M	Root	35 ppm
Barberry - Berberis Vulgaris - M	Root	34 ppm
Blessed Thistle - Cnicus Benedictus - M	Plant	34 ppm
Bayberry, Candle-Berry, Southern Bayberry, Wax Myrtle - Myrica Cerifera - E - M	Bark	34 ppm
Marshmallow, White Mallow - Althaea Officinalis - M	Root	33 ppm
Dulse - Rhodymenia Palmata - E	Plant	33 ppm
Black Cohosh, Black Snake Cimicifuga Racemosa - E - M	Root	32 ppm
Pumpkin - Cucurbita Pepo - E	Seed	32 ppm
Common thyme, Garden thyme, Thyme - Thymus Vulgaris - E - M	Leaf	16 ppm
Alholva, Bockshornklee, Fenugreek, Greek Clover, Greek Trigonella Foenum-Graecum - E - M	Seed	16 ppm
Sarsaparilla - Smilax spp - E - M	Root	31 ppm
Black Walnut - Juglans Nigra - E	Fruit	30 ppm
Chinese Ginseng, Ginseng, Korean Ginseng, Oriental Ginseng - Panax Ginseng - M	Root	25 ppm
Raspberry, Red raspberry - Rubus Idaeus - E - M	Leaf	25 ppm
Curly Dock, Lengua De Vaca, Sour Dock, Yellow Dock - Rumex Crispus - M - T	Root	25 ppm
Indian Sorrel, Jamaica Sorrel, Stevia, Sweet Leaf of Paraguay - Stevia Rebaudiana - E	Leaf	25 ppm
Barley, Barleygrass - Hordeum Vulgare - E - M	Stem	24 ppm
Emblic, Myrobalan - Phyllanthus Emblica - E	Fruit	12 ppm

SELENIUM CONTINUED

Plant	Part	ppm
Box-Holly, Butcher's broom - Ruscus aculeatus - E - M	Root	24 ppm
Aloe, Bitter Aloes - Aloe Vera - E - M	Leaf	23 ppm
Crampbark, European Cranberry bush, Guelder Rose, Snowballbush - Viburnum Opulus - E - M - T	Bark	23 ppm
Peppermint - Mentha x Piperita subsp. Nothosubsp. Piperita - E - M - T	Leaf	11 ppm
European Nettle, Stinging Nettle - Urtica Dioica - E - M	Leaf	22 ppm
Coneflower, Echinacea - Echinacea ssp - M	Root	21 ppm
SafCarthamus Tinctorius - M	Flower	20 ppm
English Hawthorn, Hawthorn, Whitethorn, Woodland Hawthorn - Crataegus Laevigata - M	Fruit	20 ppm
Chaparral, Creosote Bush - Larrea Tridentata - M	Plant	19 ppm
Irish moss - Chondrus Crispus - E	Plant	18 ppm
Gentian, Yellow Gentian - Gentiana Lutea - M	Root	18 ppm
European Grape, Grape, Grapevine, Vigne Vinifere, Wine Grape - Vitis Vinifera - E - M	Stem	18 ppm
Feverfew - Chrysanthemum Parthenium - M	Plant	17 ppm
Bladderwrack, Kelp - Fucus Vesiculosus - E - M	Plant	17 ppm
Hops - Humulus Lupulus - E - M - T	Fruit	17 ppm
Mad-Dog Skullcap, Scullcap - Scutellaria lateriflora - M	Plant	8.3 ppm
Milfoil, Yarrow - Achillea Millefolium - M	Plant	16 ppm
Garlic - Allium Sativum Bulb - E	Bulb	16 ppm
Bearberry, Uva Uursi - Arctostaphylos Uva-Ursi - M	Leaf	16 ppm
Fennel - Foeniculum Vulgare - M	Fruit	16 ppm
Hydrangea, Smooth Hydrangea - Hydrangea Arborescens - E - M	Root	16 ppm
Cowgrass, Peavine Clover, Purple Clover, Red Clover - Trifolium Pratense - E - M	Flower	7.7 ppm
Devil's claw, Grapple Harpagophytum procumbens M	Root	15 ppm
White Oak - Quercus Alba - M	Bark	15 ppm
Red Elm, Slippery Elm - Ulmus Rubra - M	Bark	15 ppm
Burdock, Gobo, Great Burdock - Arctium lappa - E - M - T	Root	14 ppm
Psyllium - Plantago Psyllium - E - M	Seed	14 ppm
European Mistletoe - Viscum Album - M - T	Leaf	14 ppm
Oats - Avena Sativa - E - M	Plant	13 ppm
Field Horsetail, Horsetail - Equisetum Arvense - M	Plant	13 ppm
Peach - Prunus Persica - E - M - T	Bark	13 ppm
Gotu Kola, Pennywort - Centella Asiatica - E - M	Leaf	12 ppm
Chinese Ephedra, Ma Huang - Ephedra Sinica - M	Plant	12 ppm
Almond - Prunus Dulcis - E - M - T	Seed	6 ppm
Cascara Buckthorn, Cascara Sagrada - Frangula Purshiana - M	Bark	11 ppm
White Willow - Salix Alba - M	Bark	11 ppm
Goldenseal - Hydrastis Canadensis - M	Root	10 ppm
Ginger - Zingiber Officinale - E	Rhizome	10 ppm
Wild Yam - Dioscorea sp. - E	Root	9.4 ppm
Banana Yucca, Blue Yucca, Spanish Bayonet, Yucca - Yucca Baccata - E - M - T	Root	9 ppm
Dandelion - Taraxacum Officinale - E - M	Root	8.6 ppm
Garden Camomile, Perennial Camomile, Roman Camomile - Chamaemelum Nobile M	Flower	7.8 ppm
Chinese Magnolia Vine, Five-Flavor-Fruit, Magnolia Vine, Schizandra, Wu Wei Zi, Wu Wei Zu - Schisandra Chinensis - M	Fruit	7.4 ppm
Damiana - Turnera Diffusa - M	Leaf	6.7 ppm
Comfrey - Symphytum Officinale - E - M - T	Root	5.7 ppm
Corn - Zea Mays - E	Silk Stigma Style	5.7 ppm
Cucumber - Cucumis Sativus - E	Fruit	2.8 ppm
Indian Tobacco, Lobelia - Lobelia Inflata - M - T	Leaf	5 ppm
Flannelleaf, Flannelplant, Great mullein, Mullein, Velvet - Verbascum Thapsus - M	Leaf	5 ppm
Eyebright - Euphrasia Officinalis - M	Plant	4.7 ppm
Chickweed, Common Chickweed - Stellaria Media - E	Plant	4.3 ppm
Chinese Angelica, Dong Gui, Dong Quai - Angelica Sinensis - M	Root	3.5 ppm
Soybean - Glycine Max - E	Seed	1.25 ppm

Common Juniper, Juniper - Juniperus Communis - E - M - T	Fruit	2.4 ppm
Pau D'Arco - Tabebuia Heptaphylla - M	Bark	2 ppm
Devil's Tongue, Elephant Yam, Konjac, Leopard Palm, Snake Palm, Umbrella Arum - Amorphophallus Konjac - E - M - T	Root	1.7 ppm
Commom Licorice, Licorice, Licorice-Root, Smooth Licorice - Glycyrrhiza Glabra - M	Root	1 ppm
Corn - Zea Mays - E	Seed	Trace
American Styrax, Sweetgum - Liquidambar Styraciflua - E - M	Plant	Trace
Willow Oak - Quercus Phellos - E - M	Stem	Trace
Cabbage, Red Cabbage, White Cabbage - Brassica Oleracea var. Capitata - E	Leaf	Trace
Smooth Sumac - Rhus Glabra - E - M	Stem	Trace
Cashew - Anacardium Occidentale - E	Seed	Trace
Buckwheat - Fagopyrum Esculentum - E	Seed	Trace
Shortleaf Pine - Pinus Echinata - M	Shoot	Trace
Asparagus bean, Pea bean, Yardlong bean - Vigna Unguiculata subsp. Sesquipedalis - E	Seed	Trace
Butternut - Juglans Cinerea - E	Seed	Trace
Pistachio - Pistacia Vera - E	Seed	Trace
Cobnut, English Filbert, European Filbert, European Hazel, Hazel - Corylus Avellana - E	Seed	Trace
Buckbush - Symphoricarpos Orbiculatus - M	Stem	Trace
Asparagus - Asparagus Officinalis - E	Shoot	Trace
Lettuce - Lactuca Sativa - E	Leaf	Trace
Spinach - Spinacia Oleracea - E	Leaf	Trace
Red Cedar - Juniperus Virginiana Amphicarpaea Bracteata- E - M - T	Shoot	Trace
Banana, Plantain - Musa x Paradisiaca - E	Fruit	Trace
Allspice, Clover-Pepper, Jamaica-Pepper, Pimenta, Pimento - Pimenta Dioica - E	Plant	Trace
White Oak - Quercus Alba - M	Stem	Trace
Post Oak - Quercus Stellata - E - M	Stem	Trace
Tomato - Lycopersicon Esculentum - E - M - T	Fruit	Trace
Rutabaga, Swede, Swedish Turnip - Brassica Napus var. Napobrassica - E	Leaf	Trace
Grape Citrus Paradisi - E	Fruit	Trace
Alfalfa, Lucerne - Medicago Sativa subsp. Sativa - E	Leaf	Trace
Cauli Brassica Oleracea var. Botrytis - E	Leaf	Trace
Brussel-Sprout - Brassica Oleracea var. Gemmifera - E	Leaf	Trace
Endive, Escarole - Cichorium Endivia - M	Leaf	Trace
Cowgrass, Peavine Clover, Purple Clover, Red Clover - Trifolium Pratense - E - M	Leaf	Trace
Parsley - Petroselinum Crispum - E	Plant	Trace
Groundnut, Peanut - Arachis Hypogaea - E - M	Seed	Trace
Pecan - Carya Illinoensis - E	Seed	Trace
Shagbark Hickory - Carya Ovata - E	Seed	Trace
Coconut, Coconut Palm - Cocos Nucifera - E	Seed	Trace
Carrot - Daucus Carota - E	Root	Trace
Black Walnut - Juglans Nigra - E	Seed	Trace
Northern Red Oak - Quercus Rubra - E - M	Seed	Trace
Cowgrass, Peavine Clover, Purple Clover, Red Clover - Trifolium Pratense - E - M	Stem	Trace
Rutabaga, Swede, Swedish Turnip - Brassica Napus var. Napobrassica - E	Stem	Trace
Cauli Brassica Oleracea var. Botrytis - E	Stem	Trace
Alfalfa, Lucerne - Medicago Sativa subsp. Sativa - E	Stem	Trace
Plum - Prunus Domestica - E - M	Fruit	Trace
Cowberry, Lingen, Lingonberry - Vaccinium Vitis-Idaea var. Minus - E - M	Fruit	Trace
Dill, Garden Dill - Anethum Graveolens - E	Plant	Trace
Brussel-Sprout - Brassica Oleracea var. Gemmifera - E	Stem	Trace
European Grape, Grape, Grapevine, Vigne Vinifere, Wine Grape - Vitis Vinifera - E - M	Fruit	Trace
Rowan Berry - Sorbus Aucubaria - E - M - T	Fruit	Trace
Horseradish - Armoracia Rusticana - E	Root	Trace

Hillman Health Food Store call 855-Amish-Dr (855-264-7437) www.emineral.info Vitamins and Minerals for Better Living

SELENIUM CONTINUED

Species	Part	Quantity	Species	Part	Quantity
Black bean, Dwarf bean, Field bean, Flageolet bean, French bean, Garden bean, Green bean, Haricot, Haricot bean, Haricot vert, Kidney bean, Navy bean, Pop bean, Popping bean, Snap bean, String bean, Wax bean - Phaseolus Vulgaris - E	Seed	Trace	Brazilnut, Brazilnut-Tree, Creamnut, Paranut - Bertholletia Eexcelsa - E	Seed	1,770 ppm
			Butternut - Juglans Cinerea - E	Seed	1,450 ppm
			Pistachio - Pistacia Vera - E	Seed	1,450 ppm
			Parsley - Petroselinum Crispum - E	Leaf	1,425 ppm
			Black Walnut - Juglans Nigra - E	Seed	1,387 ppm
Potato - Solanum Tuberosum - E	Tuber	Trace	Cashew - Anacardium Occidentale - E	Seed	1,280 ppm
Black bean, Dwarf bean, Field bean, Flageolet bean, French bean, Garden bean, Green bean, Haricot, Haricot bean, Haricot vert, Kidney bean, Navy bean, Pop bean, Popping bean, Snap bean, String bean, Wax bean - Phaseolus Vulgaris - E	Fruit	Trace	Rapini, Seven-Top Turnip, Turnip - Brassica Rapa - E	Root	1,200 ppm
			Black bean, Dwarf bean, Field bean, Flageolet bean, French bean, Garden bean, Green bean, Haricot, Haricot bean, Haricot vert, Kidney bean, Navy bean, Pop bean, Popping bean, Snap bean, String bean, Wax bean - Phaseolus Vulgaris - E	Fruit	1,200 ppm
Dog Rose, Dogbrier, Rose - Rosa Canina - E - M	Fruit	Trace			
Cantaloupe, Melon, Muskmelon, Netted Melon, Nutmeg Melon, Persian Melon - Cucumis Melo subsp. ssp Melo var.Ccantalupensis - Friut - E	Fruit	Trace	Shagbark Hickory - Carya Ovata - E	Seed	1,180 ppm
			Cucumber - Cucumis Sativus - E	Fruit	1,000 ppm
			Almond - Prunus Dulcis - E - M - T	Seed	960 ppm
Onion, Shallot - Allium Cepa - Shallot Bulb - E	Bulb	Trace	Cobnut, English Filbert, European Filbert, European Hazel, Hazel - Corylus Avellana - E	Seed	900 ppm
Peach - Prunus Persica - E - M - T	Fruit	Trace	Spinach - Spinacia Oleracea - E	Leaf	855 ppm
Chinese Cabbage - Brassica Pekinensis - E	Leaf	Trace	Lettuce - Lactuca Sativa - E	Leaf	800 ppm
Bell Pepper, Cherry Pepper, Cone Pepper, Green Pepper, Paprika, Sweet Pepper - Capsicum Annuum - E	Fruit	Trace	Dill, Garden Dill - Anethum Graveolens - E	Plant	700 ppm
			Pineapple - Ananas Comosus - E	Fruit	690 ppm
			Date Palm - Phoenix Dactylifera - E	Fruit	660 ppm
Orange - Citrus Sinensis - E	Fruit	Trace	Radish - Raphanus Sativus - E	Root	425 ppm
Strawberry - Fragaria spp. - E	Fruit	Trace			
Pea - Pisum Sativum - E	Seed	Trace	Field Horsetail, Horsetail - Equisetum Arvense - M	Plant	386 ppm
Aubergine, Egg Solanum Melongena - E	Fruit	Trace	Coconut, Coconut Palm - Cocos Nucifera - E	Seed	370 ppm
Pear - Pyrus Communis - E	Fruit	Trace	Dulse - Rhodymenia Palmata - E	Plant	368 ppm
			European Grape, Grape, Grapevine, Vigne Vinifere, Wine Grape - Vitis Vinifera - E - M	Stem	365 ppm

PLANTS CONTAINING SILICON

Species	Part	Quantity	Species	Part	Quantity
European Nettle, Stinging Nettle - Urtica Dioica - E - M	Leaf	6,500 ppm	Banana, Plantain - Musa x Paradisiaca - E	Fruit	350 ppm
Red Pignut Hickory - Carya Glabra - E	Shoot	4,180 ppm	Red Currant, White Currant - Ribes Rubrum - E	Fruit	312 ppm
Northern Red Oak - Quercus Rubra - E - M	Stem	2,442 ppm	Eyebright - Euphrasia Officinalis - M	Plant	303 ppm
Shagbark Hickory - Carya Ovata - E	Shoot	2,250 ppm	Coneflower, Echinacea - Echinacea ssp - M	Root	301 ppm
			Goldenseal - Hydrastis Canadensis - M	Root	287 ppm

Plant	Part	ppm
Ginger - Zingiber Officinale - E	Rhizome	285 ppm
Box-Holly, Butcher's broom - Ruscus aculeatus - E - M	Root	280 ppm
Strawberry - Fragaria spp. - E	Fruit	270 ppm
ElytriCouchgrass, Doggrass, Quackgrass, Twitchgrass, Wheatgrass - Elytrigia Repens - E - M	Plant	253 ppm
Corn - Zea Mays - E	Silk Stigma Style	237 ppm
Burdock, Gobo, Great Burdock - Arctium lappa - E - M - T	Root	225 ppm
Hydrangea, Smooth Hydrangea - Hydrangea Arborescens - E - M	Root	223 ppm
Ladyslipper - Cypripedium Pubescens - M	Root	222 ppm
Black Currant - Ribes Nigrum - E	Fruit	220 ppm
Common thyme, Garden thyme, Thyme - Thymus Vulgaris - E - M	Leaf	202 ppm
Pecan - Carya Illinoensis - E	Seed	200 ppm
Rhubarb - Rheum Rhabarbarum - E	Pt	200 ppm
Rowan Berry - Sorbus Aucubaria - E - M - T	Fruit	190 ppm
Oats - Avena Sativa - E - M	Plant	183 ppm
European Pennyroyal - Mentha pulegium - E - M- T	Plant	182 ppm
Commom Licorice, Licorice, Licorice-Root, Smooth Licorice - Glycyrrhiza Glabra - M	Root	158 ppm
Chickweed, Common Chickweed - Stellaria Media - E	Plant	157 ppm
Gotu Kola, Pennywort - Centella Asiatica - E - M	Leaf	140 ppm
Cowberry, Lingen, Lingonberry - Vaccinium Vitis-Idaea var. Minus - E - M	Fruit	133 ppm
Lemongrass, West indian lemongrass - Cymbopogon Citratus - E - M	Plant	132 ppm
Indian Sorrel, Jamaica Sorrel, Stevia, Sweet Leaf of Paraguay - Stevia Rebaudiana - E	Leaf	132 ppm
Cauli Brassica Oleracea var. Botrytis - E	Flower	125 ppm
Crampbark, European Cranberry bush, Guelder Rose, Snowballbush - Viburnum Opulus - E - M - T	Bark	99 ppm
Carrot - Daucus Carota - E	Root	91 ppm
Indian Sorrel, Jamaica Sorrel, Kharkadi, Red Sorrel, Sorrel - Hibiscus Sabdariffa - E	Flower	91 ppm
Cauli Brassica Oleracea var. Botrytis - E	Leaf	90 ppm
Sarsaparilla - Smilax spp - E - M	Root	88 ppm
Pau D'Arco - Tabebuia Heptaphylla - M	Bark	84 ppm
Beet, Beetroot, Garden Beet, Sugar Beet - Beta Vulgaris - E	Root	83 ppm
Bladderwrack, Kelp - Fucus Vesiculosus - E - M	Plant	76 ppm
Onion, Shallot - Allium Cepa - Shallot Bulb - E	Bulb	75 ppm
Flannelleaf, Flannelplant, Great mullein, Mullein, Velvet Verbascum Thapsus - M	Leaf	74 ppm
Bearberry, Uva Uursi - Arctostaphylos Uva-Ursi - M	Leaf	70 ppm
Apple - Malus Domestica - E	Fruit	70 ppm
Irish moss - Chondrus Crispus - E	Plant	67 ppm
Blue Cohosh - Caulophyllum Thalictroides - M	Root	63 ppm
Plum - Prunus Domestica - E - M	Fruit	62 ppm
Cloudberry - Rubus Chamaemorus - E - M	Fruit	62 ppm
Pea - Pisum Sativum - E	Seed	59 ppm
Parsnip - Pastinaca Sativa - E	Root	50 ppm
Mad-Dog Skullcap, Scullcap - Scutellaria lateriflora - M	Plant	48 ppm
SafCarthamus Tinctorius - M	Flower	47 ppm
Dandelion - Taraxacum Officinale - E - M	Root	47 ppm
Alholva, Bockshornklee, Fenugreek, Greek Clover, Greek Trigonella Foenum-Graecum - E - M	Seed	47 ppm
Feverfew - Chrysanthemum Parthenium - M	Plant	46 ppm
Milfoil, Yarrow - Achillea Millefolium - M	Plant	45 ppm
Hops - Humulus Lupulus - E - M - T	Fruit	45 ppm
Common Juniper, Juniper - Juniperus Communis - E - M - T	Fruit	45 ppm
Buchu, Honey Buchu, Mountain Buchu - Agathosma Betulina Buchu, Honey Buchu, Mountain Buchu - Agathosma Betulina - M	Leaf	43 ppm
Devil's claw, Grapple Harpagophytum procumbens - M	Root	43 ppm
Gooseberry - Ribes Uva-Crispa - E	Fruit	42 ppm
Damiana - Turnera Diffusa - M	Leaf	41 ppm

Hillman Health Food Store call 855-Amish-Dr (855-264-7437) www.emineral.info Vitamins and Minerals for Better Living

SILICON CONTINUED

Plant	Part	ppm
Bilberry, Dwarf Bilberry, Whortleberry - Vaccinium Myrtillus - E - M	Fruit	38 ppm
Comfrey - Symphytum Officinale - E - M - T	Root	35 ppm
Chinese Angelica, Dong Gui, Dong Quai - Angelica Sinensis - M	Root	34 ppm
Barley, Barleygrass - Hordeum Vulgare - E - M	Stem	34 ppm
Chinese Magnolia Vine, Five-Flavor-Fruit, Magnolia Vine, Schizandra, Wu Wei Zi, Wu Wei Zu - Schisandra Chinensis - M	Fruit	34 ppm
Bell Pepper, Cherry Pepper, Cone Pepper, Green Pepper, Paprika, Sweet Pepper - Capsicum Annuum - E	Fruit	33 ppm
Garden Camomile, Perennial Camomile, Roman Camomile - Chamaemelum Nobile M	Flower	31 ppm
Chinese Ephedra, Ma Huang - Ephedra Sinica - M	Plant	31 ppm
Chaparral, Creosote Bush - Larrea Tridentata - M	Plant	31 ppm
Sage - Salvia Officinalis - E - M	Leaf	31 ppm
Marshmallow, White Mallow - Althaea Officinalis - M	Root	30 ppm
Rutabaga, Swede, Swedish Turnip - Brassica Napus var. Napobrassica - E	Root	30 ppm
Peach - Prunus Persica - E - M - T	Fruit	30 ppm
White Willow - Salix Alba - M	Bark	29 ppm
European Grape, Grape, Grapevine, Vigne Vinifere, Wine Grape - Vitis Vinifera - E - M	Fruit	28 ppm
Black Cohosh, Black Snake - Cimicifuga Racemosa - E - M	Root	27 ppm
Cabbage, Red Cabbage, White Cabbage - Brassica Oleracea var. Capitata - E	Leaf	25 ppm
Dog Rose, Dogbrier, Rose - Rosa Canina - E - M	Fruit	25 ppm
Barberry - Berberis Vulgaris - M	Root	23 ppm
Mandarin, Tangerine - Citrus Reticulata - E	Fruit	23 ppm
Aloe, Bitter Aloes - Aloe Vera - E - M	Leaf	22 ppm
Black Walnut - Juglans Nigra - E	Fruit	22 ppm
Pear - Pyrus Communis - E	Fruit	20 ppm
Northern Red Oak - Quercus Rubra - E - M	Seed	20 ppm
Horseradish - Armoracia Rusticana - E	Root	19 ppm
White Oak - Quercus Alba - M	Bark	16 ppm
Raspberry, Red raspberry - Rubus Idaeus - E - M	Leaf	13 ppm
Curly Dock, Lengua De Vaca, Sour Dock, Yellow Dock - Rumex Crispus - M - T	Root	13 ppm
Cowgrass, Peavine Clover, Purple Clover, Red Clover - Trifolium Pratense - E - M	Flower	12 ppm
Banana Yucca, Blue Yucca, Spanish Bayonet, Yucca - Yucca Baccata - E - M - T	Root	12 ppm
Potato - Solanum Tuberosum - E	Tuber	10 ppm
Common Valerian, Garden-Heliotrope, Valerian - Valeriana Officinalis - E - M	Root	9 ppm
Indian Tobacco, Lobelia - Lobelia Inflata - M - T	Leaf	8 ppm
Fennel - Foeniculum Vulgare - M	Fruit	4.2 ppm
Celery - Apium Graveolens - E	Root	2 ppm
Black Cutch, Catechu - Acacia Catechu - M	Plant	Trace
Acacia nilotica (L.) WILLD. ex DELILE -- Babul	Plant	Trace
Garlic - Allium Sativum Bulb - E	Bulb	Trace
Devil's Tongue, Elephant Yam, Konjac, Leopard Palm, Snake Palm, Umbrella Arum - Amorphophallus Konjac - E - M - T	Root	Trace
Cayenne, Chili, Hot Pepper, Red Chili, Spur Pepper, Tabasco - Capsicum Frutescens - E	Fruit	Trace
Grape Citrus Paradisi - E	Fruit	Trace
Orange - Citrus Sinensis - E	Fruit	Trace
Blessed Thistle - Cnicus Benedictus - M	Plant	Trace
English Hawthorn, Hawthorn, Whitethorn, Woodland Hawthorn - Crataegus Laevigata - M	Fruit	Trace
Pumpkin - Cucurbita Pepo - E	Seed	Trace
Wild Yam - Dioscorea sp. - E	Root	Trace
Cascara Buckthorn, Cascara Sagrada - Frangula Purshiana - M	Bark	Trace
Soybean - Glycine Max - E	Seed	Trace
Tomato - Lycopersicon Esculentum - E - M - T	Fruit	Trace
Alfalfa, Lucerne - Medicago Sativa subsp. Sativa - E	Plant	Trace
Peppermint - Mentha x Piperita subsp. Nothosubsp. Piperita - E - M - T	Leaf	Trace

Species	Part	Quantity
Bayberry, Candle-Berry, Southern Bayberry, Wax Myrtle - Myrica Cerifera - E - M	Bark	Trace
Catnip - Nepeta Cataria - M	Plant	Trace
Chinese Ginseng, Ginseng, Korean Ginseng, Oriental Ginseng - Panax Ginseng - M	Root	Trace
American Ginseng, Ginseng - Panax Quinquefolius - M	Plant	Trace
Psyllium - Plantago Psyllium - E - M	Seed	Trace
Chinese Cornbind, Chinese Knotweed, Fleeceflower, Fo Ti, He Shou Wu - Polygonum Multiflorum - E - M - T	Root	Trace
Peach - Prunus Persica - E - M - T	Bark	Trace
Lady's Thistle, Milk Thistle - Silybum Marianum - M	Plant	Trace
Red Elm, Slippery Elm - Ulmus Rubra - M	Bark	Trace
European Mistletoe - Viscum Album - M - T	Leaf	Trace

PLANTS CONTAINING SODIUM

Species	Part	Quantity
European Nettle, Stinging Nettle - Urtica Dioica - E - M	Leaf	491,400 ppm
Olive - Olea Europaea - E	Fruit	110,092 ppm
Dulse - Rhodymenia Palmata - E	Plant	99,170 ppm
Irish moss - Chondrus Crispus - E	Plant	81,200 ppm
Bladderwrack, Kelp - Fucus Vesiculosus - E - M	Plant	56,100 ppm
New Zealand Spinach - Tetragonia Tetragonioides - E	Leaf	21,665 ppm
Bok-Choy, Celery Cabbage, Celery Mustard, Chinese Cabbage, Chinese Mustard, Chinese White Cabbage, Pak-Choi - Brassica Chinensis - E	Leaf	21,477 ppm
Lettuce - Lactuca Sativa - E	Leaf	18,560 ppm
Chinese Boxthorn, Chinese Matrimony Vine, Chinese Wolfberry - Lycium Chinense - E - M	Leaf	18,365 ppm
Celery - Apium Graveolens - E	Pt	17,135 ppm
Beet, Beetroot, Garden Beet, Sugar Beet - Beta Vulgaris - E	Leaf	16,571 ppm
Garland Chrysanthemum - Chrysanthemum Coronarium - Bud - E	Leaf	16,300 ppm
Swamp Cabbage, Water Spinach - Ipomoea Aquatica - E	Leaf	15,000 ppm
Rapini, Seven-Top Turnip, Turnip - Brassica Rapa - E	Root	11,600 ppm
Beebread, Beeplant, Borage, Talewort - Borago Officinalis - E - M - T	Plant	11,440 ppm
Spinach - Spinacia Oleracea - E	Plant	10,669 ppm
Radish - Raphanus Sativus - E	Leaf	9,565 ppm
Carrot - Daucus Carota - E	Root	9,504 ppm
Oats - Avena Sativa - E - M	Plant	9,400 ppm
Red Mangrove - Rhizophora Mangle - M	Leaf	9,200 ppm
Purple Tephrosia, Wild Indigo - Tephrosia Purpurea - M - T	Leaf	8,700 ppm
Lantana, Wild Sage - Lantana Camara - M	Leaf	8,200 ppm
Berro, Watercress - Nasturtium Officinale - E	Herb	8,200 ppm
Commom Licorice, Licorice, Licorice-Root, Smooth Licorice - Glycyrrhiza Glabra - M	Root	8,180 ppm
Chinese Parsley, Cilantro, Coriander - Coriandrum Sativum - E	Leaf	7,581 ppm
Purslane, Verdolaga - Portulaca Oleracea - E	Herb	7,400 ppm
Garland Chrysanthemum - Chrysanthemum Coronarium - Bud - E	Bud	6,990 ppm
Artichoke - Cynara Cardunculus - E	Flower	6,840 ppm
Beet, Beetroot, Garden Beet, Sugar Beet - Beta Vulgaris - E	Root	6,705 ppm
Tomato - Lycopersicon Esculentum - E - M - T	Fruit	6,600 ppm
Parsley - Petroselinum Crispum - E	Plant	5,569 ppm
European Pennyroyal - Mentha pulegium - E - M - T	Plant	5,410 ppm
Dandelion - Taraxacum Officinale - E - M	Leaf	5,278 ppm
Radish - Raphanus Sativus - E	Root	5,020 ppm
Swamp Taro - Cyrtosperma Chamissonis - E	Root	4,855 ppm
American Ginseng, Ginseng - Panax Quinquefolius - M	Plant	4,800 ppm
Snakegourd - Trichosanthes Anguina - E - M	Fruit	4,630 ppm
Dog Rose, Dogbrier, Rose - Rosa Canina - E - M	Fruit	4,600 ppm
Collards, Cow Cabbage, Spring-Heading Cabbage, Tall Kale, Tree Kale - Brassica Oleracea - E	Leaf	4,589 ppm
Endive, Escarole - Cichorium Endivia - M	Leaf	4,560 ppm

SODIUM CONTINUED

Plant	Part	ppm
Cabbage, Red Cabbage, White Cabbage - Brassica Oleracea var. Capitata - E	Leaf	4,510 ppm
Black Mustard - Brassica Nigra - E	Leaf	4,506 ppm
Indian Saffron, Turmeric - Curcuma Longa - E	Rhizome	4,290 ppm
Soybean - Glycine Max - E	Seed	3,800 ppm
Curly Kale, Kale, Kitchen Kale, Scotch Kale - Brassica Oleracea var. Sabellica l. var. Acephala - E	Leaf	3,650 ppm
Comfrey - Symphytum Officinale - E - M - T	Root	3,510 ppm
Rice - Oryza Sativa - E	Plant	3,500 ppm
Dill, Garden Dill - Anethum Graveolens - E	Plant	3,308 ppm
Clove, Clovetree - Syzygium Aromaticum - E	Flower	3,250 ppm
Cauli Brassica Oleracea var. Botrytis - E	Leaf	3,091 ppm
Wheat - Triticum Aestivum - E - M	Plant	3,000 ppm
Broadbean, Faba Bean, Habas - Vicia Faba - E	Fruit	2,980 ppm
Du Zhong, Gutta-Percha Tree, Tu Chung - Eucommia Ulmoides - M	Bark	2,820 ppm
Buchu, Honey Buchu, Mountain Buchu - Agathosma Betulina	Leaf	2,760 ppm
Buchu, Honey Buchu, Mountain Buchu - Agathosma Betulina - M		
Cassava, Tapioca, Yuca - Manihot Esculenta - E	Root	2,655 ppm
Chinese Magnolia Vine, Five-Flavor-Fruit, Magnolia Vine, Schizandra, Wu Wei Zi, Wu Wei Zu - Schisandra Chinensis - M	Fruit	2,630 ppm
Broadbean, Faba Bean, Habas - Vicia Faba - E	Seed	2,630 ppm
Garden Camomile, Perennial Camomile, Roman Camomile - Chamaemelum Nobile M	Flower	2,580 ppm
Applemint - Mentha x Rotundifolia - E - M - T	Leaf	2,520 ppm
Chicory, Succory, Witloof - Cichorium Intybus - E - M	Root	2,500 ppm
White Mulberry - Morus Alba - E - M	Fruit	2,467 ppm
Pigweed - Amaranthus sp. - E - M	Leaf	2,406 ppm
Jerusalem Artichoke - Helianthus Tuberosus E	Tuber	2,400 ppm
SafCarthamus Tinctorius - M	Flower	2,320 ppm
Cauli Brassica Oleracea var. Botrytis - E	Flower	2,300 ppm
Barley, Barleygrass - Hordeum Vulgare - E - M	Stem	2,240 ppm
Kohlrabi - Brassica Oleracea var. Gongylodes - E	Stem	2,222 ppm
Ban-Xia, Pan-Hsia - Pinellia Ternata - E - M - T	Tuber	2,200 ppm
Wheat - Triticum Aestivum - E - M	Seed	2,200 ppm
Aubergine, Egg Solanum Melongena - E	Fruit	2,150 ppm
Chinese Boxthorn, Chinese Matrimony Vine, Chinese Wolfberry - Lycium Chinense - E - M	Fruit	2,140 ppm
Onion, Shallot - Allium Cepa - Shallot Bulb - E	Bulb	2,052 ppm
Guinea Grass - Panicum Maximum - M	Leaf	0-4,100 ppm
Cumin - Cuminum Cyminum - E - M	Fruit	2,028 ppm
Brussel-Sprout - Brassica Oleracea var. Gemmifera - E	Leaf	1,990 ppm
Fennel - Foeniculum Vulgare - M	Fruit	1,980 ppm
Broomrape, Cistanchis Herba, Jou Tsung Jung - Cistanche Salsa - M	Plant	1,970 ppm
Peppermint - Mentha x Piperita subsp. Nothosubsp. Piperita - E - M - T	Leaf	1,950 ppm
Water Lotus - Nelumbo Nucifera - E - M	Rhizome	1,935 ppm
Chinese Cabbage - Brassica Pekinensis - E	Leaf	1,932 ppm
Kuan Chung, Shield Fernle - Blechnum Orientale - E - M - T	Rhizome	1,930 ppm
Rutabaga, Swede, Swedish Turnip - Brassica Napus var. Napobrassica - E	Root	1,930 ppm
Strawberry Guava - Psidium Cattleianum - E	Fruit	1,915 ppm
Celery - Apium Graveolens - E	Seed	1,900 ppm
Ben Nut, Benzolive Tree, Drumstick Tree, Horseradish Tree, Moringa, West Indian Ben - Moringa Oleifera - E	Fruit	420-3,560 ppm
Soybean - Glycine Max - E	Sprout Seedling	1,622 ppm
Oats - Avena Sativa - E - M	Seed	1,600 ppm
Burdock, Gobo, Great Burdock - Arctium lappa - E - M - T	Root	1,520 ppm
Waxgourd - Benincasa Hispida - Fruit	Fruit	1,500 ppm
Common thyme, Garden thyme, Thyme - Thymus Vulgaris - E - M	Leaf	1,490 ppm
Chickweed, Common Chickweed - Stellaria Media - E	Plant	1,470 ppm
Perilla - Perilla Frutescens - E - M - T	Leaf	1,429 ppm
Chicory, Succory, Witloof - Cichorium Intybus - E - M	Leaf	1,428 ppm

Name	Part	ppm
Emblic, Myrobalan - Phyllanthus Emblica - E	Fruit	1,384 ppm
Marshmallow, White Mallow - Althaea Officinalis - M	Root	1,370 ppm
Common thyme, Garden thyme, Thyme - Thymus Vulgaris - E - M	Plant	1,341 ppm
Chinese Licorice - Glycyrrhiza Uralensis - M	Root	1,340 ppm
Garden Cress - Lepidium Sativum - E	Leaf	1,320 ppm
Butterbur - Petasites Japonicus - T	Pt	1,270 ppm
Bitter Melon, Sorosi - Momordica Charantia - E	Leaf	1,234 ppm
Sweet Potato - Ipomoea Batatas - E	Root	1,229 ppm
Blessed Thistle - Cnicus Benedictus - M	Plant	1,220 ppm
Acerola - Malpighia Glabra - E - M	Fruit	1,219 ppm
Dandelion - Taraxacum Officinale - E - M	Root	1,130 ppm
Cantaloupe, Melon, Muskmelon, Netted Melon, Nutmeg Melon, Persian Melon - Cucumis Melo subsp. ssp Melo var.Ccantalupensis - Friut - E	Fruit	1,115 ppm
Pomarrosa, Rose Apple - Syzygium Jambos - E	Fruit	340-2,200 ppm
Sage - Salvia Officinalis - E - M	Leaf	1,080 ppm
Gotu Kola, Pennywort - Centella Asiatica - E - M	Leaf	1,040 ppm
Soursop - Annona Muricata - E	Fruit	1,035 ppm
Pumpkin - Cucurbita Pepo - E	Flower	1,030 ppm
Flax, Lin Linum Usitatissimum - E	Seed	1,014 ppm
Giant Taro - Alocasia Macrorrhiza - E	Root	1,010 ppm
Capillary Wormwood - Artemisia Capillaris - M	Plant	1,010 ppm
Okra - Abelmoschus Esculentus - Friut - E - M	Fruit	1,000 ppm
Baikal Skullcap, Chinese Skullcap, Huang Qin - Scutellaria Baicalensis - M	Root	991 ppm
Cape Jasmine, Gardenia, Jasmin, Shan-Chih-Tzu, Shan-Zhi-Zi, Zhi Zi - Gardenia Jasminoides - M	Fruit	985 ppm
Black Caraway, Black Cumin, Fennel-Flower, Nutmeg-Flower, Roman Coriander - Nigella Sativa - E - M	Seed	980 ppm
Asian Plantain - Plantago Asiatica - E - M	Plant	950 ppm
Bai-Wei, Pai-Wei - Cynanchum Atratum - E - M	Root	940 ppm
Oriental Pipewort - Eriocaulon spp. - M	Leaf	940 ppm
Rice - Oryza Sativa - E	Seed	939 ppm
Marjoram, Sweet Marjoram - Origanum Majorana - E	Plant	935 ppm
Sicklepod - Senna Obtusifolia - E - T	Seed	930 ppm
Alholva, Bockshornklee, Fenugreek, Greek Clover, Greek Trigonella Foenum-Graecum - E - M	Seed	915 ppm
Chervil - Anthriscus Cerefolium E	Leaf	895 ppm
Indian Sorrel, Jamaica Sorrel, Stevia, Sweet Leaf of Paraguay - Stevia Rebaudiana - E	Leaf	892 ppm
Salsify - Tragopogon Porrifolius - E	Root	870 ppm
Betel Nut, Pin-Lang - Areca Catechu Amphicarpaea Bracteata- E - M	Seed	867 ppm
Cornmint, Field Mint, Japanese Mint - Mentha Arvensis var. Piperascens - E - M- T	Plant	860 ppm
Rhubarb - Rheum Rhabarbarum - E	Pt	855 ppm
Allspice, Clover-Pepper, Jamaica-Pepper, Pimenta, Pimento - Pimenta Dioica - E	Fruit	842 ppm
Date Palm - Phoenix Dactylifera - E	Seed	820 ppm
Aceituna Dulce, Jambolan, Java Plum - Syzygium Cumini - E	Fruit	90-1,605 ppm
Mace, Nutmeg - Myristica Fragrans - E	Aril	800 ppm
Chinese Boxthorn, Chinese Matrimony Vine, Chinese Wolfberry - Lycium Chinense - E - M	Root Bark	793 ppm
Green Gram, Mungbean - Vigna Radiata - E	Sprout Seedling	782 ppm
Mongoloid Dandelion - Taraxacum Mongolicum - E - M	Plant	763 ppm
Alholva, Bockshornklee, Fenugreek, Greek Clover, Greek Trigonella Foenum-Graecum - E - M	Leaf	761 ppm
Bayberry, Candle-Berry, Southern Bayberry, Wax Myrtle - Myrica Cerifera - E - M	Bark	760 ppm
Large-Fruited Provision Tree - Pachira Macrocarpa - E	Seed	760 ppm
Flannelleaf, Flannelplant, Great mullein, Mullein, Velvet Verbascum Thapsus - M	Leaf	760 ppm
Corn - Zea Mays - E	Seed	757 ppm

SODIUM CONTINUED

Jew's Mallow, Mulukiya, Nalta Jute - Corchorus Olitorius - E - M	Leaf	755 ppm
Chives - Allium Schoenoprasum - E	Leaf	750 ppm
Mountain Yam - Dioscorea Pentaphylla - E	Root	750 ppm
Indian Tamarind, Kilytree, Tamarind - Tamarindus Indica - M	Fruit	743 ppm
Cayenne, Chili, Hot Pepper, Red Chili, Spur Pepper, Tabasco - Capsicum Frutescens - E	Fruit	734 ppm
Terminalia catappa L. -- Indian Almond, Malabar Almond, Tropical Almond	Seed	730 ppm
Devil's claw, Grapple Harpagophytum procumbens - M	Root	718 ppm
Cucumber - Cucumis Sativus - E	Fruit	714 ppm
Indian Fig, Nopal, Nopalito, Prickly Pear - Opuntia Ficus-Indica - E - M	Seed	714 ppm
Papaya - Carica Papaya - E - M	Leaf	711 ppm
Ginger - Zingiber Officinale - E	Rhizome	709 ppm
Black bean, Dwarf bean, Field bean, Flageolet bean, French bean, Garden bean, Green bean, Haricot, Haricot bean, Haricot vert, Kidney bean, Navy bean, Pop bean, Popping bean, Snap bean, String bean, Wax bean - Phaseolus Vulgaris - E	Fruit	707 ppm
Asparagus - Asparagus Officinalis - E	Shoot	685 ppm
Asparagus bean, Pea bean, Yardlong bean - Vigna Unguiculata subsp. Sesquipedalis - E	Shoot	685 ppm
Lemongrass, West indian lemongrass - Cymbopogon Citratus - E - M	Plant	640 ppm
Sesame - Sesamum Indicum - E - M	Seed	634 ppm
Indian Gooseberry, Otaheite Gooseberry - Phyllanthus Acidus - E	Fruit	632 ppm
Black Pepper, Pepper, White Pepper - Piper Nigrum - E - M	Fruit	627 ppm
Coconut, Coconut Palm - Cocos Nucifera - E	Seed	626 ppm
Chinese Foxglove - Rehmannia Glutinosa - M	Root	626 ppm
Bell Pepper, Cherry Pepper, Cone Pepper, Green Pepper, Paprika, Sweet Pepper - Capsicum Annuum - E	Fruit	625 ppm
Tarragon - Artemisia Dracunculus - M	Plant	620 ppm
Ajwan - Trachyspermum Ammi - E - M	Fruit	605 ppm
Luffa, Smooth Loofah, Vegetable Sponge - Luffa Aegyptiaca - E	Fruit	600 ppm
Chinese Spikenard - Nardostachys Chinensis - M	Rhizome	596 ppm
Rosemary - Rosmarinus Officinalis - E - M	Plant	592 ppm
Equatorial Ivory Palm - Phytelephas Aequatorialis - E	Mesocarp	180-1,165 ppm
Pea - Pisum Sativum - E	Fruit	578 ppm
Parsnip - Pastinaca Sativa - E	Root	575 ppm
Chayote - Sechium Edule - E - M	Fruit	570 ppm
Maracuya, Passion Passiflora Edulis - E	Fruit	280-1,124 ppm
Field Horsetail, Horsetail - Equisetum Arvense - M	Plant	560 ppm
Garlic - Allium Sativum Bulb - E	Bulb	559 ppm
Yambean - Pachyrhizus Erosus - E	Tuber	555 ppm
Papaya - Carica Papaya - E - M	Fruit	554 ppm
Lentil - Lens Culinaris - E	Sprout Seedling	545 ppm
Mamey - Mammea Americana - Fruit	Fruit	150-1,085 ppm
Psyllium - Plantago Psyllium - E - M	Seed	540 ppm
Malanga, Tannia, Yautia - Xanthosoma Sagittifolium - E	Leaf	540 ppm
Chinese Angelica, Dong Gui, Dong Quai - Angelica Sinensis - M	Root	539 ppm
Black Oak - Quercus Velutina - E - M	Stem	539 ppm
Pistachio - Pistacia Vera - E	Seed	538 ppm
Blackberry Lily, Shenan - Belamcanda Chinensis - M	Rhizome	527 ppm
White Mulberry - Morus Alba - E - M	Root Bark	520 ppm
Avocado - Persea Americana - E - M - T	Fruit	520 ppm
Pepper Elder, Yerba De La Plata - Peperomia Pelucida - Leaf	Leaf	80-1,025 ppm
Aloe, Bitter Aloes - Aloe Vera - E - M	Leaf	510 ppm
Tea - Camellia Sinensis - E	Leaf	500 ppm
Garden Sorrel - Rumex Acetosa - E - M - T	Leaf	500 ppm
Japanese Ginseng - Panax Japonicus - M	Rhizome	499 ppm
Radish - Raphanus Sativus - E	Fruit	495 ppm
Water Lotus - Nelumbo Nucifera - E - M	Seed	490 ppm

Name	Part	ppm
Taro - Colocasia Esculenta - E	Leaf	484 ppm
Elephant Garlic, Kurrat - Allium Ampeloprasum - E	Leaf	472 ppm
Balloon Flower, Chieh-Keng, Jie-Geng - Platycodon Grandiflorum - E - M - T	Root	472 ppm
Lemon - Citrus Limon - E	Fruit	470 ppm
Wu Chia Pi - Acanthopanax Gracilistylis - M	Root Bark	463 ppm
Water Chestnut - Eleocharis Dulcis - Tuber	Tuber	100-920 ppm
Calamus, Flagroot, Myrtle Flag, Sweet Calamus, Sweetflag, Sweet Acorus Calamus - M	Rhizome	459 ppm
Sugar-Apple, Sweetsop - Annona Squamosa - E	Fruit	457 ppm
Tomatillo - Physalis Ixocarpa - E	Fruit	454 ppm
European Grape, Grape, Grapevine, Vigne Vinifere, Wine Grape - Vitis Vinifera - E - M	Fruit	454 ppm
Calabash Gourd, White-Flowered Gourd - Lagenaria Siceraria - E	Fruit	450 ppm
Black Gram - Vigna Mungo - E	Seed	449 ppm
Jussiaeae Herba, Pond Dragon - Jussiaea Repens - M	Plant	438 ppm
Coca - Erythroxylum Coca var. Coca - E - M	Leaf	435 ppm
Chinese Parsley, Cilantro, Coriander - Coriandrum Sativum E	Fruit	430 ppm
Chinese Ephedra, Ma Huang - Ephedra Sinica - M	Plant	430 ppm
Asparagus Pea, Goa Bean, Winged Bean - Psophocarpus Tetragonolobus - E	Seed	429 ppm
Chai-Hu - Bupleurum - M	Root	428 ppm
Udo - Aralia Cordata - E - M	Leaf	425 ppm
Bei Sha Shen - Glehnia Littoralis - E - M	Root	425 ppm
Red Cedar - Juniperus Virginiana Amphicarpaea Bracteata- E - M - T	Shoot	422 ppm
Blueberry - Vaccinium Corymbosum - F	Fruit	414 ppm
Chaparral, Creosote Bush - Larrea Tridentata - M	Plant	410 ppm
Pear - Pyrus Communis - E	Fruit	407 ppm
Sweet Potato - Ipomoea Batatas - E	Leaf	400 ppm
Malanga, Tannia, Yautia - Xanthosoma Sagittifolium - E	Root	400 ppm
Bei-Mu, Fritillary - Fritillaria Thunbergii - Blub - E - M	Bulb	396 ppm
Northern Red Oak - Quercus Rubra - E - M	Stem	396 ppm
Jack Bean - Canavalia Ensiformis - E	Seed	394 ppm
Basil, Cuban Basil, Sweet Basil - Ocimum Basilicum - E	Plant	386 ppm
Indian Sorrel, Jamaica Sorrel, Kharkadi, Red Sorrel, Sorrel - Hibiscus Sabdariffa - E	Flower	382 ppm
Date Palm - Phoenix Dactylifera - E	Fruit	380 ppm
White Oak - Quercus Alba - M	Stem	380 ppm
Air Potato, Potato Yam - Dioscorea Bulbifera - E	Rhizome	378 ppm
Fig - Ficus Carica - E	Fruit	366 ppm
Peach - Prunus Persica - E - M - T	Fruit	366 ppm
Lentil - Lens Culinaris - E	Seed	360 ppm
Loquat - Eriobotrya Japonica - E	Fruit	351 ppm
Indian Tamarind, Kilytree, Tamarind - Tamarindus Indica - M	Leaf	351 ppm
Barberry - Berberis Vulgaris - M	Root	350 ppm
Pomegranate - Punica Granatum - E	Fruit	350 ppm
Greater Yam, Winged Yam - Dioscorea Alata - E	Root	335 ppm
Bitter Melon, Sorosi - Momordica Charantia - E	Fruit	333 ppm
Asparagus bean, Pea bean, Yardlong bean - Vigna Unguiculata subsp. Sesquipedalis - E	Fruit	333 ppm
Mat Bean, Moth Bean - Vigna Aconitifolia - E	Seed	332 ppm
Henbane - Hyoscyamus Niger - E - M	Seed	327 ppm
Potato - Solanum Tuberosum - E	Tuber	323 ppm
Mud Plantain, Tse-Hsieh, Water Plantain, Ze-Xie - Alisma Plantago-Aquatica - M	Rhizome	322 ppm
Horseradish - Armoracia Rusticana - E	Root	315 ppm
Summer Squash - Cucurbita spp. - E	Fruit	315 ppm
Green Gram, Mungbean - Vigna Radiata - E	Seed	311 ppm
Chickpea, Garbanzo - Cicer Arietinum - E	Seed	310 ppm
Opium Poppy, Poppyseed Poppy - Papaver Somniferum - E	Seed	300 ppm
Red Pignut Hickory - Carya Glabra - E	Shoot	297 ppm
Pea - Pisum Sativum - E	Seed	297 ppm
Chinese Goldthread, Huang-Lian, Huang-Lien - Coptis Chinensis - M	Rhizome	296 ppm

SODIUM CONTINUED

Name	Part	ppm
Huang-Lia, Huang-Lian, Huang-Lien, Japanese Goldthread - Coptis Japonica - M	Rhizome	296 ppm
Generic Goldthread - Coptis spp. - M	Rhizome	296 ppm
Kiwi - Actinidia Chinensis - E	Fruit	295 ppm
Garlic - Allium Sativum Bulb - E	Leaf	294 ppm
Rush - Juncus Effusus E - M - T	Pith	291 ppm
Chih-Mu, Zhi-Mu - Anemarrhena Asphodeloides - M	Rhizome	289 ppm
Cassia, Cassia Bark, Cassia Lignea, China Junk Cassia, Chinazimt, Chinese Cassia - Cinnamomum Aromaticuminnamon- E - M - T	Bark	287 ppm
Ceylon Cinnamon, Cinnamon - Cinnamomum Verum - E - M - T	Bark	287 ppm
Common Garden Peony, Peony, White Peony - Paeonia Lactiflora - M	Root	286 ppm
Cherimoya - Annona Cherimola - E	Fruit	285 ppm
Asian Wild Ginger - Asiasarum Heterotropoides - M	Root	278 ppm
Siebold's Wild Ginger - Asiasarum Sieboldii - M	Root	278 ppm
Custard Apple - Annona Reticulata - E	Fruit	275 ppm
Mai-Men-Dong, Mai-Men-Tung - Ophiopogon Japonicus - M	Tuber	273 ppm
Shagbark Hickory - Carya Ovata - E	Shoot	270 ppm
Butter Bean, Lima Bean - Phaseolus Lunatus - E	Seed	269 ppm
Averrhoa bilimbi L. -- Bilimbi, Limon chino	Fruit	40-533 ppm
Summer Savory - Satureja Hortensis - E	Plant	264 ppm
Dill, Garden Dill - Anethum Graveolens - E	Fruit	262 ppm
Groundnut, Peanut - Arachis Hypogaea - E - M	Seed	260 ppm
Bonavist Bean, Hyacinth Bean, Lablab Bean - Lablab Purpureus - E - M - T	Seed	260 ppm
Cashew - Anacardium Occidentale - E	Seed	257 ppm
Barley, Barleygrass - Hordeum Vulgare - E - M	Sprout Seedling	256 ppm
Nutsedge - Cyperus Rotundus - E - M	Rhizome	254 ppm
Desert Wormwood - Artemisia Herba-Alba - M	Plant	250 ppm
Lambsquarter - Chenopodium Album - E - M - T	Leaf	250 ppm
Genipap, Jagua - Genipa Americana - E - M	Fruit	250 ppm
Indian Tamarind, Kilytree, Tamarind - Tamarindus Indica - M	Flower	250 ppm
Quince - Cydonia Oblonga - E	Fruit	247 ppm
Chinese Senega - Polygala Tenuifolia - M	Root	247 ppm
Guavas - Psidium Guajava - E	Fruit	246 ppm
Bai-Zhu, Pai-Chu - Atractylodes Ovata - M	Rhizome	238 ppm
Watermelon - Citrullus Lanatus - E	Fruit	236 ppm
Elephant-Foot Yam - Amorphophallus Campanulatus - E - M- T	Root	233 ppm
Perejil - Peperomia Pereskiifolia - Leaf	Leaf	70-465 ppm
Common Valerian, Garden-Heliotrope, Valerian - Valeriana Officinalis - E - M	Root	230 ppm
Tian Ma - Gastrodia Elata - Rhizome	Rhizome	228 ppm
Lime - Citrus Aurantiifolia - E	Fruit	222 ppm
American Styrax, Sweetgum - Liquidambar Styraciflua - E - M	Plant	220 ppm
Sour Cherry - Prunus Cerasus - E - M - T	Plant	216 ppm
Chinese Anemone - Pulsatilla Chinensis - M	Root	213 ppm
Caraway, Carum - Carum Carvi - E	Fruit	212 ppm
Dokudami, Fishwort, Yu Xing Cao - Houttuynia Cordata - E - M	Plant	212 ppm
Mimosa - Albizia Julibrissin - E - M	Bark	211 ppm
Ben Nut, Benzolive Tree, Drumstick Tree, Horseradish Tree, Moringa, West Indian Ben - Moringa Oleifera - E	Shoot	90-420 ppm
Chinese Ginseng, Ginseng, Korean Ginseng, Oriental Ginseng - Panax Ginseng - M	Root	209 ppm
Morinda - Morinda spp. - M	Root	206 ppm
Pigeonpea - Cajanus Vajan - E	Seed	205 ppm
Common Turkish Oregano, European Oregano, Oregano, Pot Marjoram, Wild Marjoram, Wild Oregano - Origanum Vulgare - E	Plant	205 ppm
Aconite, Fu-Tsu - Aconitum Carmichaelii - E - M	Tuber	204 ppm
Perilla - Perilla Frutescens - E - M - T	Plant	204 ppm
Chaff Achyranthes Bidentata - M	Root	198 ppm

Species	Part	Quantity
Cang Zhu - Atractylodes Lancea - M	Rhizome	197 ppm
Cardamom - Elettaria Cardamomum - E - M	Seed	196 ppm
Madder - Rubia Cordifolia - M	Root	195 ppm
Pumpkin - Cucurbita Pepo - E	Seed	193 ppm
Curry Murraya spp. - E - M	Fruit	192 ppm
Chayote - Sechium Edule - E - M	Shoot	190 ppm
Bastard Cardamom, Chin Kousha, Malabar Cardamom, Tavoy Cardamom - Amomum Xanthioides - E	Seed	187 ppm
Asparagus bean, Pea bean, Yardlong bean - Vigna Unguiculata subsp. Sesquipedalis - E	Seed	186 ppm
Jih-Chiung - Cnidium Officinale - M	Rhizome	185 ppm
Crampbark, European Cranberry bush, Guelder Rose, Snowballbush - Viburnum Opulus - E - M - T	Bark	184 ppm
Pineapple - Ananas Comosus - E	Fruit	180 ppm
Evening-Primrose - Oenothera Biennis - E - M	Seed	180 ppm
Moutan, Tree Peony - Paeonia Moutan - M	Root Bark	180 ppm
Anise, Sweet Cumin - Pimpinella Anisum - E - M	Fruit	177 ppm
Buckbush - Symphoricarpos Orbiculatus - M	Stem	176 ppm
Carambola, Star Averrhoa Carambola - E	Fruit	17-351 ppm
Grape Citrus Paradisi - E	Fruit	175 ppm
Chinese Rhubarb - Rheum Palmatum - E	Rhizome	175 ppm
Alfalfa, Lucerne - Medicago Sativa subsp. Sativa - E	Plant	170 ppm
Corn Salad, Lamb's Lettuce - Valerianella Locusta - E	Plant	321-331 ppm
Genipap, Jagua - Genipa Americana - E - M	Seed	165 ppm
White Lupine - Lupinus Albus - M - T	Seed	165 ppm
American Cranberry, Cranberry, Large Cranberry - Vaccinium Macrocarpon - E	Fruit	165 ppm
Ginkgo, Maidenhair Tree - Ginkgo Biloba - Tree - E - M - T	Seed	160 ppm
Mace, Nutmeg - Myristica Fragrans - E	Seed	160 ppm
Mad-Dog Skullcap, Scullcap - Scutellaria lateriflora - M	Plant	160 ppm
Cowgrass, Peavine Clover, Purple Clover, Red Clover - Trifolium Pratense - E - M	Flower	160 ppm
Noble Dendrobium - Dendrobium Nobile - M	Stem	156 ppm
European Grape, Grape, Grapevine, Vigne Vinifere, Wine Grape - Vitis Vinifera - E - M	Stem	156 ppm
Antler Herb, Clubmoss - Lycopodium Clavatum - M - T	Plant	155 ppm
Heal-All, Self-Heal - Prunella Vulgaris - E - M	Flower	155 ppm
Mandarin, Tangerine - Citrus Reticulata - E	Fruit	154 ppm
Jack Artocarpus Heterophyllus - E	Fruit	150 ppm
Indian Tobacco, Lobelia - Lobelia Inflata - M - T	Leaf	150 ppm
Almond - Prunus Dulcis - E - M - T	Seed	147 ppm
Bai Zhi - Angelica Dahurica - M	Root	143 ppm
Mango - Mangifera Indica - E - M	Fruit	143 ppm
Guanique - Chamissoa Altissima - M	Leaf	28-280 ppm
Japanese Gentian - Gentiana Scabra - E	Root	140 ppm
Chinese Dogwood - Cornus Officinalis - E - M	Fruit	138 ppm
Cockscomb - Celosia Cristata - M	Flower	137 ppm
Chinese Birthwort - Aristolochia Debilis - E - M - T	Fruit	136 ppm
Jojoba - Simmondsia Chinensis Seed	Seed	136 ppm
Paper Mulberry - Broussonetia Papyrifera - E - M	Fruit	135 ppm

PLANTS CONTAINING STRONTIUM

Species	Part	Quantity
Red Pignut Hickory - Carya Glabra - E	Shoot	1,100 ppm
American Persimmon - Diospyros Virginiana - E - M	Leaf	1,000 ppm
Black Gum, Black Tupelo - Nyssa Sylvatica - E - M	Leaf	910 ppm
Shagbark Hickory - Carya Ovata - E	Shoot	900 ppm
Black Gum, Black Tupelo - Nyssa Sylvatica - E - M	Stem	880 ppm
Cabbage, Red Cabbage, White Cabbage - Brassica Oleracea var. Capitata - E	Leaf	870 ppm
American Styrax, Sweetgum - Liquidambar Styraciflua - E - M	Stem	840 ppm
Sassafras - Sassafras Albidum - E - M - T	Leaf	680 ppm
Smooth Sumac - Rhus Glabra - E - M	Stem	670 ppm
Lettuce - Lactuca Sativa - E	Shoot	580 ppm

STRONTIUM CONTINUED

Plant	Part	ppm
White Oak - Quercus Alba - M	Plant	532 ppm
Black Cherry, Wild Cherry - Prunus Serotina - E - M - T	Stem	480 ppm
Red Cedar - Juniperus Virginiana Amphicarpaea Bracteata - E - M - T	Shoot	440 ppm
Buckbush - Symphoricarpos Orbiculatus - M	Stem	440 ppm
Dwarf Sumac, Winged Sumac - Rhus Copallina - E - M	Stem	427 ppm
Chinese Cabbage - Brassica Pekinensis - E	Leaf	420 ppm
Parsley - Petroselinum Crispum - E	Plant	396 ppm
American Persimmon - Diospyros Virginiana - E - M	Stem	378 ppm
Sassafras - Sassafras Albidum - E - M - T	Stem	370 ppm
Northern Red Oak - Quercus Rubra - E - M	Stem	330 ppm
Dwarf Sumac, Winged Sumac - Rhus Copallina - E - M	Leaf	288 ppm
American Styrax, Sweetgum - Liquidambar Styraciflua - E - M	Leaf	246 ppm
Endive, Escarole - Cichorium Endivia - M	Shoot	240 ppm
Grape Citrus Paradisi - E	Fruit	220 ppm
Asparagus - Asparagus Officinalis - E	Shoot	200 ppm
Black Oak - Quercus Velutina - E - M	Stem	186 ppm
Onion, Shallot - Allium Cepa - Shallot Bulb - E	Bulb	162 ppm
Butterbur - Petasites Japonicus - T	Plant	160 ppm
Carrot - Daucus Carota - E	Root	148 ppm
Tomato - Lycopersicon Esculentum - E - M - T	Fruit	140 ppm
Qian Hu - Peucedanum Decursivum - M	Plant	130 ppm
Willow Oak - Quercus Phellos - E - M	Stem	126 ppm
Post Oak - Quercus Stellata - E - M	Stem	126 ppm
Giant Knotweed, Hu-Zhang, Japanese Knotweed, Mexican Bamboo - Polygonum Cuspidatum - E - M - T	Plant	120 ppm
Dandelion - Taraxacum Officinale - E - M	Plant	120 ppm
Ramie - Boehmeria Nivea - M	Plant	118 ppm
Orange - Citrus Sinensis - E	Fruit	110 ppm
Alehoof - Glechoma Hederacea - M	Plant	110 ppm
Black bean, Dwarf bean, Field bean, Flageolet bean, French bean, Garden bean, Green bean, Haricot, Haricot bean, Haricot vert, Kidney bean, Navy bean, Pop bean, Popping bean, Snap bean, String bean, Wax bean - Phaseolus Vulgaris - E	Fruit	105 ppm
Coca - Erythroxylum Coca var. Coca - E - M	Leaf	104 ppm
Butter Bean, Lima Bean - Phaseolus Lunatus - E	Seed	100 ppm
Cucumber - Cucumis Sativus - E	Fruit	98 ppm
Shortleaf Pine - Pinus Echinata - M	Shoot	84 ppm
Japanese Cinnamon - Cinnamomum Sieboldii - E - M - T	Bark	80 ppm
Ceylon Cinnamon, Cinnamon - Cinnamomum Verum - E - M - T	Bark	80 ppm
Brazilnut, Brazilnut-Tree, Creamnut, Paranut - Bertholletia Eexcelsa - E	Seed	77 ppm
Beet, Beetroot, Garden Beet, Sugar Beet - Beta Vulgaris - E	Root	70 ppm
Japanese Cinnamon - Cinnamomum Sieboldii - E - M - T	Root Bark	70 ppm
Java Cinnamon, Padang Cassia - Cinnamomum Burmannii - E - M - T	Bark	60 ppm
Chinese Polystichum - Polystichum Polyblepharum - T	Plant	60 ppm
Potato - Solanum Tuberosum - E	Tuber	60 ppm
Clove, Clovetree - Syzygium Aromaticum - E	Flower	60 ppm
Asparagus bean, Pea bean, Yardlong bean - Vigna Unguiculata subsp Sesquipedalis - E	Seed	60 ppm
Plum - Prunus Domestica - E - M	Fruit	51 ppm
Mugwort - Artemisia Vulgaris - M	Plant	50 ppm
Cassia, Cassia Bark, Cassia Lignea, China Junk Cassia, Chinazimt, Chinese Cassia - Cinnamomum Aromaticuminnamon - E - M - T	Bark	50 ppm
Peach - Prunus Persica - E - M - T	Fruit	45 ppm
Soybean - Glycine Max - E	Seed	42 ppm
European Grape, Grape, Grapevine, Vigne Vinifere, Wine Grape - Vitis Vinifera - E - M	Fruit	38.5 ppm

Species	Part	Quantity
Black bean, Dwarf bean, Field bean, Flageolet bean, French bean, Garden bean, Green bean, Haricot, Haricot bean, Haricot vert, Kidney bean, Navy bean, Pop bean, Popping bean, Snap bean, String bean, Wax bean - Phaseolus Vulgaris - E	Seed	34 ppm
Allspice, Clover-Pepper, Jamaica-Pepper, Pimenta, Pimento - Pimenta Dioica - E	Plant	20 ppm
Pear - Pyrus Communis - E	Fruit	18.5 ppm
Cantaloupe, Melon, Muskmelon, Netted Melon, Nutmeg Melon, Persian Melon - Cucumis Melo subsp. ssp Melo var.Ccantalupensis - Friut - E	Fruit	16.5 ppm
Almond - Prunus Dulcis - E - M - T	Seed	16 ppm
Corn - Zea Mays - E	Seed	14 ppm
Bell Pepper, Cherry Pepper, Cone Pepper, Green Pepper, Paprika, Sweet Pepper - Capsicum Annuum - E	Fruit	12 ppm
Pistachio - Pistacia Vera - E	Seed	10 ppm
Apple - Malus Domestica - E	Fruit	8.6 ppm
Black Walnut - Juglans Nigra - E	Seed	7.1 ppm
Aubergine, Egg Solanum Melongena - E	Fruit	5.6 ppm
Cashew - Anacardium Occidentale - E	Seed	4.2 ppm
Coconut, Coconut Palm - Cocos Nucifera - E	Seed	2.8 ppm
Pecan - Carya Illinoensis - E	Seed	2.5 ppm
Shagbark Hickory - Carya Ovata - E	Seed	2.5 ppm
Northern Red Oak - Quercus Rubra - E - M	Seed	1.3 ppm
Cobnut, English Filbert, European Filbert, European Hazel, Hazel - Corylus Avellana - E	Seed	
Spinach - Spinacia Oleracea - E	Plant	
Butternut - Juglans Cinerea - E	Seed	
Flax, Lin Linum Usitatissimum - E	Seed	
American Ginseng, Ginseng - Panax Quinquefolius - M	Plant	

PLANTS CONTAINING SULFUR

Species	Part	Quantity
Cauli Brassica Oleracea var. Botrytis - E	Leaf	11,800 ppm
Dill, Garden Dill - Anethum Graveolens - E	Plant	11,175 ppm
Parsnip - Pastinaca Sativa - E	Root	11,050 ppm
Horseradish - Armoracia Rusticana - E	Root	10,000 ppm
Garden Cress - Lepidium Sativum - E	Seed	9,545 ppm
Cabbage, Red Cabbage, White Cabbage - Brassica Oleracea var. Capitata - E	Leaf	8,750 ppm
Red Mangrove - Rhizophora Mangle - M	Leaf	7,900 ppm
Butterbur - Petasites Japonicus - T	Plant	7,300 ppm
European Nettle, Stinging Nettle - Urtica Dioica - E - M	Leaf	6,665 ppm
Snakegourd - Trichosanthes Anguina - E - M	Fruit	6,480 ppm
Purslane, Verdolaga - Portulaca Oleracea - E	Plant	6,300 ppm
Radish - Raphanus Sativus - E	Root	6,140 ppm
Black Pepper, Pepper, White Pepper - Piper Nigrum - E - M	Fruit	5,760 ppm
Spinach - Spinacia Oleracea - E	Plant	5,700 ppm
White Mulberry - Morus Alba - E - M	Leaf	5,600 ppm
Cucumber - Cucumis Sativus - E	Fruit	5,250 ppm
Qian Hu - Peucedanum Decursivum - M	Plant	5,200 ppm
Rapini, Seven-Top Turnip, Turnip - Brassica Rapa - E	Root	5,100 ppm
Rutabaga, Swede, Swedish Turnip - Brassica Napus var. Napobrassica - E	Root	5,000 ppm
Girasol, Sun Helianthus Annuus - E	Seed	4,880 ppm
Cashew - Anacardium Occidentale - E	Seed	4,800 ppm
Parsley - Petroselinum Crispum - E	Plant	4,700 ppm
Oats - Avena Sativa - E - M	Plant	4,100 ppm
Onion, Shallot - Allium Cepa - Shallot Bulb - E	Bulb	4,075 ppm
Soybean - Glycine Max - E	Seed	4,066 ppm
Indian Sorrel, Jamaica Sorrel, Kharkadi, Red Sorrel, Sorrel - Hibiscus Sabdariffa - E	Seed	4,000 ppm
Chickweed, Common Chickweed - Stellaria Media - E	Plant	3,828 ppm
Lettuce - Lactuca Sativa - E	Shoot	3,800 ppm
Ramie - Boehmeria Nivea - M	Plant	3,700 ppm
Broadbean, Faba Bean, Habas - Vicia Faba - E	Fruit	3,630 ppm
Almond - Prunus Dulcis - E - M - T	Seed	3,420 ppm

SULFUR CONTINUED

Name	Part	ppm
Alehoof - Glechoma Hederacea - M	Plant	3,400 ppm
Pawpaw - Asimina Triloba - Friut - E	Fruit	3,333 ppm
Dandelion - Taraxacum Officinale - E - M	Plant	3,300 ppm
Tomatillo - Physalis Ixocarpa - E	Fruit	3,250 ppm
Wheat - Triticum Aestivum - E - M	Seed	3,200 ppm
Oats - Avena Sativa - E - M	Seed	3,100 ppm
Wheat - Triticum Aestivum - E - M	Plant	2,900 ppm
Butternut - Juglans Cinerea - E	Seed	2,870 ppm
Pistachio - Pistacia Vera - E	Seed	2,870 ppm
Mugwort - Artemisia Vulgaris - M	Plant	2,800 ppm
Soursop - Annona Muricata - E	Fruit	2,700 ppm
Black Walnut - Juglans Nigra - E	Seed	2,652 ppm
Giant Knotweed, Hu-Zhang, Japanese Knotweed, Mexican Bamboo - Polygonum Cuspidatum - E - M - T	Plant	2,600 ppm
Cape Gooseberry, Ground Cherry - Physalis Peruviana - E	Fruit	2,515 ppm
Bell Pepper, Cherry Pepper, Cone Pepper, Green Pepper, Paprika, Sweet Pepper - Capsicum Annuum - E	Fruit	2,440 ppm
Green Gram, Mungbean - Vigna Radiata - E	Seed	2,378 ppm
Tomato - Lycopersicon Esculentum - E - M - T	Fruit	2,330 ppm
Mango - Mangifera Indica - E - M	Seed	2,300 ppm
Pea - Pisum Sativum - E	Plant	2,300 ppm
Shagbark Hickory - Carya Ovata - E	Seed	2,180 ppm
Groundnut, Peanut - Arachis Hypogaea - E - M	Seed	2,100 ppm
Chinese Polystichum - Polystichum Polyblepharum - T	Plant	2,100 ppm
Grape Citrus Paradisi - E	Fruit	2,090 ppm
Cobnut, English Filbert, European Filbert, European Hazel, Hazel - Corylus Avellana - E	Seed	2,070 ppm
Mat Bean, Moth Bean - Vigna Aconitifolia - E	Seed	2,018 ppm
Beet, Beetroot, Garden Beet, Sugar Beet - Beta Vulgaris - E	Root	2,000 ppm
Genipap, Jagua - Genipa Americana - E - M	Fruit	2,000 ppm
Black Gram - Vigna Mungo - E	Seed	1,953 ppm
Neem - Azadirachta Indica - M	Seed	1,921 ppm
Ceylon Cinnamon, Cinnamon - Cinnamomum Verum - E - M - T	Bark	1,900 ppm
Potato - Solanum Tuberosum - E	Tuber	1,900 ppm
Red Currant, White Currant - Ribes Rubrum - E	Fruit	1,782 ppm
Alholva, Bockshornklee, Fenugreek, Greek Clover, Greek Trigonella Foenum-Graecum - E - M	Plant	1,670 ppm
Carrot - Daucus Carota - E	Root	1,635 ppm
Chaparral, Creosote Bush - Larrea Tridentata - M	Plant	1,600 ppm
American Ginseng, Ginseng - Panax Quinquefolius - M	Plant	1,500 ppm
Okra - Abelmoschus Esculentus - Friut - E - M	Fruit	1,400 ppm
Black Currant - Ribes Nigrum - E	Fruit	1,385 ppm
Coconut, Coconut Palm - Cocos Nucifera - E	Seed	1,370 ppm
Chinese Cabbage - Brassica Pekinensis - E	Shoot	1,365 ppm
Genipap, Jagua - Genipa Americana - E - M	Seed	1,300 ppm
Strawberry - Fragaria spp. - E	Fruit	1,270 ppm
Rhubarb - Rheum Rhabarbarum - E	Pt	1,240 ppm
Lentil - Lens Culinaris - E	Seed	1,220 ppm
Cassia, Cassia Bark, Cassia Lignea, China Junk Cassia, Chinazimt, Chinese Cassia - Cinnamomum Aromaticuminnamon - E - M - T	Bark	1,200 ppm
Cloudberry - Rubus Chamaemorus - E - M	Fruit	1,185 ppm
Northern Red Oak - Quercus Rubra - E - M	Seed	1,160 ppm
Flax, Lin Linum Usitatissimum - E	Seed	1,147 ppm
Corn - Zea Mays - E	Fruit	1,140 ppm
Gooseberry - Ribes Uva-Crispa - E	Fruit	1,113 ppm
Bilberry, Dwarf Bilberry, Whortleberry - Vaccinium Myrtillus - E - M	Fruit	1,075 ppm
Cowberry, Lingen, Lingonberry - Vaccinium Vitis-Idaea var. Minus - E - M	Fruit	1,075 ppm
English Walnut - Juglans Rregia - E	Seed	1,040 ppm
Celery - Apium Graveolens - E	Root	1,000 ppm
Java Cinnamon, Padang Cassia - Cinnamomum Burmannii - E - M - T	Bark	1,000 ppm
Mandarin, Tangerine - Citrus Reticulata - E	Fruit	1,000 ppm
Orange - Citrus Sinensis - E	Fruit	1,000 ppm
Rice - Oryza Sativa - E	Plant	1,000 ppm
Dog Rose, Dogbrier, Rose - Rosa Canina - E - M	Fruit	1,000 ppm

Species	Part	Quantity
Greater Yam, Winged Yam - Dioscorea Alata - E	Root	990 ppm
Endive, Escarole - Cichorium Endivia - M	Shoot	912 ppm
Papaya - Carica Papaya - E - M	Fruit	900 ppm
Japanese Cinnamon - Cinnamomum Sieboldii - E - M - T	Bark	900 ppm
Guinea Grass - Panicum Maximum - M	Leaf	0-1,800 ppm
Ambarella - Spondias Dulcis - E	Seed	900 ppm
European Grape, Grape, Grapevine, Vigne Vinifere, Wine Grape - Vitis Vinifera - E - M	Fruit	888 ppm
Tea - Camellia Sinensis - E	Leaf	880 ppm
Black bean, Dwarf bean, Field bean, Flageolet bean, French bean, Garden bean, Green bean, Haricot, Haricot bean, Haricot vert, Kidney bean, Navy bean, Pop bean, Popping bean, Snap bean, String bean, Wax bean - Phaseolus Vulgaris - E	Fruit	875 ppm
Asparagus - Asparagus Officinalis - E	Shoot	864 ppm
Emblic, Myrobalan - Phyllanthus Emblica - E	Fruit	820 ppm
Rye - Secale Cereale - E	Seed	1,460-1,640 ppm
Pecan - Carya Illinoensis - E	Seed	800 ppm
Japanese Cinnamon - Cinnamomum Sieboldii - E - M - T	Root Bark	800 ppm
Elephant Garlic, Kurrat - Allium Ampeloprasum - E	Leaf	700 ppm
Peach - Prunus Persica - E - M - T	Fruit	700 ppm
Ben Nut, Benzolive Tree, Drumstick Tree, Horseradish Tree, Moringa, West Indian Ben - Moringa Oleifera - E	Fruit	0-1,370 ppm
Carambola, Star Averrhoa Carambola - E	Fruit	1,000-1,300 ppm
Indian Tamarind, Kilytree, Tamarind - Tamarindus Indica - M	Leaf	630 ppm
Mango - Mangifera Indica - E - M	Fruit	615 ppm
Sweet Potato - Ipomoea Batatas - E	Root	610 ppm
Date Palm - Phoenix Dactylifera - E	Fruit	590 ppm
Malanga, Tannia, Yautia - Xanthosoma Sagittifolium - E	Root	580 ppm
Taro - Colocasia Esculenta - E	Root	565 ppm
Elephant-Foot Yam - Amorphophallus Campanulatus - E - M - T	Root	530 ppm
Bread Artocarpus Altilis - E	Fruit	530 ppm
Banana, Plantain - Musa x Paradisiaca - E	Fruit	500 ppm
American Cranberry, Cranberry, Large Cranberry - Vaccinium Macrocarpon - E	Fruit	500 ppm
Curry Murraya spp. - E - M	Fruit	450 ppm
Pomarrosa, Rose Apple - Syzygium Jambos - E	Fruit	130-840 ppm
Giant Taro - Alocasia Macrorrhiza - E	Root	400 ppm
Plum - Prunus Domestica - E - M	Fruit	400 ppm
Aceituna Dulce, Jambolan, Java Plum - Syzygium Cumini - E	Fruit	130-800 ppm
Pear - Pyrus Communis - E	Fruit	300 ppm
Cassava, Tapioca, Yuca - Manihot Esculenta - E	Root	250 ppm
Salsify - Tragopogon Porrifolius - E	Root	250 ppm
Taro - Colocasia Esculenta - E	Leaf	240 ppm
Barley, Barleygrass - Hordeum Vulgare - E - M	Seed	200 ppm
Cantaloupe, Melon, Muskmelon, Netted Melon, Nutmeg Melon, Persian Melon - Cucumis Melo subsp. ssp Melo var. Ccantalupensis - Friut - E	Fruit	198 ppm
Swamp Taro - Cyrtosperma Chamissonis - E	Root	195 ppm
Ambarella - Spondias Dulcis - E	Fruit	180 ppm
Aubergine, Egg Solanum Melongena - E	Fruit	152 ppm
Guavas - Psidium Guajava - E	Fruit	140 ppm
Black bean, Dwarf bean, Field bean, Flageolet bean, French bean, Garden bean, Green bean, Haricot, Haricot bean, Haricot vert, Kidney bean, Navy bean, Pop bean, Popping bean, Snap bean, String bean, Wax bean - Phaseolus Vulgaris - E	Seed	137 ppm
Pomegranate - Punica Granatum - E	Fruit	120 ppm
Imbu, Umbu - Spondias Tuberosa - E	Fruit	120 ppm
Pineapple - Ananas Comosus - E	Fruit	70 ppm
Apple - Malus Domestica - E	Fruit	23 ppm

PLANTS CONTAINING VANADIUM

Species	Part	Quantity

VANADIUM CONTINUED

Species	Part	Quantity
Black bean, Dwarf bean, Field bean, Flageolet bean, French bean, Garden bean, Green bean, Haricot, Haricot bean, Haricot vert, Kidney bean, Navy bean, Pop bean, Popping bean, Snap bean, String bean, Wax bean - Phaseolus Vulgaris - E	Fruit	105 ppm
Lettuce - Lactuca Sativa - E	Leaf	20.3 ppm
Cabbage, Red Cabbage, White Cabbage - Brassica Oleracea var. Capitata - E	Leaf	14.5 ppm
Tomato - Lycopersicon Esculentum - E - M - T	Fruit	6 ppm
Black Cherry, Wild Cherry - Prunus Serotina - E - M - T	Leaf	4.8 ppm
Dwarf Sumac, Winged Sumac - Rhus Copallina - E - M	Leaf	4.8 ppm
Black Gum, Black Tupelo - Nyssa Sylvatica - E - M	Leaf	4.55 ppm
Buckbush - Symphoricarpos Orbiculatus - M	Stem	4.4 ppm
Sassafras - Sassafras Albidum - E - M - T	Leaf	3.4 ppm
Butter Bean, Lima Bean - Phaseolus Lunatus - E	Seed	3 ppm
Red Cedar - Juniperus Virginiana Amphicarpaea Bracteata - E - M - T	Shoot	2.64 ppm
Sassafras - Sassafras Albidum - E - M - T	Stem	2.59 ppm
American Styrax, Sweetgum - Liquidambar Styraciflua - E - M	Leaf	2.46 ppm
Asparagus bean, Pea bean, Yardlong bean - Vigna Unguiculata subsp. Sesquipedalis - E	Seed	2.4 ppm
Asparagus - Asparagus Officinalis - E	Shoot	2 ppm
Dwarf Sumac, Winged Sumac - Rhus Copallina - E - M	Stem	1.83 ppm
Black Cherry, Wild Cherry - Prunus Serotina - E - M - T	Stem	1.6 ppm
White Oak - Quercus Alba - M	Stem	1.52 ppm
American Persimmon - Diospyros Virginiana - E - M	Leaf	1.5 ppm
Corn - Zea Mays - E	Seed	1.35 ppm
Black Gum, Black Tupelo - Nyssa Sylvatica - E - M	Stem	1.32 ppm
Northern Red Oak - Quercus Rubra - E - M	Stem	1.32 ppm
Shortleaf Pine - Pinus Echinata - M	Shoot	1.26 ppm
Red Pignut Hickory - Carya Glabra - E	Shoot	1.1 ppm
American Persimmon - Diospyros Virginiana - E - M	Stem	1.08 ppm
Black Oak - Quercus Velutina - E - M	Stem	Trace
Pear - Pyrus Communis - E	Fruit	Trace
Allspice, Clover-Pepper, Jamaica-Pepper, Pimenta, Pimento - Pimenta Dioica - E	Plant	Trace
Black Walnut - Juglans Nigra - E	Seed	Trace
Cashew - Anacardium Occidentale - E	Seed	Trace
Butternut - Juglans Cinerea - E	Seed	Trace
American Ginseng, Ginseng - Panax Quinquefolius - M	Plant	Trace
Almond - Prunus Dulcis - E - M - T	Seed	Trace
Northern Red Oak - Quercus Rubra - E - M	Seed	Trace
Brazilnut, Brazilnut-Tree, Creamnut, Paranut - Bertholletia Eexcelsa - E	Seed	Trace
Pecan - Carya Illinoensis - E	Seed	Trace
Shagbark Hickory - Carya Ovata - E	Seed	Trace
Cobnut, English Filbert, European Filbert, European Hazel, Hazel - Corylus Avellana - E	Seed	Trace
Pistachio - Pistacia Vera - E	Seed	Trace
Coconut, Coconut Palm - Cocos Nucifera - E	Seed	Trace
Flax, Lin Linum Usitatissimum - E	Seed	Trace

PLANTS CONTAINING YTTRIUM

Species	Part	Quantity
Red Pignut Hickory - Carya Glabra - E	Shoot	55 ppm
Cabbage, Red Cabbage, White Cabbage - Brassica Oleracea var. Capitata - E	Leaf	29 ppm
American Styrax, Sweetgum - Liquidambar Styraciflua - E - M	Leaf	24.6 ppm
American Persimmon - Diospyros Virginiana - E - M	Stem	16.2 ppm
Black Cherry, Wild Cherry - Prunus Serotina - E - M - T	Leaf	14.4 ppm
Dwarf Sumac, Winged Sumac - Rhus Copallina - E - M	Leaf	14.4 ppm
Shagbark Hickory - Carya Ovata - E	Shoot	13.5 ppm
Lettuce - Lactuca Sativa - E	Leaf	8.7 ppm
Northern Red Oak - Quercus Rubra - E - M	Stem	6.6 ppm
Black Gum, Black Tupelo - Nyssa Sylvatica - E - M	Leaf	6.37 ppm
Tomato - Lycopersicon Esculentum - E - M - T	Fruit	6 ppm
Buckbush - Symphoricarpos Orbiculatus - M	Stem	4.4 ppm

Species	Part	Quantity
Dwarf Sumac, Winged Sumac - Rhus Copallina - E - M	Stem	4.27 ppm
White Oak - Quercus Alba - M	Stem	4.1 ppm
Black Cherry, Wild Cherry - Prunus Serotina - E - M - T	Stem	3.78 ppm
Black Gum, Black Tupelo - Nyssa Sylvatica - E - M	Stem	3.08 ppm
Black Oak - Quercus Velutina - E - M	Stem	2.5 ppm
Asparagus bean, Pea bean, Yardlong bean - Vigna Unguiculata subsp. Sesquipedalis - E	Seed	2.4 ppm

PLANTS CONTAINING ZINC

Species	Part	Quantity
Red Pignut Hickory - Carya Glabra - E	Shoot	1,100 ppm
Lettuce - Lactuca Sativa - E	Leaf	974 ppm
Aloe, Bitter Aloes - Aloe Vera - E - M	Leaf	770 ppm
Chinese Goldthread, Huang-Lian, Huang-Lien - Coptis Chinensis - M	Rhizome	600 ppm
Huang-Lia, Huang-Lian, Huang-Lien, Japanese Goldthread - Coptis Japonica - M	Rhizome	600 ppm
Generic Goldthread - Coptis spp. - M	Rhizome	600 ppm
Shagbark Hickory - Carya Ovata - E	Shoot	342 ppm
Red Cedar - Juniperus Virginiana Amphicarpaea Bracteata- E - M - T	Shoot	317 ppm
American Styrax, Sweetgum - Liquidambar Styraciflua - E - M	Stem	240 ppm
Black Cherry, Wild Cherry - Prunus Serotina - E - M - T	Stem	216 ppm
Smooth Sumac - Rhus Glabra - E - M	Stem	208 ppm
Black Cherry, Wild Cherry - Prunus Serotina - E - M - T	Leaf	192 ppm
Spinach - Spinacia Oleracea - E	Plant	185 ppm
White Oak - Quercus Alba - M	Stem	182 ppm
Parsley - Petroselinum Crispum - E	Plant	164 ppm
American Persimmon - Diospyros Virginiana - E - M	Stem	162 ppm
Brussel-Sprout - Brassica Oleracea var. Gemmifera - E	Leaf	157 ppm
Collards, Cow Cabbage, Spring-Heading Cabbage, Tall Kale, Tree Kale - Brassica Oleracea - E	Leaf	157 ppm
Cucumber - Cucumis Sativus - E	Fruit	157 ppm
Calabash Gourd, White-Flowered Gourd - Lagenaria Siceraria - E	Fruit	157 ppm
Dill, Garden Dill - Anethum Graveolens - E	Plant	150 ppm
Black bean, Dwarf bean, Field bean, Flageolet bean, French bean, Garden bean, Green bean, Haricot, Haricot bean, Haricot vert, Kidney bean, Navy bean, Pop bean, Popping bean, Snap bean, String bean, Wax bean - Phaseolus Vulgaris - E	Fruit	150 ppm
Endive, Escarole - Cichorium Endivia - M	Leaf	146 ppm
Northern Red Oak - Quercus Rubra - E - M	Stem	138 ppm
Sassafras - Sassafras Albidum - E - M - T	Stem	136 ppm
Black Gum, Black Tupelo - Nyssa Sylvatica - E - M	Stem	132 ppm
Plum - Prunus Domestica - E - M	Fruit	131 ppm
Opium Poppy, Poppyseed Poppy - Papaver Somniferum - E	Seed	130 ppm
Dwarf Sumac, Winged Sumac - Rhus Copallina - E - M	Stem	128 ppm
Asparagus - Asparagus Officinalis - E	Shoot	124 ppm
Tomato - Lycopersicon Esculentum - E - M - T	Fruit	120 ppm
Cauli Brassica Oleracea var. Botrytis - E	Leaf	118 ppm
American Ginseng, Ginseng - Panax Quinquefolius - M	Plant	114 ppm
Manioc Hibiscus - Abelmoschus Manihot - E - M	Leaf	108 ppm
Pigweed - Amaranthus sp. - E - M	Leaf	108 ppm
Sesame - Sesamum Indicum - E - M	Seed	102 ppm
Butter Bean, Lima Bean - Phaseolus Lunatus - E	Seed	100 ppm
American Styrax, Sweetgum - Liquidambar Styraciflua - E - M	Leaf	98 ppm
Cauli Brassica Oleracea var. Botrytis - E	Flower	97 ppm
Dwarf Sumac, Winged Sumac - Rhus Copallina - E - M	Leaf	96 ppm
European Nettle, Stinging Nettle - Urtica Dioica - E - M	Leaf	95 ppm
Bonavist Bean, Hyacinth Bean, Lablab Bean - Lablab Purpureus - E - M - T	Seed	93 ppm
Black Oak - Quercus Velutina - E - M	Stem	93 ppm

ZINC CONTINUED

Plant	Part	ppm
Swamp Cabbage, Water Spinach - Ipomoea Aquatica - E	Leaf	92 ppm
Willow Oak - Quercus Phellos - E - M	Stem	92 ppm
Buckbush - Symphoricarpos Orbiculatus - M	Stem	92 ppm
Mugwort - Artemisia Vulgaris - M	Plant	90 ppm
Soybean - Glycine Max - E	Seed	90 ppm
Evening-Primrose - Oenothera Biennis - E - M	Seed	90 ppm
Celery - Apium Graveolens - E	Seed	89 ppm
Emblic, Myrobalan - Phyllanthus Emblica - E	Fruit	89 ppm
Shortleaf Pine - Pinus Echinata - M	Shoot	88 ppm
Mad-Dog Skullcap, Scullcap - Scutellaria lateriflora - M	Plant	86 ppm
European Mistletoe - Viscum Album - M - T	Leaf	86 ppm
Buchu, Honey Buchu, Mountain Buchu - Agathosma Betulina Buchu, Honey Buchu, Mountain Buchu - Agathosma Betulina - M	Leaf	84 ppm
Pumpkin - Cucurbita Pepo - E	Seed	83 ppm
Chinese Cabbage - Brassica Pekinensis - E	Leaf	80 ppm
Carrot - Daucus Carota - E	Root	79 ppm
Bell Pepper, Cherry Pepper, Cone Pepper, Green Pepper, Paprika, Sweet Pepper - Capsicum Annuum - E	Fruit	77 ppm
Sicklepod - Senna Obtusifolia - E - T	Seed	76 ppm
European Grape, Grape, Grapevine, Vigne Vinifere, Wine Grape - Vitis Vinifera - E - M	Stem	75 ppm
Common thyme, Garden thyme, Thyme - Thymus Vulgaris - E - M	Plant	74 ppm
Chayote - Sechium Edule - E - M	Leaf	73 ppm
Radish - Raphanus Sativus - E	Root	72 ppm
Tomatillo - Physalis Ixocarpa - E	Fruit	71 ppm
Celery - Apium Graveolens - E	Root	70 ppm
Beet, Beetroot, Garden Beet, Sugar Beet - Beta Vulgaris - E	Root	70 ppm
Parsnip - Pastinaca Sativa - E	Root	70 ppm
Mud Plantain, Tse-Hsieh, Water Plantain, Ze-Xie - Alisma Plantago-Aquatica - M	Rhizome	68 ppm
Ladyslipper - Cypripedium Pubescens - M	Root	67 ppm
Dill, Garden Dill - Anethum Graveolens - E	Fruit	66 ppm
Taro - Colocasia Esculenta - E	Root	66 ppm
Mustard Greens - Brassica Juncea - E	Leaf	65 ppm
Jerusalem Artichoke - Helianthus Tuberosus E	Tuber	64 ppm
Caraway, Carum - Carum Carvi - E	Fruit	61 ppm
White Mustard - Sinapis Alba - E - M - T	Seed	61 ppm
Okra - Abelmoschus Esculentus - Friut - E - M	Fruit	60 ppm
Butterbur - Petasites Japonicus - T	Plant	60 ppm
Pea - Pisum Sativum - E	Seed	60 ppm
Chinese Polystichum - Polystichum Polyblepharum - T	Plant	60 ppm
Purslane, Verdolaga - Portulaca Oleracea - E	Shoot	60 ppm
Dandelion - Taraxacum Officinale - E - M	Root	60 ppm
Asian Wild Ginger - Asiasarum Heterotropoides - M	Root	59 ppm
Siebold's Wild Ginger - Asiasarum Sieboldii - M	Root	59 ppm
Anise, Sweet Cumin - Pimpinella Anisum - E - M	Fruit	59 ppm
Sage - Salvia Officinalis - E - M	Leaf	59 ppm
Cumin - Cuminum Cyminum - E - M	Fruit	58 ppm
Adzuki Bean - Vigna Angularis - E	Seed	58 ppm
Cashew - Anacardium Occidentale - E	Seed	57 ppm
Ginger - Zingiber Officinale - E	Rhizome	57 ppm
Pecan - Carya Illinoensis - E	Seed	56 ppm
Wild Yam - Dioscorea sp. - E	Root	56 ppm
Dokudami, Fishwort, Yu Xing Cao - Houttuynia Cordata - E - M	Plant	56 ppm
European Pennyroyal - Mentha pulegium - E - M- T	Plant	56 ppm
Black Gum, Black Tupelo - Nyssa Sylvatica - E - M	Leaf	55 ppm
Horseradish - Armoracia Rusticana - E	Root	54 ppm
Pumpkin - Cucurbita Maxima - E	Leaf	54 ppm
Girasol, Sun Helianthus Annuus - E	Seed	54 ppm
Lentil - Lens Culinaris - E	Sprout Seedling	54 ppm
Onion, Shallot - Allium Cepa - Shallot Bulb - E	Bulb	53 ppm
Brazilnut, Brazilnut-Tree, Creamnut, Paranut - Bertholletia Eexcelsa - E	Seed	53 ppm

Name	Part	ppm
Alehoof - Glechoma Hederacea - M	Plant	53 ppm
White Lupine - Lupinus Albus - M - T	Seed	53 ppm
Chinese Parsley, Cilantro, Coriander - Coriandrum Sativum E	Fruit	52 ppm
Post Oak - Quercus Stellata - E - M	Stem	52 ppm
Chickweed, Common Chickweed - Stellaria Media - E	Plant	52 ppm
Chaff Achyranthes Bidentata - M	Root	51 ppm
Giant Taro - Alocasia Macrorrhiza - E	Root	51 ppm
Coneflower, Echinacea - Echinacea ssp - M	Root	51 ppm
Asparagus Pea, Goa Bean, Winged Bean - Psophocarpus Tetragonolobus - E	Seed	51 ppm
Elephant-Foot Yam - Amorphophallus Campanulatus - E - M- T	Root	50 ppm
Chickpea, Garbanzo - Cicer Arietinum - E	Seed	50 ppm
Swamp Taro - Cyrtosperma Chamissonis - E	Root	50 ppm
Perilla - Perilla Frutescens - E - M - T	Plant	50 ppm
Black bean, Dwarf bean, Field bean, Flageolet bean, French bean, Garden bean, Green bean, Haricot, Haricot bean, Haricot vert, Kidney bean, Navy bean, Pop bean, Popping bean, Snap bean, String bean, Wax bean - Phaseolus Vulgaris - E	Seed	50 ppm
Common Turkish Oregano, European Oregano, Oregano, Pot Marjoram, Wild Marjoram, Wild Oregano - Origanum Vulgare - E	Plant	49 ppm
Giant Knotweed, Hu-Zhang, Japanese Knotweed, Mexican Bamboo - Polygonum Cuspidatum - E - M - T	Plant	49 ppm
Bastard Cardamom, Chin Kousha, Malabar Cardamom, Tavoy Cardamom - Amomum Xanthioides - E	Seed	48 ppm
Henbane - Hyoscyamus Niger - E - M	Seed	48 ppm
Green Gram, Mungbean - Vigna Radiata - E	Sprout Seedling	48 ppm
Shagbark Hickory - Carya Ovata - E	Seed	46 ppm
Black Walnut - Juglans Nigra - E	Seed	46 ppm
Rhubarb - Rheum Rhabarbarum - E	Pt	46 ppm
Potato - Solanum Tuberosum - E	Tuber	44.1 ppm
Celery - Apium Graveolens - E	Leaf	44 ppm
Irish moss - Chondrus Crispus - E	Plant	44 ppm
Ramie - Boehmeria Nivea - M	Plant	43 ppm
Marjoram, Sweet Marjoram - Origanum Majorana - E	Plant	43 ppm
Red Mangrove - Rhizophora Mangle - M	Leaf	43 ppm
Ajwan - Trachyspermum Ammi - E - M	Fruit	43 ppm
Lentil - Lens Culinaris - E	Seed	42 ppm
Qian Hu - Peucedanum Decursivum - M	Plant	42 ppm
Rice Paper Tree, Tong-Cao, Tung-Tsao - Tetrapanax Papyrifera M	Pith	42 ppm
Summer Squash - Cucurbita spp. - E	Fruit	41 ppm
Coffee Senna - Senna Occidentalis - E - T	Seed	41 ppm
Chinese Birthwort - Aristolochia Debilis - E - M - T	Fruit	40 ppm
Black Mustard - Brassica Nigra - E	Leaf	40 ppm
Japanese Cinnamon - Cinnamomum Sieboldii - E - M - T	Bark	40 ppm
Dyer's Woad - Isatis Tinctoria - M	Root	40 ppm
Jussiaeae Herba, Pond Dragon - Jussiaea Repens - M	Plant	40 ppm
Cloudberry - Rubus Chamaemorus - E - M	Fruit	40 ppm
Bilberry, Dwarf Bilberry, Whortleberry - Vaccinium Myrtillus - E - M	Fruit	40 ppm
Burdock, Gobo, Great Burdock - Arctium lappa - E - M - T	Root	39 ppm
Cockscomb - Celosia Cristata - M	Flower	39 ppm
Cobnut, English Filbert, European Filbert, European Hazel, Hazel - Corylus Avellana - E	Seed	39 ppm
Dulse - Rhodymenia Palmata - E	Plant	39 ppm
Madder - Rubia Cordifolia - M	Root	39 ppm
Pawpaw - Asimina Triloba - Friut - E	Fruit	38 ppm
Rush - Juncus Effusus E - M - T	Pith	38 ppm
Apricot - Prunus Armeniaca - E - M - T	Seed	38 ppm
Rosemary - Rosmarinus Officinalis - E - M	Plant	38 ppm

Hillman Health Food Store call 855-Amish-Dr (855-264-7437) www.emineral.info Vitamins and Minerals for Better Living

ZINC CONTINUED

Asparagus bean, Pea bean, Yardlong bean - Vigna Unguiculata subsp. Sesquipedalis - E	Seed	38 ppm
Peach - Prunus Persica - E - M - T	Fruit	37.5 ppm
Chai-Hu - Bupleurum - M	Root	37 ppm
Butternut - Juglans Cinerea - E	Seed	37 ppm
Almond - Prunus Dulcis - E - M - T	Seed	37 ppm
Cabbage, Red Cabbage, White Cabbage - Brassica Oleracea var. Capitata - E	Leaf	36 ppm
Artichoke - Cynara Cardunculus - E	Flower	36 ppm
Black Pepper, Pepper, White Pepper - Piper Nigrum - E - M	Fruit	35.7 ppm
Groundnut, Peanut - Arachis Hypogaea - E - M	Seed	35 ppm
Eyebright - Euphrasia Officinalis - M	Plant	35 ppm
Apple - Malus Domestica - E	Fruit	35 ppm
Onion, Shallot - Allium Cepa - Shallot Bulb - E	Seed	34 ppm
Pigeonpea - Cajanus Vajan - E	Seed	34 ppm
Gotu Kola, Pennywort - Centella Asiatica - E - M	Bark	34 ppm
Ceylon Cinnamon, Cinnamon - Cinnamomum Verum - E - M - T	Leaf	34 ppm
Mongoloid Dandelion - Taraxacum Mongolicum - E - M	Plant	34 ppm
Cang Zhu - Atractylodes Lancea - M	Rhizome	33 ppm
Rutabaga, Swede, Swedish Turnip - Brassica Napus var. Napobrassica - E	Root	33 ppm
Nutsedge - Cyperus Rotundus - E - M	Rhizome	33 ppm
Coca - Erythroxylum Novogranatense var. Novogranatense - E - M	Leaf	33 ppm
Fennel - Foeniculum Vulgare - M	Fruit	33 ppm
Lady's Thistle, Milk Thistle - Silybum Marianum - M	Plant	33 ppm
Corn Salad, Lamb's Lettuce - Valerianella Locusta - E	Plant	62-64.5 ppm
Bai-Zhu, Pai-Chu - Atractylodes Ovata - M	Rhizome	32 ppm
SafCarthamus Tinctorius - M	Flower	32 ppm
Sickle Senna - Cassia Tora - Sprout - Seedling - M	Seed	31 ppm
Cantaloupe, Melon, Muskmelon, Netted Melon, Nutmeg Melon, Persian Melon - Cucumis Melo subsp. ssp Melo var.Ccantalupensis - Friut - E	Fruit	31 ppm
Bai-Wei, Pai-Wei - Cynanchum Atratum - E - M	Root	31 ppm
Asian Plantain - Plantago Asiatica - E - M	Plant	31 ppm
Peach - Prunus Persica - E - M - T	Seed	31 ppm
Green Gram, Mungbean - Vigna Radiata - E	Seed	31 ppm
Tea - Camellia Sinensis - E	Leaf	30 ppm
Barley, Barleygrass - Hordeum Vulgare - E - M	Seed	30 ppm
Pistachio - Pistacia Vera - E	Seed	30 ppm
Chinese Kudzu - Pueraria Pseudohirsuta - E - M	Root	30 ppm
Clove, Clovetree - Syzygium Aromaticum - E	Flower	30 ppm
Bai Zhi - Angelica Dahurica - M	Root	29 ppm
Coca - Erythroxylum Coca var. Coca - E - M	Leaf	29 ppm
Gentian, Yellow Gentian - Gentiana Lutea - M	Root	29 ppm
Date Palm - Phoenix Dactylifera - E	Seed	29 ppm
Radish - Raphanus Sativus - E	Seed	29 ppm
Curly Kale, Kale, Kitchen Kale, Scotch Kale - Brassica Oleracea var. Sabellica l. var. Acephala - E	Leaf	28 ppm
Cardamom - Elettaria Cardamomum - E - M	Fruit	28 ppm
Loquat - Eriobotrya Japonica - E	Leaf	28 ppm
Gennoshiouko, Oriental Geranium - Geranium Thunbergii - E - M	Plant	28 ppm
Antler Herb, Clubmoss - Lycopodium Clavatum - M - T	Plant	28 ppm
Cornmint, Field Mint, Japanese Mint - Mentha Arvensis var. Piperascens - E - M- T	Plant	28 ppm
Water Lotus - Nelumbo Nucifera - E - M	Seed	28 ppm
Chinese Raspberry - Rubus Cchingii - E - M	Fruit	28 ppm
Ching-Chieh, Jing-Jie - Schizonepeta Tenuifolia - E - M	Plant	28 ppm
Alholva, Bockshornklee, Fenugreek, Greek Clover, Greek Trigonella Foenum-Graecum - E - M	Seed	28 ppm
Chih-Mu, Zhi-Mu - Anemarrhena Asphodeloides - M	Rhizome	27 ppm
Chinese Ginseng, Ginseng, Korean Ginseng, Oriental Ginseng - Panax Ginseng - M	Root	27 ppm
European Grape, Grape, Grapevine, Vigne Vinifere, Wine Grape - Vitis Vinifera - E - M	Fruit	27 ppm

Plant	Part	ppm
Pear - Pyrus Communis - E	Fruit	26.6 ppm
Noble Dendrobium - Dendrobium Nobile - M	Stem	26 ppm
Bei Sha Shen - Glehnia Littoralis - E - M	Root	26 ppm
Amur Cork Tree, Huang Bai, Huang Po, Po Mu - Phellodendron Amurense - M	Bark	26 ppm
Sarsaparilla - Smilax spp - E - M	Root	26 ppm
White Tephrosia - Tephrosia Candida - M - T	Plant	26 ppm
Aubergine, Egg Solanum Melongena - E	Fruit	25.6 ppm
American Persimmon - Diospyros Virginiana E M	Leaf	25 ppm
Chinese Parasol - Firmiana Simplex - E - M	Seed	25 ppm
Dan Zhu Ye - Lophatherum Gracile - M	Plant	25 ppm
Hsin-I, Xin-Yi - Magnolia Denudata - E - M	Flower	25 ppm
Hsin-I, Xin-Yi - Magnolia Fargesii - E - M	Flower	25 ppm
Heal-All, Self-Heal - Prunella Vulgaris - E - M	Flower	25 ppm
Coltsfoot - Tussilago Farfara - M - T	Flower	25 ppm
Cayenne, Chili, Hot Pepper, Red Chili, Spur Pepper, Tabasco - Capsicum Frutescens - E	Fruit	24 ppm
American Chestnut - Castanea Dentata - E - M	Seed	24 ppm
Lambsquarter - Chenopodium Album - E - M - T	Seed	24 ppm
Japanese Privet, Ligustri Fructus - Ligustrum Japonicum - M	Fruit	24 ppm
Chinese Privet, Glossy Privet, Ligustri Fructus, Privet, White Waxtree - Ligustrum Lucidum - M	Fruit	24 ppm
Common Garden Peony, Peony, White Peony - Paeonia Lactiflora - M	Root	24 ppm
Chinese Anemone - Pulsatilla Chinensis - M	Root	24 ppm
White Oak - Quercus Alba - M	Bark	24 ppm
Narrowleaf Sophora - Sophora Angustifolia - M - T- M - T	Root	24 ppm
Rapini, Seven-Top Turnip, Turnip - Brassica Rapa - E	Root	23 ppm
Paper Mulberry - Broussonetia Papyrifera - E - M	Fruit	23 ppm
Chinese Boxthorn, Chinese Matrimony Vine, Chinese Wolfberry - Lycium Chinense - E - M	Root Bark	23 ppm
Climbing Fern - Lygodium Japonicum - Pollen or Spore - M	Pollen Or Spore	23 ppm
Italian Stone Pine, Pignolia - Pinus Pinea - M	Seed	42-46 ppm
Dog Rose, Dogbrier, Rose - Rosa Canina - E - M	Fruit	23 ppm
Rye - Secale Cereale - E	Seed	35-45 ppm
Capillary Wormwood - Artemisia Capillaris - M	Plant	22 ppm
Indian Saffron, Turmeric - Curcuma Longa - E	Rhizome	22 ppm
Coca - Erythroxylum Novogranatense var. Truxillense - E - M	Leaf	22 ppm
Chinese Spikenard - Nardostachys Chinensis - M	Rhizome	22 ppm
Rangoon Creeper - Quisqualis Indica - E - T	Fruit	22 ppm
Desert Wormwood - Artemisia Herba-Alba - M	Plant	21 ppm
Hsin-Pa-Pi, Kisasage - Catalpa Ovata - E - M	Fruit	21 ppm
Chinese Quince, Mu-Kua - Chaenomeles Lagenaria - E	Fruit	21 ppm
Chinese Ephedra, Ma Huang - Ephedra Sinica - M	Plant	21 ppm
Oriental Pipewort - Eriocaulon spp. - M	Leaf	21 ppm
Barley, Barleygrass - Hordeum Vulgare - E - M	Stem	21 ppm
Japanese Honeysuckle - Lonicera Japonica - M	Flower	21 ppm
Psyllium - Plantago Psyllium - E - M	Seed	21 ppm
Black Currant - Ribes Nigrum - E	Fruit	21 ppm
White Willow - Salix Alba - M	Bark	21 ppm
Mat Bean, Moth Bean - Vigna Aconitifolia - E	Seed	21 ppm
Da-Zao, Jujube, Ta-Tsao - Zizyphus Jujuba - E - M	Fruit	21 ppm
Amphicarpaea Bracteata- E - M	Shoot	0-40 ppm
Jack Bean - Canavalia Ensiformis - E	Seed	20 ppm
Japanese Cinnamon - Cinnamomum Sieboldii - E - M - T	Root Bark	20 ppm
Ceylon Cinnamon, Cinnamon - Cinnamomum Verum - E - M - T	Bark	20 ppm
Adlay, Adlay Millet, Job's-Tears, Yi-Yi-Ren - Coix Lacryma-Jobi - E - M	Seed	20 ppm
Barley, Barleygrass - Hordeum Vulgare - E - M	Sprout Seedling	20 ppm
Chinese Boxthorn, Chinese Matrimony Vine, Chinese Wolfberry - Lycium Chinense - E - M	Fruit	20 ppm
Mace, Nutmeg - Myristica Fragrans - E	Aril	20 ppm

ZINC CONTINUED

Name	Part	ppm
Japanese Ginseng - Panax Japonicus - M	Rhizome	20 ppm
Allspice, Clover-Pepper, Jamaica-Pepper, Pimenta, Pimento - Pimenta Dioica - E	Fruit	20 ppm
Guavas - Psidium Guajava - E	Fruit	20 ppm
Garden Sorrel - Rumex Acetosa - E - M - T	Leaf	20 ppm
Corn - Zea Mays - E	Seed	20 ppm
Wu Chia Pi - Acanthopanax Gracilistylis - M	Root Bark	19 ppm
Cassava, Tapioca, Yuca - Manihot Esculenta - E	Root	19 ppm
Chinese Magnolia Vine, Five-Flavor-Fruit, Magnolia Vine, Schizandra, Wu Wei Zi, Wu Wei Zu - Schisandra Chinensis - M	Fruit	19 ppm
Wheat - Triticum Aestivum - E - M	Seed	19 ppm
American Cranberry, Cranberry, Large Cranberry - Vaccinium Macrocarpon - E	Fruit	19 ppm
Malanga, Tannia, Yautia - Xanthosoma Sagittifolium - E	Root	19 ppm
Equatorial Ivory Palm - Phytelephas Aequatorialis - E	Mesocarp	13-37 ppm
Guanique - Chamissoa Altissima - M	Leaf	4-36 ppm
Sheng Ma - Cimicifuga Dahurica - M	Rhizome	18 ppm
Wou Chou Yu - Euodia Rutaecarpa - E	Fruit	18 ppm
Japanese Gentian - Gentiana Scabra - E	Root	18 ppm
Devil's claw, Grapple - Harpagophytum procumbens - M	Root	18 ppm
Macadamia - Macadamia spp. - E	Seed	18 ppm
Ban-Xia, Pan-Hsia - Pinellia Ternata - E - M - T	Tuber	18 ppm
Balloon Flower, Chieh-Keng, Jie-Geng - Platycodon Grandiflorum - E - M - T	Root	18 ppm
Baikal Skullcap, Chinese Skullcap, Huang Qin - Scutellaria Baicalensis - M	Root	18 ppm
Rowan Berry - Sorbus Aucubaria - E - M - T	Fruit	18 ppm
Chinese Angelica, Dong Gui, Dong Quai - Angelica Sinensis - M	Root	17 ppm
Blackberry Lily, Shenan - Belamcanda Chinensis - M	Rhizome	17 ppm
Kuan Chung, Shield Fernle - Blechnum Orientale - E - M - T	Rhizome	17 ppm
Chinese Chestnut - Castanea Mollisima - M	Seed	17 ppm
Coconut, Coconut Palm - Cocos Nucifera - E	Seed	17 ppm
Greater Yam, Winged Yam - Dioscorea Alata - E	Root	17 ppm
Fortune's Fern - Drynaria Fortunei - M	Rhizome	17 ppm
Lian-Jiao, Lien-Chiao - Forsythia Suspensa - M	Fruit	17 ppm
Strawberry - Fragaria spp. - E	Fruit	17 ppm
Chinese Ash - Fraxinus Rhynchophylla - M - E	Bark	17 ppm
Cape Jasmine, Gardenia, Jasmin, Shan-Chih-Tzu, Shan-Zhi-Zi, Zhi Zi - Gardenia Jasminoides - M	Fruit	17 ppm
Northern Red Oak - Quercus Rubra - E - M	Seed	17 ppm
Hsi Chien, Saint Paul'Swort - Siegesbeckia Orientalis - M	Plant	17 ppm
Crampbark, European Cranberry bush, Guelder Rose, Snowballbush - Viburnum Opulus - E - M - T	Bark	17 ppm
Betel Nut, Pin-Lang - Areca Catechu Amphicarpaea Bracteata - E - M	Seed	16 ppm
Jack Artocarpus Heterophyllus - E	Fruit	16 ppm
Huang Qi, Huang-Chi - Astragalus Membranaceus - M	Root	16 ppm
Hardy Orchid, Hyacinth Bletilla, Hyacinth Orchid, Shiran - Bletilla Striata - M	Tuber	16 ppm
Bitter Orange, Petitgrain - Citrus Aurantium - E	Fruit	16 ppm
Jih-Chiung - Cnidium Officinale - M	Rhizome	16 ppm
Genipap, Jagua - Genipa Americana - E - M	Seed	16 ppm
Goldenseal - Hydrastis Canadensis - M	Root	16 ppm
Qiang Huo - Notopterygium Incisum - M	Rhizome	16 ppm
Mai-Men-Dong, Mai-Men-Tung - Ophiopogon Japonicus - M	Tuber	16 ppm
Avocado - Persea Americana - E - M - T	Fruit	16 ppm
Red Currant, White Currant - Ribes Rubrum - E	Fruit	16 ppm
Gooseberry - Ribes Uva-Crispa - E	Fruit	16 ppm
Garlic - Allium Sativum Bulb - E	Bulb	15.3 ppm
Tu Huo - Angelica Laxiflora - M	Root	15 ppm
Cherimoya - Annona Cherimola - E	Fruit	15 ppm
Sarson - Brassica Rapa - E	Seed	15 ppm
Morinda - Morinda spp. - M	Root	15 ppm
Indian Fig, Nopal, Nopalito, Prickly Pear - Opuntia Ficus-Indica - E - M	Seed	15 ppm

Name	Part	ppm
Moutan, Tree Peony - Paeonia Moutan - M	Root Bark	15 ppm
Cherokee Rose - Rosa Laevigata - E - M	Fruit	15 ppm
Ching-Feng-Teng - Sinomenium Acutum - E - M	Rhizome	15 ppm
Common thyme, Garden thyme, Thyme - Thymus Vulgaris - E - M	Leaf	15 ppm
Chinese Jack-In-The-Pulpit - Arisaema Consanguineum - E - M - T	Rhizome	14 ppm
Citron - Citrus Medica - E	Fruit	14 ppm
Hawthorn - Crataegus Cuneata - M	Fruit	14 ppm
Du Zhong, Gutta-Percha Tree, Tu Chung - Eucommia Ulmoides - M	Bark	14 ppm
Genipap, Jagua - Genipa Americana - E - M	Fruit	14 ppm
White Mulberry - Morus Alba - E - M	Root Bark	14 ppm
Chinese Foxglove - Rehmannia Glutinosa - M	Root	14 ppm
Shan Dou Gen - Sophora Subprostrata - M - T	Root	14 ppm
Cowberry, Lingen, Lingonberry - Vaccinium Vitis-Idaea var. Minus - E - M	Fruit	14 ppm
Banana Yucca, Blue Yucca, Spanish Bayonet, Yucca - Yucca Baccata - E - M - T	Root	14 ppm
Aconite, Fu-Tsu - Aconitum Carmichaelii - E - M	Tuber	13 ppm
Broomrape, Cistanchis Herba, Jou Tsung Jung - Cistanche Salsa - M	Plant	13 ppm
Orange - Citrus Sinensis - E	Fruit	13 ppm
Chinese Licorice - Glycyrrhiza Uralensis - M	Root	13 ppm
Hsuan-Shen, Yuan-Shen - Scrophularia Buergeriana - M	Root	13 ppm
Chinese Dogwood - Cornus Officinalis - E - M	Fruit	12 ppm
Air Potato, Potato Yam - Dioscorea Bulbifera - E	Rhizome	12 ppm
Bei-Mu, Fritillary - Fritillaria Thunbergii - Blub - E - M	Bulb	12 ppm
Tian Ma - Gastrodia Elata - Rhizome	Rhizome	12 ppm
Equatorial Ivory Palm - Phytelephas Aequatorialis - E	Flower	7-24 ppm
Chinese Senega - Polygala Tenuifolia - M	Root	12 ppm
Dan-Shen, Red Sage, Tan-Shen - Salvia Miltiorrhiza - E - M	Root	12 ppm
Mango - Mangifera Indica - E - M	Fruit	11.4 ppm
Sweet Potato - Ipomoea Batatas - E	Root	11 ppm
Chocolate Vine - Akebia Quinata - M	Stem	10 ppm
Chervil - Anthriscus Cerefolium - E	Leaf	10 ppm
European Chestnut - Castanea Sativa - E - M	Seed	10 ppm
Cassia, Cassia Bark, Cassia Lignea, China Junk Cassia, Chinazimt, Chinese Cassia - Cinnamomum Aromaticuminnamon- E - M - T	Bark	10 ppm
Java Cinnamon, Padang Cassia - Cinnamomum Burmannii - E - M - T	Bark	10 ppm
Russian Olive - Elaeagnus Umbellatus - E - M	Fruit	3-20 ppm
Horsetail, Scouring Rush - Equisetum Hyemale - M	Plant	10 ppm
Banana, Plantain - Musa x Paradisiaca - E	Fruit	10 ppm
Chinese Rhubarb - Rheum Palmatum - E	Rhizome	10 ppm
Lime - Citrus Aurantiifolia - E	Fruit	9 ppm
Grape Citrus Paradisi - E	Fruit	9 ppm
Chinese Magnolia, Hou Pu, Magnolia- Magnolia Officinalis - E - M	Bark	9 ppm
Mimosa - Albizia Julibrissin - E - M	Bark	8 ppm
Bread Artocarpus Altilis - E	Fruit	8 ppm
Watermelon - Citrullus Lanatus - E	Fruit	8 ppm
Mandarin, Tangerine - Citrus Reticulata - E	Fruit	8 ppm
Ma-Huang - Ephedra spp. - M	Plant	8 ppm
Ginkgo, Maidenhair Tree - Ginkgo Biloba - Tree - E - M - T	Seed	8 ppm
Chinese Cornbind, Chinese Knotweed, Fleeceflower, Fo Ti, He Shou Wu - Polygonum Multiflorum - E - M - T	Rhizome	8 ppm
Fig - Ficus Carica - E	Fruit	7 ppm
Curry Murraya spp. - E - M	Fruit	7 ppm
Sour Cherry - Prunus Cerasus - E - M - T	Fruit	7 ppm
Pau D'Arco - Tabebuia Heptaphylla - M	Bark	7 ppm
Blueberry - Vaccinium Corymbosum - E	Fruit	7 ppm
Taro - Colocasia Esculenta - E	Leaf	6.6 ppm
Pineapple - Ananas Comosus - E	Fruit	6 ppm
Carambola, Star Averrhoa Carambola - E	Fruit	1-12 ppm
Bladderwrack, Kelp - Fucus Vesiculosus - E - M	Plant	6 ppm
Basil, Cuban Basil, Sweet Basil - Ocimum Basilicum - E	Leaf	6 ppm

ZINC CONTINUED

Papaya - Carica Papaya - E - M	Fruit	5.4 ppm
Soursop - Annona Muricata - E	Fruit	4 ppm
Indian Tobacco, Lobelia - Lobelia Inflata - M - T	Leaf	4 ppm
Date Palm - Phoenix Dactylifera - E	Fruit	4 ppm
Flannelleaf, Flannelplant, Great mullein, Mullein, Velvet Verbascum Thapsus - M	Leaf	4 ppm
Commom Licorice, Licorice, Licorice-Root, Smooth Licorice - Glycyrrhiza Glabra - M	Root	3 ppm
Comfrey - Symphytum Officinale - E - M - T	Root	2.8 ppm
Scarlet Runner Bean - Phaseolus Coccineus - E	Seed	2 ppm
Salsify - Tragopogon Porrifolius - E	Root	2 ppm
Ambarella - Spondias Dulcis - E	Fruit	1.9 ppm
Imbu, Umbu - Spondias Tuberosa - E	Fruit	1.33 ppm
Milfoil, Yarrow - Achillea Millefolium - M	Plant	Trace
Calamus, Flagroot, Myrtle Flag, Sweet Calamus, Sweetflag, Sweet Acorus Calamus - M	Rhizome	Trace
Elephant Garlic, Kurrat - Allium Ampeloprasum - E	Plant	Trace
Marshmallow, White Mallow - Althaea Officinalis - M	Root	Trace
Devil's Tongue, Elephant Yam, Konjac, Leopard Palm, Snake Palm, Umbrella Arum - Amorphophallus Konjac - E - M - T	Root	Trace
Bearberry, Uva Uursi - Arctostaphylos Uva-Ursi - M	Leaf	Trace
Artemisia cina BERG. -- Levant Wormseed	Plant	Trace
Tarragon - Artemisia Dracunculus - M	Plant	Trace
Oats - Avena Sativa - E - M	Plant	Trace
Barberry - Berberis Vulgaris - M	Root	Trace
Beebread, Beeplant, Borage, Talewort - Borago Officinalis - E - M - T	Plant	Trace
Blue Cohosh - Caulophyllum Thalictroides - M	Root	Trace
Garden Camomile, Perennial Camomile, Roman Camomile - Chamaemelum Nobile M	Flower	Trace
Feverfew - Chrysanthemum Parthenium - M	Plant	Trace
Black Cohosh, Black Snake Cimicifuga Racemosa - E - M	Root	Trace
Blessed Thistle - Cnicus Benedictus - M	Plant	Trace
English Hawthorn, Hawthorn, Whitethorn, Woodland Hawthorn - Crataegus Laevigata - M	Fruit	Trace
Lemongrass, West indian lemongrass - Cymbopogon Citratus - E - M	Plant	Trace
ElytriCouchgrass, Doggrass, Quackgrass, Twitchgrass, Wheatgrass - Elytrigia Repens - E - M	Plant	Trace
Field Horsetail, Horsetail - Equisetum Arvense - M	Plant	Trace
Cascara Buckthorn, Cascara Sagrada - Frangula Purshiana - M	Bark	Trace
Indian Sorrel, Jamaica Sorrel, Kharkadi, Red Sorrel, Sorrel - Hibiscus Sabdariffa - E	Flower	Trace
Hops - Humulus Lupulus - E - M - T	Fruit	Trace
Hydrangea, Smooth Hydrangea - Hydrangea Arborescens - E - M	Root	Trace
Black Walnut - Juglans Nigra - E	Hull Husk	Trace
Common Juniper, Juniper - Juniperus Communis - E - M - T	Fruit	Trace
Chaparral, Creosote Bush - Larrea Tridentata - M	Plant	Trace
Flax, Lin Linum Usitatissimum - E	Seed	Trace
Alfalfa, Lucerne - Medicago Sativa subsp. Sativa - E	Plant	Trace
Peppermint - Mentha x Piperita subsp. Nothosubsp. Piperita - E - M - T	Leaf	Trace
Bayberry, Candle Berry, Southern Bayberry, Wax Myrtle - Myrica Cerifera - E - M	Bark	Trace
Berro, Watercress - Nasturtium Officinale - E	Plant	Trace
Catnip - Nepeta Cataria - M	Plant	Trace
Chinese Cornbind, Chinese Knotweed, Fleeceflower, Fo Ti, He Shou Wu - Polygonum Multiflorum - E - M - T	Root	Trace
Peach - Prunus Persica - E - M - T	Bark	Trace
Raspberry, Red raspberry - Rubus Idaeus - E - M	Leaf	Trace
Curly Dock, Lengua De Vaca, Sour Dock, Yellow Dock - Rumex Crispus - M - T	Root	Trace

Lancaster Agriculture Products 717-687-9222 www.lancasterag.com Naturally Interested in Your Future

Species	Part	Quantity
Box-Holly, Butcher's broom - Ruscus aculeatus - E - M	Bark	Trace
Indian Sorrel, Jamaica Sorrel, Stevia, Sweet Leaf of Paraguay - Stevia Rebaudiana - E	Leaf	Trace
Cowgrass, Peavine Clover, Purple Clover, Red Clover - Trifolium Pratense - E - M	Flower	Trace
Damiana - Turnera Diffusa - M	Leaf	Trace
Red Elm, Slippery Elm - Ulmus Rubra - M	Bark	Trace
Common Valerian, Garden-Heliotrope, Valerian - Valeriana Officinalis - E - M	Root	Trace

SOURCING THE AMINO ACIDS

PLANTS CONTAINING ALANINE

Species	Part	Quantity
Berro, Watercress - Nasturtium Officinale - E	Herb	27,400 ppm
Jew's Mallow, Mulukiya, Nalta Jute - Corchorus Olitorius - E - M	Leaf	20,840 ppm
Lambsquarter - Chenopodium Album - E - M - T	Plant	20,511 ppm
Ceratonia siliqua L. -- Carob, Locust Bean, St.John's-Bread	Seed	19,270 ppm
Soybean - Glycine Max - E	Seed	18,795 ppm
Black bean, Dwarf bean, Field bean, Flageolet bean, French bean, Garden bean, Green bean, Haricot, Haricot bean, Haricot vert, Kidney bean, Navy bean, Pop bean, Popping bean, Snap bean, String bean, Wax bean - Phaseolus Vulgaris - E	Sprout Seedling	18,710 ppm
Asparagus - Asparagus Officinalis - E	Seed	18,581 ppm
Cassie, Huisache, Opopanax, Popinac, Sweet Acacia - Acacia Farnesiana - M	Leaf	18,450 ppm
Bok-Choy, Celery Cabbage, Celery Mustard, Chinese Cabbage, Chinese Mustard, Chinese White Cabbage, Pak-Choi - Brassica Chinensis - E	Leaf	18,378 ppm
Spinach - Spinacia Oleracea - E	Plant	16,864 ppm
Pigweed - Amaranthus sp. - E - M	Leaf	16,722 ppm
Chives - Allium Schoenoprasum - E	Leaf	15,750 ppm
Watermelon - Citrullus Lanatus - E	Seed	15,000 ppm
Sesame - Sesamum Indicum - E - M	Seed	14,802 ppm
Swamp Cabbage, Water Spinach - Ipomoea Aquatica - E	Leaf	14,475 ppm
White Lupine - Lupinus Albus - M - T	Seed	14,470 ppm
Chaya - Cnidoscolus Chayamansa - E	Leaf	14,260 ppm
Butternut - Juglans Cinerea - E	Seed	14,194 ppm
Cauli Brassica Oleracea var. Botrytis - E	Flower	13,565 ppm
Adzuki Bean - Vigna Angularis - E	Seed	13,401 ppm
Purslane, Verdolaga - Portulaca Oleracea - E	Herb	13,400 ppm
Lentil - Lens Culinaris - E	Seed	13,200 ppm
White Mustard - Sinapis Alba - E - M - T	Seed	12,700 ppm
Cauli Brassica Oleracea var. Botrytis - E	Leaf	12,673 ppm
Opium Poppy, Poppyseed Poppy - Papaver Somniferum - E	Seed	12,637 ppm
Ben Nut, Benzolive Tree, Drumstick Tree, Horseradish Tree, Moringa, West Indian Ben - Moringa Oleifera - E	Shoot	5,320-24,930 ppm
Pumpkin - Cucurbita Pepo - E	Seed	12,441 ppm
Corn - Zea Mays - E	Seed	12,272 ppm
Corn Salad, Lamb's Lettuce - Valerianella Locusta - E	Plant	12,220 ppm
Butter Bean, Lima Bean - Phaseolus Lunatus - E	Seed	12,190 ppm
Groundnut, Peanut - Arachis Hypogaea - E - M	Seed	12,137 ppm
Asparagus bean, Pea bean, Yardlong bean - Vigna Unguiculata subsp. Sesquipedalis - E	Seed	12,111 ppm
Broadbean, Faba Bean, Habas - Vicia Faba - E	Seed	12,000 ppm
Lentil - Lens Culinaris - E	Sprout Seedling	11,865 ppm
Girasol, Sun Helianthus Annuus - E	Seed	11,800 ppm
Bonavist Bean, Hyacinth Bean, Lablab Bean - Lablab Purpureus - E - M - T	Seed	11,775 ppm
Cowage, Velvetbean - Mucuna Pruriens - E	Seed	11,600 ppm
Green Gram, Mungbean - Vigna Radiata - E	Seed	11,545 ppm
Pea - Pisum Sativum - E	Seed	11,353 ppm

ALANINE CONTINUED

Asparagus Pea, Goa Bean, Winged Bean - Psophocarpus Tetragonolobus - E	Seed	11,346 ppm
Alholva, Bockshornklee, Fenugreek, Greek Clover, Greek Trigonella Foenum-Graecum - E - M	Seed	11,220 ppm
Collards, Cow Cabbage, Spring-Heading Cabbage, Tall Kale, Tree Kale - Brassica Oleracea - E	Leaf	10,981 ppm
Vinespinach - Basella Alba - E - M	Leaf	10,870 ppm
Pigeonpea - Cajanus Vajan - E	Seed	10,870 ppm
Curly Kale, Kale, Kitchen Kale, Scotch Kale - Brassica Oleracea var. Sabellica l. var. Acephala - E	Leaf	10,680 ppm
Cacao - Theobroma Ccacao - E	Seed	10,400 ppm
Green Gram, Mungbean - Vigna Radiata - E	Sprout Seedling	10,399 ppm
Pistachio - Pistacia Vera - E	Seed	10,340 ppm
Black Caraway, Black Cumin, Fennel-Flower, Nutmeg-Flower, Roman Coriander - Nigella Sativa - E - M	Seed	10,255 ppm
Black bean, Dwarf bean, Field bean, Flageolet bean, French bean, Garden bean, Green bean, Haricot, Haricot bean, Haricot vert, Kidney bean, Navy bean, Pop bean, Popping bean, Snap bean, String bean, Wax bean - Phaseolus Vulgaris - E	Seed	10,171 ppm
Endive, Escarole - Cichorium Endivia - M	Leaf	9,984 ppm
Almond - Prunus Dulcis - E - M - T	Seed	9,864 ppm
Summer Squash - Cucurbita spp. - E	Fruit	9,810 ppm
Chickpea, Garbanzo - Cicer Arietinum - E	Seed	9,360 ppm
Lettuce - Lactuca Sativa - E	Leaf	9,333 ppm
Asparagus Pea, Goa Bean, Winged Bean - Psophocarpus Tetragonolobus - E	Tuber	9,319 ppm
Chinese Foxglove - Rehmannia Glutinosa - M	Root	9,000 ppm
Fennel - Foeniculum Vulgare - M	Fruit	8,655 ppm
Papaver bracteatum L. -- Great Scarlet Poppy	Seed	8,650 ppm
Black bean, Dwarf bean, Field bean, Flageolet bean, French bean, Garden bean, Green bean, Haricot, Haricot bean, Haricot vert, Kidney bean, Navy bean, Pop bean, Popping bean, Snap bean, String bean, Wax bean - Phaseolus Vulgaris - E	Fruit	8,633 ppm
Onion, Shallot - Allium Cepa - Shallot Bulb - E	Bulb	8,597 ppm
Buffalo Gourd - Cucurbita Foetidissima - E - M - T	Seed	10,130-17,100 ppm
Indian Fig, Nopal, Nopalito, Prickly Pear - Opuntia Ficus-Indica - E - M	Seed	8,480 ppm
Chayote - Sechium Edule - E - M	Fruit	8,000 ppm
Aloe, Bitter Aloes - Aloe Vera - E - M	Leaf	0-15,769 ppm
Italian Stone Pine, Pignolia - Pinus Pinea - M	Seed	12,540-15,000 ppm
Basil, Cuban Basil, Sweet Basil - Ocimum Basilicum - E	Leaf	7,470 ppm
Asparagus Pea, Goa Bean, Winged Bean - Psophocarpus Tetragonolobus - E	Leaf	7,430 ppm
Okra - Abelmoschus Esculentus - Friut - E - M	Fruit	7,300 ppm
Water Lotus - Nelumbo Nucifera - E - M	Seed	7,242 ppm
Indian Fig, Nopal, Nopalito, Prickly Pear - Opuntia Ficus-Indica - E - M	Bud	7,180 ppm
Cashew - Anacardium Occidentale - E	Seed	7,141 ppm
Buckwheat - Fagopyrum Esculentum - E	Seed	6,880 ppm
Aubergine, Egg Solanum Melongena - E	Fruit	6,815 ppm
Cayenne, Chili, Hot Pepper, Red Chili, Spur Pepper, Tabasco - Capsicum Frutescens - E	Fruit	6,691 ppm
Sicklepod - Senna Obtusifolia - E - T	Seed	6,500 ppm
Brazilnut, Brazilnut-Tree, Creamnut, Paranut - Bertholletia Eexcelsa - E	Seed	5,897 ppm
Evening-Primrose - Oenothera Biennis - E - M	Seed	5,870 ppm
Pea - Pisum Sativum - E	Fruit	5,737 ppm
Potato - Solanum Tuberosum - E	Tuber	5,700 ppm
Mango - Mangifera Indica - E - M	Fruit	5,650 ppm
Cabbage, Red Cabbage, White Cabbage - Brassica Oleracea var. Capitata - E	Leaf	5,615 ppm
Ginkgo, Maidenhair Tree - Ginkgo Biloba - Tree - E - M - T	Seed	5,352 ppm

Pawpaw - Asimina Triloba - Friut - E	Fruit	5,331 ppm
Apricot - Prunus Armeniaca - E - M - T	Fruit	4,980 ppm
Carrot - Daucus Carota - E	Root	4,830 ppm
Bell Pepper, Cherry Pepper, Cone Pepper, Green Pepper, Paprika, Sweet Pepper - Capsicum Annuum - E	Fruit	4,774 ppm
Celery - Apium Graveolens - E	Pt	4,665 ppm
Avocado - Persea Americana - E - M - T	Fruit	4,625 ppm
Cucumber - Cucumis Sativus - E	Fruit	4,557 ppm
American Chestnut - Castanea Dentata - E - M	Seed	4,395 ppm
Beet, Beetroot, Garden Beet, Sugar Beet - Beta Vulgaris - E	Root	4,338 ppm
Rapini, Seven-Top Turnip, Turnip - Brassica Rapa - E	Root	4,305 ppm
Radish - Raphanus Sativus - E	Root	4,265 ppm
Tomato - Lycopersicon Esculentum - E - M - T	Fruit	4,132 ppm
Oats - Avena Sativa - E - M	Seed	4,000 ppm
Rye - Secale Cereale - E	Seed	7,110-7,985 ppm
Bread Artocarpus Altilis - E	Seed	3,360-7,685 ppm
Orange - Citrus Sinensis - E	Fruit	3,775 ppm
Strawberry - Fragaria spp. - E	Fruit	3,677 ppm
Chinese Chestnut - Castanea Mollisima - M	Seed	3,581 ppm
Wheat - Triticum Aestivum - E - M	Seed	3,542 ppm
Yambean - Pachyrhizus Erosus - E	Tuber	3,500 ppm
Peach - Prunus Persica - E - M - T	Fruit	3,402 ppm
Macadamia - Macadamia spp. - E	Seed	3,385 ppm
Pumpkin - Cucurbita Pepo - E	Fruit	3,333 ppm
Sweet Potato - Ipomoea Batatas - E	Root	3,314 ppm
Rutabaga, Swede, Swedish Turnip - Brassica Napus var. Napobrassica - E	Root	3,190 ppm
Garlic - Allium Sativum Bulb - E	Bulb	3,168 ppm
European Chestnut - Castanea Sativa - E - M	Seed	3,036 ppm
Mountain Yam - Dioscorea Pentaphylla - E	Root	2,965 ppm
Guavas - Psidium Guajava - E	Fruit	2,952 ppm
Cassava, Tapioca, Yuca - Manihot Esculenta - E	Root	2,765 ppm
Mandarin, Tangerine - Citrus Reticulata - E	Fruit	2,740 ppm
Squaw Perideridia Gairdneri - E - M	Root	2,603 ppm
Water Lotus - Nelumbo Nucifera - E - M	Rhizome	2,585 ppm
Jerusalem Artichoke - Helianthus Tuberosus E	Tuber	2,573 ppm
Taro - Colocasia Esculenta - E	Root	2,485 ppm
American Ginseng, Ginseng - Panax Quinquefolius - M	Plant	2,250 ppm
Fig - Ficus Carica - E	Fruit	2,154 ppm
Watermelon - Citrullus Lanatus - E	Fruit	2,000 ppm
Plum - Prunus Domestica - E - M	Fruit	1,959 ppm
Calathea allouia (AUBL.) LINDL. - Leren, Lleren	Root	3,545-3,900 ppm
Blueberry - Vaccinium Corymbosum - E	Fruit	1,820 ppm
Ginger - Zingiber Officinale - E	Rhizome	1,793 ppm
Banana, Plantain - Musa x Paradisiaca - E	Fruit	1,515 ppm
Strawberry Guava - Psidium Cattleianum - E	Fruit	1,500 ppm
American Elder, American Elderberry, Elderberry, Sweet Elder - Sambucus Canadensis - E	Fruit	1,485 ppm
Curry Murraya spp. - E - M	Fruit	1,469 ppm
European Grape, Grape, Grapevine, Vigne Vinifere, Wine Grape - Vitis Vinifera - E - M	Fruit	1,440 ppm
Date Palm - Phoenix Dactylifera - E	Fruit	1,290 ppm
Pineapple - Ananas Comosus - E	Fruit	1,259 ppm
Papaya - Carica Papaya - E - M	Fruit	1,253 ppm
Burdock, Gobo, Great Burdock - Arctium lappa - E - M - T	Root	1,250 ppm
Emblic, Myrobalan - Phyllanthus Emblica - E	Fruit	1,190 ppm
Breadroot, Indian Bread-Root, Indian Turnip, Prairie Apple, Prairie Potato, Prairie Turnip - Psoralea Esculenta - E - M - T	Root	1,139 ppm
Pear - Pyrus Communis - E	Fruit	803 ppm
Apple - Malus Domestica - E	Fruit	435 ppm
Pea - Pisum Sativum - E	Shoot	313 ppm
Grape Citrus Paradisi - E	Fruit	90 ppm
Elephant Garlic, Kurrat - Allium Ampeloprasum - E	Plant	Trace
Jericho Rose - Anastatica Hierochuntica	Fruit	Trace
Tarragon - Artemisia Dracunculus - M	Plant	Trace
Tea - Camellia Sinensis - E	Plant	Trace
Jack Bean - Canavalia Ensiformis - E	Seed	Trace
Flax, Lin Linum Usitatissimum - E	Seed	Trace

ALANINE CONTINUED

Species	Part	Quantity
Antler Herb, Clubmoss - Lycopodium Clavatum - M - T	Pollen Or Spore	Trace
Sage - Salvia Officinalis - E - M	Plant	Trace
Santalum album L. -- White Sandalwood	Fruit	Trace
Common thyme, Garden thyme, Thyme - Thymus Vulgaris - E - M	Plant	Trace
Tilia sp. -- Basswood, Lime, Linden	Flower	Trace

PLANTS CONTAINING ARGININE

Species	Part	Quantity
Chinese Foxglove - Rehmannia Glutinosa - M	Root	87,000 ppm
Girasol, Sun Helianthus Annuus - E	Seed	82,000 ppm
Buffalo Gourd - Cucurbita Foetidissima - E - M - T	Seed	39,900-143,000 ppm
Ceratonia siliqua L. -- Carob, Locust Bean, St.John's-Bread	Seed	55,460 ppm
Black Caraway, Black Cumin, Fennel-Flower, Nutmeg-Flower, Roman Coriander - Nigella Sativa - E - M	Seed	53,050 ppm
Butternut - Juglans Cinerea - E	Seed	50,300 ppm
Watermelon - Citrullus Lanatus - E	Seed	46,600 ppm
White Lupine - Lupinus Albus - M - T	Seed	44,400 ppm
Pumpkin - Cucurbita Pepo - E	Seed	43,328 ppm
Cassie, Huisache, Opopanax, Popinac, Sweet Acacia - Acacia Farnesiana - M	Leaf	39,480 ppm
Aloe, Bitter Aloes - Aloe Vera - E - M	Leaf	0-78,216 ppm
Groundnut, Peanut - Arachis Hypogaea - E - M	Seed	37,022 ppm
Italian Stone Pine, Pignolia - Pinus Pinea - M	Seed	46,680-71,600 ppm
Sesame - Sesamum Indicum - E - M	Seed	34,930 ppm
Chaya - Cnidoscolus Chayamansa - E	Leaf	34,720 ppm
Soybean - Glycine Max - E	Seed	30,950 ppm
Berro, Watercress - Nasturtium Officinale - E	Herb	30,000 ppm
Alholva, Bockshornklee, Fenugreek, Greek Clover, Greek Trigonella Foenum-Graecum - E - M	Seed	27,115 ppm
Indian Fig, Nopal, Nopalito, Prickly Pear - Opuntia Ficus-Indica - E - M	Seed	27,100 ppm
Black Mustard - Brassica Nigra - E	Leaf	26,657 ppm
Cowage, Velvetbean - Mucuna Pruriens - E	Seed	26,180 ppm
Almond - Prunus Dulcis - E - M - T	Seed	26,098 ppm
Chives - Allium Schoenoprasum - E	Leaf	25,250 ppm
Brazilnut, Brazilnut-Tree, Creamnut, Paranut - Bertholletia Eexcelsa - E	Seed	24,727 ppm
Black bean, Dwarf bean, Field bean, Flageolet bean, French bean, Garden bean, Green bean, Haricot, Haricot bean, Haricot vert, Kidney bean, Navy bean, Pop bean, Popping bean, Snap bean, String bean, Wax bean - Phaseolus Vulgaris - E	Sprout Seedling	24,516 ppm
Lentil - Lens Culinaris - E	Seed	24,400 ppm
Broadbean, Faba Bean, Habas - Vicia Faba - E	Seed	24,370 ppm
Pistachio - Pistacia Vera - E	Seed	22,740 ppm
Papaver bracteatum L. -- Great Scarlet Poppy	Seed	21,650 ppm
Opium Poppy, Poppyseed Poppy - Papaver Somniferum - E	Seed	21,401 ppm
Green Gram, Mungbean - Vigna Radiata - E	Sprout Seedling	20,693 ppm
Asparagus Pea, Goa Bean, Winged Bean - Psophocarpus Tetragonolobus - E	Seed	20,576 ppm
Chickpea, Garbanzo - Cicer Arietinum - E	Seed	20,560 ppm
Lentil - Lens Culinaris - E	Sprout Seedling	20,365 ppm
Pea - Pisum Sativum - E	Seed	20,246 ppm
Jew's Mallow, Mulukiya, Nalta Jute - Corchorus Olitorius - E - M	Leaf	20,185 ppm
Swamp Cabbage, Water Spinach - Ipomoea Aquatica - E	Leaf	19,655 ppm
Bonavist Bean, Hyacinth Bean, Lablab Bean - Lablab Purpureus - E - M - T	Seed	19,365 ppm
Spinach - Spinacia Oleracea - E	Plant	19,239 ppm
White Mustard - Sinapis Alba - E - M - T	Seed	18,725 ppm
Asparagus - Asparagus Officinalis - E	Shoot	18,452 ppm
Asparagus bean, Pea bean, Yardlong bean - Vigna Unguiculata subsp. Sesquipedalis - E	Seed	18,401 ppm
Green Gram, Mungbean - Vigna Radiata - E	Seed	18,383 ppm

Flax, Lin Linum Usitatissimum - E	Seed	18,000 ppm
Bok-Choy, Celery Cabbage, Celery Mustard, Chinese Cabbage, Chinese Mustard, Chinese White Cabbage, Pak-Choi - Brassica Chinensis - E	Leaf	17,951 ppm
Cashew - Anacardium Occidentale - E	Seed	17,711 ppm
American Ginseng, Ginseng - Panax Quinquefolius - M	Plant	17,615 ppm
Onion, Shallot - Allium Cepa - Shallot Bulb - E	Bulb	17,222 ppm
Asparagus bean, Pea bean, Yardlong bean - Vigna Unguiculata subsp. Sesquipedalis - E	Fruit	16,131 ppm
Lambsquarter - Chenopodium Album - E - M - T	Plant	16,116 ppm
Cauli Brassica Oleracea var. Botrytis - E	Leaf	15,573 ppm
Butter Bean, Lima Bean - Phaseolus Lunatus - E	Seed	15,390 ppm
Taro - Colocasia Esculenta - E	Leaf	15,340 ppm
Garlic - Allium Sativum Bulb - E	Bulb	15,216 ppm
Evening-Primrose - Oenothera Biennis - E - M	Seed	15,048 ppm
Black bean, Dwarf bean, Field bean, Flageolet bean, French bean, Garden bean, Green bean, Haricot, Haricot bean, Haricot vert, Kidney bean, Navy bean, Pop bean, Popping bean, Snap bean, String bean, Wax bean - Phaseolus Vulgaris - E	Seed	15,026 ppm
Chicory, Succory, Witloof - Cichorium Intybus - E - M	Leaf	14,892 ppm
Adzuki Bean - Vigna Angularis - E	Seed	14,834 ppm
Pigweed - Amaranthus sp. - E - M	Leaf	14,556 ppm
Pigeonpea - Cajanus Vajan - E	Seed	14,530 ppm
Brussel-Sprout - Brassica Oleracea var. Gemmifera - E	Leaf	14,494 ppm
Rutabaga, Swede, Swedish Turnip - Brassica Napus var. Napobrassica - E	Root	14,310 ppm
Achiote, Annato, Annatto, Annoto, Arnato, Bija, Lipstick Pod, Lipsticktree - Bixa Orellana - E	Seed	14,260 ppm
Dill, Garden Dill - Anethum Graveolens - E	Fruit	13,678 ppm
Pea - Pisum Sativum - E	Fruit	13,254 ppm
Collards, Cow Cabbage, Spring-Heading Cabbage, Tall Kale, Tree Kale - Brassica Oleracea - E	Leaf	13,112 ppm
Oats - Avena Sativa - E - M	Seed	13,000 ppm
Corn Salad, Lamb's Lettuce - Valerianella Locusta - E	Plant	12,640 ppm
Ben Nut, Benzolive Tree, Drumstick Tree, Horseradish Tree, Moringa, West Indian Ben - Moringa Oleifera - E	Shoot	5,320-24,930 ppm
Cauli Brassica Oleracea var. Botrytis - E	Flower	12,400 ppm
Wheat - Triticum Aestivum - E - M	Seed	12,000 ppm
Buckwheat - Fagopyrum Esculentum - E	Seed	11,910 ppm
Curly Kale, Kale, Kitchen Kale, Scotch Kale - Brassica Oleracea var. Sabellica l. var. Acephala - E	Leaf	11,840 ppm
Lettuce - Lactuca Sativa - E	Leaf	11,833 ppm
Kohlrabi - Brassica Oleracea var. Gongylodes - E	Stem	11,667 ppm
Jerusalem Artichoke - Helianthus Tuberosus E	Tuber	11,627 ppm
Purslane, Verdolaga - Portulaca Oleracea - E	Herb	10,400 ppm
Water Lotus - Nelumbo Nucifera - E - M	Seed	10,242 ppm
Sicklepod - Senna Obtusifolia - E - T	Seed	10,200 ppm
Vinespinach - Basella Alba - E - M	Leaf	10,145 ppm
Endive, Escarole - Cichorium Endivia - M	Leaf	9,984 ppm
Cassava, Tapioca, Yuca - Manihot Esculenta - E	Root	9,970 ppm
Asparagus Pea, Goa Bean, Winged Bean - Psophocarpus Tetragonolobus - E	Tuber	9,671 ppm
Ginkgo, Maidenhair Tree - Ginkgo Biloba - Tree - E - M - T	Seed	9,366 ppm
Macadamia - Macadamia spp. - E	Seed	9,250 ppm
Cabbage, Red Cabbage, White Cabbage - Brassica Oleracea var. Capitata - E	Leaf	9,225 ppm
Squaw Perideridia Gairdneri - E - M	Root	8,954 ppm
Cucumber - Cucumis Sativus - E	Fruit	8,608 ppm
Okra - Abelmoschus Esculentus - Friut - E - M	Fruit	8,450 ppm
Breadroot, Indian Bread-Root, Indian Turnip, Prairie Apple, Prairie Potato, Prairie Turnip - Psoralea Esculenta - E - M - T	Root	7,976 ppm
Summer Squash - Cucurbita spp. - E	Fruit	7,910 ppm

Hillman Health Food Store call 855-Amish-Dr (855-264-7437) www.emineral.info Vitamins and Minerals for Better Living

ARGININE CONTINUED

Name	Part	ppm
Chinese Chestnut - Castanea Mollisima - M	Seed	7,852 ppm
Cayenne, Chili, Hot Pepper, Red Chili, Spur Pepper, Tabasco - Capsicum Frutescens - E	Fruit	7,834 ppm
Asparagus Pea, Goa Bean, Winged Bean - Psophocarpus Tetragonolobus - E	Leaf	7,689 ppm
Aubergine, Egg Solanum Melongena - E	Fruit	7,559 ppm
Black bean, Dwarf bean, Field bean, Flageolet bean, French bean, Garden bean, Green bean, Haricot, Haricot bean, Haricot vert, Kidney bean, Navy bean, Pop bean, Popping bean, Snap bean, String bean, Wax bean - Phaseolus Vulgaris - E	Fruit	7,503 ppm
Fennel - Foeniculum Vulgare - M	Fruit	7,460 ppm
Watermelon - Citrullus Lanatus - E	Fruit	6,949 ppm
Potato - Solanum Tuberosum - E	Tuber	6,850 ppm
American Chestnut - Castanea Dentata - E - M	Seed	6,778 ppm
Yambean - Pachyrhizus Erosus - E	Tuber	6,635 ppm
Basil, Cuban Basil, Sweet Basil - Ocimum Basilicum - E	Leaf	6,620 ppm
Pumpkin - Cucurbita Pepo - E	Fruit	6,429 ppm
Mountain Yam - Dioscorea Pentaphylla - E	Root	6,035 ppm
Bread Artocarpus Altilis - E	Seed	4,940-11,300 ppm
Bell Pepper, Cherry Pepper, Cone Pepper, Green Pepper, Paprika, Sweet Pepper - Capsicum Annuum - E	Fruit	5,592 ppm
Corn - Zea Mays - E	Seed	5,450 ppm
Chayote - Sechium Edule - E - M	Fruit	5,430 ppm
Burdock, Gobo, Great Burdock - Arctium lappa - E - M - T	Root	5,250 ppm
Indian Fig, Nopal, Nopalito, Prickly Pear - Opuntia Ficus-Indica - E - M	Bud	4,955 ppm
Orange - Citrus Sinensis - E	Fruit	4,908 ppm
Rye - Secale Cereale - E	Seed	8,130-9,130 ppm
Water Lotus - Nelumbo Nucifera - E - M	Rhizome	4,210 ppm
Celery - Apium Graveolens - E	Pt	4,105 ppm
Tomato - Lycopersicon Esculentum - E - M - T	Fruit	3,637 ppm
Mandarin, Tangerine - Citrus Reticulata - E	Fruit	3,546 ppm
Carrot - Daucus Carota - E	Root	3,520 ppm
Taro - Colocasia Esculenta - E	Root	3,510 ppm
Mango - Mangifera Indica - E - M	Fruit	3,400 ppm
Apricot - Prunus Armeniaca - E - M - T	Fruit	3,300 ppm
European Chestnut - Castanea Sativa - E - M	Seed	3,192 ppm
Calabash Gourd, White-Flowered Gourd - Lagenaria Siceraria - E	Fruit	3,140 ppm
Curry Murraya spp. - E - M	Fruit	3,111 ppm
Chaparral, Creosote Bush - Larrea Tridentata - M	Plant	3,100 ppm
Strawberry - Fragaria spp. - E	Fruit	3,084 ppm
Beet, Beetroot, Garden Beet, Sugar Beet - Beta Vulgaris - E	Root	2,997 ppm
Rapini, Seven-Top Turnip, Turnip - Brassica Rapa - E	Root	2,950 ppm
Sweet Potato - Ipomoea Batatas - E	Root	2,835 ppm
European Grape, Grape, Grapevine, Vigne Vinifere, Wine Grape - Vitis Vinifera - E - M	Fruit	2,520 ppm
Ginger - Zingiber Officinale - E	Rhizome	2,486 ppm
Pawpaw - Asimina Triloba - Friut - E	Fruit	2,336 ppm
American Elder, American Elderberry, Elderberry, Sweet Elder - Sambucus Canadensis - E	Fruit	2,326 ppm
Avocado - Persea Americana - E - M - T	Fruit	2,293 ppm
Blueberry - Vaccinium Corymbosum - E	Fruit	2,210 ppm
Date Palm - Phoenix Dactylifera - E	Fruit	2,090 ppm
Calathea allouia (AUBL.) LINDL. - Leren, Lleren	Root	3,385-3,720 ppm
Banana, Plantain - Musa x Paradisiaca - E	Fruit	1,826 ppm
Guavas - Psidium Guajava - E	Fruit	1,512 ppm
Peach - Prunus Persica - E - M - T	Fruit	1,458 ppm
Pineapple - Ananas Comosus - E	Fruit	1,333 ppm
Papaya - Carica Papaya - E - M	Fruit	895 ppm
Plum - Prunus Domestica - E - M	Fruit	878 ppm
Emblic, Myrobalan - Phyllanthus Emblica - E	Fruit	871 ppm
Fig - Ficus Carica - E	Fruit	814 ppm
Cacao - Theobroma Ccacao - E	Seed	800 ppm
Strawberry Guava - Psidium Cattleianum - E	Fruit	775 ppm
Grape Citrus Paradisi - E	Fruit	760 ppm
Carambola, Star Averrhoa Carambola - E	Fruit	110-1,210 ppm

Species	Part	Quantity
Pear - Pyrus Communis - E	Fruit	432 ppm
Apple - Malus Domestica - E	Fruit	373 ppm
Black Currant - Ribes Nigrum - E	Fruit Juice	35 ppm
Elephant Garlic, Kurrat - Allium Ampeloprasum - E	Plant	Trace
Jericho Rose - Anastatica Hierochuntica	Fruit	Trace
Sugar-Apple, Sweetsop - Annona Squamosa - E	Fruit	Trace
Horseradish - Armoracia Rusticana - E	Root	Trace
Tarragon - Artemisia Dracunculus - M	Leaf	Trace
Tea - Camellia Sinensis - E	Plant	Trace
Jack Bean - Canavalia Ensiformis - E	Seed	Trace
Shepherd's Purse - Capsella Bursa-Pastoris - E - M	Plant	Trace
Hops - Humulus Lupulus - E - M - T	Fruit	Trace
Antler Herb, Clubmoss - Lycopodium Clavatum - M - T	Pollen Or Spore	Trace
Chinaberry - Melia Azedarach - T	Seed	Trace
Spearmint - Mentha Spicata - E - M - T	Leaf	Trace
Paeonia officinalis L. -- Double Peony	Root	Trace
Ban-Xia, Pan-Hsia - Pinellia Ternata - E - M - T	Tuber	Trace
Sour Cherry - Prunus Cerasus - E - M - T	Fruit	Trace
Radish - Raphanus Sativus - E	Plant	Trace
Terminalia chebula RETZ. -- Black Myrobalan, Chebulic Myrobalan, Ink Nut, Myrobalan	Fruit	Trace
Cowgrass, Peavine Clover, Purple Clover, Red Clover - Trifolium Pratense - E - M	Plant	Trace
European Mistletoe - Viscum Album - M - T	Juice	Trace

PLANTS CONTAINING ASPARGINE

Species	Part	Quantity
White Lupine - Lupinus Albus - M - T	Seed	116,340 ppm
Commom Licorice, Licorice, Licorice-Root, Smooth Licorice - Glycyrrhiza Glabra - M	Root	40,000 ppm
Comfrey - Symphytum Officinale - E - M - T	Root	30,000 ppm
Marshmallow, White Mallow - Althaea Officinalis - M	Root	20,000 ppm
Water Lotus - Nelumbo Nucifera - E - M	Rhizome	20,000 ppm
Date Palm - Phoenix Dactylifera - E	Fruit	4,500 ppm
Orange - Citrus Sinensis - E	Fruit	1,800 ppm
Pineapple - Ananas Comosus - E	Fruit	1,251 ppm
Mandarin, Tangerine - Citrus Reticulata - E	Fruit	850 ppm
Ginger - Zingiber Officinale - E	Rhizome	500 ppm
Grape Citrus Paradisi - E	Fruit	420 ppm
Tomato - Lycopersicon Esculentum - E - M - T	Fruit	300 ppm
Apple - Malus Domestica - E	Fruit	171 ppm
Black Currant - Ribes Nigrum - E	Fruit Juice	87 ppm
Milfoil, Yarrow - Achillea Millefolium - M	Plant	Trace
Mud Plantain, Tse-Hsieh, Water Plantain, Ze-Xie - Alisma Plantago-Aquatica - M	Plant	Trace
Elephant Garlic, Kurrat - Allium Ampeloprasum - E	Plant	Trace
Onion, Shallot - Allium Cepa - Shallot Bulb - E	Bulb	Trace
Giant Taro - Alocasia Macrorrhiza - E	Plant	Trace
Sugar-Apple, Sweetsop - Annona Squamosa - E	Plant	Trace
Celery - Apium Graveolens - E	Root	Trace
Horseradish - Armoracia Rusticana - E	Root	Trace
Tarragon - Artemisia Dracunculus - M	Leaf	Trace
Asparagus lucidus LINDL. -- Lucid Asparagus	Root	Trace
Asparagus - Asparagus Officinalis - E	Shoot	Trace
Atropa bella-donna L. -- Belladonna	Root	Trace
Tea - Camellia Sinensis - E	Plant	Trace
Bell Pepper, Cherry Pepper, Cone Pepper, Green Pepper, Paprika, Sweet Pepper - Capsicum Annuum - E	Fruit	Trace
Cayenne, Chili, Hot Pepper, Red Chili, Spur Pepper, Tabasco - Capsicum Frutescens - E	Fruit	Trace
Coffee - Coffea Arabica - E - M	Seed	Trace
Convallaria majalis L. -- Lily-Of-The-Valley	Plant	Trace
Euonymus atropurpureus JACQ. -- Burning Bush, Wahoo	Bark	Trace
Strawberry - Fragaria spp. - E	Plant	Trace
Ginkgo, Maidenhair Tree - Ginkgo Biloba - Tree - E - M - T	Fruit	Trace

ASPARGINE CONTINUED

Species	Part	Quantity
Hops - Humulus Lupulus - E - M - T	Fruit	Trace
Huperzia spp -- Cutleaf Clubmoss	Plant	Trace
Chinese Boxthorn, Chinese Matrimony Vine, Chinese Wolfberry - Lycium Chinense - E - M	Leaf	Trace
Tobacco - Nicotiana Tabacum - Leaf	Leaf	Trace
Black Caraway, Black Cumin, Fennel-Flower, Nutmeg-Flower, Roman Coriander - Nigella Sativa - E - M	Seed	Trace
Rice - Oryza Sativa - E	Juice	Trace
American Ginseng, Ginseng - Panax Quinquefolius - M	Plant	Trace
Black bean, Dwarf bean, Field bean, Flageolet bean, French bean, Garden bean, Green bean, Haricot, Haricot bean, Haricot vert, Kidney bean, Navy bean, Pop bean, Popping bean, Snap bean, String bean, Wax bean - Phaseolus Vulgaris - E	Fruit	Trace
Betel Pepper - Piper Betel - E - M	Leaf	Trace
Sour Cherry - Prunus Cerasus - E - M - T	Fruit	Trace
Black Locust - Robinia Pseudoacacia - T	Leaf	Trace
Sage - Salvia Officinalis - E - M	Plant	Trace
Santalum album L. -- White Sandalwood	Fruit	Trace
Terminalia chebula RETZ. -- Black Myrobalan, Chebulic Myrobalan, Ink Nut, Myrobalan	Fruit	Trace
Tilia sp. -- Basswood, Lime, Linden	Fruit	Trace
Broadbean, Faba Bean, Habas - Vicia Faba - E	Leaf	Trace
Black Gram - Vigna Mungo - E	Seed	Trace
Green Gram, Mungbean - Vigna Radiata - E	Seed	Trace
European Mistletoe - Viscum Album - M - T	Juice	Trace
Indian Fig, Nopal, Nopalito, Prickly Pear - Opuntia Ficus-Indica - E - M	Seed	5,740 ppm
Sicklepod - Senna Obtusifolia - E - T	Seed	2,440 ppm
Buffalo Gourd - Cucurbita Foetidissima - E - M - T	Seed	2,150-3,080 ppm
Wheat - Triticum Aestivum - E - M	Seed	1,449 ppm
Date Palm - Phoenix Dactylifera - E	Fruit	1,140 ppm
Watermelon - Citrullus Lanatus - E	Fruit	236 ppm
American Ginseng, Ginseng - Panax Quinquefolius - M	Plant	200 ppm
Gum Arabic, Gum Arabic Tree, Kher, Senegal Gum, Sudan Gum Arabic - Acacia Senegal - M	Plant	Trace
Onion, Shallot - Allium Cepa - Shallot Bulb - E	Bulb	Trace
Tea - Camellia Sinensis - E	Leaf	Trace
Coffee - Coffea Arabica - E - M	Seed	Trace
Carrot - Daucus Carota - E	Tissue Culture	Trace
Ginkgo, Maidenhair Tree - Ginkgo Biloba - Tree - E - M - T	Seed	Trace
Flax, Lin Linum Usitatissimum - E	Seed	Trace
Rice - Oryza Sativa - E	Plant	Trace
Tilia sp. -- Basswood, Lime, Linden	Flower	Trace
Withania somnifera (L.) DUNAL - Ashwagandha	Fruit	Trace

PLANTS CONTAINING CYSTEINE

Species	Part	Quantity
Girasol, Sun Helianthus Annuus - E	Seed	16,000 ppm
Soybean - Glycine Max - E	Seed	6,430 ppm
Watermelon - Citrullus Lanatus - E	Seed	5,742 ppm

PLANTS CONTAINING GLUTAMIC ACID

Species	Part	Quantity
Ceratonia siliqua L. -- Carob, Locust Bean, St.John's-Bread	Seed	131,600 ppm
White Lupine - Lupinus Albus - M - T	Seed	96,985 ppm
Soybean - Glycine Max - E	Seed	77,280 ppm
Bok-Choy, Celery Cabbage, Celery Mustard, Chinese Cabbage, Chinese Mustard, Chinese White Cabbage, Pak-Choi - Brassica Chinensis - E	Leaf	76,932 ppm
Chives - Allium Schoenoprasum - E	Leaf	72,385 ppm
Groundnut, Peanut - Arachis Hypogaea - E - M	Seed	65,281 ppm
Asparagus - Asparagus Officinalis - E	Shoot	64,645 ppm
Wheat - Triticum Aestivum - E - M	Seed	63,000 ppm
Butternut - Juglans Cinerea - E	Seed	62,942 ppm

Almond - Prunus Dulcis - E - M - T	Seed	62,070 ppm
Chaya - Cnidoscolus Chayamansa - E	Leaf	58,900 ppm
Pigeonpea - Cajanus Vajan - E	Seed	56,270 ppm
Black bean, Dwarf bean, Field bean, Flageolet bean, French bean, Garden bean, Green bean, Haricot, Haricot bean, Haricot vert, Kidney bean, Navy bean, Pop bean, Popping bean, Snap bean, String bean, Wax bean - Phaseolus Vulgaris - E	Sprout Seedling	55,054 ppm
Cassie, Huisache, Opopanax, Popinac, Sweet Acacia - Acacia Farnesiana - M	Leaf	54,070 ppm
Tomato - Lycopersicon Esculentum - E - M - T	Fruit	54,053 ppm
White Mustard - Sinapis Alba - E - M - T	Seed	53,275 ppm
Watermelon - Citrullus Lanatus - E	Seed	53,000 ppm
Chinese Foxglove - Rehmannia Glutinosa - M	Root	53,000 ppm
Sesame - Sesamum Indicum - E - M	Seed	51,927 ppm
Pistachio - Pistacia Vera - E	Seed	51,139 ppm
Lentil - Lens Culinaris - E	Seed	49,000 ppm
Opium Poppy, Poppyseed Poppy - Papaver Somniferum - E	Seed	48,713 ppm
Green Gram, Mungbean - Vigna Radiata - E	Seed	46,883 ppm
Pumpkin - Cucurbita Pepo - E	Seed	46,358 ppm
Broadbean, Faba Bean, Habas - Vicia Faba - E	Seed	45,000 ppm
Pea - Pisum Sativum - E	Fruit	44,313 ppm
Alholva, Bockshornklee, Fenugreek, Greek Clover, Greek Trigonella Foenum-Graecum - E - M	Seed	43,870 ppm
Asparagus Pea, Goa Bean, Winged Bean - Psophocarpus Tetragonolobus - E	Seed	43,749 ppm
Papaver bracteatum L. -- Great Scarlet Poppy	Seed	43,200 ppm
Asparagus bean, Pea bean, Yardlong bean - Vigna Unguiculata subsp. Sesquipedalis - E	Seed	43,190 ppm
Bonavist Bean, Hyacinth Bean, Lablab Bean - Lablab Purpureus - E - M - T	Seed	42,815 ppm
Lentil - Lens Culinaris - E	Sprout Seedling	41,935 ppm
Vinespinach - Basella Alba - E - M	Leaf	41,015 ppm
Spinach - Spinacia Oleracea - E	Plant	40,735 ppm
Cowage, Velvetbean - Mucuna Pruriens - E	Seed	40,440 ppm
Cauli Brassica Oleracea var. Botrytis - E	Leaf	40,275 ppm
Jew's Mallow, Mulukiya, Nalta Jute - Corchorus Olitorius - E - M	Leaf	40,130 ppm
Cucumber - Cucumis Sativus - E	Fruit	38,987 ppm
Chickpea, Garbanzo - Cicer Arietinum - E	Seed	38,150 ppm
Barley, Barleygrass - Hordeum Vulgare - E - M	Seed	38,000 ppm
Berro, Watercress - Nasturtium Officinale - E	Herb	38,000 ppm
Indian Fig, Nopal, Nopalito, Prickly Pear - Opuntia Ficus-Indica - E - M	Seed	37,500 ppm
Black bean, Dwarf bean, Field bean, Flageolet bean, French bean, Garden bean, Green bean, Haricot, Haricot bean, Haricot vert, Kidney bean, Navy bean, Pop bean, Popping bean, Snap bean, String bean, Wax bean - Phaseolus Vulgaris - E	Seed	37,019 ppm
Cashew - Anacardium Occidentale - E	Seed	36,867 ppm
Buffalo Gourd - Cucurbita Foetidissima - E - M - T	Seed	52,800-73,530 ppm
Cabbage, Red Cabbage, White Cabbage - Brassica Oleracea var. Capitata - E	Leaf	36,099 ppm
Black Caraway, Black Cumin, Fennel-Flower, Nutmeg-Flower, Roman Coriander - Nigella Sativa - E - M	Seed	35,900 ppm
Adzuki Bean - Vigna Angularis - E	Seed	35,802 ppm
Pigweed - Amaranthus sp. - E - M	Leaf	35,128 ppm
Pea - Pisum Sativum - E	Seed	35,005 ppm
Pumpkin - Cucurbita Pepo - E	Fruit	35,000 ppm
Cauli Brassica Oleracea var. Botrytis - E	Flower	34,240 ppm
Butter Bean, Lima Bean - Phaseolus Lunatus - E	Seed	33,820 ppm
Purslane, Verdolaga - Portulaca Oleracea - E	Herb	33,792 ppm
Swamp Cabbage, Water Spinach - Ipomoea Aquatica - E	Leaf	33,465 ppm
Lambsquarter - Chenopodium Album - E - M - T	Leaf	33,188 ppm
Brazilnut, Brazilnut-Tree, Creamnut, Paranut - Bertholletia Eexcelsa - E	Seed	32,600 ppm
Fennel - Foeniculum Vulgare - M	Fruit	32,427 ppm

GLUTAMIC ACID CONTINUED

Oats - Avena Sativa - E - M	Seed	31,000 ppm
Beet, Beetroot, Garden Beet, Sugar Beet - Beta Vulgaris - E	Root	30,994 ppm
Lettuce - Lactuca Sativa - E	Leaf	30,333 ppm
Italian Stone Pine, Pignolia - Pinus Pinea - M	Seed	40,840-59,800 ppm
Water Lotus - Nelumbo Nucifera - E - M	Seed	29,000 ppm
Corn Salad, Lamb's Lettuce - Valerianella Locusta - E	Plant	28,195 ppm
Evening-Primrose - Oenothera Biennis - E - M	Seed	28,068 ppm
Okra - Abelmoschus Esculentus Friut - E - M	Fruit	27,100 ppm
Endive, Escarole - Cichorium Endivia - M	Leaf	26,731 ppm
Jerusalem Artichoke - Helianthus Tuberosus E	Tuber	26,493 ppm
Corn - Zea Mays - E	Seed	26,457 ppm
Radish - Raphanus Sativus - E	Root	25,580 ppm
Aubergine, Egg Solanum Melongena - E	Fruit	24,907 ppm
Ben Nut, Benzolive Tree, Drumstick Tree, Horseradish Tree, Moringa, West Indian Ben - Moringa Oleifera - E	Shoot	10,350-48,500 ppm
Potato - Solanum Tuberosum - E	Tuber	24,150 ppm
Curly Kale, Kale, Kitchen Kale, Scotch Kale - Brassica Oleracea var. Sabellica l. var. Acephala - E	Leaf	24,065 ppm
Buckwheat - Fagopyrum Esculentum - E	Seed	23,300 ppm
Aloe, Bitter Aloes - Aloe Vera - E - M	Leaf	0-43,256 ppm
Cayenne, Chili, Hot Pepper, Red Chili, Spur Pepper, Tabasco - Capsicum Frutescens - E	Fruit	21,542 ppm
Collards, Cow Cabbage, Spring-Heading Cabbage, Tall Kale, Tree Kale - Brassica Oleracea - E	Leaf	21,471 ppm
Rye - Secale Cereale - E	Seed	36,610-41,110 ppm
Summer Squash - Cucurbita spp. - E	Fruit	19,935 ppm
Chayote - Sechium Edule - E - M	Fruit	19,570 ppm
Garlic - Allium Sativum Bulb - E	Bulb	19,320 ppm
Black bean, Dwarf bean, Field bean, Flageolet bean, French bean, Garden bean, Green bean, Haricot, Haricot bean, Haricot vert, Kidney bean, Navy bean, Pop bean, Popping bean, Snap bean, String bean, Wax bean - Phaseolus Vulgaris - E	Fruit	19,219 ppm
Oats - Avena Sativa - E - M	Plant	19,000 ppm
Asparagus Pea, Goa Bean, Winged Bean - Psophocarpus Tetragonolobus - E	Tuber	18,779 ppm
Ginkgo, Maidenhair Tree - Ginkgo Biloba - Tree - E - M - T	Seed	18,643 ppm
Macadamia - Macadamia spp. - E	Seed	18,330 ppm
Celery - Apium Graveolens - E	Pt	18,285 ppm
Green Gram, Mungbean - Vigna Radiata - E	Sprout Seedling	16,912 ppm
Asparagus Pea, Goa Bean, Winged Bean - Psophocarpus Tetragonolobus - E	Leaf	16,803 ppm
Carrot - Daucus Carota - E	Root	16,545 ppm
Indian Fig, Nopal, Nopalito, Prickly Pear - Opuntia Ficus-Indica - E - M	Bud	16,000 ppm
Rapini, Seven-Top Turnip, Turnip - Brassica Rapa - E	Root	15,990 ppm
Basil, Cuban Basil, Sweet Basil - Ocimum Basilicum - E	Leaf	15,650 ppm
Bell Pepper, Cherry Pepper, Cone Pepper, Green Pepper, Paprika, Sweet Pepper - Capsicum Annuum - E	Fruit	15,277 ppm
Cassava, Tapioca, Yuca - Manihot Esculenta - E	Root	14,925 ppm
Rutabaga, Swede, Swedish Turnip - Brassica Napus var. Napobrassica - E	Root	13,730 ppm
Chaparral, Creosote Bush - Larrea Tridentata - M	Plant	13,600 ppm
Squaw Perideridia Gairdneri - E - M	Root	12,319 ppm
Breadroot, Indian Bread-Root, Indian Turnip, Prairie Apple, Prairie Potato, Prairie Turnip - Psoralea Esculenta - E - M - T	Root	12,319 ppm
Bread Artocarpus Altilis - E	Seed	10,360-23,690 ppm
Apricot - Prunus Armeniaca - E - M - T	Fruit	11,500 ppm
American Chestnut - Castanea Dentata - E - M	Seed	11,043 ppm
Strawberry - Fragaria spp. - E	Fruit	10,676 ppm
Pinyon Pine - Pinus Edulis	Seed	19,690-20,925 ppm
Cacao - Theobroma Ccacao - E	Seed	10,200 ppm
Chinese Chestnut - Castanea Mollisima - M	Seed	9,600 ppm
Ginger - Zingiber Officinale - E	Rhizome	9,328 ppm
Peach - Prunus Persica - E - M - T	Fruit	8,586 ppm

Species	Part	Quantity
Mountain Yam - Dioscorea Pentaphylla - E	Root	8,565 ppm
Avocado - Persea Americana - E - M - T	Fruit	8,045 ppm
Burdock, Gobo, Great Burdock - Arctium lappa - E - M - T	Root	7,850 ppm
Guavas - Psidium Guajava - E	Fruit	7,704 ppm
Yambean - Pachyrhizus Erosus - E	Tuber	7,560 ppm
Watermelon - Citrullus Lanatus - E	Fruit	7,420 ppm
Pawpaw - Asimina Triloba - Friut - E	Fruit	7,332 ppm
European Grape, Grape, Grapevine, Vigne Vinifere, Wine Grape - Vitis Vinifera - E - M	Fruit	7,099 ppm
Orange - Citrus Sinensis - E	Fruit	7,097 ppm
Mango - Mangifera Indica - E - M	Fruit	6,800 ppm
Water Lotus - Nelumbo Nucifera - E - M	Rhizome	6,650 ppm
Emblic, Myrobalan - Phyllanthus Emblica - E	Fruit	6,535 ppm
Sweet Potato - Ipomoea Batatas - E	Root	6,360 ppm
Date Palm - Phoenix Dactylifera - E	Fruit	6,160 ppm
Taro - Colocasia Esculenta - E	Root	5,925 ppm
European Chestnut - Castanea Sativa - E - M	Seed	5,628 ppm
Blueberry - Vaccinium Corymbosum - E	Fruit	5,393 ppm
Mandarin, Tangerine - Citrus Reticulata - E	Fruit	5,158 ppm
Calathea allouia (AUBL.) LINDL. - Leren, Lleren	Root	8,825-9,710 ppm
American Elder, American Elderberry, Elderberry, Sweet Elder - Sambucus Canadensis - E	Fruit	4,752 ppm
American Ginseng, Ginseng - Panax Quinquefolius - M	Plant	4,450 ppm
Banana, Plantain - Musa x Paradisiaca - E	Fruit	4,312 ppm
Carambola, Star Averrhoa Carambola - E	Fruit	770-8,480 ppm
Strawberry Guava - Psidium Cattleianum - E	Fruit	3,930 ppm
Fig - Ficus Carica - E	Fruit	3,447 ppm
Curry Murraya spp. - E - M	Fruit	3,341 ppm
Pineapple - Ananas Comosus - E	Fruit	3,333 ppm
Grape Citrus Paradisi - E	Fruit	2,800 ppm
Plum - Prunus Domestica - E - M	Fruit	2,500 ppm
Pear - Pyrus Communis - E	Fruit	1,729 ppm
Apple - Malus Domestica - E	Fruit	1,244 ppm
Black Currant - Ribes Nigrum - E	Fruit Juice	210 ppm
Pea - Pisum Sativum - E	Shoot	70 ppm
Elephant Garlic, Kurrat - Allium Ampeloprasum - E	Plant	Trace
Anabasis aphylla L. -- Anabasis	Plant	Trace
Tarragon - Artemisia Dracunculus - M	Shoot	Trace
Shepherd's Purse - Capsella Bursa-Pastoris - E - M	Plant	Trace
Papaya - Carica Papaya - E - M	Fruit	Trace
Gotu Kola, Pennywort - Centella Asiatica - E - M	Plant	Trace
Lemon - Citrus Limon - E	Plant	Trace
Alehoof - Glechoma Hederacea - M	Plant	Trace
Huperzia spp -- Cutleaf Clubmoss	Plant	Trace
Flax, Lin Linum Usitatissimum - E	Seed	Trace
Chinaberry - Melia Azedarach - T	Plant	Trace
White Mulberry - Morus Alba - E - M	Leaf	Trace
Rice - Oryza Sativa - E	Hay	Trace
Ban-Xia, Pan-Hsia - Pinellia Ternata - E - M - T	Tuber	Trace
Sour Cherry - Prunus Cerasus - E - M - T	Fruit	Trace
Castorbean - Ricinus Communis - T	Seed	Trace
Dandelion - Taraxacum Officinale - E - M	Leaf	Trace
Tilia sp. -- Basswood, Lime, Linden	Fruit	Trace
Puncture-Vine - Tribulus Terrestris - Leaf	Fruit	Trace
Cowgrass, Peavine Clover, Purple Clover, Red Clover - Trifolium Pratense - E - M	Plant	Trace

Plants Containing Glutamine

Species	Part	Quantity
Sicklepod - Senna Obtusifolia - E - T	Seed	21,300 ppm
Aloe, Bitter Aloes - Aloe Vera - E - M	Leaf	0-20,607 ppm
Date Palm - Phoenix Dactylifera - E	Fruit	870 ppm
Orange - Citrus Sinensis - E	Fruit	630 ppm
Black Currant - Ribes Nigrum - E	Fruit Juice	290 ppm
Pineapple - Ananas Comosus - E	Fruit	256 ppm
Apple - Malus Domestica - E	Plant	20 ppm

PLANTS CONTAINING GLYCINE

Species	Part	Quantity

GLYCINE CONTINUED

Plant	Part	ppm
Ceratonia siliqua L. -- Carob, Locust Bean, St.John's-Bread	Seed	24,910 ppm
Berro, Watercress - Nasturtium Officinale - E	Herb	22,400 ppm
Black Caraway, Black Cumin, Fennel-Flower, Nutmeg-Flower, Roman Coriander - Nigella Sativa - E - M	Seed	20,700 ppm
Sesame - Sesamum Indicum - E - M	Seed	19,918 ppm
Pumpkin - Cucurbita Pepo - E	Seed	19,295 ppm
Groundnut, Peanut - Arachis Hypogaea - E - M	Seed	18,993 ppm
Soybean - Glycine Max - E	Seed	18,445 ppm
Jew's Mallow, Mulukiya, Nalta Jute - Corchorus Olitorius - E - M	Leaf	17,420 ppm
Chives - Allium Schoenoprasum - E	Leaf	17,375 ppm
White Lupine - Lupinus Albus - M - T	Seed	17,185 ppm
Spinach - Spinacia Oleracea - E	Plant	15,914 ppm
Pigweed - Amaranthus sp. - E - M	Leaf	15,880 ppm
Lambsquarter - Chenopodium Album - E - M - T	Leaf	15,861 ppm
Butternut - Juglans Cinerea - E	Seed	15,601 ppm
Black bean, Dwarf bean, Field bean, Flageolet bean, French bean, Garden bean, Green bean, Haricot, Haricot bean, Haricot vert, Kidney bean, Navy bean, Pop bean, Popping bean, Snap bean, String bean, Wax bean - Phaseolus Vulgaris - E	Sprout Seedling	15,484 ppm
Girasol, Sun Helianthus Annuus - E	Seed	15,400 ppm
Cowage, Velvetbean - Mucuna Pruriens - E	Seed	15,265 ppm
Cassie, Huisache, Opopanax, Popinac, Sweet Acacia - Acacia Farnesiana - M	Leaf	14,590 ppm
Alholva, Bockshornklee, Fenugreek, Greek Clover, Greek Trigonella Foenum-Graecum - E - M	Seed	14,366 ppm
Indian Fig, Nopal, Nopalito, Prickly Pear - Opuntia Ficus-Indica - E - M	Seed	14,200 ppm
White Mustard - Sinapis Alba - E - M - T	Seed	14,038 ppm
Buffalo Gourd - Cucurbita Foetidissima - E - M - T	Seed	14,735-27,700 ppm
Swamp Cabbage, Water Spinach - Ipomoea Aquatica - E	Leaf	13,150 ppm
Almond - Prunus Dulcis - E - M - T	Seed	12,929 ppm
Asparagus - Asparagus Officinalis - E	Shoot	12,774 ppm
Asparagus Pea, Goa Bean, Winged Bean - Psophocarpus Tetragonolobus - E	Seed	12,437 ppm
Fennel - Foeniculum Vulgare - M	Fruit	12,144 ppm
Ben Nut, Benzolive Tree, Drumstick Tree, Horseradish Tree, Moringa, West Indian Ben - Moringa Oleifera - E	Shoot	5,170-24,225 ppm
Broadbean, Faba Bean, Habas - Vicia Faba - E	Seed	12,100 ppm
Opium Poppy, Poppyseed Poppy - Papaver Somniferum - E	Seed	12,047 ppm
Pistachio - Pistacia Vera - E	Seed	11,391 ppm
Bonavist Bean, Hyacinth Bean, Lablab Bean - Lablab Purpureus - E - M - T	Seed	11,345 ppm
Purslane, Verdolaga - Portulaca Oleracea - E	Herb	11,000 ppm
Corn Salad, Lamb's Lettuce - Valerianella Locusta - E	Leaf	10,970 ppm
Chaya - Cnidoscolus Chayamansa - E	Leaf	10,850 ppm
Lentil - Lens Culinaris - E	Sprout Seedling	10,635 ppm
Evening-Primrose - Oenothera Biennis - E - M	Seed	10,500 ppm
Green Gram, Mungbean - Vigna Radiata - E	Seed	10,489 ppm
Curly Kale, Kale, Kitchen Kale, Scotch Kale - Brassica Oleracea var. Sabellica l. var. Acephala - E	Leaf	10,232 ppm
Cauli Brassica Oleracea var. Botrytis - E	Leaf	10,203 ppm
Butter Bean, Lima Bean - Phaseolus Lunatus - E	Seed	10,090 ppm
Collards, Cow Cabbage, Spring-Heading Cabbage, Tall Kale, Tree Kale - Brassica Oleracea - E	Leaf	9,834 ppm
Buckwheat - Fagopyrum Esculentum - E	Seed	9,750 ppm
Vinespinach - Basella Alba - E - M	Leaf	9,710 ppm
Lettuce - Lactuca Sativa - E	Leaf	9,500 ppm
Black bean, Dwarf bean, Field bean, Flageolet bean, French bean, Garden bean, Green bean, Haricot, Haricot bean, Haricot vert, Kidney bean, Navy bean, Pop bean, Popping bean, Snap bean, String bean, Wax bean - Phaseolus Vulgaris - E	Seed	9,474 ppm

Papaver bracteatum L. -- Great Scarlet Poppy	Seed	9,350 ppm
Endive, Escarole - Cichorium Endivia - M	Leaf	9,340 ppm
Bok-Choy, Celery Cabbage, Celery Mustard, Chinese Cabbage, Chinese Mustard, Chinese White Cabbage, Pak-Choi - Brassica Chinensis - E	Leaf	9,189 ppm
Asparagus Pea, Goa Bean, Winged Bean - Psophocarpus Tetragonolobus - E	Tuber	9,155 ppm
Chickpea, Garbanzo - Cicer Arietinum - E	Seed	9,075 ppm
Pigeonpea - Cajanus Vajan - E	Seed	8,970 ppm
Adzuki Bean - Vigna Angularis - E	Seed	8,734 ppm
Pea - Pisum Sativum - E	Seed	8,704 ppm
Asparagus bean, Pea bean, Yardlong bean - Vigna Unguiculata subsp. Sesquipedalis - E	Seed	8,550 ppm
Cauli Brassica Oleracea var. Botrytis - E	Flower	8,270 ppm
Cashew - Anacardium Occidentale - E	Seed	8,169 ppm
Pumpkin - Cucurbita Pepo - E	Fruit	8,000 ppm
Italian Stone Pine, Pignolia - Pinus Pinea - M	Seed	12,230-15,000 ppm
Water Lotus - Nelumbo Nucifera - E - M	Rhizome	7,464 ppm
Pea - Pisum Sativum - E	Fruit	7,122 ppm
Orange - Citrus Sinensis - E	Fruit	7,097 ppm
Summer Squash - Cucurbita spp. - E	Fruit	6,962 ppm
Basil, Cuban Basil, Sweet Basil - Ocimum Basilicum - E	Leaf	6,900 ppm
Sicklepod - Senna Obtusifolia - E - T	Seed	6,890 ppm
Brazilnut, Brazilnut-Tree, Creamnut, Paranut - Bertholletia Eexcelsa - E	Seed	6,797 ppm
Water Lotus - Nelumbo Nucifera - E - M	Seed	6,697 ppm
Black bean, Dwarf bean, Field bean, Flageolet bean, French bean, Garden bean, Green bean, Haricot, Haricot bean, Haricot vert, Kidney bean, Navy bean, Pop bean, Popping bean, Snap bean, String bean, Wax bean - Phaseolus Vulgaris - E	Fruit	6,680 ppm
Green Gram, Mungbean - Vigna Radiata - E	Sprout Seedling	6,618 ppm
Asparagus Pea, Goa Bean, Winged Bean - Psophocarpus Tetragonolobus - E	Leaf	6,436 ppm
Chayote - Sechium Edule - E - M	Fruit	6,430 ppm
Cayenne, Chili, Hot Pepper, Red Chili, Spur Pepper, Tabasco - Capsicum Frutescens - E	Fruit	6,038 ppm
Potato - Solanum Tuberosum - E	Tuber	5,700 ppm
Wheat - Triticum Aestivum - E - M	Seed	5,635 ppm
Aubergine, Egg Solanum Melongena - E	Fruit	5,452 ppm
Onion, Shallot - Allium Cepa - Shallot Bulb - E	Bulb	5,341 ppm
Bread Artocarpus Altilis - E	Seed	4,650-10,635 ppm
Corn - Zea Mays - E	Seed	5,283 ppm
Ginkgo, Maidenhair Tree - Ginkgo Biloba - Tree - E - M - T	Seed	5,174 ppm
Mandarin, Tangerine - Citrus Reticulata - E	Fruit	5,158 ppm
Cucumber - Cucumis Sativus - E	Fruit	4,810 ppm
Garlic - Allium Sativum Bulb - E	Bulb	4,800 ppm
Indian Fig, Nopal, Nopalito, Prickly Pear - Opuntia Ficus-Indica - E - M	Bud	4,745 ppm
Okra - Abelmoschus Esculentus - Friut - E - M	Fruit	4,400 ppm
Celery - Apium Graveolens - E	Pt	4,290 ppm
Radish - Raphanus Sativus - E	Root	4,265 ppm
Bell Pepper, Cherry Pepper, Cone Pepper, Green Pepper, Paprika, Sweet Pepper - Capsicum Annuum - E	Fruit	4,228 ppm
Chaparral, Creosote Bush - Larrea Tridentata - M	Plant	4,200 ppm
American Chestnut - Castanea Dentata - E - M	Seed	4,038 ppm
Rye - Secale Cereale - E	Seed	7,010-7,870 ppm
Macadamia - Macadamia spp. - E	Seed	3,815 ppm
Tomato - Lycopersicon Esculentum - E - M - T	Fruit	3,637 ppm
Cabbage, Red Cabbage, White Cabbage - Brassica Oleracea var. Capitata - E	Leaf	3,610 ppm
Pawpaw - Asimina Triloba - Friut - E	Fruit	3,501 ppm
Chinese Chestnut - Castanea Mollisima - M	Seed	3,271 ppm
Avocado - Persea Americana - E - M - T	Fruit	3,226 ppm
Rapini, Seven-Top Turnip, Turnip - Brassica Rapa - E	Root	3,075 ppm
Date Palm - Phoenix Dactylifera - E	Fruit	3,010 ppm
Guavas - Psidium Guajava - E	Fruit	2,952 ppm

GLYCINE CONTINUED

Species	Part	Quantity
Apricot - Prunus Armeniaca - E - M - T	Fruit	2,930 ppm
Yambean - Pachyrhizus Erosus - E	Tuber	2,855 ppm
Strawberry - Fragaria spp. - E	Fruit	2,847 ppm
Sweet Potato - Ipomoea Batatas - E	Root	2,725 ppm
Rutabaga, Swede, Swedish Turnip - Brassica Napus var. Napobrassica - E	Root	2,610 ppm
Taro - Colocasia Esculenta - E	Root	2,520 ppm
Aloe, Bitter Aloes - Aloe Vera - E - M	Leaf	0-5,030 ppm
Ginger - Zingiber Officinale - E	Rhizome	2,486 ppm
Mountain Yam - Dioscorea Pentaphylla - E	Root	2,480 ppm
Jerusalem Artichoke - Helianthus Tuberosus E	Tuber	2,478 ppm
Carrot - Daucus Carota - E	Root	2,455 ppm
European Chestnut - Castanea Sativa - E - M	Seed	2,353 ppm
Beet, Beetroot, Garden Beet, Sugar Beet - Beta Vulgaris - E	Root	2,287 ppm
Calathea allouia (AUBL.) LINDL. - Leren, Lleren	Root	3,920-4,310 ppm
Cassava, Tapioca, Yuca - Manihot Esculenta - E	Root	2,030 ppm
Oats - Avena Sativa - E - M	Seed	2,000 ppm
Chinese Foxglove - Rehmannia Glutinosa - M	Root	2,000 ppm
Peach - Prunus Persica - E - M - T	Fruit	1,944 ppm
Mango - Mangifera Indica - E - M	Fruit	1,900 ppm
Squaw Perideridia Gairdneri - E - M	Root	1,842 ppm
Blueberry - Vaccinium Corymbosum - E	Fruit	1,819 ppm
American Elder, American Elderberry, Elderberry, Sweet Elder - Sambucus Canadensis - E	Fruit	1,782 ppm
Papaya - Carica Papaya - E - M	Fruit	1,611 ppm
Burdock, Gobo, Great Burdock - Arctium lappa - E - M - T	Root	1,550 ppm
American Ginseng, Ginseng - Panax Quinquefolius - M	Plant	1,540 ppm
Strawberry Guava - Psidium Cattleianum - E	Fruit	1,500 ppm
Banana, Plantain - Musa x Paradisiaca - E	Fruit	1,437 ppm
Carambola, Star Averrhoa Carambola - E	Fruit	260-2,860 ppm
Curry Murraya spp. - E - M	Fruit	1,296 ppm
Pineapple - Ananas Comosus - E	Fruit	1,259 ppm
Fig - Ficus Carica - E	Fruit	1,197 ppm
Watermelon - Citrullus Lanatus - E	Fruit	1,178 ppm
Breadroot, Indian Bread-Root, Indian Turnip, Prairie Apple, Prairie Potato, Prairie Turnip - Psoralea Esculenta - E - M - T	Root	1,097 ppm
European Grape, Grape, Grapevine, Vigne Vinifere, Wine Grape - Vitis Vinifera - E - M	Fruit	1,029 ppm
Emblic, Myrobalan - Phyllanthus Emblica - E	Fruit	980 ppm
Cacao - Theobroma Ccacao - E	Seed	900 ppm
Plum - Prunus Domestica - E - M	Fruit	811 ppm
Pear - Pyrus Communis - E	Fruit	679 ppm
Apple - Malus Domestica - E	Plant	497 ppm
Tarragon - Artemisia Dracunculus - M	Shoot	Trace
Tea - Camellia Sinensis - E	Leaf	Trace
Jack Bean - Canavalia Ensiformis - E	Seed	Trace
Gotu Kola, Pennywort - Centella Asiatica - E - M	Plant	Trace
Grape Citrus Paradisi - E	Fruit	Trace
Flax, Lin Linum Usitatissimum - E	Seed	Trace
Chinaberry - Melia Azedarach - T	Plant	Trace
Rice - Oryza Sativa - E	Plant	Trace
Ban-Xia, Pan-Hsia - Pinellia Ternata - E - M - T	Tuber	Trace
Sour Cherry - Prunus Cerasus - E - M - T	Fruit	Trace
Sage - Salvia Officinalis - E - M	Plant	Trace
Common thyme, Garden thyme, Thyme - Thymus Vulgaris - E - M	Plant	Trace
Tilia sp. -- Basswood, Lime, Linden	Fruit	Trace

PLANTS CONTAINING HISTIDINE

Species	Part	Quantity
Girasol, Sun Helianthus Annuus - E	Seed	20,000 ppm
Black bean, Dwarf bean, Field bean, Flageolet bean, French bean, Garden bean, Green bean, Haricot, Haricot bean, Haricot vert, Kidney bean, Navy bean, Pop bean, Popping bean, Snap bean, String bean, Wax bean - Phaseolus Vulgaris - E	Sprout Seedling	12,688 ppm
Ceratonia siliqua L. -- Carob, Locust Bean, St.John's-Bread	Seed	11,750 ppm
White Lupine - Lupinus Albus - M - T	Seed	11,500 ppm

Soybean - Glycine Max - E	Seed	10,770 ppm
Cassie, Huisache, Opopanax, Popinac, Sweet Acacia - Acacia Farnesiana - M	Leaf	9,870 ppm
Buffalo Gourd - Cucurbita Foetidissima - E - M - T	Seed	5,835-19,000 ppm
Bonavist Bean, Hyacinth Bean, Lablab Bean - Lablab Purpureus - E - M - T	Seed	8,986 ppm
Jew's Mallow, Mulukiya, Nalta Jute - Corchorus Olitorius - E - M	Leaf	8,950 ppm
Lentil - Lens Culinaris - E	Seed	8,900 ppm
Pigeonpea - Cajanus Vajan - E	Seed	8,655 ppm
Asparagus Pea, Goa Bean, Winged Bean - Psophocarpus Tetragonolobus - E	Leaf	8,618 ppm
Lentil - Lens Culinaris - E	Sprout Seedling	8,565 ppm
Mat Bean, Moth Bean - Vigna Aconitifolia - E	Seed	8,536 ppm
Butternut - Juglans Cinerea - E	Seed	8,359 ppm
Asparagus bean, Pea bean, Yardlong bean - Vigna Unguiculata subsp. Sesquipedalis - E	Seed	8,245 ppm
White Mustard - Sinapis Alba - E - M - T	Seed	8,153 ppm
Groundnut, Peanut - Arachis Hypogaea - E - M	Seed	8,013 ppm
Berro, Watercress - Nasturtium Officinale - E	Herb	8,000 ppm
Taro - Colocasia Esculenta - E	Leaf	7,950 ppm
Butter Bean, Lima Bean - Phaseolus Lunatus - E	Seed	7,796 ppm
Green Gram, Mungbean - Vigna Radiata - E	Seed	7,642 ppm
Spinach - Spinacia Oleracea - E	Plant	7,601 ppm
Asparagus bean, Pea bean, Yardlong bean - Vigna Unguiculata subsp. Sesquipedalis - E	Fruit	7,407 ppm
Lambsquarter - Chenopodium Album - E - M - T	Leaf	7,389 ppm
Green Gram, Mungbean - Vigna Radiata - E	Sprout Seedling	7,353 ppm
Alholva, Bockshornklee, Fenugreek, Greek Clover, Greek Trigonella Foenum-Graecum - E - M	Seed	7,350 ppm
Pumpkin - Cucurbita Pepo - E	Seed	7,316 ppm
Sesame - Sesamum Indicum - E - M	Seed	7,112 ppm
Broadbean, Faba Bean, Habas - Vicia Faba - E	Seed	7,050 ppm
Watermelon - Citrullus Lanatus - E	Seed	7,018 ppm
Cowage, Velvetbean - Mucuna Pruriens - E	Seed	6,945 ppm
Black bean, Dwarf bean, Field bean, Flageolet bean, French bean, Garden bean, Green bean, Haricot, Haricot bean, Haricot vert, Kidney bean, Navy bean, Pop bean, Popping bean, Snap bean, String bean, Wax bean - Phaseolus Vulgaris - E	Seed	6,754 ppm
Black Mustard - Brassica Nigra - E	Leaf	6,627 ppm
Pigweed - Amaranthus sp. - E - M	Leaf	6,256 ppm
Swamp Cabbage, Water Spinach - Ipomoea Aquatica - E	Leaf	6,240 ppm
Asparagus - Asparagus Officinalis - E	Shoot	6,065 ppm
Adzuki Bean - Vigna Angularis - E	Seed	6,054 ppm
Chives - Allium Schoenoprasum - E	Leaf	6,000 ppm
Oats - Avena Sativa - E - M	Seed	6,000 ppm
Chickpea, Garbanzo - Cicer Arietinum - E	Seed	6,000 ppm
Wheat - Triticum Aestivum - E - M	Seed	6,000 ppm
Almond - Prunus Dulcis - E - M - T	Seed	5,837 ppm
Opium Poppy, Poppyseed Poppy - Papaver Somniferum - E	Seed	5,664 ppm
Asparagus Pea, Goa Bean, Winged Bean - Psophocarpus Tetragonolobus - E	Tuber	5,657 ppm
Vinespinach - Basella Alba - E - M	Leaf	5,650 ppm
Pistachio - Pistacia Vera - E	Seed	5,576 ppm
Bok-Choy, Celery Cabbage, Celery Mustard, Chinese Cabbage, Chinese Mustard, Chinese White Cabbage, Pak-Choi - Brassica Chinensis - E	Leaf	5,556 ppm
Brussel-Sprout - Brassica Oleracea var. Gemmifera - E	Leaf	5,426 ppm
Cauli Brassica Oleracea var. Botrytis - E	Leaf	5,370 ppm
Purslane, Verdolaga - Portulaca Oleracea - E	Herb	5,170 ppm
Cauli Brassica Oleracea var. Botrytis - E	Flower	5,165 ppm
Pea - Pisum Sativum - E	Seed	5,061 ppm
Corn Salad, Lamb's Lettuce - Valerianella Locusta - E	Plant	5,000 ppm

HISTIDINE CONTINUED

Plant	Part	ppm
Collards, Cow Cabbage, Spring-Heading Cabbage, Tall Kale, Tree Kale - Brassica Oleracea - E	Leaf	4,917 ppm
Papaver bracteatum L. -- Great Scarlet Poppy	Seed	4,650 ppm
Ben Nut, Benzolive Tree, Drumstick Tree, Horseradish Tree, Moringa, West Indian Ben - Moringa Oleifera - E	Shoot	1,960-9,185 ppm
Curly Kale, Kale, Kitchen Kale, Scotch Kale - Brassica Oleracea var. Sabellica l. var. Acephala - E	Leaf	4,440 ppm
Brazilnut, Brazilnut-Tree, Creamnut, Paranut - Bertholletia Eexcelsa - E	Seed	4,159 ppm
Cashew - Anacardium Occidentale - E	Seed	4,059 ppm
Chinese Foxglove - Rehmannia Glutinosa - M	Root	4,000 ppm
Summer Squash - Cucurbita spp. - E	Fruit	3,955 ppm
Evening-Primrose - Oenothera Biennis - E - M	Seed	3,949 ppm
Achiote, Annato, Annatto, Annoto, Arnato, Bija, Lipstick Pod, Lipsticktree - Bixa Orellana - E	Seed	3,930 ppm
Italian Stone Pine, Pignolia - Pinus Pinea - M	Seed	5,750-7,475 ppm
Endive, Escarole - Cichorium Endivia - M	Leaf	3,704 ppm
Corn - Zea Mays - E	Seed	3,702 ppm
Lettuce - Lactuca Sativa - E	Leaf	3,667 ppm
Fennel - Foeniculum Vulgare - M	Fruit	3,631 ppm
Mandarin, Tangerine - Citrus Reticulata - E	Fruit	3,546 ppm
Black bean, Dwarf bean, Field bean, Flageolet bean, French bean, Garden bean, Green bean, Haricot, Haricot bean, Haricot vert, Kidney bean, Navy bean, Pop bean, Popping bean, Snap bean, String bean, Wax bean - Phaseolus Vulgaris - E	Fruit	3,494 ppm
Water Lotus - Nelumbo Nucifera - E - M	Seed	3,485 ppm
Chicory, Succory, Witloof - Cichorium Intybus - E - M	Leaf	3,468 ppm
Dill, Garden Dill - Anethum Graveolens - E	Fruit	3,466 ppm
Yambean - Pachyrhizus Erosus - E	Tuber	3,410 ppm
Cayenne, Chili, Hot Pepper, Red Chili, Spur Pepper, Tabasco - Capsicum Frutescens - E	Fruit	3,346 ppm
Cabbage, Red Cabbage, White Cabbage - Brassica Oleracea var. Capitata - E	Leaf	3,343 ppm
Banana, Plantain - Musa x Paradisiaca - E	Fruit	3,147 ppm
Okra - Abelmoschus Esculentus - Friut - E - M	Fruit	3,100 ppm
Aubergine, Egg Solanum Melongena - E	Fruit	3,098 ppm
Rutabaga, Swede, Swedish Turnip - Brassica Napus var. Napobrassica - E	Root	2,900 ppm
Basil, Cuban Basil, Sweet Basil - Ocimum Basilicum - E	Leaf	2,870 ppm
Buckwheat - Fagopyrum Esculentum - E	Seed	2,750 ppm
Garlic - Allium Sativum Bulb - E	Bulb	2,712 ppm
Radish - Raphanus Sativus - E	Root	2,520 ppm
Celery - Apium Graveolens - E	Pt	2,425 ppm
Bread Artocarpus Altilis - E	Seed	2,070-4,735 ppm
Bell Pepper, Cherry Pepper, Cone Pepper, Green Pepper, Paprika, Sweet Pepper - Capsicum Annuum - E	Fruit	2,319 ppm
Chayote - Sechium Edule - E - M	Fruit	2,285 ppm
Ginkgo, Maidenhair Tree - Ginkgo Biloba - Tree - E - M - T	Seed	2,275 ppm
Chinese Chestnut - Castanea Mollisima - M	Seed	2,256 ppm
American Chestnut - Castanea Dentata - E - M	Seed	2,158 ppm
Tomato - Lycopersicon Esculentum - E - M - T	Fruit	2,149 ppm
Potato - Solanum Tuberosum - E	Tuber	2,140 ppm
Kohlrabi - Brassica Oleracea var. Gongylodes - E	Stem	2,111 ppm
Onion, Shallot - Allium Cepa - Shallot Bulb - E	Bulb	2,071 ppm
Rye - Secale Cereale - E	Seed	3,670-4,120 ppm
Cucumber - Cucumis Sativus - E	Fruit	2,025 ppm
Apricot - Prunus Armeniaca - E - M - T	Fruit	1,980 ppm
Jerusalem Artichoke - Helianthus Tuberosus E	Tuber	1,906 ppm
Pumpkin - Cucurbita Pepo - E	Fruit	1,905 ppm
Curry Murraya spp. - E - M	Fruit	1,843 ppm
Water Lotus - Nelumbo Nucifera - E - M	Rhizome	1,820 ppm
Ginger - Zingiber Officinale - E	Rhizome	1,738 ppm
Macadamia - Macadamia spp. - E	Seed	1,730 ppm
Rapini, Seven-Top Turnip, Turnip - Brassica Rapa - E	Root	1,720 ppm
Pea - Pisum Sativum - E	Fruit	1,682 ppm

Lancaster Agriculture Products 717-687-9222 www.lancasterag.com Naturally Interested in Your Future

Species	Part	Quantity
Mountain Yam - Dioscorea Pentaphylla - E	Root	1,615 ppm
Beet, Beetroot, Garden Beet, Sugar Beet - Beta Vulgaris - E	Root	1,577 ppm
Burdock, Gobo, Great Burdock - Arctium lappa - E - M - T	Root	1,550 ppm
Pinyon Pine - Pinus Edulis	Seed	2,770-2,945 ppm
Cassava, Tapioca, Yuca - Manihot Esculenta - E	Root	1,430 ppm
Strawberry - Fragaria spp. - E	Fruit	1,423 ppm
Orange - Citrus Sinensis - E	Fruit	1,359 ppm
Pawpaw - Asimina Triloba - Friut - E	Fruit	1,336 ppm
Carrot - Daucus Carota - E	Root	1,310 ppm
Breadroot, Indian Bread-Root, Indian Turnip, Prairie Apple, Prairie Potato, Prairie Turnip - Psoralea Esculenta - E - M - T	Root	1,266 ppm
European Grape, Grape, Grapevine, Vigne Vinifere, Wine Grape - Vitis Vinifera - E - M	Fruit	1,235 ppm
European Chestnut - Castanea Sativa - E - M	Seed	1,218 ppm
Sweet Potato - Ipomoea Batatas - E	Root	1,200 ppm
Mango - Mangifera Indica - E - M	Fruit	1,200 ppm
Aloe, Bitter Aloes - Aloe Vera - E - M	Leaf	0-2,327 ppm
Taro - Colocasia Esculenta - E	Root	1,160 ppm
Avocado - Persea Americana - E - M - T	Fruit	1,127 ppm
American Ginseng, Ginseng - Panax Quinquefolius - M	Plant	1,100 ppm
Squaw Perideridia Gairdneri - E - M	Root	1,080 ppm
Peach - Prunus Persica - E - M - T	Fruit	1,053 ppm
Calabash Gourd, White-Flowered Gourd - Lagenaria Siceraria - E	Fruit	900 ppm
Plum - Prunus Domestica - E - M	Fruit	878 ppm
Cacao - Theobroma Ccacao - E	Seed	800 ppm
American Elder, American Elderberry, Elderberry, Sweet Elder - Sambucus Canadensis - E	Fruit	742 ppm
Blueberry - Vaccinium Corymbosum - E	Fruit	715 ppm
Watermelon - Citrullus Lanatus - E	Fruit	707 ppm
Pineapple - Ananas Comosus - E	Fruit	667 ppm
Emblic, Myrobalan - Phyllanthus Emblica - E	Fruit	658 ppm
Calathea allouia (AUBL.) LINDL. - Leren, Lleren	Root	1,080-1,190 ppm
Fig - Ficus Carica - E	Fruit	527 ppm
Guavas - Psidium Guajava - E	Fruit	504 ppm
Papaya - Carica Papaya - E - M	Fruit	448 ppm
Date Palm - Phoenix Dactylifera - E	Fruit	390 ppm
Strawberry Guava - Psidium Cattleianum - E	Fruit	260 ppm
Pear - Pyrus Communis - E	Fruit	247 ppm
Carambola, Star Averrhoa Carambola - E	Fruit	40-440 ppm
Apple - Malus Domestica - E	Fruit	187 ppm
Grape Citrus Paradisi - E	Fruit	140 ppm
Elephant Garlic, Kurrat - Allium Ampeloprasum - E	Plant	Trace
Tea - Camellia Sinensis - E	Leaf	Trace
Hemp, Indian Hemp, Marihuana, Marijuana - Cannabis Sativa - M	Seed	Trace
Soybean - Glycine Max - E	Sprout Seedling	Trace
Hops - Humulus Lupulus - E - M - T	Fruit	Trace
Flax, Lin Linum Usitatissimum - E	Seed	Trace
Antler Herb, Clubmoss - Lycopodium Clavatum - M - T	Pollen Or Spore	Trace
Cowgrass, Peavine Clover, Purple Clover, Red Clover - Trifolium Pratense - E - M	Plant	Trace

PLANTS CONTAINING ISOLECINE

Species	Part	Quantity
Girasol, Sun Helianthus Annuus - E	Seed	46,500 ppm
Buffalo Gourd - Cucurbita Foetidissima - E - M - T	Seed	9,825-44,000 ppm
Black bean, Dwarf bean, Field bean, Flageolet bean, French bean, Garden bean, Green bean, Haricot, Haricot bean, Haricot vert, Kidney bean, Navy bean, Pop bean, Popping bean, Snap bean, String bean, Wax bean - Phaseolus Vulgaris - E	Sprout Seedling	20,000 ppm
Soybean - Glycine Max - E	Seed	19,353 ppm
Bok-Choy, Celery Cabbage, Celery Mustard, Chinese Cabbage, Chinese Mustard, Chinese White Cabbage, Pak-Choi - Brassica Chinensis - E	Leaf	18,164 ppm
Taro - Colocasia Esculenta - E	Leaf	18,130 ppm

ISOLEUCINE CONTINUED

Plant	Part	ppm
White Lupine - Lupinus Albus - M - T	Seed	18,030 ppm
Jew's Mallow, Mulukiya, Nalta Jute - Corchorus Olitorius - E - M	Leaf	18,000 ppm
Bonavist Bean, Hyacinth Bean, Lablab Bean - Lablab Purpureus - E - M - T	Seed	17,972 ppm
Spinach - Spinacia Oleracea - E	Plant	17,458 ppm
Wheat - Triticum Aestivum - E - M	Plant	17,000 ppm
Ceratonia siliqua L. -- Carob, Locust Bean, St.John's-Bread	Seed	16,450 ppm
Lambsquarter - Chenopodium Album - E - M - T	Leaf	16,116 ppm
Asparagus Pea, Goa Bean, Winged Bean - Psophocarpus Tetragonolobus - E	Seed	16,016 ppm
Pea - Pisum Sativum - E	Fruit	15,925 ppm
Cowage, Velvetbean - Mucuna Pruriens - E	Seed	15,900 ppm
Cassie, Huisache, Opopanax, Popinac, Sweet Acacia - Acacia Farnesiana - M	Leaf	15,020 ppm
Chives - Allium Schoenoprasum - E	Leaf	14,875 ppm
Butter Bean, Lima Bean - Phaseolus Lunatus - E	Seed	14,785 ppm
Asparagus - Asparagus Officinalis - E	Shoot	14,452 ppm
Pigweed - Amaranthus sp. - E - M	Leaf	14,316 ppm
Lettuce - Lactuca Sativa - E	Leaf	14,000 ppm
Green Gram, Mungbean - Vigna Radiata - E	Sprout Seedling	13,866 ppm
Swamp Cabbage, Water Spinach - Ipomoea Aquatica - E	Leaf	13,810 ppm
Corn Salad, Lamb's Lettuce - Valerianella Locusta - E	Plant	13,750 ppm
Lentil - Lens Culinaris - E	Seed	13,650 ppm
Alholva, Bockshornklee, Fenugreek, Greek Clover, Greek Trigonella Foenum-Graecum - E - M	Seed	13,650 ppm
Pumpkin - Cucurbita Pepo - E	Seed	13,580 ppm
Sesame - Sesamum Indicum - E - M	Seed	13,541 ppm
Black Mustard - Brassica Nigra - E	Leaf	13,402 ppm
Broadbean, Faba Bean, Habas - Vicia Faba - E	Seed	13,210 ppm
Oats - Avena Sativa - E - M	Plant	13,000 ppm
Curly Kale, Kale, Kitchen Kale, Scotch Kale - Brassica Oleracea var. Sabellica l. var. Acephala - E	Leaf	12,675 ppm
Mat Bean, Moth Bean - Vigna Aconitifolia - E	Seed	12,600 ppm
Asparagus bean, Pea bean, Yardlong bean - Vigna Unguiculata subsp. Sesquipedalis - E	Fruit	12,346 ppm
Chicory, Succory, Witloof - Cichorium Intybus - E - M	Leaf	12,240 ppm
Butternut - Juglans Cinerea - E	Seed	12,197 ppm
Watermelon - Citrullus Lanatus - E	Seed	12,100 ppm
Wheat - Triticum Aestivum - E - M	Seed	12,000 ppm
Cauli Brassica Oleracea var. Botrytis - E	Leaf	11,707 ppm
Endive, Escarole - Cichorium Endivia - M	Leaf	11,594 ppm
White Mustard - Sinapis Alba - E - M - T	Seed	11,576 ppm
Purslane, Verdolaga - Portulaca Oleracea - E	Herb	11,400 ppm
Green Gram, Mungbean - Vigna Radiata - E	Seed	11,083 ppm
Black Caraway, Black Cumin, Fennel-Flower, Nutmeg-Flower, Roman Coriander - Nigella Sativa - E - M	Seed	10,960 ppm
Lentil - Lens Culinaris - E	Sprout Seedling	10,865 ppm
Asparagus bean, Pea bean, Yardlong bean - Vigna Unguiculata subsp. Sesquipedalis - E	Seed	10,800 ppm
Black bean, Dwarf bean, Field bean, Flageolet bean, French bean, Garden bean, Green bean, Haricot, Haricot bean, Haricot vert, Kidney bean, Navy bean, Pop bean, Popping bean, Snap bean, String bean, Wax bean - Phaseolus Vulgaris - E	Seed	10,722 ppm
Groundnut, Peanut - Arachis Hypogaea - E - M	Seed	10,680 ppm
Berro, Watercress - Nasturtium Officinale - E	Herb	10,600 ppm
Ben Nut, Benzolive Tree, Drumstick Tree, Horseradish Tree, Moringa, West Indian Ben - Moringa Oleifera - E	Shoot	4,510-21,135 ppm
Collards, Cow Cabbage, Spring-Heading Cabbage, Tall Kale, Tree Kale - Brassica Oleracea - E	Leaf	10,490 ppm
Chickpea, Garbanzo - Cicer Arietinum - E	Seed	10,320 ppm
Pistachio - Pistacia Vera - E	Seed	10,143 ppm

Asparagus Pea, Goa Bean, Winged Bean - Psophocarpus Tetragonolobus - E	Tuber	9,976 ppm
Cauli Brassica Oleracea var. Botrytis - E	Flower	9,820 ppm
Opium Poppy, Poppyseed Poppy - Papaver Somniferum - E	Seed	9,708 ppm
Chaya - Cnidoscolus Chayamansa - E	Plant	9,610 ppm
Brussel-Sprout - Brassica Oleracea var. Gemmifera - E	Leaf	9,425 ppm
Pea - Pisum Sativum - E	Seed	9,224 ppm
Adzuki Bean - Vigna Angularis - E	Seed	9,138 ppm
Almond - Prunus Dulcis - E - M - T	Seed	9,058 ppm
Oats - Avena Sativa - E - M	Seed	9,000 ppm
Chinese Foxglove - Rehmannia Glutinosa - M	Root	9,000 ppm
Asparagus Pea, Goa Bean, Winged Bean - Psophocarpus Tetragonolobus - E	Leaf	8,812 ppm
Pigeonpea - Cajanus Vajan - E	Seed	8,780 ppm
Kohlrabi - Brassica Oleracea var. Gongylodes - E	Stem	8,667 ppm
Dill, Garden Dill - Anethum Graveolens - E	Fruit	8,307 ppm
Papaver bracteatum L. -- Great Scarlet Poppy	Seed	8,300 ppm
Cabbage, Red Cabbage, White Cabbage - Brassica Oleracea var. Capitata - E	Leaf	8,156 ppm
Vinespinach - Basella Alba - E - M	Leaf	7,680 ppm
Fennel - Foeniculum Vulgare - M	Fruit	7,624 ppm
Cashew - Anacardium Occidentale - E	Seed	7,436 ppm
Calabash Gourd, White-Flowered Gourd - Lagenaria Siceraria - E	Fruit	7,400 ppm
Okra - Abelmoschus Esculentus Friut - E - M	Fruit	6,900 ppm
Chayote - Sechium Edule - E - M	Fruit	6,855 ppm
Black bean, Dwarf bean, Field bean, Flageolet bean, French bean, Garden bean, Green bean, Haricot, Haricot bean, Haricot vert, Kidney bean, Navy bean, Pop bean, Popping bean, Snap bean, String bean, Wax bean - Phaseolus Vulgaris - E	Fruit	6,783 ppm
Indian Fig, Nopal, Nopalito, Prickly Pear - Opuntia Ficus-Indica - E - M	Seed	6,775 ppm
Summer Squash - Cucurbita spp. - E	Fruit	6,645 ppm
Achiote, Annato, Annatto, Annoto, Arnato, Bija, Lipstick Pod, Lipsticktree - Bixa Orellana - E	Seed	6,380 ppm
Brazilnut, Brazilnut-Tree, Creamnut, Paranut - Bertholletia Eexcelsa - E	Seed	6,218 ppm
Water Lotus - Nelumbo Nucifera - E - M	Seed	6,212 ppm
Buckwheat - Fagopyrum Esculentum - E	Seed	6,080 ppm
Sicklepod - Senna Obtusifolia - E - T	Seed	5,960 ppm
Aubergine, Egg Solanum Melongena - E	Fruit	5,948 ppm
Basil, Cuban Basil, Sweet Basil - Ocimum Basilicum - E	Leaf	5,880 ppm
Evening-Primrose - Oenothera Biennis - E - M	Seed	5,870 ppm
Radish - Raphanus Sativus - E	Root	5,815 ppm
Potato - Solanum Tuberosum - E	Tuber	5,700 ppm
Cacao - Theobroma Ccacao - E	Seed	5,600 ppm
Corn - Zea Mays - E	Seed	5,366 ppm
Italian Stone Pine, Pignolia - Pinus Pinea - M	Seed	9,330-10,700 ppm
Cayenne, Chili, Hot Pepper, Red Chili, Spur Pepper, Tabasco - Capsicum Frutescens - E	Fruit	5,304 ppm
Garlic - Allium Sativum Bulb - E	Bulb	5,208 ppm
Common thyme, Garden thyme, Thyme - Thymus Vulgaris - E - M	Plant	5,054 ppm
Rutabaga, Swede, Swedish Turnip - Brassica Napus var. Napobrassica - E	Root	4,835 ppm
Chaparral, Creosote Bush - Larrea Tridentata - M	Plant	4,700 ppm
Eryngium creticus -- Cretan culantro	Shoot	0-9,380 ppm
Ginkgo, Maidenhair Tree - Ginkgo Biloba - Tree - E - M - T	Seed	4,661 ppm
Date Palm - Phoenix Dactylifera - E	Fruit	4,650 ppm
Onion, Shallot - Allium Cepa - Shallot Bulb - E	Bulb	4,578 ppm
Rapini, Seven-Top Turnip, Turnip - Brassica Rapa - E	Root	4,425 ppm
Cucumber - Cucumis Sativus - E	Fruit	4,303 ppm
Celery - Apium Graveolens - E	Pt	4,290 ppm
Aloe, Bitter Aloes - Aloe Vera - E - M	Leaf	0-8,526 ppm
Pawpaw - Asimina Triloba - Friut - E	Fruit	4,166 ppm
Indian Fig, Nopal, Nopalito, Prickly Pear - Opuntia Ficus-Indica - E - M	Bud	4,140 ppm

ISOLEUCINE CONTINUED

Species	Part	Quantity
Pumpkin - Cucurbita Pepo - E	Fruit	3,690 ppm
Bell Pepper, Cherry Pepper, Cone Pepper, Green Pepper, Paprika, Sweet Pepper - Capsicum Annuum - E	Fruit	3,683 ppm
Tomato - Lycopersicon Esculentum - E - M - T	Fruit	3,471 ppm
Beet, Beetroot, Garden Beet, Sugar Beet - Beta Vulgaris - E	Root	3,470 ppm
American Chestnut - Castanea Dentata - E - M	Seed	3,438 ppm
Carrot - Daucus Carota - E	Root	3,360 ppm
Jerusalem Artichoke - Helianthus Tuberosus E	Tuber	3,145 ppm
Rye - Secale Cereale - E	Seed	5,490-6,165 ppm
Sweet Potato - Ipomoea Batatas - E	Root	3,019 ppm
Apricot - Prunus Armeniaca - E - M - T	Fruit	3,000 ppm
Ginger - Zingiber Officinale - E	Rhizome	2,926 ppm
Chinese Chestnut - Castanea Mollisima - M	Seed	2,890 ppm
Yambean - Pachyrhizus Erosus - E	Tuber	2,855 ppm
Avocado - Persea Americana - E - M - T	Fruit	2,759 ppm
Water Lotus - Nelumbo Nucifera - E - M	Rhizome	2,585 ppm
Macadamia - Macadamia spp. - E	Seed	2,510 ppm
Mountain Yam - Dioscorea Pentaphylla - E	Root	2,425 ppm
Squaw Perideridia Gairdneri - E - M	Root	2,413 ppm
Watermelon - Citrullus Lanatus - E	Fruit	2,238 ppm
Bread Artocarpus Altilis - E	Fruit	2,175 ppm
Guavas - Psidium Guajava - E	Fruit	2,160 ppm
Mango - Mangifera Indica - E - M	Fruit	2,000 ppm
Cassava, Tapioca, Yuca - Manihot Esculenta - E	Root	1,935 ppm
Orange - Citrus Sinensis - E	Fruit	1,888 ppm
Calathea allouia (AUBL.) LINDL. - Leren, Lleren	Root	3,430-3,775 ppm
Taro - Colocasia Esculenta - E	Root	1,840 ppm
European Chestnut - Castanea Sativa - E - M	Seed	1,720 ppm
Strawberry - Fragaria spp. - E	Fruit	1,661 ppm
Peach - Prunus Persica - E - M - T	Fruit	1,620 ppm
Burdock, Gobo, Great Burdock - Arctium lappa - E - M - T	Root	1,500 ppm
Mandarin, Tangerine - Citrus Reticulata - E	Fruit	1,370 ppm
Blueberry - Vaccinium Corymbosum - E	Fruit	1,365 ppm
American Elder, American Elderberry, Elderberry, Sweet Elder - Sambucus Canadensis - E	Fruit	1,336 ppm
Breadroot, Indian Bread-Root, Indian Turnip, Prairie Apple, Prairie Potato, Prairie Turnip - Psoralea Esculenta - E - M - T	Root	1,308 ppm
Banana, Plantain - Musa x Paradisiaca - E	Fruit	1,282 ppm
Carambola, Star Averrhoa Carambola - E	Fruit	230-2,530 ppm
Fig - Ficus Carica - E	Fruit	1,101 ppm
Cassie, Huisache, Opopanax, Popinac, Sweet Acacia - Acacia Farnesiana - M	Seed	1,100 ppm
Strawberry Guava - Psidium Cattleianum - E	Fruit	1,085 ppm
Plum - Prunus Domestica - E - M	Fruit	1,081 ppm
Curry Murraya spp. - E - M	Fruit	1,037 ppm
Pineapple - Ananas Comosus - E	Fruit	963 ppm
Papaya - Carica Papaya - E - M	Fruit	716 ppm
Pear - Pyrus Communis - E	Fruit	679 ppm
Emblic, Myrobalan - Phyllanthus Emblica - E	Fruit	595 ppm
Apple - Malus Domestica - E	Fruit	497 ppm
American Ginseng, Ginseng - Panax Quinquefolius - M	Plant	370 ppm
European Grape, Grape, Grapevine, Vigne Vinifere, Wine Grape - Vitis Vinifera - E - M	Fruit	257 ppm
Black Currant - Ribes Nigrum - E	Fruit Juice	28 ppm
Elephant Garlic, Kurrat - Allium Ampeloprasum - E	Plant	
Hops - Humulus Lupulus - E - M - T	Fruit	
Flax, Lin Linum Usitatissimum - E	Plant	
Spearmint - Mentha Spicata - E - M - T	Leaf	
Rice - Oryza Sativa - E	Hay	
Tilia sp. -- Basswood, Lime, Linden	Flower	
Cowgrass, Peavine Clover, Purple Clover, Red Clover - Trifolium Pratense - E - M	Plant	

PLANTS CONTAINING LEUCINE

Species	Part	Quantity
Girasol, Sun Helianthus Annuus - E	Seed	35,500 ppm
Buffalo Gourd - Cucurbita Foetidissima - E - M - T	Seed	14,120-67,000 ppm

Plant	Part	ppm
Berro, Watercress - Nasturtium Officinale - E	Herb	33,200 ppm
Soybean - Glycine Max - E	Seed	32,500 ppm
Black bean, Dwarf bean, Field bean, Flageolet bean, French bean, Garden bean, Green bean, Haricot, Haricot bean, Haricot vert, Kidney bean, Navy bean, Pop bean, Popping bean, Snap bean, String bean, Wax bean - Phaseolus Vulgaris - E	Sprout Seedling	32,473 ppm
Cassie, Huisache, Opopanax, Popinac, Sweet Acacia - Acacia Farnesiana - M	Leaf	32,190 ppm
Jew's Mallow, Mulukiya, Nalta Jute - Corchorus Olitorius - E - M	Leaf	31,580 ppm
White Lupine - Lupinus Albus - M - T	Seed	30,625 ppm
Ceratonia siliqua L. -- Carob, Locust Bean, St.John's-Bread	Seed	30,550 ppm
Black Caraway, Black Cumin, Fennel-Flower, Nutmeg-Flower, Roman Coriander - Nigella Sativa - E - M	Seed	29,595 ppm
Taro - Colocasia Esculenta - E	Leaf	27,335 ppm
Asparagus Pea, Goa Bean, Winged Bean - Psophocarpus Tetragonolobus - E	Seed	27,242 ppm
Spinach - Spinacia Oleracea - E	Plant	26,483 ppm
Wheat - Triticum Aestivum - E - M	Plant	26,000 ppm
Cowage, Velvetbean - Mucuna Pruriens - E	Seed	25,175 ppm
Pigweed - Amaranthus sp. - E - M	Leaf	23,458 ppm
Lentil - Lens Culinaris - E	Seed	22,900 ppm
Butternut - Juglans Cinerea - E	Seed	22,750 ppm
Broadbean, Faba Bean, Habas - Vicia Faba - E	Seed	22,735 ppm
Sesame - Sesamum Indicum - E - M	Seed	22,586 ppm
Pea - Pisum Sativum - E	Fruit	22,552 ppm
Bonavist Bean, Hyacinth Bean, Lablab Bean - Lablab Purpureus - E - M - T	Seed	22,355 ppm
Pumpkin - Cucurbita Pepo - E	Seed	22,336 ppm
Lambsquarter - Chenopodium Album - E - M - T	Leaf	22,295 ppm
Watermelon - Citrullus Lanatus - E	Seed	21,100 ppm
Lentil - Lens Culinaris - E	Sprout Seedling	20,935 ppm
Chives - Allium Schoenoprasum - E	Leaf	20,875 ppm
Groundnut, Peanut - Arachis Hypogaea - E - M	Seed	20,653 ppm
Butter Bean, Lima Bean - Phaseolus Lunatus - E	Seed	20,595 ppm
Asparagus bean, Pea bean, Yardlong bean - Vigna Unguiculata subsp. Sesquipedalis - E	Seed	20,356 ppm
Green Gram, Mungbean - Vigna Radiata - E	Seed	20,308 ppm
Purslane, Verdolaga - Portulaca Oleracea - E	Herb	19,900 ppm
Swamp Cabbage, Water Spinach - Ipomoea Aquatica - E	Leaf	19,390 ppm
Black bean, Dwarf bean, Field bean, Flageolet bean, French bean, Garden bean, Green bean, Haricot, Haricot bean, Haricot vert, Kidney bean, Navy bean, Pop bean, Popping bean, Snap bean, String bean, Wax bean - Phaseolus Vulgaris - E	Seed	19,386 ppm
Alholva, Bockshornklee, Fenugreek, Greek Clover, Greek Trigonella Foenum-Graecum - E - M	Seed	19,327 ppm
Adzuki Bean - Vigna Angularis - E	Seed	19,270 ppm
White Mustard - Sinapis Alba - E - M - T	Seed	19,078 ppm
Bok-Choy, Celery Cabbage, Celery Mustard, Chinese Cabbage, Chinese Mustard, Chinese White Cabbage, Pak-Choi - Brassica Chinensis - E	Leaf	18,806 ppm
Ben Nut, Benzolive Tree, Drumstick Tree, Horseradish Tree, Moringa, West Indian Ben - Moringa Oleifera - E	Shoot	7,910-37,065 ppm
Corn Salad, Lamb's Lettuce - Valerianella Locusta - E	Plant	18,470 ppm
Green Gram, Mungbean - Vigna Radiata - E	Sprout Seedling	18,382 ppm
Oats - Avena Sativa - E - M	Plant	18,000 ppm
Wheat - Triticum Aestivum - E - M	Seed	18,000 ppm
Chaya - Cnidoscolus Chayamansa - E	Leaf	17,980 ppm
Pistachio - Pistacia Vera - E	Seed	17,445 ppm
Pigeonpea - Cajanus Vajan - E	Seed	17,325 ppm
Asparagus - Asparagus Officinalis - E	Shoot	17,161 ppm
Mat Bean, Moth Bean - Vigna Aconitifolia - E	Seed	17,062 ppm

LEUCINE CONTINUED

Plant	Part	ppm
Asparagus bean, Pea bean, Yardlong bean - Vigna Unguiculata subsp. Sesquipedalis - E	Fruit	16,461 ppm
Almond - Prunus Dulcis - E - M - T	Seed	16,234 ppm
Opium Poppy, Poppyseed Poppy - Papaver Somniferum - E	Seed	15,919 ppm
Collards, Cow Cabbage, Spring-Heading Cabbage, Tall Kale, Tree Kale - Brassica Oleracea - E	Leaf	15,900 ppm
Endive, Escarole - Cichorium Endivia - M	Leaf	15,781 ppm
Chickpea, Garbanzo - Cicer Arietinum - E	Seed	15,530 ppm
Asparagus Pea, Goa Bean, Winged Bean - Psophocarpus Tetragonolobus - E	Leaf	15,508 ppm
Pea - Pisum Sativum - E	Seed	15,279 ppm
Asparagus Pea, Goa Bean, Winged Bean - Psophocarpus Tetragonolobus - E	Tuber	15,023 ppm
Cauli Brassica Oleracea var. Botrytis - E	Flower	15,000 ppm
Curly Kale, Kale, Kitchen Kale, Scotch Kale - Brassica Oleracea var. Sabellica l. var. Acephala - E	Leaf	14,865 ppm
Vinespinach - Basella Alba - E - M	Leaf	14,640 ppm
Corn - Zea Mays - E	Seed	14,477 ppm
Cauli Brassica Oleracea var. Botrytis - E	Leaf	14,069 ppm
Oats - Avena Sativa - E - M	Seed	14,000 ppm
Papaver bracteatum L. -- Great Scarlet Poppy	Seed	13,550 ppm
Lettuce - Lactuca Sativa - E	Leaf	13,167 ppm
Cashew - Anacardium Occidentale - E	Seed	13,072 ppm
Indian Fig, Nopal, Nopalito, Prickly Pear - Opuntia Ficus-Indica - E - M	Seed	12,800 ppm
Brazilnut, Brazilnut-Tree, Creamnut, Paranut - Bertholletia Eexcelsa - E	Seed	12,281 ppm
Chayote - Sechium Edule - E - M	Fruit	12,000 ppm
Black bean, Dwarf bean, Field bean, Flageolet bean, French bean, Garden bean, Green bean, Haricot, Haricot bean, Haricot vert, Kidney bean, Navy bean, Pop bean, Popping bean, Snap bean, String bean, Wax bean - Phaseolus Vulgaris - E	Fruit	11,511 ppm
Black Mustard - Brassica Nigra - E	Leaf	11,192 ppm
Summer Squash - Cucurbita spp. - E	Fruit	10,920 ppm
Sicklepod - Senna Obtusifolia - E - T	Seed	10,900 ppm
Brussel-Sprout - Brassica Oleracea var. Gemmifera - E	Leaf	10,853 ppm
Basil, Cuban Basil, Sweet Basil - Ocimum Basilicum - E	Leaf	10,780 ppm
Evening-Primrose - Oenothera Biennis - E - M	Seed	10,780 ppm
Okra - Abelmoschus Esculentus Friut - E - M	Fruit	10,500 ppm
Italian Stone Pine, Pignolia - Pinus Pinea - M	Seed	17,300-20,600 ppm
Dill, Garden Dill - Anethum Graveolens - E	Fruit	10,018 ppm
Water Lotus - Nelumbo Nucifera - E - M	Seed	9,879 ppm
Chicory, Succory, Witloof - Cichorium Intybus - E - M	Leaf	8,976 ppm
Cayenne, Chili, Hot Pepper, Red Chili, Spur Pepper, Tabasco - Capsicum Frutescens - E	Fruit	8,568 ppm
Aubergine, Egg Solanum Melongena - E	Fruit	8,550 ppm
Cabbage, Red Cabbage, White Cabbage - Brassica Oleracea var. Capitata - E	Leaf	8,423 ppm
Achiote, Annato, Annatto, Annoto, Arnato, Bija, Lipstick Pod, Lipsticktree - Bixa Orellana - E	Seed	8,140 ppm
Buckwheat - Fagopyrum Esculentum - E	Seed	8,140 ppm
Calabash Gourd, White-Flowered Gourd - Lagenaria Siceraria - E	Fruit	8,070 ppm
Chaparral, Creosote Bush - Larrea Tridentata - M	Plant	7,800 ppm
Kohlrabi - Brassica Oleracea var. Gongylodes - E	Stem	7,445 ppm
Garlic - Allium Sativum Bulb - E	Bulb	7,392 ppm
Radish - Raphanus Sativus - E	Root	7,170 ppm
Potato - Solanum Tuberosum - E	Tuber	7,100 ppm
Ginkgo, Maidenhair Tree - Ginkgo Biloba - Tree - E - M - T	Seed	7,047 ppm
Celery - Apium Graveolens - E	Pt	6,530 ppm
Bread Artocarpus Altilis - E	Seed	5,630-12,875 ppm
Bell Pepper, Cherry Pepper, Cone Pepper, Green Pepper, Paprika, Sweet Pepper - Capsicum Annuum - E	Fruit	6,002 ppm
Cucumber - Cucumis Sativus - E	Fruit	5,822 ppm
Apricot - Prunus Armeniaca - E - M - T	Fruit	5,640 ppm

Rye - Secale Cereale - E	Seed	9,800-11,000 ppm
Pumpkin - Cucurbita Pepo - E	Fruit	5,476 ppm
Tomato - Lycopersicon Esculentum - E - M - T	Fruit	5,455 ppm
American Chestnut - Castanea Dentata - E - M	Seed	5,335 ppm
Pawpaw - Asimina Triloba - Friut - E	Fruit	5,002 ppm
Chinese Foxglove - Rehmannia Glutinosa - M	Root	5,000 ppm
Beet, Beetroot, Garden Beet, Sugar Beet - Beta Vulgaris - E	Root	4,968 ppm
Chinese Chestnut - Castanea Mollisima - M	Seed	4,807 ppm
Avocado - Persea Americana - E - M - T	Fruit	4,780 ppm
Macadamia - Macadamia spp. - E	Seed	4,750 ppm
Eryngium creticus -- Cretan culantro	Shoot	0-9,470 ppm
Common thyme, Garden thyme, Thyme - Thymus Vulgaris - E - M	Plant	4,644 ppm
Mountain Yam - Dioscorea Pentaphylla - E	Root	4,525 ppm
Cacao - Theobroma Ccacao - E	Plant	4,500 ppm
Onion, Shallot - Allium Cepa - Shallot Bulb - E	Bulb	4,469 ppm
Sweet Potato - Ipomoea Batatas - E	Root	4,455 ppm
Yambean - Pachyrhizus Erosus - E	Tuber	4,425 ppm
Jerusalem Artichoke - Helianthus Tuberosus E	Tuber	4,384 ppm
Ginger - Zingiber Officinale - E	Rhizome	4,257 ppm
Rapini, Seven-Top Turnip, Turnip - Brassica Rapa - E	Root	4,060 ppm
Guavas - Psidium Guajava - E	Fruit	3,960 ppm
Taro - Colocasia Esculenta - E	Root	3,780 ppm
Cassie, Huisache, Opopanax, Popinac, Sweet Acacia - Acacia Farnesiana - M	Seed	3,750 ppm
Rutabaga, Swede, Swedish Turnip - Brassica Napus var. Napobrassica - E	Root	3,675 ppm
Strawberry - Fragaria spp. - E	Fruit	3,667 ppm
Carrot - Daucus Carota - E	Root	3,520 ppm
Aloe, Bitter Aloes - Aloe Vera - E - M	Leaf	0-6,952 ppm
Squaw Perideridia Gairdneri - E - M	Root	3,366 ppm
Water Lotus - Nelumbo Nucifera - E - M	Rhizome	3,300 ppm
Peach - Prunus Persica - E - M - T	Fruit	3,240 ppm
American Elder, American Elderberry, Elderberry, Sweet Elder - Sambucus Canadensis - E	Fruit	2,970 ppm
Mango - Mangifera Indica - E - M	Fruit	2,950 ppm
Cassava, Tapioca, Yuca - Manihot Esculenta - E	Root	2,860 ppm
Banana, Plantain - Musa x Paradisiaca - E	Fruit	2,758 ppm
Blueberry - Vaccinium Corymbosum - E	Fruit	2,600 ppm
European Chestnut - Castanea Sativa - E - M	Seed	2,518 ppm
Breadroot, Indian Bread-Root, Indian Turnip, Prairie Apple, Prairie Potato, Prairie Turnip - Psoralea Esculenta - E - M - T	Root	2,448 ppm
Calathea allouia (AUBL.) LINDL. - Leren, Lleren	Root	4,440-4,885 ppm
Bread Artocarpus Altilis - E	Fruit	2,210 ppm
Carambola, Star Averrhoa Carambola - E	Fruit	400-4,400 ppm
Watermelon - Citrullus Lanatus - E	Fruit	2,120 ppm
Strawberry Guava - Psidium Cattleianum - E	Fruit	2,015 ppm
Curry Murraya spp. - E - M	Fruit	1,699 ppm
Burdock, Gobo, Great Burdock - Arctium lappa - E - M - T	Root	1,600 ppm
Fig - Ficus Carica - E	Fruit	1,580 ppm
American Ginseng, Ginseng - Panax Quinquefolius - M	Plant	1,530 ppm
Papaya - Carica Papaya - E - M	Fruit	1,432 ppm
Plum - Prunus Domestica - E - M	Fruit	1,419 ppm
Pineapple - Ananas Comosus - E	Fruit	1,407 ppm
Mandarin, Tangerine - Citrus Reticulata - E	Fruit	1,290 ppm
Pear - Pyrus Communis - E	Fruit	1,235 ppm
Date Palm - Phoenix Dactylifera - E	Fruit	1,140 ppm
Orange - Citrus Sinensis - E	Fruit	1,136 ppm
Emblic, Myrobalan - Phyllanthus Emblica - E	Fruit	1,084 ppm
Apple - Malus Domestica - E	Fruit	746 ppm
European Grape, Grape, Grapevine, Vigne Vinifere, Wine Grape - Vitis Vinifera - E - M	Fruit	720 ppm
Pea - Pisum Sativum - E	Shoot	35 ppm
Black Currant - Ribes Nigrum - E	Fruit Juice	28 ppm
Gum Arabic, Gum Arabic Tree, Kher, Senegal Gum, Sudan Gum Arabic - Acacia Senegal - M	Plant	Trace
Elephant Garlic, Kurrat - Allium Ampeloprasum - E	Plant	Trace

LEUCINE CONTINUED

Species	Part	Quantity
Tarragon - Artemisia Dracunculus - M	Shoot	Trace
Tea - Camellia Sinensis - E	Leaf	Trace
Shepherd's Purse - Capsella Bursa-Pastoris - E - M	Plant	Trace
Epazote, Worm Chenopodium Ambrosioides - E - M - T	Plant	Trace
Hops - Humulus Lupulus - E - M - T	Fruit	Trace
Huperzia spp -- Cutleaf Clubmoss	Plant	Trace
Flax, Lin Linum Usitatissimum - E	Seed	Trace
Chinaberry - Melia Azedarach - T	Seed	Trace
Spearmint - Mentha Spicata - E - M- T	Leaf	Trace
White Mulberry - Morus Alba - E - M	Leaf	Trace
Rice - Oryza Sativa - E	Hay	Trace
Sour Cherry - Prunus Cerasus - E - M - T	Fruit	Trace
Tilia sp. -- Basswood, Lime, Linden	Flower	Trace
Cowgrass, Peavine Clover, Purple Clover, Red Clover - Trifolium Pratense - E - M	Plant	Trace

PLANTS CONTAINING LYSINE

Species	Part	Quantity
Berro, Watercress - Nasturtium Officinale - E	Herb	26,800 ppm
Soybean - Glycine Max - E	Seed	26,560 ppm
Ceratonia siliqua L. -- Carob, Locust Bean, St.John's-Bread	Seed	26,320 ppm
Black bean, Dwarf bean, Field bean, Flageolet bean, French bean, Garden bean, Green bean, Haricot, Haricot bean, Haricot vert, Kidney bean, Navy bean, Pop bean, Popping bean, Snap bean, String bean, Wax bean - Phaseolus Vulgaris - E	Sprout Seedling	25,700 ppm
Lentil - Lens Culinaris - E	Sprout Seedling	23,735 ppm
Asparagus Pea, Goa Bean, Winged Bean - Psophocarpus Tetragonolobus - E	Seed	23,304 ppm
Lambsquarter - Chenopodium Album - E - M - T	Seed	22,550 ppm
Lentil - Lens Culinaris - E	Seed	22,035 ppm
White Lupine - Lupinus Albus - M - T	Seed	21,585 ppm
Black Caraway, Black Cumin, Fennel-Flower, Nutmeg-Flower, Roman Coriander - Nigella Sativa - E - M	Seed	20,700 ppm
Spinach - Spinacia Oleracea - E	Plant	20,664 ppm
Cowage, Velvetbean - Mucuna Pruriens - E	Seed	20,564 ppm
Cassie, Huisache, Opopanax, Popinac, Sweet Acacia - Acacia Farnesiana - M	Leaf	20,170 ppm
Pea - Pisum Sativum - E	Fruit	19,980 ppm
Pumpkin - Cucurbita Pepo - E	Seed	19,693 ppm
Broadbean, Faba Bean, Habas - Vicia Faba - E	Seed	19,265 ppm
Bok-Choy, Celery Cabbage, Celery Mustard, Chinese Cabbage, Chinese Mustard, Chinese White Cabbage, Pak-Choi - Brassica Chinensis - E	Leaf	19,019 ppm
Butter Bean, Lima Bean - Phaseolus Lunatus - E	Seed	19,010 ppm
Parsley - Petroselinum Crispum - E	Plant	18,724 ppm
Asparagus - Asparagus Officinalis - E	Shoot	18,710 ppm
Alholva, Bockshornklee, Fenugreek, Greek Clover, Greek Trigonella Foenum-Graecum - E - M	Seed	18,525 ppm
Green Gram, Mungbean - Vigna Radiata - E	Seed	18,296 ppm
Bonavist Bean, Hyacinth Bean, Lablab Bean - Lablab Purpureus - E - M - T	Seed	18,000 ppm
Wheat - Triticum Aestivum - E - M	Plant	18,000 ppm
Asparagus bean, Pea bean, Yardlong bean - Vigna Unguiculata subsp. Sesquipedalis - E	Seed	17,975 ppm
Jew's Mallow, Mulukiya, Nalta Jute - Corchorus Olitorius - E - M	Leaf	17,825 ppm
Green Gram, Mungbean - Vigna Radiata - E	Sprout Seedling	17,437 ppm
Adzuki Bean - Vigna Angularis - E	Seed	17,294 ppm
Taro - Colocasia Esculenta - E	Leaf	17,155 ppm
Pigeonpea - Cajanus Vajan - E	Seed	17,010 ppm

Plant	Part	ppm
Black bean, Dwarf bean, Field bean, Flageolet bean, French bean, Garden bean, Green bean, Haricot, Haricot bean, Haricot vert, Kidney bean, Navy bean, Pop bean, Popping bean, Snap bean, String bean, Wax bean - Phaseolus Vulgaris - E	Seed	16,667 ppm
Black Mustard - Brassica Nigra - E	Leaf	16,642 ppm
Buffalo Gourd - Cucurbita Foetidissima - E - M - T	Seed	10,130-33,000 ppm
White Mustard - Sinapis Alba - E - M - T	Seed	16,252 ppm
Pigweed - Amaranthus sp. - E - M	Leaf	15,278 ppm
Chaya - Cnidoscolus Chayamansa - E	Leaf	15,190 ppm
Asparagus bean, Pea bean, Yardlong bean - Vigna Unguiculata subsp. Sesquipedalis - E	Fruit	15,144 ppm
Cauli Brassica Oleracea var. Botrytis - E	Leaf	15,143 ppm
Pea - Pisum Sativum - E	Seed	14,995 ppm
Chickpea, Garbanzo - Cicer Arietinum - E	Seed	14,595 ppm
Achiote, Annato, Annatto, Annoto, Arnato, Bija, Lipstick Pod, Lipsticktree - Bixa Orellana - E	Seed	14,250 ppm
Corn Salad, Lamb's Lettuce - Valerianella Locusta - E	Plant	14,025 ppm
Oats - Avena Sativa - E - M	Plant	14,000 ppm
Lettuce - Lactuca Sativa - E	Leaf	14,000 ppm
Asparagus Pea, Goa Bean, Winged Bean - Psophocarpus Tetragonolobus - E	Tuber	13,897 ppm
Cauli Brassica Oleracea var. Botrytis - E	Flower	13,825 ppm
Mat Bean, Moth Bean - Vigna Aconitifolia - E	Seed	13,818 ppm
Pistachio - Pistacia Vera - E	Seed	13,295 ppm
Purslane, Verdolaga - Portulaca Oleracea - E	Herb	13,200 ppm
Curly Kale, Kale, Kitchen Kale, Scotch Kale - Brassica Oleracea var. Sabellica l. var. Acephala - E	Leaf	12,675 ppm
Ben Nut, Benzolive Tree, Drumstick Tree, Horseradish Tree, Moringa, West Indian Ben - Moringa Oleifera - E	Shoot	5,370-25,165 ppm
Vinespinach - Basella Alba - E - M	Leaf	12,465 ppm
Collards, Cow Cabbage, Spring-Heading Cabbage, Tall Kale, Tree Kale - Brassica Oleracea - E	Leaf	12,293 ppm
Opium Poppy, Poppyseed Poppy - Papaver Somniferum - E	Seed	11,789 ppm
Dill, Garden Dill - Anethum Graveolens - E	Fruit	11,242 ppm
Brussel-Sprout - Brassica Oleracea var. Gemmifera - E	Leaf	10,996 ppm
Groundnut, Peanut - Arachis Hypogaea - E - M	Seed	10,627 ppm
Summer Squash - Cucurbita spp. - E	Fruit	10,285 ppm
Endive, Escarole - Cichorium Endivia - M	Leaf	10,145 ppm
Girasol, Sun Helianthus Annuus - E	Seed	9,900 ppm
Asparagus Pea, Goa Bean, Winged Bean - Psophocarpus Tetragonolobus - E	Leaf	9,849 ppm
Sicklepod - Senna Obtusifolia - E - T	Seed	9,500 ppm
Black bean, Dwarf bean, Field bean, Flageolet bean, French bean, Garden bean, Green bean, Haricot, Haricot bean, Haricot vert, Kidney bean, Navy bean, Pop bean, Popping bean, Snap bean, String bean, Wax bean - Phaseolus Vulgaris - E	Fruit	9,044 ppm
Wheat - Triticum Aestivum - E - M	Seed	9,000 ppm
Watermelon - Citrullus Lanatus - E	Seed	8,932 ppm
Sesame - Sesamum Indicum - E - M	Seed	8,729 ppm
Cashew - Anacardium Occidentale - E	Seed	8,311 ppm
Papaver bracteatum L. -- Great Scarlet Poppy	Seed	8,150 ppm
Okra - Abelmoschus Esculentus - Friut - E - M	Fruit	8,100 ppm
Water Lotus - Nelumbo Nucifera - E - M	Seed	8,000 ppm
Butternut - Juglans Cinerea - E	Seed	7,966 ppm
Chicory, Succory, Witloof - Cichorium Intybus - E - M	Leaf	7,956 ppm
Cabbage, Red Cabbage, White Cabbage - Brassica Oleracea var. Capitata - E	Leaf	7,621 ppm
Watermelon - Citrullus Lanatus - E	Fruit	7,303 ppm
Cayenne, Chili, Hot Pepper, Red Chili, Spur Pepper, Tabasco - Capsicum Frutescens - E	Fruit	7,262 ppm
Buckwheat - Fagopyrum Esculentum - E	Seed	7,110 ppm
Apricot - Prunus Armeniaca - E - M - T	Fruit	7,105 ppm
Oats - Avena Sativa - E - M	Seed	7,000 ppm
Almond - Prunus Dulcis - E - M - T	Seed	6,966 ppm

LYSINE CONTINUED

Potato - Solanum Tuberosum - E	Tuber	6,800 ppm
Radish - Raphanus Sativus - E	Root	6,785 ppm
Garlic - Allium Sativum Bulb - E	Bulb	6,552 ppm
Bread Artocarpus Altilis - E	Seed	5,700-13,035 ppm
Pumpkin - Cucurbita Pepo - E	Fruit	6,429 ppm
Aubergine, Egg Solanum Melongena - E	Fruit	6,320 ppm
Indian Fig, Nopal, Nopalito, Prickly Pear - Opuntia Ficus-Indica - E - M	Seed	6,275 ppm
Kohlrabi - Brassica Oleracea var. Gongylodes - E	Stem	6,222 ppm
Basil, Cuban Basil, Sweet Basil - Ocimum Basilicum - E	Leaf	6,180 ppm
Chayote - Sechium Edule - E - M	Fruit	6,145 ppm
Onion, Shallot - Allium Cepa - Shallot Bulb - E	Bulb	6,104 ppm
Indian Fig, Nopal, Nopalito, Prickly Pear - Opuntia Ficus-Indica - E - M	Bud	6,005 ppm
Corn - Zea Mays - E	Seed	5,699 ppm
Brazilnut, Brazilnut-Tree, Creamnut, Paranut - Bertholletia Eexcelsa - E	Seed	5,597 ppm
Cucumber - Cucumis Sativus - E	Fruit	5,570 ppm
Tomato - Lycopersicon Esculentum - E - M - T	Fruit	5,455 ppm
Celery - Apium Graveolens - E	Pt	5,410 ppm
Bell Pepper, Cherry Pepper, Cone Pepper, Green Pepper, Paprika, Sweet Pepper - Capsicum Annuum - E	Fruit	5,183 ppm
Italian Stone Pine, Pignolia - Pinus Pinea - M	Seed	9,010-9,655 ppm
American Chestnut - Castanea Dentata - E - M	Seed	4,784 ppm
Calabash Gourd, White-Flowered Gourd - Lagenaria Siceraria - E	Fruit	4,700 ppm
Yambean - Pachyrhizus Erosus - E	Tuber	4,700 ppm
Ginkgo, Maidenhair Tree - Ginkgo Biloba - Tree - E - M - T	Seed	4,594 ppm
Water Lotus - Nelumbo Nucifera - E - M	Rhizome	4,500 ppm
Rapini, Seven-Top Turnip, Turnip - Brassica Rapa - E	Root	4,425 ppm
Jerusalem Artichoke - Helianthus Tuberosus E	Tuber	4,288 ppm
Beet, Beetroot, Garden Beet, Sugar Beet - Beta Vulgaris - E	Root	4,180 ppm
Chinese Chestnut - Castanea Mollisima - M	Seed	4,116 ppm
Chinese Foxglove - Rehmannia Glutinosa - M	Root	4,000 ppm
Aloe, Bitter Aloes - Aloe Vera - E - M	Leaf	0-7,748 ppm
Evening-Primrose - Oenothera Biennis - E - M	Seed	3,842 ppm
Pawpaw - Asimina Triloba - Friut - E	Fruit	3,831 ppm
Rutabaga, Swede, Swedish Turnip - Brassica Napus var. Napobrassica - E	Root	3,770 ppm
Avocado - Persea Americana - E - M - T	Fruit	3,653 ppm
Orange - Citrus Sinensis - E	Fruit	3,548 ppm
Rye - Secale Cereale - E	Seed	6,050-6,795 ppm
Burdock, Gobo, Great Burdock - Arctium lappa - E - M - T	Root	3,350 ppm
Macadamia - Macadamia spp. - E	Seed	3,330 ppm
Sweet Potato - Ipomoea Batatas - E	Root	3,280 ppm
Carrot - Daucus Carota - E	Root	3,275 ppm
Mango - Mangifera Indica - E - M	Fruit	3,200 ppm
Soursop - Annona Muricata - E	Fruit	3,180 ppm
Cassava, Tapioca, Yuca - Manihot Esculenta - E	Root	3,175 ppm
Ginger - Zingiber Officinale - E	Rhizome	3,110 ppm
Squaw Perideridia Gairdneri - E - M	Root	2,984 ppm
Strawberry - Fragaria spp. - E	Fruit	2,966 ppm
Mountain Yam - Dioscorea Pentaphylla - E	Root	2,800 ppm
Breadroot, Indian Bread-Root, Indian Turnip, Prairie Apple, Prairie Potato, Prairie Turnip - Psoralea Esculenta - E - M - T	Root	2,743 ppm
European Chestnut - Castanea Sativa - E - M	Seed	2,617 ppm
Mandarin, Tangerine - Citrus Reticulata - E	Fruit	2,579 ppm
Date Palm - Phoenix Dactylifera - E	Fruit	2,450 ppm
Waxgourd - Benincasa Hispida - Fruit	Fruit	2,305 ppm
Taro - Colocasia Esculenta - E	Root	2,280 ppm
Papaya - Carica Papaya - E - M	Fruit	2,238 ppm
Common thyme, Garden thyme, Thyme - Thymus Vulgaris - E - M	Plant	2,236 ppm
Carambola, Star Averrhoa Carambola - E	Fruit	400-4,400 ppm
American Ginseng, Ginseng - Panax Quinquefolius - M	Plant	2,100 ppm
Calathea allouia (AUBL.) LINDL. - Leren, Lleren	Root	3,810-4,190 ppm

Species	Part	Quantity
Sugar-Apple, Sweetsop - Annona Squamosa - E	Fruit	2,055 ppm
Indian Tamarind, Kilytree, Tamarind - Tamarindus Indica - M	Fruit	2,026 ppm
Eryngium creticus -- Cretan culantro	Shoot	0-3,980 ppm
Banana, Plantain - Musa x Paradisiaca - E	Fruit	1,865 ppm
Peach - Prunus Persica - E - M - T	Fruit	1,863 ppm
Pineapple - Ananas Comosus - E	Fruit	1,852 ppm
Cassie, Huisache, Opopanax, Popinac, Sweet Acacia - Acacia Farnesiana - M	Seed	1,800 ppm
Grape Citrus Paradisi - E	Fruit	1,760 ppm
Curry Murraya spp. - E - M	Fruit	1,728 ppm
Guavas - Psidium Guajava - E	Fruit	1,656 ppm
Pouteria caimito RADLK. -- Abiu, Caimito	Fruit	0-3,160 ppm
Fig - Ficus Carica - E	Fruit	1,436 ppm
Custard Apple - Annona Reticulata - E	Fruit	1,300 ppm
American Elder, American Elderberry, Elderberry, Sweet Elder - Sambucus Canadensis - E	Plant	1,287 ppm
Bread Artocarpus Altilis - E	Fruit	1,258 ppm
Lime - Citrus Aurantiifolia - E	Fruit	1,190 ppm
Emblic, Myrobalan - Phyllanthus Emblica - E	Fruit	1,168 ppm
Plum - Prunus Domestica - E - M	Fruit	1,149 ppm
Pouteria campechiana BAEHNI - - Canistel	Fruit	840-2,130 ppm
Pear - Pyrus Communis - E	Fruit	865 ppm
Strawberry Guava - Psidium Cattleianum - E	Fruit	825 ppm
Cacao - Theobroma Ccacao - E	Seed	800 ppm
Blueberry - Vaccinium Corymbosum - E	Fruit	780 ppm
European Grape, Grape, Grapevine, Vigne Vinifere, Wine Grape - Vitis Vinifera - E - M	Fruit	772 ppm
Apple - Malus Domestica - E	Fruit	746 ppm
Melicoccus bijugatas JACQ. -- Genip, Honey berry, Mamoncillo, Pitomba	Fruit	170-545 ppm
Elephant Garlic, Kurrat - Allium Ampeloprasum - E	Plant	Trace
Tarragon - Artemisia Dracunculus - M	Shoot	Trace
Tea - Camellia Sinensis - E	Leaf	Trace
Hops - Humulus Lupulus - E - M - T	Fruit	Trace
Flax, Lin Linum Usitatissimum - E	Plant	Trace
Chinaberry - Melia Azedarach - T	Seed	Trace
Spearmint - Mentha Spicata - E - M- T	Leaf	Trace
Rice - Oryza Sativa - E	Hay	Trace
Santalum album L. -- White Sandalwood	Fruit	Trace
Cowgrass, Peavine Clover, Purple Clover, Red Clover - Trifolium Pratense - E - M	Plant	Trace
Tulipa gesneriana L. -- Tulip	Stem	Trace

PLANTS CONTAINING METHIONINE

Species	Part	Quantity
Girasol, Sun Helianthus Annuus - E	Seed	20,500 ppm
Black Caraway, Black Cumin, Fennel-Flower, Nutmeg-Flower, Roman Coriander - Nigella Sativa - E - M	Seed	16,750 ppm
Brazilnut, Brazilnut-Tree, Creamnut, Paranut - Bertholletia Eexcelsa - E	Seed	10,346 ppm
Buffalo Gourd - Cucurbita Foetidissima - E - M - T	Seed	2,610-19,000 ppm
Sesame - Sesamum Indicum - E - M	Seed	9,413 ppm
Alholva, Bockshornklee, Fenugreek, Greek Clover, Greek Trigonella Foenum-Graecum - E - M	Leaf	8,830 ppm
Butternut - Juglans Cinerea - E	Seed	6,321 ppm
Spinach - Spinacia Oleracea - E	Plant	6,294 ppm
Pumpkin - Cucurbita Pepo - E	Seed	5,920 ppm
Swamp Cabbage, Water Spinach - Ipomoea Aquatica - E	Leaf	5,845 ppm
Evening-Primrose - Oenothera Biennis - E - M	Seed	5,763 ppm
Watermelon - Citrullus Lanatus - E	Seed	5,742 ppm
Taro - Colocasia Esculenta - E	Leaf	5,510 ppm
Soybean - Glycine Max - E	Seed	5,380 ppm
Jew's Mallow, Mulukiya, Nalta Jute - Corchorus Olitorius - E - M	Leaf	5,290 ppm
White Mustard - Sinapis Alba - E - M - T	Seed	5,136 ppm
Papaver bracteatum L. -- Great Scarlet Poppy	Seed	5,050 ppm
Opium Poppy, Poppyseed Poppy - Papaver Somniferum - E	Seed	5,042 ppm
Indian Fig, Nopal, Nopalito, Prickly Pear - Opuntia Ficus-Indica - E - M	Seed	4,830 ppm

METHIONINE CONTINUED

Black bean, Dwarf bean, Field bean, Flageolet bean, French bean, Garden bean, Green bean, Haricot, Haricot bean, Haricot vert, Kidney bean, Navy bean, Pop bean, Popping bean, Snap bean, String bean, Wax bean - Phaseolus Vulgaris - E	Sprout Seedling	4,731 ppm
Ceratonia siliqua L. -- Carob, Locust Bean, St.John's-Bread	Seed	4,700 ppm
Pigweed - Amaranthus sp. - E - M	Leaf	4,331 ppm
Oats - Avena Sativa - E - M	Seed	4,000 ppm
Barley, Barleygrass - Hordeum Vulgare - E - M	Seed	4,000 ppm
Berro, Watercress - Nasturtium Officinale - E	Herb	4,000 ppm
Wheat - Triticum Aestivum - E - M	Seed	4,000 ppm
Cowage, Velvetbean - Mucuna Pruriens - E	Seed	3,975 ppm
Pistachio - Pistacia Vera - E	Seed	3,963 ppm
Asparagus Pea, Goa Bean, Winged Bean - Psophocarpus Tetragonolobus - E	Seed	3,884 ppm
Pea - Pisum Sativum - E	Seed	3,879 ppm
Cassie, Huisache, Opopanax, Popinac, Sweet Acacia - Acacia Farnesiana - M	Leaf	3,860 ppm
Asparagus bean, Pea bean, Yardlong bean - Vigna Unguiculata subsp. Sesquipedalis - E	Seed	3,779 ppm
Chives - Allium Schoenoprasum - E	Leaf	3,750 ppm
Asparagus - Asparagus Officinalis - E	Shoot	3,742 ppm
Chaya - Cnidoscolus Chayamansa - E	Leaf	3,720 ppm
Alholva, Bockshornklee, Fenugreek, Greek Clover, Greek Trigonella Foenum-Graecum - E - M	Seed	3,720 ppm
Black bean, Dwarf bean, Field bean, Flageolet bean, French bean, Garden bean, Green bean, Haricot, Haricot bean, Haricot vert, Kidney bean, Navy bean, Pop bean, Popping bean, Snap bean, String bean, Wax bean - Phaseolus Vulgaris - E	Seed	3,653 ppm
Cauli Brassica Oleracea var. Botrytis - E	Leaf	3,652 ppm
Green Gram, Mungbean - Vigna Radiata - E	Sprout Seedling	3,571 ppm
Lentil - Lens Culinaris - E	Sprout Seedling	3,500 ppm
Corn Salad, Lamb's Lettuce - Valerianella Locusta - E	Plant	3,470 ppm
Collards, Cow Cabbage, Spring-Heading Cabbage, Tall Kale, Tree Kale - Brassica Oleracea - E	Leaf	3,442 ppm
Groundnut, Peanut - Arachis Hypogaea - E - M	Seed	3,430 ppm
Black Mustard - Brassica Nigra - E	Leaf	3,387 ppm
Asparagus Pea, Goa Bean, Winged Bean - Psophocarpus Tetragonolobus - E	Tuber	3,357 ppm
Fennel - Foeniculum Vulgare - M	Fruit	3,302 ppm
Asparagus bean, Pea bean, Yardlong bean - Vigna Unguiculata subsp. Sesquipedalis - E	Fruit	3,292 ppm
Green Gram, Mungbean - Vigna Radiata - E	Seed	3,145 ppm
Lambsquarter - Chenopodium Album - E - M - T	Leaf	3,121 ppm
Italian Stone Pine, Pignolia - Pinus Pinea - M	Seed	4,300-6,050 ppm
Butter Bean, Lima Bean - Phaseolus Lunatus - E	Seed	3,017 ppm
Ben Nut, Benzolive Tree, Drumstick Tree, Horseradish Tree, Moringa, West Indian Ben - Moringa Oleifera - E	Shoot	1,230-5,765 ppm
Chickpea, Garbanzo - Cicer Arietinum - E	Seed	2,860 ppm
White Lupine - Lupinus Albus - M - T	Seed	2,850 ppm
Purslane, Verdolaga - Portulaca Oleracea - E	Herb	2,814 ppm
Cashew - Anacardium Occidentale - E	Seed	2,787 ppm
Corn - Zea Mays - E	Seed	2,787 ppm
Asparagus Pea, Goa Bean, Winged Bean - Psophocarpus Tetragonolobus - E	Leaf	2,765 ppm
Vinespinach - Basella Alba - E - M	Leaf	2,755 ppm
Pigeonpea - Cajanus Vajan - E	Seed	2,720 ppm
Summer Squash - Cucurbita spp. - E	Fruit	2,690 ppm
Lettuce - Lactuca Sativa - E	Leaf	2,667 ppm
Mat Bean, Moth Bean - Vigna Aconitifolia - E	Seed	2,436 ppm
Adzuki Bean - Vigna Angularis - E	Seed	2,426 ppm
Brussel-Sprout - Brassica Oleracea var. Gemmifera - E	Leaf	2,285 ppm
Sicklepod - Senna Obtusifolia - E - T	Seed	2,270 ppm

Plant	Part	ppm
Broadbean, Faba Bean, Habas - Vicia Faba - E	Seed	2,265 ppm
Black bean, Dwarf bean, Field bean, Flageolet bean, French bean, Garden bean, Green bean, Haricot, Haricot bean, Haricot vert, Kidney bean, Navy bean, Pop bean, Popping bean, Snap bean, String bean, Wax bean - Phaseolus Vulgaris - E	Fruit	2,261 ppm
Endive, Escarole - Cichorium Endivia - M	Leaf	2,254 ppm
Date Palm - Phoenix Dactylifera - E	Fruit	2,190 ppm
Water Lotus - Nelumbo Nucifera - E - M	Seed	2,182 ppm
Bonavist Bean, Hyacinth Bean, Lablab Bean - Lablab Purpureus - E - M - T	Seed	2,105 ppm
Okra - Abelmoschus Esculentus - Friut - E - M	Fruit	2,100 ppm
Curly Kale, Kale, Kitchen Kale, Scotch Kale - Brassica Oleracea var. Sabellica l. var. Acephala - E	Leaf	2,060 ppm
Basil, Cuban Basil, Sweet Basil - Ocimum Basilicum - E	Leaf	2,020 ppm
Oats - Avena Sativa - E - M	Plant	2,000 ppm
Common thyme, Garden thyme, Thyme - Thymus Vulgaris - E - M	Plant	1,980 ppm
Cayenne, Chili, Hot Pepper, Red Chili, Spur Pepper, Tabasco - Capsicum Frutescens - E	Fruit	1,958 ppm
Bok-Choy, Celery Cabbage, Celery Mustard, Chinese Cabbage, Chinese Mustard, Chinese White Cabbage, Pak-Choi - Brassica Chinensis - E	Leaf	1,923 ppm
Indian Fig, Nopal, Nopalito, Prickly Pear - Opuntia Ficus-Indica - E - M	Bud	1,890 ppm
Garlic - Allium Sativum Bulb - E	Bulb	1,824 ppm
Chinese Chestnut - Castanea Mollisima - M	Seed	1,804 ppm
Achiote, Annato, Annatto, Annoto, Arnato, Bija, Lipstick Pod, Lipsticktree - Bixa Orellana - E	Seed	1,660 ppm
Cabbage, Red Cabbage, White Cabbage - Brassica Oleracea var. Capitata - E	Leaf	1,604 ppm
American Chestnut - Castanea Dentata - E - M	Seed	1,589 ppm
Potato - Solanum Tuberosum - E	Tuber	1,568 ppm
Dill, Garden Dill - Anethum Graveolens - E	Fruit	1,549 ppm
Orange - Citrus Sinensis - E	Fruit	1,510 ppm
Sweet Potato - Ipomoea Batatas - E	Root	1,510 ppm
Aubergine, Egg Solanum Melongena - E	Fruit	1,487 ppm
Kohlrabi - Brassica Oleracea var. Gongylodes - E	Stem	1,445 ppm
Avocado - Persea Americana - E - M - T	Fruit	1,438 ppm
Rye - Secale Cereale - E	Seed	2,480-2,785 ppm
Peach - Prunus Persica - E - M - T	Fruit	1,377 ppm
Bell Pepper, Cherry Pepper, Cone Pepper, Green Pepper, Paprika, Sweet Pepper - Capsicum Annuum - E	Fruit	1,364 ppm
Radish - Raphanus Sativus - E	Root	1,355 ppm
Rapini, Seven-Top Turnip, Turnip - Brassica Rapa - E	Root	1,350 ppm
Beet, Beetroot, Garden Beet, Sugar Beet - Beta Vulgaris - E	Root	1,341 ppm
Tomato - Lycopersicon Esculentum - E - M - T	Fruit	1,322 ppm
Pumpkin - Cucurbita Pepo - E	Fruit	1,310 ppm
Parsley - Petroselinum Crispum - E	Plant	1,282 ppm
Ginkgo, Maidenhair Tree - Ginkgo Biloba - Tree - E - M - T	Seed	1,226 ppm
Chicory, Succory, Witloof - Cichorium Intybus - E - M	Leaf	1,224 ppm
Yambean - Pachyrhizus Erosus - E	Tuber	1,200 ppm
European Grape, Grape, Grapevine, Vigne Vinifere, Wine Grape - Vitis Vinifera - E - M	Fruit	1,132 ppm
Celery - Apium Graveolens - E	Pt	1,120 ppm
Bread Artocarpus Altilis - E	Seed	960-2,195 ppm
Onion, Shallot - Allium Cepa - Shallot Bulb - E	Bulb	1,090 ppm
Pea - Pisum Sativum - E	Fruit	1,088 ppm
Water Lotus - Nelumbo Nucifera - E - M	Rhizome	1,050 ppm
Mandarin, Tangerine - Citrus Reticulata - E	Fruit	1,048 ppm
European Chestnut - Castanea Sativa - E - M	Seed	1,028 ppm
Cucumber - Cucumis Sativus - E	Fruit	1,012 ppm
Chinese Foxglove - Rehmannia Glutinosa - M	Root	1,000 ppm
Mountain Yam - Dioscorea Pentaphylla - E	Root	970 ppm
Rutabaga, Swede, Swedish Turnip - Brassica Napus var. Napobrassica - E	Root	965 ppm
Macadamia - Macadamia spp. - E	Seed	950 ppm

METHIONINE CONTINUED

Species	Part	Quantity
Calabash Gourd, White-Flowered Gourd - Lagenaria Siceraria - E	Fruit	900 ppm
Pouteria caimito RADLK. -- Abiu, Caimito	Fruit	0-1,780 ppm
Squaw Perideridia Gairdneri - E - M	Root	889 ppm
Jerusalem Artichoke - Helianthus Tuberosus E	Tuber	858 ppm
Pawpaw - Asimina Triloba - Friut - E	Fruit	836 ppm
Cassava, Tapioca, Yuca - Manihot Esculenta - E	Root	825 ppm
Pineapple - Ananas Comosus - E	Fruit	815 ppm
Calathea allouia (AUBL.) LINDL. - Leren, Lleren	Root	1,415-1,560 ppm
Waxgourd - Benincasa Hispida - Fruit	Fruit	770 ppm
Ginger - Zingiber Officinale - E	Rhizome	737 ppm
Blueberry - Vaccinium Corymbosum - E	Fruit	715 ppm
Watermelon - Citrullus Lanatus - E	Fruit	707 ppm
American Elder, American Elderberry, Elderberry, Sweet Elder - Sambucus Canadensis - E	Fruit	693 ppm
Taro - Colocasia Esculenta - E	Root	680 ppm
Carambola, Star Averrhoa Carambola - E	Fruit	110-1,210 ppm
Carrot - Daucus Carota - E	Root	575 ppm
Mango - Mangifera Indica - E - M	Fruit	550 ppm
Curry Murraya spp. - E - M	Fruit	490 ppm
Burdock, Gobo, Great Burdock - Arctium lappa - E - M - T	Root	450 ppm
Apricot - Prunus Armeniaca - E - M - T	Fruit	440 ppm
Banana, Plantain - Musa x Paradisiaca - E	Fruit	427 ppm
Plum - Prunus Domestica - E - M	Fruit	405 ppm
Soursop - Annona Muricata - E	Fruit	370 ppm
Guavas - Psidium Guajava - E	Plant	360 ppm
Emblic, Myrobalan - Phyllanthus Emblica - E	Fruit	355 ppm
Bread Artocarpus Altilis - E	Fruit	340 ppm
American Ginseng, Ginseng - Panax Quinquefolius - M	Plant	340 ppm
Pear - Pyrus Communis - E	Fruit	309 ppm
Fig - Ficus Carica - E	Fruit	287 ppm
Sugar-Apple, Sweetsop - Annona Squamosa - E	Fruit	260 ppm
Breadroot, Indian Bread-Root, Indian Turnip, Prairie Apple, Prairie Potato, Prairie Turnip - Psoralea Esculenta - E - M - T	Root	253 ppm
Grape Citrus Paradisi - E	Fruit	222 ppm
Strawberry Guava - Psidium Cattleianum - E	Fruit	205 ppm
Indian Tamarind, Kilytree, Tamarind - Tamarindus Indica - M	Fruit	204 ppm
Cassie, Huisache, Opopanax, Popinac, Sweet Acacia - Acacia Farnesiana - M	Seed	200 ppm
Papaya - Carica Papaya - E - M	Fruit	179 ppm
Lime - Citrus Aurantiifolia - E	Fruit	170 ppm
Pouteria campechiana BAEHNI - - Canistel	Fruit	130-330 ppm
Chayote - Sechium Edule - E - M	Fruit	145 ppm
Custard Apple - Annona Reticulata - E	Fruit	140 ppm
Apple - Malus Domestica - E	Plant	124 ppm
Strawberry - Fragaria spp. - E	Fruit	119 ppm
Chrysophyllum cainito RADLK. -- Caimito, Star Apple	Fruit	20-60 ppm
Elephant Garlic, Kurrat - Allium Ampeloprasum - E	Plant	Trace
Jericho Rose - Anastatica Hierochuntica	Plant	Trace
Shepherd's Purse - Capsella Bursa-Pastoris - E - M	Plant	Trace
Coffee - Coffea Arabica - E - M	Seed	Trace
Flax, Lin Linum Usitatissimum - E	Seed	Trace
Chinaberry - Melia Azedarach - T	Seed	Trace
Melicoccus bijugatas JACQ. -- Genip, Honey berry, Mamoncillo, Pitomba	Fruit	Trace
Spearmint - Mentha Spicata - E - M- T	Leaf	Trace
Rice - Oryza Sativa - E	Plant	Trace
Cowgrass, Peavine Clover, Purple Clover, Red Clover - Trifolium Pratense - E - M	Plant	Trace

PLANTS CONTAINING PHENYLALANINE

Species	Part	Quantity
Girasol, Sun Helianthus Annuus - E	Seed	48,000 ppm
Buffalo Gourd - Cucurbita Foetidissima - E - M – T	Seed	11,050-46,000 ppm
Berro, Watercress - Nasturtium Officinale - E	Herb	22,800 ppm

Black bean, Dwarf bean, Field bean, Flageolet bean, French bean, Garden bean, Green bean, Haricot, Haricot bean, Haricot vert, Kidney bean, Navy bean, Pop bean, Popping bean, Snap bean, String bean, Wax bean - Phaseolus Vulgaris - E	Sprout Seedling	22,796 ppm
Black Caraway, Black Cumin, Fennel-Flower, Nutmeg-Flower, Roman Coriander - Nigella Sativa - E - M	Seed	21,560 ppm
Soybean - Glycine Max - E	Seed	20,830 ppm
Pigeonpea - Cajanus Vajan - E	Seed	20,780 ppm
Chaya - Cnidoscolus Chayamansa - E	Leaf	18,600 ppm
Jew's Mallow, Mulukiya, Nalta Jute - Corchorus Olitorius - E - M	Leaf	17,250 ppm
Swamp Cabbage, Water Spinach - Ipomoea Aquatica - E	Leaf	16,865 ppm
Watermelon - Citrullus Lanatus - E	Seed	16,600 ppm
White Lupine - Lupinus Albus - M - T	Seed	16,025 ppm
Pigweed - Amaranthus sp. - E - M	Leaf	16,000 ppm
Green Gram, Mungbean - Vigna Radiata - E	Seed	15,865 ppm
Groundnut, Peanut - Arachis Hypogaea - E - M	Seed	15,715 ppm
Asparagus Pea, Goa Bean, Winged Bean - Psophocarpus Tetragonolobus - E	Seed	15,590 ppm
Lentil - Lens Culinaris - E	Seed	15,575 ppm
Asparagus bean, Pea bean, Yardlong bean - Vigna Unguiculata subsp. Sesquipedalis - E	Seed	15,518 ppm
Spinach - Spinacia Oleracea - E	Plant	15,320 ppm
Ceratonia siliqua L. -- Carob, Locust Bean, St.John's-Bread	Seed	15,040 ppm
Cassie, Huisache, Opopanax, Popinac, Sweet Acacia - Acacia Farnesiana - M	Leaf	15,020 ppm
Butternut - Juglans Cinerea - E	Seed	14,918 ppm
Lentil - Lens Culinaris - E	Sprout Seedling	14,735 ppm
Butter Bean, Lima Bean - Phaseolus Lunatus - E	Seed	13,760 ppm
Taro - Colocasia Esculenta - E	Leaf	13,600 ppm
Bonavist Bean, Hyacinth Bean, Lablab Bean - Lablab Purpureus - E - M - T	Seed	13,285 ppm
Pumpkin - Cucurbita Pepo - E	Seed	13,128 ppm
Black bean, Dwarf bean, Field bean, Flageolet bean, French bean, Garden bean, Green bean, Haricot, Haricot bean, Haricot vert, Kidney bean, Navy bean, Pop bean, Popping bean, Snap bean, String bean, Wax bean - Phaseolus Vulgaris - E	Seed	13,127 ppm
Asparagus bean, Pea bean, Yardlong bean - Vigna Unguiculata subsp. Sesquipedalis - E	Fruit	12,675 ppm
Corn Salad, Lamb's Lettuce - Valerianella Locusta - E	Plant	12,640 ppm
Vinespinach - Basella Alba - E - M	Leaf	12,320 ppm
Pistachio - Pistacia Vera - E	Seed	12,317 ppm
Chickpea, Garbanzo - Cicer Arietinum - E	Seed	12,290 ppm
Green Gram, Mungbean - Vigna Radiata - E	Sprout Seedling	12,290 ppm
Adzuki Bean - Vigna Angularis - E	Seed	12,153 ppm
Broadbean, Faba Bean, Habas - Vicia Faba - E	Seed	12,000 ppm
Alholva, Bockshornklee, Fenugreek, Greek Clover, Greek Trigonella Foenum-Graecum - E - M	Seed	11,980 ppm
Almond - Prunus Dulcis - E - M - T	Seed	11,642 ppm
Purslane, Verdolaga - Portulaca Oleracea - E	Herb	11,500 ppm
White Mustard - Sinapis Alba - E - M - T	Seed	11,416 ppm
Ben Nut, Benzolive Tree, Drumstick Tree, Horseradish Tree, Moringa, West Indian Ben - Moringa Oleifera - E	Shoot	4,870-22,820 ppm
Mat Bean, Moth Bean - Vigna Aconitifolia - E	Seed	11,382 ppm
Chives - Allium Schoenoprasum - E	Leaf	11,250 ppm
Wheat - Triticum Aestivum - E - M	Plant	11,000 ppm
Asparagus Pea, Goa Bean, Winged Bean - Psophocarpus Tetragonolobus - E	Tuber	10,587 ppm
Lambsquarter - Chenopodium Album - E - M - T	Leaf	10,574 ppm
Oats - Avena Sativa - E - M	Seed	10,000 ppm
Sesame - Sesamum Indicum - E - M	Seed	9,863 ppm
Black Mustard - Brassica Nigra - E	Leaf	9,720 ppm

PHENYLALANINE CONTINUED

Opium Poppy, Poppyseed Poppy - Papaver Somniferum - E	Seed	9,461 ppm
Pea - Pisum Sativum - E	Seed	9,460 ppm
Bok-Choy, Celery Cabbage, Celery Mustard, Chinese Cabbage, Chinese Mustard, Chinese White Cabbage, Pak-Choi - Brassica Chinensis - E	Leaf	9,402 ppm
Asparagus - Asparagus Officinalis - E	Shoot	9,290 ppm
Collards, Cow Cabbage, Spring-Heading Cabbage, Tall Kale, Tree Kale - Brassica Oleracea - E	Leaf	9,178 ppm
Cauli Brassica Oleracea var. Botrytis - E	Flower	9,175 ppm
Lettuce - Lactuca Sativa - E	Leaf	9,167 ppm
Bread Artocarpus Altilis - E	Seed	7,970-18,225 ppm
Cauli Brassica Oleracea var. Botrytis - E	Leaf	9,022 ppm
Pea - Pisum Sativum - E	Fruit	8,902 ppm
Wheat - Triticum Aestivum - E - M	Seed	8,694 ppm
Endive, Escarole - Cichorium Endivia - M	Leaf	8,535 ppm
Indian Fig, Nopal, Nopalito, Prickly Pear - Opuntia Ficus-Indica - E - M	Seed	8,255 ppm
Papaver bracteatum L. -- Great Scarlet Poppy	Plant	8,150 ppm
Asparagus Pea, Goa Bean, Winged Bean - Psophocarpus Tetragonolobus - E	Leaf	8,121 ppm
Cashew - Anacardium Occidentale - E	Seed	8,046 ppm
Brazilnut, Brazilnut-Tree, Creamnut, Paranut - Bertholletia Eexcelsa - E	Seed	7,718 ppm
Chayote - Sechium Edule - E - M	Fruit	7,430 ppm
Evening-Primrose - Oenothera Biennis - E - M	Seed	7,364 ppm
Dill, Garden Dill - Anethum Graveolens - E	Fruit	7,256 ppm
Fennel - Foeniculum Vulgare - M	Fruit	7,098 ppm
Brussel-Sprout - Brassica Oleracea var. Gemmifera - E	Leaf	6,997 ppm
Black bean, Dwarf bean, Field bean, Flageolet bean, French bean, Garden bean, Green bean, Haricot, Haricot bean, Haricot vert, Kidney bean, Navy bean, Pop bean, Popping bean, Snap bean, String bean, Wax bean - Phaseolus Vulgaris - E	Fruit	6,886 ppm
Sicklepod - Senna Obtusifolia - E - T	Seed	6,530 ppm
Summer Squash - Cucurbita spp. - E	Fruit	6,485 ppm
Italian Stone Pine, Pignolia - Pinus Pinea - M	Seed	9,190-12,800 ppm
Water Lotus - Nelumbo Nucifera - E - M	Seed	6,242 ppm
Corn - Zea Mays - E	Seed	6,240 ppm
Chinese Foxglove - Rehmannia Glutinosa - M	Plant	6,000 ppm
Aubergine, Egg Solanum Melongena - E	Fruit	5,700 ppm
Cacao - Theobroma Ccacao - E	Seed	5,600 ppm
Potato - Solanum Tuberosum - E	Tuber	5,550 ppm
Cabbage, Red Cabbage, White Cabbage - Brassica Oleracea var. Capitata - E	Leaf	5,214 ppm
Cayenne, Chili, Hot Pepper, Red Chili, Spur Pepper, Tabasco - Capsicum Frutescens - E	Fruit	5,059 ppm
Buckwheat - Fagopyrum Esculentum - E	Seed	5,045 ppm
Chicory, Succory, Witloof - Cichorium Intybus - E - M	Leaf	4,896 ppm
Achiote, Annato, Annatto, Annoto, Arnato, Bija, Lipstick Pod, Lipsticktree - Bixa Orellana - E	Seed	4,650 ppm
Radish - Raphanus Sativus - E	Root	4,455 ppm
Garlic - Allium Sativum Bulb - E	Bulb	4,392 ppm
Kohlrabi - Brassica Oleracea var. Gongylodes - E	Stem	4,333 ppm
Indian Fig, Nopal, Nopalito, Prickly Pear - Opuntia Ficus-Indica - E - M	Bud	4,250 ppm
Chaparral, Creosote Bush - Larrea Tridentata - M	Plant	4,200 ppm
Celery - Apium Graveolens - E	Leaf	4,105 ppm
Chinese Chestnut - Castanea Mollisima - M	Seed	3,879 ppm
Ginkgo, Maidenhair Tree - Ginkgo Biloba - Tree - E - M - T	Seed	3,813 ppm
Pumpkin - Cucurbita Pepo - E	Fruit	3,810 ppm
Apricot - Prunus Armeniaca - E - M - T	Fruit	3,810 ppm
Tomato - Lycopersicon Esculentum - E - M - T	Fruit	3,801 ppm
Rye - Secale Cereale - E	Seed	6,740-7,570 ppm
American Chestnut - Castanea Dentata - E - M	Seed	3,746 ppm
Mango - Mangifera Indica - E - M	Fruit	3,700 ppm
Sweet Potato - Ipomoea Batatas - E	Root	3,645 ppm
Aloe, Bitter Aloes - Aloe Vera - E - M	Leaf	0-7,103 ppm

Bell Pepper, Cherry Pepper, Cone Pepper, Green Pepper, Paprika, Sweet Pepper - Capsicum Annuum - E	Fruit	3,546 ppm
Calabash Gourd, White-Flowered Gourd - Lagenaria Siceraria - E	Fruit	3,365 ppm
Mountain Yam - Dioscorea Pentaphylla - E	Root	3,340 ppm
Beet, Beetroot, Garden Beet, Sugar Beet - Beta Vulgaris - E	Root	3,312 ppm
Onion, Shallot - Allium Cepa - Shallot Bulb - E	Bulb	3,270 ppm
Pawpaw - Asimina Triloba - Friut - E	Fruit	3,001 ppm
Rutabaga, Swede, Swedish Turnip - Brassica Napus var. Napobrassica - E	Root	3,000 ppm
Yambean - Pachyrhizus Erosus - E	Tuber	2,950 ppm
Taro - Colocasia Esculenta - E	Root	2,795 ppm
Macadamia - Macadamia spp. - E	Seed	2,675 ppm
Jerusalem Artichoke - Helianthus Tuberosus E	Tuber	2,668 ppm
Avocado - Persea Americana - E - M - T	Fruit	2,643 ppm
Carrot - Daucus Carota - E	Root	2,620 ppm
Common thyme, Garden thyme, Thyme - Thymus Vulgaris - E - M	Plant	2,603 ppm
Ginger - Zingiber Officinale - E	Rhizome	2,455 ppm
Orange - Citrus Sinensis - E	Fruit	2,340 ppm
Water Lotus - Nelumbo Nucifera - E - M	Rhizome	2,250 ppm
Rapini, Seven-Top Turnip, Turnip - Brassica Rapa - E	Root	2,090 ppm
American Elder, American Elderberry, Elderberry, Sweet Elder - Sambucus Canadensis - E	Fruit	1,980 ppm
Cassava, Tapioca, Yuca - Manihot Esculenta - E	Root	1,900 ppm
European Chestnut - Castanea Sativa - E - M	Seed	1,851 ppm
Calathea allouia (AUBL.) LINDL. - Leren, Lleren	Root	3,325-3,655 ppm
Peach - Prunus Persica - E - M - T	Plant	1,782 ppm
Watermelon - Citrullus Lanatus - E	Fruit	1,767 ppm
Squaw Perideridia Gairdneri - E - M	Root	1,714 ppm
Mandarin, Tangerine - Citrus Reticulata - E	Fruit	1,693 ppm
Burdock, Gobo, Great Burdock - Arctium lappa - E - M - T	Root	1,650 ppm
Blueberry - Vaccinium Corymbosum - E	Fruit	1,560 ppm
Cassie, Huisache, Opopanax, Popinac, Sweet Acacia - Acacia Farnesiana - M	Seed	1,500 ppm
Banana, Plantain - Musa x Paradisiaca - E	Fruit	1,476 ppm
Curry Murraya spp. - E - M	Fruit	1,267 ppm
Breadroot, Indian Bread-Root, Indian Turnip, Prairie Apple, Prairie Potato, Prairie Turnip - Psoralea Esculenta - E - M - T	Root	1,224 ppm
Plum - Prunus Domestica - E - M	Fruit	1,149 ppm
Carambola, Star Averrhoa Carambola - E	Fruit	190-2,090 ppm
Pineapple - Ananas Comosus - E	Fruit	889 ppm
Bread Artocarpus Altilis - E	Fruit	885 ppm
Fig - Ficus Carica - E	Fruit	862 ppm
Papaya - Carica Papaya - E - M	Fruit	806 ppm
Date Palm - Phoenix Dactylifera - E	Fruit	740 ppm
European Grape, Grape, Grapevine, Vigne Vinifere, Wine Grape - Vitis Vinifera - E - M	Fruit	720 ppm
Emblic, Myrobalan - Phyllanthus Emblica - E	Fruit	658 ppm
Apple - Malus Domestica - E	Fruit	311 ppm
Guavas - Psidium Guajava - E	Fruit	144 ppm
Strawberry Guava - Psidium Cattleianum - E	Fruit	50 ppm
Elephant Garlic, Kurrat - Allium Ampeloprasum - E	Plant	Trace
Ammi visnaga (L.) LAM. -- Visnaga	Plant	Trace
Grape Citrus Paradisi - E	Fruit	Trace
Hops - Humulus Lupulus - E - M - T	Fruit	Trace
Flax, Lin Linum Usitatissimum - E	Seed	Trace
American Ginseng, Ginseng - Panax Quinquefolius - M	Plant	Trace
Passiflora incarnata L. -- Manzana de Mayo, Mayapple, Passionflower	Fruit	Trace
Sour Cherry - Prunus Cerasus - E - M - T	Fruit	Trace
Tilia sp. -- Basswood, Lime, Linden	Flower	Trace
Cowgrass, Peavine Clover, Purple Clover, Red Clover - Trifolium Pratense - E - M	Plant	Trace
Black Gram - Vigna Mungo - E	Sprout Seedling	Trace

Plants Containing Proline

PHENYLALANINE CONTINUED

Species	Part	Quantity
Cabbage, Red Cabbage, White Cabbage - Brassica Oleracea var. Capitata - E	Leaf	31,821 ppm
Soybean - Glycine Max - E	Seed	23,344 ppm
Chives - Allium Schoenoprasum - E	Leaf	23,125 ppm
Cassie, Huisache, Opopanax, Popinac, Sweet Acacia - Acacia Farnesiana - M	Leaf	21,890 ppm
Asparagus Pea, Goa Bean, Winged Bean - Psophocarpus Tetragonolobus - E	Seed	20,991 ppm
Asparagus - Asparagus Officinalis - E	Shoot	20,903 ppm
White Mustard - Sinapis Alba - E - M - T	Seed	20,800 ppm
Wheat - Triticum Aestivum - E - M	Seed	20,447 ppm
Jew's Mallow, Mulukiya, Nalta Jute - Corchorus Olitorius - E - M	Leaf	20,052 ppm
Cowage, Velvetbean - Mucuna Pruriens - E	Seed	19,555 ppm
Berro, Watercress - Nasturtium Officinale - E	Herb	19,200 ppm
Ceratonia siliqua L. -- Carob, Locust Bean, St.John's-Bread	Seed	18,800 ppm
Black bean, Dwarf bean, Field bean, Flageolet bean, French bean, Garden bean, Green bean, Haricot, Haricot bean, Haricot vert, Kidney bean, Navy bean, Pop bean, Popping bean, Snap bean, String bean, Wax bean - Phaseolus Vulgaris - E	Sprout Seedling	18,172 ppm
Alholva, Bockshornklee, Fenugreek, Greek Clover, Greek Trigonella Foenum-Graecum - E - M	Seed	17,800 ppm
Pumpkin - Cucurbita Pepo - E	Fruit	17,100 ppm
Chickpea, Garbanzo - Cicer Arietinum - E	Seed	16,530 ppm
White Lupine - Lupinus Albus - M - T	Seed	16,480 ppm
Asparagus Pea, Goa Bean, Winged Bean - Psophocarpus Tetragonolobus - E	Tuber	15,939 ppm
Groundnut, Peanut - Arachis Hypogaea - E - M	Seed	15,362 ppm
Okra - Abelmoschus Esculentus - Friut - E - M	Fruit	14,930 ppm
Pigweed - Amaranthus sp. - E - M	Leaf	14,556 ppm
Black Caraway, Black Cumin, Fennel-Flower, Nutmeg-Flower, Roman Coriander - Nigella Sativa - E - M	Seed	14,520 ppm
Sesame - Sesamum Indicum - E - M	Seed	14,277 ppm
Lambsquarter - Chenopodium Album - E - M - T	Leaf	14,205 ppm
Asparagus bean, Pea bean, Yardlong bean - Vigna Unguiculata subsp. Sesquipedalis - E	Seed	14,050 ppm
Spinach - Spinacia Oleracea - E	Plant	13,301 ppm
Broadbean, Faba Bean, Habas - Vicia Faba - E	Seed	13,265 ppm
Lentil - Lens Culinaris - E	Seed	13,200 ppm
Purslane, Verdolaga - Portulaca Oleracea - E	Herb	13,200 ppm
Almond - Prunus Dulcis - E - M - T	Seed	13,127 ppm
Bonavist Bean, Hyacinth Bean, Lablab Bean - Lablab Purpureus - E - M - T	Seed	12,822 ppm
Butternut - Juglans Cinerea - E	Seed	12,787 ppm
Curly Kale, Kale, Kitchen Kale, Scotch Kale - Brassica Oleracea var. Sabellica l. var. Acephala - E	Leaf	12,610 ppm
Girasol, Sun Helianthus Annuus - E	Seed	12,500 ppm
Cauli Brassica Oleracea var. Botrytis - E	Leaf	12,244 ppm
Corn - Zea Mays - E	Seed	12,147 ppm
Green Gram, Mungbean - Vigna Radiata - E	Seed	12,090 ppm
Lentil - Lens Culinaris - E	Sprout Seedling	11,865 ppm
Pigeonpea - Cajanus Vajan - E	Seed	11,830 ppm
Watermelon - Citrullus Lanatus - E	Seed	11,800 ppm
Swamp Cabbage, Water Spinach - Ipomoea Aquatica - E	Leaf	11,685 ppm
Opium Poppy, Poppyseed Poppy - Papaver Somniferum - E	Seed	11,392 ppm
Cauli Brassica Oleracea var. Botrytis - E	Flower	11,110 ppm
Collards, Cow Cabbage, Spring-Heading Cabbage, Tall Kale, Tree Kale - Brassica Oleracea - E	Leaf	10,981 ppm
Butter Bean, Lima Bean - Phaseolus Lunatus - E	Seed	10,855 ppm
Corn Salad, Lamb's Lettuce - Valerianella Locusta - E	Plant	10,830 ppm
Pumpkin - Cucurbita Pepo - E	Seed	10,743 ppm

Ben Nut, Benzolive Tree, Drumstick Tree, Horseradish Tree, Moringa, West Indian Ben - Moringa Oleifera - E	Shoot	4,510-21,135 ppm
Indian Fig, Nopal, Nopalito, Prickly Pear - Opuntia Ficus-Indica - E - M	Seed	10,500 ppm
Water Lotus - Nelumbo Nucifera - E - M	Seed	10,424 ppm
Black bean, Dwarf bean, Field bean, Flageolet bean, French bean, Garden bean, Green bean, Haricot, Haricot bean, Haricot vert, Kidney bean, Navy bean, Pop bean, Popping bean, Snap bean, String bean, Wax bean - Phaseolus Vulgaris - E	Seed	10,294 ppm
Vinespinach - Basella Alba - E - M	Leaf	10,145 ppm
Adzuki Bean - Vigna Angularis - E	Seed	10,097 ppm
Fennel - Foeniculum Vulgare - M	Fruit	9,873 ppm
Pistachio - Pistacia Vera - E	Seed	9,851 ppm
Endive, Escarole - Cichorium Endivia - M	Leaf	9,500 ppm
Papaver bracteatum L. -- Great Scarlet Poppy	Seed	8,400 ppm
Rye - Secale Cereale - E	Seed	14,910-16,745 ppm
Pea - Pisum Sativum - E	Seed	8,183 ppm
Lettuce - Lactuca Sativa - E	Leaf	8,000 ppm
Brazilnut, Brazilnut-Tree, Creamnut, Paranut - Bertholletia Eexcelsa - E	Seed	7,884 ppm
Ginkgo, Maidenhair Tree - Ginkgo Biloba - Tree - E - M - T	Seed	7,738 ppm
Buffalo Gourd - Cucurbita Foetidissima - E - M - T	Seed	8,290-15,390 ppm
Apricot - Prunus Armeniaca - E - M - T	Fruit	7,400 ppm
Asparagus Pea, Goa Bean, Winged Bean - Psophocarpus Tetragonolobus - E	Leaf	7,257 ppm
Cacao - Theobroma Ccacao - E	Seed	7,200 ppm
Cayenne, Chili, Hot Pepper, Red Chili, Spur Pepper, Tabasco - Capsicum Frutescens - E	Fruit	7,099 ppm
Cashew - Anacardium Occidentale - E	Seed	7,019 ppm
Black bean, Dwarf bean, Field bean, Flageolet bean, French bean, Garden bean, Green bean, Haricot, Haricot bean, Haricot vert, Kidney bean, Navy bean, Pop bean, Popping bean, Snap bean, String bean, Wax bean - Phaseolus Vulgaris - E	Fruit	6,989 ppm
Italian Stone Pine, Pignolia - Pinus Pinea - M	Seed	12,900-13,900 ppm
Chayote - Sechium Edule - E - M	Fruit	6,855 ppm
Potato - Solanum Tuberosum - E	Tuber	6,700 ppm
Bok-Choy, Celery Cabbage, Celery Mustard, Chinese Cabbage, Chinese Mustard, Chinese White Cabbage, Pak-Choi - Brassica Chinensis - E	Leaf	6,625 ppm
Water Lotus - Nelumbo Nucifera - E - M	Rhizome	6,500 ppm
Evening-Primrose - Oenothera Biennis - E - M	Seed	6,297 ppm
Pea - Pisum Sativum - E	Fruit	6,231 ppm
Buckwheat - Fagopyrum Esculentum - E	Seed	5,965 ppm
Basil, Cuban Basil, Sweet Basil - Ocimum Basilicum - E	Leaf	5,880 ppm
Summer Squash - Cucurbita spp. - E	Fruit	5,855 ppm
Aubergine, Egg Solanum Melongena - E	Fruit	5,700 ppm
Squaw Perideridia Gairdneri - E - M	Root	5,524 ppm
Sicklepod - Senna Obtusifolia - E - T	Seed	5,360 ppm
Bell Pepper, Cherry Pepper, Cone Pepper, Green Pepper, Paprika, Sweet Pepper - Capsicum Annuum - E	Fruit	5,047 ppm
Yambean - Pachyrhizus Erosus - E	Tuber	4,330 ppm
Bread Artocarpus Altilis - E	Seed	3,690-8,440 ppm
Macadamia - Macadamia spp. - E	Seed	4,075 ppm
Onion, Shallot - Allium Cepa - Shallot Bulb - E	Bulb	4,033 ppm
Chinese Foxglove - Rehmannia Glutinosa - M	Root	4,000 ppm
Indian Fig, Nopal, Nopalito, Prickly Pear - Opuntia Ficus-Indica - E - M	Bud	3,995 ppm
American Chestnut - Castanea Dentata - E - M	Seed	3,811 ppm
Pawpaw - Asimina Triloba - Friut - E	Fruit	3,648 ppm
Radish - Raphanus Sativus - E	Root	3,490 ppm
Orange - Citrus Sinensis - E	Fruit	3,473 ppm

PHENYLALANINE CONTINUED

Emblic, Myrobalan - Phyllanthus Emblica - E	Fruit	3,225 ppm
Celery - Apium Graveolens - E	Leaf	3,208 ppm
Chaya - Cnidoscolus Chayamansa - E	Leaf	3,100 ppm
Cucumber - Cucumis Sativus - E	Fruit	3,038 ppm
Beet, Beetroot, Garden Beet, Sugar Beet - Beta Vulgaris - E	Root	2,997 ppm
Avocado - Persea Americana - E - M - T	Fruit	2,993 ppm
Chinese Chestnut - Castanea Mollisima - M	Seed	2,904 ppm
Sweet Potato - Ipomoea Batatas - E	Root	2,840 ppm
Watermelon - Citrullus Lanatus - E	Fruit	2,827 ppm
Tomato - Lycopersicon Esculentum - E - M - T	Fruit	2,810 ppm
Burdock, Gobo, Great Burdock - Arctium lappa - E - M - T	Root	2,600 ppm
Mountain Yam - Dioscorea Pentaphylla - E	Root	2,585 ppm
Jerusalem Artichoke - Helianthus Tuberosus E	Tuber	2,573 ppm
Mandarin, Tangerine - Citrus Reticulata - E	Fruit	2,499 ppm
Cassava, Tapioca, Yuca - Manihot Esculenta - E	Root	2,415 ppm
Garlic - Allium Sativum Bulb - E	Bulb	2,400 ppm
Ginger - Zingiber Officinale - E	Rhizome	2,376 ppm
Carrot - Daucus Carota - E	Root	2,375 ppm
Peach - Prunus Persica - E - M - T	Fruit	2,349 ppm
Fig - Ficus Carica - E	Fruit	2,346 ppm
Plum - Prunus Domestica - E - M	Fruit	2,297 ppm
European Chestnut - Castanea Sativa - E - M	Seed	2,222 ppm
Taro - Colocasia Esculenta - E	Root	2,045 ppm
Mango - Mangifera Indica - E - M	Fruit	2,000 ppm
Strawberry - Fragaria spp. - E	Fruit	1,898 ppm
Guavas - Psidium Guajava - E	Fruit	1,800 ppm
Aloe, Bitter Aloes - Aloe Vera - E - M	Leaf	0-3,339 ppm
Blueberry - Vaccinium Corymbosum - E	Fruit	1,624 ppm
Date Palm - Phoenix Dactylifera - E	Fruit	1,590 ppm
Banana, Plantain - Musa x Paradisiaca - E	Fruit	1,554 ppm
Curry Murraya spp. - E - M	Fruit	1,440 ppm
Calathea allouia (AUBL.) LINDL. - Leren, Lleren	Root	2,610-2,870 ppm
Carambola, Star Averrhoa Carambola - E	Fruit	260-2,860 ppm
Breadroot, Indian Bread-Root, Indian Turnip, Prairie Apple, Prairie Potato, Prairie Turnip - Psoralea Esculenta - E - M - T	Root	1,266 ppm
American Elder, American Elderberry, Elderberry, Sweet Elder - Sambucus Canadensis - E	Fruit	1,238 ppm
European Grape, Grape, Grapevine, Vigne Vinifere, Wine Grape - Vitis Vinifera - E - M	Fruit	1,132 ppm
American Ginseng, Ginseng - Panax Quinquefolius - M	Plant	1,120 ppm
Pineapple - Ananas Comosus - E	Fruit	963 ppm
Strawberry Guava - Psidium Cattleianum - E	Fruit	930 ppm
Papaya - Carica Papaya - E - M	Fruit	895 ppm
Tomato - Lycopersicon Esculentum - E - M - T	Root	725 ppm
Pear - Pyrus Communis - E	Fruit	679 ppm
Grape Citrus Paradisi - E	Fruit	590 ppm
Pea - Pisum Sativum - E	Root	575 ppm
Apple - Malus Domestica - E	Plant	435 ppm
Oats - Avena Sativa - E - M	Root	276 ppm
Barley, Barleygrass - Hordeum Vulgare - E - M	Root	219 ppm
Wheat - Triticum Aestivum - E - M	Root	173 ppm
Oats - Avena Sativa - E - M	Shoot	150 ppm
Black Currant - Ribes Nigrum - E	Fruit Juice	98 ppm
Corn - Zea Mays - E	Root	69 ppm
Pea - Pisum Sativum - E	Shoot	23 ppm
Wheat - Triticum Aestivum - E - M	Shoot	12 ppm
Corn - Zea Mays - E	Shoot	11 ppm
Elephant Garlic, Kurrat - Allium Ampeloprasum - E	Plant	Trace
Jericho Rose - Anastatica Hierochuntica	Plant	Trace
Tarragon - Artemisia Dracunculus - M	Leaf	Trace
Tea - Camellia Sinensis - E	Leaf	Trace
Shepherd's Purse - Capsella Bursa-Pastoris - E - M	Plant	Trace
Alehoof - Glechoma Hederacea - M	Plant	Trace
Hops - Humulus Lupulus - E - M - T	Fruit	Trace
Flax, Lin Linum Usitatissimum - E	Seed	Trace
Antler Herb, Clubmoss - Lycopodium Clavatum - M - T	Pollen Or Spore	Trace
Chinaberry - Melia Azedarach - T	Seed	Trace
White Mulberry - Morus Alba - E - M	Leaf	Trace

Species	Part	Quantity
Passiflora incarnata L. -- Manzana de Mayo, Mayapple, Passionflower	Plant	Trace
Sour Cherry - Prunus Cerasus - E - M - T	Fruit	Trace
Rosa damascena MILLER -- Damask Rose	Pollen Or Spore	Trace
Santalum album L. -- White Sandalwood	Fruit	Trace
Indian Tamarind, Kilytree, Tamarind - Tamarindus Indica - M	Fruit	Trace
Terminalia chebula RETZ. -- Black Myrobalan, Chebulic Myrobalan, Ink Nut, Myrobalan	Fruit	Trace

PLANTS CONTAINING SERINE

Species	Part	Quantity
Black bean, Dwarf bean, Field bean, Flageolet bean, French bean, Garden bean, Green bean, Haricot, Haricot bean, Haricot vert, Kidney bean, Navy bean, Pop bean, Popping bean, Snap bean, String bean, Wax bean - Phaseolus Vulgaris - E	Sprout Seedling	24,086 ppm
Ceratonia siliqua L. -- Carob, Locust Bean, St.John's-Bread	Seed	23,500 ppm
Soybean - Glycine Max - E	Seed	23,125 ppm
White Lupine - Lupinus Albus - M - T	Seed	20,870 ppm
Cassie, Huisache, Opopanax, Popinac, Sweet Acacia - Acacia Farnesiana - M	Leaf	17,600 ppm
Butternut - Juglans Cinerea - E	Seed	16,967 ppm
Cowage, Velvetbean - Mucuna Pruriens - E	Seed	16,220 ppm
Swamp Cabbage, Water Spinach - Ipomoea Aquatica - E	Leaf	16,200 ppm
Butter Bean, Lima Bean - Phaseolus Lunatus - E	Seed	15,900 ppm
Chives - Allium Schoenoprasum - E	Leaf	15,750 ppm
Groundnut, Peanut - Arachis Hypogaea - E - M	Seed	15,362 ppm
Asparagus - Asparagus Officinalis - E	Shoot	14,968 ppm
Lentil - Lens Culinaris - E	Sprout Seedling	14,835 ppm
Jew's Mallow, Mulukiya, Nalta Jute - Corchorus Olitorius - E - M	Leaf	14,815 ppm
Lentil - Lens Culinaris - E	Seed	14,560 ppm
Bonavist Bean, Hyacinth Bean, Lablab Bean - Lablab Purpureus - E - M - T	Seed	14,510 ppm
Pistachio - Pistacia Vera - E	Seed	14,054 ppm
Sesame - Sesamum Indicum - E - M	Seed	13,751 ppm
Watermelon - Citrullus Lanatus - E	Seed	13,700 ppm
Asparagus Pea, Goa Bean, Winged Bean - Psophocarpus Tetragonolobus - E	Seed	13,474 ppm
Cauli Brassica Oleracea var. Botrytis - E	Flower	13,440 ppm
Alholva, Bockshornklee, Fenugreek, Greek Clover, Greek Trigonella Foenum-Graecum - E - M	Seed	13,365 ppm
Pigweed - Amaranthus sp. - E - M	Leaf	13,353 ppm
Black bean, Dwarf bean, Field bean, Flageolet bean, French bean, Garden bean, Green bean, Haricot, Haricot bean, Haricot vert, Kidney bean, Navy bean, Pop bean, Popping bean, Snap bean, String bean, Wax bean - Phaseolus Vulgaris - E	Seed	13,205 ppm
Broadbean, Faba Bean, Habas - Vicia Faba - E	Seed	12,950 ppm
Green Gram, Mungbean - Vigna Radiata - E	Seed	12,930 ppm
Lambsquarter - Chenopodium Album - E - M - T	Leaf	12,740 ppm
Pea - Pisum Sativum - E	Fruit	12,364 ppm
Spinach - Spinacia Oleracea - E	Plant	12,351 ppm
Pumpkin - Cucurbita Pepo - E	Seed	12,333 ppm
Asparagus bean, Pea bean, Yardlong bean - Vigna Unguiculata subsp. Sesquipedalis - E	Seed	12,030 ppm
Berro, Watercress - Nasturtium Officinale - E	Herb	12,000 ppm
Aloe, Bitter Aloes - Aloe Vera - E - M	Leaf	0-23,540 ppm
White Mustard - Sinapis Alba - E - M - T	Seed	11,567 ppm
Pigeonpea - Cajanus Vajan - E	Seed	11,500 ppm
Girasol, Sun Helianthus Annuus - E	Seed	11,400 ppm
Adzuki Bean - Vigna Angularis - E	Seed	11,275 ppm
Chickpea, Garbanzo - Cicer Arietinum - E	Seed	11,000 ppm
Asparagus Pea, Goa Bean, Winged Bean - Psophocarpus Tetragonolobus - E	Tuber	10,892 ppm

SERINE CONTINUED

Cauli Brassica Oleracea var. Botrytis - E	Leaf	10,740 ppm
Opium Poppy, Poppyseed Poppy - Papaver Somniferum - E	Seed	10,588 ppm
Bok-Choy, Celery Cabbage, Celery Mustard, Chinese Cabbage, Chinese Mustard, Chinese White Cabbage, Pak-Choi - Brassica Chinensis - E	Leaf	10,258 ppm
Chaya - Cnidoscolus Chayamansa - E	Leaf	10,230 ppm
Black bean, Dwarf bean, Field bean, Flageolet bean, French bean, Garden bean, Green bean, Haricot, Haricot bean, Haricot vert, Kidney bean, Navy bean, Pop bean, Popping bean, Snap bean, String bean, Wax bean - Phaseolus Vulgaris - E	Fruit	10,175 ppm
Buffalo Gourd - Cucurbita Foetidissima - E - M - T	Seed	12,585-20,180 ppm
Fennel - Foeniculum Vulgare - M	Fruit	9,873 ppm
Ben Nut, Benzolive Tree, Drumstick Tree, Horseradish Tree, Moringa, West Indian Ben - Moringa Oleifera - E	Shoot	4,140-19,400 ppm
Cabbage, Red Cabbage, White Cabbage - Brassica Oleracea var. Capitata - E	Leaf	9,493 ppm
Almond - Prunus Dulcis - E - M - T	Seed	9,424 ppm
Chinese Foxglove - Rehmannia Glutinosa - M	Root	9,000 ppm
Curly Kale, Kale, Kitchen Kale, Scotch Kale - Brassica Oleracea var. Sabellica l. var. Acephala - E	Leaf	8,945 ppm
Evening-Primrose - Oenothera Biennis - E - M	Seed	8,858 ppm
Papaver bracteatum L. -- Great Scarlet Poppy	Seed	8,850 ppm
Cacao - Theobroma Ccacao - E	Seed	8,800 ppm
Corn Salad, Lamb's Lettuce - Valerianella Locusta - E	Plant	8,750 ppm
Cashew - Anacardium Occidentale - E	Seed	8,637 ppm
Pea - Pisum Sativum - E	Seed	8,562 ppm
Purslane, Verdolaga - Portulaca Oleracea - E	Herb	8,440 ppm
Vinespinach - Basella Alba - E - M	Leaf	8,260 ppm
Collards, Cow Cabbage, Spring-Heading Cabbage, Tall Kale, Tree Kale - Brassica Oleracea - E	Leaf	8,195 ppm
Endive, Escarole - Cichorium Endivia - M	Leaf	7,890 ppm
Brazilnut, Brazilnut-Tree, Creamnut, Paranut - Bertholletia Eexcelsa - E	Seed	7,718 ppm
Indian Fig, Nopal, Nopalito, Prickly Pear - Opuntia Ficus-Indica - E - M	Seed	7,665 ppm
Italian Stone Pine, Pignolia - Pinus Pinea - M	Seed	10,190-15,300 ppm
Water Lotus - Nelumbo Nucifera - E - M	Seed	7,636 ppm
Summer Squash - Cucurbita spp. - E	Fruit	7,595 ppm
Sicklepod - Senna Obtusifolia - E - T	Seed	7,590 ppm
Wheat - Triticum Aestivum - E - M	Seed	7,567 ppm
Chayote - Sechium Edule - E - M	Fruit	7,285 ppm
Buckwheat - Fagopyrum Esculentum - E	Seed	7,110 ppm
Cayenne, Chili, Hot Pepper, Red Chili, Spur Pepper, Tabasco - Capsicum Frutescens - E	Fruit	6,528 ppm
Lettuce - Lactuca Sativa - E	Leaf	6,500 ppm
Ginkgo, Maidenhair Tree - Ginkgo Biloba - Tree - E - M - T	Seed	6,467 ppm
Asparagus Pea, Goa Bean, Winged Bean - Psophocarpus Tetragonolobus - E	Leaf	6,436 ppm
Corn - Zea Mays - E	Seed	6,365 ppm
Pumpkin - Cucurbita Pepo - E	Fruit	6,100 ppm
Apricot - Prunus Armeniaca - E - M - T	Fruit	6,080 ppm
Bread Artocarpus Altilis - E	Seed	4,960-11,340 ppm
Basil, Cuban Basil, Sweet Basil - Ocimum Basilicum - E	Leaf	5,610 ppm
Aubergine, Egg Solanum Melongena - E	Fruit	5,576 ppm
Black Caraway, Black Cumin, Fennel-Flower, Nutmeg-Flower, Roman Coriander - Nigella Sativa - E - M	Seed	5,385 ppm
Potato - Solanum Tuberosum - E	Tuber	5,250 ppm
Barley, Barleygrass - Hordeum Vulgare - E - M	Seed	5,000 ppm
Bell Pepper, Cherry Pepper, Cone Pepper, Green Pepper, Paprika, Sweet Pepper - Capsicum Annuum - E	Fruit	4,638 ppm
Garlic - Allium Sativum Bulb - E	Bulb	4,560 ppm
Okra - Abelmoschus Esculentus Friut - E - M	Fruit	4,510 ppm
Yambean - Pachyrhizus Erosus - E	Tuber	4,330 ppm

Beet, Beetroot, Garden Beet, Sugar Beet - Beta Vulgaris - E	Root	4,259 ppm
Celery - Apium Graveolens - E	Pt	4,105 ppm
Radish - Raphanus Sativus - E	Root	4,070 ppm
Cucumber - Cucumis Sativus - E	Fruit	4,051 ppm
Oats - Avena Sativa - E - M	Seed	4,000 ppm
Tomato - Lycopersicon Esculentum - E - M - T	Fruit	3,967 ppm
Indian Fig, Nopal, Nopalito, Prickly Pear - Opuntia Ficus-Indica - E - M	Bud	3,830 ppm
Mountain Yam - Dioscorea Pentaphylla - E	Root	3,825 ppm
Rye - Secale Cereale - E	Seed	6,810-7,645 ppm
Onion, Shallot - Allium Cepa - Shallot Bulb - E	Bulb	3,815 ppm
American Chestnut - Castanea Dentata - E - M	Seed	3,697 ppm
Pawpaw - Asimina Triloba - Friut - E	Fruit	3,666 ppm
Macadamia - Macadamia spp. - E	Seed	3,610 ppm
Rapini, Seven-Top Turnip, Turnip - Brassica Rapa - E	Root	3,565 ppm
Green Gram, Mungbean - Vigna Radiata - E	Sprout Seedling	3,466 ppm
Sweet Potato - Ipomoea Batatas - E	Root	3,400 ppm
Rutabaga, Swede, Swedish Turnip - Brassica Napus var. Napobrassica - E	Root	3,385 ppm
Chinese Chestnut - Castanea Mollisima - M	Seed	3,255 ppm
Mango - Mangifera Indica - E - M	Fruit	3,150 ppm
Avocado - Persea Americana - E - M - T	Fruit	3,148 ppm
Taro - Colocasia Esculenta - E	Root	3,135 ppm
Grape Citrus Paradisi - E	Fruit	3,100 ppm
Jerusalem Artichoke - Helianthus Tuberosus E	Tuber	2,954 ppm
Water Lotus - Nelumbo Nucifera - E - M	Rhizome	2,870 ppm
Carrot - Daucus Carota - E	Root	2,865 ppm
Strawberry - Fragaria spp. - E	Fruit	2,728 ppm
Squaw Perideridia Gairdneri - E - M	Root	2,667 ppm
Pinyon Pine - Pinus Edulis	Seed	4,910-5,220 ppm
Ginger - Zingiber Officinale - E	Rhizome	2,596 ppm
Peach - Prunus Persica - E - M - T	Fruit	2,592 ppm
Cassava, Tapioca, Yuca - Manihot Esculenta - E	Root	2,415 ppm
Orange - Citrus Sinensis - E	Fruit	2,410 ppm
Carambola, Star Averrhoa Carambola - E	Fruit	430-4,735 ppm
European Chestnut - Castanea Sativa - E - M	Seed	2,139 ppm
Date Palm - Phoenix Dactylifera - E	Fruit	1,960 ppm
Watermelon - Citrullus Lanatus - E	Fruit	1,885 ppm
Breadroot, Indian Bread-Root, Indian Turnip, Prairie Apple, Prairie Potato, Prairie Turnip - Psoralea Esculenta - E - M - T	Root	1,857 ppm
Pineapple - Ananas Comosus - E	Fruit	1,852 ppm
Banana, Plantain - Musa x Paradisiaca - E	Fruit	1,826 ppm
Mandarin, Tangerine - Citrus Reticulata - E	Fruit	1,773 ppm
Fig - Ficus Carica - E	Fruit	1,771 ppm
Guavas - Psidium Guajava - E	Fruit	1,728 ppm
Calathea allouia (AUBL.) LINDL. - Leren, Lleren	Root	3,085-3,390 ppm
European Grape, Grape, Grapevine, Vigne Vinifere, Wine Grape - Vitis Vinifera - E - M	Fruit	1,646 ppm
Plum - Prunus Domestica - E - M	Fruit	1,351 ppm
Papaya - Carica Papaya - E - M	Fruit	1,343 ppm
Blueberry - Vaccinium Corymbosum - E	Fruit	1,300 ppm
Burdock, Gobo, Great Burdock - Arctium lappa - E - M - T	Root	1,250 ppm
American Ginseng, Ginseng - Panax Quinquefolius - M	Plant	1,240 ppm
Curry Murraya spp. - E - M	Fruit	1,181 ppm
Emblic, Myrobalan - Phyllanthus Emblica - E	Fruit	905 ppm
Strawberry Guava - Psidium Cattleianum - E	Fruit	880 ppm
Pear - Pyrus Communis - E	Fruit	865 ppm
Apple - Malus Domestica - E	Fruit	497 ppm
Black Currant - Ribes Nigrum - E	Fruit Juice	60 ppm
Flax, Lin Linum Usitatissimum - E	Seed	Trace
Gum Arabic, Gum Arabic Tree, Kher, Senegal Gum, Sudan Gum Arabic - Acacia Senegal - M	Plant	Trace
Elephant Garlic, Kurrat - Allium Ampeloprasum - E	Plant	Trace
Tarragon - Artemisia Dracunculus - M	Shoot	Trace
Tea - Camellia Sinensis - E	Leaf	Trace
Jack Bean - Canavalia Ensiformis - E	Seed	Trace
Carrot - Daucus Carota - E	Plant	Trace
Soybean - Glycine Max - E	Plant	Trace
Hops - Humulus Lupulus - E - M - T	Fruit	Trace

SERINE CONTINUED

Species	Part	Quantity
Chinaberry - Melia Azedarach - T	Seed	Trace
Rice - Oryza Sativa - E	Plant	Trace
Ban-Xia, Pan-Hsia - Pinellia Ternata - E - M - T	Tuber	Trace
Sour Cherry - Prunus Cerasus - E - M - T	Fruit	Trace
Sage - Salvia Officinalis - E - M	Plant	Trace
Santalum album L. -- White Sandalwood	Fruit	Trace
Tilia sp. -- Basswood, Lime, Linden	Flower	Trace
Cowgrass, Peavine Clover, Purple Clover, Red Clover - Trifolium Pratense - E - M	Plant	Trace

PLANTS CONTAINING THREONINE

Species	Part	Quantity
Berro, Watercress - Nasturtium Officinale - E	Herb	26,600 ppm
Black bean, Dwarf bean, Field bean, Flageolet bean, French bean, Garden bean, Green bean, Haricot, Haricot bean, Haricot vert, Kidney bean, Navy bean, Pop bean, Popping bean, Snap bean, String bean, Wax bean - Phaseolus Vulgaris - E	Sprout Seedling	18,925 ppm
Swamp Cabbage, Water Spinach - Ipomoea Aquatica - E	Leaf	18,590 ppm
Soybean - Glycine Max - E	Seed	17,330 ppm
Ceratonia siliqua L. - Carob, Locust Bean, St.John's-Bread	Seed	16,920 ppm
Oats - Avena Sativa - E - M	Plant	16,000 ppm
Chinese Foxglove - Rehmannia Glutinosa - M	Root	16,000 ppm
Watermelon - Citrullus Lanatus - E	Seed	15,300 ppm
White Lupine - Lupinus Albus - M - T	Seed	14,860 ppm
Spinach - Spinacia Oleracea - E	Plant	14,489 ppm
Chives - Allium Schoenoprasum - E	Leaf	13,875 ppm
Jew's Mallow, Mulukiya, Nalta Jute - Corchorus Olitorius - E - M	Leaf	13,350 ppm
Cowage, Velvetbean - Mucuna Pruriens - E	Seed	13,250 ppm
Buffalo Gourd - Cucurbita Foetidissima - E - M - T	Seed	4,605-26,000 ppm
Asparagus Pea, Goa Bean, Winged Bean - Psophocarpus Tetragonolobus - E	Seed	12,863 ppm
Sesame - Sesamum Indicum - E - M	Seed	12,396 ppm
Pigweed - Amaranthus sp. - E - M	Leaf	11,910 ppm
Bonavist Bean, Hyacinth Bean, Lablab Bean - Lablab Purpureus - E - M - T	Seed	11,789 ppm
White Mustard - Sinapis Alba - E - M - T	Seed	11,720 ppm
Taro - Colocasia Esculenta - E	Leaf	11,645 ppm
Lentil - Lens Culinaris - E	Seed	11,325 ppm
Asparagus - Asparagus Officinalis - E	Shoot	10,968 ppm
Broadbean, Faba Bean, Habas - Vicia Faba - E	Seed	10,950 ppm
Lentil - Lens Culinaris - E	Sprout Seedling	10,935 ppm
Cassie, Huisache, Opopanax, Popinac, Sweet Acacia - Acacia Farnesiana - M	Leaf	10,730 ppm
Asparagus Pea, Goa Bean, Winged Bean - Psophocarpus Tetragonolobus - E	Tuber	10,587 ppm
Bok-Choy, Celery Cabbage, Celery Mustard, Chinese Cabbage, Chinese Mustard, Chinese White Cabbage, Pak-Choi - Brassica Chinensis - E	Leaf	10,471 ppm
Corn Salad, Lamb's Lettuce - Valerianella Locusta - E	Plant	10,415 ppm
Lambsquarter - Chenopodium Album - E - M - T	Leaf	10,383 ppm
Butter Bean, Lima Bean - Phaseolus Lunatus - E	Seed	10,320 ppm
Chaya - Cnidoscolus Chayamansa - E	Leaf	10,230 ppm
Black bean, Dwarf bean, Field bean, Flageolet bean, French bean, Garden bean, Green bean, Haricot, Haricot bean, Haricot vert, Kidney bean, Navy bean, Pop bean, Popping bean, Snap bean, String bean, Wax bean - Phaseolus Vulgaris - E	Seed	10,216 ppm
Asparagus bean, Pea bean, Yardlong bean - Vigna Unguiculata subsp. Sesquipedalis - E	Seed	10,112 ppm
Alholva, Bockshornklee, Fenugreek, Greek Clover, Greek Trigonella Foenum-Graecum - E - M	Seed	9,880 ppm
Lettuce - Lactuca Sativa - E	Leaf	9,833 ppm
Girasol, Sun Helianthus Annuus - E	Seed	9,806 ppm
Pea - Pisum Sativum - E	Fruit	9,792 ppm
Cauli Brassica Oleracea var. Botrytis - E	Leaf	9,773 ppm
Butternut - Juglans Cinerea - E	Seed	9,725 ppm

Black Mustard - Brassica Nigra - E	Leaf	9,720 ppm
Opium Poppy, Poppyseed Poppy - Papaver Somniferum - E	Seed	9,708 ppm
Pumpkin - Cucurbita Pepo - E	Seed	9,701 ppm
Ben Nut, Benzolive Tree, Drumstick Tree, Horseradish Tree, Moringa, West Indian Ben - Moringa Oleifera - E	Shoot	4,110-19,260 ppm
Pea - Pisum Sativum - E	Seed	9,603 ppm
Groundnut, Peanut - Arachis Hypogaea - E - M	Seed	9,570 ppm
Curly Kale, Kale, Kitchen Kale, Scotch Kale - Brassica Oleracea var. Sabellica l. var. Acephala - E	Leaf	9,460 ppm
Purslane, Verdolaga - Portulaca Oleracea - E	Herb	9,400 ppm
Cauli Brassica Oleracea var. Botrytis - E	Flower	9,300 ppm
Collards, Cow Cabbage, Spring-Heading Cabbage, Tall Kale, Tree Kale - Brassica Oleracea - E	Leaf	9,014 ppm
Green Gram, Mungbean - Vigna Radiata - E	Seed	8,598 ppm
Pigeonpea - Cajanus Vajan - E	Seed	8,580 ppm
Brussel-Sprout - Brassica Oleracea var. Gemmifera - E	Leaf	8,568 ppm
Asparagus bean, Pea bean, Yardlong bean - Vigna Unguiculata subsp. Sesquipedalis - E	Fruit	8,560 ppm
Green Gram, Mungbean - Vigna Radiata - E	Sprout Seedling	8,192 ppm
Black bean, Dwarf bean, Field bean, Flageolet bean, French bean, Garden bean, Green bean, Haricot, Haricot bean, Haricot vert, Kidney bean, Navy bean, Pop bean, Popping bean, Snap bean, String bean, Wax bean - Phaseolus Vulgaris - E	Fruit	8,119 ppm
Chickpea, Garbanzo - Cicer Arietinum - E	Seed	8,090 ppm
Endive, Escarole - Cichorium Endivia - M	Leaf	8,051 ppm
Vinespinach - Basella Alba - E - M	Leaf	7,970 ppm
Asparagus Pea, Goa Bean, Winged Bean - Psophocarpus Tetragonolobus - E	Leaf	7,862 ppm
Papaver bracteatum L. -- Great Scarlet Poppy	Seed	7,800 ppm
Adzuki Bean - Vigna Angularis - E	Seed	7,787 ppm
Almond - Prunus Dulcis - E - M - T	Seed	7,730 ppm
Achiote, Annato, Annatto, Annoto, Arnato, Bija, Lipstick Pod, Lipsticktree - Bixa Orellana - E	Seed	7,600 ppm
Pistachio - Pistacia Vera - E	Seed	7,511 ppm
Indian Fig, Nopal, Nopalito, Prickly Pear - Opuntia Ficus-Indica - E - M	Seed	7,330 ppm
Aloe, Bitter Aloes - Aloe Vera - E - M	Leaf	0-14,652 ppm
Oats - Avena Sativa - E - M	Seed	7,000 ppm
Fennel - Foeniculum Vulgare - M	Fruit	6,604 ppm
Okra - Abelmoschus Esculentus - Friut - E - M	Fruit	6,500 ppm
Chayote - Sechium Edule - E - M	Fruit	6,285 ppm
Dill, Garden Dill - Anethum Graveolens - E	Fruit	6,227 ppm
Water Lotus - Nelumbo Nucifera - E - M	Seed	6,060 ppm
Cayenne, Chili, Hot Pepper, Red Chili, Spur Pepper, Tabasco - Capsicum Frutescens - E	Fruit	6,038 ppm
Cashew - Anacardium Occidentale - E	Seed	6,022 ppm
Wheat - Triticum Aestivum - E - M	Seed	6,000 ppm
Ginkgo, Maidenhair Tree - Ginkgo Biloba - Tree - E - M - T	Seed	5,976 ppm
Sicklepod - Senna Obtusifolia - E - T	Seed	5,940 ppm
Basil, Cuban Basil, Sweet Basil - Ocimum Basilicum - E	Leaf	5,880 ppm
Buckwheat - Fagopyrum Esculentum - E	Seed	5,850 ppm
Chicory, Succory, Witloof - Cichorium Intybus - E - M	Leaf	5,712 ppm
Radish - Raphanus Sativus - E	Root	5,620 ppm
Cabbage, Red Cabbage, White Cabbage - Brassica Oleracea var. Capitata - E	Leaf	5,615 ppm
Kohlrabi - Brassica Oleracea var. Gongylodes - E	Stem	5,445 ppm
Corn - Zea Mays - E	Seed	5,366 ppm
Aubergine, Egg Solanum Melongena - E	Fruit	4,957 ppm
Brazilnut, Brazilnut-Tree, Creamnut, Paranut - Bertholletia Eexcelsa - E	Seed	4,759 ppm
Evening-Primrose - Oenothera Biennis - E - M	Seed	4,600 ppm
Rutabaga, Swede, Swedish Turnip - Brassica Napus var. Napobrassica - E	Root	4,445 ppm
Summer Squash - Cucurbita spp. - E	Fruit	4,430 ppm

THREONINE CONTINUED

Bread Artocarpus Altilis - E	Seed	3,850-8,800 ppm
Potato - Solanum Tuberosum - E	Tuber	4,300 ppm
Bell Pepper, Cherry Pepper, Cone Pepper, Green Pepper, Paprika, Sweet Pepper - Capsicum Annuum - E	Fruit	4,228 ppm
Celery - Apium Graveolens - E	Pt	4,105 ppm
Italian Stone Pine, Pignolia - Pinus Pinea - M	Seed	7,610-8,190 ppm
Calabash Gourd, White-Flowered Gourd - Lagenaria Siceraria - E	Fruit	4,035 ppm
Indian Fig, Nopal, Nopalito, Prickly Pear - Opuntia Ficus-Indica - E - M	Bud	3,845 ppm
Cucumber - Cucumis Sativus - E	Fruit	3,797 ppm
Garlic - Allium Sativum Bulb - E	Bulb	3,768 ppm
Tomato - Lycopersicon Esculentum - E - M - T	Fruit	3,637 ppm
Beet, Beetroot, Garden Beet, Sugar Beet - Beta Vulgaris - E	Root	3,470 ppm
Pumpkin - Cucurbita Pepo - E	Fruit	3,452 ppm
Apricot - Prunus Armeniaca - E - M - T	Fruit	3,445 ppm
Jerusalem Artichoke - Helianthus Tuberosus E	Tuber	3,431 ppm
American Chestnut - Castanea Dentata - E - M	Seed	3,389 ppm
Black Caraway, Black Cumin, Fennel-Flower, Nutmeg-Flower, Roman Coriander - Nigella Sativa - E - M	Seed	3,345 ppm
Yambean - Pachyrhizus Erosus - E	Tuber	3,225 ppm
Chinese Chestnut - Castanea Mollisima - M	Seed	3,214 ppm
Watermelon - Citrullus Lanatus - E	Fruit	3,180 ppm
Carrot - Daucus Carota - E	Root	3,110 ppm
Rapini, Seven-Top Turnip, Turnip - Brassica Rapa - E	Root	3,075 ppm
Onion, Shallot - Allium Cepa - Shallot Bulb - E	Bulb	3,052 ppm
Sweet Potato - Ipomoea Batatas - E	Root	3,019 ppm
Rye - Secale Cereale - E	Seed	5,320-5,975 ppm
Pawpaw - Asimina Triloba - Friut - E	Fruit	2,812 ppm
Common thyme, Garden thyme, Thyme - Thymus Vulgaris - E - M	Plant	2,722 ppm
Macadamia - Macadamia spp. - E	Seed	2,705 ppm
Avocado - Persea Americana - E - M - T	Fruit	2,565 ppm
Mountain Yam - Dioscorea Pentaphylla - E	Root	2,530 ppm
Eryngium creticus -- Cretan culantro	Shoot	0-5,045 ppm
Water Lotus - Nelumbo Nucifera - E - M	Rhizome	2,440 ppm
Squaw Perideridia Gairdneri - E - M	Root	2,413 ppm
Taro - Colocasia Esculenta - E	Root	2,350 ppm
Strawberry - Fragaria spp. - E	Fruit	2,254 ppm
Mango - Mangifera Indica - E - M	Fruit	2,250 ppm
Guavas - Psidium Guajava - E	Fruit	2,232 ppm
Peach - Prunus Persica - E - M - T	Fruit	2,187 ppm
Cassava, Tapioca, Yuca - Manihot Esculenta - E	Root	2,065 ppm
Ginger - Zingiber Officinale - E	Rhizome	2,057 ppm
Pinyon Pine - Pinus Edulis	Seed	3,670-3,900 ppm
Bread Artocarpus Altilis - E	Fruit	1,770 ppm
European Chestnut - Castanea Sativa - E - M	Seed	1,604 ppm
Calathea allouia (AUBL.) LINDL. - Leren, Lleren	Root	2,815-3,095 ppm
Breadroot, Indian Bread-Root, Indian Turnip, Prairie Apple, Prairie Potato, Prairie Turnip - Psoralea Esculenta - E - M - T	Root	1,477 ppm
Cacao - Theobroma Ccacao - E	Seed	1,400 ppm
American Elder, American Elderberry, Elderberry, Sweet Elder - Sambucus Canadensis - E	Fruit	1,336 ppm
Banana, Plantain - Musa x Paradisiaca - E	Fruit	1,321 ppm
Burdock, Gobo, Great Burdock - Arctium lappa - E - M - T	Root	1,300 ppm
Carambola, Star Averrhoa Carambola - E	Fruit	230-2,530 ppm
Blueberry - Vaccinium Corymbosum - E	Fruit	1,170 ppm
Fig - Ficus Carica - E	Fruit	1,149 ppm
Strawberry Guava - Psidium Cattleianum - E	Fruit	1,140 ppm
Orange - Citrus Sinensis - E	Fruit	1,132 ppm
Cassie, Huisache, Opopanax, Popinac, Sweet Acacia - Acacia Farnesiana - M	Seed	1,100 ppm
Pouteria caimito RADLK. -- Abiu, Caimito	Fruit	0-2,190 ppm
Plum - Prunus Domestica - E - M	Fruit	1,081 ppm
American Ginseng, Ginseng - Panax Quinquefolius - M	Plant	1,070 ppm
Papaya - Carica Papaya - E - M	Fruit	985 ppm

Date Palm - Phoenix Dactylifera - E	Fruit	980 ppm
Curry Murraya spp. - E - M	Fruit	979 ppm
European Grape, Grape, Grapevine, Vigne Vinifere, Wine Grape - Vitis Vinifera - E - M	Fruit	926 ppm
Pineapple - Ananas Comosus - E	Fruit	859 ppm
Mandarin, Tangerine - Citrus Reticulata - E	Fruit	806 ppm
Emblic, Myrobalan - Phyllanthus Emblica - E	Fruit	668 ppm
Pear - Pyrus Communis - E	Fruit	618 ppm
Apple - Malus Domestica - E	Fruit	435 ppm
Grape Citrus Paradisi - E	Fruit	100 ppm
Black Currant - Ribes Nigrum - E	Fruit Juice	17 ppm
Elephant Garlic, Kurrat - Allium Ampeloprasum - E	Plant	Trace
Jericho Rose - Anastatica Hierochuntica	Plant	Trace
Tea - Camellia Sinensis - E	Leaf	Trace
Hops - Humulus Lupulus - E - M - T	Fruit	Trace
Flax, Lin Linum Usitatissimum - E	Seed	Trace
Chinaberry - Melia Azedarach - T	Seed	Trace
Spearmint - Mentha Spicata - E - M- T	Leaf	Trace
Rice - Oryza Sativa - E	Hay	Trace
Sour Cherry - Prunus Cerasus - E - M - T	Fruit	Trace
Cowgrass, Peavine Clover, Purple Clover, Red Clover - Trifolium Pratense - E - M	Plant	Trace

PLANTS CONTAINING TRYPTOPHAN

Evening-Primrose - Oenothera Biennis - E - M	Seed	16,000 ppm
Girasol, Sun Helianthus Annuus - E	Seed	15,900 ppm
Asparagus Pea, Goa Bean, Winged Bean - Psophocarpus Tetragonolobus - E	Seed	8,313 ppm
Bonavist Bean, Hyacinth Bean, Lablab Bean - Lablab Purpureus - E - M - T	Seed	7,255 ppm
Berro, Watercress - Nasturtium Officinale E	Herb	6,000 ppm
Asparagus Pea, Goa Bean, Winged Bean - Psophocarpus Tetragonolobus - E	Tuber	5,915 ppm
White Mustard - Sinapis Alba - E - M - T	Seed	5,628 ppm
Asparagus Pea, Goa Bean, Winged Bean - Psophocarpus Tetragonolobus - E	Leaf	5,011 ppm
Chickpea, Garbanzo - Cicer Arietinum - E	Seed	4,970 ppm
Sesame - Sesamum Indicum - E - M	Seed	4,969 ppm
Black bean, Dwarf bean, Field bean, Flageolet bean, French bean, Garden bean, Green bean, Haricot, Haricot bean, Haricot vert, Kidney bean, Navy bean, Pop bean, Popping bean, Snap bean, String bean, Wax bean - Phaseolus Vulgaris - E	Sprout Seedling	4,731 ppm
Spinach - Spinacia Oleracea - E	Plant	4,632 ppm
Pumpkin - Cucurbita Pepo - E	Seed	4,630 ppm
Alholva, Bockshornklee, Fenugreek, Greek Clover, Greek Trigonella Foenum-Graecum - E - M	Seed	4,300 ppm
Vinespinach - Basella Alba - E - M	Leaf	4,060 ppm
Jew's Mallow, Mulukiya, Nalta Jute - Corchorus Olitorius - E - M	Leaf	4,000 ppm
Black Mustard - Brassica Nigra - E	Leaf	3,976 ppm
Green Gram, Mungbean - Vigna Radiata - E	Sprout Seedling	3,886 ppm
Chives - Allium Schoenoprasum - E	Leaf	3,875 ppm
Asparagus - Asparagus Officinalis - E	Shoot	3,871 ppm
Butternut - Juglans Cinerea - E	Seed	3,786 ppm
Almond - Prunus Dulcis - E - M - T	Seed	3,745 ppm
Pigweed - Amaranthus sp. - E - M	Leaf	3,729 ppm
Chicory, Succory, Witloof - Cichorium Intybus - E - M	Leaf	3,672 ppm
Corn Salad, Lamb's Lettuce - Valerianella Locusta - E	Plant	3,610 ppm
Purslane, Verdolaga - Portulaca Oleracea - E	Herb	3,400 ppm
Ben Nut, Benzolive Tree, Drumstick Tree, Horseradish Tree, Moringa, West Indian Ben - Moringa Oleifera - E	Shoot	1,440-6,745 ppm
Cauli Brassica Oleracea var. Botrytis - E	Flower	3,360 ppm
Taro - Colocasia Esculenta - E	Leaf	3,345 ppm
Groundnut, Peanut - Arachis Hypogaea - E - M	Seed	3,321 ppm

TRYPTOPHAN CONTINUED

Species	Part	ppm
Collards, Cow Cabbage, Spring-Heading Cabbage, Tall Kale, Tree Kale - Brassica Oleracea - E	Leaf	3,278 ppm
Asparagus bean, Pea bean, Yardlong bean - Vigna Unguiculata subsp. Sesquipedalis - E	Seed	3,276 ppm
White Lupine - Lupinus Albus - M - T	Seed	3,225 ppm
Bok-Choy, Celery Cabbage, Celery Mustard, Chinese Cabbage, Chinese Mustard, Chinese White Cabbage, Pak-Choi - Brassica Chinensis - E	Leaf	3,206 ppm
Cauli Brassica Oleracea var. Botrytis - E	Leaf	3,115 ppm
Butter Bean, Lima Bean - Phaseolus Lunatus - E	Seed	3,024 ppm
Oats - Avena Sativa - E - M	Seed	3,000 ppm
Barley, Barleygrass - Hordeum Vulgare - E - M	Seed	3,000 ppm
Wheat - Triticum Aestivum - E - M	Seed	3,000 ppm
Broadbean, Faba Bean, Habas - Vicia Faba - E	Seed	2,950 ppm
Pistachio - Pistacia Vera - E	Seed	2,944 ppm
Black bean, Dwarf bean, Field bean, Flageolet bean, French bean, Garden bean, Green bean, Haricot, Haricot bean, Haricot vert, Kidney bean, Navy bean, Pop bean, Popping bean, Snap bean, String bean, Wax bean - Phaseolus Vulgaris - E	Seed	2,877 ppm
Green Gram, Mungbean - Vigna Radiata - E	Seed	2,859 ppm
Lentil - Lens Culinaris - E	Seed	2,826 ppm
Fennel - Foeniculum Vulgare - M	Fruit	2,775 ppm
Buffalo Gourd - Cucurbita Foetidissima - E - M - T	Seed	1,840-5,472 ppm
Opium Poppy, Poppyseed Poppy - Papaver Somniferum - E	Seed	2,735 ppm
Brazilnut, Brazilnut-Tree, Creamnut, Paranut - Bertholletia Eexcelsa - E	Seed	2,690 ppm
Pea - Pisum Sativum - E	Fruit	2,671 ppm
Brussel-Sprout - Brassica Oleracea var. Gemmifera - E	Leaf	2,642 ppm
Asparagus bean, Pea bean, Yardlong bean - Vigna Unguiculata subsp. Sesquipedalis - E	Fruit	2,634 ppm
Curly Kale, Kale, Kitchen Kale, Scotch Kale - Brassica Oleracea var. Sabellica l. var. Acephala - E	Leaf	2,575 ppm
Lambsquarter - Chenopodium Album - E - M - T	Leaf	2,421 ppm
Cashew - Anacardium Occidentale - E	Seed	2,411 ppm
Pigeonpea - Cajanus Vajan - E	Seed	2,370 ppm
Potato - Solanum Tuberosum - E	Tuber	2,250 ppm
Basil, Cuban Basil, Sweet Basil - Ocimum Basilicum - E	Leaf	2,210 ppm
Adzuki Bean - Vigna Angularis - E	Seed	2,207 ppm
Sicklepod - Senna Obtusifolia - E - T	Seed	2,180 ppm
Cayenne, Chili, Hot Pepper, Red Chili, Spur Pepper, Tabasco - Capsicum Frutescens - E	Fruit	2,122 ppm
Buckwheat - Fagopyrum Esculentum - E	Seed	2,065 ppm
Common thyme, Garden thyme, Thyme - Thymus Vulgaris - E - M	Plant	2,009 ppm
Oats - Avena Sativa - E - M	Plant	2,000 ppm
Black bean, Dwarf bean, Field bean, Flageolet bean, French bean, Garden bean, Green bean, Haricot, Haricot bean, Haricot vert, Kidney bean, Navy bean, Pop bean, Popping bean, Snap bean, String bean, Wax bean - Phaseolus Vulgaris - E	Fruit	1,953 ppm
Celery - Apium Graveolens - E	Pt	1,865 ppm
Eryngium creticus -- Cretan culantro	Shoot	0-3,715 ppm
Onion, Shallot - Allium Cepa - Shallot Bulb - E	Bulb	1,853 ppm
Jerusalem Artichoke - Helianthus Tuberosus E	Tuber	1,811 ppm
Pumpkin - Cucurbita Pepo - E	Fruit	1,800 ppm
Water Lotus - Nelumbo Nucifera - E - M	Seed	1,788 ppm
Pea - Pisum Sativum - E	Seed	1,750 ppm
Summer Squash - Cucurbita spp. - E	Fruit	1,740 ppm
Chayote - Sechium Edule - E - M	Fruit	1,715 ppm
Okra - Abelmoschus Esculentus - Friut - E - M	Fruit	1,710 ppm
Achiote, Annato, Annatto, Annoto, Arnato, Bija, Lipstick Pod, Lipsticktree - Bixa Orellana - E	Seed	1,680 ppm
Indian Fig, Nopal, Nopalito, Prickly Pear - Opuntia Ficus-Indica - E - M	Seed	1,665 ppm
Mat Bean, Moth Bean - Vigna Aconitifolia - E	Seed	1,628 ppm
Italian Stone Pine, Pignolia - Pinus Pinea - M	Seed	3,030-3,250 ppm

Cabbage, Red Cabbage, White Cabbage - Brassica Oleracea var. Capitata - E	Leaf	1,604 ppm
Garlic - Allium Sativum Bulb - E	Bulb	1,584 ppm
Ginkgo, Maidenhair Tree - Ginkgo Biloba - Tree - E - M - T	Seed	1,583 ppm
Bell Pepper, Cherry Pepper, Cone Pepper, Green Pepper, Paprika, Sweet Pepper - Capsicum Annuum - E	Fruit	1,500 ppm
Lettuce - Lactuca Sativa - E	Leaf	1,500 ppm
Bread Artocarpus Altilis - E	Seed	1,230-2,815 ppm
Cassava, Tapioca, Yuca - Manihot Esculenta - E	Root	1,365 ppm
Beet, Beetroot, Garden Beet, Sugar Beet - Beta Vulgaris - E	Root	1,341 ppm
Rutabaga, Swede, Swedish Turnip - Brassica Napus var. Napobrassica - E	Root	1,255 ppm
Aubergine, Egg Solanum Melongena - E	Fruit	1,239 ppm
Tomato - Lycopersicon Esculentum - E - M - T	Fruit	1,157 ppm
Kohlrabi - Brassica Oleracea var. Gongylodes - E	Stem	1,110 ppm
Rapini, Seven-Top Turnip, Turnip - Brassica Rapa - E	Root	1,100 ppm
Apricot - Prunus Armeniaca - E - M - T	Fruit	1,100 ppm
Cucumber - Cucumis Sativus - E	Fruit	1,012 ppm
American Chestnut - Castanea Dentata - E - M	Seed	957 ppm
Corn - Zea Mays - E	Seed	957 ppm
Water Lotus - Nelumbo Nucifera - E - M	Rhizome	955 ppm
Carrot - Daucus Carota - E	Root	900 ppm
Chinese Chestnut - Castanea Mollisima - M	Seed	874 ppm
Rye - Secale Cereale - E	Seed	1,540-1,730 ppm
Strawberry - Fragaria spp. - E	Fruit	830 ppm
Watermelon - Citrullus Lanatus - E	Fruit	825 ppm
Avocado - Persea Americana - E - M - T	Fruit	816 ppm
Endive, Escarole - Cichorium Endivia - M	Leaf	805 ppm
Sweet Potato - Ipomoea Batatas - E	Root	800 ppm
Taro - Colocasia Esculenta - E	Root	785 ppm
Radish - Raphanus Sativus - E	Root	775 ppm
Squaw Perideridia Gairdneri - E - M	Root	762 ppm
Papaya - Carica Papaya - E - M	Fruit	716 ppm
Mango - Mangifera Indica - E - M	Fruit	700 ppm
Ginger - Zingiber Officinale - E	Rhizome	693 ppm
Orange - Citrus Sinensis - E	Fruit	680 ppm
Calabash Gourd, White-Flowered Gourd - Lagenaria Siceraria - E	Fruit	675 ppm
Date Palm - Phoenix Dactylifera - E	Fruit	645 ppm
Breadroot, Indian Bread-Root, Indian Turnip, Prairie Apple, Prairie Potato, Prairie Turnip - Psoralea Esculenta - E - M - T	Root	633 ppm
Mountain Yam - Dioscorea Pentaphylla - E	Root	595 ppm
Soursop - Annona Muricata - E	Fruit	585 ppm
American Elder, American Elderberry, Elderberry, Sweet Elder - Sambucus Canadensis - E	Fruit	559 ppm
Pawpaw - Asimina Triloba - Friut - E	Fruit	536 ppm
Waxgourd - Benincasa Hispida - Fruit	Fruit	515 ppm
Guavas - Psidium Guajava - E	Fruit	504 ppm
European Chestnut - Castanea Sativa - E - M	Seed	485 ppm
Mandarin, Tangerine - Citrus Reticulata - E	Fruit	484 ppm
Banana, Plantain - Musa x Paradisiaca - E	Fruit	466 ppm
Cassie, Huisache, Opopanax, Popinac, Sweet Acacia - Acacia Farnesiana - M	Seed	450 ppm
Curry Murraya spp. - E - M	Fruit	432 ppm
Sugar-Apple, Sweetsop - Annona Squamosa - E	Fruit	375 ppm
Pouteria campechiana BAEHNI - Canistel	Fruit	280-710 ppm
Burdock, Gobo, Great Burdock - Arctium lappa - E - M - T	Root	300 ppm
Fig - Ficus Carica - E	Fruit	287 ppm
Indian Tamarind, Kilytree, Tamarind - Tamarindus Indica - M	Fruit	262 ppm
Strawberry Guava - Psidium Cattleianum - E	Fruit	260 ppm
Lime - Citrus Aurantiifolia - E	Fruit	255 ppm
Custard Apple - Annona Reticulata - E	Fruit	245 ppm
Russian Olive - Elaeagnus Umbellatus - E - M	Fruit	90-485 ppm
Melicoccus bijugatas JACQ. -- Genip, Honey berry, Mamoncillo, Pitomba	Fruit	140-450 ppm
Carambola, Star Averrhoa Carambola - E	Fruit	40-440 ppm
Grape Citrus Paradisi - E	Fruit	220 ppm

TRYPTOPHAN CONTINUED

Species	Part	Quantity
Blueberry - Vaccinium Corymbosum - E	Fruit	195 ppm
Peach - Prunus Persica - E - M - T	Fruit	162 ppm
European Grape, Grape, Grapevine, Vigne Vinifere, Wine Grape - Vitis Vinifera - E - M	Fruit	154 ppm
Emblic, Myrobalan - Phyllanthus Emblica - E	Fruit	131 ppm
Apple - Malus Domestica - E	Fruit	124 ppm
Chrysophyllum cainito RADLK. -- Caimito, Star Apple	Fruit	40-120 ppm
Elephant Garlic, Kurrat - Allium Ampeloprasum - E	Plant	Trace
Hemp, Indian Hemp, Marihuana, Marijuana - Cannabis Sativa - M	Seed	Trace
Hops - Humulus Lupulus - E - M - T	Fruit	Trace
Flax, Lin Linum Usitatissimum - E	Seed	Trace
Alfalfa, Lucerne - Medicago Sativa subsp. Sativa - E	Plant	Trace
Spearmint - Mentha Spicata - E - M - T	Leaf	Trace
Black Caraway, Black Cumin, Fennel-Flower, Nutmeg-Flower, Roman Coriander - Nigella Sativa - E - M	Seed	Trace
Rivea corymbosa HALL. f. -- Snakeplant	Seed	Trace
Tecoma stans (L.) HBK -- Yellow Elder	Plant	Trace
Cowgrass, Peavine Clover, Purple Clover, Red Clover - Trifolium Pratense - E - M	Plant	Trace

PLANTS CONTAINING TYROSINE

Species	Part	Quantity
Water Lotus - Nelumbo Nucifera - E - M	Rhizome	2,901,390 ppm
Black Mustard - Brassica Nigra - E	Leaf	19,440 ppm
Cowage, Velvetbean - Mucuna Pruriens - E	Seed	16,907 ppm
Black Caraway, Black Cumin, Fennel-Flower, Nutmeg-Flower, Roman Coriander - Nigella Sativa - E - M	Seed	16,530 ppm
Ceratonia siliqua L. -- Carob, Locust Bean, St.John's-Bread	Seed	16,450 ppm
Asparagus Pea, Goa Bean, Winged Bean - Psophocarpus Tetragonolobus - E	Seed	15,896 ppm
Black bean, Dwarf bean, Field bean, Flageolet bean, French bean, Garden bean, Green bean, Haricot, Haricot bean, Haricot vert, Kidney bean, Navy bean, Pop bean, Popping bean, Snap bean, String bean, Wax bean - Phaseolus Vulgaris - E	Sprout Seedling	15,484 ppm
White Lupine - Lupinus Albus - M - T	Seed	15,185 ppm
Soybean - Glycine Max - E	Seed	15,090 ppm
Oats - Avena Sativa - E - M	Seed	14,000 ppm
Groundnut, Peanut - Arachis Hypogaea - E - M	Seed	13,198 ppm
Spinach - Spinacia Oleracea - E	Plant	12,826 ppm
Bonavist Bean, Hyacinth Bean, Lablab Bean - Lablab Purpureus - E - M - T	Seed	12,788 ppm
Berro, Watercress - Nasturtium Officinale - E	Herb	12,600 ppm
Taro - Colocasia Esculenta - E	Leaf	12,415 ppm
Cassie, Huisache, Opopanax, Popinac, Sweet Acacia - Acacia Farnesiana - M	Leaf	12,010 ppm
Jew's Mallow, Mulukiya, Nalta Jute - Corchorus Olitorius - E - M	Leaf	11,965 ppm
Sesame - Sesamum Indicum - E - M	Seed	11,818 ppm
Lambsquarter - Chenopodium Album - E - M - T	Leaf	11,148 ppm
Pumpkin - Cucurbita Pepo - E	Seed	10,948 ppm
Chaya - Cnidoscolus Chayamansa - E	Leaf	10,850 ppm
Swamp Cabbage, Water Spinach - Ipomoea Aquatica - E	Leaf	10,625 ppm
Broadbean, Faba Bean, Habas - Vicia Faba - E	Seed	10,315 ppm
Watermelon - Citrullus Lanatus - E	Seed	10,200 ppm
Chives - Allium Schoenoprasum - E	Leaf	10,125 ppm
Butternut - Juglans Cinerea - E	Seed	10,108 ppm
Pea - Pisum Sativum - E	Fruit	9,792 ppm
Pigweed - Amaranthus sp. - E - M	Leaf	9,624 ppm
Asparagus bean, Pea bean, Yardlong bean - Vigna Unguiculata subsp. Sesquipedalis - E	Fruit	9,465 ppm
Wheat - Triticum Aestivum - E - M	Seed	9,000 ppm
Okra - Abelmoschus Esculentus - Friut - E - M	Fruit	8,700 ppm

Asparagus bean, Pea bean, Yardlong bean - Vigna Unguiculata subsp. Sesquipedalis - E	Seed	8,584 ppm
Butter Bean, Lima Bean - Phaseolus Lunatus - E	Seed	8,450 ppm
Lentil - Lens Culinaris - E	Seed	8,445 ppm
Alholva, Bockshornklee, Fenugreek, Greek Clover, Greek Trigonella Foenum-Graecum - E - M	Seed	8,400 ppm
Asparagus Pea, Goa Bean, Winged Bean - Psophocarpus Tetragonolobus - E	Tuber	8,286 ppm
Ben Nut, Benzolive Tree, Drumstick Tree, Horseradish Tree, Moringa, West Indian Ben - Moringa Oleifera - E	Shoot	3,470-16,260 ppm
Papaver bracteatum L. -- Great Scarlet Poppy	Seed	8,100 ppm
White Mustard - Sinapis Alba - E - M - T	Seed	7,961 ppm
Green Gram, Mungbean - Vigna Radiata - E	Seed	7,850 ppm
Curly Kale, Kale, Kitchen Kale, Scotch Kale - Brassica Oleracea var. Sabellica l. var. Acephala - E	Leaf	7,530 ppm
Pistachio - Pistacia Vera - E	Seed	7,427 ppm
Almond - Prunus Dulcis - E - M - T	Seed	7,374 ppm
Opium Poppy, Poppyseed Poppy - Papaver Somniferum - E	Seed	7,305 ppm
Girasol, Sun Helianthus Annuus - E	Seed	7,037 ppm
Vinespinach - Basella Alba - E - M	Leaf	6,955 ppm
Collards, Cow Cabbage, Spring-Heading Cabbage, Tall Kale, Tree Kale - Brassica Oleracea - E	Leaf	6,884 ppm
Buffalo Gourd - Cucurbita Foetidissima - E - M - T	Seed	11,350-13,680 ppm
Black bean, Dwarf bean, Field bean, Flageolet bean, French bean, Garden bean, Green bean, Haricot, Haricot bean, Haricot vert, Kidney bean, Navy bean, Pop bean, Popping bean, Snap bean, String bean, Wax bean - Phaseolus Vulgaris - E	Seed	6,833 ppm
Adzuki Bean - Vigna Angularis - E	Seed	6,828 ppm
Cauli Brassica Oleracea var. Botrytis - E	Leaf	6,766 ppm
Indian Fig, Nopal, Nopalito, Prickly Pear - Opuntia Ficus-Indica - E - M	Seed	6,590 ppm
Endive, Escarole - Cichorium Endivia - M	Leaf	6,441 ppm
Bok-Choy, Celery Cabbage, Celery Mustard, Chinese Cabbage, Chinese Mustard, Chinese White Cabbage, Pak-Choi - Brassica Chinensis - E	Leaf	6,197 ppm
Asparagus - Asparagus Officinalis - E	Shoot	6,194 ppm
Pigeonpea - Cajanus Vajan - E	Seed	6,015 ppm
Barley, Barleygrass - Hordeum Vulgare - E - M	Seed	6,000 ppm
Italian Stone Pine, Pignolia - Pinus Pinea - M	Seed	8,780-11,400 ppm
Cacao - Theobroma Ccacao - E	Seed	5,700 ppm
Cauli Brassica Oleracea var. Botrytis - E	Flower	5,555 ppm
Green Gram, Mungbean - Vigna Radiata - E	Sprout Seedling	5,462 ppm
Asparagus Pea, Goa Bean, Winged Bean - Psophocarpus Tetragonolobus - E	Leaf	5,443 ppm
Chickpea, Garbanzo - Cicer Arietinum - E	Seed	5,415 ppm
Pea - Pisum Sativum - E	Seed	5,345 ppm
Lettuce - Lactuca Sativa - E	Leaf	5,333 ppm
Corn - Zea Mays - E	Seed	5,117 ppm
Pumpkin - Cucurbita Pepo - E	Fruit	5,000 ppm
Chayote - Sechium Edule - E - M	Fruit	5,000 ppm
Corn Salad, Lamb's Lettuce - Valerianella Locusta - E	Plant	5,000 ppm
Cashew - Anacardium Occidentale - E	Seed	4,995 ppm
Summer Squash - Cucurbita spp. - E	Fruit	4,905 ppm
Brazilnut, Brazilnut-Tree, Creamnut, Paranut - Bertholletia Eexcelsa - E	Seed	4,728 ppm
Fennel - Foeniculum Vulgare - M	Fruit	4,498 ppm
Sicklepod - Senna Obtusifolia - E - T	Seed	4,420 ppm
Purslane, Verdolaga - Portulaca Oleracea - E	Herb	4,400 ppm
Basil, Cuban Basil, Sweet Basil - Ocimum Basilicum - E	Leaf	4,320 ppm
Black bean, Dwarf bean, Field bean, Flageolet bean, French bean, Garden bean, Green bean, Haricot, Haricot bean, Haricot vert, Kidney bean, Navy bean, Pop bean, Popping bean, Snap bean, String bean, Wax bean - Phaseolus Vulgaris - E	Fruit	4,317 ppm
Potato - Solanum Tuberosum - E	Tuber	3,900 ppm

TYROSINE CONTINUED

Evening-Primrose - Oenothera Biennis - E - M	Seed	3,629 ppm
Aubergine, Egg Solanum Melongena - E	Fruit	3,593 ppm
Macadamia - Macadamia spp. - E	Seed	3,465 ppm
Cayenne, Chili, Hot Pepper, Red Chili, Spur Pepper, Tabasco - Capsicum Frutescens - E	Fruit	3,427 ppm
Indian Fig, Nopal, Nopalito, Prickly Pear - Opuntia Ficus-Indica - E - M	Bud	3,220 ppm
Onion, Shallot - Allium Cepa - Shallot Bulb - E	Bulb	3,161 ppm
Chaparral, Creosote Bush - Larrea Tridentata - M	Plant	3,100 ppm
Water Lotus - Nelumbo Nucifera - E - M	Seed	3,030 ppm
Chinese Foxglove - Rehmannia Glutinosa - M	Root	3,000 ppm
Sambucus nigra L. -- Black Elder, Elder, European Alder, European Elder, European Elderberry	Fruit	2,900 ppm
American Chestnut - Castanea Dentata - E - M	Seed	2,822 ppm
Cabbage, Red Cabbage, White Cabbage - Brassica Oleracea var. Capitata - E	Leaf	2,807 ppm
Beet, Beetroot, Garden Beet, Sugar Beet - Beta Vulgaris - E	Root	2,760 ppm
Buckwheat - Fagopyrum Esculentum - E	Seed	2,750 ppm
Chinese Chestnut - Castanea Mollisima - M	Seed	2,735 ppm
Common thyme, Garden thyme, Thyme - Thymus Vulgaris - E - M	Plant	2,603 ppm
Aloe, Bitter Aloes - Aloe Vera - E - M	Leaf	0-5,073 ppm
American Elder, American Elderberry, Elderberry, Sweet Elder - Sambucus Canadensis - E	Fruit	2,524 ppm
Radish - Raphanus Sativus - E	Root	2,520 ppm
Sweet Potato - Ipomoea Batatas - E	Root	2,504 ppm
Tomato - Lycopersicon Esculentum - E - M - T	Fruit	2,479 ppm
Bell Pepper, Cherry Pepper, Cone Pepper, Green Pepper, Paprika, Sweet Pepper - Capsicum Annuum - E	Fruit	2,455 ppm
Cucumber - Cucumis Sativus - E	Fruit	2,278 ppm
Rutabaga, Swede, Swedish Turnip - Brassica Napus var. Napobrassica - E	Root	2,225 ppm
Apricot - Prunus Armeniaca - E - M - T	Fruit	2,125 ppm
Yambean - Pachyrhizus Erosus - E	Tuber	2,120 ppm
Garlic - Allium Sativum Bulb - E	Bulb	1,944 ppm
Squaw Perideridia Gairdneri - E - M	Root	1,905 ppm
Avocado - Persea Americana - E - M - T	Fruit	1,904 ppm
Rye - Secale Cereale - E	Seed	3,390-3,800 ppm
Breadroot, Indian Bread-Root, Indian Turnip, Prairie Apple, Prairie Potato, Prairie Turnip - Psoralea Esculenta - E - M - T	Root	1,899 ppm
Mountain Yam - Dioscorea Pentaphylla - E	Root	1,885 ppm
Taro - Colocasia Esculenta - E	Root	1,875 ppm
Celery - Apium Graveolens - E	Pt	1,865 ppm
Date Palm - Phoenix Dactylifera - E	Fruit	1,730 ppm
Jerusalem Artichoke - Helianthus Tuberosus E	Tuber	1,715 ppm
Carrot - Daucus Carota - E	Root	1,640 ppm
Rapini, Seven-Top Turnip, Turnip - Brassica Rapa - E	Root	1,600 ppm
Mango - Mangifera Indica - E - M	Fruit	1,600 ppm
Fig - Ficus Carica - E	Fruit	1,532 ppm
Pawpaw - Asimina Triloba - Friut - E	Fruit	1,501 ppm
Peach - Prunus Persica - E - M - T	Fruit	1,458 ppm
Watermelon - Citrullus Lanatus - E	Fruit	1,413 ppm
Ginkgo, Maidenhair Tree - Ginkgo Biloba - Tree - E - M - T	Seed	1,360 ppm
Cassava, Tapioca, Yuca - Manihot Esculenta - E	Root	1,270 ppm
Carambola, Star Averrhoa Carambola - E	Fruit	230-2,530 ppm
European Chestnut - Castanea Sativa - E - M	Seed	1,251 ppm
Orange - Citrus Sinensis - E	Fruit	1,208 ppm
Ginger - Zingiber Officinale - E	Rhizome	1,122 ppm
Calathea allouia (AUBL.) LINDL. - Leren, Lleren	Root	1,805-1,985 ppm
Banana, Plantain - Musa x Paradisiaca - E	Fruit	932 ppm
Curry Murraya spp. - E - M	Fruit	922 ppm
Burdock, Gobo, Great Burdock - Arctium lappa - E - M - T	Root	900 ppm
Pineapple - Ananas Comosus - E	Fruit	889 ppm
Mandarin, Tangerine - Citrus Reticulata - E	Fruit	887 ppm
Guavas - Psidium Guajava - E	Fruit	720 ppm
Bread Artocarpus Altilis - E	Fruit	645 ppm
European Grape, Grape, Grapevine, Vigne Vinifere, Wine Grape - Vitis Vinifera - E - M	Fruit	617 ppm

Species	Part	Quantity
Emblic, Myrobalan - Phyllanthus Emblica - E	Fruit	575 ppm
Blueberry - Vaccinium Corymbosum - E	Fruit	520 ppm
Papaya - Carica Papaya - E - M	Fruit	448 ppm
Plum - Prunus Domestica - E - M	Fruit	405 ppm
Strawberry Guava - Psidium Cattleianum - E	Fruit	360 ppm
Apple - Malus Domestica - E	Fruit	249 ppm
Pear - Pyrus Communis - E	Fruit	185 ppm
Grape Citrus Paradisi - E	Fruit	61 ppm
Elephant Garlic, Kurrat - Allium Ampeloprasum - E	Plant	Trace
Tarragon - Artemisia Dracunculus - M	Shoot	Trace
Alehoof - Glechoma Hederacea - M	Plant	Trace
Hops - Humulus Lupulus - E - M - T	Fruit	Trace
Flax, Lin Linum Usitatissimum - E	Seed	Trace
Rice - Oryza Sativa - E	Plant	Trace
American Ginseng, Ginseng - Panax Quinquefolius - M	Plant	Trace
Passiflora incarnata L. -- Manzana de Mayo, Mayapple, Passionflower	Leaf	Trace
Plantago major L. -- Common Plantain	Plant	Trace
Plantago ovata FORSSK. -- Blond Psyllium, Indian Plantago, Ispaghula, Psyllium, Spogel Seeds	Seed	Trace
Sour Cherry - Prunus Cerasus - E - M - T	Fruit	Trace
Sage - Salvia Officinalis - E - M	Plant	Trace
Tilia sp. -- Basswood, Lime, Linden	Fruit	Trace
Cowgrass, Peavine Clover, Purple Clover, Red Clover - Trifolium Pratense - E - M	Plant	Trace

PLANTS CONTAINING VALINE

Species	Part	Quantity
Girasol, Sun Helianthus Annuus - E	Seed	50,000 ppm
Berro, Watercress - Nasturtium Officinale - E	Herb	27,400 ppm
Pea - Pisum Sativum - E	Fruit	27,003 ppm
Buffalo Gourd - Cucurbita Foetidissima - E - M - T	Seed	11,665-48,000 ppm
Black bean, Dwarf bean, Field bean, Flageolet bean, French bean, Garden bean, Green bean, Haricot, Haricot bean, Haricot vert, Kidney bean, Navy bean, Pop bean, Popping bean, Snap bean, String bean, Wax bean - Phaseolus Vulgaris - E	Sprout Seedling	23,226 ppm
Pumpkin - Cucurbita Pepo - E	Seed	21,186 ppm
Ceratonia siliqua L. -- Carob, Locust Bean, St.John's-Bread	Seed	20,680 ppm
Jew's Mallow, Mulukiya, Nalta Jute - Corchorus Olitorius - E - M	Leaf	20,185 ppm
Soybean - Glycine Max - E	Seed	19,910 ppm
Spinach - Spinacia Oleracea - E	Plant	19,120 ppm
Cowage, Velvetbean - Mucuna Pruriens - E	Seed	18,232 ppm
Swamp Cabbage, Water Spinach - Ipomoea Aquatica - E	Leaf	17,930 ppm
Taro - Colocasia Esculenta - E	Leaf	17,850 ppm
White Lupine - Lupinus Albus - M - T	Seed	16,860 ppm
Cassie, Huisache, Opopanax, Popinac, Sweet Acacia - Acacia Farnesiana - M	Leaf	16,740 ppm
Asparagus Pea, Goa Bean, Winged Bean - Psophocarpus Tetragonolobus - E	Seed	16,692 ppm
Pigweed - Amaranthus sp. - E - M	Leaf	16,481 ppm
Butternut - Juglans Cinerea - E	Seed	15,942 ppm
Lentil - Lens Culinaris - E	Seed	15,675 ppm
Sesame - Sesamum Indicum - E - M	Seed	15,527 ppm
Chives - Allium Schoenoprasum - E	Leaf	15,500 ppm
Asparagus - Asparagus Officinalis - E	Shoot	15,226 ppm
Chaya - Cnidoscolus Chayamansa - E	Leaf	15,190 ppm
Pistachio - Pistacia Vera - E	Seed	14,688 ppm
Broadbean, Faba Bean, Habas - Vicia Faba - E	Seed	14,420 ppm
Lambsquarter - Chenopodium Album - E - M - T	Leaf	14,396 ppm
Butter Bean, Lima Bean - Phaseolus Lunatus - E	Seed	14,370 ppm
Ben Nut, Benzolive Tree, Drumstick Tree, Horseradish Tree, Moringa, West Indian Ben - Moringa Oleifera - E	Shoot	6,110-28,630 ppm

VALINE CONTINUED

Black Mustard - Brassica Nigra - E	Leaf	14,286 ppm
White Mustard - Sinapis Alba - E - M - T	Seed	14,178 ppm
Bok-Choy, Celery Cabbage, Celery Mustard, Chinese Cabbage, Chinese Mustard, Chinese White Cabbage, Pak-Choi - Brassica Chinensis - E	Leaf	14,104 ppm
Asparagus Pea, Goa Bean, Winged Bean - Psophocarpus Tetragonolobus - E	Tuber	14,061 ppm
Opium Poppy, Poppyseed Poppy - Papaver Somniferum - E	Seed	13,806 ppm
Corn Salad, Lamb's Lettuce - Valerianella Locusta - E	Plant	13,750 ppm
Cauli Brassica Oleracea var. Botrytis - E	Leaf	13,747 ppm
Bonavist Bean, Hyacinth Bean, Lablab Bean - Lablab Purpureus - E - M - T	Seed	13,670 ppm
Green Gram, Mungbean - Vigna Radiata - E	Sprout Seedling	13,655 ppm
Asparagus bean, Pea bean, Yardlong bean - Vigna Unguiculata subsp. Sesquipedalis - E	Fruit	13,333 ppm
Lentil - Lens Culinaris - E	Sprout Seedling	13,300 ppm
Purslane, Verdolaga - Portulaca Oleracea - E	Herb	13,200 ppm
Cauli Brassica Oleracea var. Botrytis - E	Flower	12,920 ppm
Black bean, Dwarf bean, Field bean, Flageolet bean, French bean, Garden bean, Green bean, Haricot, Haricot bean, Haricot vert, Kidney bean, Navy bean, Pop bean, Popping bean, Snap bean, String bean, Wax bean - Phaseolus Vulgaris - E	Seed	12,699 ppm
Asparagus bean, Pea bean, Yardlong bean - Vigna Unguiculata subsp. Sesquipedalis - E	Seed	12,688 ppm
Collards, Cow Cabbage, Spring-Heading Cabbage, Tall Kale, Tree Kale - Brassica Oleracea - E	Leaf	12,620 ppm
Groundnut, Peanut - Arachis Hypogaea - E - M	Seed	12,437 ppm
Dill, Garden Dill - Anethum Graveolens - E	Fruit	12,130 ppm
Alholva, Bockshornklee, Fenugreek, Greek Clover, Greek Trigonella Foenum-Graecum - E - M	Seed	12,120 ppm
Oats - Avena Sativa - E - M	Plant	12,000 ppm
Adzuki Bean - Vigna Angularis - E	Seed	11,818 ppm
Lettuce - Lactuca Sativa - E	Leaf	11,667 ppm
Curly Kale, Kale, Kitchen Kale, Scotch Kale - Brassica Oleracea var. Sabellica l. var. Acephala - E	Leaf	11,645 ppm
Pea - Pisum Sativum - E	Seed	11,116 ppm
Brussel-Sprout - Brassica Oleracea var. Gemmifera - E	Leaf	11,067 ppm
Oats - Avena Sativa - E - M	Seed	11,000 ppm
Almond - Prunus Dulcis - E - M - T	Seed	10,752 ppm
Papaver bracteatum L. -- Great Scarlet Poppy	Seed	10,600 ppm
Asparagus Pea, Goa Bean, Winged Bean - Psophocarpus Tetragonolobus - E	Leaf	10,583 ppm
Cashew - Anacardium Occidentale - E	Seed	10,580 ppm
Indian Fig, Nopal, Nopalito, Prickly Pear - Opuntia Ficus-Indica - E - M	Seed	10,500 ppm
Pigeonpea - Cajanus Vajan - E	Seed	10,480 ppm
Watermelon - Citrullus Lanatus - E	Seed	10,200 ppm
Chickpea, Garbanzo - Cicer Arietinum - E	Seed	10,150 ppm
Endive, Escarole - Cichorium Endivia - M	Leaf	10,145 ppm
Fennel - Foeniculum Vulgare - M	Fruit	10,037 ppm
Chayote - Sechium Edule - E - M	Fruit	9,860 ppm
Brazilnut, Brazilnut-Tree, Creamnut, Paranut - Bertholletia Eexcelsa - E	Seed	9,425 ppm
Vinespinach - Basella Alba - E - M	Leaf	9,420 ppm
Black bean, Dwarf bean, Field bean, Flageolet bean, French bean, Garden bean, Green bean, Haricot, Haricot bean, Haricot vert, Kidney bean, Navy bean, Pop bean, Popping bean, Snap bean, String bean, Wax bean - Phaseolus Vulgaris - E	Fruit	9,250 ppm
Chicory, Succory, Witloof - Cichorium Intybus - E - M	Leaf	9,180 ppm
Okra - Abelmoschus Esculentus - Friut - E - M	Fruit	9,100 ppm
Barley, Barleygrass - Hordeum Vulgare - E - M	Seed	9,000 ppm
Wheat - Triticum Aestivum - E - M	Seed	9,000 ppm
Evening-Primrose - Oenothera Biennis - E - M	Seed	8,645 ppm
Summer Squash - Cucurbita spp. - E	Fruit	8,385 ppm

Black Caraway, Black Cumin, Fennel-Flower, Nutmeg-Flower, Roman Coriander - Nigella Sativa - E - M	Seed	8,325 ppm
Buckwheat - Fagopyrum Esculentum - E	Seed	8,140 ppm
Mat Bean, Moth Bean - Vigna Aconitifolia - E	Seed	8,127 ppm
Water Lotus - Nelumbo Nucifera - E - M	Seed	8,061 ppm
Achiote, Annato, Annatto, Annoto, Arnato, Bija, Lipstick Pod, Lipsticktree - Bixa Orellana - E	Seed	7,730 ppm
Corn - Zea Mays - E	Seed	7,696 ppm
Italian Stone Pine, Pignolia - Pinus Pinea - M	Seed	12,410-15,300 ppm
Sicklepod - Senna Obtusifolia - E - T	Seed	7,420 ppm
Basil, Cuban Basil, Sweet Basil - Ocimum Basilicum - E	Leaf	7,170 ppm
Aubergine, Egg Solanum Melongena - E	Fruit	7,063 ppm
Chinese Foxglove - Rehmannia Glutinosa - M	Root	7,000 ppm
Garlic - Allium Sativum Bulb - E	Bulb	6,984 ppm
Cabbage, Red Cabbage, White Cabbage - Brassica Oleracea var. Capitata - E	Leaf	6,952 ppm
Cayenne, Chili, Hot Pepper, Red Chili, Spur Pepper, Tabasco - Capsicum Frutescens - E	Fruit	6,854 ppm
Potato - Solanum Tuberosum - E	Tuber	6,450 ppm
Aloe, Bitter Aloes - Aloe Vera - E - M	Leaf	0-12,769 ppm
Ginkgo, Maidenhair Tree - Ginkgo Biloba - Tree - E - M - T	Seed	6,311 ppm
Radish - Raphanus Sativus - E	Root	6,200 ppm
Bread Artocarpus Altilis - E	Seed	5,350-12,235 ppm
Calabash Gourd, White-Flowered Gourd - Lagenaria Siceraria - E	Fruit	6,055 ppm
Cacao - Theobroma Ccacao - E	Seed	5,700 ppm
Celery - Apium Graveolens - E	Pt	5,600 ppm
Eryngium creticus -- Cretan culantro	Shoot	0-11,200 ppm
Kohlrabi - Brassica Oleracea var. Gongylodes - E	Stem	5,555 ppm
Indian Fig, Nopal, Nopalito, Prickly Pear - Opuntia Ficus-Indica - E - M	Bud	5,485 ppm
Common thyme, Garden thyme, Thyme - Thymus Vulgaris - E - M	Plant	5,422 ppm
Bell Pepper, Cherry Pepper, Cone Pepper, Green Pepper, Paprika, Sweet Pepper - Capsicum Annuum - E	Fruit	4,910 ppm
Rutabaga, Swede, Swedish Turnip - Brassica Napus var. Napobrassica - E	Root	4,640 ppm
American Chestnut - Castanea Dentata - E - M	Seed	4,622 ppm
Cucumber - Cucumis Sativus - E	Fruit	4,304 ppm
Ginger - Zingiber Officinale - E	Rhizome	4,202 ppm
Chaparral, Creosote Bush - Larrea Tridentata - M	Plant	4,200 ppm
Rye - Secale Cereale - E	Seed	7,470-8,390 ppm
Pumpkin - Cucurbita Pepo - E	Fruit	4,167 ppm
Beet, Beetroot, Garden Beet, Sugar Beet - Beta Vulgaris - E	Root	4,100 ppm
Jerusalem Artichoke - Helianthus Tuberosus E	Tuber	4,098 ppm
Chinese Chestnut - Castanea Mollisima - M	Seed	3,976 ppm
Sweet Potato - Ipomoea Batatas - E	Root	3,976 ppm
Yambean - Pachyrhizus Erosus - E	Tuber	3,870 ppm
Tomato - Lycopersicon Esculentum - E - M - T	Fruit	3,801 ppm
Avocado - Persea Americana - E - M - T	Fruit	3,770 ppm
Rapini, Seven-Top Turnip, Turnip - Brassica Rapa - E	Root	3,690 ppm
Pawpaw - Asimina Triloba - Friut - E	Fruit	3,661 ppm
Carrot - Daucus Carota - E	Root	3,600 ppm
Apricot - Prunus Armeniaca - E - M - T	Fruit	3,445 ppm
Macadamia - Macadamia spp. - E	Seed	3,300 ppm
Squaw Perideridia Gairdneri - E - M	Root	3,175 ppm
Peach - Prunus Persica - E - M - T	Fruit	3,078 ppm
Orange - Citrus Sinensis - E	Fruit	3,020 ppm
Onion, Shallot - Allium Cepa - Shallot Bulb - E	Bulb	2,943 ppm
Mountain Yam - Dioscorea Pentaphylla - E	Root	2,910 ppm
Taro - Colocasia Esculenta - E	Root	2,790 ppm
Date Palm - Phoenix Dactylifera - E	Fruit	2,710 ppm
Mango - Mangifera Indica - E - M	Fruit	2,700 ppm
Water Lotus - Nelumbo Nucifera - E - M	Rhizome	2,630 ppm
Calathea allouia (AUBL.) LINDL. - Leren, Lleren	Root	4,585-5,040 ppm
Cassava, Tapioca, Yuca - Manihot Esculenta - E	Root	2,510 ppm

VALINE CONTINUED

European Chestnut - Castanea Sativa - E - M	Seed	2,378 ppm		Grape Citrus Paradisi - E	Fruit	240 ppm
Mandarin, Tangerine - Citrus Reticulata - E	Fruit	2,176 ppm		Black Currant - Ribes Nigrum - E	Fruit Juice	170 ppm
Strawberry - Fragaria spp. - E	Fruit	2,135 ppm		American Ginseng, Ginseng - Panax Quinquefolius - M	Plant	82 ppm
Guavas - Psidium Guajava - E	Fruit	2,016 ppm		Pea - Pisum Sativum - E	Shoot	33 ppm
Watermelon - Citrullus Lanatus - E	Fruit	1,885 ppm		Gum Arabic, Gum Arabic Tree, Kher, Senegal Gum, Sudan Gum Arabic - Acacia Senegal - M	Plant	Trace
Banana, Plantain - Musa x Paradisiaca - E	Fruit	1,826 ppm		Mud Plantain, Tse-Hsieh, Water Plantain, Ze-Xie - Alisma Plantago-Aquatica - M	Rhizome	Trace
Blueberry - Vaccinium Corymbosum - E	Fruit	1,820 ppm				
Breadroot, Indian Bread-Root, Indian Turnip, Prairie Apple, Prairie Potato, Prairie Turnip - Psoralea Esculenta - E - M - T	Root	1,730 ppm		Elephant Garlic, Kurrat - Allium Ampeloprasum - E	Plant	Trace
				Tarragon - Artemisia Dracunculus - M	Leaf	Trace
Cassie, Huisache, Opopanax, Popinac, Sweet Acacia - Acacia Farnesiana - M	Seed	1,650 ppm		Tea - Camellia Sinensis - E	Leaf	Trace
				Alehoof - Glechoma Hederacea - M	Plant	Trace
Burdock, Gobo, Great Burdock - Arctium lappa - E - M - T	Root	1,650 ppm		Hops - Humulus Lupulus - E - M - T	Fruit	Trace
				Flax, Lin Linum Usitatissimum - E	Seed	Trace
American Elder, American Elderberry, Elderberry, Sweet Elder - Sambucus Canadensis - E	Fruit	1,634 ppm		Antler Herb, Clubmoss - Lycopodium Clavatum - Pollen Or Spore - M - T	Pollen Or Spore	Trace
				Spearmint - Mentha Spicata - E - M- T	Leaf	Trace
Bread Artocarpus Altilis - E	Fruit	1,600 ppm		Rice - Oryza Sativa - E	Hay	Trace
Carambola, Star Averrhoa Carambola - E	Fruit	260-2,860 ppm		Passiflora incarnata L. -- Manzana de Mayo, Mayapple, Passionflower Leaf	Leaf	Trace
Fig - Ficus Carica - E	Fruit	1,340 ppm				
Curry Murraya spp. - E - M	Fruit	1,325 ppm				
Plum - Prunus Domestica - E - M	Fruit	1,284 ppm				
Pineapple - Ananas Comosus - E	Fruit	1,185 ppm		Plantago ovata FORSSK. -- Blond Psyllium, Indian Plantago, Ispaghula, Psyllium, Spogel Seeds Plant	Plant	Trace
Strawberry Guava - Psidium Cattleianum - E	Fruit	1,035 ppm				
European Grape, Grape, Grapevine, Vigne Vinifere, Wine Grape - Vitis Vinifera - E - M	Fruit	926 ppm		Sour Cherry - Prunus Cerasus - E - M - T	Fruit	Trace
				Tilia sp. -- Basswood, Lime, Linden Fruit	Fruit	Trace
Papaya - Carica Papaya - E - M	Fruit	895 ppm		Cowgrass, Peavine Clover, Purple Clover, Red Clover - Trifolium Pratense - E - M	Plant	Trace
Pear - Pyrus Communis - E	Fruit	865 ppm				
Emblic, Myrobalan - Phyllanthus Emblica - E	Fruit	785 ppm				
Apple - Malus Domestica - E	Fruit	560 ppm				

INDEX

7-beta-casomorphin, 89
Aba bean, 191
abnormal heart rhythm, 42, 78
Abortifacient, 644
abscesses, 141, 503, 505, 522
Abscesses, 644
ABSCESSES, 619
Absorbent, 644
ACE inhibitors, 237
Acerola, 59
acetaminophen, 562
acetylcholine, 187, 242, 299
aching muscles, 509
Achiote, 130
Achy muscles, 117
acid phosphatase, 236
acne, 41, 492, 504, 513, 516, 601, 628
Acne, 152
Acorus calamus, 599
Acrochordons, 644
Actaea racemosa L. var. racemosa aka black bugbane, 483
Acute hunger, 184, 185
ADD, 475, 573
adenosine monophosphate, 197
ADHD, 573
adrenal glands, 45, 241, 540
Aegopodium podagraria, 482
Aesculus hippocastanum, 547
aggregation of platelets, 513
Aging, 53
AGING, 617
Ague gue, 644
AIDS, 186, 188, 191, 236, 304
Aikal Skullcaps, 475
ALA, 196, 197, 508

Alanine, 176, 177, 309, 313, 318, 325, 331, 355, 364, 371, 374, 376, 381, 401, 418, 423, 459, 463, 465, 553
alcohol, 27, 46, 53, 110, 115, 134, 180, 189, 227, 228, 242, 483, 487, 496, 503, 543, 550, 555, 562, 598, 604, 633
Alcohol, 47, 88, 191
alcoholism, 42, 109, 115, 181, 483, 487, 496, 524, 555
Alcoholism, 53, 181
Alexiteric, 644
alkaline phosphatase, 89
alkaloid, 600
allergies, 33, 34, 35, 38, 183, 226, 300, 479, 500, 502, 506, 537, 584
ALLERGY, 617
Allspice, 81, 102, 151
Almond, 81, 92, 102, 106, 132, 136, 143, 149, 151, 178, 181, 182, 189, 193, 309, 549, 623
Aloe, 139, 153, 178, 182, 619, 624, 625
aloe vera gel, 618
Alopecia, 644
Alpha-linolenic acid, 196
Alpha-lipoic, 196
alpha-lipoic acid, 197
Alternative Medicine Digest, 305, 306
Althea officinalis, 560
ALTITUDE SICKNESS, 617
aluminum, 73, 74, 101, 114, 133, 142, 309, 310, 312, 313, 328, 352, 355, 359, 364, 370, 381, 401, 406, 409, 418, 423, 450, 458, 471
Aluminum, 70, 73, 74, 101, 237, 459, 493, 502, 513, 531, 535, 540, 549, 553, 561, 565, 574, 592, 605
Alzheimer's disease, 46, 51, 73, 115, 142, 242, 535, 556, 636
ALZHEIMER'S DISEASE, 617
Amaranthus hybridus, 586
Amazon Center for Environmental Education and Research, 305
Amebic dysentery, 644
amenorrhea, 572
AMENORRHEA, 617
American Botanical Council, 304, 305
American Health, Business of Herbs, 306
American Health, the Center for Alternative Medicine in Women's Health, 305
American Herb Association, 304
American persimmon, 81, 83, 110, 147
American Society of Pharmacognosy, 304
Amish Burn Ointment, 618
Ammi visnaga, 554
AMP, 197
Amphiachyris dracunculoides, 489

817

Amygdalitis, 644
Amylase Inhibitors, 198
analgesic, 484, 501, 502, 508, 517, 523, 547, 561
Ananas comosus, 574
anemia, 51, 75, 95, 104, 108, 109, 150, 183, 185, 497, 508, 536, 549
Anemia, 49, 98, 108, 182, 183, 186
anencephaly, 49
Anesthetic, 644
Angelica, 506, 512, 607, 617, 619, 621, 622
Angelica sinensis, 506, 512
angina, 236, 240, 544, 554
ANGINA, 617
angina pectoris, 236, 554
Anise, 477, 617, 618, 620
ANKYLOSING SPONDYLITIS, 617
Anodyne, 644
anorexia, 534
Anorexia, 116, 152
Anthocyanins, 69
Antiallergic, 69
antibacterial, 293, 480, 522, 527, 533, 635
antibiotic, 37, 68, 492, 521, 522, 635, 638
Anticaking agents, 73
Anticarcinogenic, 69, 138
Anticholinergic, 644
anti-clotting medications, 62
anticonvulsant, 291
anticonvulsive, 556
antifungal, 293, 480, 522, 527, 635
Antihelmintic, 644
Antihepatotoxin, 644
anti-inflammatory, 152, 196, 236, 238, 289, 475, 493, 494, 499, 502, 503, 507, 517, 532, 534, 537, 547, 567, 598, 604, 609, 628, 637, 639
Antiinflammatory, 69
Anti-inflammatory, 69
Anti-inflammatory, 98
Anti-inflammatory, 137
Anti-inflammatory, 138
Anti-inflammatory, 153
Anti-inflammatory, 581
antimicrobial, 37, 638
antimony, 75
Antimony, 70, 75, 553
antioxidant, 51, 53, 62, 98, 99, 120, 128, 137, 138, 148, 153, 196, 197, 226, 238, 240, 243, 296, 300, 301, 499, 598, 604, 612, 642
antioxidants, 37, 58, 62, 141, 153, 196, 292, 482, 503, 507, 515, 567, 579, 592, 604, 636, 637, 639, 641
antiperspirants, 73
Antirheumatic, 644
Antiscorbutic, 644, 645

antiseptic, 481, 482, 494, 503, 513, 516, 519, 522, 523, 527, 533, 534, 601
antispasmodic, 480, 494, 508, 527, 609
Antithrombogenic, 69
Antitussive, 645
Antivinous, 645
antiviral, 293, 522, 527, 628, 635
Antiviral, 69, 138, 619
Antler herb, 79
anxiety, 105, 188, 192, 243, 475, 502, 515, 517, 536, 546, 556, 573, 598
Anxiety, 116, 117, 181
Aperitive, 645
aphrodisiac, 566, 571, 573, 588
Aphrodisiac, 456, 645
Aphthae, 645
Apium graveolens, 501
Apoplexy, 434, 645
Apostemes, 645
appetite loss, 566
appetite stimulant, 508
Apple, 59, 79, 81, 83, 102, 106, 136, 179, 182, 562, 563, 620, 625
Apricot, 53, 59, 83, 106
Apricot kernels, 53
Apricot Kernels, 54
Apricots, 41, 69
Arctium lappa, 492
Arctostaphylos uva-ursi, 481
Arginine, 176, 177, 178, 309, 313, 318, 321, 325, 331, 339, 355, 359, 364, 371, 372, 374, 376, 381, 401, 418, 423, 459, 463, 465, 553
Argon, 70
arishtha, 566
ark, 440, 469
Armoracia rusticana, 548
Arnica, 478, 618, 625
Arnica Montana, 478
Arrhythmias, 134, 135
arsenic, 77, 78, 79
Arsenic, 70, 77, 79, 553
arterial plaque, 58, 554
arteriosclerosis, 53, 554
arthritic, 48, 188, 497, 557, 566
arthritis, 99, 183, 234, 236, 291, 478, 479, 481, 484, 497, 499, 500, 501, 506, 509, 517, 549, 557, 563, 574, 604, 609
Arthritis, 98, 120, 152
ARTHRITIS, 617
Artichoke, 99, 121, 145
as ascorbic acid, 58
Ascites, 645
Ascorbic Acid, 58
Ashwagandha, 180

Asparagus, 41, 49, 74, 81, 83, 92, 99, 115, 118, 129, 132, 135, 136, 147, 151, 153, 177, 178, 179, 181, 182, 183, 184, 185, 186, 187, 188, 189, 190, 191, 193, 194, 195
Aspartic Acid, 179, 553
Aspidosperma quebracho-blanco, 581
Association for Tropical Biology (Life), Council of Agricultural Science and Technology (Cornerstone Life Member), Herb Research Foundation, 304
asthma, 33, 34, 138, 226, 236, 477, 483, 484, 487, 502, 506, 526, 527, 535, 536, 537, 545, 550, 552, 560, 566, 581, 589, 599, 639
ASTHMA, 617
Astragalus, 456, 479, 622, 624
Astragalus mongholicus, 479
astringent, 508, 509, 517, 526, 527, 592, 611
Astringent, 645
Atheroma, 645
atherosclerosis, 58, 89, 228, 238, 289
Atherosclerosis, 56, 645
athlete's foot, 494, 503, 601
ATHLETE'S FOOT, 617
Atitiperiodic, 645
atropine, 243
Atropine, 402, 645
Aubrey Hampton, 293
Autism, 33, 53
Avidin, 67
Avocado, 59, 479, 621, 622, 623, 624
Avocados, 44, 62, 479
Azadirachta indica, 566
B. subtilis, 36
Bacillus subtilis, 36
Bacillus Subtilis, 36
back pain, 141, 147, 534, 573
BACKACHE, 618
bacteria, 33, 34, 35, 36, 37, 38, 39, 45, 47, 52, 68, 227, 235, 239, 243, 297, 302, 479, 509, 522, 601, 604, 634, 638
bactericide, 524
bad breath, 59, 238, 601
BAD BREATH, 618
Baked beans, 49
Baking powder, 73
BALDNESS, 618
Ballota nigra, 485
Banana, 59, 79, 92, 136, 143, 625, 626
Bananas, 47
Barberry, 90, 94, 110, 139
barium, 80, 81, 146
Barium, 70, 80, 81, 553
barley, 227, 315, 344, 634, 641
Barley, 49, 94, 132, 139, 187, 407
Barrenness, 645
Basil, 90, 480, 622

Battelle Columbus Laboratories, 304
Bay, 480, 542, 621, 625
Bayberry, 94
bdellium, 307
bead tree, 566
beans, 198, 228, 325, 407, 530, 641
Beans, 42, 45, 297, 620, 622
Bearberry, 94, 481, 618
Bee Balm, 608
Bee Pollen, 226
Beef blood, 53
beefsteak plant, 507
beehives, 226
beeswax, 618, 637, 638
Beet, 81, 83, 115, 130, 135, 136, 145, 149
Beetroot, 81, 83, 115, 130, 132, 135, 136, 145, 149
Beggar - Lice, 481, 621
Bell pepper, 81, 99, 102, 115, 129, 130, 136, 149, 179
Belpharitis, 645
benzethonium chloride, 293
Benzoin, 419, 645
berberine, 615
Beryllium, 70, 553
Beta - carotene, 505, 522, 523
Beta-carotene, 226, 553, 606
beta-glucan, 227
Betaine, 228
Beta-sitosterol, 228
Bible, 304
Bifidobacterium bifidum, 35
Bifidobacterium Bifidum, 36
Bifidobacterium infantis, 36
Bifidobacterium Infantis, 36
Bifidobacterium Longum, 36
Bilberries, 482
bilberry, 640
Bilberry, 59, 69, 121, 136, 482, 617, 619, 620, 621, 623
bile, 38, 39, 237, 506, 566, 604, 615
Biliousness, 645
bilirubin, 615
Biotin, 47, 66, 67
birth control, 118, 499, 566, 609
birth defects, 46, 49, 51, 75, 152, 303
Bishop's Weed, 482, 624
Bismuth, 70, 553
Bitter Gourd, 483, 620
bitter herbs, 338, 351, 401, 439, 462
Bitter melon, 132, 135
bitter tonic, 508, 524, 534
Black bean, 74, 81, 90, 99, 102, 110, 115, 118, 121, 129, 130, 132, 135, 143, 147, 151, 153, 177, 178, 181, 182, 183, 184, 185, 186, 187, 188, 189, 190, 191, 193, 194, 195

Black caraway, 178, 179, 182, 185, 186, 187, 188, 189, 194
Black cherry, 74, 81, 83, 90, 99, 110, 118, 129, 147, 151, 153
Black cohosh, 94, 139
Black Cohosh, 483, 484, 623, 625
Black cumin, 179, 182, 185, 186, 189, 194
black currant, 233, 291
Black currant, 83, 102, 136, 179
Black Haw, 484, 623, 624
Black Horehound, 485, 623
Black mustard, 145, 178, 184, 193, 194, 195, 320, 321
Black Nightshade, 485, 625
Black pepper, 92, 106, 149
Black walnut, 81, 102, 106, 139, 143, 149, 151
Black Walnut, 486, 621
Blackberry, 486, 620
Blackcurrant, 59
Blackcurrants, 69
bladder, 78, 79, 238, 481, 531, 534, 537, 548, 549, 551, 554
BLADDER INFECTIONS, 618
Bladderwrack, 79, 90, 106, 118, 139, 145
bleeding, 59, 62, 69, 108, 110, 120, 141, 236, 455, 484, 510, 521, 549, 576, 585, 611
bleeding gums, 59, 141
Blessed thistle, 94, 139
bloating, 477, 502, 504, 578, 635, 639, 641
blood cleaner, 492
blood pressure, 69, 80, 84, 88, 116, 117, 144, 145, 150, 196, 484, 501, 513, 517, 532, 554, 584, 587, 600, 604, 609, 615
blood purifier, 503, 600
Bloodroot, 487, 621, 625, 626
bloody stools, 584
Blue cohosh, 94, 110, 121, 139
Blue Cohosh, 487, 624
Blueberry, 59, 488, 618, 623
BODY ODOR, 618
boils, 483, 500, 503, 533
Boils, 646
Bok, 135, 145, 181, 184, 186, 191, 195
Bonavist bean, 153, 177, 181, 182, 183, 184, 185, 186, 188, 190, 191, 193, 194
bone disease, 59, 74
Bone loss, 117
bones, 58, 60, 68, 74, 80, 88, 89, 98, 117, 131, 132, 135, 140, 141, 146, 150, 177, 185, 186, 238, 297, 549
Borage, 118, 135, 145, 233, 488, 489, 624
borage oil, 233, 289
Borago officinalis, 488

boron, 82, 309, 312, 338, 349, 351, 352, 355, 359, 364, 372, 373, 381, 401, 409, 416, 418, 423, 428, 450, 452, 458, 464, 482
Boron, 82, 83, 237, 513, 529, 531, 535, 553, 569, 586, 604
Boswellia, 377
Botanical Products International, 305
bottled water, 75
Bovine Cartilage, 234
Bovine Colostrum, 234
bowel gas, 497, 531, 608
BPH, 152, 624
brain food, 49
Bran, 50, 68, 297
Brassica juncea, 565
Brazil nut, 617, 619, 624
Brazil nuts, 80, 136, 138
Brazilnut, 81, 92, 102, 106, 139, 143, 151, 178, 187
breast cancer, 60, 508
BREAST ENLARGEMENT, 618
breast milk, 74
breastfeeding, 74, 293, 532, 627, 638
BREAST-FEEDING PROBLEMS, 618
breath freshener, 571
Breathlessness, 108
Brewer's yeast, 46, 47, 48, 49, 53, 235
Brittle hair, 104, 153
brittle nails, 47
Broad bean, 106, 177, 178, 190
Broadbean, 79, 92, 181, 182, 183, 184, 185, 186, 189, 190, 194, 195
Broccoli, 41, 43, 45, 47, 59, 68, 69, 226, 606, 621
bromelain, 236, 575, 639
Bromelain, 236
Bromine, 70, 84, 339, 351, 359, 401, 418, 450, 458
bronchitis, 141, 483, 487, 519, 522, 524, 527, 534, 535, 599
Bronchitis, 646
BRONCHITIS, 618
Broom weed, 489
brown rice, 53, 118, 138, 297
Brown rice, 49
bruises, 478, 480, 494, 500, 505, 571, 592, 611
BRUISES, 618
bruising, 68, 78, 510
Brussel sprouts, 49
Brussels sprouts, 59, 83
Buchu, 121
Buckwheat, 69, 92, 106, 129
Buffalo gourd, 178, 180, 182, 183, 184, 185, 187, 188, 191, 195
BUGBITES, 622
Bugleweed, 621
BUNIONS, 618
Burdock, 99, 139, 143, 492, 493, 505, 622, 624

burdock leaves, 618
Burnet - Saxifrage, 493, 625
Burnet Saxifrage, 493
Burning bush, 179
burns, 84, 152, 485, 494, 503, 505, 513, 527, 535, 540, 611
BURNS, 618
BURSITIS, 619
Butcher's Broom, 494, 621, 626
Butter, 41, 74, 110, 118, 129, 132, 147, 151, 153, 177, 183, 184, 185, 186, 188, 190, 191, 195
Butterbur, 81, 90, 92, 106, 110, 136, 147, 149
Butternut, 81, 92, 102, 106, 143, 149, 151, 177, 178, 181, 182, 183, 185, 187, 188, 190, 193, 194, 195
Cabbage, 45, 59, 68, 81, 99, 102, 129, 130, 135, 149, 151, 177, 182, 184, 187, 188, 189, 191, 192, 194, 195, 623, 625
Cacao, 99
Cachexia, 646
Cacoethes, 646
Cadmium, 70, 553
Caffeine, 88
calcium, 25, 36, 52, 53, 60, 82, 88, 89, 90, 92, 99, 116, 117, 131, 133, 135, 136, 140, 146, 179, 186, 235, 236, 297, 298, 309, 310, 312, 313, 317, 320, 325, 328, 338, 339, 349, 351, 352, 355, 358, 359, 364, 370, 372, 373, 374, 376, 381, 382, 401, 406, 409, 416, 418, 423, 426, 428, 442, 446, 450, 458, 462, 464, 465, 471, 473, 494, 505, 522, 523, 549, 554, 633, 634, 641, 642
Calcium, 52, 70, 88, 89, 117, 132, 179, 237, 459, 475, 493, 502, 513, 529, 531, 535, 540, 549, 553, 561, 565, 569, 574, 584, 586, 592, 604, 605, 606, 612
Calendula, 494, 618, 619, 622, 624, 625
Calendula officinalis, 494
calming, 192, 500, 501, 505, 516, 556, 573, 600, 605
camels, 369
Camu Camu, 59
Camu-Camu, 495, 496, 620
cancer, 35, 50, 58, 60, 62, 75, 78, 79, 81, 95, 101, 103, 118, 135, 138, 140, 144, 145, 150, 151, 178, 226, 227, 238, 239, 240, 243, 289, 291, 296, 297, 300, 301, 455, 499, 501, 503, 508, 533, 534, 561, 574, 582, 599, 604, 612, 627, 636, 639, 640, 642
Cancer, 41, 78, 79, 81, 188, 304, 619, 646
cancer cells, 58, 612
CANCER PREVENTION, 619
candida, 494
Candida, 37, 481
candidiasis, 293
CANKER SORES, 619
Cankerroot, 496, 619
Cantaloupe, 41, 81, 115, 226

Capers, 496, 497, 619
capillary, 69, 292
Capillary fragility, 69
Capparis spinosa, 496
Capsaicin, 236, 237
capsaicinoids, 236
carbohydrates, 26, 43, 45, 47, 117, 131, 140, 226, 295, 483, 552, 578, 612, 638
Carbon, 70
Carbon Dioxide, 70
carbon monoxide, 53
carbuncles, 533
Carbuncles, 646
Cardamom, 497, 620, 621, 622, 625
cardec, 243
CARDIAC ARRHYTHMIA, 619
Cardiotonic, 646
cardiovascular disease, 44, 94, 301, 566
Carminative, 620, 646
Carob, 177, 178, 181, 182, 183, 184, 185, 186, 187, 188, 189, 190, 191, 194, 195, 498, 620
Caroba jacaranda procera, 498
carotenes, 567, 579
Carotenes, 301
carotenoids, 236, 300
CARPAL TUNNEL SYNDROME, 619
carrot, 482
Carrot, 59, 74, 79, 81, 102, 115, 135, 136, 145, 147, 180, 619, 620, 623, 625, 626
Carrots, 41, 226
Carthamus tinctorius, 587
cartilage, 99, 120, 146, 150, 177, 180, 189, 234, 238
Cashew, 81, 92, 99, 102, 106, 136, 143, 149, 151
cassia, 345, 435, 457
Cat's Claw, 499, 621, 623, 625
Cataplasm, 646
cataracts, 43, 62, 153, 300, 604, 639
CATARACTS, 619
catarrh, 141, 608
Catechins, 69
Cathartic, 646
Catnip, 94, 110, 121, 139, 499, 619
cattle, 485
Cauliflower, 42, 57, 59, 67, 83, 90, 99, 102, 129, 130, 132, 135, 136, 149, 153, 177, 190, 193, 622
Caulophyllum thalictroides, 487
Cayenne, 179, 236, 237
Celandine, 501, 619, 621, 626
Celery, 83, 90, 135, 145, 153, 179, 501, 617, 620, 621, 622
Celiac disease, 33
Cenestin, 298
Center for Mind-Body Medicine, Center for Plant Conservation, 305
Cephaelis acuminata, 550

821

Hillman Health Food Store call 855-Amish-Dr (855-264-7437) www.emineral.info Vitamins and Minerals for Better Living

Index

Cereals, 42
Cerium, 70
Cesium, 70, 553
Chamomile, 502, 503, 573, 617, 619, 620, 621, 622, 624, 625
Chamomile tea, 502, 503
Chancre, 646
Chaparral, 92, 139, 503, 625
Chaste berry, 504
Chasteberry, 617, 618, 623, 624
Chaya, 178, 181, 187, 194
Checkered Skipper Butterflies, 489
Checkered Skipper Butterfly, 489
Cheese, 43, 49, 51
Chelidonium majus, 501
Chemical poisonings, 53
Chenopodium ambrosioides, 613
Cherries, 69
Cherry, 59, 81, 99, 102, 115, 129, 130, 136, 149, 179
chest pain, 534, 555, 557
chestnut tree, 424, 547
chew sticks, 455
Chicken, 44, 49
Chickpea, 178, 189, 193
Chickpeas, 49
Chickweed, 74, 92, 94, 110, 149, 504, 505, 623
Chicory, 90, 193, 505, 621
Chilblains, 646
childbirth, 484, 512, 532, 572
Chili, 59, 179
Chili pepper, 59
chills, 500, 526
Chinese Angelica, 506, 512, 622, 623, 624
Chinese boxthorn, 179
Chinese cabbage, 81, 115, 147
Chinese foxglove, 178, 181, 191
Chinese matrimony vine, 179
Chinese wolfberry, 179, 612
Chiropractors, 26
Chiso, 507, 508, 621
chitin, 237
Chitosan, 237
Chives, 118, 177, 178, 181, 182, 184, 185, 187, 189, 190, 191, 193, 194, 195
Chlorine, 70, 309, 312, 325, 339, 351, 355, 370, 372, 376, 401, 426, 450, 459
Chlorophyll, 238
Chokecherry, 59
Cholecalciferol, 60
cholesterol, 37, 44, 45, 47, 53, 62, 69, 94, 120, 150, 187, 192, 196, 227, 228, 237, 238, 243, 289, 290, 292, 501, 513, 516, 554, 567, 579, 581, 587, 598, 604, 609, 628, 633, 634, 637, 639, 641
choline, 56, 187, 228, 299

Choline, 56, 340, 553
chondroitin, 180, 238, 239
Chondroitin, 238, 239
chondroitin sulfate, 180, 238, 239
Chorea, 646
chromium, 26, 94, 95, 235, 328, 339, 349, 351, 352, 359, 364, 370, 376, 381, 401, 406, 409, 418, 428, 450, 458, 471
Chromium, 51, 70, 94, 237, 459, 493, 502, 513, 529, 535, 540, 549, 553, 561, 565, 574, 592, 604, 605
Chronic fatigue, 181, 182, 185, 193
CHRONIC FATIGUE SYNDROME, 619
chronic hepatitis, 52
chronic lower back pain, 58
Cicatrizant, 647
Cichorium intybus, 505
Cilantro, 94, 118, 135, 145
Cinchona, 508, 619, 621, 622, 647
Cinchona officinalis, 508
Cinnamomum Zeylanicum, 509
Cinnamon, 81, 85, 92, 94, 106, 121, 136, 336, 435, 509, 621, 623
circulation, 53, 105, 142, 236, 509, 513, 547, 554, 566, 608
cirrhosis, 191, 193, 615
citric acids, 486
Citron, 510
Citronella, 509, 510, 622
Citrus aurantifolia, 510
Citrus australasica, 511
Citrus australis, 511
Citrus fruits, 49, 68, 69
Citrus halimii, 511
Citrus indica, 511
Citrus maxima, 510
Citrus medica, 510
Citrus reticulata, 510
citrus seed extract, 293
Citrus trifoliata, 510
CLA, 239
Clams, 51
clostridium difficile, 235
clothing, 84, 85
Cloudberry, 59, 136
Clove, 121, 513, 617, 623, 625, 626
Clover, 81, 102, 151, 582, 623, 624
Clubmoss, 79, 179
cobalt, 26, 97, 349, 352, 359, 364, 370, 372, 376, 381, 401, 406, 409, 418, 428, 450, 458, 471
Cobalt, 70, 237, 459, 493, 502, 513, 529, 535, 540, 549, 553, 561, 565, 574, 592, 604, 605
Coca, 81, 83, 106, 132, 147
Cocoa, 513, 626
Coconut, 92, 99, 102, 106, 136, 143, 151
Cod, 51, 241

codeine, 243
Coenzyme Q10, 240
Coffee, 179, 180, 617, 620
Cold intolerance, 105
COLD SORES, 621
colds, 41, 59, 455, 483, 493, 500, 509, 521, 522, 524, 527, 529, 533, 537, 546, 561, 566, 574, 610, 611
COLDS, 619
colic, 484, 500, 502, 509, 517, 526, 534, 562, 609
Colic, 647
colitis, 494
collagen, 58, 98, 99, 140, 141, 177, 186, 188, 189, 191
Collagen, 99, 140, 141, 148, 647
Collard greens, 41
Collards, 90, 99, 145, 153, 193
Collinsonia canadensis, 547
Collyrium, 647
Coloring agents, 73
Comfrey, 145, 179, 515, 618, 619, 621, 625
comfrey root, 618
Common Checkered Skipper Butterfly, 489
Common thyme, 110, 115, 139
Common-thyme, 74
Complementary Medicine for the Physician, 306
Condyloma, 647
Condylomata, 647
Cone pepper, 81, 102, 115, 129, 130, 136, 149, 179
Coneflower, 110, 139, 143
confusion, 242, 475, 627
congestion, 144, 524, 558, 566, 581
conjugated linoleic acid, 239
Conjunctivitis, 647
Conrad Elvehjem, 44
constipation, 39, 141, 291, 494, 497, 505, 575, 578, 585, 639
Constipation, 38, 104, 117, 134
CONSTIPATION, 619
Consumption, 647
Contagion, 647
convulsions, 484, 536
Convulsions, 647
copper, 26, 78, 89, 90, 98, 99, 100, 117, 128, 136, 154, 309, 310, 312, 313, 320, 325, 328, 339, 349, 351, 355, 358, 359, 364, 370, 372, 373, 381, 401, 409, 418, 423, 426, 428, 434, 442, 446, 450, 452, 458, 462, 464, 473, 482, 488, 642
Copper, 51, 70, 98, 99, 100, 128, 459, 475, 493, 535, 553, 569, 584, 586, 592, 612
Coptis trifolia, 496
CoQ$_{10}$, 240
Cordial, 647
coriander, 342, 516
Coriander, 94, 515, 516, 618, 622

Coriandrum sativum, 515
Corn, 42, 79, 81, 83, 92, 106, 110, 129, 143, 151, 177, 184, 188, 191, 195, 228, 617
Corn salad, 193
cornea, 549
Cornmeal, 49
corns, 78
Corns, 648
CORNS, 619
cortisone, 45
Couchgrass, 516, 618, 621
cough, 84, 141, 237, 477, 486, 524, 526, 534, 550, 558, 566, 600, 610, 616
COUGHING, 619
coughs, 485, 489, 493, 500, 524, 529, 546, 560, 564, 590, 600
Country Mallow, 517, 620, 624
Cowage, 178, 185, 186, 189, 190, 191, 194, 195
cow's milk, 89, 138
Crabapple, 59
Cradle Cap, 66
Crampbark, 90, 139
Cramps, 88
Cranberry, 59, 121, 626
Crataegus oxyacantha, 543
Cravings, 120
CRC Handbook (and Database) of Biological Activities of Phytochemicals, 305
CRC Handbook (and database) of Phytochemical Constituents of GRAS Herbs and Other Economic Plants, 305
CRC Handbook of Agricultural Energy Potential for Developing Countries, 305
CRC Handbook of Alternative Cash Crops, 306
CRC Handbook of Edible Weeds, 305
CRC Handbook of Medicinal Herbs, 305
CRC Handbook of Nuts, 305
CRC Handbook of Proximate Analysis Tables of Higher Plants, 305
Cream, 41
Cretinism, 104
Crocus sativus, 588
Crohn's disease, 131, 289
Cubeb, 519, 622
Cucumber, 59, 74, 79, 81, 99, 115, 118, 129, 130, 132, 135, 136, 143, 147, 149, 153, 626
Cucurbita pepo, 579
cumin, 516
Cumin, 83, 182, 185, 186, 187, 188, 189, 194, 618, 619
Curcuma longa, 604
Curly dock, 139
Curly kale, 99, 145
curry, 295, 604
Cut leaf, 179

823

Hillman Health Food Store call 855-Amish-Dr (855-264-7437) www.emineral.info Vitamins and Minerals for Better Living

cuts, 437, 505, 548, 564
CUTS, 619
Cyanocobalamin, 51
Cyanogenetic, 648
Cymbopogon citratus, 556
Cymbopogon nardus, 509
Cyperus rotundus, 567
cystic fibrosis, 536
Cystine, 180, 553
cystitis, 505, 549
Cystitis, 648
Daemonorops Draco, 521
daidzein, 297
Damiana, 622
Dandelion, 81, 83, 90, 92, 94, 106, 110, 135, 136, 145, 147, 149, 617, 623, 624
DANDRUFF, 619
Date Palm, 180
Dates, 49
deafness, 555
Decoction, 312, 341, 365, 388, 450, 648
decongestant, 527, 547
Dehydration, 144
Delirium, 648
DELIVERY, 624
dementia, 46, 132, 535
Demulcent, 648
Dental cavities, 117
Deobstruent, 648
deodorant, 527
Depilatory creams, 648
Depressed mood, 94, 104
depression, 43, 46, 114, 136, 191, 192, 196, 241, 242, 529, 536, 539, 546, 556, 598, 627, 636
Depression, 116, 152, 185, 188, 191, 192, 193
DEPRESSION, 136, 620
Depurative, 648
dermatitis, 39, 47, 233, 552, 560, 613, 639
DERMATOSES, 624
Designer Food Program, 304
Desmodium styracifolium, 481
detoxification, 35, 53, 137, 177, 505
Detoxification, 137
Devil's claw, 74, 94, 110
Devil's Claw, 621
DHA, 240, 241, 289, 290
DHEA, 241, 242
DHEA sulfate, 241
diabetes, 44, 53, 69, 116, 117, 137, 142, 150, 151, 196, 198, 233, 240, 289, 290, 291, 479, 481, 482, 483, 488, 505, 509, 516, 532, 536, 555, 566, 615, 634, 637, 639, 641
Diabetes, 66, 152, 177, 184
DIABETES, 620
diabetics, 197, 198, 483, 509

Diaphoretic, 648
diarrhea, 35, 37, 38, 44, 45, 58, 59, 62, 75, 78, 80, 83, 91, 105, 119, 134, 141, 144, 198, 234, 236, 293, 298, 299, 455, 480, 482, 483, 486, 489, 500, 508, 509, 526, 534, 555, 557, 561, 569, 574, 578, 585, 599, 604, 635
Diarrhea, 88, 108, 139, 150
DIARRHEA, 620
digestion, 34, 35, 51, 89, 91, 92, 236, 291, 297, 300, 482, 483, 493, 494, 509, 532, 546, 562, 566, 571, 578
Dill, 83, 90, 102, 118, 121, 130, 135, 153, 358, 617, 621
dimethylaminoethanol, 242
Dioestrus, 648
Dioscorea villosa, 609
Dioscorides, 564, 596
diphtheria, 522
disambiguation, 605
Discutient, 648
disinfectant, 526, 527
Disorientation, 134, 135
diuretic, 141, 481, 487, 489, 492, 493, 498, 499, 501, 505, 515, 519, 524, 531, 533, 537, 548, 549, 551, 561, 596, 609
Diuretic, 648
Diversity, Economic Botany, 306
DIVERTICULITIS, 620
dizziness, 88, 234, 536, 543, 555, 581, 592, 633, 637
Dizziness, 100, 134
DIZZINESS, 620
DMAE, 242, 243
docosahexaenoic acid, 240, 289
Dogwood, 79
dopamine, 46, 99, 121, 193
Dorothy Hodgkin, 51
Dr Linus Pauling, 58
Dr. Herb Pierson, 304
Dr. Jacob Harich, 293
Dr. Mark Holbreich, 33
Dragon's Blood, 521, 625, 626
Dropsy, 648
Drug addiction, 53, 193
DRY MOUTH, 620
dry skin, 289, 592
Dry skin, 104
Duke's Herbal Vineyard, 304, 305
Dull hair, 98, 120
Dulse, 79, 94, 139, 143, 145
Dwarf bean, 74, 81, 90, 102, 110, 115, 118, 121, 129, 130, 132, 135, 143, 147, 151, 153, 177, 178, 181, 182, 183, 184, 185, 186, 187, 188, 189, 190, 191, 193, 194, 195
Dwarf sumac, 81, 121, 147

Dyschezia, 648
dysentery, 480, 482, 497, 534, 549, 555, 599, 639
DYSLACTEA, 618
DYSMENORRHEA, 623
DYSPEPSIA, 622
Dysuria, 648
E. T. Krebs, 50
earache, 293, 522
EARACHE, 620
earaches, 605
ebony, 356, 362
Ecbolic, 648
Echinacea, 74, 94, 110, 139, 143, 521, 522, 523, 617, 618, 619, 620, 621, 622, 623, 624, 625, 626
Echinacea angustifolia, 521
eczema, 38, 289, 492, 503, 505, 537, 552, 560, 611
EGCG, 243
egg, 43, 47, 299
Eggplant, 59, 81, 92, 110, 523, 625
Eggs, 41, 43, 44, 45, 47, 51, 68
Egilops, 648
Egypt, 304, 409, 417, 464, 509, 531
eicosapentaenoic acid, 289
Elderberry, 59, 524, 619, 625
Elecampane, 524, 622
Elephant garlic, 179
Elletaria cardamom, 497
Elmer V. McCollum, 40
Elymus repens, 516
Emetic, 648
Emmenagogue, 648
emollient, 517, 532
Emollient, 648
EMPHYSEMA, 620
Endive, 81, 115, 129, 135, 145, 147, 153
ENDOMETRIOSIS, 620
English filbert, 106, 136, 149, 151
English Walnut, 526
Enterococcus Faecium, 36, 37
Ephedra, 526, 578, 617, 620
Ephedra sinica, 526
ephedrine, 243
epigallocatechin gallate, 243
epilepsy, 242, 289, 291, 475, 487, 498, 539, 601
Epstein Barr virus, 186
Equisetum arvense, 549
ERECTION PROBLEMS, 620
Ergot, 649
Ergotism, 649
Ernst Krebs, 54
Erysipelas, 649
essential fatty acid, 196, 239
essential fatty acids, 196, 240, 567, 612, 642
essential oil, 477, 513, 557, 601
Essiac Tea, 439

Estratab, 298
Estrogen, 69
Eucalyptus, 527, 618, 620, 624, 625
Eucalyptus globulus, 527
Evening Primrose, 193, 289, 528, 529, 617, 620, 621, 623, 624, 625
excessive menstruation problems, 587
expectorant, 519, 527, 532, 547, 551, 596
Expectorant, 649
eye, 43, 152, 153, 304, 395, 455, 483, 493, 500, 503, 526, 549, 566, 596, 601, 611
eye ailments, 395
Eyebright, 143
eyewash, 482
Ezekiel, 314, 328, 335, 356, 362, 407, 457
Faba bean, 79, 92, 177, 178, 181, 182, 183, 184, 185, 186, 189, 190, 194, 195
facial paralysis, 517
fainting, 487, 550
FAINTING, 620
Father Nature's Farmacy, 304
fatigue, 53, 62, 78, 83, 177, 179, 186, 302, 487, 504, 505, 510, 512, 521, 535, 536, 544, 592, 635
Fatigue, 91, 98, 104, 105, 108, 109, 116, 117, 132, 134, 139, 144, 145, 148, 153, 176, 184, 186, 192
fat-soluble, 25, 40, 62, 237, 299, 301, 598, 636
Fava bean, 106, 530, 620, 623
Fava Bean, 530
Febrifuge, 649
fennel, 482
Fennel, 99, 106, 121, 139, 178, 179, 182, 183, 185, 186, 187, 188, 189, 194, 531, 618, 621
fenugreek, 532
Fenugreek, 370, 532, 618, 619, 620, 622
fero-coumarins, 608
fever, 194, 502, 504, 508, 517, 522, 524, 526, 527, 531, 533, 536, 555, 557, 566, 611
FEVER, 620
Feverfew, 94, 139, 532, 617, 621
fevers, 58, 455, 489, 499, 500, 522, 549, 566, 569, 574, 605, 616
Fiber, 297, 641
fibromyalgia, 302, 536, 627, 635
Field bean, 74, 81, 90, 99, 102, 110, 115, 118, 121, 129, 130, 132, 135, 143, 147, 151, 153, 177, 178, 181, 182, 183, 184, 185, 186, 187, 188, 189, 190, 191, 193, 194, 195
Field Guide to Medicinal Plants, 305
Fig, 59, 83, 180, 619
Filbert, 81, 92, 99
Filipendula ulmaria, 561
fish, 26, 77, 80, 82, 178, 181, 196, 228, 240, 241, 289, 290, 370, 380, 409, 417, 464, 497
Fish, 51, 289, 290
fissures, 578

Flageolet bean, 74, 81, 90, 99, 102, 110, 115, 118, 121, 129, 130, 132, 135, 143, 147, 151, 153, 177, 178, 181, 183, 184, 185, 186, 187, 188, 189, 190, 191, 193, 194, 195
flatulence, 292, 562, 578, 635, 641
FLATULENCE, 620
Flavanones, 69
Flavones, 69
flavonoids, 293, 482, 513, 579, 600, 638, 639
Flavonoids, 69, 293, 504, 628
Flax, 92, 118, 132, 180, 196, 619, 620
Flaxseed oil, 196
Flour, 73, 133
flu, 58, 509, 521, 522, 524, 549, 555, 566, 599
FLU, 619
fluid retention, 104, 547
Fluid retention, 104
fluorine, 26, 101, 102, 359, 401, 418, 458
Fluorine, 70, 535
Foeniculum vulgare, 531
Folate, 49
Folic Acid, 49
folk remedy, 496, 549, 552, 615
Forsythia, 533, 619, 620, 625
Forsythia suspensa, 533
fractures, 58, 60, 68, 140, 146, 147, 298, 478
free radicals, 48, 62, 137, 187, 226, 292, 598
French bean, 74, 81, 90, 99, 102, 110, 115, 118, 129, 130, 132, 135, 143, 147, 151, 153, 177, 178, 181, 182, 183, 184, 185, 186, 187, 188, 189, 190, 191, 193, 194, 195
FRIGIDITY, 622
frostbite, 526, 547
Fructooligosaccharides, 35
Fucus vesiculosus, 553
Fumaric Acid, 290
fungal diseases, 483
FUNGAL INFECTIONS, 621
fungi, 33
fungus, 503, 583, 601
gallbladder, 226, 501, 533, 609
Gallium, 70, 401
GALLSTONES, 621
gamma oryzanol, 634
Gamma-linolenic, 291
gamma-linolenic acid, 291
Gangrene, 649
Ganoderma lyceum, 583
Garbanzo, 178, 189, 193
garcinia cambogia, 295, 296
Garden bean, 74, 81, 90, 99, 102, 110, 115, 118, 121, 129, 130, 132, 135, 143, 147, 151, 153, 177, 178, 181, 182, 183, 184, 185, 186, 187, 188, 189, 190, 191, 193, 194, 195
Garden beet, 81, 115, 130, 132, 135, 136, 145, 149

Garden dill, 102, 121, 130, 135, 136, 143, 149, 153
Garden thyme, 110, 115, 139, 177
Garden-thyme, 74
Garlic, 59, 94, 106, 139, 380, 381, 617, 618, 619, 620, 621, 622, 623, 624, 625, 626
gas, 84, 130, 235, 500, 502, 531, 534, 557, 600, 613, 639
gastric lipase, 300
Gaultheria procumbens, 610
genetically modified foods, 33
genital herpes, 601, 638
GENITAL HERPES, 621
Gentian, 139, 534, 620, 622
Gentiana lutea, 534
Germanium, 51, 103, 381, 535, 612
Giant taro, 179
Ginger, 79, 94, 102, 110, 121, 130, 143, 179, 312, 534, 617, 618, 619, 620, 621, 622, 623, 625, 626
gingivitis, 59, 638
GINGIVITIS, 621
Ginkgo, 69, 179, 180, 535, 617, 620, 621, 622, 623, 624, 625, 626
Ginkgo biloba, 535
Ginseng, 79, 83, 94, 106, 121, 129, 139, 145, 151, 153, 180, 535, 536, 617, 619, 620, 622
Ginseng, a Concise Handbook, 305
GLA, 233, 291, 642
glaucoma, 196, 197, 551, 552
GLAUCOMA, 621
glucomannan, 291, 292
Glucomannan, 291, 292
glucosamine, 238
Glutamate, 309, 313, 318, 325, 331, 355, 364, 371, 372, 374, 376, 381, 401, 423, 459, 463, 465
Glutamic Acid, 180, 553
Gluten, 606
Glycine, 176, 182, 309, 313, 318, 325, 331, 355, 364, 371, 372, 374, 376, 381, 401, 418, 423, 459, 463, 465, 553
glycosaminoglycans, 238
Glycyrrhiza glabra, 557
Goa bean, 181, 182, 184, 187, 188, 189, 190, 191, 193, 195
Goiter, 104, 649
Goji, 59, 612
Golden rod, 537
Goldenseal, 143, 539, 615, 617, 619, 620, 622, 624, 625, 626
Gonorrhea, 649
Gotu kola, 74, 94
Gotu Kola, 539, 617, 619, 625
gout, 44, 48, 145, 480, 482, 497, 501, 503, 531, 537, 639
GOUT, 621
Goutweed, 482

Grains, 50
Grape, 59, 74, 79, 81, 83, 121, 139, 143, 292, 293, 513, 621
grapefruit, 301, 510, 632, 633
Grapefruit, 59, 79, 81, 115, 136, 147, 149, 179
Grapefruit seed extract, 293, 294, 295
Grapes, 69, 641
Grapple plant, 94
Gravel, 649
GRAVES' DISEASE, 621
graying hair, 49
Green bean, 74, 81, 90, 99, 102, 110, 115, 118, 121, 129, 130, 132, 135, 143, 147, 151, 153, 177, 178, 181, 182, 183, 184, 185, 186, 187, 188, 189, 190, 191, 193, 194, 195
Green gram, 183, 184, 185, 186, 190, 193
Green leafy vegetables, 62, 68
Green pepper, 81, 102, 115, 129, 130, 136, 149, 179
Green Pepper, 69
green tea, 243, 527, 640
Green tea, 69
growth hormones, 234
growth impairment, 49
Gruel, 649
GSE, 293, 294, 295
Guava, 59, 542, 543, 622
gums, 58, 600, 641
H. pylori, 38, 235
Habas, 92, 181, 186, 194
Hafnium, 70
hair loss, 45, 47, 104, 152, 493, 628
Hair loss, 108, 139, 186
hallucinogen, 616
Hamamelis virginiana, 611
Handbook of Legumes of World Economic Importance, 305
Handbook of Northeastern Indian Medicinal Plants, 305
HANGOVER, 621
hardening of the arteries, 40, 547
Haricot, 74, 81, 90, 99, 102, 110, 115, 118, 121, 129, 130, 132, 135, 143, 147, 151, 153, 177, 178, 181, 182, 183, 184, 185, 186, 187, 188, 189, 190, 191, 193, 194, 195
Haricot vert, 81, 121, 129, 143, 177, 178
Hawthorn, 69, 79, 139, 543, 544, 619, 621, 622
headache, 84, 88, 142, 233, 484, 503, 512, 526, 534, 536, 543, 555, 581, 600, 605, 610
Headache, 100, 108
HEADACHE, 621
headaches, 43, 44, 115, 192, 196, 226, 236, 395, 475, 480, 500, 502, 503, 504, 532, 548, 550, 608, 627, 637
heart, 42, 46, 47, 51, 52, 58, 62, 75, 78, 80, 89, 114, 116, 117, 134, 135, 136, 138, 145, 150, 178, 189, 196, 197, 226, 236, 240, 241, 290, 293, 297, 484, 487, 489, 492, 499, 512, 513, 533, 540, 544, 547, 554, 555, 571, 587, 604, 609
heart disease, 46, 51, 58, 62, 114, 138, 150, 178, 196, 226, 241, 290, 293, 297, 484, 544, 587, 604
Heart disease, 53, 240
HEART DISEASE, 621
Heart's Ease, 571
heartburn, 298, 502, 585, 599
HEARTBURN, 621
heaven, 320
Helianthus annuus, 598
Helium, 70
hemlock, 387, 482
Hemlock, 482
Hemoglobin, 98, 108
hemorrhage, 499, 550
hemorrhages, 59
hemorrhoids, 69, 481, 494, 500, 526, 537, 547, 549, 566, 578, 585, 611, 639
Hemorrhoids, 650
HEMORRHOIDS, 621
hepatitis, 484, 540
HEPATOSIS, 623
Herb Research Foundation, 305
herbal tea, 524, 548, 551
hernia, 502
Herpes, 178, 186
herpes simplex, 197
herpes zoster, 197
hexacosanol, 637
hiccups, 566
high blood pressure, 142, 193, 236, 240, 243, 291, 479, 482, 506, 512, 526, 530, 540, 555, 556, 557, 586, 615, 633
High blood pressure, 53, 88, 188
HIGH BLOOD PRESSURE, 621
HIGH CHOLESTEROL, 622
histamines, 69
Histidine, 183, 309, 313, 321, 325, 331, 339, 355, 359, 364, 371, 372, 374, 376, 381, 401, 418, 423, 459, 463, 465
Histopathology, 27
HIV INFECTION, 622
hives, 226, 638, 639, 640
HIVES, 622
HMB, 295
holy tree, 566
homocysteine, 46, 51, 228
honey, 309, 314, 331, 423, 479, 483, 498, 500, 561, 571, 638
Honey, 74, 139, 432, 618
Honeysuckle, 545, 620, 624, 625
Hops, 139, 179, 546, 622
Horehound, 485, 546, 622

827

Horse Chestnut, 547, 621, 626
Horsebalm, 547, 617, 619
Horsemint, 608
Horseradish, 102, 106, 130, 149, 179, 182, 193, 195, 548, 617, 624
Horsetail, 79, 90, 95, 110, 132, 139, 143, 549, 618
hot flashes, 484, 504, 599
Hot pepper, 179
human carcinogen, 78
Humphrey Davy, 88, 91, 116, 134, 144
Humulus lupulus, 546
Hyacinth, 153, 177, 181, 182, 183, 184, 185, 186, 188, 190, 191, 193, 194
Hydrocotyle asiatica, 539
Hydrogen, 70
Hydroxycitric Acid, 295
hydroxyl-beta-methylbultyrate, 295
Hypericum perforatum, 598
Hyperinulinemia, 184
hypertension, 53, 69, 89, 117, 142, 240, 483, 527, 530, 552
Hypoglycemia, 176, 182, 190
Hypotension, 119
HYPOTHYROIDISM, 622
hysteria, 43, 475, 487
IBS, 622
Idiocy, 650
Ignatius Kaim, 120
Immune System, 33
impaired memory, 46, 132
impatiens capensis, 551
IMPOTENCE, 620
incense, 329, 404
Indian mustard, 565
indigestion, 233, 234, 298, 477, 501, 508, 527, 531, 534, 561, 562
Indigestion, 88
INDIGESTION, 622
Indole, 296
indole-3-carbinol, 296
Indolent, 650
inducing labor, 484
infections, 33, 35, 38, 39, 105, 141, 152, 176, 226, 235, 241, 302, 475, 479, 481, 488, 494, 497, 499, 503, 509, 512, 517, 519, 522, 523, 524, 533, 534, 536, 540, 549, 555, 567, 601, 635
INFERTILITY, 622
inflammation, 26, 38, 39, 88, 137, 141, 142, 233, 234, 236, 484, 497, 500, 501, 505, 512, 523, 524, 532, 537, 549, 557, 558, 576, 581, 592, 599, 604, 608, 609, 637, 638, 642
INFLAMMATORY BOWEL DISEASE, 622
INHIBITED SEXUAL DESIRE IN WOMEN, 622
Inositol, 48
Inositol Hexaphosphate, 48

insanity, 517
insect bites, 478, 556, 571
INSECT BITES, 622
insect repellent, 510, 566, 586
Insipid, 650
Insolation, 650
Insoluble Fiber, 297
insomnia, 142, 243, 475, 515, 556, 573, 599, 600, 605
Insomnia, 88, 192
INSOMNIA, 622
insulin, 48, 94, 148, 150, 152, 153, 176, 177, 184, 185, 194, 483, 509, 516, 641
INTERMITTENT CLAUDICATION, 622
International Association of Plant Taxonomists, 305
International Expeditions, 305
International Society for Tropical Root Crops, 305
International Weed Science Society, 305
intestinal gas, 509
INTESTINAL PARASITES, 622
Inula helenium, 524
Inulin, 35, 505, 635
inulin oligosaccharides, 634
iodine, 26, 101, 104, 105, 106, 107, 309, 312, 325, 339, 351, 355, 381, 423, 428, 553
Iodine, 70, 104, 105, 553
IP-6, 636
Ipecac, 550, 622
Ipriflavone, 297, 298
Irish moss, 79, 90, 95, 118, 139, 145
iron, 26, 36, 90, 99, 108, 109, 110, 121, 122, 136, 140, 238, 243, 309, 310, 312, 313, 317, 320, 325, 328, 338, 339, 351, 352, 355, 358, 359, 364, 370, 372, 373, 376, 381, 401, 406, 409, 416, 418, 423, 426, 428, 442, 446, 450, 457, 458, 462, 464, 465, 471, 473, 482, 488, 505, 522, 523, 637, 642
Iron, 51, 70, 98, 108, 109, 133, 150, 237, 475, 483, 493, 502, 513, 526, 529, 531, 535, 540, 549, 553, 561, 565, 569, 574, 584, 586, 592, 604, 605, 606, 612
Irregular heartbeat, 88
irregular heartbeats, 508
irritability, 45, 484, 634
irritable bowel syndrome, 298, 578, 639
Isoleucine, 184, 185, 309, 313, 318, 321, 325, 331, 339, 355, 359, 364, 371, 372, 374, 376, 381, 401, 418, 423, 459, 463, 465, 553
Isthmian Ethnobotanical Dictionary, 304, 305
itching, 68, 289, 483, 505, 601, 611
Ivy, 552
Jaborandi, 551, 620, 621
Jacques Cartier, 58
Japanese cinnamon, 81
Japanese plant, 291
jaundice, 496, 505, 531, 533, 569, 575

Jaundice, 650
Jewelweed, 551, 552, 622, 624
John Keim, 618
joint pain, 563, 566
Joseph Black, 116
Journal of Optimal Nutrition, 306
Journal or Aromatherapy, 306
Judas tree, 395
Juglans nigra, 486
Juglans regia L, 526
juniper, 95, 397, 437, 468
Kakadu plum, 59
Kale, 41, 59, 99, 145
Kava, 573
Kelp, 79, 85, 90, 106, 118, 139, 145, 553, 621, 622
Khella, 554, 619
khellin, 554
kidney, 61, 73, 74, 79, 84, 99, 103, 134, 135, 141, 178, 198, 242, 290, 298, 479, 481, 493, 497, 503, 505, 510, 517, 522, 537, 544, 548, 549, 554, 636
Kidney bean, 74, 81, 90, 99, 102, 110, 115, 118, 121, 129, 130, 132, 135, 143, 147, 151, 153, 177, 178, 181, 182, 183, 184, 185, 186, 187, 188, 189, 190, 191, 193, 194, 195
kidney failure, 61
KIDNEY STONES, 621
kidneys, 80, 89, 90, 91, 92, 94, 116, 119, 134, 136, 142, 144, 145, 149, 150, 152, 609, 613
Kinesiopathology, 26
Kitchen kale, 99, 145
Knotweed, 79, 147
konjac root, 291
Krypton, 70
Kudzu, 79, 555, 617, 621
Kuhn, Gyorgi, 43
Kumquats, 511
Kwashiorkor, 184, 194
Lablab bean, 153, 181, 183, 184, 185, 186, 188, 190, 191, 193, 194
Labor, 650
labor pains, 484, 545
Lactase, 298
lactic acid, 37, 38, 39, 48, 53
Lactobacillus acidophilus, 35
Lactobacillus Acidophilus, 37
Lactobacillus brevis, 37
Lactobacillus Brevis, 37
Lactobacillus bulgaricus, 37
Lactobacillus Bulgaricus, 36, 37
Lactobacillus Casei, 36, 37
Lactobacillus plantarum, 37
Lactobacillus Plantarum, 36, 37
Lactobacillus rhamnosus, 38
Lactobacillus Rhamnosus, 36, 38
Lactobacillus Salivarius, 38

lactose intolerance, 38, 39, 89, 298
Lady's Thumb, 571
Lady's thistle, 139, 143
Ladyslipper, 121, 139
laetrile, 54
Laetrile, 54
Lamb's lettuce, 83, 110, 177, 184, 191, 193
Lambs quarter, 132, 135, 177, 182, 183, 184, 185, 186, 189, 190, 191, 194, 195
lanolin, 618
Lanthanum, 70
large intestines, 36
Larrea divaricata, 503
LARYNGITIS, 622
Laurus nobilis, 480
Lavandula Angustifolia, 555
Lavender, 555, 556, 622, 625
laxative, 292, 486, 492, 494, 502, 505, 533, 535, 566
Laxative, 292, 651
laxatives, 135
L-Dopa, 530
lead, 43, 44, 47, 48, 52, 77, 78, 92, 94, 99, 102, 108, 119, 121, 139, 141, 145, 146, 150, 179, 187, 196, 198, 240, 241, 243, 291, 544, 641
Lead, 70
Leafy green vegetables, 46
Leafy vegetables, 41
Leaky Gut, 34
Lean beef, 47
Lecithin, 57, 132, 299
leg cramps, 508
leg vein, 547
Lemon balm, 556, 621, 622, 624, 626
Lemon Balm, 573
Lemongrass, 95, 139, 556, 617, 621
lemons, 510
Lentil, 92, 106, 177, 178, 181, 183, 184, 185, 186, 188, 189, 190, 191, 195
lentils, 400, 407
Lentils, 49
leprosy, 483, 566, 616
Leprosy, 651
Leptospermum scoparium, 600
Lesser Periwinkle, 557, 625
Lettuce, 59, 79, 81, 83, 90, 92, 95, 99, 102, 115, 118, 121, 129, 130, 132, 135, 143, 145, 147, 149, 151, 153, 184, 188, 191, 195
Leucine, 185, 310, 313, 318, 321, 325, 331, 339, 355, 359, 364, 371, 372, 374, 376, 381, 401, 418, 423, 459, 463, 465, 553
libido, 539, 616
lice, 509, 571, 601
LICE, 623

Licorice, 79, 90, 95, 118, 145, 179, 557, 558, 617, 618, 619, 620, 621, 622, 623, 624, 625, 626
ligaments, 26, 27, 58, 120, 186, 189
Lily, 179
Lima bean, 74, 110, 118, 129, 132, 147, 151, 153, 177, 183, 184, 185, 186, 188, 190, 195
limau kedut kera, 511
Lime, 59, 180, 510, 511
limejuice, 483
limes, 58, 510, 511
Limeys, 58
linen, 346, 375, 548
linoleic acid, 239, 299
linoment, 478
Linseed, 93, 118, 132, 180, 196
Linseed oil, 196
Lipase, 300
Lithium, 70, 114, 115, 237, 364, 376, 401, 409, 418, 458, 553
lithium orotate, 114, 115
liver, 44, 45, 50, 52, 53, 60, 62, 68, 75, 78, 79, 98, 99, 104, 109, 110, 115, 120, 136, 138, 148, 151, 152, 177, 178, 179, 187, 189, 191, 193, 194, 195, 197, 226, 227, 228, 233, 240, 241, 242, 290, 299, 300, 302, 475, 479, 483, 484, 494, 497, 501, 503, 508, 517, 529, 531, 534, 562, 566, 589, 592, 604, 615
Liver, 41, 50, 53, 150, 189, 191
liver poisoning, 562
LIVER PROBLEMS, 623
Living Liqueurs, 305
lobelia, 618
lockjaw, 484
Locust bean, 178, 181, 183, 187
Loganberry, 59
lomotil, 243
Lonicera caprifolium, 545
loose teeth, 59
lotions, 503, 508, 510, 611
Low body temperature, 98
low sperm count, 566
Lucid asparagus, 179
Lucy Willis, 49
lumbago, 508
Lupine chaya, 177
lutein, 300, 301, 501, 567, 579
Lutein, 300
Lycium barbarum, 612
Lycopene, 301
LYME DISEASE, 623
Lysine, 176, 185, 186, 310, 313, 318, 321, 325, 331, 339, 355, 359, 364, 371, 372, 374, 376, 381, 401, 418, 423, 459, 463, 465, 553
M.A. Boas, 47
Mackerel, 196
macro minerals, 89, 117

macula, 300
MACULAR DEGENERATION, 623
magnesium, 25, 36, 52, 82, 88, 89, 90, 92, 116, 117, 118, 119, 120, 133, 136, 140, 179, 238, 289, 291, 302, 309, 312, 320, 325, 328, 338, 339, 351, 352, 355, 358, 359, 364, 370, 372, 373, 376, 381, 401, 406, 409, 418, 423, 426, 428, 442, 446, 450, 458, 462, 464, 471, 473, 505, 522, 523, 580, 598, 634, 641
Magnesium, 52, 70, 116, 117, 237, 459, 475, 487, 493, 502, 513, 529, 535, 539, 540, 549, 553, 561, 565, 569, 574, 586, 592, 605, 606
Magnolia vine, 79
malaria, 508, 534, 566, 599
malic acid, 290, 302, 486
Malic Acid, 302
mallow, 139, 182, 183, 184, 560
Mallows, 622
Mandarin orange, 59, 510
manganese, 26, 120, 121, 122, 309, 310, 312, 313, 320, 328, 339, 349, 352, 355, 358, 359, 364, 370, 372, 373, 376, 381, 401, 406, 409, 418, 423, 428, 434, 442, 446, 450, 452, 458, 462, 464, 471, 482, 488, 505, 522, 523, 642
Manganese, 51, 70, 120, 121, 122, 237, 459, 475, 487, 493, 502, 513, 529, 535, 539, 540, 549, 553, 561, 565, 569, 574, 586, 592, 604, 605
Mango, 41, 59, 90, 93, 106, 149
Mangrove, 106, 118, 121, 145
Mannose, 302
margosa, 566
Marigold, 494
Marjoram, 83, 90, 110
Marrubium vulgare, 546
Marsh Mallow, 625
marshmallow, 560, 618
Marshmallow, 95, 110, 139, 179, 560, 617, 618
Masticatory, 651
Matricaria chamomilla, 502
Matricaria recutita, 502
Meadowsweet, 561, 620
Meats, 51
Medical Advisory Board of Herbalife, 305
Medicinal Plant Adviser to Reader's Digest and Time-Life, 305
Medicinal Plants of China, 305
Medicinal Plants of the Bible, 305
medicine, 34, 75, 136, 302, 304, 305, 395, 470, 475, 483, 485, 492, 497, 498, 499, 506, 507, 508, 512, 515, 516, 517, 519, 521, 522, 524, 534, 535, 536, 548, 550, 551, 555, 556, 557, 561, 573, 575, 576, 581, 583, 585, 586, 587, 588, 591, 592, 596, 605, 608
Mediterranean diet, 567
Medlar, 59

Melaleuca tree, 601
Melancholy, 651
melatonin, 46, 627
Melatonin, 627
Melissa officinalis, 556
Melon, 41, 59, 81, 115
memory, 51, 74, 95, 132, 188, 299, 531, 535, 539, 557, 566
menaquinones, 68
Menest, 298
menopause, 140, 141, 297, 484, 494, 555, 599, 609
MENOPAUSE, 623
menstrual cramps, 494, 503, 506, 562, 588
MENSTRUAL CRAMPS, 623
menstrual cycle, 484
menstrual pain, 484, 502
menstruation, 504, 512, 569
mental retardation, 61, 137
Mentha apicata, 563
Mentha piperita, 563
Mentha suaveolens, 563
Mercury, 70
methionine, 51, 53, 128, 137, 148, 187, 310, 313, 318, 321, 325, 331, 339, 359, 364, 371, 372, 374, 376, 381, 401, 418, 423, 459, 463, 465
Methionine, 176, 186, 187, 355, 553
Methoxyisoflavone, 628
Mica Muro, 59
micro flora, 33
micro mineral, 89, 117, 120, 137
Microbotanica, the Scientific Advisory Team of Shaman Pharmaceuticals, 305
migraine, 43, 192, 196, 503, 532, 534, 555
Milfoil, 139, 179
Milk, 43, 45, 47, 51, 68, 69, 95, 110, 562, 617, 623
millet, 407
Mind-Body Connection, 306
miscarriage, 475, 484, 572, 587
miscarriages, 69
Mitchella repens, 572
Molasses, 50
molybdenum, 26, 128, 129, 352, 359, 364, 376, 401, 409, 418, 450, 458
Molybdenum, 128, 553
Momordica charantia, 483
Monarda fistulosa, 608
monoglycerides, 300
morning sickness, 509, 534
Moses, 378, 435
mosquito plant, 509
mosquitoes, 510
motion sickness, 485, 534
MOTION SICKNESS, 623
Mountain Mint, 563, 622, 623, 624
mouth infection, 480

mouthwash, 503, 569, 601
mucilage, 576, 595, 600, 639
Mucilage, 651
Mucilaginous, 456, 651
Mugwort, 81, 93, 95, 106, 121, 136, 149, 153
Mulberry, 79, 90
Mullein, 74, 95, 110, 564, 618, 619, 620, 622
multiple sclerosis, 48, 52, 196, 299, 535
MULTIPLE SCLEROSIS, 623
mumps, 523, 533
Mung bean, 178
Mungbean, 93, 181, 183, 184, 186, 188, 190, 193
muscle aches, 478, 610
Muscle cramping, 116, 134
muscle pain, 58, 75, 484, 555
mushrooms, 77, 227, 562
Mushrooms, 47
Muskmelon, 81, 115
Mustard, 565, 566, 622, 624
MYCOSES, 621
myelin, 51, 190, 241
Myopathology, 26
Myrciaria dubia, 495
myrrh, 309, 311, 345, 361, 369, 377, 410, 423, 456, 618
Myrrh, 619
Myxedema, 104
Narcissus, 413, 651
Narcotic, 324, 651
Naringin, 632, 633
National Cancer Institute, 304
National College of Phytotherapy, 305
Natural Health, 306
Nature's Herbs, 305
nausea, 37, 44, 62, 78, 83, 84, 91, 116, 233, 234, 236, 299, 477, 485, 501, 503, 509, 534, 550, 562, 574, 581, 599
NAUSEA, 623
Navy bean, 74, 81, 90, 99, 102, 110, 115, 118, 121, 129, 130, 132, 135, 143, 147, 151, 153, 177, 178, 181, 182, 183, 184, 185, 186, 187, 188, 189, 190, 191, 193, 194, 195
Neem, 90, 118, 566, 567, 623, 624
Neon, 70
neotropical ethnobotany, 304
nerve pain, 512, 536
nerve tonic, 481, 485
nerves, 45, 51, 131, 135, 190, 485, 501, 502, 573, 599
Nervine, 651
nervous disorders, 241, 517, 539, 573
nervous system, 26, 46, 73, 114, 121, 190, 191, 484, 498, 517, 526, 532, 533, 578, 592, 605
Nettle, 431, 450
neuralgia, 547, 586

neuritis, 483
Neuropathology, 26
neurotransmitter, 121, 150, 177, 181, 182, 187, 191, 192, 299
News from the Herbal Village, 305, 306
niacin, 44
Niacin, 44
Nickel, 51, 70, 237, 349, 351, 352, 359, 364, 372, 376, 381, 401, 409, 418, 450, 458, 513, 535, 553, 604
night blindness, 40, 41, 226, 482
Night blindness, 152
night sweats, 484, 504
nightshade, 485
nimba, 566
Niter, 652
nitrilosides, 54
Nitrogen, 40, 70, 130, 237, 309, 310, 312, 313, 320, 325, 328, 338, 339, 355, 358, 359, 364, 370, 372, 373, 376, 381, 382, 401, 406, 409, 416, 418, 423, 426, 428, 434, 450, 458, 462, 464, 465, 471, 473, 487, 493, 502, 512, 513, 529, 531, 535, 539, 540, 549, 561, 565, 569, 574, 586, 592, 604
Noah, 469
Nobel Prize, 58, 103, 140
Non GMO soybean oil, 68
Nosebleed, 69
nosebleeds, 509, 566
Numbness, 66, 116
Nut grass, 567
Nutmeg, 95
nutritive, 532
Nuts, 42, 44, 47, 62, 567, 622, 637
Nutsedge, 567
Oatmeal, 42
Oats, 93, 95, 99, 106, 110, 118, 121, 132, 139, 145, 149, 187, 192, 194
Obesity, 184, 188, 194
OBESITY, 623
Ocimum basilicum, 480
Octacosanol, 633
ocular irritations, 611
Oenothera Biennis, 528
Oily fish, 51
ointment, 236, 478, 529, 537
ointments, 236, 336, 503, 527, 548
Okra, 189
Old Testament, 526
oleuropein, 635
Oligoneuron Small, 537
oligosaccharides, 35, 634, 635
Oligosaccharides, 634, 635
Olive, 145, 635
olive oil, 618
omega-3 fatty, 196, 289, 508, 567, 579

Onion, 59, 115, 129, 147, 149, 179, 180, 617, 620, 622, 624
Onions, 69, 418
Ophir, 430
Orange, 59, 79, 81, 93, 115, 147, 179, 182, 510, 511
oranges, 302, 501, 510
Oregano, 90, 569, 621, 622, 624
Organic Gardening, 306
Organization for Tropical Studies, 305
Oriental Healing Arts Society, 305
Origanum vulgare, 569
Orotic acid, 52
Oryzanol, 634
osteoarthritis, 82, 142, 146, 238, 239, 479, 499, 599
osteomalacia, 60, 88
Osteoporosis, 88, 140
OSTEOPOROSIS, 623
Oswego tea, 608
OTALGIA, 620
OVERWEIGHT, 623
oxygen, 35, 48, 77, 103, 104, 108, 109, 120, 240, 302
Oxygen, 70, 99, 108, 109
PABA, 50
PAIN, 623
painful joints, 527
painful periods, 572
Paliurus, 347
Pallor, 108
palm, 92, 106, 143, 179, 182, 327, 354, 423, 547, 590
Palpitations, 91
Panax ginseng, 535, 536
pancreatic lipase, 300
pangamate, 53
Pangamic Acid, 53
panic, 116, 181, 502
panic attacks, 502
Panic disorder, 184, 188
Pansy, 570, 621
Pantotene, 553
pantothen, 45
Pantothenic Acid, 45
Papaya, 41, 59, 90, 622, 626
Paprika, 81, 102, 115, 129, 130, 136, 149, 179
Para-aminobenzoic acid, 50
parasites, 75, 505, 571, 608, 613
Parkinson's disease, 46, 132, 530, 633
PARKINSON'S DISEASE, 623
Parsley, 59, 79, 83, 102, 115, 121, 129, 130, 135, 136, 143, 145, 147, 149, 153, 186, 571, 618, 622, 623
parsnip, 482
Parsnip, 136, 149
Partridge Berry, 572, 624

Passiflora incarnata, 573
Passion fruit, 59
Passionflower, 573, 622, 623, 624
Pasta, 49
pasteurized milk, 89
Pathophysiology, 27
Pau – D'arco, 574, 621
Pau D'Arco, 90
Paul Gregory, 46
Paul Gyorgi, 43
Pausinystalia yohimbe, 616
Pawpaw, 59
Pea, 74, 81, 83, 93, 106, 129, 130, 136, 149, 151, 177, 178, 181, 182, 183, 184, 185, 186, 187, 188, 189, 190, 191, 194, 195
Pea bean, 81, 83, 93, 129, 136, 151, 177
Peach, 59, 74, 83, 95, 99, 115, 139, 623
Pear, 59, 81, 83, 136, 151, 180
Peas, 41
Pecan, 81, 93, 102, 106, 136, 151
pectin, 486
Pennyroyal, 74, 110, 139, 145, 624
Peppermint, 139, 562, 563, 618, 620, 621, 622, 623, 624
perfume, 447, 498
Perilla frutescens, 507
periodontitis, 58
perioxidase, 236
Peripheral Neuropathy, 66
Persea Americana, 479
Persian lilac, 566
Persimmon, 59
Petroselinum crispum, 571
pharyngeal lipase, 300
Phenylalanine, 188, 193, 310, 313, 318, 321, 325, 331, 339, 355, 359, 364, 371, 372, 374, 376, 381, 401, 418, 423, 459, 463, 465
Phi Beta Kappa, Sigma Xi, Smithsonian Institution, 305
phlegm, 550, 566, 592
Phosphatidylserine, 636
phospholipid, 131, 132, 636
phospholipids, 131, 132, 299, 636
phosphoric acid, 131, 299
Phosphorous, 89, 131, 133
Phosphorus, 70, 131, 132, 505, 522, 523, 553, 584, 606
photosynthesis, 238
phthisis, 517
Phthisis, 652
Phytic Acid, 636
Pigeon pea, 181
Pigweed, 177, 182, 184, 185, 187, 189, 191, 192, 193, 587, 617, 621, 623, 625
piles, 517, 605, 611
Pilocarpus microphyllus, 551
Pimpinella anisum, 477
Pimpinella saxifraga, 493
pineal gland, 627
Pineapple, 59, 93, 106, 121, 130, 143, 179, 182, 562, 574, 575, 617, 618, 619, 623, 625, 626
pins and needles, 78
Piper cubeba, 519
Pistachio, 93, 99, 102, 106, 143, 149, 151, 178, 181, 182, 187, 188, 191, 195
Pistachios, 81
Plant Genome Project, 304
Plantago major, 575
Plantago psyllium, 578
Plantain, 575, 576, 578, 621, 622, 623, 624, 625
Plectranthus esculentus, 552
pleurisy, 551, 605
Plum, 59, 79, 81, 83, 99, 115, 129, 136, 154
PMS, 504, 588, 624
pneumonia, 508
PNEUMONIA, 624
PODAGRIA, 621
poison, 78, 482, 551, 552
poison ivy, 482, 551, 552
POISON IVY, 624
POISON OAK, 624
POISON SUMAC, 624
poisonous, 177, 482, 485, 503, 522, 523, 534, 589
Policosanol, 637
pollutants, 53
polyphenol, 243
polyphenols, 243
Pomelo, 510
poor vision, 482
Pop bean, 74, 90, 99, 102, 110, 115, 118, 121, 129, 130, 132, 135, 143, 147, 151, 154, 177, 178, 181, 182, 183, 184, 185, 186, 187, 188, 189, 191, 192, 193, 194, 195
Popping bean, 74, 90, 99, 102, 110, 130, 143, 151, 154, 178, 181, 182, 183, 184, 185, 186, 187, 188, 189, 191, 192, 193, 194, 195
Poppy seed, 178
Poppyseed, 83, 95, 99, 118, 132, 154, 177, 181, 182, 195
porridge, 586
Portulaca oleracea, 580
post-partum bleeding, 521
potassium, 25, 91, 104, 114, 116, 134, 135, 136, 144, 180, 309, 310, 312, 313, 317, 320, 325, 328, 338, 339, 349, 351, 352, 355, 358, 359, 364, 372, 373, 376, 381, 401, 406, 409, 416, 418, 423, 426, 428, 442, 446, 450, 458, 462, 464, 471, 473, 488, 505, 522, 523, 580
Potassium, 52, 70, 130, 134, 135, 237, 459, 475, 487, 493, 502, 512, 513, 529, 531, 535, 539, 540,

549, 553, 561, 565, 569, 574, 584, 586, 592, 604, 605, 606
Potato, 59, 79, 81, 93, 106, 129, 136, 552, 618, 621, 625
Potatoes, 47
Poultice, 652
poultry, 26, 77, 178, 181
Prebiotics, 652
pregnancy, 49, 74, 89, 103, 104, 121, 152, 240, 484, 485, 572, 578, 587, 592
PREGNANCY, 624
Premarin, 298
premature aging, 52, 53, 140, 141, 539
Premature aging, 137
premenstrual syndrome, 46, 233, 291, 484, 529, 588, 598
PREMENSTRUAL SYNDROME, 624
primrose plant, 289
Probiotic, 34, 35, 36, 652
probiotics, 34, 35, 634
Procuring, 652
Proline, 189, 310, 313, 318, 325, 331, 355, 364, 371, 372, 374, 376, 381, 401, 418, 423, 459, 463, 465, 553
Propolis, 638
prostaglandins, 289, 291
prostate, 60, 151, 152, 228, 239, 242, 300, 301, 519, 549, 567, 580, 581, 583
prostatic enlargement, 572
PROSTATITIS, 624
Protactinium, 70
protease inhibitors, 236
protein, 26, 48, 51, 58, 68, 89, 94, 98, 99, 104, 108, 109, 120, 121, 140, 141, 148, 149, 152, 176, 177, 186, 189, 192, 194, 235, 295, 497, 567, 579, 612, 638, 642
proteins, 26, 45, 46, 47, 50, 51, 68, 89, 91, 104, 117, 130, 137, 143, 148, 196, 226, 234, 236, 243, 295, 593, 611, 638, 642
Prunella vulgaris, 592
Prunus africana, 580
pruritis, 236
pseudoephedrine, 243
Psidium guava, 542
psoriasis, 234, 236, 290, 483, 492, 505, 555
PSORIASIS, 624
Psyllium, 139, 578, 619, 620, 621, 622, 638, 639
Pueraria lobata, 555
Pumpkin, 41, 53, 95, 99, 132, 139, 154, 177, 178, 181, 182, 183, 184, 185, 186, 187, 188, 189, 191, 193, 194, 195, 579, 620, 624, 626
Pumpkins, 196, 579
Purgative, 653
Purslane, 177, 189, 580, 619, 620, 621, 622, 623, 624, 626

Putrid, 653
Pycnanthemum virginianum, 563
Pygeum, 580, 581, 624
Pyridoxine, 46
quercetin, 639, 640
Quercetin, 639, 640
Quevrancho, 581, 622
Quevrancho blanco, 581
Quevrancho Colorado, 581
Quinine, 508
Rabbit Eye Blueberry (Vaccinium virgatum), 488
rabies, 475
radiation, 105, 141, 180, 503, 562
Radish, 83, 90, 130, 132, 135, 136, 143, 145, 149, 622
Radium, 70
Radon, 70
Raisin, 59
rapid heartbeat, 484, 487, 556
rash, 197, 484, 502, 505, 555, 575, 584, 601
rashes, 494, 505, 529, 533, 551, 552, 608
Raspberry, 59, 95, 110, 121, 139, 623, 624
rattlesnake's bites, 576
RAYNAUD'S DISEASE, 624
Recommended Dietary Allowances, 90, 105, 106, 110, 118, 138, 154
red blood cells, 43, 49, 50, 51, 62, 108, 238, 596
Red cabbage, 81, 83, 99, 102, 115, 129, 130, 136, 145, 147, 149, 151
Red chili, 179
Red clover, 95, 110, 118, 121, 582
Red currant, 79, 83, 93, 102, 136, 143
Red mangrove, 83
Red pepper, 59, 617, 618, 619, 620, 621, 622, 623, 624, 625
Red wine, 69
Redcurrant, 59
reed, 334, 382
Refrigerant, 653
Reishi, 583, 584, 617
resin, 521, 600
respiratory infections, 41, 59
respiratory problems, 555, 561, 600
restlessness, 556
resveratrol, 470, 567, 640, 641
Resveratrol, 640, 641
Rheum rhabarbarum, 585
rheumatism, 142, 480, 481, 484, 487, 503, 505, 517, 534, 540, 547, 551, 561, 605, 609, 610
Rheumatism, 653
rheumatoid, 45, 183, 226, 233, 241, 289, 499, 500, 566, 599, 638
rheumatoid arthritis, 45, 183, 226, 233, 241, 289, 500, 599, 638
Rheumatology Unit, 305

rhinitis, 236, 483
Rhubarb, 90, 102, 135, 136, 585, 619
Riboflavin, 43
Rice, 49, 79, 180, 228
richweed, 547
rickets, 60, 526, 599
ringworm, 483, 485, 503, 557
Road bean, 192
Robert Burns Woodward, 51
Rodale Press, 305, 306
Roger Williams, 45
Rose, 59, 69
Rose hip, 59
Rose hips, 69
Rosemary, 562, 586, 617, 618, 619, 620, 626
Rosenthal Center for Alternative/Complementary Medicine, 305
Rosmarinus officinalis, 586
rotaviral, 38
rotavirus, 37, 38, 234
Rough Pig Weed, 586
Rough skin, 120
Rubefacient, 653
Rubidium, 70, 136, 339, 352, 359, 418, 450, 458, 553
Rubus fructicosus, 486
Ruscus aculeatus, 494
Rutabaga, 83, 130, 136, 149
Rye, 106
Safflower, 79, 95, 110, 139, 587, 618
Saffron, 121, 130, 588, 621
Sage, 121, 145, 588, 589, 617, 618, 621, 625, 626
saliva, 550
Salmon, 44, 196
salmonella, 302, 604
Salvia officinalis, 588
Sambucus nigra, 524
Sanguinaria Candensis, 487
Saponaria, 596
Sardines, 51
Sarsaparilla, 95, 139
Sassafras, 74, 81, 99, 110, 118, 121, 147, 151, 154
Saw Palmetto, 590, 618, 624
scabies, 483
SCABIES, 624
scalp irritations, 500
scarlet, 178, 187, 399, 494
Schisandra, 591, 592, 623
Schisandra chinensis, 591
schizophrenia, 181, 289, 475, 529, 627
Schizophrenia, 53
sciatica, 508, 517
Sciatica, 612, 653
SCIATICA, 624
scleroderma, 297, 540, 641

Scotch kale, 99, 145
SCRAPES, 619
Scrofula, 653
scurvy, 58, 136, 510
Scurvy, 58, 59
Scutellaria L, 475
Seabuckthorn, 59
seafood, 75, 77, 110, 138
Seafood, 49
seaweed, 80, 104, 553
Seborrheic Dermatitis, 66
Sedative, 653
seizures, 103, 116, 289, 573, 589
selenium, 26, 117, 137, 138, 139, 150, 151, 328, 352, 359, 364, 370, 381, 401, 406, 409, 418, 450, 458, 471, 505, 522, 523, 598, 642
Selenium, 70, 137, 138, 237, 459, 487, 493, 502, 512, 535, 539, 540, 549, 553, 561, 565, 574, 584, 605
Self – Heal, 592, 621
Self-heal, 592
senility, 53, 181, 539
Serenoa repens, 590
Serine, 190, 310, 313, 318, 325, 331, 355, 364, 371, 372, 374, 376, 381, 401, 418, 423, 459, 463, 465, 553
serotonin, 46, 192
Sesame, 99, 106, 132, 154, 177, 178, 181, 182, 183, 184, 185, 187, 189, 191, 192, 193, 194, 195, 593, 618, 619, 625
sesame oil, 517
Sesamum orientale, 593
shingles, 197
SHINGLES, 624
Shittah, 411, 469
Shittin tree, 469
shock, 551, 599
Sialogogue, 653
sickle cell anemia, 43
Sickle pod, 180, 182
Sida cordifolia, 517
Silica, 140, 141, 142, 143, 237, 309, 312, 328, 352, 355, 359, 381, 401, 406, 418, 423, 450, 458, 459, 471, 487, 502, 505, 506, 512, 517, 522, 523, 531, 535, 539, 540, 549, 561, 565, 574, 592, 605
silicoaluminate, 73, 106
Silicon, 70, 140
Silver, 70, 364, 370, 376, 401, 409, 418, 458, 553
Silybum Marianum, 562
SINUSITIS, 624
skin ailments, 537, 587
skin cleaner, 481, 484, 485, 486, 505, 524, 547, 549
Skin diseases, 53
skin disorders, 41, 513, 566
skin grafting, 618

835

Hillman Health Food Store call 855-Amish-Dr (855-264-7437) www.emineral.info Vitamins and Minerals for Better Living

skin inflammations, 494, 524, 611
skin lesions, 197, 233, 500, 611
SKIN PROBLEMS, 624
skin rashes, 43, 68, 83, 233, 497, 503, 638
Skipper Butterfly, 489
Skull Cap, 573
Skullcap, 79, 118, 475, 624
sleep aid, 187, 192, 502, 546
sleep cycle, 627
Sleep disturbance, 104
sleep problems, 556
Slippery elm, 139
Slippery Elm, 595, 619, 620, 625
smallpox, 523
SMOKING, 624
Smooth sumac, 74, 81, 95
snakebites, 503, 523, 534
Snap bean, 74, 90, 99, 102, 110, 115, 118, 129, 130, 132, 135, 143, 147, 151, 154, 177, 178, 181, 182, 183, 184, 185, 186, 187, 188, 189, 191, 192, 193, 194, 195
soap, 84, 486, 596
soaps, 508, 519, 535, 536, 571, 586, 589, 596
Soapwort, 596, 624
Society for Conservation Biology, 305
Society for Economic Botany, 305
soda pop, 84, 144
Sodium, 70, 144, 145, 237, 309, 310, 312, 313, 317, 320, 325, 328, 338, 349, 351, 352, 355, 358, 359, 364, 370, 372, 373, 376, 381, 401, 406, 409, 416, 418, 423, 426, 428, 442, 446, 450, 458, 459, 462, 464, 471, 473, 487, 502, 505, 506, 512, 513, 517, 522, 523, 529, 531, 535, 539, 540, 549, 553, 561, 565, 569, 574, 586, 592, 604, 605
Solanum melongena, 523
Solanum nigrum, 485
Solomon, 365, 388, 392, 402, 403, 425, 434, 445, 456, 472, 526
sore breasts, 500
sore throat, 480, 493, 523, 557, 560
SORE THROAT, 625
sores, 494, 496, 503, 505, 523, 527, 556, 569, 585, 589, 600, 615, 639
SORES, 625
sorrel, 139
Sorrel, 95, 106, 121, 130, 149
Sour cherry, 83
Southern Appalachian Botanical Club, 305
Soybean, 81, 93, 145, 154, 180, 181, 182, 191, 619, 620, 623
spasm, 26, 500, 502, 592
spasms, 26, 116, 134, 192, 475, 484, 485, 487, 501, 571
Spearmint, 562, 563
spina bifida, 49

Spinach, 41, 43, 49, 57, 59, 68, 79, 93, 99, 102, 106, 118, 121, 130, 135, 136, 143, 145, 149, 154, 177, 182, 183, 184, 185, 186, 187, 188, 189, 191, 192, 193, 194, 195, 606, 619, 622, 624, 625
Spirulina, 642
spleen, 75, 110, 136, 505, 508, 529, 531, 609
sprains, 478, 480, 611
Spur pepper, 179
St. John's Wort, 598
St. Johns Wort, 573
St. John's-Wort, 620, 622, 623
staph infection, 522
Staphylococcus aureus, 37
Starvation, 177, 182, 185
Stellaria media, 504
sterols, 228, 242, 634
Stevia, 95
STIES, 625
Stiff joints, 120
stimulant, 480, 485, 497, 508, 519, 523, 524, 527, 532, 551, 552, 562, 566, 581, 613, 616
Stinging nettle, 93, 102, 118, 121, 130, 136, 139, 143, 145, 149, 154, 617, 618, 619, 622, 623, 624
stings, 510, 638
STINGS, 622
stomach, 35, 38, 39, 44, 45, 47, 74, 75, 78, 80, 92, 108, 141, 226, 227, 236, 239, 291, 292, 300, 482, 483, 484, 487, 496, 499, 502, 509, 513, 524, 534, 543, 548, 555, 557, 558, 562, 566, 581, 585, 599, 600, 604, 608, 609, 615, 637, 641
stomach ache, 78
stomach aches, 497, 500, 608
stomach aid, 524, 534
stomach cramps, 562
Stomachic, 654
Stone Root, 547
Strangury, 654
Strawberry, 59, 83, 106, 143, 179
Streptococcus thermophilus, 38
Streptococcus Thermophilus, 36, 38
String bean, 74, 90, 99, 102, 110, 115, 118, 129, 130, 132, 135, 143, 147, 151, 154, 177, 178, 181, 182, 183, 184, 185, 186, 187, 188, 189, 191, 192, 193, 194, 195
STROKE, 625
Strontium, 70, 146, 147, 352, 364, 376, 401, 409, 418, 459, 513, 553
stunted growth, 61
stupor, 475, 581
Styptic, 654
Sudorific, 654
Sugar beet, 81, 83, 115, 130, 132, 135, 136, 145, 149, 179
Sulforaphane, 642, 643

Sulfur, 70, 148, 309, 312, 325, 352, 355, 359, 364, 372, 376, 401, 409, 418, 423, 426, 450, 459
Sulphur, 553
Sumac, 121, 147
SUNBURN, 625
Sunflower, 42, 62, 106, 149, 177, 178, 180, 182, 183, 184, 185, 187, 188, 193, 195, 598, 599, 622
sunflower seeds, 53, 598
Sunflower seeds, 42, 62, 598, 599
Supplements/ Dietary Advisory Board, 305
Suppurative, 654
Swamp cabbage, 106, 132, 154, 178, 182, 184, 187, 191, 192, 194, 195
Sweet acacia, 177, 178, 181, 183, 184, 185, 186, 187, 188, 189, 191, 192, 194
sweet cane, 451
Sweet flag, 599
Sweet Leaf, 608
Sweet marjoram, 83
Sweet pepper, 81, 115, 129, 136, 149, 179
Sweet potato, 106
Sweet potatoes, 41, 45
Sweet Violet, 600
Sweetflag, 129, 623
Sweetgum, 81, 83, 147
swelling, 80, 109, 110, 134, 141, 142, 144, 236, 478, 482, 485, 557, 592
Swelling, 91, 134, 145
SWELLING, 625
swellings, 489, 494, 500, 531, 549, 610
swine flu, 555
swollen joints, 610
Swordfish, 44
Symphytum officinale, 515
SYNCOPE, 620
Syndrome Gulf War Syndrome, 193
syphilis, 498, 522, 574, 600
systemic lupus erythematosus, 241
Syzygium aromatic, 513
Tabasco, 179
Tabebuia avellanedae, 574
Table salt, 92, 145
Tanacetum parthenium, 532
Tangerine, 59, 79, 93, 179
tannins, 592, 611, 638
Tantalum, 70
Tarragon, 179
Tea, 179, 180, 482, 513, 600, 601, 617, 619, 620, 622, 625
Tea tree, 600, 601
teeth, 60, 80, 82, 88, 89, 101, 116, 131, 132, 141, 497, 513
Tellurium, 381
TENDINITIS, 619
Tenesmus, 654

Tertian, 654
Thallium, 70
The Environmentarian, HerbalGram, Herbs for Health, 306
The International Permaculture Species Yearbook, 306
The Journal of Alternative & Complementary Medicine, 306
theobroma cacao, 513
theophylline, 243
Thiamine, 42
third degree burns, 618
thirst, 134, 487, 550, 555
Thistle, 562, 617
Thorium, 70
thorn bush, 455
Threonine, 176, 191, 310, 313, 318, 321, 325, 331, 339, 355, 359, 364, 371, 372, 374, 376, 381, 401, 418, 423, 459, 463, 465, 553
throat, 142, 475, 494, 496, 497, 508, 517, 557, 560, 564, 589, 635
throat infections, 293
thrush, 496, 509, 601
Thyme, 90, 95, 110, 115, 139, 601, 618, 625
Thymus vulgaris, 601
Tin, 70, 328, 352, 370, 376, 381, 406, 450, 459, 471, 487, 502, 506, 512, 517, 531, 535, 539, 540, 553, 561, 565, 574, 592, 605
tingling, 44, 66, 94, 116
TINNITUS, 625
tiredness, 45, 49, 234, 479, 634
Titanium, 70, 237, 352, 364, 376, 401, 409, 459
TMG, 228
tobacco, 46, 47, 576, 642
Tocopherol, 62
tokos, 62
Tomato, 59, 74, 81, 83, 90, 93, 99, 102, 106, 115, 129, 130, 135, 136, 145, 147, 149, 151, 154, 179, 181, 621
Tomatoes, 47, 69, 301
tongue, 49, 104, 550, 589
tonic, 475, 477, 479, 486, 487, 496, 502, 503, 505, 508, 517, 522, 524, 526, 531, 532, 533, 534, 536, 539, 547, 548, 592, 596, 599, 600, 615
tonsillitis, 493, 500, 533, 557
TONSILLITIS, 625
TOOTH DECAY, 625
toothache, 513, 557
TOOTHACHE, 625
toothaches, 493, 523, 534, 566
toothbrushes, 455, 566
toothpaste, 101, 106, 144
toothpastes, 101, 610
Touch-Me-Not's, 552
toxins, 27, 34, 35, 128, 524, 566, 608

Traveler's diarrhea, 38
Trifolium pratense, 582
triglyceride, 44, 150, 186, 241, 634
triglycerides, 94, 241, 289, 292
Trigonella foenum-graecum, 532
trimethylglycine, 228
Trimethylglycine, 56
triocontanol, 637
Tryptophan, 192, 310, 313, 318, 321, 325, 339, 355, 364, 371, 372, 374, 376, 381, 401, 418, 423, 459, 463, 465
tuberculosis, 497, 524, 537, 549, 611
TUBERCULOSIS, 625
tumors, 103, 105, 108, 177, 234, 289, 291, 455, 499, 503, 556, 561, 571, 611, 636, 639, 642
Tungsten, 70
Turmeric, 145, 604, 617, 618, 619, 621, 625
Turnip greens, 68
turpentine, 350
twitching, 475
typhoid, 508
Tyrosine, 188, 193, 310, 313, 318, 321, 325, 331, 355, 364, 371, 374, 376, 381, 401, 418, 423, 429, 459, 463, 465
ulcer, 180, 480, 502
ulcerative colitis, 560
ulcers, 38, 44, 75, 108, 141, 235, 485, 486, 494, 496, 499, 509, 524, 526, 527, 534, 540, 547, 549, 561, 566, 567, 605, 615
ULCERS, 625
Ulmus rubra, 595
ultraviolet radiation, 60, 300
Uncaria tomentosa, 499
universal antioxidant, 196
upper respiratory infections, 45
Uranium, 70
uric acid, 48, 128
urinary tract infection, 522
urinary tract infections, 481
uterine inflammation, 487
uterotonic, 615
Vaccines, 73
Vaccinium angustifolium, 488
Vaccinium corymbosum, 488
Vaccinium myrtillus, 482
vaginal disorders, 481
vaginal dryness, 484
vaginal tract, 36, 38
VAGINITIS, 625
Valerian, 95, 139, 573, 605, 619, 622
Valeriana officinalis, 605
Valine, 185, 194, 195, 310, 313, 318, 321, 325, 331, 339, 355, 364, 371, 372, 374, 376, 401, 418, 423, 455, 459, 463, 465, 553
vanadium, 150, 151

Vanadium, 51, 70, 150, 151, 376, 401, 553
varicose veins, 494, 508, 540, 547
VARICOSE VEINS, 626
vasodilator, 44
Veal, 44
Velvet bean, 183, 184, 185, 186, 189, 191, 192, 194, 195, 620, 623
venereal diseases, 498, 540
Venery, 655
Verbascum Thapsus, 564
Verbena, 605, 621
Vermifuge, 655
vertebra, 26
Vertebral Subluxation Complex, 26
vertigo, 142, 613
VERTIGO, 620
Vervain, 655
Viburnum prunifolium, 484
Vicia faba, 530
Vinca minor, 557
Viola odorata, 600
Viola tricolor, 570
viral hepatitis, 562
viral infections, 58
VIRAL INFECTIONS, 626
vitamin A, 40, 41, 53, 152, 226, 483, 488, 552, 579
Vitamin A, 40, 153, 351, 505, 522, 523, 553, 582
Vitamin B, 148, 185, 584
vitamin B_1, 42, 43, 148, 505, 522, 523, 553
Vitamin B1, 42
Vitamin B_{10}, 50
Vitamin B_{12}, 51, 606
vitamin B_{13}, 52
Vitamin B_{13}, 52
vitamin B_{15}, 53
Vitamin B17, 54
vitamin B_2, 43, 45, 505, 522, 523
Vitamin B_2, 43
vitamin B_3, 44, 46, 94, 192, 291, 488, 505, 522, 523, 553
Vitamin B_3, 44
vitamin B_5, 45
Vitamin B_5, 45
vitamin B_6, 46, 193, 289, 291, 488
Vitamin B_6, 46, 191
vitamin B_7, 47, 148, 197
Vitamin B_7, 47
vitamin B_8, 48, 299, 636
Vitamin B_8, 48
vitamin B_9, 49, 51, 52, 228, 488
Vitamin B_9, 49
Vitamin B_p, 56
Vitamin C, 58, 186, 189, 495, 496, 505, 522, 523, 553, 606
vitamin D, 60, 61, 82, 88, 89, 117, 131, 290, 553

Vitamin D, 60, 88, 132, 584
vitamin E, 53, 62, 109, 153, 196, 290, 488, 553, 598
Vitamin E, 62, 109, 137, 138, 580, 593, 598, 606
Vitamin H, 66
Vitamin K, 68
Vitamin P, 69
Vitex agnus-castus, 504
Voluptuousness, 655
vomiting, 75, 78, 80, 83, 84, 91, 116, 134, 139, 144, 234, 236, 299, 485, 487, 500, 509, 534, 536, 550, 555, 562, 569, 581
Vulnerary, 655
Wagner-Jauregg, 43
walnut, 526
Walnuts, 196, 526
warfarin, 68, 243, 637
warts, 78, 501
WARTS, 626
Washington Academy of Sciences, 305
Water lotus, 79, 179, 194
water retention, 516, 557
Water spinach, 106, 132, 154, 183, 184, 187, 192, 194, 195
Watercress, 90, 132, 135, 145, 177, 178, 183, 185, 186, 187, 188, 189, 192, 193, 194, 195
Watermelon, 59, 132, 177, 178, 180, 181, 183, 185, 187, 188, 191, 192, 194
water-soluble, 25, 42, 43, 44, 45, 46, 47, 50, 51, 291, 293, 297, 628, 632, 641
Wax bean, 74, 90, 99, 102, 110, 115, 118, 129, 130, 132, 135, 143, 147, 151, 154, 177, 178, 181, 183, 184, 185, 186, 187, 188, 189, 191, 192, 193, 194, 195
weakness, 26, 49, 58, 80, 91, 117, 119, 134, 534, 544
Wheat, 50, 93, 118, 149, 180, 181, 184, 185, 186, 187, 189, 194, 228, 606, 620
Wheat germ, 50, 228
wheat germ oil, 618, 633
Wheatgrass, 95, 118, 143, 606, 619
White cabbage, 81, 83, 99, 102, 129, 130, 136, 145, 147, 149, 151
White currant, 79, 83, 102, 136, 143
White lupine, 178, 183, 191, 192, 194
White mustard, 95, 177, 181, 183, 187, 189, 192, 193, 195
white oak bark, 618
White pepper, 93, 106, 149
White potatoes, 45
Whole grains, 45, 49, 53, 138
Wild Bergamot, 608, 625
Wild cherry, 74, 81, 83, 90, 99, 110, 121, 129, 147, 151, 154
Wild Foods Forum, 306
Wild indigo, 145

Wild yam, 95, 609
Wild Yam, 609, 618, 620
Willow, 81, 147, 617, 618, 619, 620, 621, 623, 624, 625
Willow oak, 81, 147
Winged bean, 181, 183, 184, 185, 186, 187, 188, 189, 191, 192, 193, 194, 195
Winged sumac, 81, 147
Winter squash, 41
Wintergreen, 610, 619, 621, 624
Witch Hazel, 611, 618, 621, 624, 626
Wolfberry, 59, 79, 90, 145, 612, 623
World Health Organization, 37, 305
worms, 486, 552, 566, 576, 613
WORMS, 626
wormseed, 613
Wormseed, 613, 626
wormwood, 316, 473, 618
Wormwood, 473
wound healing, 152, 177, 234, 478, 523, 540, 557, 586
wounds, 58, 238, 493, 494, 499, 501, 503, 505, 523, 527, 529, 537, 548, 571, 592, 638
WRINKLES, 626
xanthenes, 579
Xanthorhiza simplicissima, 615
Xenon, 70
Xeon, 70
Yardlong bean, 76, 83, 93, 129, 132, 136, 154, 177, 181, 183, 185, 186, 187, 188, 189, 194
Yarrow, 69, 95, 179
Yeast, 50, 235
YEAST INFECTIONS, 626
Yellow squash, 41
Yellowroot, 615, 625
Yogurt, 43, 51, 618
Yohimbe, 616, 620, 622
yolks, 62, 299
Yttrium, 71, 401
Zellwegger's syndrome, 241
zinc, 26, 36, 88, 89, 90, 99, 117, 136, 152, 153, 183, 289, 291, 309, 310, 312, 313, 320, 349, 352, 355, 358, 359, 364, 370, 372, 373, 376, 381, 401, 406, 409, 423, 428, 442, 446, 450, 459, 462, 464, 471, 473, 488, 505, 522, 523, 529, 642
Zinc, 51, 71, 152, 153, 154, 237, 475, 487, 502, 506, 512, 513, 517, 529, 531, 535, 539, 540, 553, 561, 565, 569, 574, 586, 589, 592, 605, 618
Zingiber officinale, 534
Zirconium, 71

Hillman Health Food Store call 855-Amish-Dr (855-264-7437) www.emineral.info Vitamins and Minerals for Better Living